Stanhope and Lancaster's

COMMUNITY HEALTH NURSING IN CANADA

Stanhope and Lancaster's
COMMUNITY HEALTH NURSING IN CANADA

FOURTH EDITION

Sandra A. **MacDonald, RN, PhD**
Professor and Associate Dean of Undergraduate Programs
Faculty of Nursing
Memorial University of Newfoundland
St. John's, Newfoundland

Sonya L. **Jakubec, RN, PhD**
Professor
School of Nursing and Midwifery
Mount Royal University
Calgary, Alberta

U.S. Authors
Marcia **Stanhope, PhD, RN, FAAN**
Education and Practice Consultant and
Professor Emeritus
College of Nursing
University of Kentucky
Lexington, Kentucky

Jeanette **Lancaster, RN, PhD, FAAN**
Sadie Heath Cabiness Professor and Dean Emeritus
School of Nursing
University of Virginia
Charlottesville, Virginia
Associate, Tuft & Associates, Inc.

ELSEVIER

ELSEVIER

Library of Congress Control Number: 2021944941

Managing Director, Global ERC: Kevonne Holloway
Senior Content Strategist (Acquisitions, Canada): Roberta A. Spinosa-Millman
Director, Content Development Manager: Laurie Gower
Content Development Specialist: Martina van de Velde
Publishing Services Manager: Deepthi Unni
Senior Project Manager: Manchu Mohan
Design Direction: Bridget Hoette

Printed in the United States of America.

Last digit is the print number: 9 8 7 6 5 4 3 2 1

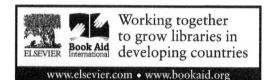

I would like to dedicate this book to the unsung heroes at the front lines of the COVID-19 pandemic—the community health nurses—who keep us safe through their planning, response, and protection of individuals, families, and communities across Canada. Thank you for all you do!

—*Sandra A. Macdonald*

For the communities—the leaders, practitioners, activists, organizations, families, and individuals—in the cities and small towns in western Canada and West Africa where I have worked and witnessed the triumphs and tragedies of community health and well-being. I have learned from and continue to be inspired by you all—people walking the talk.

—*Sonya L. Jakubec*

Mary Lou Batty, RN, BN, BA, MN, PhD
Senior Teaching Associate
Faculty of Nursing
University of New Brunswick
Fredericton, New Brunswick

R. Lisa Bourque-Bearskin, RN, PhD
Associate Professor
School of Nursing
Thompson Rivers University
Kamloops, British Columbia
    Past President
Indigenous Nurses Association of Canada
Ottawa, Ontario

Elizabeth (Liz) Diem, RN, PhD
Assistant Professor
Faculty of Health Sciences
School of Nursing
University of Ottawa
Ottawa, Ontario

Manon Lemonde, RN, PhD
Associate Professor
Faculty of Health Sciences
University of Ontario Institute of Technology
Oshawa, Ontario

Victoria Morley, RN, BScN, MEd
Faculty Clinical Advisor
Laurentian University
Sudbury, Ontario

Alwyn Moyer, RN, PhD
Adjunct Professor
University of Ottawa
Ottawa, Ontario
Self-employed Health Consultant

Ivana Zuliani, RN, BScN, MScN
Nurse Consultant
Workplace Safety and Insurance Board
Sudbury, Ontario

REVIEWERS

Mary Lou Batty, RN, BN, BA, MN, PhD
Senior Teaching Associate
Faculty of Nursing
University of New Brunswick
Fredericton, New Brunswick

Dr Sylvane Filice, RN, HBScN, MPH(N), PhD
Assistant Professor
School of Nursing
Lakehead University
Thunder Bay, Ontario

Kelly Fleming, RN, BN, MSN
Instructor
School of Nursing and Midwifery
Faculty of Health and Community Studies
Mount Royal University
Calgary, Alberta

Kathryn Halverson, RN, BScN, MSN
Faculty Lecturer
School of Nursing
Lakehead University
Thunder Bay, Ontario

Frances Legault, RN, BScN, MSN, PhD
Assistant Professor Nursing (Retired)
School of Nursing
University of Ottawa
Ottawa, Ontario

Manon Lemonde, RN, PhD
Associate Professor
Faculty of Health Sciences
University of Ontario Institute of Technology
Oshawa, Ontario

Natalie McMullin, RN, BScN, MN
Nursing Instructor
Nursing and Allied Health Studies
Keyano College
Fort McMurray, Alberta

Grace Ross, BScN, MSc, RN, RP
Sessional Lecturer
School of Nursing
Faculty of Health
York University
Toronto, Ontario

People are profoundly influenced by one another and their social contexts. Determinants of health, such as income and social status, social environments, and social support networks, directly affect the health of Canadians. Macro-level factors, such as poverty and unemployment, and micro-level factors, such as lifestyle, also influence the health of Canadians. Therefore, to protect and promote the health of Canadians, it is important to address the individual as well as the social, political, and economic conditions that negatively influence health.

Community health nursing supports the health of a variety of patients—individuals, families, groups or aggregates, communities, populations, or society. It emphasizes health promotion; disease prevention; health protection; health maintenance, restoration, and palliation; health education, cultural safety, advocacy, coordination, management, and care evaluation. The community health nurse (CHN) builds capacity in patients by collaborating with them to build on their strengths, skills, and knowledge and ensure resources and services are distributed equally to reach those most in need.

CHNs provide health services to all age groups in a variety of public and private settings. One of the challenges for community health nursing is to facilitate and identify strategies that meet the demands of a constantly changing health care system within ever-evolving social contexts. CHNs need to be visionaries in designing their roles and identifying their practice areas. To do so effectively, they need to understand the concepts and theories of public health, changing health care systems and social realities, the roles and responsibilities of CHNs and other health care providers, the importance of prevention and health protection, and the need to engage with other health care providers and patients as partners in assessing, planning, implementing, and evaluating community health care efforts.

Disease prevention and health protection strategies designed to address the determinants of health are most effective when they are developed through professional relationships and partnerships among government, businesses, voluntary organizations, patients, communities, and health care providers. These partnerships aim to eliminate health disparities among Canadians by focusing on community health care for children, minorities, older persons, and other vulnerable groups in order to increase the lifespan and quality of Canadians' lives. CHNs have a collaborative role in these partnerships, identifying and planning programs and policies that are acceptable to partners and responsive to patients' needs. CHNs develop professional relationships and partnerships to create healthy public policy that supports better health care, improved health education, healthy environments, and addresses issues related to the determinants of health.

Compared with other developed countries, community health nursing in Canada has traditionally placed greater emphasis on the determinants of health as factors that influence health; the Ottawa Charter for Health Promotion, specifically on equity in health and health promotion strategies; Epp's health promotion framework; population health; the Canadian Community Health Nursing Standards of Practice; and the development of the certification process for community health nursing. Unfortunately, in recent years, Canada has been falling behind in addressing the determinants of health and health inequities.

In this text, the term *community health nursing* encompasses a variety of practitioners, such as public health nurses (PHNs); home health nurses (HHNs); occupational health nurses (OHNs); and primary health care nurse practitioners (PHCNPs), who practise in a variety of settings in the community. This text focuses on the evidence, processes, and practices CHNs employ to protect and promote patient health.

CHNs are ideally positioned to work with communities to promote health, because they are aware of the many factors that interact to influence health. They engage in "upstream thinking" when approaching community health interventions, which involves consideration of the determinants of health and other relevant economic, political, and environmental factors that may influence the health of the patient. CHNs strive to use the strategies and approaches for health promotion outlined in the Ottawa Charter to promote and preserve the health of Canadians.

This fourth edition of *Community Health Nursing in Canada* provides a comprehensive approach to community health nursing concepts, skills, and practice. This text presents readers with historical, conceptual, and theoretical perspectives in content areas that are necessary for novice practitioners in community health nursing practice. It also identifies the increasing importance of social justice and the impact of society on individual health, which expresses a shift from individual-centred care to population- and community-centred care.

This edition has been extensively revised. Examples have been updated using current Canadian research and statistics, including some references to the COVID-19 pandemic and Black Lives Matter movement that emerged during the later development phase of this edition. Readers are directed to the most current Canadian websites for further information on a variety of topics. Regardless of the examples given, this edition maintains a population-based approach; a socio-environmental, equity, and social justice perspective; and a behavioural perspective.

The authors and contributors of the text recognize and acknowledge the diverse histories of the First Peoples of the lands now referred to as Canada. It is recognized that individual communities identify themselves in various ways. At the time of writing, the recommendations of the Truth and Reconciliation Commission (TRC) and the United Nations Declaration on the Rights of Indigenous Peoples (UNDRIP) (adopted by Canada in 2016) were in the early phases of implementation by various levels of government to address many years of legislated wrongs and inequities against Indigenous people. It is too early to report how the TRC recommendations and UNDRIP will influence community health policy and practice. However, they have influenced the terms used to refer to the diverse Indigenous populations in Canada and highlighted current inequities. The terms *Indigenous people(s)* and *Indigenous health*, used throughout this text, acknowledge the inherent rights and political views of the diverse groups of original peoples with historical and cultural ties to Canada. *Indigenous* is distinct from *Aboriginal*, which is a broad term that does not account for the various original peoples (First Nations people, Métis, and Inuit) in the country. Community health nursing practice should be informed by an understanding of and respect for the rights of Indigenous people to claim their identity according to their original names as a form of resistance to the legislated terms that have created inequity and harm over many years. The context and considerations surrounding acceptable terminology when referring to Indigenous people and inequities shaping their community health experiences are discussed in greater depth in Chapters 7 and 14.

This text also recognizes that language is fluid and ever-evolving. The authors recognize that childbirth is not only experienced by women but may be experienced by others who do not identify as female or who find the term *woman* to not be representative of how they identify themselves. The terms *patient*, *person*, or *parent* are used when possible in the text. *Woman/women* is used when the research is specifically done with a population that identifies as a woman.

A list of additional resources for more in-depth exposure to certain topics is included in each chapter. Students are required to incorporate prior learning in such areas as physiology, psychology, sociology, research, and ethics. Nursing program graduates can further develop their knowledge and skills in community health nursing practice as they apply the Canadian Community Health Nursing Standards of Practice.

Learning is a lifelong adventure, and it is our hope that graduates will continue to develop their knowledge and skills in community health nursing through curiosity, experience, continuing education, and, for some, through further academic learning, such as master's and doctoral programs.

TEXT ORGANIZATION

This text's 18 chapters are organized into four units for ease of use by students and faculty. The ordering of the chapters is a suggestion only. Each chapter stands alone, so the ordering can be modified by individual faculty.

Chapters begin with a list of numbered **Objectives** that guide student learning and assist faculty in knowing what students should gain from the content and reflect what are sometimes referred to in the field of nursing education as "ends in view." The **Chapter Outline** alerts students to the structure and content of the chapter. **Key Terms** are identified at the beginning of the chapter, and the definitions are provided, in alphabetical order for quick reference, in a Glossary at the end of the text to help students understand unfamiliar terminology. The key terms are bolded in the text.

CLASSIC FEATURES

- **Determinants of Health** boxes relate the chapter content to the determinants of health as supported by the literature. Ideas about the meaning of the facts presented expand on their possible impact. The information presented in these boxes is intended to stimulate further class discussion about the determinants of health, their impact, and further implications.
- **How To …** boxes provide specific, application-oriented information.
- **Evidence-Informed Practice** boxes illustrate the application of the latest research findings in nursing and community health nursing and include critical thinking questions for reflection and discussion.
- **Levels of Prevention** boxes provide examples of primary, secondary, and tertiary prevention related to community health nursing practice specific to the chapter.
- **Ethical Considerations** boxes provide examples of ethical situations and the relevant principles involved. Questions are raised for student and faculty reflection and discussion.
- **Student Experience** boxes assist students to apply and reflect on specific content areas in each chapter. Questions encourage students to use their critical thinking skills and, often, to share findings for discussion and debate with classmates.
- The **Chapter Summary** at the end of each chapter is organized around the numbered learning objectives and provides a summary of the most important points made in the chapter.
- The **Tool Box** section at the end of each chapter directs students to excellent sources of supplemental information, including appendices that are relevant to the chapter content and specific links to websites with practical tools, such as checklists or guides, that will assist students in applying chapter-related content. The Tool Box links can be accessed on the text's accompanying Evolve website at https://evolve.elsevier.com/Canada/Stanhope/community/. At the time of publication, these links were active and were selected on the basis of such factors as source, authorship, affiliation, and currency. Users are encouraged to evaluate web resources for these and other factors. One example of a resource that could be used to evaluate web resources is https://www.lib.berkeley.edu/TeachingLib/Guides/Internet/Evaluate.html.
- **Appendices:** There are 10 appendices at the end of the text, and six more can be accessed on the Evolve website. The majority of these appendices are Canadian and are referred to in the chapters throughout the text. They provide a more in-depth look at primary sources, such as the Canadian Community Health Nursing Standards of Practice, the Ottawa Charter for Health Promotion, the Giger and Davidhizar Transcultural Assessment Model, and the Calgary Family Assessment Model.

- Many acronyms and abbreviations are used throughout the chapters, and a list of commonly used **Abbreviations** is provided on the inside back cover of this text for easy reference.

FEATURES OF THE FOURTH EDITION

- *Chapter 15: Working With People Who Experience Structural Vulnerabilities* has been thoroughly revised and refocused to view vulnerable populations through a social justice lens.
- Greater coverage is provided throughout the textbook regarding global health, global issues, and the global environment.
- All references to the Canadian Community Health Nursing Standards of Practice (and Appendix A, which lists the standards) have been updated to reflect the latest edition published in 2019.

Evolve Resources

Information that is available at the text's Evolve website has been expanded and is accessible at https://evolve.elsevier.com/Canada/Stanhope/community/. Students and instructors are advised to establish access to the Evolve website as soon as they purchase their textbook.

For Students

- Appendices
- Chapter Summaries
- Glossary
- Learning Objectives
- Next-Generation NCLEX (NGN)-Style Case Studies
- Review Questions (multiple choice NCLEX examination format)
- Toolbox (access to the links in the Tool Box sections for each chapter)
- Weblinks

For Instructors

TEACH for Nurses, including Nursing Curriculum Standards, Teaching Activities, and Case Studies
Additional Case Studies, with suggested answers
Critical Analysis Questions, with suggested answers
Critical Thinking Activities
Critical View Questions
Image Collection, with all images from the book
Lecture slides, in PowerPoint
Test Bank, with more than 270 questions in NCLEX examination format
Next-Generation NCLEX (NGN)-Style Case Studies for Community Health Nursing

NEXT-GENERATION NCLEX (NGN)

The National Council for the State Boards of Nursing (NCSBN) is a not-for-profit organization whose members include nursing regulatory bodies. In empowering and supporting nursing regulators in their mandate to protect the public, the NCSBN is involved in the development of nursing licensure examinations, such as the NCLEX-RN. In Canada, the NCLEX-RN was introduced in 2015 and is, as of the writing of this text, the recognized licensure exam required for practising RNs in Canada.

The NCLEX-RN as of 2023 will be changing to ensure that its item types adequately measure clinical judgement, critical thinking, and problem-solving skills on a consistent basis. The NCSBN will also be incorporating into the examination what they call the Clinical Judgement Measurement Model (CJMM), which is a framework the NCSBN has created to measure a novice nurse's ability to apply clinical judgement in practice.

These changes to the examination come as a result of findings indicating that novice nurses have a much higher than desirable error rate with patients (errors causing patient harm) and upon NCSBN's investigation discovering that the overwhelming majority of these errors were caused by failures of clinical judgement.

Clinical judgement has been a foundation underlying nursing education for decades, based on the work of a number of nursing theorists. The theory of clinical judgement that most closely aligns to what NCSBN is basing their CJMM is the work by Christine A. Tanner.

The new version of the NCLEX-RN is identified loosely as the "Next-Generation NCLEX" or "NGN" and will feature:

- Six key skills in the CJMM: recognizing cues, analyzing cues, prioritizing hypotheses, generating solutions, taking actions, and evaluating outcomes.
- Approved item types as of March 2021: multiple response, extended drag and drop, cloze (drop-down), enhanced hot-spot (highlighting), matrix/grid, bowtie, and trend. More question types may be added.
- All new item types are accompanied by mini-case studies with comprehensive patient information—some of it relevant to the question, and some of it not.
- Case information may present a single, unchanging moment in time (a "single episode" case study) or multiple moments in time as a patient's condition changes (an "unfolding" case study).
- Single-episode case studies may be accompanied by one to six questions; unfolding case studies are accompanied by six questions.

For more information (and detail) regarding the NCLEX-RN and changes coming to the exam, visit the NCSBNs website: https://www.ncsbn.org/11447.htm and https://ncsbn.org/Building_a_Method_for_Writing_Clinical_Judgment_It.pdf.

For further NCLEX-RN examination preparation resources, see *Elsevier's Canadian Comprehensive Review for the NCLEX-RN Examination*, Second Edition, ISBN 9780323709385.

Prior to preparing for any nursing licensure examination, please refer to your provincial or territorial nursing regulatory body to determine which licensure examination is required in order for you to practice in your chosen jurisdiction.

LIST OF BOXED FEATURES

CHN IN PRACTICE: A CASE STUDY

Identifying Health Inequities, 6
Ethical Principles, 7
Upstream, Midstream, and Downstream Approaches, 13
Identifying Levels of Prevention, 13
Collaborative Community Health Practice, 25
Historical Reflection for Contemporary Practice, 44
Discharge Planning for Postcerebrovascular Accident Care, 52
Case Management and Decision Making in Northern Manitoba, 56
Complex Urban Home Care, 58
Sexual Assault Nurse Examiner Practice in the Emergency Department, 74
Rural Palliative Care Practice, 78
Health Promotion Strategies, 112
Expanding Clinic Services, 126
Ethical Considerations in Planning Care, 141
Interpretation in the Home Visit, 169
Cultural Competence and the Home Visit, 171
Epidemiology, 185
Foodborne Illness, 200
Caring for Older Persons in the Community, 224
Community Asset Mapping, 224
Health Promotion Program for Mill Employees, 242
Older Persons' Issues, 271
Adolescent Prenatal Community Nursing: A Family Assessment, 297
Mutual Goal Setting and Problem Solving During Prenatal Community Health Nursing, 304
Supporting a Family—and the Wider Community—Through Difficult News, 306
Group Work With the Parents of Teenagers Who Have Discipline Problems, 321
Sarah's Developing Indigenous Community Health Practice, 345
"Buns in the Oven": A Prenatal Nutrition Program, 354
CHN Support and Care for a Family Living With Poverty, 357
Street Outreach to King Street Supported Housing Units, 359
Home Care for a High-Priority Family, 375
A Program for Young Parents, 377
High-Priority Pregnancy Care in the Community, 385
Ebola, 412
Tuberculosis, 421
Fishing for Answers in Corner Brook, 429
Understanding Patterns of Air Pollution and Dermatitis, 437
Bringing Environmental Care to the Clinic, 441
Managing Soil and Water Contamination in the Community, 447
A Community Health Nurse Is Challenged in a Tornado Zone, 465

LEVELS OF PREVENTION

Related to Public Health Nursing, 13
Related to Health Education, 52
Related to Home Health Nursing, 60
Related to Public Health Nursing, 65
Related to Occupational Health Nursing, 68
Related to Rural and Outpost Nursing, 72
Related to Nurse Practitioner Practice, 73
Related to Corrections Nursing, 73
Related to Community Health Education, 107
Related to Ethical Decision Making, 138
Related to Culture and Literacy, 167
Related to Cardiovascular Disease, 197
Related to Health Program Planning and Evaluation, 241
Related to Families Experiencing Violence or Abuse, 300
Related to Structurally Vulnerable Populations, 383
Related to Communicable Disease Interventions, 398
Related to Unhealthy Environments, 438
Related to Environmental Health, 446
Related to Disaster Management, 464

ETHICAL CONSIDERATIONS

These boxes appear in the following chapters:
Chapter 4: Health Promotion, 87
Chapter 5: Evidence-Informed Practice in Community Health Nursing, 121
Chapter 9: Working With the Community, 205
Chapter 10: Health Program Planning and Evaluation, 237
Chapter 11: Working With the Individual as Patient: Health and Wellness Across the Lifespan, 268
Chapter 13: Working With Groups, Teams, and Partners, 316
Chapter 16: Communicable and Infectious Disease Prevention and Control, 396
Chapter 17: Environmental Health, 434
Chapter 18: Pandemic Preparedness, 459

CULTURAL CONSIDERATIONS

Community Inclusion, 105
A Systematic Review of Motor Vehicle Crashes in Indigenous Populations in Canada, 123
Using Participatory Action Research, 124
Layers of Mental Health Promotion and Support for Syrian Refugees, 168
Community Wisdom, 206
Caregiving Patterns and Toxic Stress in Children, 263
South Asian Men's View of Physical Activity, 264
Culture, Food, and Family Health, 293
Indigenous Ways of Knowing and Being, 326
Social Justice and Equity Considerations in Disaster Planning for Higher Risk Groups, 458

HOW TO ...

Distinguish Public Health Nursing, 12

Apply the Utilitarian Ethics Decision Process, 132

Apply the Deontological Ethics Decision Process, 132

Apply the Principlism Ethics to the Decision Process, 134

Apply the Virtue Ethics Decision Process, 135

Apply the Ethics of Care Decision Process, 137

Apply the Process of Relational Practice to Working With Patients, 166

Select and Use an Interpreter, 169

Identify a Key Informant for Interviews, 215

Obtain a Quick Assessment of a Community, 217

Plan for the Assessment Process, 290

Set an Appointment With the Family, 290

Prepare for the Home Visit, 291

Handle Group Conflict, 316

Evaluate the Concept of Homelessness, 359

Identify Warning Signs for Needed Support and Early Intervention to Prevent Child Abuse, 363

Recognize Actual or Potential Child Abuse, 363

Assess Socioeconomic Concerns Resulting From Substance Use Disorders, 374

Assess Structural Vulnerability, 378

Intervene With Structurally Vulnerable Patients, 379

Care Navigation for People Experiencing Structural Vulnerabilities, 381

Support Care Navigation in Working With People Experiencing Structural Vulnerabilities, 381

Apply the Community Health Nursing Process to Environmental Health, 437

DETERMINANTS OF HEALTH

Literacy, 107

Diversity, 157

Community-Level Determinants of Health, 207

Family-Level Determinants of Health, 279

Income, Age, Gender, Racism, and Biology, 355

Mental Health, 369

The Influence of the Determinants of Health on Communicable and Infectious Diseases, 393

Physical and Psychosocial Environments, 428

EVIDENCE-INFORMED PRACTICE

Chapter 1: [Stadjuhar, K.I., Mollison, A., Giesbrecht, M., et al. (2019)], 15

Chapter 2: [Sanders, T., O'Mahony, J., Duncan, S., Mahara, S., Pitman, V., Ringstad, K., & Weatherman, K. (2019)], 30

Chapter 2: [MacDougall, H. (2009)], 32

Chapter 3: [Whelan, N., Steenbeek, A., Martin-Misener, R., et al. (2014)], 64

Chapter 4: [Cusack, C., Hall, W., Scruby, L., et al. (2008)], 110

Chapter 5: [Rice, V. H., & Stead, L. F. (2006)], 122

Chapter 6: [Oberle, K., & Tenove, S. (2000)], 138

Chapter 6: [Flicker, S., & Guta, A. (2008)], 139

Chapter 7: [McCabe, J., & Holmes, D. (2014)], 158

Chapter 7: [Khanlou, N., Haque, N., Mustafa, N., Vazquez, L., Mantini, A., & Weiss, J. (2017)], 164

Chapter 8: [Issekutz, Graham, Prasad, et al. (2005)], 182

Chapter 8: [Fantus, D., Shah, B. R., Qiu, F., et al. (2009)], 198

Chapter 9: [Horton, J., & MacLeod, M. (2008)], 211

Chapter 10: [Campbell, R., Patterson, D., Adams, A. E., et al. (2008)], 239

Chapter 11: [Bird, S., Wiles, J., Okalik, L., et al. (2008)], 262

Chapter 12: [Campbell, K., MacKinnon, K., Dobbins, M., Van Borek, N., & Jack, S. (2019)], 288

Chapter 13: [McCallin, A., & Bamford, A. (2007); Canadian Public Health Association (2010)], 310

Chapter 15: [Coulombe, S., Pacheco, T., Cox, E., Khalil, C., Doucerain, M.M., et al. (2020), 354; [Carter-Snell, C., Jakubec, S.L., & Hagen, B. (2020)], 365

Chapter 16: [Hislop, T. G., Teh, C., Low, A., et al. (2007)], 411

Chapter 17: [Kovesi, T., Creery, D., Gilbert, N. L., et al. (2006)], 442

Chapter 18: [Tolomiczenko, G. S., Kahan, M., Ricci, M., et al. (2005)], 457, [Parry, 2003], 457; [Booth, Matukas, Tomlinson, et al., 2003], 457; [Dwosh, Hong, Austgardan, et al., 2003], 457

ACKNOWLEDGEMENTS

First and foremost, we want to thank our immediate and extended families for their patience, love, and support, particularly during times they had to adjust plans and endure our states of distraction through the intense writing and editing process. We also thank our friends and colleagues for their words of encouragement.

We would like to acknowledge and thank all the reviewers who have inspired new directions and enhancements in this edition. Our appreciation goes to our colleagues at Memorial University of Newfoundland and Mount Royal University in Calgary, and community health research collaborators across the country who have encouraged and supported us during the writing of this text. In particular, we wish to thank our copy editors, Sarah McSwiney and Stephanie Bishop, who provided numerous insights, essential updates, and key contributions to the text, and Dr. Lisa Bourque-Bearskin, who specifically and importantly updated our chapters on diversity and Indigenous health with careful attention to the current discourse and issues.

We wish to thank Marcia Stanhope and Jeanette Lancaster and acknowledge their contributions over many years and many editions of community health nursing texts and the contributors to *Foundations of Nursing in the Community*, the original U.S. text from which this latest Canadian edition has evolved. Heather Jessup-Falcioni and Gloria A. Viverais-Dresler were the first Canadian authors to work on the Canadian edition, and we gratefully acknowledge their foundational work that has made this text possible. We also want to thank our team at Elsevier, especially Tamara Myers, director of education content, for her excellent leadership; Roberta Spinosa-Millman, senior content strategist (acquisitions editor), for her capable direction; and Martina van de Velde, content development specialist, for her dedication to the task, attention to detail, added clarity, enduring support, and encouragement. We also extend our gratitude to Manchu Mohan for her commitment to quality and meticulous consolidation of edits for a polished, final production-ready textbook. Finally, we wish to acknowledge each other and our effective and energizing editorial collaboration across the east and west of this country through many hurdles and life's circumstances—we love it when a plan comes together!

Sandra A. MacDonald, RN, PhD

Sandra A. MacDonald is currently a professor of nursing and the Associate Dean of Undergraduate Programs at the Faculty of Nursing at Memorial University of Newfoundland (MUN), Canada. She has served for over 30 years as a faculty member and researcher, as well as president of the Association of Registered Nurses of Newfoundland and Labrador (ARNNL), and board member of the Canadian Nurses Association. Dr. MacDonald is a faculty associate with the Centre for Collaborative Health Professional Education and teaches in adult medical–surgical nursing, including clinical teaching in the areas of intensive care, coronary care, and emergency. Her publications and research have been in primary care, community health assessment, program evaluation, and simulation-based education. Dr. MacDonald holds a diploma in nursing from the Salvation Army Grace General Hospital, BSc and MSc degrees of Nursing from MUN, and a PhD in Health Services from Walden University, Minneapolis, Minnesota. Dr. MacDonald is the coauthor for another Elsevier publication: *Mosby's Canadian Manual of Diagnostic and Laboratory Tests.* Dr. MacDonald received the Award for Excellence in Nursing Education in 2010 from the ARNNL and the MUN President's Award for Distinguished Teaching in 2012. She was awarded the Primary Care Researcher of the Year Award twice from the Primary Health Care Unit at MUN for her research on community health needs and resources, and age-friendly communities.

Sonya L. Jakubec, RN, PhD

Sonya L. Jakubec is a professor with the Faculty of Health and Community Studies at Mount Royal University, Calgary, Alberta. Her area of practice and research is community mental health across the lifespan, with a focus on social interventions and health promotion. Her clinical practice has involved rural/northern community mental health in Canada and West Africa, teaching and training for preservice and inservice, refugee care, crisis and emergency mental health, as well as teaching and research. Dr. Jakubec has a 30 year background in community mental health nursing, with practice, leadership and research in rural/remote and global health contexts. Her research concentrates on health promotion across the lifespan including palliative and grief care, with a particular interest in health and environment connections. Dr. Jakubec has researched and published in the areas of community mental health services; older persons and community health; mental health and sexual assault/intimate partner violence in rural communities; and community recreation (including outdoor nature interventions and community gardening) and social inclusion in mental health promotion.

Marcia Stanhope, RN, DSN, FAAN

Marcia Stanhope is an education and practice consultant for nursing education programs in the United States, an Associate with Tuft & Associates, Inc., an executive search firm in Chicago, Illinois; and Professor Emeritus from the University of Kentucky, College of Nursing, Lexington, Kentucky. She received the Provost Public Scholar award for contributions to the communities of Kentucky. She was appointed to the Good Samaritan Endowed Chair in Community Health Nursing and held the position for 12 years. She has practised community and home health nursing, has served as an administrator and consultant in home health, and has been involved in the development of a number of nurse-managed centres as well as the doctorate of nursing practice program nationally. She has taught community health, public health, epidemiology, primary care nursing, policy, and administration courses. Dr. Stanhope was the former Associate Dean and formerly directed the Division of Community Health Nursing and Administration at the University of Kentucky. She has been responsible for both undergraduate and graduate courses in population-centred, community-oriented nursing. She has also taught at the University of Virginia and the University of Alabama, Birmingham. Her presentations and publications have been in the areas of home health, community health and community-focused nursing practice, nurse-managed centres, primary care nursing, and the doctorate of nursing practice. Dr. Stanhope holds a diploma in nursing from the Good Samaritan Hospital, Lexington, Kentucky, and a BS in Nursing from the University of Kentucky. She has an MS in Public Health Nursing from Emory University in Atlanta, and a PhD in Nursing from the University of Alabama, Birmingham. Dr. Stanhope is the coauthor of four other Elsevier publications: *Handbook of Community-Based and Home Health Nursing Practice*; *Public and Community Health Nurse's Consultant*; *Case Studies in Community Health Nursing Practice: A Problem-Based Learning Approach*; and *Public Health Nursing: Population-Centered Health Care in the Community.*

Jeanette Lancaster, RN, PhD, FAAN

Jeanette Lancaster often serves as a visiting professor in both Taiwan and Hong Kong. She is an associate with Tuft & Associates, Inc. She served for 19 years as the Sadie Heath Cabaniss Professor of Nursing and Dean at the University of Virginia School of Nursing in Charlottesville, Virginia. When Dr. Lancaster stepped down as dean at the University of Virginia, a professorship, grant program for faculty, office suite, and the street in front of the school were named in her honour. From 2008 to 2009 she served as a visiting professor in the School of Nursing at the University of Hong Kong. In Spring 2013 and Fall 2014, she served as a professor with Semester at Sea and taught cross-cultural health promotion and nutrition as the students, faculty, staff, and life-long learners sailed around the world for 4 months.

Dr. Lancaster also served as president of the American Association of Colleges of Nursing. She has practised psychiatric nursing and taught both psychiatric and community health nursing. She formerly directed the master's program in community health nursing at the University of Alabama, Birmingham, and served as dean of the School of Nursing at Wright State University in Dayton, Ohio. Her publications and presentations have been largely in the areas of community and public health nursing, leadership and change, and the significance of nurses to effective primary health care. Dr. Lancaster is a graduate of the University of Tennessee Health Sciences Center, College of Nursing. She holds an MS in Psychiatric Nursing from Case Western Reserve University in Cleveland, Ohio, and a PhD in Public Health from the University of Oklahoma. Dr. Lancaster is the author of another Mosby/Elsevier publication, *Nursing Issues in Leading and Managing Change*, and coauthor (with Dr. Stanhope) of *Public Health Nursing: Population-Centered Health Care in the Community*.

UNIT I Background and Roles for Community Health Nursing, 1

1 Community Health Nursing, 2
- Health Care in Canada, 3
  - *Canadian Community Health Agencies: Health Canada and the Public Health Agency of Canada, 3*
- Population Health and the Determinants of Health, 3
  - *Social Determinants of Health, 5*
- Ethics, Equity, Social Justice, and Human Rights, 6
  - *Ethics, 6*
  - *Equity, 7*
  - *Social Justice, 7*
- Primary Health Care, 9
  - *Principles of Primary Health Care, 9*
- Public Health Practice, 11
  - *Principles of Public Health Practice: Levels of Intervention and Prevention, 12*
  - *The Community Health Patient, 14*
  - *Populations and Aggregates, 14*
  - *Collaborating in Interprofessional Teams, 14*
- Community Health Nursing Practice, 15
  - *Community Health Nursing Roles and Functions, 16*
  - *Areas of Community Health Nursing Practice, 16*
- Canadian Community Health Nursing Standards of Practice, 20
  - *Approaches to Practice: Health Promotion, Empowerment, Capacity Building, and Population Health, 21*
  - *Chapter Summary, 25*

2 The Evolution of Community Health Nursing in Canada, 29
- The Global Historical Roots of Public Health, 31
- Early Public Health Efforts in Canada, 32
- Milestones in Community Health Nursing in Canada, 33
  - *The Late 1800s to the Early 1900s, 34*
  - *Remarkable Legacies, 35*
  - *Post–World War I: 1918 to the Early 1940s, 35*
  - *Post–World War II: 1945 to 1970, 37*
  - *1970 to 1999, 38*
  - *2000 to the Present, 39*
  - *Chapter Summary, 44*

3 Community Health Nursing in Canada: Settings, Functions, and Roles, 47
- General Community Health Nursing Functions and Practices, 48
  - *Care and Counselling, 48*
  - *Continuity of Care, 49*
  - *Referral, 49*
  - *Health Education, 52*
  - *Team Building, Community Development, and Collaboration, 53*
- Settings, Functions, and Roles of Community Health Nurses in Canada, 57
  - *The Home Health Nurse, 58*
  - *The Public Health Nurse, 62*
  - *The Occupational Health Nurse, 65*
  - *Rural and Outpost Nurses, 68*
  - *The Nurse Practitioner, 72*
  - *The Corrections Nurse, 73*
  - *The Forensic Nurse, 73*
  - *Other Community Health Nurses, 75*
  - *Chapter Summary, 77*

UNIT II Community Health Foundations and Principles, 83

4 Health Promotion, 84
- Promotion of Health, 85
  - *Development of the Concept of Health, 85*
  - *Foundational Concepts in Health Promotion, 86*
- Evolution of Health Promotion, 90
  - *Lalonde Report, 90*
  - *Alma-Ata Declaration, 90*
  - *World Health Organization Principles of Health Promotion, 92*
  - *Ottawa Charter for Health Promotion, 92*
  - *Epp Report: A Canadian Framework for Health Promotion, 93*
  - *Developments in Health Promotion, 93*
  - *Population Health Promotion Model, Revisited, 94*
  - *International Health Promotion Conferences, 95*
  - *Summary of the Evolution of Health Promotion, 96*
- Health Promotion Models, Theories, and Frameworks, 96
  - *Individual-Focused Perspectives, 97*
  - *Community-Focused Perspectives, 98*
  - *Public Policy–Focused Perspectives, 100*
  - *Ecological Models, 100*
  - *Existential and Humanistic Theoretical Perspectives, 101*
- Health Promotion Approaches, 101
  - *Biomedical Approach, 101*
  - *Behavioural Approach, 101*
  - *Socioenvironmental Approach, 101*

Health Promotion Strategies, 102
  Strengthening Community Action, 103
  Building Healthy Public Policy, 105
  Creating Supportive Environments, 106
  Developing Personal Skills, 106
  Health Literacy, 107
  Reorienting Health Services, 108
  Activities to Facilitate Health Promotion
    Strategies, 108
  Mutual Aid, 109
  Advocacy, 109
Health Promotion Skills, 109
  Working With Focus Groups, 110
  Preparing Funding Applications, 110
  Developing Health Promotion Capacity, 110
  Chapter Summary, 112

5 Evidence-Informed Practice in Community Health
   Nursing, 117
Evidence-Informed Practice, 117
The Evidence-Informed Practice Process, 118
  Formulating the Clinical Question, 119
  Gathering and Assessing Evidence, 121
  Determining Which Evidence Is Best to Inform
    Practice, 125
  Chapter Summary, 126

6 Ethics in Community Health Nursing Practice, 128
History of Nursing and Ethics, 129
Ethical Decision Making, 129
Ethics, 130
  Definitions, Theories, and Principles, 130
  Rule Ethics, 131
  Ethical Principles, 132
  Virtue Ethics, 135
  Relational Ethics, 136
  Ethics of Care, 136
Nursing Code of Ethics, 137
Nursing Code of Ethics and Community Health
  Nursing, 138
Advocacy and Ethics, 139
  Definitions, Codes, and Standards, 139
  Conceptual Framework for Advocacy, 140
  Practical Framework for Advocacy, 140
Principles for the Justification of Public Health
  Interventions, 140
  Chapter Summary, 141

7 Diversity and Relational Practice in Community Health
   Nursing, 145
Diversity, Culture, Race, and Ethnicity, 146
Key Demographic Groups for Community Health
  Nursing in Canada, 147
  An Aging Population, 147
  Indigenous Peoples, 148
  Immigrant Population, 148
Types of Diversity, 149
  Ethnic Diversity, 149
  Multiculturalism, 152
  Linguistic Diversity, 152

  Religious Diversity, 153
  Sexual Diversity, 153
  Disability/Diverse Abilities, 154
Diversity, Inequities, and the Determinants of
  Health, 156
Approaches to Diversity in Community Health
  Nursing Practice, 157
Cultural Competence, 159
  Developing Culturally Responsive Care, 160
  Inhibitors to Culturally Responsive Care, 160
Cultural Safety, 163
  Cultural Humility, 164
Cultural Nursing Assessment, 165
  Relational Practice: Assessment and Intervening
    Processes, 165
Applying Cultural Skills in Community Health
  Practice, 167
  Working With Immigrant and Refugee
    Populations, 167
  Using an Interpreter, 168
  Chapter Summary, 170

8 Epidemiological Applications, 176
Epidemiology: An Overview, 177
History of Epidemiology, 178
Common Epidemiological Measures in
  Community Health Nursing, 180
  Measures of Morbidity and Mortality, 180
Epidemiological Models and Approaches, 185
  The Epidemiological Triangle, 185
  The Web of Causation, 186
  The Life Course Approach, 188
Levels of Prevention, 189
  Primary Prevention, 189
  Secondary Prevention, 189
  Tertiary Prevention, 189
  The Natural History of Disease Related to Levels
    of Prevention, 189
Screening, 189
  Reliability and Validity, 191
The Basics of Epidemiological Research, 192
  Types of Epidemiological Studies, 192
  Sources of Data, 195
  Age-Adjusted Death Rates, 196
  Comparison Groups, 196
How Community Health Nurses use
  Epidemiology, 196
  Chapter Summary, 199

9 Working With the Community, 202
What Is a Community?, 203
The Community as Partner, 204
  Community and the Determinants of Health, 206
Characteristics of Community Health Nursing
  Practice, 207
  Community Health, 207
  Strategies to Improve Community Health, 209
  Healthy Communities, 209
  Community Partnerships and Coalitions, 210

Community Development, 211
Community Capacity Building, 211
Outcomes of Community Development, 212
Assessing Community Health, 213
Data Collection and Interpretation, 213
Data-Collection Methods, 214
Identifying Community Health Concerns, 218
Planning for Community Health, 218
Analyzing Health Concerns, 218
Identifying Health Concern Priorities, 219
Establishing Goals and Objectives, 220
Identifying and Prioritizing Intervention
Activities, 221
Implementation in the Community, 221
The Community Health Nurse's Role, 221
The Community Health Concern and the
Community Health Nurse's Role, 222
The Social Change Process and the Community
Health Nurse's Role, 222
Evaluating the Intervention for Community
Health, 222
Chapter Summary, 223

10 Health Program Planning and Evaluation, 227
The Health Program Management Process, 227
Health Program Planning for Community Health
Nursing, 228
Health Program Planning Models, 229
Program Logic Model, 229
PRECEDE-PROCEED Model, 230
The Health Program Planning Process, 232
Assessing and Defining the Patient Health
Concern, 233
Identifying Health Program Goals and Objectives,
234
Planning for Implementation, 236
Weighing Health Concern Solution Options, 237
Choosing the Best Solution, 237
The Health Program Evaluation Process, 237
Health Program Evaluation Sources, 238
Health Program Evaluation Criteria, 239
Chapter Summary, 241

UNIT III Stakeholders and Populations of
Community Health Practice, 245

11 Working With the Individual as Client: Health and
Wellness Across the Lifespan, 246
Healthy Living Approach, 246
Early Child Development as a Determinant of
Health, 247
Child and Adolescent Health, 248
Overweight and Obesity, 251
Physical Activity, 252
Nutrition, 252
The Comprehensive School Health Approach, 254
Unintentional Injuries and Accidents, 256

Tobacco Use, 257
Immunization, 258
Adult Health, 259
Women's Health, 259
Men's Health, 264
Older Persons' Health, 266
The Role of the Community Health Nurse in
Caring for Older Persons, 268
Resources for Community Health Nurses, 270
Chapter Summary, 271

12 Working With Families, 275
Family Nursing in the Community, 276
The Canadian Family, 277
Definition of Family, 277
Family Demography, 277
Family Structure, 278
Determinants of Health, 278
Family Health, 280
Family Health and Functionality, 280
Four Approaches to Family Nursing, 281
Theoretical Frameworks for Family Nursing, 281
Family Assessment Models and Approaches, 287
Friedman Family Assessment Model (Short
Form), 287
Calgary Family Assessment Model, 287
McGill Model of Nursing, 287
McMaster Model of Family Functioning, 288
Relational Practice, 288
Family Home Visits, 290
Planning for Home Visits, 290
Engagement, 291
Family Assessment, 293
Interventions, 294
Termination and Evaluation, 294
Postvisit Documentation, 295
Appraisal of Family Health Risks and Capacity, 295
Biological Risk Assessment, 295
Environmental Risk Assessment, 297
Behavioural Risk Assessment, 299
Family Interventions, 299
Calgary Family Intervention Model, 300
Family Health Risk Reduction, 301
Family Empowerment, 302
Family Resiliency, 302
Care Planning With Families, 303
Advantages and Challenges of Mutual Goal
Setting, 303
Clinical Judgement, 304
Community Resources, 305
Chapter Summary, 305

13 Working With Groups, Teams, and Partners, 309
Groups, Teams, and Partners, 309
Principles of a Group Process, 311
A Model for Group Development, 312
Task and Maintenance Roles, 313
Group Rules and Standards, 313
Leadership Behaviours, 314

Conflict Transformation, 315
Group Evaluation, 317
Working With Health Care Teams and Partners, 317
Team Building in the Community, 317
Forming Community Partnerships, 319
Interprofessional Partnerships, 319
Interprofessional Education, 320
Chapter Summary, 321

14 Indigenous Health: Working With First Nations People, Inuit, and Métis, 324
Indigenous Peoples in Canada: Definitions, 325
Population Snapshot of Indigenous Peoples, 325
The Health Status of Indigenous People, 326
The Historical and Legislative Context of Indigenous Health Issues, 327
Precolonization and Colonization, 327
Key Events and Legislation, 328
First Nations Peoples Treaties, 328
The Indian Act, 330
The Consequences of Colonization and Historical Trauma, 330
Residential School Legacy, 330
The Sixties Scoop, 332
Indigenous Health Advocacy Actions, 332
Indigenous Nursing in Canada, 332
The Truth and Reconciliation Commission of Canada, 333
Decolonization, 333
Indigenous Determinants of Health, 334
Proximal Determinants of Health, 334
Intermediate Determinants of Health, 335
Distal Determinants of Health, 335
CHN in Practice: a Comprehensive Case Study, 336
Developing an Exercise and Wellness Program for Indigenous Women in Northern Creek, 336
Background, 336
Community Health Assessment, 336
Planning for a Community Health Nursing Intervention, 337
Chapter Summary, 345

15 Working With People Who Experience Structural Vulnerabilities, 351
Vulnerability: Definition and Influencing Factors, 352
Determinants of Health, 355
Factors Predisposing People to Vulnerability (Health Inequities), 355
Poverty, 356
Poverty and Health, 356
Homelessness and Housing Instability, 358
Understanding the Concept of Homelessness, 358
Effects of Housing Instability on Health, 359
Homelessness and At-Risk Populations, 359
Violence, 360
Homicides, 360
Social and Community Factors That Influence Violence, 360

Violence as a Form of Abuse, 361
Assault, 364
Community Mental Health, 366
At-Risk Populations for Mental Illness, 367
Determinants of Mental Health, 369
The Community Health Nurse's Collaborative Role in Community Mental Health Care, 369
Substance Use and Community Health, 372
Promotion of Healthy Lifestyles and Resiliency Factors, 373
Harm Reduction in Prevention Strategies, 373
Vulnerability of Children and Youth, 375
Adolescent Sexual Behaviour and Pregnancy, 375
Community Health Nurses Caring for People Experiencing Structural Vulnerabilities: Roles and Levels of Prevention, 377
The Roles of the Community Health Nurse, 380
Levels of Prevention and the Community Health Nurse, 383
Chapter Summary, 384

UNIT IV Specific Domains of Community Health Practice, 389

16 Communicable and Infectious Disease Prevention and Control, 390
Historical Perspectives, 391
Determinants of Health, 392
Communicable Diseases, 394
Agent, Host, and Environment, 394
Modes of Transmission, 395
Disease Development, 395
Disease Spectrum, 395
Surveillance of Communicable Diseases, 396
List of Notifiable Diseases, 396
Primary, Secondary, and Tertiary Prevention, 397
The Role of Community Health Nurses in Disease Prevention and Control, 398
Vaccine-Preventable Diseases, 398
Non–Vaccine-Preventable Diseases, 404
Sexually Transmitted Infections, 405
Infectious Diseases, 410
Viral Hepatitis, 410
Ebola Virus Disease, 411
Waterborne and Foodborne Diseases, 412
Vectorborne Diseases, 414
Diseases of Travellers, 415
Zoonoses, 416
Parasitic Diseases, 416
The Community Health Nurse's Role in Providing Preventive Care, 416
Primary Prevention, 416
Secondary Prevention, 418
Tertiary Prevention, 419
Chapter Summary, 420

17 Environmental Health, 425

    Environmental Concepts and Principles, 426

        Environmental Risk Factors and Health, 426

        Principles of Environmental Health, 427

    The Environment as a Determinant of Health, 428

        Environmental Risk Factors, 428

        Environmental Pollutants, 429

    Environmental Health Management in Canada, 430

        Governmental Protection of Environmental Health, 430

        Canada's Ecological Footprint, 433

        Canada's Greenhouse Gas Emissions Targets, 433

        Key Areas of Environmental Health Concern: Air, Water, and Food, 433

    Environmental Epidemiology, 435

    Environmental Health Assessment, 436

        Community Health Nursing Assessment and Referral Practices, 437

        Risk Assessment, 439

        Risk Communication, 440

    Reducing Environmental Health Risks, 441

        Risk Management, 441

    The Environment and Children's Health, 442

    Community Health Nurses' Roles in Environmental Health, 444

        Environmental Ethics and Environmental Justice, 444

        Environmental Advocacy, 445

        The Community Health Nurse and Environmental Health Policy, 445

        Chapter Summary, 446

18 Emergency Management and Disaster Preparedness, 451

    Types of Disasters, 452

        Natural Disasters, 452

        Human-Made Disasters, 453

        Biological Disasters, 453

    Canada's Emergency Management Framework, 455

    Disaster Prevention and Mitigation, 455

    Disaster Preparedness, 456

        Personal Preparedness, 456

        Professional Preparedness, 456

        Community Preparedness, 457

        Influenza Pandemic Preparedness, 459

        Public Health Nurses and the H1N1 Outbreak, 460

    Disaster Response, 462

        The Role of the Community Health Nurse in Disaster Response, 463

        Emergency Lodging After a Disaster, 463

    Disaster Recovery, 464

        Chapter Summary, 465

Glossary, 468

List of Appendices, 478

Appendix 1: Canadian Community Health Nursing Standards of Practice (Chapters 1, 3, 4, 6, 7, 9, 10, 11, 13, 15, 16), 478

Appendix 2: CNA Position Statement: Social Determinants of Health (Chapters 1, 14), 482

Appendix 3: Declaration of Alma-Ata (Chapters 1, 4), 485

Appendix 4: Ottawa Charter for Health Promotion (Chapters 1, 4), 487

Appendix 5: The Giger and Davidhizar Transcultural Assessment Model (Chapter 7), 490

Appendix 6: Community-as-Partner Model (Chapter 9), 493

Appendix 7: The Calgary Family Assessment Model and the Calgary Family Intervention Model (Chapter 12), 495

Appendix 8: CNA Position Statement: "Nurses and Environmental Health" (Chapter 17), 504

Appendix 9: Non–Vaccine-Preventable Infectious Diseases (Chapter 16), 508

Appendix 10: Viral Hepatitis Profiles (Chapter 16), 514

Index, 518

Background and Roles for Community Health Nursing

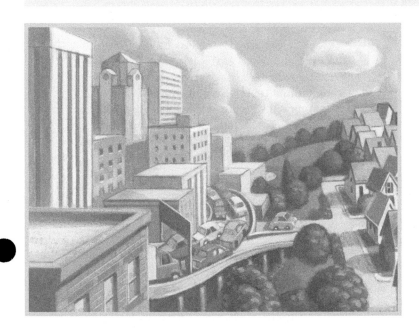

1

Community Health Nursing

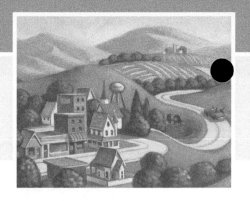

OUTLINE

Health Care in Canada, 3
  Canadian Community Health Agencies: Health Canada
    and the Public Health Agency of Canada, 3
Population Health and the Determinants of Health, 3
  Social Determinants of Health, 5
Ethics, Equity, Social Justice, and Human Rights, 6
  Ethics, 6
  Equity, 7
  Social Justice, 7
Primary Health Care, 9
  Principles of Primary Health Care, 9
Public Health Practice, 11

Principles of Public Health Practice: Levels of
    Intervention and Prevention, 12
The Community Health Patient, 14
Populations and Aggregates, 14
Collaborating in Interprofessional Teams, 14
Community Health Nursing Practice, 15
  Community Health Nursing Roles and Functions, 16
  Areas of Community Health Nursing Practice, 16
**Canadian Community Health Nursing Standards of
  Practice, 20**
  Approaches to Practice: Health Promotion,
    Empowerment, Capacity Building, and Population
    Health, 21

OBJECTIVES

After reading this chapter, you should be able to:
1.1 Describe the general structure of Canada's health care
    system.
1.2 Describe the population health promotion model and
    explain the determinants of health.
1.3 Explain the importance of ethics, equity, social justice,
    and human rights in community health nursing.

1.4 Identify and describe the principles of primary health
    care.
1.5 Discuss the principles of public health practice.
1.6 Explain community health nursing practice.
1.7 Discuss the Canadian Community Health Nursing
    Standards of Practice.

KEY TERMS*

aggregates, 14
Canadian Nurses Association (CNA), 8
capacity building, 15
collaboration, 15
community, 14
community health nursing, 3
determinants of health, 4
downstream thinking, 13
empowerment, 21
equality, 7
equity, 7
family, 6
global health, 8
health promotion, 21
midstream thinking, 13
patient, 6
population, 14

population health, 14
population-focused practice, 4
primary care, 9
primary health care, 9
primary prevention, 13
primordial prevention, 13
public health, 11
public health nursing, 12
secondary prevention, 13
social determinants of health, 5
social justice, 7
society, 6
subpopulations, 14
tertiary prevention, 13
United Nations Children's Emergency Fund (UNICEF), 8
upstream thinking, 13
World Health Organization (WHO), 8

*See the Glossary on page 468 for definitions.

Community health nursing is a term that applies to all nurses who work in and with the community in a variety of practice areas, such as public health, home health, occupational health, and other similar fields. In recent years, community health nursing has become a more visible field of practice in Canada. The number of recognized community health nursing specialties has increased, and community health nurses (CHNs) (who comprise close to 16% of the nursing workforce) have increasingly become a vital part of the Canadian health care landscape (Canadian Institute for Health Information, 2017). While many nurses working in community health do not identify themselves as CHNs, the variety of settings in which nurses practise within the community has expanded, as has the scope of the community nursing role. First adopted in 2003, the *Canadian Community Health Nursing Professional Practice Model and Standards of Practice* (Community Health Nurses of Canada, 2019) has further reinforced the status of community health nursing as a specialty field of practice within the discipline of nursing (refer to Appendix 1).

Recognizing that health status is influenced by determinants such as income, employment, education, gender, race, and social environment, CHNs aim to improve the health of all persons by addressing these determinants and minimizing health disparities wherever possible. They also consider that lifestyle choices (e.g., tobacco, alcohol, drug use, diet, physical activity, sexual practices) influence health as well. The relationship of policy and health status makes policy influence and development an important priority for CHNs.

CHNs continue to make a difference through their work in areas such as population health, "upstream thinking," evidence-informed nursing practice, the determinants of health, and the Ottawa Charter for Health Promotion—areas that will be explored in this text. Chapter 1 briefly introduces the reader to some of the key community health nursing concepts, such as the determinants of health, public health, primary health care, social justice, and community health nursing. These concepts are elaborated on in distinct units and chapters throughout this text.

HEALTH CARE IN CANADA

Canada is a bilingual country that is geographically vast, covering diverse types of terrain over 10 provinces and three territories and comprising many Indigenous and immigrant cultural groups that reside in both urban and rural settings. In order to create a more equitable national health care system for all Canadians, the federal government created the *Canada Health Act*, which was enacted in 1984. The five principles of this Act are (1) universality, (2) accessibility, (3) comprehensiveness of services, (4) portability, and (5) public administration (Health Canada, 2018).

The federal government's roles in health care include establishing and administering national principles under the *Canada Health Act* as well as providing financial support to the provinces and territories that ultimately legislate, organize, and deliver services. The federal government also funds and/or delivers primary and supplementary services

to specific groups, including First Nations people living on reserves; Inuit; members of the Canadian Forces and some veterans; inmates in federal penitentiaries; and some groups of refugee claimants (Health Canada, 2019).

Since the 1990s, reform has taken place at various levels in the Canadian health care system, and different restructuring models have been adopted across the provinces and territories (National Collaborating Centre for Healthy Public Policy, 2018). One example of these changes was the establishment of community health centres across Canada with the goal of improving access to health care and, in underserviced regions, providing such access. Although local and regional differences in management or services exist, there are similarities among community health centres in these key goals (Canadian Association of Community Health Centres, 2019). CHNs need to be prepared to address health concerns and population health care issues locally or regionally, provincially or territorially, nationally, and globally within the context of the health care reform initiatives.

Canadian Community Health Agencies: Health Canada and the Public Health Agency of Canada

Health Canada, which has regional offices across Canada, is a Canadian umbrella agency for many health care portfolios, such as the Public Health Agency of Canada (PHAC); Canadian Institutes of Health Research (CIHR); Health Products and Food Branch (HFPB); First Nations and Inuit Health Branch (FNIHB); and Healthy Environments and Consumer Safety Branch (HECSB). Health Canada safeguards the population's health through surveillance, prevention, legislation, and research in such areas as environmental health, disease outbreaks, drug products, and food safety (Health Canada, 2020).

Following the 2003 severe acute respiratory syndrome (SARS) outbreak, the PHAC was established in 2004 to revitalize and support sustainability of the Canadian public health system. Led by a chief public health officer, this agency provides opportunities for collaboration between the federal government and the provinces and territories. The chief public health officer communicates important public health issues in an annual report and provides national health advisories and recommendations for issues such as the coronavirus disease (COVID-19). These reports are instrumental tools in community health and will be referenced throughout this text to highlight key issues that affect the health of Canadians.

POPULATION HEALTH AND THE DETERMINANTS OF HEALTH

In traditional health care, the individual is the focus, and the approach is curative or rehabilitative, whereas in population health, the population or aggregates (groups that form a population) are the focus, and importance is given to the influence of the determinants of health. Traditional health care provides treatment to individuals with an illness, whereas population health advocates for disease prevention and health promotion among groups or populations (Bourgeault, Labonté, Packer, & Runnels, 2017). **Population-focused practice** directs community health nursing practice; in contrast to individual-focused health care, it emphasizes reducing the health inequities of a defined population or aggregate. Critics can be found for the individual lifestyle perspective, population health practice (Morrison, Gagnon, Morestin, et al., 2014), and even the basic assumptions of public and population health (Mykhalovskiy, Frohlich, Poland, et al., 2019). Nonetheless, the origins and principles of population health practice are briefly introduced here and further elaborated in Chapter 4.

A New Perspective on the Health of Canadians (the Lalonde Report) (Lalonde, 1974) first initiated the shift from primarily curative aspects of care to holistic health care and provided the foundation for health promotion (MacDougall, 2007). The Ottawa Charter for Health Promotion (World Health Organization [WHO], 1986) identified the prerequisites for health as peace, shelter, education, food, income, a stable ecosystem, sustainable resources, social justice, and equity, which established the roots of the current determinants of health in Canada. *Achieving Health for All* (the Epp Report) (Epp, 1986) identified reducing inequities, increasing prevention, and enhancing coping skills as specific challenges to achieving health; these challenges are also recognized in the determinants of health.

Socioecological frameworks, adopted by some health care researchers and practitioners, also established a model of interconnectedness among the determinants of health (National Collaborating Centre for Determinants of Health, 2020). In their population health promotion model (discussed further in Chapter 4), Hamilton and Bhatti (1996) identify nine determinants of health (see Fig. 1.1). This model does not include gender and culture (unmodifiable factors) among the determinants, nor does it include the broad concept of "environment." However, it remains an important organizing framework in the evolving understanding of population health. The Government of Canada (2019) identifies 12 determinants of health, including gender and culture, and separates "environment" into "social environment" and "physical environment."

The 12 **determinants of health** that affect the health of patients (Government of Canada, 2019) are presented in the list that follows. These factors directly determine the risk for or distribution of health outcomes such as disability, disease, and death. CHNs need to consistently consider these factors in their day-to-day work.

1. *Income and social status* have regularly been shown in the literature to be the most important determinants of health: as income and social status rise, the health status of Canadians improves. Since 2005, there have consistently been great disparities in income-related health and life expectancy in Canada (Bushnik, Tjepkema, & Martel, 2020). A CHN working with low-income families may consider lobbying for their access to subsidized housing.

2. *Employment/working conditions* are associated with improved health because better economic conditions support health. Being gainfully employed also provides

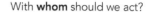

With **whom** should we act?

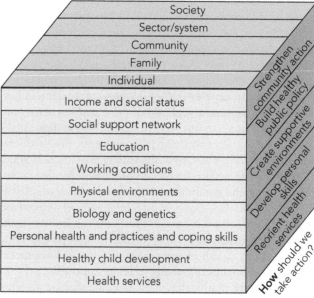

On **what** should we take action?

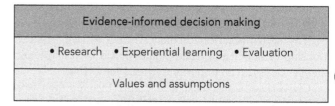

Fig. 1.1 Population Health Promotion Model. (*Source*: Public Health Agency of Canada. [2001]. *Population health promotion: An integrated model of population health and health promotion.* Adapted and reproduced with permission from the Minister of Health, 2016.)

a sense of purpose and other influences on psychological well-being.

3. *Education and literacy* are part of socioeconomic status and significantly contribute to better health outcomes since health status improves with higher levels of education. A CHN working with patients who have literacy challenges could refer these patients to community literacy programs.

4. *Childhood experiences* implies consideration of prenatal and early childhood exposures and experiences that may contribute to a variety of chronic conditions and to the development of physical and emotional health outcomes later in life. A CHN working with a group of first-time mothers could help them identify concerns that they may have about parenting and provide educational support and referral when necessary.

5. *Physical environments* refers to human-built environments (e.g., housing, playgrounds, workplaces, neighbourhoods, public transit) as well as the pollutants in the environment that affect the quality of air, water, food, and soil. A CHN working with schools could advocate for safe playground equipment on school property.

6. *Social supports and coping skills* are associated with improved health; it has been suggested that poor social relationships may, in fact, be as important a risk factor as smoking or obesity. The ability to cope with health outcomes relies heavily on social care and community support. A CHN working with self-help groups could provide support to group members through group facilitation.
7. *Healthy behaviours* include lifestyle choices and individual activities such as physical activity habits and other practices.
8. *Access to health services* is essential to all for health maintenance, promotion, protection, disease prevention, and treatment if population health is to be achieved. A CHN could assist a family experiencing poverty gain access to health services, such as eye care, by using service clubs in the community to provide funding for eyeglasses for family members with vision problems.
9. *Biology and genetic endowment* predispose some individuals to certain illnesses, such as Down syndrome, Huntington's disease, cystic fibrosis, and sickle-cell anemia.
10. *Gender* indicates that some health problems and health practices are gender specific; for example, men are more likely than women to die prematurely from heart disease, and women are more likely than men to experience sexual assault in their lifetime. Gender discrimination and inequality are also determinants of health that expose people at risk of physical and mental health problems. A CHN could work with other health care providers and local women to help the community develop a better understanding of sexual assault, access comprehensive services, and enhance trauma-informed care and other interventions in the community.
11. *Culture* may predispose some groups to certain diseases, such as sickle cell anemia and thalassemia. Culture may also have implications for access to care. A CHN working with new Canadians could partner with multicultural associations in the community to provide access to interpreters when new immigrant groups are trying to use community health services.
12. *Race/racism* is recognized as a key social determinant of health and driver of health inequities. People exposed to racism have poorer health outcomes (particularly for mental health), as well as poor access to health care and poorer health care experiences (Stanley et al., 2019). CHNs in any capacity can ask important questions about how racism visibly and invisibly operates within health services, can include racialized people in planning care with awareness of the impact of racism on health, and can advocate for equitable and acceptable services.

Social Determinants of Health

The **social determinants of health** are the social conditions and broader forces (e.g., politics and economics) that interact to influence risks to health and well-being and affect how vulnerable or resilient people are to disease and injury (National Collaborating Centre for Determinants of Health, 2020). Table 1.1 presents various Canadian and international conceptualizations of the social determinants of health. Note that Indigenous status, social safety net, and health services are not included in most older conceptualizations (Raphael, 2016). Mikkonen and Raphael (2010) later added race and disability to their model and assert that 14 social determinants influence the health of Canadians: (1) income and income distribution, (2) education, (3) employment and working conditions, (4) early life, (5) food insecurity, (6) housing,

TABLE 1.1 Various Conceptualizations of the Social Determinants of Health

Ottawa Charter	Dahlgren and Whitehead (1992)	Health Canada (1998)	World Health Organization (1986)	Centers for Disease Control and Prevention (2005)	Raphael, Bryant, and Curry-Stevens (2004)
Peace	Agriculture and food production	Income and social status	Social gradient	Socioeconomic status	Indigenous status
Shelter	Education	Social support networks	Stress	Transportation	Early life
Education	Work environment	Education, employment, and working conditions	Early life	Housing	Education
Food	Unemployment		Social exclusion	Access to services	Employment and working conditions
Income	Water and sanitation	Physical and social environments	Work	Discrimination by social grouping	Food security
Stable ecosystem	Health care services	Healthy child development	Unemployment	Social or environmental stressors	Gender
Sustainable resources	Housing	Health services	Social support		Health care services
Social justice		Gender	Addiction		Housing
Equity (WHO, 1986)		Culture	Food		Income and its distribution
			Transport (Wilkinson & Marmot, 2003)		Social safety net
					Social exclusion
					Unemployment and employment security

Source: Raphael, D. (2012). Critical perspectives on the social determinants of health. In E. McGibbon (Ed.), *Oppression: A social determinant of health.* Fernwood.

(7) health services, (8) social exclusion, (9) social safety net, (10) health services, (11) Indigenous status, (12) gender, (13) race, and (14) disability (p. 9). About 75% of health status is influenced by these factors that influence experiences of trauma, stigma, and discrimination, impacting access to care and other aspects of inequities (BC Centres for Disease Control Foundation for Public Health, 2020); these topics are further explored in Chapters 14 and 15.

Raphael (2016, 2019) and others (Bryant, Raphael, Schrecker, et al., 2011; Pederson & Machado, 2019; Canadian Council on Social Determinants of Health, 2015) have conducted extensive research on the social determinants of health and their applications within health care policy, particularly in Canada. Because social determinants of health have such profound impacts on all of society (National Collaborating Centre for Determinants of Health, 2020), efforts to improve health and reduce health inequities will require more upstream approaches. Indigenous determinants of health focus on multiple determinants of health that also include colonialism, geography, land and environmental rights, and policies for their impacts on the health of Indigenous peoples in Canada (Greenwood, de Leeuw, & Lindsay, 2018).

The World Health Organization (WHO) publication *Social Determinants of Health: The Solid Facts* (Wilkinson & Marmot, 2003; see the link on the Evolve website) provides an excellent introduction to the social determinants of health as identified at the time, with evidence to explain each of them and a discussion of policy considerations. In 2005, WHO established the Commission on Social Determinants of Health to provide recommendations on how to address the social factors contributing to health inequities (WHO, 2021). The final WHO report, *Closing the Gap in a Generation: Health Equity Through Action on the Social Determinants of Health,* included the following three recommendations with corresponding principles of action: improve daily living conditions; tackle the inequitable distribution of power, money, and resources; and understand the problem and assess the impact of action (WHO, 2008). For further information on the global issues in reference to the social determinants of health, and to review the corresponding principles of action for these recommendations, see the Evolve website. Another document, *Key Health Inequalities in Canada: A National Portrait* (PHAC, 2018), provides further information on the determinants of health, particularly inequities in health outcomes, daily living conditions, and structural drivers, with examples of their application to patient care. (Throughout this text, the term **patient** refers to the individual, **family**, group or aggregate, community, population, or **society**.)

Despite the fact that Canada is a recognized leader in the health promotion movement, Canadian decision makers have been slow to develop public health policy based on research evidence (Bryant et al., 2011). At a practical level, work to identify social determinants and inequities is explored in the "CHN in Practice: A Case Study, Identifying Health Inequities" box.

 CHN IN PRACTICE: A CASE STUDY

Identifying Health Inequities
You are joining CHN Kristin as an additional CHN at the community health centre in Houston, a small town in northern British Columbia with a population of approximately 3 200 people. Key activities in the surrounding area are fishing and other outdoor recreation, and the main industries are tourism, mining, and forestry. Keep in mind that all communities have some health inequities.

Think About It
What information would you need to explore in your new community in order to identify the possibility of health inequities? Provide rationales for your choices.

The determinants of health will be discussed throughout the text, including in "Determinants of Health" boxes in select chapters that highlight the influences of some of the determinants on the health of Canadians. The determinants of health are also highlighted in specific appendices found in this text. For example, the Canadian Nurses Association (CNA, 2018a) position statement *Social Determinants of Health* (see Appendix 2) explains why social determinants are important and directly related to the health and health inequities of individuals, groups, and all Canadians. It also lists and explains some of the most important social determinants of health noted by WHO—poverty, economic inequality, social status, stress, education and care in early life, social exclusion, employment and job security, social support, and food security. CHNs are continually reminded of how the social determinants of health can predict the health of populations, and that healthy public policy includes the social determinants of health. The position of the CNA sets out an active and ambitious position for the profession.

ETHICS, EQUITY, SOCIAL JUSTICE, AND HUMAN RIGHTS

When differences in determinants of health and health status within or between groups are shown to be systematic and avoidable, they are unfair and are called *health inequities* (PHAC, 2018). Lack of fairness in the distribution of opportunities or services impacts communities and societies and is a global concern (CNA, 2019). The topics of ethics, equity, social justice, and human rights are introduced here and discussed in further detail in Chapter 6.

Ethics

Witnessing health inequities in a community health practice founded on public health (or "health for all") poses inherent ethical dilemmas for CHNs. Regardless of his or her area of practice, every nurse encounters ethical dilemmas and must address them skillfully. CHNs experience ethical challenges that are unique to their community and patient population. For example, inequitable access to resources features in the life of a new mother attempting to care for her newborn and a toddler for whom she cannot afford additional day care;

people struggling with homelessness in urban centres; and those who have suffered a disability or other losses from an environmental disaster. Ethical practice is central to the concepts of equity and social justice, which are the foundations of community health practice. See the "CHN in Practice: A Case Study, Ethical Principles" box.

CHN IN PRACTICE: A CASE STUDY

Ethical Principles

Kristin works with Geoff, a 51-year-old single man who works seasonally picking mushrooms and resides in a pickers' campsite during the summer season. Geoff's summer work is complete, and he has found temporary shelter "squatting" in an unoccupied cabin in Houston, British Columbia, where he has resided for the past five years on and off, preferring to live "off the grid." Geoff's temporary employer has alerted the Houston community health centre that Geoff was diagnosed with tuberculosis but has not received treatment. His employer reported that during the last few weeks of the picking season, Geoff had a persistent, productive, blood-streaked cough, excessive sweating, and considerable weight loss.

Kristin visited Geoff's cabin and invited him to the health centre with a plan to convince him to get treatment in the hospital one hour away and arrange transportation for him to get there. Geoff is a self-professed loner who tends to be suspicious of others and does not want to be part of the "system" or be confined to a hospital. Kristin is attentive to his perspective, but she is also aware of her role in protecting the health of the public, and Geoff's active illness is contagious. The ethical principle most relevant to this situation is the *harm principle*, which is described by John Stuart Mill as follows: "The only purpose for which power can be rightfully exercised over any member of a civilized community, against his will, is to prevent harm to others. His own good, either physical or moral, is not a sufficient warrant."*

While Geoff refuses to be hospitalized, the concern is not for his welfare (he is not refusing treatment) but for the welfare of the public's health. Temporarily restricting Geoff's freedom by arranging for his treatment in hospital would be for the prevention of harm to others. If the restriction were only for the perceived welfare of Geoff as an individual, it would be considered paternalistic and a violation of the harm principle. (See Box 6.2 on page 130 for the International Council of Nurses code of ethics for nurses.)

Think About It
1. Is there a way to find a compromise?
2. How can Kristin explain the ethical rationale for hospital treatment to Geoff in a way that preserves his dignity?
3. How can Kristin maintain Geoff's dignity even if she has to exercise power over him to get treatment in hospital for the public good?

*Mill, J. (1959). On liberty. In B. Wishy (Ed.), *Prefaces to liberty: Selected writings of John Stuart Mill*. University Press America.

Equity

Differences in social status within and between populations have a significant impact on the health status of the larger community within which those differences occur. If the gap is large, the health status of the overall population decreases, health care costs increase, and the disharmony associated with exclusion is fostered. Inequity disadvantages everyone, not just those living with the least advantages (Mikkonen & Raphael, 2010; Wilkinson & Pickett, 2009). Improving the health of the whole population by advancing health **equity** is a core function of public health practice in Canada and globally. WHO's Commission on Social Determinants of Health noted that "action on social determinants of health empowers people, communities and countries" (WHO, 2008).

The commission recommended three principles of action to advance health equity:
1. Improve the conditions of daily life, i.e., the circumstances in which people are born, grow, live, work, and age.
2. Tackle the inequitable distribution of power, money, and resources—the structural drivers of those conditions of daily life—globally, nationally, and locally.
3. Measure the problem, evaluate action, expand the knowledge base, develop a workforce trained in the social determinants of health, and raise public awareness about the social determinants of health. (WHO, 2008).

Social Justice

CNA (2009) defines **social justice** as "the fair distribution of society's benefits, responsibilities and their consequences. It focuses on the relative position of one social group in relationship to others in society as well as on the root causes of disparities and what can be done to eliminate them" (p. 2). In the context of primary health care practice, social justice refers to ensuring fairness and equality in health services so that all members of society have equal access to health care. Distinct from equity, *equality* is the state or quality of being equal in quantity, degree, value, rank, or ability in a measurable way (CNA, 2009). Box 1.1 lists the defining attributes of social justice.

Working for social justice as a CHN involves two guiding principles: recognizing inequities and taking action to eliminate them. Recognizing inequities means identifying, understanding, and being able to describe inequities or injustices,

BOX 1.1 Ethical Responsibilities to Uphold Principles of Justice

- Not discriminating based on race, gender, or any attribute
- Respecting the history of Indigenous people
- Refraining from judging, labelling, or any stigmatizing behaviour toward anyone
- Refraining from lying, punishing, torture, or any form of inhumane treatment
- Providing care for all people (victim or perpetrator) and refraining from workplace bullying
- Making fair decisions about access to resources
- Advocating for evidence in decision making and all policies
- Working collaboratively to develop moral community

Source: Based on Canadian Nurses Association. (2017). *Code of ethics for registered nurses* (pp. 15-16). https://www.cna-aiic.ca/html/en/Code-of-Ethics-2017-Edition/files/assets/basic-html/page-22.html

the reasons for their presence, and how they affect population subgroups (including nurses). Responsible action to eliminate inequities means advocating for the reduction of the sources of oppression and working toward parity and fairness (CNA, 2009; Davison, Edwards, Webber, et al., 2006). In short, CHNs acknowledge injustice and differences and, rather than trying to treat everyone equally, work to reduce systemic inequity. The CNA document *Code of Ethics* (2017 edition; CNA, 2017) provides a more detailed discussion of the justice and ethical considerations for nurses.

Equity and Social Justice in Global Health

Around the world, the poorest of the poor tend to have the worst health. The factors that lead to the outcomes of inequities in wealth are not just the problem of the poor. Wilkinson and Pickett (2009) assert that the negative effects of inequality, such as physical and mental illness, pervade all levels of society and that more equal societies fare better than those with greater inequities. CNA (2009), in its position statement on global health and equity (see the link on the Evolve website), supports global health and equity within the context of social justice.

Brown, Cueto, and Fee (2006) provide a historical perspective on the transformation of the term *international health* to *global health*. These authors indicate that *global health* "implies consideration of the health needs of the people of the whole planet above the concerns of particular nations" (p. 62). Koplan, Bond, Merson, et al. (2009) define **global health** as "an area for study, research, and practice that places a priority on improving health and achieving equity in health for all people worldwide" (p. 1995). Koplan et al. (2009) provide an excellent comparison of the concepts of global health, international health, and public health and emphasize that global health addresses transnational health issues such as environmental health, climate change, human immunodeficiency virus (HIV), acquired immune deficiency syndrome (AIDS), and determinants of health such as poverty and education; involves an interprofessional approach with populations; and includes prevention, treatment, and care. Extending the evolving global public health discourse, Bosurgi (2019) further distinguishes between public health, global health, and planetary health, stating that public health is concerned with health protection and health promotion within the health systems, global health undertakes to improve health of populations worldwide, and planetary health looks at societies, civilizations, and the ecosystems on which they depend. Planetary health has expanded from other conceptualizations of EcoHealth and One Health that stressed the interactions of human, animal, and environmental health. It focuses on both the effects of environmental change on human health as well as the political, economic, and social systems that shape those effects (Rabinowitz, Pappaioanou, Bardosh, et al., 2018). CHNs are becoming more involved in working in global and planetary health, and in the social and political change movements to address the factors influencing health at systemic levels. See Box 1.2 for key organizations involved in global health efforts.

BOX 1.2   Key Organizations Involved in Global Health Efforts

- **Canadian Nurses Association (CNA)** is the national voice for provincial and territorial Canadian nursing associations and colleges. One of its goals is to influence global health and equity. See https://cna-aiic.ca/international-work.
- **International Council of Nurses (ICN)** is a federation of more than 130 national nurses' associations worldwide. It represents nursing as a profession internationally and influences health policy globally. Its vision is to improve health for all. See http://www.icn.ch.
- **World Health Organization (WHO)** is a leading international health organization involved in global health issues. See http://www.who.int/about/en. WHO regularly published a world health report up to 2013. *The World Health Report 2013: Research for Universal Health Coverage* is available at http://www.who.int/whr/2013/report/en/. WHO now publishes a report on world health statistics annually, available at https://www.who.int/gho/publications/en/.
- **Global Health Council** is a group of health care providers and government and nongovernmental organizations and institutions that work to achieve equity in global health. The council addresses global health issues such as women's health, children's health, HIV/AIDS, infectious diseases, and health systems. See http://www.globalhealth.org.
- **United Nations Children's Emergency Fund (UNICEF)** is an international organization that focuses on child survival and development, basic education and gender equality, HIV/AIDS and children, child protection, and policy advocacy and partnerships. See http://www.unicef.org/whatwedo/.

Note: The links that appear in this box are also available at the Evolve website for this text.

Human Rights and Community Health

A human rights approach to community health is a critical component of addressing health inequities (Rioux, 2019). This approach draws on the rule of law and national and international declarations and conventions in order to advocate for fair and just conditions for health and health care. Engaging with Indigenous peoples' perspectives, strengthening care for people with disabilities, providing reproductive health care services, and making HIV/AIDS treatment accessible are examples of the application of a human rights approach to community health (Grodin, Tarantola, Annas, et al., 2013). Freidman and Gostin (2013) propose a four-part strategy to accelerate progress toward the right to health for groups and populations:

1. Incorporate the right-to-health principles and priorities into national laws and policies.
2. Use creative strategies to increase the impact of national right-to-health litigation.
3. Empower communities and civil society groups to claim their rights to health.
4. Bring the right to health to the centre of global health governance.

The CNA position is that nurses must safeguard and uphold access to health care and all human rights as a right. The role of the profession in holding agencies and governments to account is named in the position statement (CNA, 2018b).

PRIMARY HEALTH CARE

In the early 1970s, the medical model, which focused on treatment and cure in institutions, was the most commonly used model in health care. The Lalonde Report (Lalonde, 1974) started the shift in thinking toward a population health promotion approach that considered factors influencing health, such as lifestyle. In 1978, at the International Conference on Primary Health Care held in Alma-Ata, USSR, participating countries, organizations, and WHO committed to a goal to achieve "health for all" by the year 2000 (WHO, 1978). The Declaration of Alma-Ata is recognized as part of the shift toward primary health care. The primary health care model put forward at Alma-Ata articulated the need for a comprehensive health strategy that not only provided health services (e.g., essential medications) but also addressed the underlying social, economic, and political causes of poor health (e.g., restricted educational opportunities).

Primary health care, an integrated health care delivery system and a formalized way of promoting health, was the international strategy chosen to achieve the goal of health for all (PHAC, 2011). The Lalonde Report and the Alma-Ata conference and their influence on health promotion as well as the principles of primary health care are discussed in Chapter 4. WHO, an umbrella organization of the United Nations established in 1948, aims to achieve the optimal level of health for all peoples globally (see the link for WHO on the Evolve website). This organization, which has played a key role in the development of health and health promotion approaches, provides many primary health care resources.

It is necessary to distinguish between *primary care* and *primary health care*. **Primary care** refers to the first contact between individuals and the health care system (health care providers). It usually relates to the curative treatment of disease (CNA, 2015), rehabilitation, and preventive measures, such as immunization, smoking cessation, and dietary changes. Primary care is not necessarily comprehensive care, nor is it necessarily intersectoral. *Primary health care* has a broader meaning. WHO (1978) has defined *primary health care* as "essential health care based on practical, scientifically sound, and acceptable methods and technology made universally accessible to individuals and families in the community through their full participation and at a cost that the community and country can afford to maintain at every stage of their development in the spirit of self-reliance and self-determination" (p. 2). The current definition of **primary health care** is comprehensive care that includes disease prevention, community development, a wide spectrum of services and programs, working in interprofessional teams, and intersectoral collaboration for healthy public policy (CNA, 2015). This comprehensive primary health care model endeavours to address the issues of ethics, social justice, and equity introduced earlier. The professional practice model and standards of practice for community health nursing in Canada (Community Health Nurses of Canada, 2019) have their

underpinnings in primary health care principles. Refer specifically to Standard 6: Access and Equity.

Primary health care is especially relevant to CHNs for the following reasons (CNA, 2015):
- It provides essential health services in the community.
- It considers the determinants of health.
- It focuses on health promotion, disease prevention, and protection.
- It includes therapeutic, curative, and rehabilitative care.
- It promotes coordination and interprofessional collaboration.
- It focuses on the patient as an equal partner in health with health care providers.

Principles of Primary Health Care

CHNs should be aware of the principles of primary health care as they conduct their practice. Primary health care, as a philosophy of health care, includes the following five principles, adopted at the Alma-Ata international conference (WHO, 1978):
- *Accessibility,* which means that essential health services should be equitably distributed to all populations to provide access to health services for all, including those living in rural, remote, and urban communities (CNA, 2015). Essential health services must be equitably shared among all persons, regardless of factors such as geographical location, culture, and income. This principle indicates that vulnerable groups (e.g., the homeless, persons with HIV/AIDS, persons with hepatitis) should have equal access to the health system. At present, many people do not have equal access. CHNs provide care in the community to such vulnerable populations and play a vital role in facilitating access to needed health services in their communities.
- *Health promotion,* which emphasizes services that are preventive and promotive rather than curative, such as health education and immunization (Calnan & Lemire Rodger, 2002). It also emphasizes the need for health care systems to promote health and prevent disease so that their focus is on health maintenance rather than a curative approach to care.

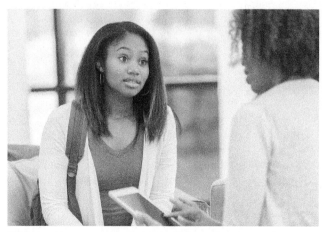

Public health nurses may be involved in health screening or education, among the many activities that fall under health promotion and disease prevention. (iStockphoto/SDI Productions)

- *Public participation,* which means that individuals and communities should be involved in the planning and design of health services that affect their health (Calnan & Lemire Rodger, 2002; CNA, 2003). This principle emphasizes that communities need to be encouraged and supported to participate in developing and managing their health care (e.g., through community partnerships and empowerment).
- *Intersectoral collaboration,* which emphasizes the integration of health development with social and economic development. Intersectoral collaboration involves different professionals across sectors working together to identify and develop sustainable health programs supported by policy (PHAC, 2016). Professionals from the health sector work interdependently with professionals from other sectors, such as agriculture, food, industry, and housing, as well as with community members to promote the health of the community.
- *Appropriate technology,* which is concerned with the appropriate use of health care resources, including human resources, equipment, and technology (CNA, 2003). This principle calls for finding the most cost-effective ways to provide appropriate health care to everyone in the community.

Table 1.2 provides examples of community health nursing responses to each of the primary health care principles.

As members of a primary health care interprofessional team, CHNs are well positioned to address the social determinants of health and health inequities that affect their

patients. However, the work of primary health care and the concerns of social determinants of health are necessarily collaborative and intersectoral in nature. The terms *interprofessional* (work among different professional practitioners), *interdisciplinary* (work among different academic disciplines or training areas), and *intersectoral* (work among distinct management or governing agencies or sectors) are all used to describe collaborative community health practice. Interaction among all sectors that impact determinants of health (health, education, housing, environment, employment, food safety, and so on) is essential for comprehensive community health service (WHO, 2008). Six principles of interprofessional collaboration in primary health care are listed in Box 1.3.

CHNs need to consider the principles in Box 1.3 as a whole when participating in interprofessional collaborative efforts in primary health care in Canada (Enhancing Interdisciplinary Collaboration in Primary Health Care Initiative Steering Committee, 2005). Factors that have been found to motivate or facilitate intersectoral action include the nature and complexity of the issue, a history of working intersectorally, political will, central agency support, expectations for improved service efficiency and effectiveness, and an established information and knowledge base. Factors that have served as barriers to intersectoral action include limited models with which to organize action, resource issues (e.g., insufficient time, personnel, and money), multiple mandates, a lack of leadership, changes in government, and a public denial of the social issue (Nelson et al., 2014).

TABLE 1.2	**Principles of Primary Health Care and Community Health Nursing Responses**
Primary Health Care Principle	**Example of Community Health Nursing Responses**
Accessibility	Cathy Crowe, a CHN who works as a public health nurse (PHN), advocates for people who are homeless in Toronto, Ontario (see http://rabble.ca/blogs/bloggers/cathycrowe).
Health promotion	CHNs have worked alongside people with low incomes to support health promotion and disease prevention by, for instance, supporting education and demonstration programs for healthy eating on a restricted budget. In some communities, these services have involved grocery store tours, community gardens, and cooking classes and interesting projects such as "Eat Well, Spend Less" in Kitchener, Ontario (see http://kdchc.org/wp-content/uploads/2010/09/Flyer-EWSL2.pdf).
Public participation	Many CHNs are involved in and establish advisory groups for the programs they are initiating in order to gather opinions and build on the wisdom and resources of service users and other stakeholders. The James Bay Community Project is an innovative example in Victoria, British Columbia, where community involvement in the planning and operation of services is designed at every step (see http://jbcp.bc.ca).
Intersectoral collaboration	CHNs have worked collaboratively with businesses, community institutions, and professionals from other sectors (e.g., at municipal and provincial levels) to develop and implement policies regarding contraband tobacco, smoking in public buildings and other locations, and displays of tobacco products (see http://rnao.ca/policy/speaking-notes/bill-186-submission-supporting-smoke-free-ontario-reducing-contraband-tobacco-).
Appropriate technology	Primary health care nurse practitioners in Ontario have helped reduce demands on the health care system by using their skills and abilities in the prevention and treatment of many chronic health conditions encountered in clinics; evidence is particularly promising in rural and northern communities. In Nigeria, community health workers trained by CHNs have distributed a treatment for river blindness to over 75 million people in over 15 African countries (see "All the Talents" at http://www.who.int/workforcealliance/knowledge/resources/Allthetalents_fullReport.pdf).

BOX 1.3 **Six Principles of Interprofessional Collaboration in Primary Health Care**

1. Patient/patient engagement
2. Population health approach
3. Best possible care and services
4. Access
5. Trust and respect
6. Effective communication

Source: Based on Virani, T. (2012). *Interprofessional collaborative teams.* Canadian Nurses Association. https://www.cna-aiic.ca/-/media/cna/page-content/pdf-en/interprofteams-virani-en-web.pdf?la=en&hash=8D073AA4883C9D0AFBD4433D8E02190233BEAC3B

PUBLIC HEALTH PRACTICE

Within the framework of "health for all," Canada has set the overarching goal of holistic health for its citizens; that every person will be as physically, mentally, emotionally, and spiritually healthy as they can be (PHAC, 2008a). To reach this overarching goal, the federal, provincial, and territorial ministers of health agreed in 2005 on the following health goals for Canada: (1) basic needs (social and physical environments); (2) belonging and engagement; (3) healthy living; and (4) a system for health (PHAC, 2008a).

According to the PHAC (2021), **public health** is defined as follows:

... an organized activity of society to promote, protect, improve, and when necessary, restore the health of individuals, specified groups, or the entire population. It is a combination of sciences, skills, and values that function through collective societal activities and involves programs, services, and institutions aimed at protecting and improving the health of all people. The term "public health" can describe a concept, a social institution, a set of scientific and professional disciplines and technologies, and a form of practice. It is a way of thinking, a set of disciplines, an institution of society, and a manner of practice. It has an increasing number and variety of specialized domains and demands of its practitioners an increasing array of skills and expertise.

This definition was developed to complement the core competencies for public health in Canada (PHAC, 2008b). The core competencies and specific public health nursing practices will be discussed in further detail in Chapters 2 and 3.

Public health aims to keep communities and populations healthy and safe through activities in the following six areas: health protection, health promotion, population health assessment, health surveillance, disease and injury prevention, and emergency preparedness and response (CPHA, 2019; PHAC, 2019). More specifically:

- *Health protection programs* are concerned with preventing physical, psychological, environmental, and sociological conditions that may put health at risk. Examples include programs such as those that address the safety of food and drinking water; the management of environmental risks such as toxic-waste handling, air pollution, and second-hand smoke; public sanitation; the spread of rabies; and communicable diseases.
- *Health promotion programs* are concerned with changing people's and societies' attitudes toward and practices regarding lifestyle choices. Examples include educational programs on tobacco use, nutrition, physical activity, injury prevention, reproductive health, the prevention of sexually transmitted infections (including HIV/AIDS), and breastfeeding.
- *Population health assessment* includes a range of methods of scanning the needs and strengths of a community. In response to the population health information gathered, analyzed, and interpreted, actions may then be taken that have a direct impact on the provision of public health programs and services. At the level of CHN practice, a community mental health nurse would assess the assets and needs of family caregivers to provide advice to a community program or service seeking to establish a respite care facility.
- *Health surveillance programs* are aimed at early detection of illness for specific asymptomatic individuals within groups for whom the early detection of an illness or problem can lead to significant improvements in health. Examples of such programs are developmental milestone screening in well-child clinics, dental examinations for school-aged children, and screening for breast and colorectal cancer.
- *Disease and injury prevention* includes a wide range of activities (also referred to as *interventions*) that are concerned with reducing risks or threats to health and promoting resilience against these threats. It may involve preventing disease or injury before it even occurs (such as legislation to ban a toxic product), reducing the potential impact of disease or injury (such as implementing a modified return-to-work program for someone recovering from an injury), and managing longer-term impacts of disease or injury (e.g., a support group for living well with Parkinson's disease).
- *Emergency preparedness and response* includes the delivery of emergency health care services in communities at all points along the continuum: prevention, preparedness, response, and recovery. For example, CHNs may collect emergency supplies and provide education on preparation for an influenza outbreak anticipated in a community; assist in the communication strategy for a disaster response; or assist in a response such as quarantine or other direct care.

In many ways, public health is considered a "success story." The dramatic increase in life expectancy among Canadians from the early 1900s to the present has been primarily the result of improvements in sanitation, the control of infectious diseases through education and immunization, and other preventive population health activities. These activities have also significantly reduced health care costs for Canadians (CPHA, 2019). Although the health of Canada's population is considered to be very good, differing rates of death, disease, and disability among various groups demonstrates that some experience worse health and a lower quality of life and life expectancy than do others (PHAC, 2018). These experiences and outcomes are related to a number of factors, including stigma and discrimination in the forms of racism, misogyny, xenophobia, homophobia and gender discrimination; the trauma caused by this discrimination is widely felt (PHAC, 2019).

At least 33% of Canadians (about 9 million) are affected by one or more of the following chronic illnesses: arthritis, hypertension, heart disease, cancer, chronic obstructive pulmonary disease, diabetes mellitus, and mood disorders (Broemeling, Watson, & Prebtani, 2008). Behavioural risk factors, such as smoking, unhealthy eating habits, obesity, and physical inactivity; societal forces, such as improved life expectancy; and unfavourable determinants of health contribute to the development of many chronic illnesses. Moreover, the number of chronic illnesses experienced per individual increases with age (PHAC, 2013a). The combined greater prevalence of chronic illnesses and increased life expectancy in society has major implications for primary health care teams (Health Council of Canada, 2009). With the successes and concerns of the public's health in mind, the emphasis in public health has shifted from the management of communicable diseases to the prevention and management of chronic illness (CHNC, 2012; PHAC, 2013a, 2013b).

CHNs who work in public health are called *public health nurses* (PHNs). PHNs acquire specialized knowledge and skills for working with different populations. **Public health nursing** is community health nursing with a distinct focus and scope of practice. (See the "How to … Distinguish Public Health Nursing" box.)

✳ HOW TO …

Distinguish Public Health Nursing

- *Population-focused:* Primary emphasis on *populations* that live in the community, as opposed to those that are institutionalized.
- *Community as context:*
  - Concern for the connection between the health status of the population and the environment in which the population lives (i.e., physical, biological, sociocultural).
  - An imperative to work *with* the members of the community to carry out public health functions.
- *Health and prevention focused:* Predominant emphasis on strategies for health promotion, health maintenance, and disease prevention, particularly primary and secondary prevention.
- *Interventions at the community and population level:* The use of political processes to affect public policy as a major intervention strategy for achieving goals.
- *Concern for the health of all members of the population or community, particularly vulnerable subpopulations.*
- *Consideration of the influence of the determinants on the health of patients.*

The knowledge and skills necessary for public health nursing are outlined in both the entry-to-practice public health nursing competencies of the Canadian Association of Schools of Nursing (CASN, 2014) and *Public Health Nursing Discipline Specific Competencies Version 1.0* of CHNC (2009). These competencies, which are elaborated on in Chapter 3, are discipline specific and identify the skills, knowledge, attitudes, beliefs, and values necessary for competent public health nursing practice in Canada.

Principles of Public Health Practice: Levels of Intervention and Prevention

When working with patients and their health concerns, CHNs need to determine whether upstream, midstream, or downstream interventions—or multiple levels of interventions—are required. The following classic public health parable helps illustrate the difference between downstream and upstream thinking. It is credited to medical sociologist, Irving Zola (McKinlay, 2019/1975):

> [A] witness sees a man caught in a river current. The witness saves the man, only to be drawn to the rescue of more drowning people. After many have been rescued, the witness walks upstream to investigate why so many people have fallen into the river. The story illustrates the tension between public health's protection mandates to respond to emergencies (help people caught in the current), and its prevention and promotion mandates (stop people from falling into the river). (National Collaborating Centre for Determinants of Health, 2014, p. 2)

As this parable suggests, creating the conditions for good health requires an exploration of different levels of intervention. When working with patients and their health concerns, CHNs must not only focus on the individual but also look further upstream for forces that may influence the individual's health: for example, access to the determinants of health, and economic, sociopolitical, and environmental factors (Martins, 2018; Lind & Baptiste, 2020). Additionally, CHNs need to ask, "How could this health issue have been prevented?" CHNs ask different questions at the downstream, midstream, and upstream levels to identify a broad range of interventions. Box 1.4 explores the focus of and questions related to each level of thinking.

In most situations, CHNs need to take an upstream-thinking approach. Community health interventions often have powerful impacts at the individual level, and when people act from an equity perspective, the impact can ripple out to create broader change. For example, a downstream program like an asthma treatment clinic for recent immigrants can have broader consequences if participants are encouraged to use the space to create other supports, such as a parent discussion group. The "CHN in Practice: A Case Study, Upstream, Midstream, and Downstream Approaches" box shows how interventions and outcomes do not fit easily into categories.

BOX 1.4 Upstream, Midstream, and Downstream Thinking

- **Upstream thinking** looks beyond the individual to take a macroscopic, big-picture population focus. It also includes a primary prevention perspective and is a population health approach. At this level, CHNs ask, "How can we change the 'causes of the causes,' or the conditions that set up the conditions for the illness or injury?"
- **Midstream thinking** addresses the micropolicy level: regional, local, community, or organizational. At this level, CHNs ask, "How can we change the causes of the illness or injury?"
- **Downstream thinking** refers to taking an individual curative focus, a view that does not consider economic, sociopolitical, and environmental factors. At this level, CHNs ask, "How can the illness and its consequences be treated?"

Source: National Collaborating Centre for Determinants of Health. (2014). *Let's talk: Moving upstream.* http://nccdh.ca/resources/entry/lets-talk-moving-upstream

CHN IN PRACTICE: A CASE STUDY

Upstream, Midstream, and Downstream Approaches
In January, Kristin notices a spike in the numbers of patients attending the community health centre with complaints of colds and respiratory irritation or seeking allergy and asthma treatment. Assessing these individuals, she notices a commonality. Many workers in the community, attempting to save money, reside in overcrowded rented cabins during the winter while off work and away from seasonal work camps that provide housing at mining, forestry, or fishing work sites during the spring, summer, and fall.

Think About It
Reflecting on possible levels of intervention—upstream, midstream, and downstream—how could Kristin address this issue?

Another public health focus of community health nursing intervention is disease prevention, which is typically divided into three levels: primary, secondary, and tertiary prevention. Another level of intervention, primordial prevention, was developed in the latter part of the twentieth century. **Primordial prevention** includes broader activities that focus on preventing the emergence of risk factors that are known to create the conditions for disease. Specifically, it involves actions to inhibit social, economic, and environmental factors that are known health hazards. Examples of primordial prevention are national policies and programs on obesity and nutrition involving the agricultural sector, the food industry, and the food import–export sector.

Primary prevention activities seek to prevent the occurrence of a disease (based on the natural history of a disease) or an injury. Examples of primary prevention include administering individual and mass immunizations, organizing community vaccination programs for influenza, and educating a community about the importance of handwashing to prevent the spread of infection.

Secondary prevention activities seek to detect a disease early in its progression (early pathogenesis), before clinical

signs and symptoms become apparent, to make a diagnosis and begin treatment. Examples of secondary prevention include conducting health screening programs to assess vision and hearing or to detect breast cancer, cervical cancer, hypertension, and scoliosis.

Tertiary prevention activities begin once a disease has become obvious; the goals are to interrupt the course of the disease, reduce the amount of disability that might occur, and begin rehabilitation. An example of tertiary prevention would be cardiac rehabilitation at a local wellness centre for groups of patients who have been recently discharged from hospital following a cardiovascular event.

The "Levels of Prevention" box illustrates the levels of primary, secondary, and tertiary prevention in relation to public health.

LEVELS OF PREVENTION

Related to Public Health Nursing
Primary Prevention
A CHN provides an influenza vaccination program in a retirement community.

Secondary Prevention
A CHN organizes an infant and child car seat safety screening program (based on Transport Canada's child car seat regulations) for a group of parents in a low-income housing complex.

Tertiary Prevention
A CHN provides education to individuals and families in a community who are coping with the effects of brain injury.

The primary, secondary, and tertiary levels of prevention are categorized into two levels of care: episodic care and distributive care. *Episodic care* refers to the curative and restorative aspect of practice (secondary and tertiary prevention), and *distributive care* refers to health maintenance, disease prevention, and health promotion (primary prevention) (Martin & Bowles, 2014; Martins, 2018). The "CHN in Practice: A Case Study, Identifying Levels of Prevention" box illustrates these two levels of care in community health nursing. This case involves home health care arrangements.

CHN IN PRACTICE: A CASE STUDY

Identifying Levels of Prevention
Mr. Yablonzski, a 75-year-old retired miner, was discharged from the hospital in Smithers, British Columbia, with a referral from the Houston community health centre for home health care services at his home in Houston. This referral was made to assess his respiratory status following a diagnosis of chronic obstructive pulmonary disease (COPD).

Episodic care from CHN Kristin involves teaching Mr. and Mrs. Yablonzski about Mr. Yablonzski's medications and how to implement healthy lifestyle patterns. Because Mr. Yablonzski lives with his wife and his daughter, Kristin conducts a family nursing assessment (see Chapter 12) to determine the family's current health status, its health concerns, and its strengths and capacities. The family's psychosocial adaptation and the patient's level of self-care and adjustment are also assessed. Based on her assessment, Kristin identifies health-enhancing behaviours such as smoking cessation, nutrition, moderate exercise, stress management, and immunization, especially flu vaccines. She also assesses Mr. Yablonzski's rehabilitation to help him reach his optimal level of functioning.

Distributive care from Kristin involves teaching Mr. Yablonzski ways to prevent exacerbating his condition (e.g., medical follow-up and lifestyle adaptations to increase his adherence to the programs set up for him) so that he can achieve his optimal level of functioning.

Think About It
What levels of prevention do medical follow-up, smoking cessation, and moderate exercise reflect?

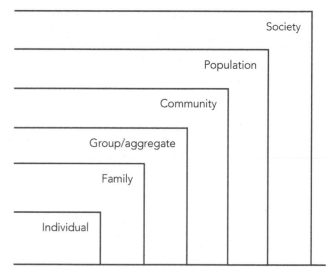

Fig. 1.2 The Community Health Nursing Patient.

The Community Health Patient

It is important to consider what the word *community* in the term *community health nursing* means. **Community** may be defined as people and the relationships that emerge among them as they develop and commonly share agencies, institutions, or a physical environment. Members of a community can be defined in terms of either geography (e.g., a city or town, a group of cities or towns that form a region, district, or province) or a common interest or focus (e.g., children attending a particular school).

Does the CHN work *in* the community or *with* the community? When the CHN provides health care to individuals and families, the focus is on health promotion and disease prevention, and the CHN views the community as a resource; therefore, the CHN is said to be working *in* the community. When the CHN views the community itself as the patient and applies the community health nursing process to the whole community, the CHN is said to be working *with* the community. This concept of working with the community is explored further in Chapter 9.

Populations and Aggregates

In Canada, community health nursing practice emphasizes population health promotion, disease prevention, and health protection. CHNs work with various types of patients, as illustrated in Fig. 1.2. CHNs bring people together, such as community members who know what it takes to make their community healthy, at the same time always ensuring that they are responsive to the current available evidence relevant to CHN practice.

Although it is hoped that all direct care providers contribute to the community's health, in the broadest sense, not all are primarily concerned with the population focus, or the "big picture." All CHNs in a given community, including those working in hospitals, physicians' offices, and health clinics, should contribute positively to the health of the community. Examples of community settings for health promotion, disease prevention, and treatment for individuals include ambulatory surgery, outpatient clinics, physician and advanced-practice nursing clinics, employment and school

sites, preschool programs, housing projects, and summer camps. These sites often provide individual-focused health care services, in contrast to population-focused services.

The terms *population* and *aggregates* are sometimes used interchangeably, but differences do exist. A **population** refers to a large group of people who share one or more personal or environmental characteristics. Generally, **subpopulations** are referred to as *aggregates* within the larger population (Savage, 2020). Therefore, **aggregates** are defined as groups within a population. Examples of a subpopulation, or aggregate, within a population include high-risk infants younger than 1 year of age, unmarried pregnant adolescents, and individuals exposed to a particular harmful incident, such as a chemical spill.

Population health refers to the health outcomes of a population as measured by the determinants of health and health status indicators. CHNs, other health care providers, and government policymakers use health status indicators and health patterns to determine the health of a community (McEwen & Nies, 2018).

The PHAC (2013b) developed a population health approach whose goals are to maintain and improve the health of populations and decrease health inequities between populations. The approach comprises eight key elements:
1. Focus on the health of populations.
2. Address the determinants of health and their interactions.
3. Base decisions on evidence.
4. Increase upstream investments.
5. Apply multiple interventions and strategies.
6. Collaborate across sectors and levels.
7. Employ mechanisms for public involvement.
8. Demonstrate accountability for health outcomes. (PHAC, 2013b)

Population health is covered in further detail in Chapter 4.

Collaborating in Interprofessional Teams

CHNs cannot be expected to be experts in all areas and aspects of complex community health work. Thus, interprofessional collaboration and partnership development are essential in community health nursing practice. It is critical that clear boundaries be in place to ensure positive, successful, and collaborative partnerships and that CHNs and other health care providers become comfortable with a blurring of roles and responsibilities (although CHNs always work in their scope of practice). At the same time, it is important for CHNs to recognize the value of their generalist health care knowledge, which enables them to address diverse and complex community health care concerns. The *Canadian Community Health Nursing: Professional Practice Model and Standards of Practice* is a helpful guide that facilitates the practice of CHNs in Canada as they work within the principles of primary health care to promote and preserve the health of populations (CHNC, 2019).

Within their practice, CHNs often work as part of a team with physicians, social workers, nutritionists, physiotherapists, occupational therapists, epidemiologists, researchers, and other health care providers. The patient, the focus of care, is also a team member and participates in shared decision making with regard to his or her health concerns. All team members are valued for their individual expertise, and trust among them is essential, as is sharing of power in the decision-making process. Collaboration among members of the interprofessional team contributes to ensuring that the patient receives the best care possible. **Collaboration** refers to the commitment of two or more partners (e.g., agency, patient, professional) to work together to address identified patient health concerns (College of Registered Nurses of Manitoba, 2019; RNAO, 2012). Groups and teams are discussed further in Chapter 13.

An example of a collaborative activity is the Canadian Collaborative Mental Health Initiative, whose mission is to enhance collaboration between mental health care providers and primary care providers (see the link on the Evolve website). A number of projects within this latter initiative employ a collaborative model, with a focus on improving access to services, mental health care, disease prevention, and health promotion.

The CNA (2019) position statement on facilitating interprofessional collaboration in primary health care is based on the following eight principles: (1) patient-centred care, (2) evidence-informed decision-making for quality care, (3) access, (4) epidemiology, (5) ethics, (6) communication, (7) social justice and equity, and (8) cultural safety. The research example in the "Evidence-Informed Practice" box shows how an access to care and social justice equity approach to population health is informing broader collaboration for end-of-life care for people experiencing homelessness.

COMMUNITY HEALTH NURSING PRACTICE

The role of the CHN has changed over the years, mainly in response to changes in health care, priorities for health care funding, the needs of the population, the educational preparation of CHNs, and the community health nursing standards of practice.

EVIDENCE-INFORMED PRACTICE

Stadjuhar, Mollison, Giesbrecht, et al. (2019) undertook to explore the needs and health access experiences of this specific target group (people at the end of life who have experienced structural vulnerabilities) in Victoria, British Columbia. The study involved completing over 300 hours of observations of people in the community and their caregivers, along with in-depth interviews.

Five significant barriers to accessing care at end of life were identified: (1) A survival imperative, such that structurally vulnerable people were just too busy trying to meet basic needs of shelter, food, and so on, to seek end-of-life health care; (2) There existed a normalization of dying with distress for both people at end of life and social care workers who were in the midst of ongoing drug overdoses, neglect, and often violent deaths routinely; (3) A problem of identifying people at end of life who could benefit from palliative care existed, with most care being provided by outreach and street-level workers outside the formal health care system; (4) Professional risk management also interrupted access and, in some cases, care was completely restricted except when individual homecare providers went against institutional policies to provide care "off the grid" to people living in camps, on the street, or in precarious housing situations; and finally (5) There was a barrier of cracks of a "siloed" care system. In most cases, needs were obvious; however, responsibility and accountability to step up to meet the needs was less clear for professionals and community workers alike. Together, findings unveiled an understanding of inequities in accessing care at the end of life. Guided by the determinants of health, this approach to understanding inequitable access and social needs has shed the light on widespread community

capacity building and support needs. A community collaborative group, Equity in Palliative Approaches to Care, has now formed to conduct further research and to develop outreach-oriented health navigation, training, and more for people experiencing structural vulnerabilities in Victoria. Members of this collaborative work together to conduct research with local, national, and international partners, and develop resources and tools, programs, and services aimed at improving access to quality care for people facing the end of life and who also face inequities like homelessness, poverty, isolation, racism, and stigma.

Application for CHNs:
It is important for CHNs to consider the population in any assessment and to customize the planning and implementation of community action projects for various aggregates in the community. According to the CCHN Standard 5, **capacity building** is the process of actively involving individuals, groups, organizations, and communities in all phases of planned change for the purpose of increasing their skills, knowledge, and willingness to take action on their own in the future.* A population health approach, concern with social determinants of health, and assessment of needs and barriers are important considerations in addressing the health care concerns of patients in their communities.

Questions for Reflection and Discussion
1. Which determinants of health are evident in this study? What other determinants could influence the health of these patients?
2. What other actions might the CHN implement to ensure improved outcomes?

*Community Health Nurses of Canada, 2019.
Source: Stadjuhar, K. I., Mollison, A., Giesbrecht, M., et al. (2019). *"Just too busy living in the moment and surviving"*: Barriers to accessing health care for structurally vulnerable populations at end-of-life. *BMC Palliative Care, 18,* 11. https://doi.org/10.1186/s12904-019-0396-7

Community Health Nursing Roles and Functions

CHNs focus on a number of specific populations and activities depending on their areas of practice, roles, and functions. The primary focus of public health nursing, for example, is on populations and the health of the community, whereas home health care nursing tends to focus on the health of individuals and families. Therefore, the CHN practising as a home health nurse (HHN) is more likely to give direct care to people than are other CHNs. The HHN assesses patient health concerns as well as the services that are available in order to plan the most appropriate course of action for a particular patient, such as an individual or a family. Throughout care delivery, the HHN educates and counsels patients so that they can learn better ways of taking care of themselves. Many private agencies, such as the Victorian Order of Nurses (VON), employ HHNs in the community. For historical and current information on the VON, a nonprofit organization based in Ontario and Nova Scotia, see the VON link on the Evolve website.

Other examples of CHNs are occupational health nurses, nurse practitioners, outpost nurses, military nurses, forensic nurses, telenurses, corrections nurses, nurse entrepreneurs, parish nurses, and street or outreach nurses. Refer to Table 1.3 for further information on all of these and additional community health nursing practice areas. Chapter 3 provides in-depth information on each of these community health nursing specialties, their practice settings, and their roles.

CHNs have various opportunities to assume many different roles at different times, depending on the patient and practice settings (Table 1.4). Not every CHN will actually take on all of the roles presented in Table 1.4 during their practice. The function and activities related to the roles of advocate, collaborator, educator, facilitator, and researcher often depend on the resources available and factors such as the patient's needs, availability, commitment, culture, and health beliefs. Many CHNs have a considerable amount of professional autonomy when they perform these diverse roles in community practice settings. While this professional autonomy can be very exciting, it is accompanied by responsibility and accountability, as indicated in Standard 8 of the CCHN Standards: "professional responsibility and accountability" (CHNC, 2019).

CHNs are mostly involved in providing family-centred care to individuals, families, and groups across the lifespan of patients, but their practice also includes identifying high-risk groups in the community. Once such groups are identified, the CHN can work with others to develop appropriate policies and interventions to reduce the risk and to provide beneficial services. In the course of their practice, CHNs must remain constantly aware of diversity in the community and provide care that is appropriate to address the health care needs of diverse patients. Diversity (see Chapter 7) and all of the concepts introduced here will be explored in further depth throughout this text.

Areas of Community Health Nursing Practice

Community health nursing can be thought of as an umbrella term that covers the various nursing specialties and roles of nurses who work in and with the community. Fig. 1.3 presents the most common specialties encompassed by the term and some of the usual roles assumed by CHNs. The terms *community health nurse* and *public health nurse* have often been used interchangeably; however, the CCHN Standards differentiate among the various community health nursing specialties. The differences among all community health nursing specialties, such as public health nursing, home health nursing, and parish nursing are their unique practice settings, roles, beliefs, and philosophies about community health nursing practice.

Table 1.3 lists some of the most common CHN practice areas in Canada. CHNs working as HHNs and PHNs practise in diverse settings. These specialties share many similarities in their community health nursing practice, including use of strategies for health promotion, prevention, and protection (Community Health Nurses of Canada [CHNC], 2019). Even though the location and unit of care, the practice and goals of care, and specific nursing activities vary, all CHNs are expected to meet the eight CCHN Standards.

While Table 1.3 presents examples of the most common practice specialty areas, Table 1.5 presents examples of patients that CHNs may work with and examples of CHN roles and practices based on specialty area. Patient types and community specialty areas are discussed further in Chapter 3.

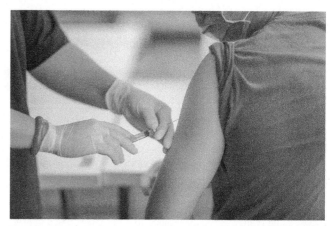

Community health nurses work with patients in many different practice settings. Here, a community health nurse provides a health care worker with a vaccine during an occupational health clinic's staff vaccination event. (iStockphoto/Udom Pinyo)

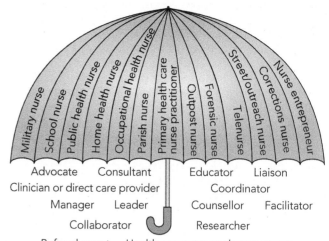

Fig. 1.3 Community Health Nursing Umbrella: Specialties and Roles.

TABLE 1.3 Examples of Community Health Nursing Practice Areas

Community Health Nurses (CHNs)	Definition	Practice Settings	Patient Group	Educational Preparation	Examples of Roles and Activities	Funding
Public health nurse (PHN)	A nurse who uses knowledge of nursing, social sciences, and public health sciences for the promotion and protection of health and for the prevention of disease among population	• Community groups • Community health centres • Workplaces • Street clinics • Schools • Outpost settings • Homes	• Population • Aggregates or groups • Communities • Families • Individuals	• Baccalaureate degree in nursing or registered or licensed practical nurse (RPN or LPN)*	• Health promotion • Disease prevention • Patient advocacy • Education • Direct care in clinics	• Provincial and municipal government funding
Home health nurse (HHN)	A nurse who uses knowledge and skills to provide direct care and treatment for individuals to maintain and restore health or to provide palliation during illness	• Patients' homes • Schools • Clinics • Workplaces • Transition services (from hospital to home) • Older adults' housing programs • Shelter or safe house program	• Individuals • Families • Caregivers	• Registered nurse (RN) or RPN or LPN*	• Direct patient care • Disease prevention • Health promotion with individual patients	• Public or private funding
Occupational health nurse (OHN)	A nurse who specializes in workplace health and safety, health promotion, disease prevention, and rehabilitation for workers	• Workplace	• Employees (individuals, groups)	• RN with certificate in occupational health	• Direct care • Assessment of the workplace • Education of employees on health and safety issues	• Employer
Parish nurse	A nurse who serves the health and wellness needs of faith community members	• Patients' homes • Places of worship • Hospitals	• Individuals • Families • Groups	• RN	• Health promotion • Health counsellor • Liaison • Health advocate • Integrator of faith and health	• Religious or faith community funding
Primary health care nurse practitioner (PHCNP)	A nurse with advanced-practice education, which allows for an expanded role, such as diagnosing episodic illnesses, prescribing medication, and ordering diagnostic tests	• Community health centres • Clinics • Physicians' offices • Emergency departments in hospitals • Nursing stations • Long-term care facilities	• Individuals • Families • Groups • Communities	• Baccalaureate degree in nursing, minimum of post-baccalaureate diploma with licensing in extended class (EC)	• Direct care (i.e., health assessment; diagnosis and treatment of episodic illness) • Health promotion • Disease prevention • Community development and planning	• Public or private funding

Continued

TABLE 1.3   Examples of Community Health Nursing Practice Areas—cont'd

Community Health Nurses (CHNs)	Definition	Practice Settings	Patient Group	Educational Preparation	Examples of Roles and Activities	Funding
Outpost nurse	A nurse who works in an outpost or rural setting that is often geographically separated from face-to-face physician contact	• Nursing stations • Patients' homes • Community	• Individuals • Families • Groups • Rural communities	• RN	• Direct care • Health promotion • Liaison with other health care providers • Referral	• Provincial or federal funding
Military nurse	A nurse and nursing officer who is employed by the Canadian Armed Forces Health Services	• Military hospitals • Military outpatient centres • Civilian tertiary care facilities • Military operational units	• Individuals • Families	• Baccalaureate degree in nursing	• Direct patient care • Disease prevention • Occupational health care • Environmental health care	• Federal funding
Forensic nurse	A nurse who has completed continuing education programs in the area of forensic science	• Sexual assault treatment setting, often in hospital emergency departments	• Adults and children who are victims of acute sexual assault and survivors of domestic violence or intimate partner abuse	• RN or registered psychiatric nurse	• Direct patient care for collection of physical evidence • Crisis response, such as counselling and referral	• Provincial funding
Telenurse	A nurse who provides nursing service over the telephone	• Community agencies	• Individuals • Families • Caregivers	• RN	• Telephone advice • Telehealth network (live video links for nurse-led telehealth clinics)	• Provincial funding provided to private companies
Corrections nurse	A nurse who works in a correctional facility	• Correctional facilities	• Inmates (individuals, groups) • Correctional facility staff	• RN	• Direct care • Health promotion • Disease prevention • Inmate advocate • Crisis intervention	• Provincial or federal funding
Nurse entrepreneur	A nurse who is self-employed in the provision of nursing services	• Home • Variety of workplace settings	• Individuals • Families • Groups • Communities	• RN or RPN or LPN*	• Direct patient care as contracted • Consultant • Advocate • Health promotion • Disease prevention	• Private funding
Street or outreach nurse	A nurse who serves the health and wellness needs of marginalized populations living on the streets	• Community streets	• Individuals • Families • Communities	• RN	• Direct patient care (i.e., wound care; drug overdose treatment) • Disease prevention • Health promotion • Patient advocate • Political activist	• Provincial or municipal funding

*Some Canadian provinces and territories designate registered practical nurses (RPNs) or licensed practical nurses (LPNs) to work in some settings such as home health nursing and public health nursing. Note: In some provinces, *RPN* refers to *registered psychiatric nurse;* however, in this table, the abbreviation designates *registered practical nurse.*

TABLE 1.4 Common Roles, Functions, and Activities in Community Health Nursing

Role	Function/Activities	Examples
Advocate	Provides a voice to patient concerns when necessary	• Networking with other community members on behalf of homeless people • Participating in a community action group for provision of accessible transit choices • Initiating contact with community stakeholders
Clinician or direct care provider	Provides hands-on care to the patient	• Providing wound care on a diabetic patient's foot • Doing a prenatal assessment • Working in sexually transmitted infections (STI) clinics • Working in immunization clinics
Collaborator	Involves the patient and interprofessional team members or interagency groups working together toward improving patient health	• Working with a nutritionist, physiotherapist, and patient to address patient obesity • Working with health care providers in a long-term care facility to explore feeding options • Being a member of coalitions, such as heart health groups
Consultant	Provides advice and information to patients, health care providers, and agencies to assist in meeting patients' health care concerns	• Providing information to a family that is considering the use of complementary therapies • Providing information to school administrators about bullying
Counsellor	Provides support to patients to facilitate their decision making in reference to emotional challenges	• Working with a family and the family member with a new diagnosis of cancer • Working with a pregnant adolescent to explore birth choices
Educator	Facilitates patient learning through teaching that is appropriate to a patient's situation to meet his or her cognitive, affective, and psychomotor needs	• Educating a worker about back safety in the workplace • Educating a new mother on the care of her newborn
Facilitator	Works with patients and others to set and fulfill health goals	• Facilitating a self-help group for smoking cessation • Facilitating a community focus group to improve neighbourhood safety
Health promoter or change agent	Assists patients to acknowledge need for lifestyle changes and take responsibility for working toward identified change	• Working with children with obesity problems to identify the physical activity changes required • Helping patients identify stressors and stress management strategies to deal with these stressors
Leader	Guides and encourages patients to take the initiative to explore options and make decisions to enable goal achievement	• Helping a low-income neighbourhood formulate a plan to present traffic safety proposals to a local municipal council • Assisting a school board in developing a school policy on food vending machine options
Liaison	Acts as an intermediary between patients and agencies and other health care providers	• Organizing referrals to cardiac rehabilitation after surgery • Working with hospital staff to arrange for home support and follow-up for a high-risk mother
Manager	Plans and directs patient care	• Organizing home care support for a newly discharged older adult patient • Organizing a family planning clinic • Organizing sexual health clinics
Referral agent	Directs patients to additional appropriate resources in the community	• Referring community stakeholders to a health promotion consultant • Referring patients to a child car seat safety inspection clinic
Researcher	Investigates phenomena related to health and identifies opportunities for research	• Identifying increased cases of measles in a specific community • Identifying increased numbers of snowmobile injuries

Community health nursing includes various functions. It is a specialty nursing practice that involves working with patients to preserve, protect, promote, and maintain health. CHNs work *with* the patient, not just *for* the patient, in their approach to assessment, planning, intervention, and evaluation. Working *with* the patient involves establishing a partnership with the patient and building community capacity.

Although CHNs work independently as they practise in the community, they also work with other health care providers in community partnerships and as members of various interprofessional teams. The principles of primary health care and population health approaches are important, therefore, regardless of the CHN role or the individuals, groups, or populations the nurse is working alongside.

CANADIAN COMMUNITY HEALTH NURSING STANDARDS OF PRACTICE

The CCHN Standards were initially adopted by the Community Health Nurses Association of Canada (CHNAC) in 2003. The CHNAC underwent a name change in June 2009 and is now known as Community Health Nurses of Canada (CHNC). CHNC has developed a conceptual model of the Canadian community health nursing practice standards, the context of practice, foundational values and beliefs, and the community health nursing process (see Fig. 1.4). The eight CCHN Standards are listed in Table 1.6, and the complete text of the standards is provided in Appendix 1. Further explanation of this model is available through the CHNC link on the Evolve website.

Whatever their practice title and setting, within 2 years of beginning community nursing practice, CHNs are expected to meet the requirements in knowledge, skills, and abilities outlined in the CCHN Standards (CHNC, 2019). Since 2006, CNA has offered certification for Canadian community health nurses (CNA, 2020). This certification is voluntary and provides an opportunity for further professional development and the demonstration of competency and currency in community health nursing. Table 1.6 provides community health nursing practice examples applied to each of the CCHN Standards for PHNs, HHNs, and nurses working in health promotion in the community (NHPs). The CCHN Standards are referred to throughout this text.

TABLE 1.5   Community Health Nursing Patients, Roles, and Practice Examples

Patient	Role Example	Practice Example
Society Society is defined as the systems that incorporate the social, political, economic, and cultural infrastructure to address issues of concern	Advocate	A street nurse advocates for affordable housing for people who are homeless in Canada
Population A *population* is a large group of people who have at least one characteristic in common and who reside in a community (e.g., adolescents residing in Regina, mothers with newborns)	Advocate	A team of CHNs consisting of a parish nurse, a public health nurse, and a nurse practitioner have identified the need for options in the community that would provide adolescents enhanced opportunities for physical activity. The team has approached the city council requesting designated times for "adolescent-only" access to the facilities at the local sports complex
Community *Community* may be defined as people and the relationships that emerge among them as they develop and commonly share agencies, institutions, or a physical environment. Members of a community can be defined in terms of either geography (e.g., residents of Regina, Saskatchewan) or a shared status or special interest group (e.g., lone parents)	Educator	A group of public health nurses (PHNs) organize a community health fair at the local shopping centre to inform the community about diabetes
Group or Aggregate *Aggregates* are defined as groups within a population (e.g., adolescents with diabetes mellitus, high-risk newborns)	Educator	A nurse practitioner (NP) employed at a local diabetic education centre holds monthly diabetes education sessions with a small group of adolescents with diabetes mellitus. These interactive sessions provide an opportunity for group members to share challenges related to having diabetes as a teenager and ideas on how to manage these challenges
Family Family is defined as two or more individuals who depend on one another for emotional, physical, or financial support or a combination of these (e.g., Sally, adolescent diabetic, and her family)	Counsellor	A home health nurse (HHN) visits Sally and her family (parents and younger brother). At this visit, the HHN talks with the family to explore their concerns about their ability to support Sally in the management of her diabetes
Individual An *individual* is one human being (e.g., Sally, adolescent diabetic)	Liaison and referral agent	Sally is a 13-year-old newly diagnosed with type 1 diabetes mellitus. John, a community care case manager, assesses Sally in the hospital and determines that she requires assistance with the management of her diabetes. John makes a referral to a home health care agency, requesting that an HHN visit Sally within 24 hours of her discharge to address her health care needs

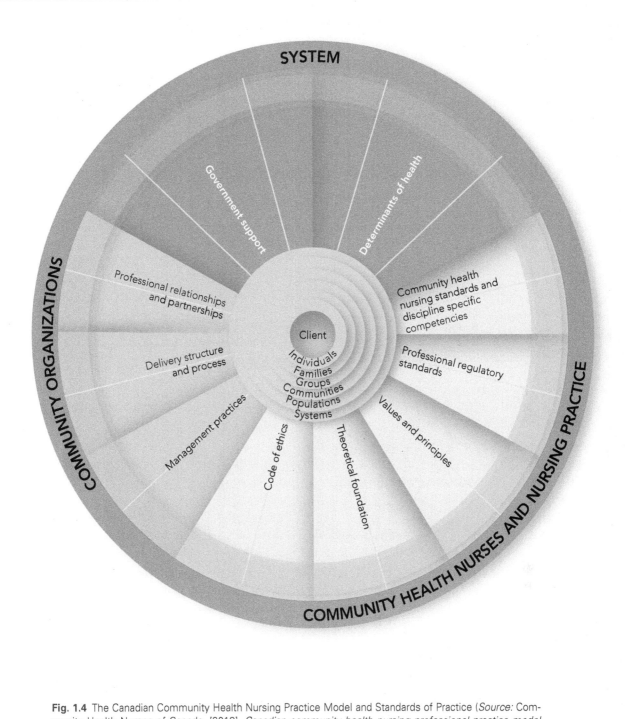

Fig. 1.4 The Canadian Community Health Nursing Practice Model and Standards of Practice (*Source:* Community Health Nurses of Canada. [2019]. *Canadian community health nursing professional practice model and standards of practice.* Community Health Nurses of Canada. https://www.chnc.ca/en/standards-of-practice. Reprinted with permission. Further reproduction prohibited.)

Approaches to Practice: Health Promotion, Empowerment, Capacity Building, and Population Health

Community health nursing practice places emphasis on health promotion, disease prevention, and health protection. **Health promotion** is the process of empowering people to increase control over and improve their health

(WHO, 1986). In community health nursing, **empowerment** refers to actively engaging the patient (which may be an individual, family, group, or the larger population) to gain greater control and involves "political efficacy, improved quality of community life and social justice" (CHNAC, 2011, pp. 24-25). The CHNAC (2011) describes *empowerment* as "not something that can be done 'to' or 'for' people—it involves people discovering and using their

TABLE 1.6   Application of the Canadian Community Health Nursing Standards of Practice*

Standard	Public Health Nurses (PHNs)	Home Health Nurses (HHNs)	Nurses Working in Health Promotion in the Community (NHPs)†
Standard 1: Health Promotion	• PHNs work with a community and use social marketing to promote the development of more recreational spaces and activities for families • PHNs promote physical activity and healthy eating through such programs as the Supermarket Safari and the Schools Awards Program	• HHNs encourage families dealing with a chronic illness to participate in regular physical and social activities	• NHPs encourage families dealing with a chronic illness to participate in regular physical and social activities
Standard 2: Prevention and Health Protection	• PHNs track immunization schedules for each child so that families and practitioners can access information when needed (in case of an outbreak, travel, school records, etc.) • PHNs work with HHNs and NHPs to develop and distribute information that is appropriate in terms of culture and reading level on identifying and reducing risk factors, such as falls, medication errors, and communicable diseases • PHNs work with parents' organizations, parent resource centres, and the police to promote proper installation of car seats through the media and conduct several clinics to provide one-on-one assessment and teaching	• HHNs work with PHNs to develop and distribute information that is appropriate in terms of culture and reading level on identifying and reducing risk factors, such as falls, communicable diseases, and low immunization rates • When HHNs observe high rates of smoking among caregivers and patients, they raise a concern, and a task group is formed to find ways to address the issue	• NHPs work with PHNs to develop and distribute information that is appropriate in terms of culture and reading level on identifying and reducing risk factors, such as falls, communicable diseases, and low immunization rates • When NHPs observe high rates of smoking within a particular patient group, they bring it to the attention of the practice team, and a plan is developed to find ways to address the issue
Standard 3: Health Maintenance, Restoration, and Palliation	• PHNs provide ongoing nursing care to families with infants and children who are experiencing difficulties. Care may be provided directly or through supervised unregulated care providers. This may include telephone follow-up, home visits, or referrals to other community-based services	• HHNs adapt the care provided to acute-care and long-term care patients and their families based on the patients' choices, their own personal skills, and the resources available in the setting and community • HHNs provide long-term nursing care—in the home, school, or work—for children, youth, and adults for conditions such as acquired brain injury. Collaboration is required with the patient, unregulated care providers, family, teachers, and employers to promote capabilities, prevent secondary illness, and improve response to treatment	• NHPs provide ongoing nursing care or care coordination to individuals and families who are experiencing poor health. Care may be provided directly or through telephone follow-up, home visits, or referrals to other community-based services

TABLE 1.6   Application of the Canadian Community Health Nursing Standards of Practice—cont'd

Standard	Public Health Nurses (PHNs)	Home Health Nurses (HHNs)	Nurses Working in Health Promotion in the Community (NHPs)[†]
Standard 4: Professional Relationships	• PHNs are selected to coordinate heart health coalitions because they are able to communicate effectively and regularly with community members and are able to help find a goal that everyone believes in • PHNs working with families experiencing childcare difficulties identify that postnatal visits based on issues or tasks do not allow them to develop a continuing relationship with families. They bring their concern to the attention of management	• HHNs and management work together to provide a "continuity of care" so that the majority of patients have the same nurse most of the time	• NHPs in the primary health care team ask to be assigned to work with a defined case load of patients rather than being assigned each day to different tasks. This arrangement allows them more opportunity to develop an ongoing relationship with patients • NHPs provide options and ask patients and caregivers how they want to learn about coping with an acute or long-term illness or disability • NHPs initiate mother-to-mother groups for women in a specific linguistic group so that they can share resources and experiences in raising children
Standard 5: Capacity Building	• PHNs encourage a school to form a school health committee that includes students, parents, teachers, administrators, and community partners. Committee members identify the school community's strengths and needs and prioritize, plan, implement, evaluate, and celebrate action for a healthier school. The school community's capacity to take its own action for health is enhanced by the formation of a sustainable structure (the committee), with the PHN as a partner in the process	• HHNs provide training and encouragement for people in the home to carry out care for a family member. For example, a mother and teenaged children would be supported in developing and carrying out a schedule for range-of-motion (ROM) exercises for a grandmother living with them • HHNs teach patients and family members how to change dressings and assess for deterioration and healing of a wound. Within a short period, the patients and the families take over the dressing changes and report steady improvement • HHNs working in palliative care listen to the concerns of stressed and exhausted caregivers and support them in making decisions about respite and hospice care	• NHPs ensure that patients and family members living with diabetes receive education and ongoing support on monitoring blood sugar, taking medication, exercising, and moderating diet. Depending on the individual and family, they may provide the service themselves on an individual basis or in a group, or refer patients to another community program
Standard 6: Health Equity	• PHNs identify that new immigrants are especially vulnerable to communicable diseases (such as tuberculosis) and make limited use of prevention services. The PHNs decide to work with the teachers in English as a second language classes and the staff in immigrant assistance centres to develop and provide health information and services at those locations • A PHN works with business owners and volunteer community groups to promote breastfeeding-friendly businesses and public places	• HHNs and case managers work together to advocate for families caring for medically fragile children by: • seeking respite care for families exhausted by the required intense care • contacting the local provincial/territorial member of Parliament to encourage enhanced funding for respite services • planning for a resolution through the provincial/territorial RN association • HHNs are joined by PHNs and NHPs to lobby for retaining home visits and case management by RNs for people living with mental illness	• NHPs and case managers work together to support immigrant families by: • hosting multicultural celebrations featuring foods from different cultural groups served by their organization • lobbying municipal councillors for funding for community gardens and food banks • planning for a resolution on health literacy at the provincial/territorial RN association • NHPs organize exercise classes at suitable times and places for workers, caregivers, or older adults

Continued

TABLE 1.6   Application of the Canadian Community Health Nursing Standards of Practice—cont'd

Standard	Public Health Nurses (PHNs)	Home Health Nurses (HHNs)	Nurses Working in Health Promotion in the Community (NHPs)[†]
Standard 7: Evidence-Informed Practice	• When managing mass virus screening at an occupational health site, PHNs use personal protective equipment to prevent contacting or spreading the virus according to best evidence • Confronted with a new pattern of gastrointestinal illness in their rural community, PHNs gather data and seek data from changes in the environment including food supply • PHNs working in a rural community implement guidelines for a smoking cessation clinic using readiness-for-change tools	• An urban HHN is increasingly referred to patients whose homes are precarious (i.e., shelters, street camps, tent cities, and temporary housing). The HHN searches the literature on street family and optimal care when home is the street, in order to understand a best approach and plan care • HHNs providing palliative care during the COVID-19 pandemic implement best practices, balancing the need for prevention of spread of the virus with knowledge of psychological safety for family and patients seeking visits and supportive care from loved ones	• Part of a shared care school-based mental health promotion program, an NHP is conducting an evaluation of a mindfulness program that has been implemented for several years without any knowledge about its effectiveness • NHPs working with a cancer survivors support group expand their peer support model upon finding strong systematic reviews about the long-term benefits of short- and long-term peer support for cancer survivors
Standard 8: Professional Responsibility and Accountability	• PHNs are assigned to work in needle exchange programs based on harm reduction. When a PHN has difficulty accepting the tenets of harm reduction, reflective practice alone and with the supervisor can help the PHN understand the program and change assumptions • PHNs work together to identify how they can incorporate the CCHN Standards in their provincial/territorial RN associations' continuing competence or quality assurance program • The nursing or professional practice council initiates action on integrating the CCHN Standards of Practice by following the steps in the CCHN Standards Toolkit[‡]: (1) forming a committee to work on the initiative; (2) conducting a stakeholder and environmental scan; and (3) developing a plan after determining that staff and management want an orientation, policies, and professional development based on the standards	• When an HHN is asked by an amyotrophic lateral sclerosis (ALS) patient to be present during removal of the bi-level positive airway pressure (Bi-PAP) machine, which will result in death, the nurse explores the patient's reasons for this decision and discusses the ethics of responding to this request with the health care team as well as the nursing practice advisor at their provincial/territorial RN association • HHNs work together to identify how they can incorporate the CCHN Standards in their provincial/territorial RN association continuing competence or quality assurance program • A group of nurses in the organization initiates action on integrating the CCHN Standards by following the steps in the CCHN Standards Toolkit: (1) organizing themselves; (2) conducting a stakeholder and environmental scan; and (3) developing a plan after determining that staff and management want an orientation, policies, and professional development based on the standards	• NHPs work in clinics serving the homeless. When an NHP has difficulty accepting the harm reduction approach adopted by the clinic, the NHP uses reflective practice alone and with the supervisor to understand the approach and change assumptions • NHPs work together to identify how they can incorporate the CCHN Standards in their provincial/territorial RN association continuing competence or quality assurance program • A group of NHPs in the organization initiates action on integrating the CCHN Standards by following the steps in the CCHN Standards Toolkit: (1) organizing themselves; (2) conducting a stakeholder and environmental scan; and (3) developing a plan after determining that staff and management want an orientation, policies, and professional development based on the standards

*The Canadian Community Health Nursing (CCHN) Standards, 2003, revised in 2008, 2011, and again in 2019, have been promoted throughout Canada by the Community Health Nurses of Canada (CHNC). Part of the promotion strategy was the development of a tool kit in March 2006. This tool kit was developed for CHNC and the Public Health Agency of Canada (PHAC) with funding received from the PHAC.

[†]The label "nurses working in health promotion" (NHP) was coined to include nurses who practise health promotion in a variety of community settings. The settings could include community health care centres, primary care clinics, family practice, care or case management centres, streets, schools, workplaces, and churches.

[‡]Community Health Nurses Association of Canada. (2007). Canadian community health nursing standards of practice (CCHN standards) toolkit. https://www.chnc.ca/en/membership/documents/loadDocument?id=521&download=1#!upload/membership/document/2016-07/2012maychnccdpreport.pdf

Sources: Adapted from Diem, E. (2007.; Revised 2019). Practice examples of application of the Canadian community health nursing standards of practice. Table presented at the First National Conference for Community Health Nurses, Toronto, Ontario. Reprinted with permission.

own strengths" (pp. 24-25). CHNs partner with patients to build capacity for community health at multiple levels of intervention and to shape empowering environments. When patients are empowered, the power shifts from health care providers to patients in the identification, prioritization, and addressing of their own health concerns. The strategies of advocacy and empowerment contribute, in turn, to capacity building (CHNC, 2011).

The PHAC developed a Community Capacity Building Tool that CHNs working on health promotion projects can use to assess the status of a project and plan to build community capacity for the project. The tool has nine features that describe community capacity. Each feature includes a set of related questions that are meant to help users reflect on how they can plan to build community capacity for their project (see the link on the Evolve website). Empowerment and capacity building will be discussed in further detail in Chapters 4 and 9. The CCHN Standards in Appendix 1 provide examples of the actions CHNs take in their advocacy role to build capacity.

STUDENT EXPERIENCE

The Rural Social Determinants of Health Game Toolkit was developed in 2017-2018 by the Cultural Competency Team, an inter-office collaboration between Colorado Community Health Network (CCHN) and Community Health Association of Mountain/Plains States (CHAMPS). The purpose of the Toolkit is to educate healthcare professionals about the ways that social, cultural, economic, environmental, and other factors impact the health and well-being of rural patients.

Activity
1. Log on to the following website: http://champsonline.org/tools-products/quality-improvement-resources/social-determinants-of-health-resources#RuralSDOHGame.
2. Download the resources at the links.
3. Follow the directions for the game.

Questions
1. What have you learned from playing this game?
2. How would you use this information as a community health nurse?

CHAPTER SUMMARY

1.1 The structure of the Canadian health care system, administering agencies, and official governance provide an organizing framework for CHN practice. The federal government administers the *Canada Health Act* and provides financial support to the provinces and territories that legislate, organize, and deliver services. Health Canada is an umbrella agency for other health agencies and branches such as the PHAC.

1.2 Population-focused practice emphasizes health protection, health promotion, and disease prevention. The social determinants of health are highly relevant to population health. These determinants include: (1) income and income distribution, (2) education, (3) employment and working conditions, (4) early life, (5) food insecurity, (6) housing, (7) health services, (8) social exclusion, (9) social safety net, (10) health services, (11) Indigenous status, (12) gender, (13) race, and (14) disability.

1.3 Principles of ethics, equity, social justice, and human rights inform CHN practice, ensuring fairness and equality in health services. Practising with these principles in focus, CHNs are becoming more involved in the intersections of environmental health and global health, known as planetary health.

1.4 *Primary health care* refers to comprehensive care that includes disease prevention, community development, a wide spectrum of services and programs, working in interprofessional teams, and intersectoral collaboration for healthy public policy. It is a philosophy of care and is composed of five important principles: (1) accessibility, (2) health promotion, (3) public participation, (4) intersectoral collaboration, and (5) appropriate technology.

1.5 *Public health* is the collective effort of the members of a society to ensure that existing conditions promote health for all in the community.

1.6 *Community health nursing* is an umbrella term used to define nursing specialties and applies to all nurses who work *in* and *with* the community. CHNs work in diverse settings and perform a variety of roles.

1.7 The CCHN Standards comprise eight standards that are intended to guide and facilitate the practice of CHNs in Canada as they work within the principles of primary health care to promote and preserve the health of populations.

CHN IN PRACTICE: A CASE STUDY

Collaborative Community Health Practice
In the town of Houston, British Columbia, Kristin has established collaborations with several CHNs and other practitioners, including home health services, a contracted substance use and addictions service social worker, the region's Northern Society for Domestic Peace, as well as the environmental health officer and community mental health nurse in the bigger town that is approximately one hour away. A recent resurgence of the mining and natural resource industries has added to community prosperity. It has also led to an increase in transient workers and greater disposable income for people in the town—with added concerns of substance use and violence in the community.

Think About It
To what extent do you think that practices of collaboration can be used in Kristin's CHN practice in Houston to address her current concerns?

📶 TOOL BOX

The Tool Box contains useful resources that can be applied to community health nursing practice. These resources are found either in the appendices at the back of this text or on the Evolve website at http://evolve.elsevier.com/Canada/Stanhope/community/.

Appendices

- Appendix 1: Canadian Community Health Nursing Professional Practice Model and Standards of Practice
- Appendix 2: CNA Position Statement: "Social Determinants of Health"
- Appendix 3: Declaration of Alma-Ata
- Appendix 4: Ottawa Charter for Health Promotion

Tools

Public Health Agency of Canada. Community Capacity Building Tool.

This tool can be used by health promotion project groups to determine current project status and options for growth in building community capacity for the project. The tool contains nine categories, with specific questions in each category that encompass planning for building community capacity.

REFERENCES

BC Centres for Disease Control Foundation for Public Health. (2020). *Decoding public health*. BCCDC Foundation for Public Health. https://bccdcfoundation.org/all-resources/decoding-public-health/.

Bosurgi, R. (2019). Climate crisis: Healthcare is a major contributor, global report finds. *BMJ, 366*, l5560. https://doi.org/10.1136/bmj.l5560.

Bourgeault, I., Labonté, R., Packer, C., et al. (2017). *Population health in Canada: Issues, research, and action*. Canadian Scholars' Press.

Broemeling, A., Watson, D. F., & Prebtani, F. (2008). Population patterns of chronic health conditions, co-morbidity and healthcare use in Canada: Implications for policy and practice. *Healthcare Quarterly, 11*(3), 70–76.

Brown, T. M., Cueto, M., & Fee, E. (2006). The World Health Organization and the transition from international to global public health. *American Journal of Public Health, 96*(1), 62–72.

Bryant, T., Raphael, D., Schrecker, T., et al. (2011). Canada: A land of missed opportunity for addressing the social determinants of health. *Health Policy, 101*(1), 44–58.

Bushnik, T., Tjepkema, M., & Martel, L. (2020). *Socioeconomic disparities in life and health expectancy among the household population in Canada*. Statistics Canada. https://www150.statcan.gc.ca/n1/pub/82-003-x/2020001/article/00001-eng.htm.

Calnan, R., & Lemire Rodger, G. (2002). *Primary health care: A new approach to health care reform*. Canadian Nurses Association.

Canadian Association of Community Health Centres. (2019). *Healthy people healthy communities: 2019 infographic. About community health centres*. CACHC. https://www.cachc.ca/about-chcs/.

Canadian Association of Schools of Nursing. (2014). *Entry-to-practice public health nursing competencies for undergraduate nursing education*. CASN.

Canadian Council on Social Determinants of Health. (2015). *A review of frameworks on the determinants of health*. CCSDH. http://ccsdh.ca/publications/.

Canadian Institute for Health Information. (2017). *Regulated nurses, 2016*. CIHI. https://www.cihi.ca/sites/default/files/document/regulated-nurses-2016-highlights_en-web.pdf.

Canadian Nurses Association. (2003). Primary health care—the time has come. *Nursing Now, 6*, 1–4.

Canadian Nurses Association. (2009). *Position statement: Global health and equity*. https://www.cna-aiic.ca/-/media/cna/page-content/pdf-en/ps106_global_health_equity_aug_2009_e.pdf.

Canadian Nurses Association. (2015). *Position statement: Primary health care*. https://www.cna-aiic.ca/-/media/cna/page-content/pdf-en/primary-health-care-position-statement.pdf.

Canadian Nurses Association. (2017). *Code of ethics for registered nurses* (pp. 15–16). https://www.cna-aiic.ca/html/en/Code-of-Ethics-2017-Edition/files/assets/basic-html/page-22.html.

Canadian Nurses Association. (2018a). *Position statement: Social determinants of health*. https://www.cna-aiic.ca/-/media/cna/page-content/pdf-en/social-determinants-of-health-position-statement_2018_e.pdf.

Canadian Nurses Association. (2018b). *Position statement: Nurses, health and human rights*. https://www.cna-aiic.ca/-/media/cna/page-content/pdf-en/nurses-health-and-human-rights-position-statement_dec-2018.pdf?la=en&hash=F3E784558F08815146C4472003CBCA6434468226.

Canadian Nurses Association. (2019). *Position statement: Interprofessional collaboration*. https://www.cna-aiic.ca/-/media/cna/page-content/pdf-en/cna-position-statement_interprofessional-collaboration.pdf?la=en&hash=E1177042D65084A8792865A62E2003D0C78B46F87287.

Canadian Nurses Association. (2020). *CNA certification program*. https://www.cna-aiic.ca/en/certification.

Canadian Public Health Association (CPHA). (2019). *Public health in the context of health system renewal in Canada: Background document*. https://www.cpha.ca/public-health-context-health-system-renewal-canada.

Centers for Disease Control and Prevention. (2005). *Social determinants of health*. https://www.cdc.gov/socialdeterminants/.

College of Registered Nurses of Manitoba. (2019). *Interprofessional collaborative care: Practice direction*. https://www.crnm.mb.ca/uploads/document/document_file_261.pdf?t=1561125779.

Community Health Nurses of Canada. (2009). *Public health nursing discipline specific competencies version 1.0*. CHNC. https://www.chnc.ca/en/competencies.

Community Health Nurses Association of Canada. (2011). *Canadian community health nursing standards of practice*. CHNC. https://www.chnc.ca/en/publications-resources.

Community Health Nurses of Canada. (2012). *Public health nursing: Primary prevention of chronic diseases*. https://www.chnc.ca/en/membership/documents/loadDocument?id=521&download=1#upload/membership/document/2016-07/2012maychnccdpreport.pdf.

Community Health Nurses of Canada. (2019). *Canadian community health nursing professional practice model and standards of practice*. https://www.chnc.ca/standards-of-practice.

Dahlgren, G., & Whitehead, M. (1992). *Policies and strategies to promote equity in health*. WHO Regional Office for Europe.

Davison, C. M., Edwards, N., Webber, J., et al. (2006). Development of a social justice gauge and its use to review the Canadian Nurses Association's code of ethics for registered nurses. *Advances in Nursing Science, 29*(4), E13–E26.

Enhancing Interdisciplinary Collaboration in Primary Health Care Initiative Steering Committee. (2005). *The principles and* framework for interdisciplinary collaboration in primary health care.

Epp, J. (1986). *Achieving health for all: A framework for health promotion*. Government of Canada, Minister of Supply and Services.

Freidman, E. A., & Gostin, L. O. (2013). Pillars for progress on the right to health: Harnessing the potential of human rights through a framework convention on global health. In M. Grodin, D. Tarantola, G. Annas, et al. (Eds.), *Health and human rights in a changing world* (pp. 232–246). Routledge.

Government of Canada. (2019). *Social determinants of health and health inequalities*. https://www.canada.ca/en/public-health/services/health-promotion/population-health/what-determines-health.html.

Greenwood, M., de Leeuw, S., & Lindsay, N. M. (Eds.). (2018). *Determinants of Indigenous peoples' health in Canada: Beyond the social*. Canadian Scholars' Press.

Grodin, M., Tarantola, D., Annas, G., et al. (Eds.). (2013). *Health and human rights in a changing world*. Routledge.

Hamilton, N., & Bhatti, T. (1996). *Population health promotion: An integrated model of population health and health promotion*. Health Canada: Health Promotion Development Division. http://www.phac-aspc.gc.ca/ph-sp/php-psp/index-eng.php.

Health Canada. (1998). *Taking action on population health: A position paper for health promotion and programs branch staff*. Health Canada.

Health Canada. (2018). *Health care system: Canada health act*. https://www.canada.ca/en/health-canada/services/health-care-system/canada-health-care-system-medicare/canada-health-act.html.

Health Canada. (2019). *Health care system: Canada's health care system*. https://www.canada.ca/en/health-canada/services/health-care-system/reports-publications/health-care-system/canada.html.

Health Canada. (2020). *Health Canada's organizational structure*. https://www.canada.ca/en/health-canada/corporate/organizational-structure.html.

Health Council of Canada. (2009). *Getting it right: Case studies of effective management of chronic disease using primary health care teams*. https://publications.gc.ca/collections/collection_2012/ccs-hcc/H174-31-2009-eng.pdf.

Koplan, J. P., Bond, T. C., Merson, M. H., et al. (2009). Towards a common definition of global health. *Lancet, 373*(9679), 1993–1995.

Lalonde, M. (1974). *A new perspective on the health of Canadians: A working document*. Government of Canada.

Lind, C., & Baptiste, L. (2020). Health promotion. In L. L. Stamler, L. Yiu, A. Dosani, et al. (Eds.), *Community health nursing: A Canadian perspective* (5th ed., pp. 137–167). Pearson Education Canada.

MacDougall, H. (2007). Reinventing public health: A new perspective on the health of Canadians and its international impact. *Journal of Epidemiology & Community Health, 61*(11), 955–959. https://doi.org/10.1136/jech.2006.046912.

Martin, K. S., & Bowles, K. H. (2014). The nurse in home health and hospice. In M. Stanhope, & J. Lancaster (Eds.), *Foundations of nursing in the community: Community-oriented practice*. Elsevier.

Martins, D. C. (2018). Thinking upstream: Nursing theories and population-focused nursing practice. In M. A. Nies, & M. McEwen (Eds.), *Community/public health nursing: Promoting the health of populations* (7th ed., pp. 36–49). Elsevier.

McEwen, M., & Nies, M. A. (2018). Health: A community view. In M. A. Nies, & M. McEwen (Eds.), *Community/public health nursing: Promoting the health of populations* (7th ed., pp. 1–18). Elsevier.

McKinlay, J. B. (2019/1975). *A case for refocusing upstream: The political economy of illness. Applying behavioral science to cardiovascular risk: Proceedings of a conference*. American Heart Association, 7–17. https://iaphs.org/wp-content/uploads/2019/11/IAPHS-McKinlay-Article.pdf.

Mikkonen, J., & Raphael, D. (2010). *Social determinants of health: The Canadian facts*. Toronto: York University School of Health Policy and Management. http://www.thecanadianfacts.org.

Mill, J. (1959). On liberty. In B. Wishy (Ed.), *Prefaces to liberty: Selected writings of John Stuart Mill*. University Press America.

Morrison, V., Gagnon, F., Morestin, F., et al. (2014). *Keywords in healthy public policy*. National collaborating centre for healthy public policy. http://www.ncchpp.ca/165/Publications.ccnpps?id_article=1206.

Mykhalovskiy, E., Frohlich, K., Poland, B., et al. (2019). Critical social science *with* public health: Agonism, critique and engagement. *Critical Public Health, 29*(5), 522–533. https://doi.org/10.1080/09581596.2018.1474174.

National Collaborating Centre for Determinants of Health. (2014). *Let's talk: Moving upstream*. http://nccdh.ca/resources/entry/lets-talk-moving-upstream.

National Collaborating Centre for Determinants of Health. (2020). *About determinants of health*. http://nccdh.ca/resources/about-social-determinants-of-health/.

National Collaborating Centre for Healthy Public Policy. (2018). *Structural profile of public health in Canada*. http://www.ncchpp.ca/710/Structural_Profile_of_Public_Health_in_Canada.ccnpps.

Nelson, S., Turnbull, J., Bainbridge, L., et al. (2014). *Optimizing scopes of practice: New models for a new health care system*. Canadian Academy of Health Sciences. https://www.cahs-acss.ca/wp-content/uploads/2014/08/Optimizing-Scopes-of-Practice_REPORT-English.pdf.

Pederson, A., & Machado, S. (2019). Shifting vulnerabilities: Gender, ethnicity, race, and health inequalities in Canada. In T. Bryant, D. Raphael, & M. Rioux (Eds.), *Staying alive: Critical perspectives on health, illness, and health care* (3rd ed., pp. 199–232). Canadian Scholars' Press.

Public Health Agency of Canada. (2001). *Population health promotion: An integrated model of population health and health promotion*. https://www.canada.ca/en/public-health/services/health-promotion/population-health/population-health-promotion-integrated-model-population-health-health-promotion.html.

Public Health Agency of Canada. (2008a). *Health goals for Canada: A federal, provincial and territorial commitment to Canadians*. http://www.phac-aspc.gc.ca/cphorsphc-respcacsp/2008/fr-rc/cphorsphc-respcacsp10a-eng.php#3.

Public Health Agency of Canada. (2008b). *Core competencies for public health in Canada: Release 1.0*. http://www.phac-aspc.gc.ca/php-psp/ccph-cesp/pdfs/cc-manual-eng090407.pdf.

Public Health Agency of Canada. (2011). *Reducing health inequalities: A challenge for our times*. http://publications.gc.ca/collections/collection_2012/aspc-phac/HP35-22-2011-eng.pdf.

Public Health Agency of Canada. (2013a). *The chief public health officer's report on the state of public health in Canada 2013: Infectious disease—the never-ending threat*. http://www.phac-aspc.gc.ca/cphorsphc-respcacsp/index-eng.php.

Public Health Agency of Canada. (2013b). *Population health approach: The organizing framework.* http://cbpp-pcpe.phac-aspc.gc.ca/population-health-approach-organizing-framework/.

Public Health Agency of Canada. (2016). *Canadian best practice portal: Key element 6: Collaborate across sectors and levels.* https://cbpp-pcpe.phac-aspc.gc.ca/population-health-approach-organizing-framework/key-element-6-collaborate-sectors-levels/.

Public Health Agency of Canada. (2018). *Key health inequalities in Canada: A national portrait.* https://www.canada.ca/content/dam/phac-aspc/documents/services/publications/science-research/key-health-inequalities-canada-national-portrait-executive-summary/hir-full-report-eng.pdf.

Public Health Agency of Canada. (2019). *The chief public health officer's report on the state of public health in Canada 2019: Addressing stigma in Canada's health system.* https://www.canada.ca/en/public-health/corporate/organizational-structure/canada-chief-public-health-officer/addressing-stigma.html.

Public Health Agency of Canada. (2021). *Public health practice: Glossary of terms.* https://www.canada.ca/en/public-health/services/public-health-practice/skills-online/glossary-terms.html.

Rabinowitz, P., Pappaioanou, M., Bardosh, K., et al. (2018). A planetary vision for one health. *BMJ Global Health, 3*(5), e001137. https://doi.org/10.1136/bmjgh-2018-001137.

Raphael, D. (2016). *Social determinants of health: Canadian perspectives* (3rd ed.). Canadian Scholars' Press.

Raphael, D. (2019). Social determinants of health. In T. Bryant, D. Raphael, & M. Rioux (Eds.), *Staying alive: Critical perspectives on health, illness, and health care* (3rd ed., pp. 138–170). Canadian Scholars' Press.

Raphael, D., Bryant, T., & Curry-Stevens, A. (2004). Toronto Charter outlines future health policy directions for Canada and elsewhere. *Health Promotion International, 19*(2), 269–273. https://doi.org/10.1093/heapro/dah214.

Registered Nurses Association of Ontario. (2012). *Best practice guidelines: Developing and sustaining interprofessional health care: Optimizing patients/patients, organizational, and system outcomes.* https://rnao.ca/bpg/guidelines/interprofessional-team-work-healthcare.

Rioux, M. (2019). The right to health: Human rights approaches to health. In T. Bryant, D. Raphael, & M. Rioux (Eds.), *Staying alive: Critical perspectives on health, illness, and health care* (3rd ed., pp. 84–112). Canadian Scholars' Press.

Savage, C. L. (2020). *Public/community health nursing practice: Caring for populations* (2nd ed.). F. A. Davis.

Stadjuhar, K. I., Mollison, A., Giesbrecht, M., et al. (2019). *"Just too busy living in the moment and surviving"*: Barriers to accessing health care for structurally vulnerable populations at end-of-life. *BMC Palliative Care, 18*, 11. https://doi.org/10.1186/s12904-019-0396-7.

Stanley, J., Harris, R., Cormack, D., et al. (2019). The impact of racism on the future health of adults: Protocol for a prospective cohort study. *BMC Public Health, 19*, 346. https://doi.org/10.1186/s12889-019-6664-x.

Wilkinson, R., & Marmot, M. (2003). *Social determinants of health: The solid facts* (2nd ed.). WHO Regional Office for Europe. http://www.euro.who.int/__data/assets/pdf_file/0005/98438/e81384.pdf.

Wilkinson, R., & Pickett, K. (2009). *The spirit level: Why more equal societies almost always do better.* Allen Lane.

World Health Organization. (1978). *Declaration of Alma-Ata.* http://www.who.int/publications/almaata_declaration_en.pdf.

World Health Organization. (1986). *The Ottawa charter for health promotion.* http://www.who.int/healthpromotion/conferences/previous/ottawa/en/.

World Health Organization. (2008). *Closing the gap in a generation: Health equity through action on the social determinants of health.* https://www.who.int/social_determinants/thecommission/finalreport/en/.

World Health Organization. (2021). *Social determinants of health.* https://www.who.int/health-topics/social-determinants-of-health#tab=tab_1.

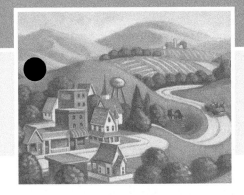

2

The Evolution of Community Health Nursing in Canada

OUTLINE

The Global Historical Roots of Public Health, 31
Early Public Health Efforts in Canada, 32
Milestones in Community Health Nursing in Canada, 33
   The Late 1800s to the Early 1900s, 34
   Remarkable Legacies, 35

Post–World War I: 1918 to the Early 1940s, 35
Post–World War II: 1945 to 1970, 37
1970 to 1999, 38
2000 to the Present, 39

OBJECTIVES

After reading this chapter, you should be able to:

2.1 Explain significant global historical events that led to the development of the modern concept of public health.

2.2 Describe early public health efforts in Canada.

2.3 Discuss some of the historical milestones in the development of community health nursing in Canada.

KEY TERMS*

Canadian Nurses Association (CNA), 29
Canadian Public Health Association (CPHA), 34
Canadian Red Cross, 36
demonstration project, 36

district nursing, 32
outpost nursing, 36
visiting nurse associations, 36
visiting nurses, 36

*See the Glossary on page 468 for definitions.

In Canada, nursing began with providing care in the community and then later concentrated on acute care in hospitals. More recently, the focus of nursing has started to shift back to the community. In 2019, close to 40% of all nurses in Canada worked outside of the hospital setting, in community health services, long-term care, or other environments that serve the community health sector (CNA, 2020). Gaining a better understanding of and appreciation for community health nursing today requires knowledge of the past. Lessons learned through history provide direction for current and future community health nursing practice. For example, lessons learned from the global outbreak of severe acute respiratory syndrome (SARS) in 2003 led to a renewed emphasis on public health and efforts to deal with pandemic threats such as avian flu, H1N1 flu, Middle East respiratory syndrome coronavirus (MERS-CoV), Ebola virus, and coronavirus disease (COVID-19) to manage the global threat of these diseases. A comprehensive understanding of the evolution of the profession of nursing allows community health nurses (CHNs) to function effectively in the current sociopolitical and economic environments. The **Canadian Nurses Association (CNA)**, the national voice for provincial and territorial Canadian nursing associations and colleges, encourages nurses to understand, consider, collect, and preserve their nursing history (see the link to the CNA's [2008] *Position Statement: The Value of Nursing History Today* on the Evolve website). This was reinforced in 2015 in the National Nursing Education Framework developed by the Canadian Association of Schools of Nursing, where history was identified as an essential component of an undergraduate nursing education (CASN, 2015).

As noted in Chapter 1, the term *community health nursing,* as it is used today, is the umbrella term for nurses who work in and with the community in a variety of practice areas, such as home health nursing, public health nursing, occupational health nursing, forensic nursing, parish nursing, and as nurse practitioners (CHNC, 2019). Specific roles and functions have continued to evolve in the community, including the role of the public health nurse (PHN) and advanced practice nurse (APN). In the past, public health nursing was considered separate from community health nursing, but today in Canada it is considered to be one of the practice areas for CHNs. Home visiting nurses such as the Victorian Order of Nurses (VON) also offered a variety of different nursing services and provided care in the home.

For more than 120 years, CHNs in Canada have made significant contributions to solving public health problems. Although only a few historical figures are highlighted in this chapter, many nurse leaders, milestone events, and landmark decisions have played a part in building organizations and providing services to shape public health and community health nursing practice. Effective planning for the future is built on these foundations, on critique, and on lessons learned.

Over the years, CHNs have demonstrated knowledge, skills, flexibility, and creativity, as well as the ability to work with diverse patients and other health care providers. Leaders in community health nursing have worked to improve the health status of individuals, families, and populations. Many have endeavoured to learn about the contexts and conditions that shape inequity and vulnerability, and to challenge injustices. Many of the diverse and challenging formal community health roles that exist today can be traced back to historic periods when public health efforts focused on environmental factors, such as sanitation and the control of communicable diseases; education for health promotion and the prevention of disease and disability; and care of sick people in their homes. In more recent Canadian history, CHNs contributed to transformation change and deinstitutionalization of mental health care in the 1960s and 1970s (Boschma, 2012).

Although community health nurses have contributed to positive change in the health care system, historical initiatives in public health have reflected colonialism, oppression, and racism, and resulted in harmful practices in Canada and elsewhere (Smith, 2020; Grypma, 2017). One historical example of oppression includes the systemic exclusion of Black nurse applicants from nursing education programs and practice in Canada during the first half of the 1900s (Flynn, 2009). Between the 1930s and into the 1970s, Indigenous people in Canada received separate community health services, including tuberculosis (TB) treatments and practices that left Indigenous people more vulnerable to disease, both through the residential school system and what was then called the Indian Health Service (MacCallum, 2017; Meijer Drees, 2014). In the later 1970s until the 1990s, community health nursing's preoccupation with personal lifestyle factors as a determinant of health also entrenched the field in systematic victim-blaming, counter to good public health practice (Smith, 2020). This chapter begins here, looking at the wide canvas of the history of community health nursing, the triumphs, and the shame that have influenced the evolution of community health nursing.

EVIDENCE-INFORMED PRACTICE

Historically, community-based PHNs have played a significant role in disease prevention and health promotion, with strong interests in early interventions for children and youth. Well-baby clinics, school vaccination programs, sexual health education, and family planning have been traditional activities of community-based PHNs. Engaging with school communities to promote child and youth health has been a long-time task of PHNs in Canada and elsewhere. School nursing was one of the areas of specialty work of community health nursing in Canada early in the twentieth century. Over several decades, the nursing connection with schools has become more tenuous, even if intersectoral and interdisciplinary comprehensive school health models have emerged as strong examples of disease prevention with school populations.

It is this role and engagement of PHNs in school health teams that was the topic of Sanders, O'Mahony, Duncan, et al.'s (2019) participatory action research project. In a thematic analysis of two schools' engagement processes with a PHN, discoveries included facilitators and barriers to public health nursing engagement, and the influences of community context on engagement. School contexts where there were existing health committees or some existing focus on health facilitated the effectiveness of the PHN activities and health promotion outcomes. Regardless of the context, relationships were essential to the effective health work of PHNs. In this analysis, it became clear that the PHN role in schools needs development and optimization to sustain the vital link between health promotion, disease prevention, and schools.

Application for CHNs:

Community health nursing continues to evolve to ensure that promotion and disease prevention are addressed, which are often the result of early interventions such as fundamental work with children and youth. Collaboration and relationships are essential to community health nursing practice. The context and environment can influence CHN practice.

Questions for Reflection and Discussion

1. If school contexts are important sites of community health nursing practice, what historical and contextual factors might have contributed to decreased development and support of school nursing in Canada?
2. What search words would you use to find out more about these influences, and how school nursing and other areas of community health nursing have been prioritized or not?

Source: Sanders, T., O'Mahony, J., Duncan, S., Mahara, S., Pitman, V., Ringstad, K., & Weatherman, K. (2019). Opening the doors for school health—An exploration of public health nurses' capacities to engage in comprehensive school health programs. *Public Health Nursing, 36*(3), 348–356. https://doi.org/10.1111/phn.12607

THE GLOBAL HISTORICAL ROOTS OF PUBLIC HEALTH

Throughout history, people have worked to understand, prevent, and control disease, illness, and injury. Their ability to preserve health and treat health conditions has depended on their understanding of history, engagement in politics, knowledge of science, the use and availability of technologies, and the degree of coordination and resources assigned to the health concerns of the day. For example, Indigenous people in Canada and elsewhere historically viewed the ecosystem as the centre of health, with social and environmental care being required for well-being and sustainability (Parkes, 2011). Ancient Babylonians understood the importance of hygiene, and historical records indicate they also had some medical skills and knew how to use medicine to treat the sick. Egyptian people circa 1000 BCE developed a variety of pharmaceutical preparations and became known for their remarkable construction of earth privies and public drainage systems. Ancient Greek people were more concerned with personal health than community health, practising many health-promoting behaviours and linking health to the environment in ways that are now considered vital for good health. Classical Roman civilization viewed medicine from the perspective of community health and social medicine. It placed great emphasis on the regulation of medical practice and punishment for negligence; provision of clean water through a complex system of settling basins, aqueducts, and reservoirs; establishment of sewage systems and drainage of swamps; and supervision of street cleaning and public food preparation (Pellegrino, 1963). Certain values, principles, and practices took dominance at different times in the history of public health, and aligned with other political, economic, and environmental activities.

The decline of the Greco–Roman civilization led to the decay of urban culture and the disintegration of community health organization and practice (Rosen, 1958). During the Middle Ages, between 500 and 1500 CE, European cities suffered high population density, lacked clean water, and had inefficient systems to dispose of refuse and body wastes. Poor sanitary conditions and residential crowding caused increases in communicable diseases, such as cholera, smallpox, and bubonic plague. Most people had to secure their own health care services; however, religious institutions, such as convents and monasteries, began to establish hospitals to care for the sick, poor, and neglected, including the aged, disabled, and orphaned (Rosen, 1958). Later in the Middle Ages, an interest in health education and the promotion of personal hygiene and healthy living grew, and moderate eating was encouraged. In the eleventh century, similar forces guided the work of Muslim nurses in what is now Saudi Arabia. Rufaida Al-Asalmiya cared for injured soldiers, established a school of nursing for women, and developed a code for nursing conduct and ethics (Jan, 1996). During the Renaissance (from the fourteenth through the sixteenth centuries), health practices were influenced by a recognition of human dignity and worth (Kalisch & Kalisch, 1995). Table 2.1 summarizes the historical roots of public

TABLE 2.1 **The Historical Roots of Western Public Health, Public Health Nursing, and Community Health Nursing**

Year	Milestone
1601	Elizabethan *Poor Law* enacted
1617	Sisterhood of the Dames de Charité organized in France by St. Vincent de Paul
1789	Baltimore Health Department established
1798	Marine Hospital Service established in the United States; later became Public Health Service
1812	Sisters of Mercy established in Dublin, Ireland; nuns visited the poor
1813	Ladies Benevolent Society of Charleston, South Carolina, founded
1836	Lutheran deaconesses made home visits in Kaiserswerth, Germany
1851	Florence Nightingale visited Kaiserswerth, Germany, for 3 months of nurse training
1855	Quarantine Board established in New Orleans, Louisiana; beginning of tuberculosis eradication campaign in the United States
1859	District nursing established in Liverpool, England, by William Rathbone
1860	Florence Nightingale Training School for Nurses established at St. Thomas Hospital in London, England
1864	Founding of American Red Cross
1895	Founding of Canadian Red Cross

health efforts, public health nursing, and community health nursing in Western Europe and North America.

The Industrial Revolution in nineteenth-century Europe led to social changes, including great advances in transportation, communication, and other forms of technology. Previous caregiving structures, which relied on families, neighbours, and friends, had by then become inadequate because of increased migration, urbanization, and higher populations. During this period, small numbers of Roman Catholic and Protestant religious women provided nursing care in institutions and in people's homes (Kalisch & Kalisch, 1995).

Many women who performed informal nursing functions in almshouses and early hospitals in Great Britain were poorly educated and untrained. As the practice of medicine became more complex in the mid-1800s, hospital work required a more skilled caregiver, and physicians and hospital administrators sought to improve the quality of nursing services. Early experimental efforts led to some improvement in care, and the groundbreaking work of Florence Nightingale, discussed briefly in this chapter, later revolutionized public health care. Through these efforts, both public health and the discipline of nursing came into their own, focused on principles of public health.

During the Crimean War (1854–1856), the British military established hospitals for the sick and wounded soldiers in Scutari (the former name for Üsküdar, a municipality of Istanbul). These hospitals were crowded, and plagued by poor

EVIDENCE-INFORMED PRACTICE

MacDougall (2009) describes the deep historical roots involved in the creation of twenty-first century pandemic preparation plans; for example, allocating personnel, facilities, vaccines, and equipment; addressing and discussing ethical issues; and determining whether preventive or curative measures would be most effective.

The first cholera epidemic in Canada was in 1832 in Ontario and Quebec, and it provided guidance for disease prevention and control when cholera reoccurred in 1834, 1849, 1854, and 1866. The governing bodies identified the importance of strong leadership at central and local levels; clear communication about the disease and its nature; clear information on the steps required to prevent or control the disease; and adequate legal and financial support for front-line workers and volunteers. They also recognized that each outbreak would spawn a response from society based on the society's cultural values and perceptions of danger. These principles remain the foundation for current programs and policies pertaining to disease prevention and were seen being exercised in the COVID-19 pandemic response in 2020.

Application for CHNs

The importance of history to present-day pandemic response and community health nursing practice is well stated. CHNs use lessons learned from the past and apply them to current practices. When considering changes to health care practices, it is often valuable to conduct a historical review to identify past lessons learned.

Questions for Reflection and Discussion

1. Consider the flu, measles, coronaviruses, and other potential pandemics. What trends, developments, and historical events have changed the societal response to pandemics?
2. What roles might CHNs assume in a pandemic?

Source: MacDougall, H. (2009). "Truly alarming": Cholera in 1832. *Canadian Journal of Public Health, 100*(5), 333–336.

sanitation, lice, and rats. They also provided insufficient food and medical supplies, and, overall, poor care (Kalisch & Kalisch, 1995). The British public demanded improved conditions, and Florence Nightingale asked to be sent to work in Scutari. Her personal wealth, social and political connections, and knowledge of hospitals influenced the British government, and along with 40 other women, 117 hired nurses, and 15 paid servants, Nightingale went to Scutari. There, she succeeded in significantly improving the soldiers' health using an approach that included better environmental conditions and excellent nursing care. Using simple charts and measures to track patterns of disease and death, she documented a decrease in mortality rate from 415 per 1 000 at the beginning of the war to 11.5 per 1 000 at the end (Cohen, 1984). Following the example of Nightingale in Scutari, nurses practising community health care start by identifying health care needs that affect the entire population. They then organize themselves and the community and mobilize resources to meet these needs in ways that are adapted to the environment broadly as well as to its local districts.

After the Crimean War, Nightingale returned to England in 1856, having established a strong reputation. She went on to organize hospital nursing practice and nursing education in hospitals in England, replacing untrained lay nurses with trained "Nightingale nurses." Believing that nursing should not only promote health but also prevent illness, she focused on both hospital and community nursing that emphasized the importance of nutrition, rest, sanitation, and hygiene (Nightingale, 1894, 1946). Nightingale's work marks the beginning of community health nursing practice as we know it today. In Canada, some of the hospital nursing programs established in the late 1950s and early 1960s adopted Nightingale's philosophy of nursing; that is, that healing processes can be facilitated or hindered by nursing interventions (Allemang, 2000).

In 1859 in Liverpool, England, British philanthropist William Rathbone founded the first association for **district nursing,** a system in which a nurse was assigned to each district in a town to provide a wide variety of health services to people in need. Based on the success of these "friendly visitors" (Kalisch & Kalisch, 1995), Florence Nightingale and William Rathbone made recommendations for providing nursing in the home that established district and visiting nursing throughout England (Nutting & Dock, 1935).

EARLY PUBLIC HEALTH EFFORTS IN CANADA

Early public health efforts in Canada were driven by the need to deal with epidemics. Before 1900, Canada did not have Europe's problems of overcrowded cities and had the advantage of alternating hot and cold seasons, reducing disease-causing organisms in the environment. However, devastating epidemics did occur, typically coinciding with the arrival of new immigrants from Europe on crowded, unsanitary ships carrying such highly contagious diseases as smallpox, typhus, cholera, and influenza. The diseases spread quickly and particularly wrought havoc among Indigenous people in Canada, who were introduced to harmful conditions and pathogens during colonization (Cadotte & James-Abra, 2015; Rutty & Sullivan, 2010). The impact of colonization and the historical Indigenous understanding of health and care of the community are discussed in further detail in Chapter 14.

With colonization and industrialization, rapid population growth in the cities led to inadequate housing and poor sanitation, thus causing epidemics of diseases such as smallpox, yellow fever, cholera, typhoid, and typhus. Tuberculosis (TB) was always present, and infant mortality rates continued to rise as did concern regarding the health of the public (Vukic & Dilworth, 2019). In short, from the seventeenth to the nineteenth centuries, epidemics ravaged towns and cities in Canada, killing tens of thousands of people. Smallpox (and other epidemics) set the stage for the reshaping of well-being and health practices from Indigenous practices to the health practices of colonizers. To prevent the devastation caused by such outbreaks, Canadian authorities began to establish programs intended to protect public health, although such programs in Indigenous communities failed to acknowledge Indigenous understandings of healing and community health (Bourque Bearskin, Cameron, King, et al., 2016).

The intent of the various authorities who attempted to respond to illness and suffering in Indigenous communities at the time was likely not malicious. However, disregard for the long-standing Indigenous society, knowledge, and culture in community health care practices created an additional layer of suffering for Indigenous people and contributed to the destruction of community wellness (Grypma, 2019). This approach set the stage for years of grief for and disregard of Indigenous people, the fallout of which continues to this day.

Vaccination programs were introduced as early as the end of the eighteenth century and, in some cases, were mandatory. In 1882, Ontario passed legislation for the establishment of the first Board of Health, which reported to municipal councils and assumed responsibility for educating the public about health matters (Allemang, 2000). Soon after, Boards of Health were established in other provinces to deal with the problem of frequent epidemics and the incidence and prevalence of communicable diseases as well as to ensure support and enforcement of public health efforts.

In western Canada, formal health care programs and systems of care were established much later because the population was sparse prior to 1890. Health care in the West was largely provided by family, neighbours, and Indigenous women. Even following first contact with settlers, many people could not afford the medical services that had been established, and Indigenous women played a major role in the health care of their communities and for new settlers, serving predominantly as midwives and providing local plant-based medicinal healing (Burnett, 2008, 2010). While these practices were at odds with the prevailing beliefs and values of the settlers (missionaries, government leaders, and community members alike), all employed their services. The role of Indigenous women healers was valued socially and monetarily at the time (Burnett, 2008, 2010), though disregard for Indigenous knowledge and practices prevailed.

MILESTONES IN COMMUNITY HEALTH NURSING IN CANADA

Many of the changes to public health and the conditions and profession of nursing in general during the nineteenth and twentieth centuries affected and shaped the development of community health nursing. Nightingale's vision of trained nurses and her model of nursing education influenced the development of professional nursing and, indirectly, home care and community health nursing in the United States and in Canada.

In the early years of North American colonization, nursing care was typically informal, provided in the home by the women of the household. Early care was often provided with support from Indigenous women healers who had a strong social structure of caring for the ill, injured, birthing, and dying, and knowledge of plants and herbs used for their healing properties (Burnett, 2008, 2010; Grypma, 2019). From the early seventeenth century onward, women and other groups, such as religious orders and wealthy philanthropists, saw the need to take care of those who could not afford to hire caregivers; these compassionate caregivers laid the foundations for contemporary community health nursing. Table 2.2

TABLE 2.2   Milestones in the Early Evolution of Community Health Nursing in Canada: 1617–1898

Year	Milestone
1617	Marie Rollet Hébert became the first laywoman to care for the sick in her own home and in other homes in the community in Quebec.
1629	First nurses (male attendants) worked with the sick in what resembled a modern community clinic in Acadia. Jesuit priests also cared for the sick.
1639	The Duchesse d'Aiguillon arranged for three nuns to settle in Quebec and establish a mission (later known as Quebec's first hospital—Hôtel-Dieu); these nuns also cared for the sick in the community.
1641	Jeanne Mance arrived in Ville-Marie (later Montreal) and established the first Hôtel-Dieu hospital there. Being the first lay nurse in North America, she cared for those wounded in battle and also took on a major leadership role in the community and became very involved in political activities to improve life within the colony.
1737	Marguerite d'Youville founded the order of the Grey Nuns; in Canada, they became the first nurses who visited and cared for the sick in their own homes and developed community hospitals for the care of the acutely and chronically ill regardless of their race, culture, religion, or social status. Hardill identifies these home visits as the initiation of community visits to the sick poor and states that this was the beginning of "the practical origins of modern Canadian outreach nursing."*
1845–1895	The Grey Nuns founded community hospitals and made home visits to the poor in Ottawa, Ontario; St. Boniface, Manitoba; Edmonton, Alberta; and northern native settlements in Saskatchewan.
1859	Florence Nightingale published her "Notes on Nursing," which influenced the philosophy of nursing, including community health nursing, in Canada.
1898	Lady Aberdeen, wife of the Governor General of Canada, recognized the need for specialized health services for women, especially during childbirth, and for health care for the poor living near railways and in mining areas in isolated communities. She founded the Victorian Order of Nurses (VON) in Canada. VON nurses provided home care in urban and isolated rural areas.

Sources: Allemang, 2000; Canadian Nurses Association, 2016; Hardill, 2007; Astle et al., 2019; Grypma, 2019.
*Hardill, 2007, p. 91.

presents significant milestones in the development of community health nursing practice in Canada from its beginnings in 1617 to 1898.

The Late 1800s to the Early 1900s

A significant development in the nursing profession during the late nineteenth and early twentieth centuries was the institution of various professional nursing bodies. The International Council of Nurses (ICN) was founded in 1899, becoming the first professional nursing organization. Great Britain, the United States, and Germany were charter members; Canada was also represented in the organization. In 1908, a national organization of nurses was established in Canada as the Provisional Society of the Canadian National Association of Trained Nurses (CNATN), which became a member of the ICN in 1909. By 1924, the CNATN membership had expanded considerably, and the association was renamed the Canadian Nurses Association (CNA). In 1930, CNA brought provincial nursing associations under its umbrella (McLeary & McParland, 2020). These and other nursing organizations continue to develop and advance the profession of nursing and advocate the importance of nursing in the community.

The early 1900s marked the introduction of organized public health nursing as a major component of public health programs. For example, PHNs employed by the Toronto Department of Health made home visits for all cases of TB (also referred to as *consumption*), unless the physicians-in-charge indicated visits were not necessary (Royce, 1983). The purpose of these home visits was to teach the person with TB self-care and inform family members of ways to prevent the spread of infection throughout the household. The Department of Health maintained records of children who had been exposed to TB in the home. When people infected with TB had to be moved away from their homes or schools, PHNs arranged and oversaw complete fumigation of the house. PHNs also established separate schools or camps for children with TB and arranged entirely separate treatment for Indigenous people, as was the norm (Meijer Drees, 2014).

In 1906, the Montreal Board of Health implemented a program of medical inspection of schoolchildren with nurses from the VON conducting home visits to families with newborns and visits to children at schools (Duncan, Leipert, & Mill, 1999). Around this time, school nurses were also hired to work in Hamilton and Toronto schools. Just prior to World War I, the focus shifted to maternal–child health, resulting in expanded roles for PHNs. However, some specialized nursing roles, such as that of the "TB nurse," were maintained. In 1910, the **Canadian Public Health Association (CPHA)** was founded to deliver and support national and international health and social service programs (CPHA, 2020; Rutty & Sullivan, 2010).

Lillian Wald

Public health nursing made significant strides in the United States in the late nineteenth and early twentieth centuries,

largely because of the work of a nurse and social reformer named Lillian Wald. Wald recognized that sickness should be considered within its social and economic context. Her visionary work is recognized in three critical areas: the invention of public health nursing; the establishment of an American insurance system for home-based care, and the creation of an American public health nursing service (Buhler-Wilkerson, 1993).

In 1909, Wald, along with Lee Frankel, who oversaw the welfare department of the Metropolitan Life Insurance Company, established the first public health nursing program for the life insurance policyholders of that company, believing that keeping workers healthy would increase their productivity. Wald proposed that nurses assess illness, teach health practices, and collect data from policyholders in place of insurance company nurses (Hamilton, 1992). According to Frachel (1988), Wald's program made several contributions to public health nursing, including the following:

- Providing home nursing care on a fee-for-service basis
- Establishing an effective cost-accounting system for visiting nurses
- Using advertisements in newspapers and on the radio to recruit nurses
- Reducing mortality rates from infectious diseases

In 1909 the Metropolitan Life Insurance Company implemented a program using visiting nurse organizations to provide care for sick policyholders. By 1918, Metropolitan Life calculated an average 7% decrease in the mortality rate of policyholders and almost a 20% decrease in the mortality rate of children younger than 3 years. The insurance company attributed this improvement, as well as its own reduced costs, to the work of visiting nurses. In the 1920s, the Canadian Metropolitan Life Insurance Company provided home nursing services for policyholders who became ill and required in-home care.

Eunice Dyke

In the early 1900s, a Canadian nurse named Eunice Dyke became interested in the public health issues in Ontario. Dyke attended the Johns Hopkins Training School for Nurses in Baltimore, Maryland, where her district nursing experiences as a student incited in her a deep interest in public health issues. She returned to Canada and worked at the Toronto Department of Health, where she implemented her vision for public health nursing and emerged as a leading Canadian figure in the field for several decades. In 1911, she became the first director of Public Health Nursing in the Toronto Department of Health. Many noteworthy developments in public health nursing occurred during Dyke's nursing leadership (see Box 2.1).

Kate Brighty Colley

In 1917, Manitoba became the first province in Canada to establish a public health nursing service (Stewart, 1979). In 1919, following a 2-month diploma program in public health nursing at the University of Alberta, Kate Brighty Colley started working as a public health district nurse with Alberta's

BOX 2.1   Eunice Dyke: Public Health Nurse Pioneer in Canada

Public health nursing evolved in Canada in the late nineteenth and early twentieth centuries, largely because of the pioneering work of Eunice Dyke. In 1914, Dyke played a key role in decentralizing public health nursing. Before this time, PHNs worked in specialized areas of nursing (e.g., TB care), but they began to assume a more generalist role (although they did not provide bedside nursing care in the home as CHNs or visiting nurses would). Dyke's philosophy was that family, home, and community represented essential parts of the work of PHNs, so public health nursing should be generalized and connected to community agencies. This philosophy represented a fundamental shift from specialist public health nursing—which focused on the individual—to community health. Dyke ensured better care for new immigrants by hiring nurses who could speak foreign languages. Finally, she introduced the placement of PHNs in Toronto schools through the Board of Health.*

Dyke kept a journal, referred to as the "Brown Book," where she described the contents of a PHN's black bag, a useful aid that she initiated and that would become a symbol of public health nursing. The contents of the bag, which were organized to ensure cleanliness, included equipment for assessment and care of the patient in the home. The contents of a PHN's black bag as listed in Dyke's journal are as follows[†]:

Nursing Supplies

Castor oil	Green soap	Mouthwash
Vaseline tube	Thermometers: rectal	Instruments:
Bags: absorbent	and mouth	scissors and
cotton, rectal	Hand towel	forceps
tube, and funnel	Bichloride tablets	Gown
Book	Talcum powder	Olive oil
Alcohol	Bandages—1 and	Basin
Safety pins	2 inch	

Literature on Tuberculosis and Child Welfare

Care of baby—2	Diet slips—2	Prenatal care—2
City order	Birth registration	
papers—2	cards—2	

Sanitary Supplies

Spectum outfit	Refills
Handkerchiefs	Paper bags

For further discussion on the historical significance of a PHN's bag, refer to the article "The Public Health Nursing Bag as Tool and Symbol."[‡]
Sources: *MacQueen, 1997. [†]Royce, 1983, p. 40. [‡]Abrams, 2009.

Department of Public Health (Stewart, 1979; University of Calgary, 2018). District nurses worked in isolated rural communities where no other medical services were available. Colley temporarily left that position to return in 1923 to establish a district long-term care facility in Alberta in two areas without road access, travelling to communities via horse-drawn carriage or sled. Colley contributed to community health nursing by establishing many district long-term care facilities in Alberta and was appointed superintendent of PHNs in Alberta. Additionally, she provided health information to community residents through radio broadcasts. This method of delivering health information was especially effective for those living in isolated communities.

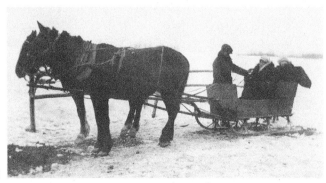

District nurses starting out on visit (Kate Brighty Colley is driving the horse-drawn sled), Onaway, Alberta, 1919. (Glenbow Archives, NA-3956-1)

Remarkable Legacies

The remarkable legacies of early leaders, such as Florence Nightingale, Lillian Wald, Eunice Dyke, and Kate Brighty Colley continue to inspire practice in the present and for the future. These nurses demonstrated an exceptional ability to develop approaches and programs to solve the health care and social problems of their times. The emphasis of community health nursing has changed over the years; however, from its inception, community health nursing practice has included health teaching as well as disease prevention. MacQueen (1997) explained that "it was when prevention became a goal that home nursing became public health nursing" (p. 51). Proactive interventions by community members led to improvements in sanitation, economic conditions, and nutrition. These interventions were credited with reducing the incidence of acute communicable diseases.

Post–World War I: 1918 to the Early 1940s

The years 1918 to the early 1940s marked several major milestones in the development of nursing and public health nursing in Canada. The first Canadian hospital diploma nursing school opened in 1874 in St. Catharines, Ontario (Grypma, 2019). It was recognized that nurses working in communities needed more knowledge and skills in disease prevention and health promotion beyond their basic education and training (Duncan et al., 1999). In 1919, the University of British Columbia (UBC) established Canada's first 5-year baccalaureate degree program in nursing, with the last year of the program including a specialty course in public health nursing (Allemang, 2000). E. Kathleen Russell, director of Public Health Nursing at the University of Toronto, proposed that additional knowledge and skills for nursing could best be provided through university education. In 1920, she was instrumental in establishing the first integrated basic degree nursing program (a major milestone in nursing education in the province), which included public health nursing education.

Early in the 1920s, the Canadian Red Cross provided financial support for public health nursing certificate courses at Dalhousie University, McGill University, University of Alberta, UBC, University of Toronto, and University of Western Ontario.

In these early days, trained graduate nurses worked in private-duty nursing or held the few hospital administrator or instructor positions that were available. Private-duty nurses often lived with the families of patients receiving care. It was expensive to hire private-duty nurses (and to receive other medical services) during the period before formalized Medicare in Canada, and only the affluent could afford such services. Subsequently, the introduction of community health nursing and home visiting contributed to urban health needs, especially for the disadvantaged.

After World War I, greater emphasis was placed on the health of aggregates, particularly infants and children. **Visiting nurses,** who provided care wherever the patient was located—at home, work, or school—took care of several families in 1 day (rather than only one patient or family, as the private-duty nurse did), making their care more economical. The movement grew, and the next few years saw the establishment of **visiting nurse associations,** agencies that provided visiting nurses.

During the same period, several voluntary organizations, including the **Canadian Red Cross** (a national organization founded to reduce human suffering through various health, safety, and disaster-relief programs), in affiliation with the International Red Cross, worked with PHNs to ensure the availability of services in communities. The focus of this initiative was to prevent disease, promote health, and provide support for those experiencing stress and suffering (Allemang, 2000; Duncan et al., 1999). The VON also contributed to public health development in Canada. The VON, through its home health nurse visiting program and preventive work, was able to demonstrate that nursing care in the community effectively addressed public health concerns (Pringle & Roe, 1992). In Canada, the VON recognized the importance of and opportunities for health promotion by nurses in all nursing work settings (Allemang, 2000).

From 1918 to 1939, disease screening programs, environmental health attention, and personal nursing care became the focus of public health nursing responsibilities (Grypma, 2019). **Outpost nursing**—that is, nursing care provided in rural and remote communities—which began in Canada in the late 1800s, gained momentum in the 1920s as a growing number of PHNs chose to work in this field. In the 1920s, the Canadian Red Cross established outpost nursing stations in Canada's north to meet the needs of Indigenous people and

new settlers in remote parts of Canada (Canadian Museum of History, n.d.). Demonstration projects, in which the Canadian Red Cross provided financial support to PHNs, made it possible for public health nursing services to be provided in rural communities in Nova Scotia and New Brunswick (Allemang, 2000). A **demonstration project** is a project funded externally to promote the testing of ideas and hunches. The Red Cross–funded projects were so successful that government, public, and private funding enabled their sustainability.

Historically, outpost nurses worked autonomously and had the responsibility of looking after populations in areas where residents had only minimal access to medical care. These nurses encountered many challenges, such as having to travel long distances, working in isolation, and communicating through language and cultural differences. Currently, even though nurses working in isolated areas continue to face many challenges, technological advances and the introduction of medical directives (the delegation of certain medical acts to nurses working in outpost settings) have made their work more rewarding and somewhat less overwhelming and isolated (McBain, 2012; Rutherdale, 2010).

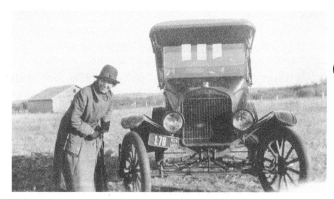

Helen Anderson, a district nurse, is shown here in 1921 beside her automobile, which she used to conduct school visits. (Glenbow Archives, NA-3956-2)

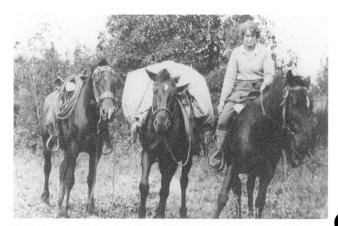

Early Canadian outpost nurses had to contend with many challenges, such as travelling long distances to visit the sick. A nurse uses pack horses to bring supplies to her station in Slave Lake, Alberta, during the 1930s. (Glenbow Archives, NA-3283-2)

In the early 1920s, a public health nursing practice section of the CNATN was formally recognized (Duncan et al., 1999). This association had leadership representation from across the country, and these public health nurse leaders and other nurses published and communicated developments in public health nursing in Canada, identifying important and emerging issues.

From the 1920s to the 1940s, nurses specializing in TB care were replaced by PHNs because of the belief that visiting nurses would be more effective and efficient if they moved to general nursing care (Toth, Fackelmann, Pigott, et al., 2004). Therefore, PHNs became specialists in TB education, prevention, and treatment.

UBC Professor G. M. Weir's 1932 report on nursing education and public health nursing recommended that public health nursing become a specialty area in advanced education (Allemang, 2000). Weir's report highlighted that 1 521 PHNs held positions such as staff nurse, supervisor, visiting nurse, school nurse, industrial nurse, and VON nurse (Allemang, 2000). The report explored the challenges these nurses faced in practice, such as transportation to rural and remote areas; some physician resistance due to lack of understanding of the PHN's role; poor compensation; and lack of advanced skill and nursing experience for working in rural settings. This report concluded that a disproportionate number of graduating nurses focused on hospital nursing rather than public health nursing, and projected that between the years 1937 and 1942, the number of PHNs would have to double to meet the needs of the Canadian population (Allemang, 2000).

The Great Depression of the 1930s led Canadians to two significant realizations: (1) that they wanted government to take responsibility for health care and (2) that poverty was not the result of personal weakness but a consequence of sociopolitical factors (Vukic & Dilworth, 2019). As an outcome of these realizations the federal government began social assistance, and provincial governments focused on public health programs, such as immunization, improved sewage systems, and clean water (Allemang, 2000; Vukic & Dilworth, 2019).

Post–World War II: 1945 to 1970

From 1945 to 1970, the vision for public health expanded beyond the maintenance and control of the physical environment to include the prevention of diseases with screening, treatment, and health education (Duncan et al., 1999). At the same time, significant advances were being made in pharmacology, especially in antibiotics to treat many infectious diseases, vaccines to prevent some communicable diseases, and other highly effective medications to treat various illnesses. These pharmacological advances shifted the previous focus on prevention and "care" to a medical focus of "cure" (Allemang, 2000).

During the 1950s and 1960s, PHNs moved from specialized nursing services in the community to generalized nursing services. The responsibilities of the PHN were often described as caring for patients from "womb to tomb," through all developmental ages and stages, starting with prenatal care. PHNs regularly visited patients in their homes, in schools, and in clinics (e.g., immunization clinics and well-baby clinics) and provided other services (e.g., hospital liaison to arrange for continuity of care). The focus of public health nursing was disease prevention and health promotion, especially through health education. While PHNs did not provide direct nursing care, the VON did provide direct nursing services in the home. In some areas of Canada, boards of education hired nurses to provide school health programs, working directly in the schools and delivering services such as screening for vision and hearing problems, checking for and monitoring communicable diseases, counselling, and individual and classroom-based health education.

The emergence of public insurance was another notable shift in the history of public health in Canada. This system of public medical insurance began in Saskatchewan in 1960 with the re-election of Tommy Douglas and his pro-public insurance platform (Rutty & Sullivan, 2010). Pharmacological advances and publicly funded medical care radically shifted the delivery of health care in Canada. The administration and education of nurses, previously guided by Nightingale's philosophy, was reformed to follow an apprenticeship and service model. Hospital care in this era was reformed to follow the biomedical and business models that predominate today (Chinn & Kramer, 2019).

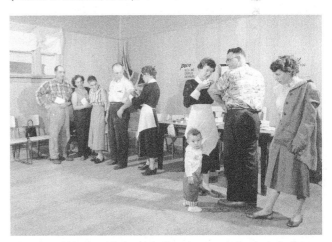

After World War II, public health in Canada expanded to include disease prevention and health education. In this photo, public health nurses are giving polio vaccinations to residents of Southey, Saskatchewan, in the 1950s. (Provincial Archives of Saskatchewan [R-A13590-3])

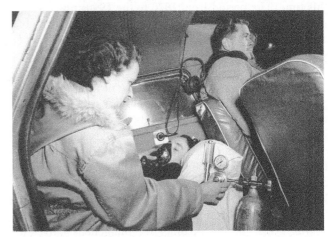

The outpost nurse is shown accompanying a young patient to hospital by air ambulance in 1952. (Provincial Archives of Saskatchewan [R-A11751])

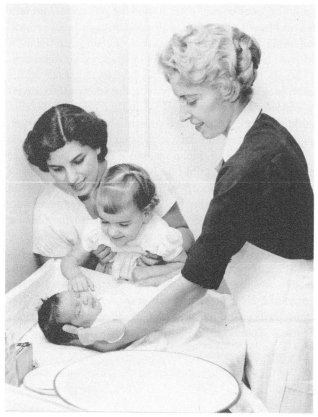

A Victorian Order of Nurses nurse visits a mother with a newborn, circa 1960. (Canada Department of Manpower and Immigration/ Library and Archives Canada)

1970 to 1999

The Lalonde Report (Lalonde, 1974) of the mid-1970s initiated the health promotion movement in Canada, which focused on healthy individual lifestyles. Canada led the worldwide effort in health promotion initiatives through written documents, such as the Epp Report (Epp, 1986) and the development of population health and the determinants of health, which are discussed further in Chapter 4.

Public health trends and the community health nursing practice environment saw considerable evolution during this time. The period from 1970 to the 1990s saw a surge in information and technology use, greater globalization, and the adoption of new forms of service organization and management centred on efficiency. In the 1970s specifically, public health departments focused on reducing morbidity and mortality from chronic illnesses and injuries, representing a shift from traditional programs (Vukic & Dilworth, 2019). At various times since the 1970s, Canada's provinces and territories placed greater emphasis on home care because of the shift from institutional care to community care brought on by such factors as fiscal concerns, patient preferences, and technology (Fournier & Karachiwalla, 2020).

In 1975, the Registered Nurses of Canadian Indian Ancestry was formed in order for Indigenous nurses to come together as a professional group and play a key role in dealing with issues and health disparities experienced in First Nations communities. In 1992, this professional association was renamed the Aboriginal Nurses Association of Canada.

In the 1980s, mothers and their newborns were discharged from hospitals shortly after birth, making the PHN's liaison role more prominent because of the need to ensure effective follow-up care (Vukic & Dilworth, 2019). The PHN's role in the prevention of chronic illnesses resulted in community development and community-based health promotion activities becoming part of public health strategies. PHNs contributed to community development by working with other community members to develop, facilitate, and implement health programs. In the late 1980s and into the 1990s, PHNs further expanded their skills in community development, capacity building, and group work by developing and supporting relevant partnerships and coalitions that included research and evaluation.

Parish nursing associations became structured as organizations unto themselves in the 1980s, due in large part to the financial crises of the times and an increased emphasis on management in all aspects of health care. Since then, parish nursing services and community programs have remained strong across the country and in a variety of faith communities. These associations often work in larger communities for vulnerable groups. For example, the Salvation Army has programs and parish nurses who work in many urban shelters, hospices, and nursing home facilities.

Escalating health care costs in the 1980s resulted in some significant reforms to Canadian health care systems. Health promotion and disease prevention programs received less financial support, whereas more funding was directed to acute hospital care, medical procedures, and institutional long-term care. Reduced federal and provincial funds led to a decrease in the number of nurses in some public health agencies. Despite the risk of reduction in the reimbursement of costs, the role of home care increased, and the specialty of occupational health nursing was established in 1982. Individuals and families began to assume more responsibility for their own health; thus, health education—always a part of community health nursing—became more popular. At this time, Ontario established the new position of "health educator" in public health units for the coordination of the province's health promotion initiatives. Possibly in response to such initiatives, consumer and professional advocacy groups urged the enactment of laws to prohibit health-harming practices (e.g., smoking, driving under the influence of alcohol). Governmental and managerial emphasis on linking policy, politics, and health care has continued to this day, various examples of which will be discussed throughout this text.

In 1987, the Community Health Nurses Association of Canada (CHNAC), an interest group of CNA, was formed (CHNAC, 2003). In the late 1980s and early 1990s, debates surfaced around the definition of the terms *community health nursing* and *public health nursing*, which were being used interchangeably and at times causing confusion. King, Harrison, and Reutter (1995) helped clarify that *community health nursing* was the broader term and encompassed "sub-specialties" such as public health nursing, home care nursing, and occupational health nursing. Also, in the 1990s, the primary health care nurse practitioner role and designation were established in several provinces.

Alongside the developments in community health and public health nursing during this period, training innovations continued in community health in Canada. In 1967, Dalhousie University in Halifax, Nova Scotia, offered the first nurse practitioner program for northern nurses (Worster, Sarco, Thrasher, et al., 2005). During the 1970s, nurses made many contributions to improving the health care of communities, including participating in the hospice movement and the development of birthing centres, daycare for older adults and disabled persons, substance use treatment programs, and rehabilitation services in long-term care. These contributions influenced training programs as well as practice. Also during this period, in Ontario, the nurse practitioner model for alternative health care delivery was initiated with an educational program offered by McMaster University. However, this program was short-lived because of a perceived duplication of services and a lack of career opportunities for nurse practitioners, due in part to an overabundance of primary care physicians in urban areas (Harper-Femson, 1998).

2000 to the Present

In 2001, researchers demonstrated that home care for older adults cost less than institutional care (Chappell, Havens, Hollander, Miller et al., 2004; Hébert, Dubuc, Buteau, et al., 2001). The Romanow Report (Commission on the Future of Health Care in Canada, 2002) identified home care as the most rapidly growing area of community health care.

In 2003, the CHNAC developed and released the Canadian Community Health Nursing Standards of Practice (CCHN Standards), as discussed in Chapter 1. The CCHN Standards defined the minimum scope of practice for CHNs. It also defined *community health nursing* as the umbrella term for community health nursing specialties such as home health nursing, public health nursing, occupational health nursing, forensic nursing, parish nursing, and nurse practitioners. It is important to note that in the United States, *community health nursing* and *public health nursing* are discussed as two distinct entities. Also in the United States, reference is often made to community-*oriented* care versus community-*based* care.

In 2006, the Canadian Nurses Association offered the first certification in community health nursing practice in Canada. That certification credential is part of a national certification program that recognizes nurses who are qualified, competent, and current in the practice of community health nursing. CHNs who have successfully passed the national practice and knowledge requirements of the certification exam can use the

official designation letters of CCHN(C) after their name (see https://www.chnc.ca/en/certification).

The CHNAC was renamed in June 2009 and is now known as Community Health Nurses of Canada (CHNC). Interest in the planning and direction of community health care in Canada has grown over the past decade. In 2005, a joint task force released a report pertaining to the Canadian public health workforce. The report identified many unique health human resources planning challenges, such as the overlapping of functions among a variety of public health care providers and the fact that public health has more regulated and unregulated care providers than do other health care workforces (Public Health Agency of Canada [PHAC], 2005). The report stressed the importance of a collaborative planning process to facilitate the tasks of the public health workforce across Canada. As a result, core competencies for PHNs were developed and released in 2008 across Canada. In 2009, core competencies for PHNs across Canada were formulated in *Public Health Nursing Discipline Specific Competencies Version 1.0* of CHNC (2009). Home health nursing competencies were developed in 2010. CHNC's "Blueprint for Action for Community Health Nursing in Canada" was developed in 2011 and its CCHN Standards were revised in 2011, then again in 2019 (CHNC, 2011a,b; 2019; Granger, Schofield, Fox, et al., 2018).

Community health nursing is receiving greater attention in today's health care system. This mounting interest may be the result of recent major public health events, such as an increase in climate-change-related disasters; the SARS outbreak; outbreaks of avian flu, measles, and H1N1; the 2014 Ebola virus epidemic; and the COVID-19 pandemic. Another contributing factor may be the creation in 2004 of the Public Health Agency of Canada, which included the appointment of a chief medical officer of health. The renewed emphasis on community health nursing as a key element of health care is due to a number of additional factors. Disparities and health inequities have been recognized in various groups—particularly in First Nations, Métis, and Inuit populations (Browne, 2017; Hajizadeh, Hu, Bombay, et al., 2018). The *Truth and Reconciliation Commission Final Report* (Government of Canada, 2015) recommended that governments recognize and implement the health care rights of Indigenous people. British Columbia's First Nations Health Authority (FNHA) was established in 2013 to reform the delivery of health care to BC First Nations to improve their health (FNHA, n.d.). The CHNC has been a prominent advocate for community health nursing and health promotion across Canada since 1987, and an increase in chronic illness and an aging population with greater demands for home health nursing care, along with the emphasis on population health and the social determinants of health, have contributed to this stronger focus on community health care.

Villeneuve and MacDonald (2006), in their report *Toward 2020: Visions for Nursing* (see the Evolve website), predicted that by the year 2020 most of health care, including nursing care, would take place in the patient's home or in the community on an outpatient basis. Extending from this vision, Schofield, Ganann, Brooks, et al. (2011) sought to study priority issues, identifying recommendations for common definitions, aggressive planning for primary health care, comprehensive social marketing strategy, refocusing undergraduate nursing education toward community health, enhancing research capacity, and establishing a community health nursing centre of excellence. This vision has both stalled and been tested over time by key challenges such as funding priorities, an aging population and, most recently, the COVID-19 pandemic when public health and home care requirements were accelerated as part of the response. It remains to be seen which community health nursing progress will and will not be sustained following the pandemic. Regardless, the move toward care in the community is supported by the expansion of trauma-informed care and cultural safety (described further in Chapter 14), the use of advanced technology, and the enhancement of resources to better support families to care for the patient at home. Interprofessional teams working across sectors will become increasingly essential and will put a greater focus on primary services and preventive programs.

Today, CHNs look to the history of public health and community health nursing for inspiration, explanation, and prediction. These lessons learned, new information and advocacy are used to promote a comprehensive approach to addressing the multiple needs of the diverse populations served. CHNs seek to learn from the past and to avoid known pitfalls as they search for successful strategies to meet the complex needs of today's populations. As plans for the future are made and as unmet community health challenges are acknowledged, the vision of what nurses in community health can accomplish serves as a sustaining force.

More than 100 years of combined efforts in the field of public health have resulted in improved health for individual Canadians, their families, and many communities. The development and availability of vaccinations, clean water, the pasteurization process, and improved living conditions in the past century have resulted in a markedly increased life expectancy and improved health status and quality of life for most Canadians. These efforts have also led to the development of community health nursing practice. In recent years, health promotion efforts have contributed to a decrease in suffering and the costs related to the treatment of illnesses. It is worth noting that relative to many other nations, Canada has a healthier population (Public Health Agency of Canada [PHAC], 2019). Table 2.3 highlights many of the key milestones in the history of public health and community health nursing.

TABLE 2.3 Milestones in the History of Public Health and Community Health Nursing	
Public Health	**Community Health Nursing**
1800s	
• 1800s: Recurrent and devastating epidemics, e.g., smallpox and tuberculosis (TB), killed thousands in Canada—accelerated by migration and colonization • 1832: Cholera epidemic killed millions worldwide and thousands in Canada • 1882: First permanent provincial Board of Health was established in Ontario • 1884: *Public Health Act* was introduced to establish municipal Boards of Health in Ontario; other provinces followed suit • Late 1800s: discovery of disease-causing bacteria led to a focus on disease prevention, including vaccination of school-aged children	• 1800s: Indigenous midwives and other lay healers cared for the sick in their homes • 1840: Elizabeth Fry founded a Protestant order of visiting nurses in London • 1860s: William Rathbone instituted district nursing in Liverpool, England, by dividing the city into districts and hiring nurses to work in them • Mid–late 1800s: Religious orders helped with care of "destitute immigrants" • 1861–1897: In England, Nightingale developed the early principles of public health nursing: disease prevention through teaching cleanliness and sanitation • 1874: Rathbone and Nightingale hired Florence Lee to study nursing needs in London; she highlighted the need for district nursing training • 1887: Florence Nightingale founded the Queen's Nursing Institute of visiting nurses; she fought for specific training and appropriate salaries for nurses • 1897: Victorian Order of Nurses (VON) in Canada founded by Lady Aberdeen; the VON focused on public health, TB prevention and care, and maternity care • Late 1800s: Private-duty nurses lived with patients in their homes and were paid well by patients • Late 1800s: Pioneer public health nurses (PHNs) were dependent on assistance from communities • Late 1800s: Rathbone, Nightingale, and Lee established community health nursing, initially in England, based on the district nursing concepts of professionalism, accountability, and use of research

TABLE 2.3   Milestones in the History of Public Health and Community Health Nursing—cont'd

Public Health	Community Health Nursing
1900–1909 • 1901: TB was the leading cause of death in Canadian cities, especially among the poor, with a mortality rate of 180 per 100 000 Canadians • Early 1900s: Major threats to public health included TB, influenza, and syphilis • Early 1900s: Infant mortality rates continued to climb in Canadian cities • 1906: Montreal became the first city in Canada to legislate medical inspection of schoolchildren	• 1905: Ms. E. C. Rayside became the first home visiting TB nurse in Ottawa • 1907: Elizabeth Lindsay became the first city nurse on the city of Toronto, Ontario, payroll • 1907: Christina Mitchell became the first home visiting TB nurse employed by the Toronto Health Department • 1908: The first public health nursing training program began at the University of British Columbia (UBC) with the financial support of the Canadian Red Cross • 1909: Canada's first school nurse was appointed in Hamilton
1910–1919 • 1911: *School Medical Inspection Act* was passed in British Columbia • 1918: Spanish influenza epidemic affected one-sixth of the Canadian population and killed approximately 30 000 Canadians • 1919: The Federal Department of Health was established in Canada • 1919: British Columbia was the first province to have a health centre with public health nurses	• 1910: Well-baby clinics were established in Toronto • 1911: Eunice Dyke became the first director of public health nursing in Toronto • 1911–1918: Metropolitan Life Insurance Company proved the effectiveness of visiting nurses in decreasing infant mortality rates • 1913: Blanche Swan became the first provincial school nurse in British Columbia • 1914: Metropolitan Life insisted that public health and visiting nurses be included on health research teams funded by the agency • 1919: The University of Alberta offered its first public health nursing course • 1919: UBC established the first baccalaureate nursing program • 1919: The Canadian Red Cross offered financial assistance to universities and scholarships to nurses to study public health nursing
1920–1929	• 1920: VON and Metropolitan Life nurses provided home nursing for the sick, education for prevention, prenatal and postnatal care, and well-baby clinics across Ontario • 1920: In Ontario, the Red Cross established nursing outposts • 1920: School boards across Ontario employed nurses, usually as PHNs, in the school setting • 1920: Urban public health departments employed nurses as specialists in school nursing, TB nursing, and maternal–child nursing areas; public health nursing was well established in major cities • 1920s: The VON stopped training its own nurses to support the development of Canadian public health nursing programs • 1920s: Private-duty nurses in Nova Scotia worked autonomously in the community • 1921: UBC graduated 56 PHNs • 1928: British Columbia Provincial Board of Health ruled all PHNs must complete a university course in public health nursing
1930–1939 • 1930s: Beginning of the Great Depression—no unemployment insurance or social assistance; outbreaks of communicable disease	• 1930s: The VON focused on home nursing care of the sick • 1930s: Most private-duty nurses were unemployed • 1930s: Public health nursing programs provided most preventive and educative public health work • 1930s: In Canada, Edna L. Moore, a nurse, advocated for generalized, rather than specialized, public health nursing, which led to the acceptance of generalized activities (as opposed to specialized activities such as TB care) for all age groups in public health nursing • 1932: The Weir Report raised concerns about and made recommendations for public health nursing (e.g., doubling the number of PHNs and raising their salaries); it also recognized public health nursing as a specialty area requiring advanced education

Continued

TABLE 2.3   Milestones in the History of Public Health and Community Health Nursing—cont'd

Public Health	Community Health Nursing
1940–1949	
• 1940: Men and women joined military service or worked in war-related industries—unemployment ceased	• 1941: In Manitoba, the Buck Commission recommended reorganization of visiting nurse programs
• 1945–1949: Industrialization and populations grew in urban centres, which provided conditions conducive to the spread of contagions	• 1943: Prenatal, postnatal, and child health programs were transferred from the VON to the provincial health department/authority
• 1947: The Saskatchewan government, led by Tommy Douglas, introduced the first provincial hospital insurance program in Canada	• 1943: PHNs assumed full responsibility for prenatal, postnatal, and child health programs from the VON
	• 1945: PHNs were the first nurses in Canada to administer immunizations
	• 1946: Registered Nurses of British Columbia (RNBC) became the first provincial nursing association certified under the *Labor Relations Act* as the bargaining agent for nurses
	• 1948: The *Hospital Insurance Act* gave hospital care to all BC residents
1950–1959	
• 1950–1960s: A nursing shortage was evident	• 1950: The Baillie–Creelman Report, a Canada-wide study, examined the roles of nurses and physicians and explored recruitment and retention of public health staff
• 1957: The Government of Canada introduced a national hospital insurance program	• 1950s: Prevention programming became the focus of PHNs' attention
	• 1950s: Nursing programs began including public health nursing content
1960–1969	
• 1966: The federal government created a national Medicare program, with the national system paying 50% of provincial health costs	• 1965: Paralytic polio was eradicated as a result of provincial vaccination campaigns
	• 1967: Dalhousie University in Nova Scotia offered the first program to train northern nurses as nurse practitioners
1970–1979	
• 1973: The Pickering Report recommended that the VON be mandated to deliver home care programs	• Early 1970s: The VON evolved to include home care for older adults and the chronically ill
• 1974: The Lalonde Report proposed that certain factors determine the health of Canadians: human biology, environment, lifestyle, and health care organization; over time, additional determinants of health were added to this list	• 1970s: In Canada, PHNs increased their focus on health promotion, in addition to disease prevention
	• 1974: The VON became the first publicly funded provincial home care program in Manitoba; this trend continued throughout Canada as a result of the Pickering Report.
• 1978: Primary health care was defined by the Declaration of Alma-Ata	• Mid-1970s: McMaster University in Ontario offered a primary health care nurse practitioner program
	• 1979: The federal government developed the Indian Health Policy, which was the first official recognition by the government of health disparities among Indigenous people
1980–1989	
• 1980s: Sexually transmitted infections became a concern	• 1980s: Health care spending constraints began to lead to reduction in programs
• 1984: The *Canada Health Act* was adopted	• 1980s: Parish nursing was formalized in response to health reforms
• 1986: The Ottawa Charter for Health Promotion identified the prerequisites for health	• 1982: Occupational health nursing was established
1990–1999	
• 1990s: TB re-emerged as a leading threat to global health	• 1990s: Primary health care nurse practitioner programs were established in most provinces across Canada
	• 1990s: With public health reorganization, public health nursing visits to patient homes were greatly reduced

TABLE 2.3   Milestones in the History of Public Health and Community Health Nursing—cont'd

Public Health	Community Health Nursing
2000–2009	
• 2000: An outbreak of *Escherichia coli* took place in Walkerton, Ontario	• 2001: Studies demonstrated that providing home care to older adults costs less than institutional care
• 2003: A SARS outbreak took place in Toronto, Ontario	• 2002: The Romanow Report identified home care as the most rapidly growing area of community health nursing
• 2004: A 10-year action plan to establish public health goals for Canada was signed by the prime minister and the premiers	• 2003: Public health nursing was placed under the umbrella term "community health nursing"
• 2004: The Public Health Agency of Canada and the position of Canada's chief public health officer were created	• 2003: The Canadian Community Health Nursing Standards of Practice (CCHN Standards) were implemented
• 2006: Research continued to support the extent of contributions to the 12 determinants of health	• 2003: PHNs anticipated and planned for handling tropical diseases, SARS, and influenza
• 2006: A joint task force released its report on public health human resources; it identified the presence of many planning challenges	• 2004: The Canadian Institute for Health Information (CIHI), based on research and consultation, developed a common set of home care indicators
• 2006: A Senate Standing Committee formed the Mental Health Commission of Canada to formulate a national mental health strategy	• Mid-2000s: PHNs continued health promotion and re-established home visiting to all mothers and their newborns
• 2007: Core competencies for public health workforce in Canada were introduced	• Mid-2000s: Health care cutbacks led to a shift back to home care
• 2008: The chief public health officer's report on the state of public health in Canada addressed health inequities	• Mid-2000s: Untrained family members often cared for the ill
• 2008: A Listeriosis outbreak in Canada was linked to packaged meat products	• 2005: *Blueprint on Aboriginal Health: A 10-Year Transformative Plan* provided an updated document to close the gap on health disparities
• 2009: An H1N1 (swine flu) outbreak took place in Canada	• 2006: The Ontario Community Health Nursing Study found that fewer CHNs were working in the community sector despite the shift to community care
	• 2006: Canadian community health nurse certification became available
	• 2009: Core competencies for PHNs were released
	• 2009: Community Health Nurses Association of Canada (CHNAC) changed its name to Community Health Nurses of Canada (CHNC)
2010–Present	
• 2014: A measles outbreak took place in Canada—in particular in western Canada	• 2010: Core competencies for home health nursing were developed by CHNC
• 2015: The Truth and Reconciliation Commission (Government of Canada) made recommendations on racial inequality and the effects of traumatic history	• 2011: The CCHN Standards were revised
	• 2011: *The Blueprint for Action for Community Health Nursing in Canada* was released
• 2020: The COVID-19 pandemic was experienced around the world	• 2013: The First Nations Health Authority was created in British Columbia
	• 2019: Revision and release of *Canadian Community Health Nursing Professional Practice Model & Standards of Practice*

Sources: Allemang, 2000; Commission on the Future of Health Care in Canada, 2002; Duncan, Leipert, & Mill, 1999; Government of Canada, 2015; Granger, Schofield, Fox, et al., 2018; Green, 1984; Hébert, Dubuc, Buteau, et al., 2001; Keddy & Dodd, 2005; MacQueen, 1997; Mansell, 2003; McKay, 2009; Mount Saint Vincent University Archives, 2005; Public Health Agency of Canada, 2020; Rutty & Sullivan, 2010; Vukic & Dilworth, 2019.

👤 STUDENT EXPERIENCE

What do you know about the history of community health and public health in your province or territory?

Activity

Add to your knowledge about public health in your province or territory by accessing the Canadian Public Health Association's History of Public Health e-book at https://www.cpha.ca/history-e-book.

Questions

1. Which particular topics and areas of development were essential milestones in the development of community health nursing in your province or territory? Which events do you relate to most? Explain.

2. What changes might you anticipate in community health nursing in your province or territory during your nursing career? And further into the future?

CHAPTER SUMMARY

2.1 A historical approach can be used to increase understanding of community health nursing in the past, as well as its current and future challenges. The global roots of public health can be traced to uncover early mechanisms of environmental health, family, and home care, as well as surveillance techniques. Community health nursing is a product of social, economic, and political forces that continue to evolve.

2.2 Early public health efforts in Canada were shaped by epidemics that, as part of colonization efforts, devastated Indigenous people in Canada, who were introduced to harmful conditions and pathogens. The increasing acceptance of public roles for women permitted community health nursing employment for nurses, which also shaped the evolution of public health in Canada.

2.3 A number of milestones mark the evolution of community health nursing in Canada. Lillian Wald's work dramatically shaped public health nursing practice and influenced the Canadian Metropolitan Life Insurance Company that began a visiting home nursing service in the 1920s. Eunice Dyke, a public health nursing pioneer in Canada in the early 1900s, played a key role in shaping public health nursing in Canada. The Weir Report of 1932 moved nursing education forward and addressed several areas related to public health nursing practice. During the 1950s and 1960s, PHNs moved from specialized nursing services to generalized nursing services. Later, in 1987, the CHNAC was formed. Primary health care nurse practitioner programs were established in several provinces across Canada in the 1990s. In 2003, the CHNAC published the CCHN Standards. In 2008, the core competencies for PHNs in Canada were released.

 CHN IN PRACTICE: A CASE STUDY

Historical Reflection for Contemporary Practice

CHNs in a suburban community health centre are incorporating historical reflection in their team meetings to better understand their practice in the context of a changing environment. Radical changes to community health care delivery are underway in their suburb because a long-standing community health care provider (the VON) is closing its local operations after nearly 100 years. Questioning how to move forward, the CHNs have been using historical reflection to examine how the CHN role and institutions have evolved and how they hope to shape the next stages of development of community health care in their neighbourhoods.

Think About It

1. What are some questions a diverse group of suburban nurses can bring to their team meetings to explore history and inform their future practice?
2. How might historical reflection be useful in your future practice?

Source: Smith, K. M., Brown, A., & Crookes, P. A. (2015). History as reflective practice: A model for integrating historical studies into nurse education. *Collegian (Royal College of Nursing, Australia), 22*(3), 341–347.

 TOOL BOX

The Tool Box contains useful resources that can be applied to community health nursing practice. These resources are found on the Evolve website at http://evolve.elsevier.com/Canada/Stanhope/community/.

Tools

This Is Public Health, A Canadian History. (https://www.cpha.ca/history-e-book)

This engaging resource was produced by the Canadian Public Health Association for a broad audience. It is available in a printable format or an online, interactive format.

REFERENCES

Abrams, S. E. (2009). The public health nursing bag as tool and symbol. *Public Health Nursing, 26*(1), 106–109.

Allemang, M. M. (2000). Development of community health nursing in Canada. In M. J. Stewart (Ed.), *Community nursing: Promoting Canadians' health* (pp. 4–32). Saunders.

Astle, B. J., Duggleby, W., Potter, P. A., et al. (Eds.). (2019). *Canadian fundamentals of nursing* (6th ed.). Elsevier Canada.

Boschma, G. (2012). Community mental health nursing in Alberta, Canada: An oral history. *Nursing History Review, 20*(1), 103–135.

Bourque Bearskin, R., Cameron, B., King, M., et al. (2016). Mâmawoh Kamâtowin, "coming together to help each other in wellness": Honouring indigenous nursing knowledge. *International Journal of Indigenous Health, 11*(1). https://doi.org/10.18357/ijih111201615024

Browne, A. (2017). Moving beyond description: Closing the health equity gap by redressing racism impacting Indigenous populations. *Social Science & Medicine, 184*, 23–26.

Buhler-Wilkerson, K. (1993). Public health then and now. Bringing care to the people: Lillian Wald's legacy to public health nursing. *American Journal of Public Health, 83*(12), 1778–1786.

Burnett, K. (2008). The healing work of Aboriginal women in indigenous and newcomer communities. In J. Elliott, M. Stuart, & C. Toman (Eds.), *Place and practice in Canadian nursing history* (pp. 40–52). Vancouver, BC: UBC Press.

Burnett, K. (2010). *Taking medicine: Women's healing work and colonial contact in southern Alberta, 1880–1930*. Vancouver, BC: UBC Press.

Cadotte, M., & James-Abra, E. (2015). Epidemics in Canada. *The Canadian encyclopedia.* https://www.thecanadianencyclopedia.ca/en/article/epidemic.

Canadian Association of Schools of Nursing. (2015). *National nursing education framework: Final report.* https://www.casn.ca/wp-content/uploads/2014/12/Framwork-FINAL-SB-Nov-30-20151.pdf.

Canadian Museum of History. (n.d.). *Canadian nursing history collection online.* https://www.historymuseum.ca/cmc/exhibitions/tresors/nursing/ncmen01e.html.

Canadian Nurses Association. (2016). *Jeanne Mance award.* https://www.cna-aiic.ca/en/about-cna/awards-and-recognition/jeanne-mance-award.

Canadian Nurses Association. (2020). *The practice of nursing: Health human resources: Nursing statistics.* https://www.cna-aiic.ca/en/nursing-practice/the-practice-of-nursing/health-human-resources/nursing-statistics.

Canadian Public Health Association. (2020). *About CPHA: Vision and mission.* https://www.cpha.ca/vision-and-mission.

Chappell, N., Dlitt, B. H., Hollander, M. J., et al. (2004). Comparative of costs of home care and residential care. *The Gerontologist, 44*(3), 389–400.

Chinn, P. L., & Kramer, M. K. (2019). *Knowledge development in nursing* (10th ed.). Elsevier.

Cohen, I. B. (1984). Florence nightingale. *Scientific American, 3,* 128–137.

Commission on the Future of Health Care in Canada. (2002). *Building on values: The future of health care in Canada—Final report.* http://publications.gc.ca/collections/Collection/CP32-85-2002E.pdf.

Community Health Nurses Association of Canada. (2003). *Canadian community health nursing standards of practice.*

Community Health Nurses of Canada. (2009). *Public health nursing discipline specific competencies version 1.0.* https://www.chnc.ca/en/competencies.

Community Health Nurses of Canada. (2011a). *Blueprint for action for community health nursing in Canada.* https://neltoolkit.rnao.ca/sites/default/files/A%20Blueprint%20for%20Action%20for%20Community%20Health%20Nursing%20in%20Canada%20March%202011.pdf.

Community Health Nurses of Canada. (2011b). *Canadian community health nursing: Professional practice model and standards of practice.* https://www.chnc.ca/en/publications-resources.

Community Health Nurses of Canada. (2019). *Canadian community health nursing professional practice model and standards of practice.* https://www.chnc.ca/standards-of-practice.

Duncan, S. M., Leipert, B. D., & Mill, J. E. (1999). Nurses as health evangelists: The evolution of public health nursing in Canada, 1918–1939. *Advances in Nursing Science, 22*(1), 40–51.

Epp, J. (1986). *Achieving health for all: A framework for health promotion.* Government of Canada, Minister of Supply and Services.

First Nations Health Authority. (n.d.). *FNHA overview.* https://www.fnha.ca/about/fnha-overview.

Flynn, K. (2009). Beyond the glass wall: Black Canadian nurses, 1940–1970. *Nursing History Review, 7*(1), 129–152.

Fournier, B., & Karachiwalla, F. (2020). *Shah's public health and preventive health care in Canada* (6th ed.). Elsevier.

Frachel, R. R. (1988). A new profession: The evolution of public health nursing. *Public Health Nursing, 5*(2), 86–90.

Government of Canada. (2015). *Truth and Reconciliation Commission final report.* https://www.rcaanc-cirnac.gc.ca/eng/1450124405592/1529106060525.

Granger, M., Schofield, R., Fox, J., et al. (2018). Three decades of professional nursing leadership: The impact of the community health nurses of Canada. *Nursing Leadership, 31*(4), 63–73. https://doi.org/10.12927/cjnl.2019.25754

Green, M. (1984). *Through the years with public health nursing: A history of public health nursing in the provincial government jurisdiction of British Columbia.* Canadian Public Health Association.

Grypma, S. (2017). Historically-informed nursing: The untapped potential of history in nursing education. *Quality Advancement in Nursing Education – Avancees en formation infirmiere, 3*(1), Article 5. http://qane-afi.casn.ca/journal/vol3/iss1/2/.

Grypma, S. (2019). The development of nursing in Canada. In B. J. Astle, W. Duggleby, P. A. Potter, et al. (Eds.), *Canadian fundamentals of nursing* (6th ed., pp. 35–47). Elsevier Canada.

Hajizadeh, M., Hu, M., Bombay, A., et al. (2018). Socioeconomic inequalities in health among Indigenous peoples living off-reserve in Canada: Trends and determinants. *Health Policy, 122*(8), 854–865.

Hamilton, D. (1992). Research and reform: Community nursing and the Framingham tuberculosis project, 1914–1923. *Nursing Research, 41*(1), 8–13.

Hardill, K. (2007). From the grey nuns to the streets: A critical history of outreach nursing in Canada. *Public Health Nursing, 24*(1), 91–97.

Harper-Femson, L. A. (1998). *Nurse practitioners' role satisfaction.* (Toronto, ON): Doctoral thesis, University of Toronto. http://www.collectionscanada.ca/obj/s4/f2/dsk2/tape17/PQDD_0012/NQ35403.pdf.

Hébert, R., Dubuc, N., Buteau, M., et al. (2001). Resources and costs associated with disabilities of elderly people living at home and in institutions. *Canadian Journal on Aging, 20*(1), 1–22.

Jan, R. (1996). Rufaida Al-Asalmiya, the first Muslim nurse. *Image, 28*(3), 267–268.

Kalisch, P. A., & Kalisch, B. J. (1995). *The advance of American nursing* (3rd ed.). Lippincott.

Keddy, B., & Dodd, D. (2005). The trained nurse: Private duty and VON home nursing (late 1800s to 1940s). In C. Bates, D. Dodd, & N. Rousseau (Eds.), *On all frontiers: Four centuries of Canadian nursing* (pp. 43–56). University of Ottawa Press.

King, M., Harrison, M. J., & Reutter, L. I. (1995). Public health nursing or community health nursing: What's in a name? In M. J. Stewart (Ed.), *Community nursing: Promoting Canadians' health* (pp. 400–412). W. B. Saunders.

Lalonde, M. (1974). *A new perspective on the health of Canadians: A working document.* Government of Canada.

MacCallum, M. J. L. (2017). *Twice as good: A history of aboriginal nurses.* Aboriginal Nurses Association of Canada. Retrieved from a web page formerly available at http://www.arnbccommunitiesofpractice.ca/ahnn/wp-content/uploads/2017/02/Twice-As-Good_A_History-of-Aboriginal-Nurses.pdf.

MacDougall, H. (2009). "Truly alarming": Cholera in 1832. *Canadian Journal of Public Health, 100*(5), 333–336.

MacQueen, J. M. (1997). *Public health nursing in Sudbury, 1920–1956 (Master's thesis).* Laurentian University.

Mansell, D. (2003). *Forging the future: A history of nursing in Canada.* Thomas Press.

McBain, L. (2012). Pulling up their sleeves and getting on with it: Providing health care in a northern remote region. *Canadian Bulletin of Medical History, 29*(2), 309–328.

McKay, M. (2009). Public health nursing in early 20th century Canada. *Canadian Journal of Public Health, 100*(4), 249–250.

McLeary, L., & McParland, T. (2020). *Ross-Kerr and Wood's Canadian nursing: Issues & perspectives* (6th ed.). Elsevier.

Meijer Drees, L. (2014). *Healing histories: Stories from Canada's Indian hospitals.* University of Alberta Press.

Mount Saint Vincent University Archives. (2005). *Nursing history digitization project: Nursing education in Nova Scotia.*

Nightingale, F. (1894). Sick nursing and health nursing. In J. S. Billings, & H. M. Hurd (Eds.), *Hospitals, dispensaries, and nursing.* Johns Hopkins Press. (Reprinted New York: Garland, 1984).

Nightingale, F. (1946). *Notes on nursing: What it is, and what it is not.* Lippincott.

Nutting, M. A., & Dock, L. L. (1935). *A history of nursing.* GP Putnam's Sons.

Parkes, M. (2011). *Ecohealth and aboriginal health: A review of common ground.* https://www.ccnsa-nccah.ca/docs/emerging/FS-EcohealthAboriginalHealth-Parkes-EN.pdf.

Pellegrino, E. D. (1963). Medicine, history, and the idea of man. *Annals of the American Academy of Political and Social Sciences, 346,* 9–20.

Pringle, D. M., & Roe, D. I. (1992). Voluntary community agencies: VON Canada as example. In A. J. Baumgart, & J. Larsen (Eds.), *Canadian nursing faces the future* (2nd ed., pp. 611–626). Mosby.

Public Health Agency of Canada. (2005). *Building the public health workforce for the 21st century: A pan-Canadian framework for public health human resources planning.* http://www.ciphi.ca/pdf/ccworkforce.pdf.

Public Health Agency of Canada. (2019). *The chief public health officer's report on the state of public health in Canada 2019: Addressing stigma: Towards a more inclusive health system.* https://www.canada.ca/en/public-health/corporate/publications/chief-public-health-officer-reports-state-public-health-canada.html.

Public Health Agency of Canada. (2020). *Chief public health officer of Canada.* https://www.canada.ca/en/public-health/corporate/organizational-structure/canada-chief-public-health-officer.html.

Rosen, G. (1958). *A history of public health.* MD Publications.

Royce, M. (1983). *Eunice Dyke: Health care pioneer.* Dundurn Press.

Rutherdale, M. (2010). *Caregiving on the periphery. Historical perspectives on nursing and midwifery in Canada.* McGill-Queen's University Press.

Rutty, C., & Sullivan, S. C. (2010). *This is public health: A Canadian history.* Canadian Public Health Association. https://www.cpha.ca/history-e-book.

Sanders, T., O'Mahony, J., Duncan, S., et al. (2019). Opening the doors for school health–An exploration of public health nurses' capacities to engage in comprehensive school health programs. *Public Health Nursing, 36*(3), 348–356. https://doi.org/10.1111/phn.12607

Schofield, R., Ganann, R., Brooks, S., et al. (2011). Community health nursing vision for 2020: Shaping the future. *Western Journal of Nursing Research, 33*(8), 1047–1068.

Smith, K. (2020). Facing history for the future of nursing. *Journal of Clinical Nursing, 29*(9–10), 1429–1431.

Smith, K. M., Brown, A., & Crookes, P. A. (2015). History as reflective practice: A model for integrating historical studies into nurse education. *Collegian (Royal College of Nursing, Australia), 22*(3), 341–347.

Stewart, I. (1979). *These were our yesterdays: A history of district nursing in Alberta.* D. W. Friesen and Sons.

Toth, A., Fackelmann, J., Pigott, W., et al. (2004). Tuberculosis prevention and treatment: Occupational health, infection control, public health, general duty staff, visiting, parish nursing or working in a physician's office—all nursing roles are key to improving tuberculosis control. *Canadian Nurse, 100*(9), 27–32.

Underwood, J. M., Mowat, D. L., Meagher-Stewart, D. M., et al. (2009). Building community and public health nursing capacity: A synthesis report of the national community health nursing study. *Canadian Journal of Public Health, 100*(5), I1–I11.

University of Calgary. (2018). *Kate Shaw Brightly Colley fonds.* https://searcharchives.ucalgary.ca/kate-shaw-brighty-colley-fonds.

Villeneuve, M., & MacDonald, J. (2006). *Toward 2020: Visions for nursing.* Canadian Nursing Association.

Vukic, A., & Dilworth, K. (2019). The history of community health nursing in Canada. In L. L. Stamler, L. Yiu, A. Dosani, et al. (Eds.), *Community health nursing: A Canadian perspective* (5th ed., pp. 1–17). Pearson Canada.

Weir, G. M. (1932). *Survey of nursing education in Canada.* University of Toronto Press.

Worster, A., Sarco, A., Thrasher, C., et al. (2005). Understanding the role of nurse practitioners in Canada. *Canadian Journal of Rural Medicine, 10*(2), 89–94.

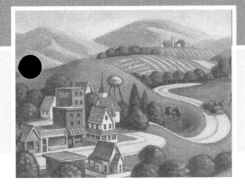

3

Community Health Nursing in Canada: Settings, Functions, and Roles

OUTLINE

General Community Health Nursing Functions and
  Practices, 48
  Care and Counselling, 48
  Continuity of Care, 49
  Referral, 49
  Health Education, 52
  Team Building, Community Development, and
    Collaboration, 53
Settings, Functions, and Roles of Community Health
  Nurses in Canada, 57

The Home Health Nurse, 58
The Public Health Nurse, 62
The Occupational Health Nurse, 65
Rural and Outpost Nurses, 68
The Nurse Practitioner, 72
The Corrections Nurse, 73
The Forensic Nurse, 73
Other Community Health Nurses, 75

OBJECTIVES

After reading this chapter, you should be able to:

3.1 Describe the various care and counselling functions of the community health nurse (CHN).

3.2 Explain the principles and steps of the referral process (including discharge planning) in relation to providing continuity of care.

3.3 Develop an awareness of the CHN's role in health promotion and disease prevention.

3.4 Describe the collaborative practice and team-building functions of the CHN.

3.5 Explain the CHN functions of consultation, decision making, and leadership.

3.6 Describe the research and evaluation functions (such as screening and surveillance) of the CHN.

3.7 Explain the CHN's advocacy function.

3.8 Define *case management* and describe a case manager's roles and activities.

3.9 Identify the roles, settings, and functions of the home health nurse.

3.10 Identify the roles, settings, and functions of the public health nurse.

3.11 Identify the roles, settings, and functions of the occupational health nurse.

3.12 Explain the distinctions between *rural* and *urban* in CHN practice and issues related to delivering services to rural, underserved populations.

3.13 Identify the roles, settings, and functions of the primary health care nurse practitioner.

3.14 Identify the roles, settings, and functions of the corrections nurse.

3.15 Identify the roles, settings, and functions of the forensic nurse.

3.16 Develop an awareness of other community health nursing specialties.

KEY TERMS*

care coordination, 60
care planning, 60
case management, 54
case manager, 55
certification, 57
contracting, 60
corrections nurse, 73
discharge planning, 50
educator, 64
evidence-informed practice, 64
faith communities, 76
family caregiving, 59

First Nations nurses, 76
forensic nurses, 73
harm reduction, 75
health advocacy, 54
health education, 52
health literacy, 53
holistic care, 76
hospice, 61
hospice care, 61
interprofessional collaboration, 62
nurse entrepreneur, 76
nurse practitioner, 72

occupational and environmental health history, 67
outpost nurses, 68
palliative approach, 61
palliative care, 61
parish nurse, 76
parish nursing, 76
pastoral care staff, 76
primary caregiver, 64
referral process, 49

risk communication, 49
rural, 70
sexual assault nurse examiners (SANEs), 73
telehealth, 75
telenurses, 75
urban, 69
virtual care, 75
work–health interactions, 65
work-site walk-through, 68

*See the Glossary on page 468 for definitions.

As noted in Chapter 1, the number of community health nursing specialties has grown in recent years. The scope of community health nursing has expanded to include nontraditional specialties including nurse practitioners (NPs) and nurse entrepreneurs. Increasingly, CHNs are also employed as community leaders in nongovernmental organizations such as community support organizations for disability, housing, and addictions services. CHN practice settings also continue to evolve. For example, CHNs today are employed in correctional, forensic, and urban street settings, as well as schools. Moreover, an increasing number are becoming involved in rural, remote practice, including global health activities. Some aspects of the CHN's role have also evolved with the growing focus on determinants of health. For example, today there is greater emphasis than ever before on the role of CHN as advocate for policy change and as activist on social justice issues pertaining to the determinants of health.

The first half of this chapter introduces several community health nursing functions and practices, whereas the second half presents the main community health nursing specialties.

GENERAL COMMUNITY HEALTH NURSING FUNCTIONS AND PRACTICES

Community health nursing requires knowledge of primary health care and population health; health promotion and levels of prevention; determinants of health; equity and social justice; epidemiology; and evidence-informed practice. CHNs must also have in-depth knowledge of the community they work in to function effectively.

To maintain a holistic focus in their community health nursing practice, CHNs raise certain questions when working in and with a patient or community. Ideally, these questions can be addressed in a collaborative, patient-centred process (directly with the community and stakeholder groups) and using best evidence (based on secondary sources such as reports, statistical analyses, and so on). Following are some questions for CHNs to consider:

- What does the community believe about its health, needs, and strengths?
- What determinants of health are relevant to the community?
- What are the sociopolitical, cultural, and ecological contexts?
- Are there any ethical issues that need to be considered and addressed?

- What determinants of health may be relevant to population health?
- What possible population health issues exist for the community?
- What are the epidemiological considerations?
- What health promotion issues need to be addressed in this community and for populations, aggregates, families, and individuals?
- What do I know and believe about the community? What do I *not* know about the community but need to know?
- Who are the stakeholders and informants I must learn from?
- How can I use the available evidence to inform my nursing practice?
- Given the setting I work in, what nursing roles might I assume as a CHN?

Beyond knowing about the health issues and the particular patient, community, or setting, all CHNs (regardless of their specialization) must be able to perform the general functions and nursing practices that follow.

Care and Counselling

In their community health nursing practice, CHNs are called upon to establish a therapeutic relationship with individuals, families, groups, communities, and populations that is based on trust, respect, caring, and listening. CHNs must employ clinical skills using the nursing process to incorporate health promotion as well as illness and injury prevention techniques that are patient centred, patient driven, culturally safe, and strengths based. With careful establishment of professional boundaries, CHNs help patients appreciate the assets and resources available in their community, draw on their strengths, and take charge of their health and well-being.

Sometimes, the CHN may provide direct care and counselling (e.g., for a patient with a complex wound needing care or other complex disease management needs; a professional receiving methadone maintenance treatment for opiate addiction; or for a patient and family receiving home hospice/palliative care at the end stages of a glioblastoma brain cancer). Other times, the CHN may have a more instructive role (e.g., teaching the patient, family member, or community the practices they can manage in the community, such as blood sugar monitoring, self-help group leadership, or even more complex advocacy and letter-writing activities). Increasingly, self-management programs are being implemented throughout the country, for example with the Department of Health and Community Services of Newfoundland and Labrador (2019). These programs are employed to support chronic illness management and the interests of many older adults to remain at home as they age (Hyman, Gucciardi, Patychuk, et al., 2014). *Self-management* refers to the work a person must undertake to live well with one or more chronic conditions. Self-management involves gaining confidence to deal with health services, changing roles, and emotional management (Franek, 2013). Specific techniques of care and counselling as well as self-management and self-care are addressed throughout this text in relation to distinct areas of community health nursing practice.

Risk Assessment and Response

In their care and counselling role, CHNs support the early identification of a disease or health threat by gathering data from many sources at the same time (to understand the cause, natural course, and expected outcomes of the disease or health threat). CHNs engage in this assessment and intervention practice at the individual, group, and population level. They also employ effective risk communication techniques. **Risk communication** is a strategic health education intervention that involves exchanging information on the potential harm of health or environmental hazards to risk assessors and managers, the general public, news media, social media, and interest groups. Although the use of social media is growing as a method of sharing knowledge and expertise, it cannot replace the direct hands-on care provided by CHNs (Peate, 2013). Social media is an alternative method of communication that could be used in combination with other methods of communication by CHNs to help meet the demands of community health nursing.

Risk communication is a means of mitigating risk or preventing harm. An example of risk communication is educating family members of schoolchildren about vaccine safety through information provided in the consent forms for children to receive a vaccine at school. Another example could be a social media campaign on Facebook or Twitter that is used to supplement health information on the risk for transmission of communicable diseases such as COVID-19. Further afield, a CHN with a nongovernmental agency such as the International Red Cross or Médecins Sans Frontières/Doctors Without Borders may facilitate risk communication by establishing psychosocial rehabilitation activities in postconflict or disaster areas.

Outreach

As part of their practice of care and counselling, CHNs use community assessment data to determine population health needs and design activities to address the unique features of the population of interest. Outreach practices serve to meet some of the unique access challenges faced by patients. For example, some patients may have mobility concerns resulting from a physical disability; situational barriers such as having a newborn or living in a remote geographical location; or cultural, social, or language barriers to service. CHNs design and implement strategies to engage with people where they live,

work, learn, worship, or play to make care and counselling a community experience rather than something housed in a clinic set apart from the realities of patients' lives.

In their strategic and evidence-informed practice, CHNs build trusting relationships with patients and engage them in identifying and resolving health issues from patients' unique locations. Those locations are diverse and include the home, schools, shopping malls, or the site of a community event. One such initiative is Calgary's Prostate Cancer Centre's MAN VAN program. The program's mobile units operate in both urban and rural areas. They offer on-the-spot prostate-specific antigen testing and information on the importance of early detection for prostate cancer (Fig. 3.1 presents the program's logo).

The strategic use of outreach practices employs a holistic approach that includes finding creative solutions to patient engagement and service-access barriers. Early involvement of key stakeholders is one of many proven approaches to developing effective outreach plans (Canadian Public Health Association [CPHA], 2010).

Continuity of Care

The ability to provide a continuum of care has been hindered by the closure of many small hospitals in the past two decades. This trend further supports the need for CHNs to build and sustain strong community partnerships with other health care providers as well as patients and community organizations. CHNs act as a referral agent and discharge planner to facilitate the provision of continuity of care to patients, so it is important for CHNs to become familiar with the principles and steps of the referral process and discharge planning. In the referral process, CHNs must always consider resource and patient barriers and seek to facilitate a seamless referral to community agencies or discharge from the CHN's care.

Referral

The **referral process** is the systematic process of directing a patient to another source of assistance when the patient or

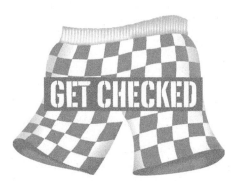

Fig. 3.1 Mobile Prostate-Specific Antigen Screening Promotional Logo. The MAN VAN program increases awareness of the importance of early detection of prostate cancer. It also measures and raises awareness about body mass index, blood pressure, and blood glucose in men. This type of program not only provides cancer screening but also serves to re-engage men with the health care system. (*Source:* Prostate Cancer Centre. [2016]. *The ManVan.* http://www.prostatecancercentre.ca/manvan/)

CHN is unable to address the patient's issue (Nies & McEwan, 2019). Hospital discharge planning frequently requires referral to community services. Therefore, the discharge planner needs to be familiar with the referral process (i.e., the principles and steps necessary to ensure an efficacious referral) and the community resources available. Referral processes can take many forms. The choice of referral process depends on the patient's needs, the availability and sustainability of local assets, and the capacity of the referring organization and the service to which the patient is being directed to at the time. Table 3.1 provides a list of the principles and steps of the referral process.

Referrals can be made by telephone, face to face, through written communication (including email, texts, or other tech-mediated formats), or through a combination of these channels. The CHN's assessment of community strengths and assets will support community connections and the effective use of local resources. In this strengths-based model, the inventory of community assets stands in contrast to the referral needs to demonstrate and mobilize the power within the community (McKnight & Block, 2010). Asset-based community development strategies are discussed further in Chapter 4. The CHN must be conscious of how

resource and patient barriers may prevent the use of community assets (see Table 3.2) and examine ways to mitigate potential barriers.

Discharge Planning

In discharge planning, the CHN often works with a community case manager to facilitate the transition of the patient into the community. Regardless of who facilitates the transition, or if there is a formal liaison, transition, or discharge service or program established to support this planning, the principles are the same and the patient and family all need to be included in the discharge process as partners. In all areas of community practice, the referral process is implemented with patient and family participation and, ideally, with a collaborative team meeting process. Such meetings can be complex. The best outcomes are found to depend on communication, effective teaching about the process, and coaching about the realities of the anticipated transition experiences, bringing together the information necessary for decision making (i.e., functional assessments, medication information, history), and evaluation with follow-up (RNAO, 2014).

Discharge planning is a process that connects patients and services to ensure an appropriate flow or continuity of care after hospital and in the community (Health PEI, 2020). Discharge planning, which requires interprofessional collaboration, aims to maximize the quality of care so that the transfer of patients from hospital to community is smooth and capitalizes on the available health care resources (Health PEI, 2020). The term is also used to refer to the process of discharging a patient from a community agency or service. Discharge planning is not a new concept; we know that the best outcomes happen with discharge planning as an early intervention. Yet, models and practices of discharge planning are not always implemented, and discharge planning does not always occur early enough in the process (Holland, Knafl, & Bowles, 2013). One study of an "in reach" (rather than outreach) model of discharge planning explored intensive and early discharge planning with community nurses going into the hospital to work with patients and interprofessional team members. The project found that early implementation of planning and the change of model reaching into the acute care mental health setting to plan discharge resulted in a significant decrease in readmission rates following discharge (Jensen, Forchuk, Seymour, et al., 2009). A study of mental health discharge planning from outpatient services to community confirmed these results, with an emphasis on the CHN and patient relationship, knowledge sharing, and advocacy for resources (Noseworthy et al., 2014).

Currently, most hospital patients are discharged after short periods of acute care and require a variety of community supports to prevent unnecessary hospital readmission; they benefit from the continuity of care facilitated by early discharge planning with a clear plan that is established well before the ultimate transfer or discharge home (Durocher, Kinsella, Gibson, et al., 2019). Many collaborative practice models are

TABLE 3.1	**The Principles and Steps of the Referral Process**
Principles	**Steps**
The referral should be appropriate.	Establish a therapeutic relationship with the patient and the need for a referral, based on assessment with referral criteria, as well as self-assessment of desire and readiness.
The referral should be practical.	Evaluate whether the patient could use the referral efficiently and effectively.
The referral should be individualized to the patient and sustainable.	Evaluate the local community assets and match with individual needs. Set realistic objectives for the referral so that the resource may be available in a sustained manner.
The referral should be timely.	Explore the suitability of resources for the specific needs and schedule of the patient.
The referral should be coordinated with other activities.	Examine the timing of other treatments or personal life events for the patient to determine feasibility.
The referral should incorporate the patient and family into planning and implementing.	Make the referral to available resources and follow up with the patient and family to determine the feasibility of the referral.
The patient should have the right to refuse the referral.	Acknowledge the patient's right to use or not use the referral for any reason.

Source: Nies & McEwan (2019), p. 165.

TABLE 3.2   Needs, Barriers, and Patient/Community Assets in the Referral Process

Referral Need	Examples of Community Resource Barriers	Patient and Community Assets
Communication with health care provider; knowledge and understanding	Attitude of health care provider (e.g., the health care provider uses medical terminology without explanation, answers patient questions abruptly, or shows an attitude of disrespect and a lack of courtesy in patient interactions)	Expert health care providers; translators/interpreters; plain language resources; volunteers and family caregivers
Access to referral site	Limited physical accessibility of resources (e.g., the local clinic has limited hours of access [daytime-only hours] and is not wheelchair accessible; transportation costs to get there are high due to travel or parking costs)	A specialized clinic is available; linkage through telehealth is available; a local agency can support travel costs and provide a volunteer for assistance
Specialist consultation or treatment	Cost of resource services (e.g., patient perceives a referral to a specialist as prohibitive because of having heard that the recommended treatments [e.g., medications] are extremely costly and not covered by the health plan)	System of referrals is in place
Preventive services	Patient priorities: the patient perceives basic needs for food, shelter, and clothing as higher priority than preventive health services (e.g., dental care)	Autonomy and choices; identification of priorities with the patient
Interventions for preventive health care or treatment	Motivation: patient is aware of a need for care but is not ready to accept the suggested intervention and take action (e.g., patient who has been referred to a dietitian for weight loss acknowledges the need to lose weight but does not follow through with the scheduled appointment)	Patient consciousness of needs; CHNs and other community supports employ motivational strategies
Initiating and engaging with services and supports	Resistance: patient had a negative experience with a community service or with a resources professional (e.g., a child was previously removed from the home by a community agency)	Patient has sought community support in the past; CHNs and other community supports employ motivational strategies
Information about available resources	Lack of knowledge about available resources: the volume of information provided (e.g., services available through genetic counselling) is either too high or too low to make clear choices	A variety of information and services are available to the patient; CHNs and others in the community can support interpretation of information
Value for the importance and urgency of prevention or treatment	Lack of understanding regarding need for referral: the patient makes assumptions based on previous experience of good health—does not recognize the importance and the consequences of the suggested referral (e.g., a sexually active teenage female may not know that a Papanicolaou test is important and may not understand the possible consequences if this test is not done as recommended; therefore, she may not follow through on the referral to her family physician or sexual health clinic)	Previous good health; youthful activity and diversions; interest in continued activities; specialized youth-oriented programs and approaches (e.g., peer-led support or social media reminders)
Initiating community health care	Patient self-image (e.g., a patient with a low self-image or who has experienced weight bias avoids seeking care because of feelings of unworthiness or judgement)	Personal and emotional connection to community health; relational practices; environmental and peer supports
Understanding and being understood in communication with care providers	Cultural factors (e.g., a patient who recently immigrated to Canada has previously experienced discrimination from health care practitioners and so resists seeing another practitioner; a patient is concerned that medical information may prevent successful immigration)	Experiences from other countries and ways of being; cultural safety and trauma-informed perspectives; cultural ambassadors and bridges in communities; interpreters and translation services
Adaptive equipment, supplies, or services	Finances (e.g., a patient does not have the monetary resources necessary to obtain equipment, supplies, or services [e.g., the patient cannot pay for an assistive device such as a motorized wheelchair])	Adaptive equipment and supplies are available in the community; creative and locally relevant innovations are designed; community agencies provide support, loans, sliding scale fees, or donations of adaptive equipment
The right services at the right time	Accessibility (e.g., a patient cannot access the necessary care because of limited available services or health care providers—rural settings, in particular, are often underserviced)	There are known ways of caring for the patient's needs; innovations and adaptations are available to bridge location and time barriers; volunteers and community groups can assist

Source: Adapted from Nies & McEwan (2019).

interested in integration and continuity of care with specific attention to the needs of rural individuals. In Ontario, the Rural Health Hub model works towards establishing more accessible and coordinated care for rural hospitals and communities (Ontario Hospital Association, 2017).

CHNs must also consider how and when to discharge patients from their care or service in the community. For instance, after a period of community care following cardiac rehabilitation or acute psychiatric illness, a CHN will have to decide if, and when, other referral agencies may be more appropriate options for the patient. Discussions about discharge, referrals, and next steps always take place in collaboration with the patient and are based on assessment of the needs of the patient. The "CHN in Practice: A Case Study, Discharge Planning for Postcerebrovascular Accident Care" box looks at creating a case management plan for a patient who has had a cerebrovascular accident (CVA).

CHN IN PRACTICE: A CASE STUDY

Discharge Planning for Postcerebrovascular Accident Care

During her visit to the regularly scheduled blood pressure clinic in a local apartment complex, Brigit, a 45-year-old woman, complained of feeling dizzy and forgetful. She could not remember which of her six medications she had taken during the past few days. Her blood pressure readings on reclining, sitting, and standing revealed gross elevation. The CHN and Brigit discussed the danger of Brigit's present status and her need to seek medical attention. Brigit called her physician from her apartment and agreed to be transported to the emergency department in the local hospital.

While in the emergency department, Brigit manifested the progressive signs and symptoms of a CVA (i.e., a stroke). During hospitalization, she lost her capacity for expressive language and demonstrated hemiparesis and a loss of bladder control. Her cognitive function became intermittently confused, and she was slow to recognize her physician and neighbours who came to visit. The hospital discharge planning nurse contacted the community case manager to screen and assess for the continuum of care needs as early as possible because Brigit lived alone and family members resided out of town, resulting in intermittent family support at home. Brigit had residual functional and cognitive deficits that would demand longer-term care.

Think About It

If you were Brigit's community case manager, which of the following steps would you take to construct a case management plan for her?

- Discuss with the family members their schedule of availability to offer care in the patient's home.
- Call the patient and introduce yourself as a prelude to working with her.
- Obtain information on the scope of services covered by your patient's employee benefit plan.
- Arrange a community placement facility site visit for the patient and family.

Health Education

Generally, **health education** involves strategic practices to inform people about health promotion, illness prevention, and treatment; it is a common function and practice of CHNs in any number of roles and settings (Stanhope & Lancaster, 2019). At times, the CHN may provide health education to a patient, family member, community, or population, depending on the issue and selected intervention. It is widely accepted that caregiver involvement in discharge planning is crucial for information and knowledge sharing, for facilitation of transitions, as well as for direct care and prevention at home or in the community. However, there continues to be a shortfall in caregiver involvement in the process (Hahn-Goldberg, Jeffs, Troup, et al., 2018). The CHN role in needs assessment, patient and caregiver engagement, and health education must not be underestimated. Regardless of his or her target or level of prevention, the CHN needs to understand many of the basic skills of an effective educator.

LEVELS OF PREVENTION

Related to Health Education

Primary Prevention

A CHN provides health education at a job site regarding safety and protective equipment.

Secondary Prevention

A CHN provides health education at a family health fair regarding early diagnosis and treatment of postpartum depression—with the goal of screening and early intervention.

Tertiary Prevention

A CHN provides health education at a cardiac rehabilitation day program to support individuals who have had cardiac events and surgery to rehabilitate and maximize functioning.

The CHN must understand both the community health issues and the educational principles of teaching and learning to be able to design, implement, and evaluate health education activities at any level of intervention. An effective educator must identify educational needs, establish educational goals and objectives, select appropriate methods and materials for education, and implement strategies to evaluate learning. Understanding the health education needs of a person, group, or population also requires an analysis of potential barriers to learning—the CHN must inquire if any age-related, language, or even competing community or personal interests will present barriers to learning.

Literacy and Health Literacy Assessment

Literacy assessment is a component of community health nursing. Many individuals are limited in their ability to read, write, and communicate clearly; however, being illiterate does not equate to cognitive or intellectual disability. A poor literacy level may result from restricted educational opportunities or may be indicative of the length of time an immigrant has been in Canada. Individuals attending a physician's office, clinic, or hospital may, on initial assessment, be clean and neatly dressed and appear well cared for at home; however, these same individuals may not be able to read, answer the assessment questions, or explain their actual living conditions, which could differ greatly from how things look on the surface. It is important that the CHN become conscious of the cultural and religious influences on the health literacy concerns of patients, along with having an awareness of the influences of racism and discrimination on health. Culture and racism are highly consequential to CHN practice (see Chapter 7). CHNs need to take a comprehensive and active approach to gaining awareness, remain humble and curious in their assessments, and ensure that someone knowledgeable is available to support a comprehensive assessment, especially when there are barriers to communication or potential for bias.

Health literacy is another component of literacy the CHN must assess. It is defined as "the ability to access, comprehend, evaluate and communicate information as a way to promote, maintain and improve health in a variety of settings across the life-course" (Public Health Agency of Canada [PHAC], 2018). An intersectoral appraisal of health literacy out of British Columbia in 2012 identified that more than 60% of adults and 88% of older persons in Canada are not considered to be health literate, which creates barriers to the use of everyday health information that is routinely available in their communities (Public Health Association of BC, 2012). Low health literacy is associated with poorer health outcomes and the inappropriate use of emergency department services and lower health screening and preventive practices (Hoffman-Goetz, Donelle, & Ahmed, 2014).

With the consequences of misunderstanding or miscommunication being so great, CHNs must not assume that a patient's nod of the head means that he or she understands what has been said. The patient may just be anxious to please the health care provider or embarrassed to admit a lack of understanding. It is important for the CHN to assess literacy and health literacy, and to clarify what the patient understands. The CHN should seek information from family and other professional or community supports to better understand the literacy and health literacy needs of the patient.

Direct health education is always tailored to the patient, group, or population being cared for. Consider the following guidelines when planning any educational strategy:
1. Gain the attention of the learner.
2. Clearly explain the objectives of instruction.
3. Inquire about the learner's previous knowledge.
4. Present the essential material in a clear, organized, and simple manner that is consistent with the learner's needs, situation, and application. Demonstrate the knowledge or skill, if possible.
5. Help the learner apply the knowledge to his or her unique situation.
6. Seek demonstration of the knowledge or skill from the learner.
7. Seek feedback on the learning experience and provide feedback on your observations.

The teaching and learning process is as important as the content being demonstrated or presented. Carefully attending to the needs of the learner and following a strategic, sequential process will maximize the value of the learning experience.

More detailed practices for the development and delivery of health education are discussed in Chapter 4. Many excellent examples of health education fact sheet resources are available (see the Registered Nurses' Association of Ontario health education fact sheets link on the Evolve website).

Team Building, Community Development, and Collaboration

The CHN uses techniques that foster team building, mutual respect, and joint decision making in all interactions with colleagues, educators, nursing students, other health care providers, and the public. At times, the CHN may employ mediation skills to facilitate interagency and intergovernmental cooperation. Similarly, the CHN may act as a catalyst and mediator to resolve issues or concerns by the community in relation to a planned health intervention or initiative.

Community Development

CHNs apply their knowledge of community assessment and community development models to support public participation in identifying and resolving health issues. As mentioned earlier, CHNs draw upon a strengths-based approach to support capacity building and empowerment in the community. They recognize the value of community wisdom and support community-generated plans for economic development, environmental improvement, or other community-based plans. Fostering interagency linkages, CHNs assist in the development of health care services and programs based on community assessments to meet the health needs of the community.

CHNs encourage and support the community to be active in stating and taking ownership of health issues that need to be resolved; they may work with community members to help them develop skills in how to identify community assets, access resources, develop social networks, and learn from the efforts of others (McKnight & Block, 2010). Cormack Russell, a leader in asset-based community development, explains that if we want to help people in a way that does not harm them and their capacities in their communities, the best place is to start "with what is strong within them, and within their communities, and not what is wrong" (Nurture Development, 2020, n.p.). In this work, CHNs may also seek to understand and support community members to discover the political process related to community health issues and ways they can become active in decisions about health issues.

Consultation, Decision Making, Leadership, and Followership

The roles of consultant and community decision maker are considered vital in the profession (Stanhope & Lancaster, 2019). CHNs use knowledge and expertise in public health, especially in health promotion, disease and injury prevention, epidemiology, and emergency preparedness to inform patients, community volunteers, nursing students, colleagues, other health care providers, professional associations, nonprofit agencies, organizations, institutions, the public, and all levels of government. CHNs are called upon to act as a resource person to communities, groups, and individuals; to link those needing services to the correct community resources; and to collaborate with the patient and service providers to determine options for change and improvement.

CHNs must also balance leadership and follower roles within an interprofessional team. Sometimes, a CHN may have an explicit leadership role on a team; perhaps he or she is the case manager for a patient, the manager of a program, or a project leader for an initiative. Other times, a CHN may need to be a collaborator and follower; perhaps he or she is the sexual assault nurse examiner (SANE) who is part of a large committee working on a demonstration project to develop more comprehensive services in the community. Whether a CHN is in a leadership or follower role, he or she draws on knowledge and the collaborative relationship with the patient and community to support decision making and effective community health leadership and action.

CHNs function to clarify how leadership and guidance will work and support development of agreed-upon roles, rules, and procedures. Systematic problem solving using the nursing process and strategic processes such as values clarification and the generation of alternatives through brainstorming are basic practices of the leadership role (Stanhope & Lancaster, 2019). CHNs may also employ skills in conflict management in their decision-making and leadership roles. Case managers frequently assist patients or service collaborators/providers in managing conflicting needs and scarce resources. For CHNs, the goals of conflict management are the support of community health and the preservation of dignity of all involved. At times, negotiation and mediation skills are important features of CHN practice.

Research and Evaluation

Research and evaluation are active components of CHN practice. CHNs in all roles engage in research and evaluation activities to investigate issues in and approaches to community health and wellness. In community health nursing practice, multiple ways of knowing (i.e., empirical, aesthetic, personal, ethical, and sociopolitical) are valued. Integrating knowledge of a variety of forms into practice, CHNs are part of knowledge creation and the critical examination of evidence-informed practice. Through appreciation and critical appraisal of diverse forms of knowledge, CHNs can integrate and draw on evidence in their work (Community Health Nurses of Canada [CHNC], 2019). By evaluating patient and program outcomes, and the conditions and contexts of community nursing work, CHNs are able to question the status quo, support change in practice, and co-create relevant and effective action for community health.

In community health nursing practice, community-consciousness-raising methods such as participatory research methodology are often used to involve community members in planning or carrying out research. Action research methodology that allows for implementation of findings and changes to the process of research may also be employed. CHNs will

also share the synthesis of research and program evaluation information with colleagues, educators, nursing students, other health care providers, and the public in an effort to support evidence-informed best practices and promote an understanding of the issues. In addition to direct involvement in research, CHNs may provide patients, communities, and decision makers an understanding of the issues from on the ground to identify program areas or practices that need to be studied or changed. Research and evidence-informed practice are explored in more depth in Chapter 5.

Screening and Surveillance

CHNs also participate in evidence-informed community health nursing practice through ongoing health screening and data gathering and monitoring practices (e.g., with screening and surveillance for certain infectious or noncommunicable diseases) (Stanhope & Lancaster, 2019). In this practice, the CHN ensures the patient understands why screening is necessary, how the procedure is done, and that follow-up is available. CHNs who engage in general practice use screening activities as an opportunity to provide health education and counselling to patients. CHNs interpret and share surveillance data with those who may be able to use them and in ways that decision makers, the community, and the public can understand (CPHA, 2010).

Health Advocacy

Advocacy helps individuals, families, and groups become aware of issues that may affect their health. It also works to develop patients' capacity to speak for themselves (CPHA, 2010). Health advocacy is a foundational and general function of CHNs in any role and in all levels of intervention in direct practice. The World Health Organization (WHO, 2004) defines **health advocacy** as a combination of individual and social actions designed (either on behalf of or with others) to gain political and community support of the conditions which promote health. The steps a CHN takes as a health advocate are discussed further in Chapter 4. The International Council of Nurses (2010) framework for health advocacy is summarized in Box 3.1.

As health advocates, CHNs collaborate and demonstrate commitment to equity, social justice, and policymaking activities. They take a leadership role or work to build the capacity of other leaders. They use advertising and media in skillful ways. Finally, they promote resource development that will lead to equal access to health and health-related services (CPHA, 2010).

Case Management

Case management is a system, a clinical decision-making process, a technology, a role, and a service for community health care in Canada. The literature uses numerous definitions of case management. This text uses the definition for **case management** provided by the Canadian Home Care Association (2012): "Case management is a collaborative strategy undertaken by health professionals and patients to maximize the patient's ability and autonomy through advocacy,

BOX 3.1 The International Council of Nurses 10-Step Advocacy Framework

Advocacy is about:

1. Taking action—overcoming obstacles to action
2. Selecting your issue—identifying and drawing attention to an issue
3. Understanding your political context—identifying the key people you need to influence
4. Building your evidence base—doing your homework on the issue and mapping the potential roles of relevant players
5. Engaging others—winning the support of key individuals/organizations
6. Developing strategic plans—collectively identifying goals and objectives and best ways to achieve them
7. Communicating messages and implementing plans—delivering your messages and counteracting the efforts of opposing interest groups
8. Seizing opportunities—timing interventions and actions for maximum impact
9. Being accountable—monitoring and evaluating process and impact; and
10. Taking a development approach—building sustainable capacity throughout the process

Source: International Council of Nurses. (2010). *Promoting health: Advocacy guide for health professionals.* http://www.whcaonline.org/uploads/publications/ICN-NEW-28.3.2010.pdf

communication, education, identification of and access to requisite resources, and service coordination" (p. 15). Herleman (2008) identified five key components of case management for community health nursing: (1) coordinating care; (2) ensuring continuity of care; (3) identifying changes in the patient's condition; (4) evaluating the care being delivered in association with health care team members; and (5) being aware of and understanding the financial implications of the care plan. Case management settings may include home care (community care access centres), the Workplace Safety and Insurance Board, the Canadian Armed Forces (Canadian Armed Forces Case Management Program), mental health and addictions, and Veterans Affairs Canada. Case managers may assume roles such as clinician or direct care provider, collaborator, liaison, facilitator, negotiator, monitor, supporter, advocate, coordinator, manager, educator, or researcher. Various models of case management exist.

Historical perspective. Canada's case management strategy, influenced by the movement in the United States (where case management was primarily community based—e.g., home care services), was driven by the need to reduce health care spending while at the same time maintain and improve the quality of patient care (Canadian Home Care Association, 2012; Kelly et al., 2018). Health care restructuring in the 1990s placed an emphasis on early hospital discharge to community care, which led to a need for increased coordination to ensure continuity of care (Daiski, 2000). A reduction in the number of nurses in the workforce, along with other cost-cutting measures, further contributed to the creation of the new strategy referred to as *case management.* CHNs and other

health care team members involved in facilitating access to and coordinating care acquired the new title of *case manager,* and the delivery of services became known as *managed care* (Daiski, 2000). Although case management took different forms across Canada, it consistently focused on the advocacy role (Canadian Home Care Association, 2012).

Case management models and strategies. Case management models are applied in communities across Canada. Home care services are an example of a case management model and include community care access centres in Ontario and Saskatchewan and continuing care programs in Nova Scotia. In Ontario, for example, community care access centres organize access to long-term care, arrange and authorize visiting health care and personal support services in people's homes, authorize services for special needs children in schools, authorize admissions to long-term care facilities, and provide information and referrals to the public about other community agencies and services (Ontario Ministry of Health and Long-Term Care, 2018a). Across the country, various agencies provide similar community access services to patient groups.

The **case manager** advocates for the patient, advises the patient, coordinates and facilitates access to suitable health care services in a timely manner, and ensures continuity of care for the patient. Regardless of the definition and implementation of case management, all CHNs involved in case management perform the following central activities, which can be translated to the nursing process: targeting, assessment, care planning, implementation, monitoring, and reassessment (National Case Management Network, 2009; Yoder-Wise et al., 2020) (see Table 3.3). Patients are usually individuals experiencing complex health challenges that require long-term interventions and various health care services.

The following are examples of the knowledge and skills required by CHNs in a case management role in the community:

- Knowledge of community resources and ability to identify best resources for the desired outcomes
- Knowledge and skills in cultural competency and safety.
- Knowledge and skills to apply the referral process
- Written and oral communication skills that facilitate collaboration
- Negotiation and conflict-resolution skills
- Critical-thinking processes to identify and prioritize health concerns from the provider and patient views
- Skill in the application of evidence-informed practice in provision of care
- Advocacy skills
- Knowledge and skill in the application of discharge planning
- Knowledge and skill in meeting the legal and professional requirements when documenting and reporting

Case management in rural settings is often more complex than in urban settings, partly because of patient differences in values and beliefs, geographical challenges, different organizational contexts, and fewer available community services and resources. See the "CHN in Practice: A Case Study, Case Management and Decision Making in Northern Manitoba" box.

TABLE 3.3   Key Case Management Activities With Examples

Key Case Management Activities	Description of Activities	Examples
Targeting	The identification of patients who require case management services	A hospital discharge planner refers the patient to a community care access centre case manager, who then contacts the chronic care patient and family in the community. An occupational health nurse in industry makes a referral to the Workplace Safety and Insurance Board case manager, who then contacts the patient.
Assessment	The process used to gather relevant assessment data appropriate to the patient situation in order to establish patient health concerns and to prioritize services required; interprofessional team assessments are ideal and therefore encouraged	The CHN, physiotherapist, occupational therapist, physician, and social worker conduct physical, cognitive, psychosocial, functional, caregiver support system, and financial assessments in the home to determine the patient's health concerns and the community services required. The CHN conducts an assessment focused on how to facilitate a patient's return to work based on the patient's abilities and disabilities, the patient's health concerns, and the available community resources required.
Care planning	The integration of assessment data into an interprofessional plan of care so that patient health concerns are addressed through the appropriate use of services and resources	Based on individualized patient assessment data and knowledge of available services and resources, the case manager develops an interprofessional care plan.
Implementation	The carrying out of the care plan through arrangements made with formal and informal support systems to provide the required services to the patient; the case manager approves services, assigns resources, and coordinates care	The case manager approves services such as Meals on Wheels and home care and assigns resources such as a home care visiting nurse, homemaker, and physiotherapist. The case manager approves services such as return-to-work programs and assigns resources such as an ergonomist, occupational therapist, and physiotherapist.
Monitoring	The observation of the patient situation for changes and the observation of the services provided to ensure that required patient outcomes will be met	The case manager monitors the patient situation, services, and resources for changes since all systems are dynamic. In this manner, the case manager can respond quickly to changes as needed.
Reassessment	A review of the extent to which goals have been met and of the effectiveness of the plan that has been implemented; also, in consultation with other team members (including the patient as a team member), the identification of services still required and of any other changes needed	Keeping resources in mind, case managers review patient situations in consultation with the patient, family, and service providers. The case manager assesses the patient's situation on a regular basis and makes changes to the care plan as needed. For example, if a caregiver becomes ill, additional services and resources may be required. If a new informal support person comes to reside with the patient, then certain services and resources may no longer be needed.

Source: Based on Yoder-Wise et al. (2020).

 CHN IN PRACTICE: A CASE STUDY

Case Management and Decision Making in Northern Manitoba

Initiating, monitoring, and evaluating resources are essential components of nursing case management. You are the new CHN based in the small northern Manitoba town of The Pas. While new to the role, you are one of only two CHNs in the town and surrounding smaller villages. Leadership and decision making are requirements in your role from day one on the job.

Think About It

As the nurse in a lead case management role with The Pas's Primary Health Care Centre, you must identify the resources available inside and outside of your community that would

facilitate your community health nursing care. How would you undertake this task for the following patients?

• A patient needing cardiac rehabilitation following discharge from the closest larger urban health centre over 600 km south of The Pas

• An older adult patient who has been cared for by family in the community with some home support worker assistance but who will require long-term care in the closest facility, which is a 90-minute drive away in Flin Flon

• A young male patient from The Pas who is referred to an orthopedic clinic in the nearest urban centre for rehabilitation due to a work-related accident with a local forestry company that has impaired his ability to walk or stand for long periods of time

SETTINGS, FUNCTIONS, AND ROLES OF COMMUNITY HEALTH NURSES IN CANADA

As discussed in Chapter 1, most CHNs work in primary health care; however, not all CHNs work intensely in the area of community development and planning, and not all use a population-based focus. Some CHNs focus mainly on the individual and family as patients. In community health nursing, the practice settings also vary, but there is some consistency in roles and functions. The model and standards of practice for all CHNs are identified by the Canadian Community Health Nursing Standards of Practice (CCHN Standards) (Community Health Nurses of Canada [CHNC], 2019). The CCHN Standards were initially published in 2003 and updated in 2008, 2011, and 2019 (they are presented in Appendix 1). These standards are discussed throughout this text. Prior to the establishment of the CCHN Standards, the CPHA published *Community Health—Public Health Nursing in Canada: Preparation and Practice* in 1990 (CPHA, 1990). For many years, this publication defined the activities of public health nurses (PHNs) and outlined their roles, functions, qualifications, and responsibilities. At that time, the emphasis in community health nursing care was on a needs approach, and the umbrella term *community health nurse* was not used.

Therefore, there were *PHNs* and *visiting nurses* from agencies such as the Victorian Order of Nurses (VON).

Elements of the current CCHN Standards are an expansion of the roles and activities outlined in the 1990 CPHA publication, and some community health nursing specialties have developed, or are in the process of developing, their own specific competencies with certification through the Canadian Nurses Association (CNA). Competencies describe the activities that a nurse engages in to meet a standard or set of standards (see the CNA link on the Evolve website). **Certification** is a mechanism that provides an indication, usually by means of written examination, of professional competence in a specialized area of practice.

Fig. 3.2 illustrates the broad range of community health nursing specialty areas, settings, and roles when working with the patient and some key concepts used in community health nursing practice.

In short, community health nursing involves working with a variety of patients, fulfilling various roles, and practising in diverse settings, the extent of which are determined by the area of specialty under the umbrella term *community health nursing*. The specialty areas of community health nursing, their practice settings and patients, and their functions and roles are described next.

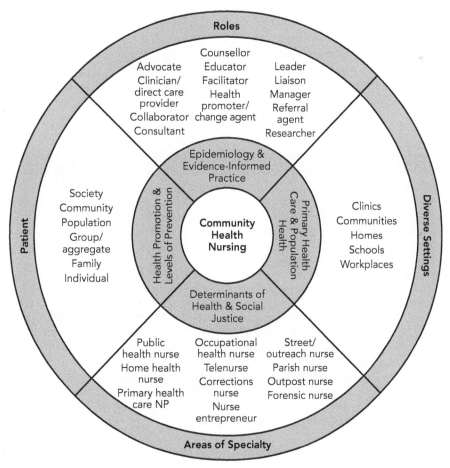

Fig. 3.2 Community Health Nursing Practice Components. *NP*, Nurse practitioner.

The Home Health Nurse

Home health care is the most rapidly expanding health care field (Canadian Home Care Association, 2019). Its growth is due to the following factors:

- Increased government or organizational demands for cost-effectiveness of services
- Shorter hospital stays
- Consumer preferences
- Technological advances such as personal-digital-assistant software for monitoring changes in condition (i.e., blood glucose monitors)
- Proven quality of service of home health care nurses
- Aging Canadian population

Home care offers patients the benefits of familiarity and being surrounded by family, friends, and pets in a setting that is interactional and conducive to expressions of caring and concern. At home, patients have an increased array of choices of food, treatments, medication schedules, and interactions with family and friends, empowering them and providing a feeling of security and well-being.

Within community health nursing, home health nursing is an important nursing specialty, of which hospice palliative care is considered a specialty. Home health providers such as home health nurses (HHNs) and homemakers usually practise in the patient's home environment, although this is not always the case. HHNs function as generalists, incorporating knowledge specialization and skills in areas such as home chemotherapy, enterostomal therapy, mental health, and continence management (Victorian Order of Nurses [VON], 2020). Across Canada, privately operated home health nursing agencies have emerged, and new agencies continue to emerge to meet the demand for home health nursing due to shortened hospital stays. Saint Elizabeth Health Care, a Canadian nonprofit organization,

was established more than 100 years ago and continues to provide home and community health care in settings across Ontario, Alberta, and Nova Scotia (Saint Elizabeth Health Care, 2020).

When working in a patient's home, the CHN is a guest (Öresland, Lutzén, Norberg, et al., 2013) and to be effective, must earn the trust of the family. The CHN must also assess and respond to the patient and setting (e.g., driving conditions, unfamiliar neighbourhoods, aggressive pets, visitors in the home). In the community setting, CHNs have the opportunity to observe family life (a privilege usually reserved for family and friends), including family dynamics, lifestyle choices, communication patterns, coping strategies, responses to health and illness, and the presence of social, cultural, spiritual, and economic issues. The "CHN in Practice: A Case Study, Complex Urban Home Care" box shows some of the complexities that can arise in home care practice.

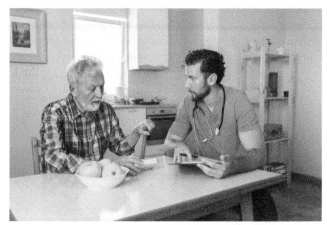

In home care practice, patients are empowered to make decisions with clear and honest information. (iStockphoto/PixelsEffect)

CHN IN PRACTICE: A CASE STUDY

Complex Urban Home Care

Stephanie is an HHN working with Darlene, a 56-year-old patient who lives independently but who requires assessment, postoperative wound care, support, and teaching following cardiac bypass surgery. Darlene lives in an urban high-rise apartment in downtown Vancouver with an excellent adapted transit system, but her mobility challenges due to chronic muscular dystrophy coupled with fatigue and restrictions related to postoperative protocols necessitate home nursing care. Stephanie collaborates with Darlene to understand her needs beyond just the postoperative protocols from the surgical team. She assists Darlene in interpreting and understanding the protocols, and in adapting the restrictions and progressive activities to her own abilities. Darlene has a weekly home support worker who provides basic homemaking services (including some assistance with meal preparation) and bathing assistance. Otherwise, Darlene manages independently at home with some adapted equipment including a walker and other aids in her kitchen and bathroom. Stephanie is proposing that Darlene consider

an additional day or two per week of home support. However, Darlene refuses, claiming that the cost will strain her already limited budget. She adds, "I can manage for the short term. Maybe I will call my sister who lives in the suburbs and ask her to come and stay with me for a week or two."

Think About It

Stephanie assesses that Darlene's recovery may already be prolonged due to her mobility challenges. Stephanie clarifies Darlene's home support needs and discusses options and ideas from social services aid to crisis/temporary home support.

1. How can Stephanie conduct her assessment and planning in ways that are respectful and supportive of Darlene's choices in relation to her own nursing goals, plans, and realities?
2. Stephanie assesses that Darlene's recovery may already be prolonged due to her mobility challenges. How can Stephanie ensure that best practices and referral for support information is thoroughly discussed to aid decision making with the patient?

Definitions in Home Health Nursing

Home health nursing in today's society cannot be defined simply as "care at home." Home health nursing includes an arrangement of disease prevention, health promotion, and episodic illness-related services provided to people in their places of residence. HHNs have the same primary preventive focus of care of aggregates, as all CHNs have. Home health nursing also involves the secondary and tertiary prevention focuses of care of individuals in collaboration with the family and other caregivers.

HHNs typically work with the family in providing care to an individual patient and in advocating for needs and rights. *Family* is self-defined, consisting of individuals who depend on one another for emotional, physical, or financial support, and includes any significant person who assists the patient in need of care at home. **Family caregiving** includes support by family members in the home (which may be paid or unpaid) to meet the patient's basic needs such as personal hygiene, meal preparation, and, in some cases, medication preparation. HHNs will advocate for the family and patient to ensure this form of care meets the needs and desires of all involved, perhaps recommending the addition of external home supports or other caregivers to provide direct care, such as when respite is needed for the family members. At-home caregivers are essential not only in providing the needed maintenance care between the skilled visits of the health care provider (a CHN, physician, or other professional practitioner) but also in providing the HHN with insight into what additional support and services may be crucial to optimal care.

Practice Settings for Home Health Nurses

The practice setting for home health nursing is usually the patient's home, but whenever a patient requires direct nursing care, the HHN visits the patient in his or her current setting, possibly a school, a shelter, a group residence, or the street (Gilmour, 2018). Each patient's place of residence has its own uniqueness for providing care and depends on where the person calls home. Home may be a house, apartment, trailer, boarding home, care home, daycare or school setting, shelter, vehicle, makeshift shelter under a bridge, or cardboard box. The HHN meets patients wherever they are, and at the same time considers what services might be available and might work for a patient if alternative shelter is desirable. Balancing patient choice and the availability of warm, acceptable, and safe shelter may be an important feature of the HHN's assessment and work with patients and community.

Some of the challenges of home care nursing include meeting the privacy needs of the patient and family and adapting as necessary to the family's lifestyle. Some families may view having CHNs, or professional caregivers, in the home as an intrusion of privacy that disrupts the normal daily routine. Families may have to make spatial adjustments in their home because of medical equipment needs.

CHNs in the home setting practise autonomously with little structure. The home environment lacks many resources typically found in health care institutions. Supporting and advocating for additional services, resources, equipment, and so on, also requires a highly individualized planning process with patients, families, and other support agencies. In response to these unique conditions, CHNs need to have good organizational skills, be adaptable to different settings, and demonstrate interpersonal savvy for working with the diverse needs of unique patients in their homes (Bjornsdottir, 2018).

The patient population that HHNs work with is changing. Formerly, most home care patients were older persons; however, younger patients now also present with myriad health care challenges, often a result of the social determinants of health. Increasingly, children with complex care needs are living at home with care from a multidisciplinary team, including HHNs.

Functions and Roles of Home Health Nurses

HHN competencies comprise: assessment, monitoring, and clinical decision making; care planning and care coordination; health maintenance, restoration, and palliation; teaching and education; communication; relationships; access and equity; and building capacity (CHNC, 2010). Optimizing the role of home health nursing requires ongoing policy shifts to fully resource and locate nursing work to the full scope of practice and competencies within the home setting. The policy change requires renewed understanding of the value in this scope of practice for a patient-centred approach (Canadian Nurses Association, 2013).

HHNs aim to help prevent the occurrence of illness and promote the patient's well-being. In the home care setting, patients possess more control and determine their own health care needs. The effectiveness of service depends on the patient's active involvement in and understanding of plans established jointly by the patient and the HHN. Patient goals are always related to the principles of health promotion, maintenance, and restoration. By maximizing a patient's level of independence, HHNs help patients function at their highest possible level and prevent their dependence on others. To achieve this, HHNs do the following:

- Provide a combination of direct care (i.e., wound care, PICC line management, medication management), counselling, and health education
- Enhance self-care skills
- Link the patient with community services that provide limited assistance to enable the patient to stay at home, if this is the goal
- Work to prevent complications in chronically ill persons
- Help to minimize the effects of disability and illness

A common misconception of home health nursing is that it is "custodial" care (or unskilled personal care concentrating on activities of daily living); however, it is important to remember that home health nursing is part of community health nursing. Thus, health promotion and disease prevention activities are fundamental components of practice. Because home health care is often intermittent, a primary objective of the HHN is to facilitate self-care and self-management. *Self-care* is described as "the practice of activities that individuals initiate and perform on their own behalf in maintaining life, health, and well-being" (Orem, 1995, p. 104). HHNs are concerned with self-management for all patients, regardless of the patients' abilities. For example, a patient recuperating at home after suffering a CVA may be unable to perform activities of daily living without assistance. Such patients can be taught to perform certain activities in a modified form. They can thereby regain control over their life and self-care activities and prevent possible losses in other self-care areas.

Contracting, or making an agreement between two or more parties, is a vital component of many HHN roles. Constantly evolving arrangements with third-party payers and contracted providers of home support or homemaking services, the high risk of liability, and the level of HHN autonomy make the work of home health contracts an important function of the home care service environment. Contracting is further discussed in Chapter 12.

LEVELS OF PREVENTION

Related to Home Health Nursing
Primary Prevention
An HHN visits an older patient for wound care and to assess the home for safety.

Secondary Prevention
An HHN provides dietary counselling and education on insulin injections to a newly diagnosed diabetic patient and his family in a rural community.

Tertiary Prevention
An HHN provides direct care (suture removal and blood pressure assessment) to a patient who has experienced a CVA to avoid complications.

Home health nursing is interprofessional care, and an important function of the HHN is **care coordination** of an interprofessional health care team, or case management practice. The HHN organizes team conferences, which offer an ideal opportunity for increasing coordination and continuity of services for optimal patient care and use of resources and services. For example, the HHN shares information on patients with complex conditions or inadequate home support with the team; this sharing of information invites joint care planning and problem solving. **Care planning** refers to the HHN, patients, and interprofessional team members working together to ensure adequate health care service at home. Most often, a referral for home care nursing for a patient is due to a physician's referral for posthospital or follow-up care for a specific concern. That concern and the patient's needs and context will largely dictate the plan of care. The HHN has a collaborative role in the patient's interprofessional team, which is established before the first visit (in most cases). Although referrals can be made by other health care providers, most often they are physician generated.

Once the referral for home health nursing is generated, the HHN meets with the patient and discusses the possible need for resources such as a home care support worker, special equipment to facilitate patient mobility, or the involvement of community agencies such as Meals on Wheels. The HHN, along with the interprofessional team, organizes the delivery of the required resources. The individual, family, and HHN set mutual goals and establish a plan of nursing care and the promotion of self-care with the complement of supports and resources best able to meet the home health needs of the patient. While HHN visits can be friendly, social, and caring experiences, they are always goal directed. For example, during an initial home visit, the HHN gathers data and determines an action plan for care by establishing a plan of care with the individual and family. Care plans can be formal (written) or informal (verbal), depending on the patient's needs. In either case, the HHN records the plan and any potential additional contracted service agreements in the patient's chart. The most important aspect of the care plan is the patient's active participation in developing, implementing, and evaluating the plan. To avoid home visits that have no predetermined goal or outcome, the HHN must establish both short-term and long-term goals with individuals and families. The goals provide for continuity of care and state the criteria for evaluating the patient's condition and progress toward an optimum level of self-care.

Home health nursing involves a number of care and counselling and other supportive functions. When performing these functions, the HHN assumes a variety of roles, including that of case manager as part of an interprofessional team.

The HHN models positive health behaviours, follows agency policies, and performs clinical skills with competence, often independently. Depending on education and experience, the HHN may engage in the roles of clinician or direct care provider, educator, researcher, manager, referral agent, consultant in home health care, or a combination of any of these. HHNs provide *care and counselling* to individuals and families. They are *educators* because they educate individuals and families on the "how" and "why" of self-care. They may also provide health education classes to community groups.

The care and counselling HHNs typically provide include the following:
- Observing and evaluating the patient's health status and condition
- Administering direct care such as rehabilitative exercises, medications, catheter insertion, colostomy irrigation, and wound care
- Helping the patient and family develop positive coping behaviours
- Educating the patient and family how and when to give treatments and medications
- Educating the patient and family to carry out physicians' orders such as treatments, therapeutic diets, or medication administration
- Reporting changes in the patient's condition to the patient's physician and arranging for medical follow-up as indicated
- Helping the individual and family identify resources that will help the patient attain a state of optimal functioning

As well, HHNs participate in the ongoing education of their colleagues as mentors, both formally, providing in-service education, and informally, as team members. The shortening of hospital stays and the trend toward in-home palliative care have contributed to a growth in importance of the *researcher* role in home health nursing. Potential research areas abound in the home health care setting, and to maintain quality and cost-effectiveness of care, research must remain a priority in the future. As *consultants,* HHNs may provide advice and counsel to patients and others, such as health care providers. Consultative practices of the HHN may include the following:

- Consulting with other nurses and health care providers
- Organizing and participating in patient care conferences
- Advocating for patients within the health care system
- Obtaining results of diagnostic tests
- Documenting care

Hospice Palliative Care

The development of hospice palliative care programs has improved the quality of care for terminally ill persons. **Palliative care** is holistic caring (i.e., physical, psychosocial, and spiritual support) that may include end-of-life care for those facing life-threatening illnesses and for the dying (and their families) so that they experience quality of life through symptom management and supportive care (Canadian Hospice Palliative Care Association [CHPCA] & CNA, 2015; Health Canada, 2018; WHO, 2020). Estimates suggest that only 15% of Canadians have access to or receive hospice palliative and end-of-life care services—depending on where they live in Canada—and even fewer receive grief and bereavement services (Costante, Lawand, & Cheng, 2019). In Canada, access to hospice palliative care has been challenged for a number of reasons: health care restructuring and the resultant limited service availability; accessibility, especially for those living in remote and rural areas and for persons with severe disabilities; the preference of many Canadians to die at home; inadequate government funding, which places an additional burden on family and informal caregivers; inadequate physician education on palliative care pain management; and underfunding for education of other health disciplines such as nursing and social work (Health Canada, 2018).

Hospice palliative care can be delivered in the home, in a specially designated palliative care unit in a hospital, or in a hospice facility. A **hospice** is a designated place where health care is provided to terminally ill persons. **Hospice care** refers to the delivery of palliative care of the very ill and dying, offering both respite and comfort. If the individual and family agree, hospice care can be comfortably delivered at home with family involvement under the direction and supervision of health care providers, especially an HHN. In 2006, The Canadian Hospice Palliative Care Association (CHPCA) published *The Pan-Canadian Gold Standard for Palliative Home Care* (see the link on the Evolve website). The standards proposed in this report were developed in partnership with the CHPCA and the Canadian Home Care Association, based on expert input from various health care providers, with the goal of ensuring that all Canadians have equitable access to the highest possible quality end-of-life care in relation to case management, nursing, palliative-specific pharmaceuticals, and personal care at the end of life (CHPCA, 2006).

Hospice care may be provided in a designated palliative care unit or in a hospice facility when a patient experiences severe complications of terminal illness or when the family becomes too exhausted to care for the patient in the home. Some communities are adopting a broader **palliative approach,** emphasizing that comfort care and quality-of-life approaches to care must begin at the point of diagnosis of a life-limiting or chronic illness rather than in the final weeks of life. A palliative approach paradigm of care would ensure that all patients who need comfort care would receive it early on, while they were still receiving curative therapies, on an as-needed but planned basis (CHPCA & CNA, 2015).

Canadian Hospice Palliative Care Nursing, or CHPCN(C), is an area of nursing practice that has certification status through CNA. This nursing specialization requires specific cognitive, psychomotor, and affective skills. Box 3.2 lists the hospice palliative care nurse competency categories. Palliative care nursing competencies that lead to certification can be found on the CNA website (see the link on the Evolve website).

Reducing pain and suffering is the goal of hospice palliative care. In both home and hospice settings, HHNs continually do the following:

- Assess the patient's response to treatment
- Report their findings to the patient's physician
- Collaborate to modify the treatment plan as needed

As the patient's level of dependence increases, his or her need for service increases. Agencies that are obligated to maintain quality care and provide for continuity coordinate health care services, which are tailored to any patient health concern. Thus, the range of services provided in home health nursing is extensive. As a result of the palliative approach, persons with terminal diseases now have the option of dying at home with support services available. In addition to prescribed home health nursing services, core services unique to the hospice include the following:

- Volunteers
- Chaplain support

BOX 3.2 Hospice Palliative Care Nurse Competency Categories

1. Care of the Person and Family
2. Pain Assessment and Management
3. Symptom Assessment and Management
4. Last Days/Hours/Imminent Death Care
5. Loss, Grief, and Bereavement Support
6. Interprofessional/Collaborative Practice
7. Education
8. Ethics and Legal Issues
9. Professional Development and Advocacy

Source: Grantham, D., O'Brien, L. A., Widger, K., et al. (2009). *Canadian hospice palliative care nursing competencies case examples.* https://www.virtualhospice.ca/Assets/Canadian%20Hospice%20Palliative%20Care%20Nursing%20Competencies%20Case%20Examples-Revised%20Feb%202010_20100211150854.pdf

- Respite care
- Financial help with medicines and equipment
- Bereavement support for the family after the family member's death

HHNs act as members of palliative interprofessional teams with experience in caring for the terminally ill and working with their families. This team may consist of the patient's family physician, specialist physicians, social workers, pharmacists, pastoral support workers, personal care workers, volunteers, the patient, and his or her family. **Interprofessional collaboration,** a necessity in home health and hospice settings, is a working agreement in which health care team members carefully analyze their practice roles and work together to determine the best plan for a patient's care. Without effective collaboration between workers from different disciplines and sectors, the patient's palliative care program would be fragmented, offering decreased or no continuity of care.

The Public Health Nurse

In 2005, the Federal, Provincial, and Territorial Joint Task Group on Public Health Human Resources developed a draft set of core competencies for public health practice in Canada in consultation with leaders in the public health community. The Public Health Agency of Canada (PHAC) assumed the lead in this effort, in collaboration with many partners, and public health nursing core competencies became available in 2009 (CHNC, 2009). Box 3.3 lists the Canadian public health nursing competency categories. (For more on the public health core competencies and a history of their development, see the PHAC link on the Evolve website.)

In Canada, public health takes a population health approach to protecting and promoting health and preventing disease for all Canadians. PHNs work with many partners, both within the public health unit or health authority (e.g., nutritionists, epidemiologists, dental hygienists, health inspectors) and external to the public health unit or health authority (e.g., community coalitions for heart health, cancer screening, diabetes, and obesity prevention; school and hospital administrators; regional planners; social service and childcare workers; lobbyists for health issues such as antismoking legislation and homelessness).

BOX 3.3 Canadian Public Health Nursing Competency Categories

1. Public Health and Nursing Sciences
2. Assessment and Analysis
3. Policy and Program Planning, Implementation and Evaluation
4. Partnerships, Collaboration, and Advocacy
5. Diversity and Inclusiveness
6. Communication
7. Leadership
8. Professional Responsibility and Accountability

Source: Community Health Nurses of Canada. (2009). *Public health nursing discipline specific competencies version 1.0.* https://www.chnc.ca/en/competencies

---

PHNs foster partnerships and collaboration among groups and build the capacity of community leaders to address health issues effectively. These liaison and support activities are much more powerful in making changes that will have an impact on the health of community members than work in isolation or with individual patients only. Consider the case of a depressed mother who is having difficulty coping with the activities and responsibilities of daily living and needs counselling. She presents a significant public health concern because her, her children's, and her family's health needs are not being met. Often, these health concerns are not obvious to the health care provider who sees an individual for the first time. However, the PHN has the knowledge and skills to identify the strengths of the woman and her family, the health concerns present, and the challenges involved. The PHN is also well positioned to identify the impact that all of these factors may have on the broader community. In this example, the PHN would consider the following:

- The children may grow to be adults with developmental or mental health concerns.
- The community mental health and social services may not be able to respond to this increased demand on resources.
- The children may become depressed or violent adults, resulting in a need for more health and corrections facilities.
- The mother may need additional mental health and social services.
- The children may be absent from school often and may not be able to complete their education.
- As adults, this mother's children may remain unemployed or be nonproductive in the workplace because their absences from school led to limited or poor job and literacy skills.
- The increased burden of care on the health care and other publicly funded systems leads to increased costs and taxes.

Definitions in Public Health Nursing

In public health nursing, the *patient* is defined as the individual, family, group or aggregate, community, population, or society. Public health nursing practice involves primary, secondary, and tertiary prevention. Using population health determinants based on sound knowledge that includes nursing science, public health science, and social sciences (CPHA, 2010), PHNs provide services such as health promotion, health protection, disease and injury prevention, and surveillance (Savage, 2020). The minimum educational preparation of PHNs is a baccalaureate degree in nursing with curriculum content in community health nursing, epidemiology, research, management, and leadership. PHNs can be involved with community health development (described earlier in the chapter), or they can implement public health interventions, including programs and policies that are provincial or Canada-wide. The immunization program is one such initiative that has both provincial and Canada-wide directives.

Practice Settings for Public Health Nurses

PHNs work for an official public health agency referred to as a health department, health unit, or regional health authority. The official agency is governed by a board of health and funded by provincial or territorial and municipal governments that develop legislation, such as a public health act, that outlines the requirements for the delivery of programs and services. For example, in Ontario, the *Health Protection and Promotion Act* directs and identifies the roles of public health agencies, and the Ontario Public Health Standards (Ontario Ministry of Health and Long-Term Care, 2018b) outline the mandate and core functions for public health practice.

The practice settings for PHNs vary and may include home, school, workplace, community health centre, and clinical settings. Historically, PHNs spent a great deal of time visiting patients in their home and students in schools. Currently, differences exist across Canada as to the extent of public health nursing involvement in schools. However, there is a movement toward comprehensive school health (see the Healthy School Communities Concept Paper link on the Evolve website). In schools, PHNs encourage the development of school health committees and promote health through collaboration with principals, teachers, families, and students. PHNs are very much involved in providing clinic services such as those for influenza prevention, family planning, travel health, immunization, sexual health, breastfeeding, and well babies. PHNs work with a variety of groups, including expectant and new parents to promote healthy pregnancy and parenting, smoking cessation and hepatitis C support groups, older persons' centres, and a range of self-help groups dealing with health issues. PHNs working with the community as patient contribute to community and workplace health promotion strategies with a focus on, for example, health issues (e.g., heart health, cancer screening initiatives), childhood obesity, and environmental health issues. More recently, some PHNs have begun working with nontraditional partners such as regional planners, developers, environmentalists, and traffic demand managers to provide consultation and awareness regarding the health impacts of the built environment in an effort to promote the development of healthy communities. They also work with at-risk populations such as the homeless and immigrants in a variety of settings that may include settlement and outreach centres.

Functions and Roles of Public Health Nurses

PHNs have many functions and roles, depending on the needs and resources of an area. Among these roles is advocate. As an advocate, the PHN collects, monitors, and analyzes data and identifies, along with the patient (e.g., an individual, family, or community), which services and programs best meet the patient's needs. The PHN and the patient then develop the most effective plan and approach to the health issue. The plan may include activities, alone or in combination, related to education and awareness, personal skills development, the creation of supportive environments, policy development,

and community action mobilization. For example, a PHN will work with a patient who wants to quit smoking by helping him or her develop the knowledge and skills related to cessation and providing support as the patient implements a plan based on motivational and change theory. With the PHN's help, the patient can increase his or her confidence, take ownership of his or her health, and become more independent in making decisions and obtaining the services necessary to stop smoking.

The PHN may also assume the role of manager with specific aggregate groups and, in this role, assess, plan, implement, and evaluate outcomes to meet patients' needs. As a leader and consultant, the PHN builds and maintains partnerships with community leaders and key stakeholders to identify community needs (e.g., playground safety, access to physical activity opportunities, hand hygiene, pedestrian safety, safer-sex practices), to develop and implement plans to meet these needs, and to identify and implement strategies that promote the adoption of health behaviours over time. Communicating complex information clearly is another important component of patient management and may involve engaging family members, translators, or religious leaders as the PHN works toward developing the care plan. Other health and social agency participants may not be as familiar as the PHN with the dynamics of family relationships, the family's financial situation, or their living conditions. It is the PHN who has been there, observed the living conditions, and assessed the family's strengths and health concerns, and can support and assist the patient to tell their story. The PHN as manager assists patients in determining the services they need most and identifies the most effective means of accessing them. For example, a PHN may go into the home to visit a new mother and her baby. Upon assessment, the PHN may find that the mother needs help finding a job, childcare, and a pediatrician. The PHN helps the mother in the following ways:

- Assists with prioritizing health concerns
- Reviews research related to how best to address her health concerns and analyzes community data to identify available and accessible resources within the mother's community
- Ensures that resources and services are culturally sensitive and delivered in the appropriate language, literacy level, and environment for the patient
- Develops a plan for resolving the health concerns, in partnership with the mother, to identify and work with her strengths
- Supports and encourages the mother to contact other agencies related to employment and childcare
- Refers the patient to an appropriate community resource or agency as needed
- Follows up with the mother to evaluate her progress and to revise the plan as needed to ensure that her health concerns are being resolved
- Follows up with agencies, such as social services, and shares information with the mother

Being both consultants and specialists, PHNs know how to access and analyze relevant data from a variety of sources. These data often include information related to the determinants of health (e.g., housing, income, employment, literacy, culture), which provide PHNs with a comprehensive understanding of the health of their community. PHNs then use this knowledge and skill at community forums and coalitions to facilitate the planning of a variety of health initiatives that may include, for example, communication or social media campaigns, health fairs for new immigrants, or community mobilization to promote safe routes to schools or increased access to clinical services.

PHNs' knowledge of the community also makes them a major referral resource. They maintain or know how to access current information about the health and social needs and the services available within the community. They know what resources a patient will find acceptable (e.g., within the social and cultural norms for his or her group). PHNs provide patients with education and skills-building opportunities to build their capacity, to enable them to access and use the resources in their community, and to learn self-care. PHNs also provide counselling and refer patients to other services in their area, just as other services refer patients to PHNs for care or follow-up. For example, a community agency or hospital may refer a new mother and her baby to a PHN for postnatal care, which would require the PHN to do a postpartum home visit follow-up, or a workplace may contact a PHN for information on how to plan a health fair and flu clinic for its employees, which would require the PHN to provide information on how to access the appropriate community agencies and resources to meet employees' health needs.

The "Evidence-Informed Practice" box discusses the roles and function of PHNs in education, raising awareness, care, and counselling.

A PHN uses an evidence-informed approach to practice when identifying the most effective strategies for changing health behaviours. **Evidence-informed practice** (sometimes called *evidence-based practice*) combines the best evidence from research with clinical practice, knowledge and expertise, and patient preferences or choices when making clinical decisions (Canadian Nurses Association [CNA], 2018; National Collaborating Centre for Methods and Tools, 2020; Jakubec & Astle, 2017). Drawing on evidence, a PHN is also an educator and a counsellor. As an **educator,** the PHN identifies the patient's learning needs and uses a variety of culturally appropriate and relevant teaching strategies to ensure that information received is information the patient can use. The PHN identifies and analyzes the resources available in the community that would best meet the needs of the patient. The PHN may have to revise or adapt an existing resource or may have to identify the most appropriate media channel to reach the target population. To this end, the PHN may have to develop skills and experience in video- and teleconferencing, arranging radio or TV advertisements, creating online resources, and conducting marketing campaigns. As a counsellor, a PHN encourages patients, reinforces their positive behaviours, and continually assesses their needs in order to develop a relationship of mutual trust and respect and to help patients increase their knowledge and skills and adopt the behaviours necessary to manage their health and self-care.

Along with education, the PHN plan will include strategies that focus on creating supportive environments, mobilizing the community, developing personal health management skills, and developing policies. PHNs act as direct primary caregivers in places such as public health clinics and in community activities such as new-baby visits. A **primary caregiver** is the health care provider who is primarily responsible for providing for the health care needs of patients. PHNs provide primary care where needed, as determined by

---

⑤ EVIDENCE-INFORMED PRACTICE

Whelan, Steenbeek, Martin-Misener, and colleagues (2014) undertook a study to determine the relationship between school-based PHN strategies and uptake of human papillomavirus (HPV) vaccine. Nova Scotia has the highest rate of cervical cancer in Canada and most of these cases are attributed to the HPV. In 2007, the vaccine Gardasil was approved and implemented in a successful school-based HPV immunization program. A retrospective, exploratory correlation study was conducted with results showing that HPV vaccine initiation was significantly associated with PHN reminder calls for: consent return and missed school clinic, HPV education to teachers, and a thank-you note to teachers. Completion of the full vaccine series was associated with student consents being returned to the teacher, and a PHN being assigned to the school in a formal relationship with defined health education and counselling roles.

Application for CHNs

Female high school students are at risk for sexually transmitted infections (STIs). CHNs working with this aggregate need to consider all aspects of vaccine uptake. The PHN role in health education, awareness, care, and counselling—and in relationship with schools and community groups—cannot be overestimated.

Questions for Reflection and Discussion

1. What particular roles and functions are important for PHNs who work with vaccination programs?
2. What unique considerations might there be for a PHN working with school groups?
3. Where could a PHN working with high school students seek evidence to inform practice?

Source: Whelan, N., Steenbeek, A., Martin-Misener, R., Scott, J., Smith, B., & D'Angelo-Scott, H. (2014). Engaging parents and schools improves uptake of the human papillomavirus (HPV) vaccine: Examining the role of the public health nurse. *Vaccine, 32*(36), 4665–4671.

community assessment. Such assessments identify gaps to which the private sector is unable to respond and also determine the impact the identified gap in services has on the health of the population. The types of primary care PHNs provide include the following:

- Prenatal services
- Postnatal visits to high-risk mothers
- Breastfeeding clinics
- Immunization services for targeted populations
- Directly observed therapy for patients with active tuberculosis (TB)
- Assessment and treatment of STIs

Essential and unique roles for PHNs also exist in the area of communicable disease control. Community health nursing skills are necessary for education, prevention, surveillance, and outbreak investigation. PHNs can do the following in their practice at a number of levels of prevention for public health:

- Find infected individuals
- Notify the contacts of infected individuals
- Input disease identification findings into regional, provincial, or territorial databases
- Refer patients to other health care providers or agencies for care and treatment as needed
- Educate individuals, families, communities, professionals, and populations about communicable diseases
- Act as advocates for public health and individual patient health
- Provide resources to reduce the rate of communicable disease in the community

Finally, PHNs also take on multiple roles in emergency preparedness and planning (further elaborated in Chapter 18). PHNs' roles in emergency preparedness and relief include:

- Providing education that will prepare communities to cope with disasters
- Establishing mass dispensing clinics
- Conducting enhanced communicable disease surveillance
- Working with environmental health specialists to ensure safe food and water for disaster victims and emergency workers
- Serving on the local emergency planning committee (CPHA, 2010)

The Occupational Health Nurse

Most adult Canadians spend a good portion of their day in a workplace setting. All CHNs need to have some basic knowledge about workforce populations, work-related hazards, and methods to control hazards and improve health.

Work–health interactions (the influence of work on health based on statistics) will continue to grow in importance, affecting how work is done, how hazards are controlled or minimized, and how health care is managed and integrated in workplace health delivery strategies. In Canada, each of the provinces and territories, as well as the federal government, has its own occupational health and safety legislation. This legislation outlines the general rights and responsibilities of the employer, the supervisor, and the worker.

An individual with a work-related health problem will often see an occupational health nurse (OHN) before seeing any other health care provider. Consequently, OHNs are in a key position to intervene with working populations at all levels of prevention. They perform critical roles in planning and delivering work-site health and safety services and psychologically safe workplace standards such as the National Standard of Canada for Psychological Health and Safety in the Workplace (Mental Health Commission of Canada, 2013). In addition, the ongoing increase in health care costs and concern about health care quality have prompted health care access for nonwork-related health concerns such as counselling and mental health support in workplaces. Examples of health service programs include smoking cessation programs, cardiac rehabilitation programs, and weight management programs.

Definition of Occupational Health Nursing

Occupational health nursing focuses on workplace health and safety, specifically the delivery of integrated health and safety services and wellness programs to individual employees and employee groups. It encompasses health promotion, maintenance, and restoration as well as the prevention of illness and injury (Canadian Occupational Health Nurses Association, 2018).

Practice Settings for Occupational Health Nurses

OHNs work in a variety of settings, including manufacturing companies, corporations, health care facilities, construction

---

⬛ LEVELS OF PREVENTION

Related to Public Health Nursing

Primary Prevention

- A PHN advocates for a member of Parliament to address issues such as refugee access to health care.
- A PHN conducts ongoing disease surveillance for communicable diseases.

Secondary Prevention

- A PHN conducts contact tracing for individuals exposed to a patient with an active case of COVID-19 or an STI. The PHN provides directly observed therapy (DOT) for patients with COVID-19.

- A PHN participates in screening programs for genetic disorders or metabolic deficiencies in newborns; breast, cervical, and testicular cancers; diabetes; hypertension; and sensory impairments in children. The PHN ensures follow-up services for patients with positive test results.

Tertiary Prevention

- A PHN provides case management services that link patients with chronic illnesses, such as diabetes, to health care and community support services.

sites, and government settings. Their scope of practice is broad and includes:

- Worker and workplace assessment and surveillance
- Primary care
- Case management
- Counselling
- Health promotion and protection
- Administration and management
- Research
- Legal and ethical monitoring
- Community orientation

CHNs apply their knowledge in occupational health and safety to the workforce aggregate. OHNs have a built-in conflict of interest that they must balance because the employer has different concerns from the employee, who is the patient. OHNs can be caught between being a company nurse and a patient advocate. The College of Registered Nurses of British Columbia recognizes that OHNs are in a potential conflict-of-interest situation and provide the following advice: "If you are an occupational health nurse, avoid conflict of interest situations by clarifying with your employer and patients that your primary responsibility is to your patients" (College of Registered Nurses of British Columbia, 2016).

Today, the greatest proportion of paid employment is in the following occupations: service work (e.g., health care, information processing, banking, insurance); professional technical work (e.g., managers, computer specialists); and clerical work (e.g., data entry clerks, secretaries). Examples of occupational hazards employees may encounter at work include the following:

- Complex chemicals
- Nonergonomic workstation design (i.e., workstation set-ups that do not meet the employee's health and safety needs)
- Job stress
- Burnout
- Exhaustion

Through its services, programs, and legislation for accident and injury prevention, the Canadian government recognizes the importance of a healthy, safe workplace for all employees.

The epidemiological triangle (see Fig. 3.3), discussed more extensively in Chapter 8, can be used to explain the relationship between work and health (Campos-Outcalt, 1994). Using the employed population as an example, the *host* is any individual susceptible to being infected by or affected by an agent. Because of the nature of work-related hazards, OHNs must assume that all employed individuals and groups are at risk of exposure to occupational hazards. The *agent* is a factor associated with illness and injury; occupational agents are classified as *biological and infectious, chemical, enviro-mechanical, physical,* or *psychosocial* hazards (see Box 3.4). Finally, the environment in the epidemiological triangle refers to those external and contextual factors that cause or allow injury or disease transmission. Environmental factors may be physical or social. For example, working in extreme heat (a physical factor) or crowded conditions (a social factor) can impact the risks workers may be exposed to in the performance of their

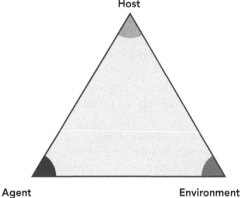

All susceptible people:
Workers
Workers' families

Host

Agent
Workplace hazards:
  Biological
  Chemical
  Ergonomic
  Physical
  Psychosocial

Environment
All other external
factors that influence
host–agent interactions:
  Physical
  Social

Fig. 3.3 The Epidemiological Triangle.

BOX 3.4   Categories of Work-Related Hazards

- *Biological and infectious hazards:* infectious or biological agents, such as bacteria, viruses, fungi, and parasites, that may be transmitted to others via contact with infected individuals or contaminated body secretions or fluids
- *Chemical hazards:* various forms of chemicals, including medications, solutions, gases, vapours, aerosols, and particulate matter, that are potentially toxic or irritating to the body system
- *Enviro-mechanical hazards:* factors encountered in the work environment that cause or potentiate accidents, injuries, strain, or discomfort (e.g., unsafe or inadequate equipment or lifting devices, slippery floors, workstation deficiencies)
- *Physical hazards:* agents within the work environment, such as radiation, electricity, extreme temperatures, and noise, that can cause tissue trauma
- *Psychosocial hazards:* factors and situations encountered or associated with one's job or work environment that create or potentiate stress, emotional strain, or interpersonal problems

Source: Rogers, B. (2007). *Occupational and environmental health nursing: Concepts and practice.* W. B. Saunders.

duties. Table 3.4 lists some of the more common workplace exposures, their known health effects, and the types of jobs associated with these exposures.

OHNs usually have additional educational preparation and experience in promoting the health and safety of workers. Many OHNs have completed continuing education programs in occupational health and safety at a certificate, diploma, or degree level. Courses taken in these programs help registered nurses (RNs) to gain further knowledge and skills related to workplace topics such as ergonomics,

TABLE 3.4   Select Job Categories, Exposures, and Associated Work-Related Diseases and Conditions

Job Categories	Exposures	Work-Related Diseases and Conditions
All workers	Workplace stress	Hypertension, mood disorders, cardiovascular disease
Agricultural workers	Pesticides, infectious agents, gases, sunlight	Pesticide poisoning, "farmer's lung," skin cancer
Anaesthetists	Anaesthetic gases	Reproductive effects, cancer
Automobile workers	Asbestos, plastics, lead, solvents	Asbestosis, dermatitis
Butchers	Vinyl plastic fumes	Meat wrapper's asthma
Caisson workers	Pressurized work environments	Caisson disease, "the bends"
Carpenters	Wood dust, wood preservatives, adhesives	Nasopharyngeal cancer, dermatitis
Cement workers	Cement dust, metals	Dermatitis, bronchitis
Ceramic workers	Talc, clays	Pneumoconiosis
Demolition workers	Asbestos, wood dust	Asbestosis
Drug manufacturers	Hormones, nitroglycerine, etc.	Reproductive effects
Dry cleaners	Solvents	Liver disease, dermatitis
Dye workers	Dyestuffs, metals, solvents	Bladder cancer, dermatitis
Embalmers	Formaldehyde, infectious agents	Dermatitis
Felt makers	Mercury, polycyclic hydrocarbons	Mercury poisoning
Foundry workers	Silica, molten metals	Silicosis
Glass workers	Heat, solvents, metal powders	Cataracts
Hospital workers	Infectious agents, cleansers, radiation	Infections, latex allergies, unintentional injuries
Insulators	Asbestos, fibrous glass	Asbestosis, lung cancer, mesothelioma
Jackhammer operators	Vibration	Raynaud's phenomenon
Lathe operators	Metal dusts, cutting oils	Lung disease, cancer
Office computer workers	Repetitive wrist motion, eye strain	Tendonitis, carpal tunnel syndrome, tenosynovitis

BOX 3.5   Occupational Health Nursing Competency Categories

1. Occupational Health Nursing Practice
2. Identification, Evaluation, and Control of Workplace Hazards
3. Health Surveillance
4. Assessment, Care, and Case Management of Injuries and Illnesses
5. Health, Safety, and Wellness Promotion
6. Health, Safety, and Wellness Management

Source: Canadian Nurses Association. (2013). *Exam blueprint and specialty competencies introduction—Blueprint for the Occupational Health Nursing Certification Exam.* https://www.mycna.ca/~/media/nurseone/files/en/occupational_health_blueprint_and_competencies_e.pdf#page=8?la=en

audiometric testing, and toxicology. CNA has recognized occupational health nursing as a specialty with official certification. Occupational health nursing competencies that lead to certification can be found on the CNA website (see the link on the Evolve website). Categories of OHN competencies are listed in Box 3.5.

Functions and Roles of Occupational Health Nurses

OHNs collaborate with a community physician or occupational medicine physician, who provides consultation and accepts referrals when medical intervention is needed. This collaboration may occur primarily through telephone contact, or the physician may be under contract with the workplace to spend a certain amount of time on-site each week.

Larger workplaces may employ other professionals such as ergonomists, safety professionals, consultant physicians and psychiatrists, employee assistance program counsellors, physiotherapists, health educators, wellness or fitness specialists, and toxicologists.

Generally, the goals of OHNs are:
- To maintain and promote health and safety in the workplace so that patients maximize their work capacity
- To improve the workplace environment by making it healthy and safe
- To enhance population health through healthy and safe work environments
- To work at the systems level to create a workplace atmosphere that contributes to a productive and comfortable psychosocial work environment

Box 3.6 lists a number of the services provided by OHNs.

OHNs practise all levels of prevention (Rogers, 2007). The initial step of assessment involves the traditional history and physical assessment but emphasizes exposure to occupational hazards and individual characteristics that may predispose a patient in a certain job to an increased health risk. Because work is a part of life for most people, the occupational and environmental health history is an indispensable component of the health assessment of individuals (Rogers, 2007) (see Appendix E.1, "Comprehensive Occupational and Environmental Health History," on the Evolve website). An **occupational and environmental health history** contains questions that provide the data necessary to rule out or confirm job-induced conditions and health concerns.

LEVELS OF PREVENTION

Related to Occupational Health Nursing

Primary Prevention

An OHN provides education to a group of new employees about safety in the workplace to prevent injury.

Secondary Prevention

An OHN provides a mass screening clinic for hearing loss resulting from noise levels in the workplace.

Tertiary Prevention

An OHN educates workers with gradual return-to-work strategies following knee replacement surgery in order to support rehabilitation goals and to avoid lost workdays.

OHNs administer individual- and workplace-level health assessments. Including occupational health, data in patient assessments recognize that a relationship might exist between the patient's health and occupational factors. Questions about the patient's occupational history can be included in a short assessment tool. Patient assessments aim to identify agent and host factors that could place the employee at risk and to determine preventive steps that can be taken to eliminate or minimize exposure and the potential health concern. When the health data from patient assessments are analyzed collectively, they may reveal patterns in risk factors associated with the occurrence of work-related injuries and illnesses in the total population of workers. For example, an NP in a clinic noted a dramatic increase in the number of cases of bladder cancer among her patients. When she looked at factors these individuals had in common, she determined that they all worked at a company that used benzidine dyes, which are known bladder carcinogens. She worked with the union and the company to assess the environmental exposure to the employees. This occupational health nursing intervention led to a safer work environment and a decrease in bladder cancer among this population group. Such an approach can be used at the company, industry, and community levels. Collecting data and questioning workplace exposures are vital steps for any intervention.

The OHN may conduct a similar assessment of the workplace itself. The purpose of this assessment, known as a **worksite walk-through** or survey, is to learn about the following (Rogers, 2007):

- The work processes and the materials
- The requirements of various jobs
- The presence of actual or potential hazards
- The work practices of employees

A systematic approach to evaluating the potential for workplace exposures is the most effective intervention for detecting and preventing occupational health risks. Appendix E.2, "Work-Site Assessment Guide," on the Evolve website, is a brief assessment tool that an OHN can incorporate into a routine history-taking.

Rural and Outpost Nurses
Definitions of Rural and Outpost Nurses

Rural and outpost nurses are RNs who work in a community health nursing role to provide comprehensive primary health care to patients in rural, remote, and northern outpost communities, often with a focus on advancing access to care and other social justice and environmental issues related to the contexts (MacLeod, Kulig & Stewart, 2019). These nurses usually have experience working in the community and may have additional education, such as a diploma in advanced practice as a primary health care nurse practitioner. **Outpost nurses** work in northern and remote communities, often with diverse indigenous populations. As introduced in Chapter 1 and elaborated in Chapter 7, the systematic oppression and discrimination endured by Indigenous peoples and the barriers encountered in addressing needs are at a crisis state. The need for enhanced access to programs and initiatives for Indigenous people living outside urban centres (where most health programs and services are located) is well documented (Garasia & Dobbs, 2019). The Canadian Indigenous Nurses Association (CINA) advocates for a concerted effort to increase the number of Indigenous nurses and for expanded services with remote nursing stations. Only select nursing schools have Indigenous-specific access/bridging/transition programs that increase Indigenous student enrollment.

The CINA asserts that increasing the number of Indigenous nurses will promote retention in rural and outpost communities and ultimately improve the health status of these communities (Canadian Indigenous Nurses Association, 2019).

Geographically isolated practice areas require considerable independence and autonomy, with telephone backup available from physicians and specialists. Outpost nurses reside in the community where they provide care, and they actively involve community members in the planning and development of community health programs and strategies. Outpost nurses self-reported that they "work with individuals and communities to solve problems collaboratively within a spirit of partnership" (Misener, MacLeod, Banks et al., 2008, p. 57). They practise as generalists across the lifespan and have as their main focus health promotion, disease prevention, medical diagnoses, and treatment of illness and injury (Misener et al., 2008). Additionally, they have on-call responsibilities and accompany patients who require evacuation. In an interpretative study by Tarlier, Johnson, and Whyte (2003), outpost nurses in northern Canada were asked to describe their community health nursing practice experiences in narrative form. Four main themes emerged from the data: (1) nurses evolve into the outpost role; (2) experienced outpost nurses build and maintain responsive relationships with the community; (3) primary care competencies are fundamental to outpost practice; and (4) experienced outpost nurses become comfortable with the autonomy and responsibility of practice. Box 3.7 summarizes some of the key study findings for each of the four themes.

Practice Settings for Rural and Outpost Nurses

Over the past two decades, the health of rural Canadians has captured the attention of researchers, government, and health care advocates, primarily as a result of research demonstrating the specific health needs of this population (MacLeod, Kulig, & Stewart, 2019).

Accessibility to health care in rural areas is related to geographical distance from urban centres (CIHI, 2020). In rural areas of Canada, residents are generally older, live in poorer socioeconomic conditions; attain lower levels of formal education; have less healthy personal health practices (e.g., increased smoking, unhealthy eating, sedentary lifestyle); and suffer increased overall mortality rates than urban Canadians (Wilson, Rourke, Oandasan et al., 2020). However, residents in rural areas of Canada also experience less stress and perceive a stronger sense of community belonging (Stackhouse, 2019). Although the many health needs of rural populations are not all unique, they differ from those of **urban** populations. Urban populations live in geographical areas described as nonrural and having a higher population density. Statistics Canada's annual Canadian Community Health Survey (Statistics Canada, 2014) provides data that can be used to compare crucial health indicators between rural and urban areas in Canada (see Box 3.8). Research data suggest that rural people have increased health risks such as being overweight or obese, higher rates of smoking, higher prevalence of heart disease, higher than average likelihood of mental illness

---

BOX 3.7   Key Findings About Outpost Nursing in Northern Canada

1. Nurses evolve into the outpost role:
   - They need to adapt to different cultures (Indigenous and northern cultures).
   - They need to adapt to geographical, personal, and professional isolation.
   - They need to shift the focus of care from acute to primary health.
   - They need to engage in upstream thinking (i.e., "the bigger picture").
2. Experienced outpost nurses build and maintain responsive relationships with the community:
   - They need to develop trust, respect, and acceptance with the community.
   - They need to foster responsive relationships to effect positive community health outcomes.
3. Primary care competencies are fundamental to outpost practice:
   - Nurses need to have advanced assessment and treatment skills.
   - Nurses need to address episodic curative situations.
   - Nurses need to focus on teaching, supporting, and counselling skills to influence health outcomes.
4. Experienced outpost nurses become comfortable with the autonomy and responsibility of practice:
   - They need to recognize and accept the extent of autonomy and responsibility of the practice setting.
   - They need to recognize the complex interplay between "autonomy, authority, power, ethics, responsibility and reciprocity of relationships" (p. 183).

Source: Tarlier, D., Johnson, J., & Whyte, N. (2003). Voices from the wilderness: An interpretive study describing the role and practice of outpost nurses. *Canadian Journal of Public Health, 94*(3), 180–184.

BOX 3.8   A Comparison of Canadian Rural Health and Urban Health Data

In rural Canada, health differs from urban Canada in the following ways:
- Mortality rates due to motor vehicle injuries for all ages are two to three times higher.
- Rural workers have higher levels of occupational hazards.
- Residents under 20 years of age have the highest risk of dying from suicide.
- Rural students have higher rates of substance use.
- Mortality rates for specific cancers (e.g., breast cancer in women over 45 years of age) are lower.
- Poorer self-reports of health quality of life and self-rated health.
- Increased morbidity from circulatory diseases and hypertension.
- Increased rates of diabetes, arthritis, and obesity.

Sources: McInnis, O.A., Young, M.M., Saewyc, E., et al. (2015). *Urban and rural student substance use.* Canadian Centre on Substance Abuse. https://apsc-saravyc.sites.olt.ubc.ca/files/2018/04/CCSA-Urban-Rural-Student-Substance-Use-Report-2015-en.pdf; Stackhouse, M.J. (2019). *The Canadian urban-rural health disparity: The role of health lifestyles and an alternative explanation for rurality's higher BMI rates.* Electronic Thesis and Dissertation Repository. 6469. https://ir.lib.uwo.ca/etd/6469

(especially depression), and higher than average incidence of hypertension and arthritis (MacLeod, Kulig, & Stewart, 2019; Stackhouse, 2019).

Community nursing practice, then, is shaped by these needs and settings, where distance, weather, limited resources and supports shape day-to-day practice. The Nursing Practice in Rural and Remote Canada study and the Centre for Rural and Northern Health Research links on the Evolve website provide a more detailed listing of publications and presentations on issues pertaining to rural and remote health care in Canada.

For generations, a scarcity of health care providers, poverty, limited access to services, limited literacy, and physical isolation have plagued many rural communities and contributed to poor health. Ninety-five percent of Canada's land mass is considered rural (Ministerial Advisory Council on Rural Health, 2002). While just over 18% of the total population (just over 6 million) resides in Canada's rural settings, only 8% of the country's physicians practice in rural communities (Wilson et al., 2020). The overall proportion of the population living in rural areas was highest in the Atlantic provinces and in the territories. Provinces in which the proportion of the population living in rural regions was close to or lower than the national average include Quebec (19.4%), Ontario (14.1%), Alberta (16.9%), and British Columbia (13.8%) (Statistics Canada, 2018).

Generally, **rural** is defined either in terms of the geographical location and population density or the distance from or the time needed (e.g., 40 km or 30 minutes) to commute to an urban centre. Some consider rural to be a state of mind. For the more affluent, *rural* may call to mind images of a recreational, retirement, or resort community located in the mountains or in lake country where one can relax and participate in outdoor activities, such as skiing, fishing, hiking, and hunting. For those with fewer resources, the term can evoke desolate scenes.

Travelling time and distance to ambulatory care services affect access to care for both rural and urban residents. For rural people, the difficulty may result from the distance they must travel. For urban people, the difficulty may not result from the distance as much as from the travel time due to traffic. Both groups tend to spend the same length of time waiting once they arrive at a clinic or a physician's office.

Functions and Roles of Rural and Outpost Nurses

From 2008 to 2012, the proportion of regulated nurses working in rural and remote areas remained stable at approximately 13% (Canadian Institute for Health Information [CIHI], 2020). According to CIHI (2020), the number of nurses in rural Canada is inadequate. Low staff turnover and a lack of supervision can be an issue in attracting new nurses to certain rural regions. However, some rural health care providers remain in a community for decades and provide care to people in several surrounding districts. A limited number of CHNs, such as PHNs and NPs, may offer a full range of services to residents in a specified area, which may span more than 150 km. Consequently, rural physicians and

CHNs provide care to individuals and families with all kinds of conditions, in all stages of life, across great distances, and in all regions of Canada.

In the more than 600 First Nations communities across the country, nurses are often the main point of contact with the health care system. There are 76 nursing stations and over 195 health centres in these communities. In about half of these health centres, RNs are employed by Health Canada through its First Nations and Inuit Health Branch. The nurses in other communities are employed by the band council or British Columbia's First Nations Health Authority, because these communities are responsible for health care services through a transfer agreement (Government of Canada, 2020).

Since 2000, research into community health nursing in Canada has found gaps in the continuum of rural mental health services, which, ideally, should include preventive education, anticipatory guidance, early intervention programs, crisis and acute care services, and follow-up care. As with other aspects of health care, CHNs in rural areas play an important role in community health education, case finding, advocacy, and case management. Although rewarding, the experience of living and working as a CHN in a rural or remote area is complex and presents many challenges (Canadian Association for Rural and Remote Nursing, 2020; MacLeod, Kulig, & Stewart, 2019; Martin-Misener, MacLeod, Wilson, et al., 2020). Some of these challenges are outlined in Box 3.9.

BOX 3.9 Rural and Remote Settings: Possible Community Health Nursing Challenges

- Autonomous practice with minimal support
- Complex and variable situations
- Limited number of clinical support resources
- Increased demand for functioning in an expanded role
- Difficulty maintaining the nursing workforce
- Difficulty separating personal and professional roles
- Fewer nurses per capita
- Additional recruitment and retention challenges due to isolation or lack of urban amenities
- Limited opportunity for involvement in research and more effort required to obtain information about evidence-informed practice

Sources: Kosteniuk, J., Stewart, N. J., Wilson, E. C., Penz, K. L., Martin-Misener, R., Morgan, D. G., MacLeod, M. D. P. (2019). Communication tools and sources of education and information: A national survey of rural and remote nurses. *Journal of the Medical Library Association, 107*(4); MacLeod, M., Kulig, J., & Stewart, N. (2019). Lessons from 20 years of research on nursing practice in rural and remote Canada. *Canadian Nurse.* https://www.canadian-nurse.com; Martin-Misener, R., MacLeod, M. L. P., Wilson, E. C., Kosteniuk, J. G., Penz, K. L., Stewart, N. J., Olynick, J., & Karunanayake, C. P. (2020). The mosaic of primary care nurses in rural and remote Canada: Results from a national survey. *Healthcare Policy, 15*(3), 63–75; Penz, K. L., Stewart, N. J., Karunanayake, C. P., Kosteniuk, J. G., & MacLeod, M. L. P. (2019). Competence and confidence in rural and remote nursing practice: A structural equation modelling analysis of national data. *Journal of Clinical Nursing, 6,* 348–366.

Confidence and competence in rural and remote nursing practice are supported in a number of ways, including mentoring, as well as exposure to rural nursing opportunities, establishing a networked work environment, identifying and growing inclusive community factors, and personal indicators of professional well-being (i.e., work engagement, burnout, perceived stress) (Penz Stewart, Karunanayake, et al., 2019).

Four high-risk industries found primarily in rural areas are forestry, mining, fishing, and agriculture. Rural CHNs need to know the exposures and hazards within their communities and refer to the most recent research evidence in order to advocate for patients and initiate appropriate nursing strategies to maintain and promote health and prevent disease.

Barriers to health care may include the availability, accessibility, affordability, and acceptability of services and health care providers to rural patients. *Availability* implies that health care services exist and employ the necessary personnel to provide the services. The sparseness of a population limits the number and array of health care services offered in a given geographical region since the cost of providing special services to a few people is often prohibitive. Additionally, where services and personnel are scarce, they must be allocated wisely. *Accessibility* implies that a person has logistical access to, and the ability to purchase, needed services. Associated with both availability and accessibility, *affordability* implies that services come at a reasonable cost and that a family has sufficient resources to purchase them when needed. *Acceptability* of care means that a particular service is appropriate and offered in a manner that corresponds with the values of a target population. Acceptability can be hampered by both the patient's cultural preferences and the urban orientation of health professions (see Box 3.10).

CHNs' attitudes, insights, and knowledge about rural populations are important to their success in working with those populations. A demeaning attitude, lack of accurate knowledge about rural populations, or insensitivity about the rural lifestyle can diminish a CHN's ability to relate to patients. Moreover, insensitivity generates mistrust, which may cause rural patients to view health care providers as outsiders to the community. On the other hand, some rural CHNs express feelings of being professionally isolated and perceive community nonacceptance. In addressing these rural issues, nursing faculty members can expose students in community health nursing courses to the rural environment by offering rural clinical experiences to help these future health care providers gain insight about rural community health nursing practice.

CHNs need to have an accurate understanding of rural patients. To design community health programs that are available, accessible, affordable, and acceptable, CHNs need to plan strategies and implement interventions that mesh with patients' belief systems. The implication is that family and community actively contribute to the planning and delivery of care as well as advocacy for and the informal case management of a member who needs it. Although the importance of forming partnerships and collaborative practices within a rural community is obvious, most research on rural communities has been a part of policy mandates or stipulations for program funding—without in-depth integration. Currently, minimal empirical data are available on rural family systems in terms of their health beliefs, values, perceptions of illness, health care–seeking behaviours, and beliefs about what constitutes appropriate care. Therefore, CHNs need to assume a more active role in promoting research on the nursing needs of rural populations to expand the profession's theoretical base, to implement empirically based clinical interventions, and to advocate for best practices in rural community health.

Because of the distance, isolation, and sparse resources they encounter, rural residents often develop independent and creative ways to cope. Some prefer to seek help through their informal networks, such as neighbours, extended family, church, and community associations or clubs before seeking care from a health care provider. CHNs describe some interesting differences between working in rural and urban areas. The boundaries between home and work may blur for rural CHNs because they may go to the same church, shop at the same stores, and have children in the same schools as their patients. Thus, CHNs in rural settings personally know many, if not all, patients as neighbours, friends, immediate family members, or part of their extended family. Small towns foster both a social informality and a corresponding lack of anonymity. Some rural CHNs say, "I never really feel like I am off duty because everybody in the area knows me through my work." In part, this may be because community members highly regard CHNs and view them as experts on health and illness. Residents may ask health-related questions when they see the CHN in a grocery store, at a service station, at a basketball game, or at a local function. Rural CHNs may also be expected to know something about everything, which can be demanding. Some of the challenges of rural nursing practice are professional isolation, difficulty separating personal and professional roles, limited opportunities for continuing education, heavy workloads, having to function well in several clinical areas, and the lack of anonymity (MacLeod, Kulig, & Stewart, 2019). Many CHNs value the close relationships they develop with patients and coworkers, the diverse clinical experiences that evolve from caring for patients of all ages with a variety of health concerns, the ability to care for patients

BOX 3.10 Barriers to Health Care in Rural Areas

- Need to travel great distances to obtain services
- Lack of personal transportation
- Limited public transportation
- Lack of telephone services
- Unavailable outreach services
- Unpredictable weather and travel conditions
- Lack of know-how to procure entitlements and services
- Poor health care provider attitudes and understanding about rural populations
- Language barriers (caregivers not linguistically competent)
- Lack of culturally appropriate care and services

for long periods (in some cases, across several generations), greater autonomy, and the pleasures of living in a rural area. CHNs can often keep a finger on the pulse of the community by becoming active in the political, social, religious, and employment activities that affect their patients, and they can work toward change, act as community educators, and educate others on how to find resources and services.

In summary, considering the unique characteristics of rural communities, strategies such as the following are needed to build rural and remote community health nursing practice capacity:

- Ensuring policymakers and managers of community health nursing organizations appreciate CHNs' practice realities
- Developing and implementing interprofessional practice models that build on the varied assets and community resources
- Involving CHNs working in Indigenous communities in the development of strategies
- Implementing ways of ensuring continuity of care and culturally appropriate care in Indigenous communities
- Ensuring undergraduate and postgraduate educational programs prepare nursing students for the realities of community health nursing practice
- Strategically planning continuing education opportunities (mycna.ca/ lists a number of options)
- Addressing the issue of CHNs leaving rural communities
- Improving identifiers used in databases so that rural and remote settings can be distinguished (Penz et al., 2019)

LEVELS OF PREVENTION

Related to Rural and Outpost Nursing
Primary Prevention
A CHN provides reports and works on an advocacy strategy to coordinate for subsidized and affordable fresh vegetables and fruit in the remote community.

Secondary Prevention
A CHN arranges for a plant medicine and food foraging specialist to lead a workshop or local food class in the remote community.

Tertiary Prevention
A CHN provides diabetes teaching and follow-up care in the small town and surrounding community for those diagnosed with type 2 diabetes.

The Nurse Practitioner

Throughout Canada, various team-based primary health care initiatives have been designed and implemented to improve access to and the continuity of care (Côté, Freeman, Jean, et al., 2019). A **nurse practitioner** is an RN with a minimum of graduate-level academic education in advanced-practice nursing. NPs represent the fastest-growing advanced-practice nursing role in Canada (CIHI, 2020).

NPs work collaboratively in health care teams. They may practise as acute care nurse practitioners (ACNPs) or primary

health care nurse practitioners (PHCNPs), although the majority of the approximately 2 500 NPs in the country are PHCNPs (CNA, 2020a). ACNPs specialize in acute care areas, such as cardiology, pediatrics, and oncology, and may provide care at the tertiary level of disease prevention in settings such as outpatient clinics. PHCNPs may have specialized education and training in a particular population, such as family or older persons and work in the community. PHCNPs have been an important part of improving access to health care in communities.

Practice Settings for Primary Health Care Nurse Practitioners

All provinces and territories now have legislation in place for NPs. PHCNPs work in both urban and rural or remote regions of the country in a variety of settings such as community health centres, clinics, urban street projects, outpost stations, urgent care centres, public health units, and long-term care facilities.

Functions and Roles of Nurse Practitioners

In Canada, NPs function in advanced nursing practice roles (CNA, 2020a). NPs' scope of practice includes assessment, diagnosis, and management of patient care for common episodic conditions across the lifespan. These advanced-practice nurses work with families, implement health promotion and disease prevention strategies (primary, secondary, and some tertiary), and participate in community development and planning (CNA, 2020a). Also, they manage and monitor patients with chronic illnesses who reside either in their own homes or in institutions such as long-term care facilities. Each province and territory has implemented or is currently working on implementing NP legislation and regulations and amendments to the nurses' acts to give NPs the authority to independently perform additional controlled acts, such as prescribing certain medications and ordering particular diagnostic and screening tests. It is important to note that NPs complement rather than replace the roles of other health care providers (Côté, Freeman, Jean, et al., 2019). They work in collaboration with patients and with family physicians but practise autonomously. NPs assume the roles of educator, health promoter, collaborator, researcher, consultant, and leader (Marceau, Hunter, Montesanti, et al., 2020).

Entry-level competency categories for Canadian NPs are listed in Box 3.11.

BOX 3.11 Canadian Nurse Practitioner Core Competency Categories

1. Patient Care
2. Quality Improvement and Research
3. Leadership
4. Education

Source: Canadian Nurses Association. (2020). *Nurse practitioners.* https://cna-aiic.ca/en/nursing-practice/the-practice-of-nursing/advanced-nursing-practice/nurse-practitioners

LEVELS OF PREVENTION

Related to Nurse Practitioner Practice
Primary Prevention
An urban clinic NP provides counselling and support for STI prevention in a mobile street clinic available to sex workers and people using intravenous drugs in the urban core.

Secondary Prevention
An urban clinic NP provides a routine screening clinic for hepatitis B and other intravenous or sexually transmitted infections.

Tertiary Prevention
An urban clinic NP provides treatment for sex workers who have hepatitis B and other STIs or skin infections acquired from contaminated intravenous drug paraphernalia.

The Corrections Nurse
Definition of Corrections Nurse

A **corrections nurse** is an RN who works in clinics within correctional facilities. Corrections nurses provide community health nursing interventions that include direct care, health promotion, disease prevention, inmate advocacy, and crisis intervention (Canadian Nurses Association, 2020b). These nursing interventions contribute to the inmates' rehabilitation and successful reintegration into the community.

Practice Settings for Corrections Nurses

Corrections nurses practise in provincial and federal remand centres, forensic psychiatric assessment centres, prisons that involve all levels of security, as well as the minimum and medium security health lodges/centres for Indigenous people who have committed crimes (Correctional Service Canada, 2019). Occasionally, they are involved in international transfer activities for correctional services (e.g., deporting an inmate to another country).

Functions and Roles of Corrections Nurses

The focus of care of corrections nurses is health promotion. A challenge corrections nurses face is ensuring the safety and security of all patients, including both correctional staff and inmates, at all times prior to health care delivery (Cox, 2015). Some of the other challenges of working with this population include maintaining dignity, confidentiality, and therapeutic relationships; addressing complex health issues (e.g., dementia, chronic physical and mental illness/addictions, terminal illnesses); challenging systemic and institutionalized disadvantages (e.g., related to aging, LGBTQ2 experiences, homelessness, and limited literacy or health literacy); and advocating for patients in correctional settings (Cox, 2015; Potter, 2018). Specialized services provided by corrections nurses reflect the needs of the incarcerated population and focus on mental health and substance use interventions (including suicide prevention and methadone programs), infectious

disease prevention and control, enhanced case management, and discharge planning. Corrections nurses work autonomously but collaborate with corrections facility employees and other health care providers (Correctional Service Canada, 2019).

LEVELS OF PREVENTION

Related to Corrections Nursing
Primary Prevention
The corrections nurse supports and refers new inmates to the Elizabeth Fry Society's social support and advocacy program.

Secondary Prevention
The corrections nurse facilitates an emotional regulation group for inmates identified as having chronic distress and emotional deregulation.

Tertiary Prevention
The corrections nurse provides suicide watch protocols and psychiatric medication to an inmate.

The Forensic Nurse
Definition of Forensic Nurse

Forensic nursing is an emerging specialty in Canadian community health nursing. Although CNA does not currently offer certification for this specialty, forensic nurses have had their own interest group within CNA since 2007 (Canadian Forensic Nurses Association, 2020). **Forensic nurses** are RNs who have additional education in forensic science in order to provide specialized care to persons who have experienced trauma or death from violence, criminal activity, or traumatic accidents such as disasters (Valentine, 2014).

Practice Settings for Forensic Nurses

Forensic nurses provide care in general or psychiatric hospitals, health science centres, correctional institutions, or clinics (Valentine, 2014). In Canada, forensic nurses also work as sexual assault nurse examiners. **Sexual assault nurse examiners (SANEs)** are RNs who have completed specialized education in forensic science. They assume a wide range of roles and responsibilities in response to the physical, emotional, and psychological needs of persons who have experienced sexual assault, regardless of age or gender. SANEs provide crisis intervention, assess injuries, provide pregnancy prevention by offering the morning-after pill, test for and treat STIs, and collaborate with community partners (Kagan-Krieger & Rehfeld, 2000).

The first SANE program began in Winnipeg, Manitoba, in 1993, and similar programs have since opened across Canada. In the absence of national standards of practice for SANEs, provincial and program standards have been developed using templates from the International Association of Forensic Nursing for comprehensive sexual assault response in communities (Lynch & Duval, 2011).

Alberta established its first sexual assault response team in Edmonton in 2000. The team comprises 11 nurses with SANE training who are on call 24 hours a day in emergency departments. SANEs conduct sexual assault assessments and collect evidence using a sexual assault evidence kit (Kent, 2000). This kit is a standard tool to collect and handle forensic evidence of deoxyribonucleic acid (DNA). Collection must be completed in a timely and nonjudgemental manner, and SANEs must ensure impartial, precise, and credible documentation of personal assault injury for use in court. See the "CHN in Practice: A Case Study, Sexual Assault Nurse Examiner Practice in the Emergency Department" box. Additionally, the Antigonish Women's Resource Centre website (see the link on the Evolve website) provides further information about a SANE program. SANE education programs, as well as development for various configurations of sexual assault response teams, have emerged throughout Canada, in both urban and rural settings (Carter-Snell, Jakubec, & Hagen, 2020).

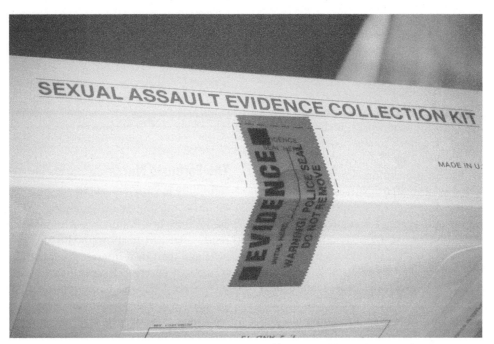

The sexual assault evidence kit includes the following to enable the collection of forensic evidence: bags to collect clothing; oral swabs; envelopes to collect fingernail scrapings or clippings; skin swabs; envelopes for hair samples; blood and urine collection containers; envelopes for the collection of foreign matter (such as condoms and tampons); external, vaginal, and rectal swabs; and a patient DNA kit. (Phototake/THE CANADIAN PRESS)

📋 CHN IN PRACTICE: A CASE STUDY*

Sexual Assault Nurse Examiner Practice in the Emergency Department

Sarah, a 20-year-old female, presents at the emergency department at 5 a.m. She tells the triage nurse that she thinks she was sexually assaulted. The SANE is notified and arrives in a timely manner. The triage nurse has determined that Sarah does not require emergency medical attention. The SANE escorts Sarah to a private and secure location and obtains the following history. Sarah states that she was at a dorm party earlier in the evening. She recalls having two beers and denies any use of illegal substances. Sarah states that she remembers feeling "woozy" and then waking up 3 hours later in her room, naked and alone. She recalls a thick white substance on her inner right thigh and is complaining of genital "soreness." Sarah is nauseated and appears exceptionally anxious as she is unable to recall a portion of the evening's events. Sarah has a steady boyfriend and is sexually active. She has no known allergies, is not on medication, and has a current immunization status.

Think About It

1. What are three primary concerns that Sarah may have?
2. What can a forensic nurse (i.e., a SANE) offer Sarah?
3. What might be an advantage of having a forensic nurse care for Sarah?

*Case study developed by Nancy Horan.

Functions and Roles of Forensic Nurses

Forensic nurses work in four subspecialties—as forensic psychiatric nurses, forensic correctional nurses, forensic nurse examiners, or death investigators working with medical examiners (Lynch & Duval, 2011; Valentine, 2014). Forensic nurses work with victims and perpetrators of violence, especially sexual assault, criminal activity such as physical assault, and traumatic accidents such as suspicious injuries, relationship and family violence, as well as child and elder abuse.

Other Community Health Nurses

The field of community health nursing is expansive and includes many nurses with other designations who practise primary health care, such as street or outreach nurses, telenurses, parish nurses, and nurse entrepreneurs.

The Street or Outreach Nurse

Street nurses are RNs with community health nursing experience. Often PHNs or NPs, these CHNs usually work in community health centres or public health units or authorities, providing extensive outreach to other community sites of care such as shelters or drug and alcohol detoxification centres. These CHNs work with people in urban centres, people of all ages who experience structural vulnerabilities or risks to health related to systemic oppression through power hierarchies, institutional barriers, and economic barriers. Some of the effects of structural vulnerability result in difficulty accessing traditional health care services, homelessness, substance use disorders, and mental illness (Bourgois, Holmes, Sue, et al., 2017). Community mental health and palliative care, as well as acute alcohol or drug detoxification and recovery services are all areas in which CHNs may be employed in street outreach work. These concerns exist in all regions and communities in Canada and affect individuals across the lifespan. The related roles and functions of community mental health nursing are addressed further in Chapter 15.

Street or outreach nurses provide services such as first aid; counselling; referral to community resources such as food banks; needle exchange; immunizations; wound care; testing for STIs; health education and promotion; and advocacy for social issues such as affordable housing, improved social programs to address poverty, and equitable access to health care. Harm reduction approaches are often employed in this work. **Harm reduction** is a strategy used widely in health policy and practice in order to reduce harm to an individual or society by modifying hazardous behaviours that are difficult, and in some cases impossible, to prevent. Harm reduction is discussed further in Chapter 15.

While there are many urban community health centres with street-level services across the country, perhaps one of the best known is the Insite clinic in the downtown East side of Vancouver. Insite is operated by the regional health authority in partnership with a nonprofit community services agency and provides a range of community health care services, including needle exchange, safe injection supervision with harm reduction education, primary nursing care, health and social care referrals, and addiction treatment. The clinic operates daily with an integrated team of RNs, registered psychiatric nurses, mental health workers, and peer workers, and it provides health and social care to thousands of patients per day (Lightfoot, Panessa, Hayden, et al., 2009). Expanding work in this area, harm reduction activist and CHN scholar Marilou Gagnon advocates for safe drug supply across the country, along with improved health and social care for all people who use substances. As a result of her expertise, she has been invited to consult on policy and practice internationally and has won a Registered Nurses Association of Ontario political action award for her efforts (RNAO, 2018).

Cathy Crowe is a street nurse who is well known for her work of more than 30 years in the greater Toronto area in Ontario. Her efforts as a social justice activist have earned her several awards, including the Atkinson Charitable Foundations Economic Justice Award, which funds efforts to reduce poverty (Crowe, 2019), to further develop initiatives for the homeless in Toronto, and to advocate for national housing policies. The Homeless Hub website is also a key resource for street and outreach nurses and includes homelessness information from across Canada. For Homeless Hub infographics on the history and current state of street nursing initiatives in Canada, see the Homeless Hub link on the Evolve website.

The Telenurse

Virtual care has been defined as any interaction between patients and members of their circle of care, occurring remotely, using any forms of communication or information technologies with the aim of facilitating or maximizing the quality and effectiveness of care (Shaw, Jamieson, Agarwal, et al., 2018). The global expansion of virtual care has increased and the tools and technologies put to widespread use during the COVID-19 pandemic.

Telehealth refers to the use of information technology to deliver health care services at a distance. Technology includes telephones and computers (e.g., email, and audio and video conferencing). Consider the example of a patient with later stage cancer who lives in a remote village in western Newfoundland. Telehealth would give her the opportunity to have a consultation with an oncologist using video conferencing without having to bear the expense and suffering of travel to an urban centre. Home health or palliative nurses may be able to participate in the conferencing, and the interprofessional team can collaborate on a plan of care (Sevean, Dampier, Spadoni, et al., 2009).

In Canada, telenursing refers to the use of virtual care technologies for triaging, delivering nursing care, and managing and coordinating health care and services using protocols (College of Nurses of Ontario, 2020; Rush, Hatt, Janke, et al., 2018). According to CNA (2017, p. 1), nursing practice in telehealth includes all patient-centred forms of nursing practice and the provision of information and education for health care professionals occurring through, or facilitated by, the use of telecommunications or electronic means. **Telenurses** are RNs who require specific nursing knowledge and skill that includes enhanced assessment skills and strong clinical knowledge necessary to provide nursing service to patients using only information technology (College of Nurses of Ontario, 2020).

Proven cost-effective in countries such as the United States and Japan, telehealth is emerging rapidly in Canada, as it serves to address the accessibility and availability issues in our geographically vast country (Gagnon, Paré, Pollender, et al., 2011). CHNs working in telenursing use evidence-informed protocols and technology-based, standardized responses to address patient health concerns. One of the challenges for telenurses is the fact that among their patients are persons travelling outside of their home province or territory, which means that telenurses frequently serve persons who are not in the same province or territory. Since provincial and territorial practice standards vary, possible inconsistencies, inaccuracies, and liability issues arise. This state of cross-jurisdictional health care is being discussed across Canada. The College of Nurses of Ontario (2020) advises telenurses to ensure clear, complete documentation that demonstrates their decision making since they may be required to testify in another jurisdictional community. In 2003, the National Initiative for Telehealth developed a framework of recommendations including telehealth policies, procedures, guidelines, and standards for various Canadian health care provider organizations. The guidelines and principles for telenursing practice standards developed by the College of Registered Nurses of British Columbia and the College of Registered Nurses of Nova Scotia are available through links on the Evolve website.

The First Nations Nurse

First Nations nurses practise in urban settings as well as semirural, rural, and remote settings. This role is distinct from that of the outpost nurse (which is more defined by distance, technology, resource scarcity, and so on). Rather, First Nations nurses are defined by cultural and organizational/sociopolitical concerns and resource allocation, related public health issues, and a population facing community health situations shaped by colonization and intergenerational trauma and grief (explored further in Chapter 14) (National Collaborating Centre for Indigenous Health, 2015). The outpost nurse works directly with Indigenous patients as well as non-Indigenous patients who live in a remote town or region. By contrast, the First Nations nurse works first and foremost with the band. First Nations nurses may be employed by Health Canada, directly by the band (through transfer payments from the federal government), or in British Columbia by the First Nations Health Authority. CHNs in this capacity work in First Nations communities to provide evidence-informed and culturally safe nursing practice to enhance the health of First Nations people (Government of Canada, 2020).

The Parish Nurse

A **parish nurse** is "a registered nurse with specialized knowledge, who is called to ministry and affirmed by a faith community to promote health, healing and wholeness" (Canadian Association for Parish Nursing Ministry [CAPNM], 2015). Parish nurses usually have additional education in pastoral care and social sciences and use all the knowledge and skills of this community health nursing specialty to provide effective services. Parish nurses strive for a truly caring congregation that supports healthy, spiritually fulfilling lives.

Members of faith congregations, like other people, experience life events such as birth, death, acute and chronic illness, stress, dependency concerns, challenges of life transitions, growth and development, and decisions regarding healthy lifestyle choices. **Faith communities** are distinct groups of people who acknowledge specific faith traditions and gather in churches, cathedrals, synagogues, or mosques. Parish nurses work within faith congregations, including communities that serve diverse cultures. They also serve faith communities in other countries. **Parish nursing** is nursing care provided in the faith community to promote whole-person health among parishioners (CAPNM, 2015).

A parish nurse views **holistic care** as the interaction of the body, mind, and spirit in the promotion of holistic wellness. Parish nurses respond to the health and wellness needs of populations of faith communities and are partners with the church in fulfilling the mission of health ministry. The Canadian Association for Parish Nursing Ministry (CAPNM, 2015) has developed core competencies for parish nursing as guidelines for practice. Currently, CNA does not offer certification status to parish nurses. Parish nurses work closely with other health care providers, **pastoral care staff** (faith community leaders, including clergy, nurses, and educational and youth ministry staff), and lay volunteers who represent various aspects of the life of the congregational community.

In addition to serving congregations in the community, parish nurses may be employed by older-adult living complexes and long-term care facilities that offer a spiritual focus to the nursing practice. Some of the usual functions of parish nurses include providing personal health counselling and health education, acting as a liaison between the faith community and the local community, facilitating activities, and providing pastoral care. They make visits to homes, hospitals, and long-term care facilities, and see persons in the faith community's house of worship. Some parish nurses have designated offices; others work in a variety of locations in response to patient needs.

The Nurse Entrepreneur

The **nurse entrepreneur** is an RN who is self-employed in the provision of nursing services to patients in the community or in a variety of settings such as workplaces, government agencies, nonprofit agencies, and private businesses. Nurse entrepreneurs may be generalists (e.g., a primary health care nurse practitioner working in an independent practice) or specialists (e.g., a nurse offering foot-care clinics, insurance company health assessments, or medical-legal consulting). The College of Nurses of Ontario (2019) identifies the following key practice components nurse entrepreneurs in independent practice must consider:

- Scope of service
- Conflict of interest
- Endorsement
- Advertising
- Fees
- Informed consent
- Documentation
- Confidentiality
- Other issues and resources (business considerations)

STUDENT EXPERIENCE

The Evolve website includes seven blogs* by a variety of CHNs about their typical day of practice. The CHNs showcased work in a variety of urban and rural settings, including a public health unit, a home care agency (e.g., Victorian Order of Nurses or Community Care Access), a workplace, and an outpatient clinic. As you read these blogs, identify and compare their roles, functions, and scope of practice, and relate their experience to what you have read about their specialization in this text. Select two of the blogs and answer the following questions:

1. What clinical setting does this CHN work in?
2. What are the educational qualifications for this CHN position?
3. What are examples of this CHN's activities that demonstrate the three levels of prevention (if applicable)?
4. What roles does this CHN have?

5. How do this CHN's roles differ from acute-based nursing practice roles?
6. What skills are required for this CHN role?
7. How are the CHN's roles of collaboration and coordination visible in the scenarios presented?
8. To what extent does this CHN provide care for individual, family, and group patients?
9. State one research question pertaining to community health nursing that arose based on the CHN's experiences and your readings. For example, a research question might be: Does a mother who breastfeeds bond faster with her new baby than a mother who does not breastfeed? Select one refereed journal article that addresses your research question. Reflect on and document the relevance of this article to a community experience that you have had or that you have read about in the blogs.

*The blogs in this exercise were developed for the Laurentian University School of Nursing Distance Education Program.

CHAPTER SUMMARY

3.1 The care and counselling functions of community health nursing include risk assessment and response, supportive counselling, and a variety of skilled therapeutic interventions.

3.2 Continuity of care is a goal of community health nursing. It requires making linkages with services to improve the patient's health status. CHNs need to be aware of the principles, steps, and barriers in the referral process. Discharge planning and the referral process promote continuity of care for all patients in the community.

3.3 Health education and literacy and health literacy assessment are undertaken by the CHN to promote, maintain, and improve health.

3.4 CHNs collaborate with many partners using a population health approach to protect and promote health and prevent disease in populations. Team building and collaboration are functions of community development. In collaborating, health care providers should be attentive to options for change and improvement and adjust the plan of care as required.

3.5 Consultation with a range of stakeholders and decision makers are both central CHN leadership activities.

3.6 Research and evaluation (such as screening and surveillance) are important functions of the CHN in all roles and settings. CHN practice is evidence-informed and continually evolving.

3.7 Health advocacy involves creating awareness of health issues by interacting with patients and families, as well as other health care providers, and working through the broader health system.

3.8 Case management involves coordinating care; ensuring continuity of care; identifying changes in the patient's condition; evaluating the care being delivered in association with health care team members; and being aware

of and understanding the financial implications of the care plan. Case management is typically an interprofessional process in which the patient is the focus of the care plan.

3.9 HHNs usually provide care in the patient's home environment. Family forms an integral part of home health nursing and includes any caregiver or significant person who takes responsibility in assisting a patient in need of care at home. Interprofessional collaboration is also critical in the home health care and hospice settings.

3.10 PHNs work in a variety of settings and have many functions and roles such as those of advocate, manager, educator, consultant, and facilitator. Public health is focused on societal health.

3.11 OHNs focus on worker and workplace assessment and surveillance, case management, health promotion, primary care, management or administration, and evidence-informed practice. Workplace hazards include exposure to biological and infectious, chemical, enviro-mechanical, physical, and psychosocial hazards.

3.12 Rural and outpost nurses work in a community health nursing role to provide comprehensive primary health care to patients in rural, remote, and northern outpost communities. The health status of rural populations depends on genetic, social, environmental, economic, and political factors that are shaped by different conditions than those of urban populations. Barriers to rural health care include a lack of availability, affordability, accessibility, and acceptability of services.

3.13 PHCNPs have been an important part of the development of improving access to health care in communities.

They provide a full range of comprehensive health services within a designated community area.

3.14 Corrections nurses work in clinics within correctional facilities. They provide community health nursing interventions to patients who are remanded, incarcerated, or paroled.

3.15 Forensic nurses work with victims and perpetrators of violence, especially sexual assault, criminal activity such as physical assault, and traumatic accidents.

3.16 Other examples of CHN roles are street or outreach nurses, telenurses, First Nations nurses, parish nurses, and nurse entrepreneurs.

CHN IN PRACTICE: A CASE STUDY

Rural Palliative Care Practice

Sally is in the terminal stages of breast cancer and lives on a farm in a small rural community. You have been visiting Sally weekly for the past 6 weeks. Sally is a 30-year-old married mother of a 10-year-old daughter named Brittney. You are the HHN who has been the direct care provider for Sally in her home. The following palliative care team members are also involved with the family: palliative care volunteers and a homemaker, physiotherapist, chaplain, family physician, pharmacist, dietitian, and social worker.

Sally has been told that there are no new options for palliative treatment, and she is preparing to die at home with the support of you, her palliative care team, community members, and family. While Sally accepts the terminal condition, she is experiencing stress and sadness that you are discussing it with her for her own problem solving and reflection.

Think About It

1. Reflect on the experiences you have had with death and dying. What values and beliefs do you hold about death and dying? How can you interact with Sally in a way that demonstrates your self-awareness while still holding Sally's situation as the primary focus of your care?
2. Based on this situation, what possible family health concerns can you identify? How might you support the family in the end-of-life experience?
3. Consider the roles of each of the palliative care team members, the family, and community members. How will you work collaboratively with this team?

TOOL BOX

The Tool Box contains useful resources that can be applied to community health nursing practice. These resources appear either in the appendices at the back of this text or on the Evolve website at http://evolve.elsevier.com/Canada/Stanhope/community/.

Appendices

- Appendix 1: Canadian Community Health Nursing Standards of Practice
- Appendix E.1: Comprehensive Occupational and Environmental Health History
- Appendix E.2: Work-Site Assessment Guide

Tools

ActNow BC. Creating a Healthy Workplace Environment Workbook and Toolkit. (https://www.health.gov.bc.ca/library/publications/year/2006/Creating-healthy-workplace-environment-workbook.pdf)

This resource assists health care providers in developing activities to improve the health of workers in their workplaces.

Institute for Work and Health. MSD Prevention Guideline. (https://www.iwh.on.ca/publications/msd-prevention-series)

This site provides information on the prevention and reduction of musculoskeletal disorders (MSD); guidelines for employers are available.

REFERENCES

Bjornsdottir, K. (2018). "I try to make a net around each patient": Home care nursing as relational practice. *Scandinavian Journal of Caring Sciences, 32*(1), 177–185.

Bourgois, M., Holmes, M., Sue, M., et al. (2017). Structural vulnerability: Operationalizing the concept to address health disparities in clinical care. *Academic Medicine, 92*(3), 299–307.

Campos-Outcalt, D. (1994). Occupational health epidemiology and objectives for the year 2000: Primary care, clinics in office practice. *Occupational Health, 21*(20), 213 [Seminal Reference].

Canadian Association for Parish Nursing Ministry. (2015). *Standards of practice.* https://www.capnm.ca/about/standards/.

Canadian Association for Rural and Remote Nursing. (2020). *About.* https://www.carrn.com/index.php/about.

Canadian Forensic Nurses Association. (2020). *About.* http://forensicnurse.ca/about/.

Canadian Home Care Association. (2012). *Health systems integration: Synthesis report.* http://www.cdnhomecare.ca.

Canadian Home Care Association. (2019). *Home care lens for policy and program: Facilitating collaboration and integrating care.* https://cdnhomecare.ca/wp-content/uploads/2020/03/CHCA-HomeCareLens_2020.pdf.

Canadian Hospice Palliative Care Association. (2006). *The pan-Canadian gold standard for palliative home care: Toward equitable access to high quality hospice palliative and end-of-life care at home.* https://www.chpca.ca/wp-content/uploads/2019/12/Gold_Standards_Palliative_Home_Care.pdf.

Canadian Hospice Palliative Care Association & Canadian Nurses Association. (2015). *Joint position statement: The palliative approach to care and the role of the nurse.* https://www.cna-aiic.ca/~/media/cna/page-content/pdf-en/the-palliative-approach-to-care-and-the-role-of-the-nurse_e.pdf.

Canadian Indigenous Nurses Association. (2019). *About us.* https://indigenousnurses.ca/about.

Canadian Institute for Health Information. (2020). *Nursing in Canada, 2019.* https://www.cihi.ca/en/nursing-in-canada-2019.

Canadian Nurses Association. (2013). *Optimizing the role of nursing in home health.* https://cna-aiic.ca/~/media/cna/page-content/pdf-en/optimizing_the_role_of_nursing_in_home_health_e.pdf?la=en.

Canadian Nurses Association. (2017). *Fact sheet: Telehealth.* https://www.cna-aiic.ca/-/media/cna/page-content/pdf-en/telehealth-fact-sheet.pdf?la=en&hash=AB1B315626AF74B3A3E1A2D7DB46001BE23E2238.

Canadian Nurses Association. (2018). *Position statement: Evidence-based decision-making and nursing practice.* https://www.cna-aiic.ca/-/media/cna/page-content/pdf-en/evidence-informed-decision-making-and-nursing-practice-position-statement_dec-2018.pdf.

Canadian Nurses Association. (2020a). *Nurse practitioners.* https://cna-aiic.ca/en/nursing-practice/the-practice-of-nursing/advanced-nursing-practice/nurse-practitioners.

Canadian Nurses Association. (2020b). *Nursing in Canada's correctional system.* https://www.cna-aiic.ca/en/nursing-practice/evidence-based-practice/nursing-in-canadas-correctional-system.

Canadian Occupational Health Nurses Association. (2018). *Information booklet.* http://cohna-aciist.ca/wp-content/uploads/2018/09/COHNA-ACIIST-Information-Booklet-E-2018.pdf.

Canadian Public Health Association. (1990). *Community health—public health nursing in Canada: Preparation and practice.*

Canadian Public Health Association. (2010). *Public Health—community health nursing practice in Canada: Roles and activities* (4th ed.). https://www.cpha.ca/sites/default/files/assets/pubs/3-1bk04214.pdf.

Carter-Snell, C., Jakubec, S., & Hagen, B. (2020). Collaboration with rural and remote communities to improve sexual assault services. *Journal of Community Health, 45*(2), 377–387.

College of Nurses of Ontario. (2019). *Practice guideline: Independent practice.* https://www.cno.org/globalassets/docs/prac/41011_fsindepprac.pdf.

College of Nurses of Ontario. (2020). *Practice guideline: Telepractice.* https://www.cno.org/globalassets/docs/prac/41041_telephone.pdf.

College of Registered Nurses of British Columbia. (2016). *Conflict of interest.* https://www.crnbc.ca/Standards/PracticeStandards/pages/conflictofinterest.aspx.

Community Health Nurses of Canada. (2009). *Public health nursing discipline specific competencies version 1.0.* https://www.chnc.ca/en/competencies.

Community Health Nurses of Canada. (2010). *Home health nursing competencies version 1.0.* https://www.chnc.ca/en/competencies.

Community Health Nurses of Canada. (2019). *Canadian community health nursing professional practice model and standards of practice.* https://www.chnc.ca/en/standards-of-practice.

Correctional Service Canada. (2019). *Correctional Services Canada healing lodges.* https://www.csc-scc.gc.ca/aboriginal/002003-2000-en.shtml.

Costante, A., Lawand, C., & Cheng, C. (2019). Access to palliative care in Canada. *Healthcare Quarterly, 21*(4), 10–12.

Côté, N., Freeman, A., Jean, E., et al. (2019). New understanding of primary health care nurse practitioner role optimisation: The dynamic relationship between the context and work meaning. *BMC Health Services Research, 19*(1), 882.

Cox, S. (2015). Nursing on the inside. *Let's Talk, 29*(3). https://www.csc-scc.gc.ca/text/pblct/lt-en/2004/no3/33-eng.shtml.

Crowe, C. (2019). *A knapsack full of dreams: Memoirs of a street nurse.* Friesen Press.

Daiski, J. (2000). The road to professionalism in nursing: Case management or practice based in nursing theory. *Nursing Science Quarterly, 13*(1), 74–79.

Department of Health and Community Services of Newfoundland and Labrador. (2019). *Chronic disease self-management program for Newfoundland and Labrador.* https://www.health.gov.nl.ca/health/chronicdisease/cdcontrol.html#self.

Durocher, E., Kinsella, E., Gibson, B., et al. (2019). Engaging older adults in discharge planning: Case studies illuminating approaches adopted by family members that promote relational autonomy. *Disability & Rehabilitation, 41*(25), 3005–3015.

Franek, J. (2013). *Self-management support interventions for persons with chronic disease: An evidence-based analysis.* Health Quality Ontario. https://www.ncbi.nlm.nih.gov/pmc/articles/PMC3814807/.

Gagnon, M., Paré, G., Pollender, H., et al. (2011). Supporting work practices through telehealth: Impact on nurses in peripheral regions. *BMC Health Services Research, 11*(1), 27. https://doi.org/10.1186/1472-6963-11-27.

Garasia, S., & Dobbs, G. (2019). Socioeconomic determinants of health and access to health care in rural Canada. *University of Toronto Medical Journal, 96*(2), 44–46.

Gilmour, H. (2018). *Formal home care use in Canada.* Statistics Canada. https://www150.statcan.gc.ca/n1/en/pub/82-003-x/2018009/article/00001-eng.pdf?st=O2meAtvq.

Government of Canada. (2020). *Indigenous health.* https://www.sac-isc.gc.ca/eng/1569861171996/1569861324236.

Hahn-Goldberg, S., Jeffs, L., Troup, A., et al. (2018). "We are doing it together"; the integral role of caregivers in a patients' transition home from the medicine unit. *PloS One, 13*(5), e0197831. https://doaj.org/article/4fa80ebac37540aba64ae5f2c6af7c5b.

Health Canada. (2018). *Framework on palliative care in Canada.* https://www.canada.ca/content/dam/hc-sc/documents/services/health-care-system/reports-publications/palliative-care/framework-palliative-care-canada/framework-palliative-care-canada.pdf.

Health Prince Edward Island. (2020). *Improving the flow and care of patients.* https://www.princeedwardisland.ca/en/information/health-pei/improving-the-flow-and-care-of-patients.

Herleman, L. (2008). Home care primary nurse case management model. *Home Health Care Management & Practice, 20*(3), 235–244 [Seminal Reference].

Hoffman-Goetz, L., Donelle, L., & Ahmed, R. (2014). *Health literacy in Canada: A primer for students.* Canadian Scholars' Press.

Holland, D., Knafl, G., & Bowles, K. (2013). Targeting hospitalised patients for early discharge planning intervention. *Journal of Clinical Nursing, 22*(19–20), 2696–2703.

Hospital Association, O. (2017). *Rural health hub implementation guide.* https://www.oha.com/health-system-transformation/rural-health-hubs.

Hyman, I., Gucciardi, E., Patychuk, D., et al. (2014). Self-management, health service use and information seeking for diabetes care among Black Caribbean immigrants in Toronto. *Canadian Journal of Diabetes, 38*(1), 32–37.

International Council of Nurses. (2010). *Promoting health: Advocacy guide for health professionals.* [Seminal Reference]. http://www.whcaonline.org/uploads/publications/ICN-NEW-28.3.2010.pdf.

Jakubec, S. L., & Astle, B. J. (2017). *Research literacy for health and community practice.* Canadian Scholars' Press.

Jensen, E., Forchuk, C., Seymour, B., et al. (2009). *An evaluation of community based discharge planning –SEEI Phase II report.* https://collections.ola.org/mon/23010/294290.pdf.

Kagan-Krieger, S., & Rehfeld, G. (2000). The sexual assault nurse examiner. *Canadian Nurse, 96*(6), 20–25.

Kelly, P., Vottero, B., & Christie-McAuliffe, C. (2018). *Introduction to quality and safety education for nurses: Core competencies for nursing leadership and management* (2nd ed.). Springer.

Kent, H. (2000). SANE nurses staff Alberta's sexual assault response team. *Canadian Medical Association Journal, 162*(5), 683–684.

Kosteniuk, J., Stewart, N. J., Wilson, E. C., et al. (2019). Communication tools and sources of education and information: A national survey of rural and remote nurses. *Journal of the Medical Library Association, 107*(4).

Lightfoot, B., Panessa, C., Hayden, S., et al. (2009). Gaining Insite: Harm reduction in nursing practice. *Canadian Nurse, 105*(4), 16–22.

Lynch, V. A., & Duval, J. B. (2011). *Forensic nursing science.* Elsevier/Mosby.

MacLeod, M., Kulig, J., & Stewart, N. (2019). *Lessons from 20 years of research on nursing practice in rural and remote Canada.* Canadian Nurse. https://www.canadian-nurse.com/en/articles/issues/2019/may-2019/lessons-from-20-years-of-research-on-nursing-practice-in-rural-and-remote-canada.

Marceau, R., Hunter, K., Montesanti, S., et al. (2020). Sustaining primary health care programs and services: A scoping review informing the nurse practitioner role in Canada. *Policy, Politics, & Nursing Practice,* 1527154420923738. https://doi.org/10.1177/1527154420923738.

Martin-Misener, R., MacLeod, M. L. P., Wilson, E. C., et al. (2020). The mosaic of primary care nurses in rural and remote Canada: Results from a national survey. *Healthcare Policy, 15*(3), 63–75.

McInnis, O. A., Young, M. M., Saewyc, E., et al. (2015). *Urban and rural student substance use.* Canadian Centre on Substance Abuse. https://apsc-saravyc.sites.olt.ubc.ca/files/2018/04/CCSA-Urban-Rural-Student-Substance-Use-Report-2015-en.pdf.

McKnight, J., & Block, P. (2010). The *abundant community: Awakening the power of families and neighborhoods.* Berrett-Koehler.

Mental Health Commission of Canada. (2013). *National standard of Canada for psychological health and safety in the workplace.* http://www.mentalhealthcommission.ca/English/issues/workplace/national-standard.

Ministerial Advisory Council on Rural Health. (2002). *Rural health in rural hands: Strategic directions for rural, remote, northern and Aboriginal communities.* https://publications.gc.ca/collections/Collection/H39-657-2002E.pdf.

Misener, R. M., MacLeod, M. L. P., Banks, K., et al. (2008). There's rural, and then there's "rural": Advice from nurses providing primary healthcare in northern remote communities. *Nursing Leadership, 21*(3), 54–63 [Seminal Reference].

National Case Management Network. (2009). *Canadian standards of practice for case management.* http://www.ncmn.ca/resources/documents/english%20standards%20for%20web.pdf.

National Collaborating Centre for Indigenous Health. (2015). *Review of core competencies for public health: An Aboriginal public health perspective.* https://www.nccih.ca/495/Review_of_Core_Competencies_for_Public_Health__An_Aboriginal_Public_Health_Perspective.nccih?id=145.

National Collaborating Centre for Methods and Tools. (2020). *About us.* https://www.nccmt.ca/.

Nies, M. A., & McEwan, M. (2019). *Community/public health nursing: Promoting the health of populations.* Elsevier.

Noseworthy, A., Sevigny, E., Laizner, A., et al. (2014). Mental health care professionals' experiences with the discharge planning process and transitioning patients attending outpatient clinics into community care. *Archives of Psychiatric Nursing, 28*(4), 263–271.

Nurture Development. (2018). *About ABCD.* https://www.nurturedevelopment.org/about-abcd/.

Ontario Ministry of Health and Long-Term Care. (2018a). *Home and community care.* http://www.health.gov.on.ca/en/public/programs/lhin/.

Ontario Ministry of Health and Long-Term Care. (2018b). *Ontario public health standards.* http://www.health.gov.on.ca/en/pro/programs/publichealth/oph_standards/docs/protocols_guidelines/Ontario_Public_Health_Standards_2018_en.pdf.

Orem, D. E. (1995). *Nursing: Concepts of practice* (3rd ed.). Mosby. [Seminal Reference].

Öresland, S., Lutzén, K., Norberg, A., et al. (2013). Nurses as "guests"– a study of a concept in light of Jacques Derrida's philosophy of hospitality. *Nursing Philosophy, 14*(2), 117–126.

Peate, I. (2013). The community nurse and the use of social media. *British Journal of Community Nursing, 18*(4), 180–185. https://doi.org/10.12968/bjcn.2013.18.4.180. https://www.magonlinelibrary.com/doi/abs/10.12968/bjcn.2013.18.4.180.

Penz, K. L., Stewart, N. J., Karunanayake, C. P., et al. (2019). Competence and confidence in rural and remote nursing practice: A structural equation modelling analysis of national data. *Journal of Clinical Nursing, 6,* 348–366.

Potter, R. H. (2018). Why are we (still) discussing correctional health and the community? *Journal of Health and Human Services Administration, 41*(3), 285.

Public Health Agency of Canada. (2018). *Health literacy and public health.* https://www.cpha.ca/health-literacy-and-public-health.

Public Health Association of BC. (2012). *An inter-sectoral approach for improving health literacy for Canadians.* http://phabc.org/wp-content/uploads/2015/09/IntersectoralApproachforHealthLiteracy-FINAL.pdf.

Registered Nurses Association of Ontario. (2014). *Clinical best practice guidelines: Care transitions.* https://rnao.ca/sites/rnao-ca/files/Care_Transitions_BPG.pdf.

Registered Nurses Association of Ontario. (2018). *RNAO leadership award in political action: Marilou Gagnon.* https://rnao.ca/content/rnao-leadership-award-political-action-marilou-gagnon.

Rogers, B. (2007). *Occupational and environmental health nursing: Concepts and practice.* W. B. Saunders. [Seminal Reference].

Rush, K., Hatt, L., Janke, R., et al. (2018). The efficacy of telehealth delivered educational approaches for patients with chronic diseases: A systematic review. (Report). *Patient Education and Counseling, 101*(8), 1310–1321.

Saint Elizabeth Health Care. (2020). *Our history.* https://sehc.com/about/our-history.

Savage, C. (2020). *Public/community health and nursing practice: Caring for populations* (2nd ed.). F.A. Davis Company.

Sevean, P., Dampier, S., Spadoni, M., et al. (2009). Patients and families experiences with video telehealth in rural/remote communities in Northern Canada. *Journal of Clinical Nursing, 18*(18), 2573–2579 [Seminal Reference].

Shaw, J., Jamieson, T., Agarwal, P., et al. (2018). Virtual care policy recommendations for patient-centred primary care: Findings of a consensus policy dialogue using a nominal group technique. *Journal of Telemedicine and Telecare, 24*(9), 608–615.

Stackhouse, M. J. (2019). *The Canadian urban - rural health disparity: The role of health lifestyles and an alternative explanation for rurality's higher BMI rates*. Electronic Thesis and Dissertation Repository. 6469. https://ir.lib.uwo.ca/etd/6469.

Stanhope, M., & Lancaster, J. (2019). *Public health nursing: Population-centred health care in the community* (10th ed.). Mosby.

Statistics Canada. (2014). *Canadian community health survey, 2014*. http://www12.statcan.gc.ca/census-recensement/2011/as-sa/98-310-x/98-310-x2011001-eng.cfm.

Statistics Canada. (2018). *Canada megatrends: Canada goes urban*. https://www150.statcan.gc.ca/n1/pub/11-630-x/11-630-x2015004-eng.htm.

Tarlier, D., Johnson, J., & Whyte, N. (2003). Voices from the wilderness: An interpretive study describing the role and practice of outpost nurses. *Canadian Journal of Public Health*, *94*(3), 180–184 [Seminal Reference].

Valentine, L. (2014). Why we do what we do: A theoretical evaluation of the integrated practice model for forensic nursing science. *Journal of Forensic Nursing, 10*(3), 113–119.

Victorian Order of Nurses. (2020). *More than a century of caring*. https://www.von.ca/en/history.

Whelan, N., Steenbeek, A., Martin-Misener, R., et al. (2014). Engaging parents and schools improves uptake of the human papillomavirus (HPV) vaccine: Examining the role of the public health nurse. *Vaccine, 32*(36), 4665–4671.

Wilson, C., Rourke, J., Oandasan, I., et al. (2020). Progress made on access to rural health care in Canada. *Canadian Family Physician, 66*(1), 31–36.

World Health Organization. (2004). *A glossary of terms for community health care and services for older persons*. [Seminal Reference] http://www.who.int/kobe_centre/ageing/ahp_vol5_glossary.pdf.

World Health Organization. (2020). *WHO definition of palliative care*. https://www.who.int/cancer/palliative/definition/en/.

Yoder-Wise, P., Waddel, J. I., & Walton, N. A. (2020). *Yoder-Wise's leading and managing in Canadian nursing* (2nd ed.). Elsevier.

Community Health Foundations and Principles

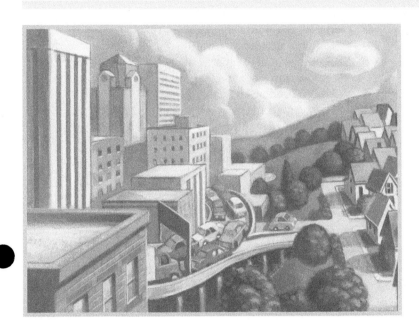

4

Health Promotion

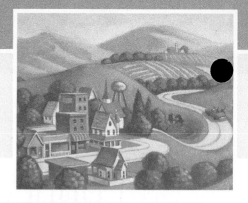

OUTLINE

Promotion of Health, 85
   Development of the Concept of Health, 85
   Foundational Concepts in Health Promotion, 86
Evolution of Health Promotion, 90
   Lalonde Report, 90
   Alma-Ata Declaration, 90
   World Health Organization Principles of
     Health Promotion, 92
   Ottawa Charter for Health Promotion, 92
   Epp Report: A Canadian Framework for Health
     Promotion, 93
   Developments in Health Promotion, 93
   Population Health Promotion Model, Revisited, 94
   International Health Promotion Conferences, 95
   Summary of the Evolution of Health Promotion, 96
Health Promotion Models, Theories, and Frameworks, 96
   Individual-Focused Perspectives, 97
   Community-Focused Perspectives, 98
   Public Policy–Focused Perspectives, 100
   Ecological Models, 100

Existential and Humanistic Theoretical Perspectives, 101
Health Promotion Approaches, 101
   Biomedical Approach, 101
   Behavioural Approach, 101
   Socioenvironmental Approach, 101
Health Promotion Strategies, 102
   Strengthening Community Action, 103
   Building Healthy Public Policy, 105
   Creating Supportive Environments, 106
   Developing Personal Skills, 106
   Health Literacy, 107
   Reorienting Health Services, 108
   Activities to Facilitate Health Promotion Strategies, 108
   Mutual Aid, 109
   Advocacy, 109
Health Promotion Skills, 109
   Working With Focus Groups, 110
   Preparing Funding Applications, 110
   Developing Health Promotion Capacity, 110

OBJECTIVES

After reading this chapter, you should be able to:

4.1 Describe the development of the concept of health and distinguish between foundational concepts in health promotion.

4.2 Identify significant Canadian and international milestones in the development of health promotion.

4.3 Describe key health promotion models, theories, and frameworks, and explain their use in community health nursing.

4.4 Compare the biomedical, behavioural, and socioenvironmental approaches to health promotion.

4.5 Identify health promotion strategies and how, when, and where they would be used.

4.6 Describe health promotion skills that community health nurses can develop and use in their practice.

KEY TERMS*

advocacy, 109
capacity building, 104
community development, 103
community mobilization, 103
disease, 86
disease course, 86
disease prevention, 86
enabling, 85
harm reduction, 88
health, 86
health enhancement, 87

health literacy, 107
health protection, 86
healthy public policy, 87
illness, 86
injury prevention, 86
protective factors, 89
resiliency, 89
risk avoidance, 87
risk factors, 89
risk reduction, 87

*See the Glossary on page 468 for definitions.

Over the past four decades, the approach to health taken in Canada has changed from a biomedical approach to a population health promotion model. Canada has received recognition as a leader in the health promotion movement globally, a process that started with the release of *A New Perspective on the Health of Canadians,* commonly referred to as the Lalonde Report (Lalonde, 1974), followed by the framework by Epp (1986) titled *Achieving Health for All. Health promotion,* as outlined in the Ottawa Charter for Health Promotion, is a strategy to improve health and is defined as "enabling people to increase control over, and to improve, their health" (World Health Organization [WHO], 1986). As recently as 2010, Canada reinforced its commitment to a health promotion model when all 14 of Canada's health ministers collectively declared their vision to work together with "non-profit, municipal, academic and community sectors and with First Nations, Inuit and Metis peoples to … promote health and wellness…so that Canadians can enjoy good health for years to come" (PHAC, 2010, p. 1). Health promotion applies to the patient as individual, family, aggregate or group, population, community, or society and involves enabling the patient to stay healthy. The use of the term *enabling* marked the beginning of the conceptualization of empowerment (discussed in Chapter 1) as a component of health promotion. **Enabling**, within health promotion, refers to taking action with patients to empower them to gain control over their health and environment with the goal of improving their health.

Optimizing population health and maintaining healthy environments that support the achievement of patient health goals require the implementation of health promotion strategies such as strengthening community action, building healthy public policy, creating supportive environments, developing personal skills, and reorienting health services. Health promotion models, frameworks, and activities such as advocacy, health communication and social marketing, and mutual aid are some of the tools community health nurses (CHNs) use to implement these strategies.

This chapter discusses the concept of health promotion and its use by CHNs. It also introduces select health promotion theories, frameworks, models, strategies, and tools. The topic of health promotion is extensive; for the purposes of this text, the areas in which CHNs play key roles will be discussed, including healthy public policy, community-based action, public participation and advocacy or action on the determinants of health, and health equity (CPHA, 2010).

PROMOTION OF HEALTH

CHNs promote health in environmental, political, and social contexts. CHNs use the nursing process to assess, plan, intervene, and evaluate their practice from a micro level (i.e., individual and family) to a macro level (i.e., systems and society). In their values and beliefs, CHNs incorporate caring, principles of primary health care, multiple ways of knowing, individual and community partnerships, environmental influence, and empowerment. As well, CHNs use the *Canadian Community Health Nursing Professional Practice Model and Standards of Practice* (CCHN Standards) in all community health nursing

practice settings. The CCHN Standards are health promotion; prevention and health protection; health maintenance, restoration, and palliation; professional relationships; capacity building; access and equity; and professional responsibility and accountability (see Appendix 1).

Throughout this text, the term *community health nursing process* is used to refer to the process by which CHNs make their community health nursing decisions. The community health nursing process combines judgement, action, responsibility, and accountability when planning care. The CHN's role in health promotion includes assisting the patient to take responsibility for their health as well as encouraging the development of healthy public policy, community-based action, public participation, and advocacy (CPHA, 2010). Therefore, it is critical for CHNs to have an in-depth understanding of the concept of health and health promotion as they make nursing decisions and conduct the community health nursing process.

Development of the Concept of Health

Understanding health promotion requires an exploration of the development of the concept of health. The conceptualization of health has changed over time, with many debates occurring over its definition. In the early to mid-1900s, the medical approach dominated, and *health* was therefore defined as the absence of disease. That definition of *health* led to the view of health and illness as two opposing ends on a continuum and with health being measured by indicators of disease, such as morbidity and mortality statistics (Vollman, Anderson, & McFarlane, 2017). As well, that definition focused primarily on disease in individuals rather than families, groups, communities, populations, or systems.

In 1947, the World Health Organization (WHO) amended its definition of *health* from "the absence of disease or infirmity" to "health as a state of complete physical, mental, and social well-being, and not merely the absence of disease or infirmity" (WHO, 1947). This expanded definition led to the view of health as a balance between physical, mental, and social well-being, which led to a holistic approach to health.

Other definitions of *health* followed to include facets such as the environment and predisposing factors such as heredity and family composition. The influence of epidemiology led to the consideration of aggregates as well as individuals in the definition of *health*. Dunn (1959) described health as ever-changing, overlapping levels of wellness (i.e., physical, biological, social, cultural) within the context of the environment. Within the definition of health developed by Dunn (1959), high-level wellness can occur only in a favourable environment.

The perspective of health as a process was introduced in the 1960s by Dewey (1963), Erikson (1963), and Piaget (1963), with further development by Havighurst in 1972 and Duvall in 1985 (Sheinfeld Gorin & Arnold, 1998). These developmental theorists viewed health as an ongoing process throughout the lifespan influenced by several factors, including lifestyle choices. Other health perspectives include health as functionality, goodness of fit, transcendence, a sense of well-being, wholeness (holistic), and empowerment (Sheinfeld Gorin & Arnold, 1998). The last three factors are part of the concept of health promotion.

This text uses the Ottawa Charter definition of *health*: "to reach a state of complete physical, mental and social wellbeing, an individual or group must be able to identify and to realize aspirations, to satisfy needs, and to change or cope with the environment" (WHO, 1986). WHO thereby identified **health** as a positive resource for everyday living that is holistic—that is, it includes physical, social, and personal capabilities. This distinction no longer presents health as an outcome (or a state to be reached); rather, health becomes incorporated into one's activities of daily living. Therefore, a patient requires health to live his or her life to its fullest potential. Today, Canada continues to embrace the Ottawa Charter definition of *health*. Viewing health as a resource suggests that communities and individuals can use this resource to manage and even change their surroundings (Health Canada, 2004). Globally, no consensus exists on what constitutes good health; however, greater consensus exists on what constitutes poor health (Maville & Huerta, 2008).

Foundational Concepts in Health Promotion

Questions often arise about the differences among various health promotion concepts, such as injury prevention, disease, disease course, illness, illness trajectory, disease prevention, health protection, risk avoidance, risk reduction, health enhancement, and harm reduction. These concepts are often used in discussions about health and health promotion, so it is important for CHNs to be able to distinguish among them.

Injury prevention refers to the use of strategies to help patients prevent and reduce the risk of injury. Injury prevention occurs at the primary, secondary, and tertiary levels. An example of injury prevention at the primary level is the use of bicycle helmets to prevent head injuries. Adams, Drake, Dang, et al. (2014) evaluated the effectiveness of a student-nurse administered school helmet program and found that it not only improved knowledge but also increased the use of helmets after participation in the program. An example of secondary prevention is the provision of a bicycle safety program for youths who have experienced head injuries. An example of tertiary prevention is the provision of rehabilitation after a head injury resulting from a bicycle accident.

Disease refers to the presence of abnormal alterations in the structure or functioning of the human body that fit within the medical model (Lubkin & Larsen, 2009). When an individual experiences a disease, it usually follows an identifiable progression known as the **disease course**. For example, the labels *monophasic, polycyclic,* and *persistent* are frequently used to describe the disease course for patients with juvenile idiopathic arthritis (Singh-Grewal , Schnieder, Bayer, et al., 2006). Health practitioners take into consideration the natural history of a disease within the context of the signs and symptoms of the disease that are experienced by the patient to help to identify the disease course.

Illness is an individual's personal experience of, perception of, and reaction to a disease, whereby he or she is unable to function at the desired "usual" level (Lubkin & Larsen, 2009). Chronic illness follows a particular trajectory. Specifically, it follows expected short- and long-term courses over time with a degree of uncertainty about the disease course that requires the affected patient, the family, and involved health care providers to adjust to associated changes; this path is referred to as the **illness trajectory** (Lubkin & Larsen, 2009). For example, a patient living with juvenile idiopathic arthritis will suffer degenerative physical changes as the disease progresses, possibly requiring assistance from others to adapt and manage activities of daily living such as mobility, bathing, and dressing. Patients adapt differently to acute and chronic illnesses.

Disease prevention refers to the activities undertaken by the health sector to prevent the occurrence of disease (primary prevention), to detect and stop disease development in those at risk (secondary prevention), and to reduce the negative effects once a disease has established itself (tertiary prevention) (Maville & Huerta, 2008). These activities relate specifically to illness and disease. Disease prevention focuses on individuals and populations that have identifiable risk factors such as genetic predisposition or involvement in risky behaviours such as practising unsafe sex. An example of disease prevention at the primary level is the administration of the H1N1 influenza vaccine to the Canadian population or administration of the seasonal influenza vaccine to the older person aggregate. An example of disease prevention at the secondary level is the screening for cervical cancer in all sexually active females using the Papanicolaou (Pap) test. An example of disease prevention at the tertiary level is the provision of speech therapy for aphasic patients following a cerebrovascular accident (CVA).

Whereas disease prevention focuses on anticipation and avoidance of immediate health risks, **health protection** focuses on health maintenance by dealing with the immediate health risks (Health Canada, 2005a). Health Canada has the responsibility of protecting the Canadian population from current and emerging health threats. With eight regional offices across Canada, Health Canada safeguards the population's health through surveillance, prevention, legislation, and research in areas such as environmental health, disease outbreaks, drug and health products, and food safety. Understanding these concepts will assist CHNs as they discuss health and health promotion approaches for various patient populations.

In 2005, WHO redefined *health promotion* as the process of enabling people to increase control over the determinants of health and thereby improve their health (Tang, Beaglehole, & O'Byrne, 2005). This definition, developed from that of the Ottawa Charter (WHO, 1986), specifies particular factors that affect health, that is, the determinants of health. The determinants of health are discussed in Chapter 1 and throughout the text. Health promotion moves beyond health maintenance to incorporate improvements in health that result in health gains (Health Canada, 2005a). It is critical that CHNs involve patients in decisions about all aspects of their health to effect improvements.

Using the health issue of adolescent obesity, the following examples show health promotion in action at individual, family, aggregate, and community levels. At an individual level, the adolescent is empowered to make healthy food choices when the school cafeteria offers reasonably priced fresh fruit and vegetable options. The CHN could advocate on behalf of students to ensure healthier food choices are made available in the school cafeteria and other community eating establishments. The CHN could educate the adolescent's family about meal planning so that family members could plan and implement healthy meals and snacks. The CHN could enable families to purchase healthy foods by providing information on how to read nutrition labels and increase families' awareness of community resources, such as community gardens and food banks. At an aggregate level, self-help groups initiated in the school could facilitate adolescents' meeting and sharing ideas on how to promote a healthy weight (the "Ethical Considerations" box presents an example of health promotion to this same aggregate, but on the issue of smoking). The CHN might advocate for the establishment of life-skills classes that focus on inexpensive healthy food preparation. Within the community, community leaders, adolescents, parents, teachers, and health care providers could work together to establish community recreational opportunities that facilitate physical activity, such as skateboard parks; walking, hiking, and biking trails; and cross-country ski trails and hills.

Health promotion activities at the community level to address the issue of adolescent obesity could also involve the CHN advocating for healthy public policy that could support funding opportunities for trail development, lighting for walkways, or tax incentives for enrollment in physical activity programs. Public policy directs or guides the actions or decisions of public or private stakeholders authorized to act on behalf of the public good (Morrison, Gagnon, Morestin & Keeling, 2014). **Healthy public policy** incorporates the definition of public policy, but also includes policy developed with the intent of having a positive effect on or promoting health, for example, funding for outdoor walkways and trails.

Risk avoidance is a disease prevention strategy used to avoid health problems and to remain at a low-risk level (placing the patient at no risk or low risk on the continuum). **Risk reduction** is a disease prevention strategy used to reduce or alter health concerns so that any disease is detected and treated early to prevent moving to a high-risk level (placing the patient at low to moderate risk). The risk continuum is often used with patients who have substance use or abuse problems, but it can be used with any group of patients: for example, populations who are at a high risk for becoming infected with the Ebola virus disease. **Health enhancement** is a health promotion strategy that is used to increase health and resiliency to promote optimal health and well-being (the patient can be at any point on the risk continuum).

Disease prevention and health promotion are foundational to community health nursing practice. Primary-prevention community health nursing interventions would aim at preventing illness or injuries from happening. Secondary-prevention community health nursing interventions would assess and support individuals and populations when risk factors are present so that screening for early detection and treatment occurs. The Canadian Task Force on Preventive Health Care develops evidence-informed guidelines for the prevention of diseases such as hypertension, cervical cancer, diabetes, and breast cancer. These guidelines can be found on the Canadian Task Force on Preventive Health Care website (see the link on the Evolve website). The CCHN Standards also provide direction for CHNs dealing with disease prevention (see Appendix 1, specifically standards 1, 2, 4, and 6). See Box 4.1 for excerpts from Standard 2, "Prevention and Health Protection."

Different strategies are available to affect the health behaviours of individuals or populations at various levels of risk. Fig. 4.1 depicts the health risk continuum and its

ETHICAL CONSIDERATIONS

A CHN assigned to a high school has noticed that many of the teenagers smoke, and starts an after-school smoking cessation program targeting the smokers; however, some students just do not want to come. Several students who want to come cannot because they take the bus right after school.
Ethical principles (see Chapter 6, Box 6.4) that apply to this scenario are as follows:
- *Distributive justice.* The benefits of the program are not equally available to all because the bused students cannot attend.
- *Autonomy.* The PHN cannot force students to come to the program if they choose not to.
- *Promoting health and well-being* (CNA *Code of Ethics for Registered Nurses*). Promoting health and well-being is a primary ethical value for CHNs. The CHN must explore other options for those students who want to come but cannot attend (e.g., social media campaign).

Questions to Consider
1. a. How does a CHN address negative aspects of health behaviours while maintaining respect for patient autonomy?
   b. What could the CHN in this situation do to maintain respect for patient autonomy and address the negative health behaviour of smoking?
2. What is the CHN's responsibility to provide programming for patients who do not yet smoke, that is, to promote patient health at a primary level of prevention?

BOX 4.1 Canadian Community Health Nursing Standards of Practice

Excerpts from Standard 2: Prevention and Health Protection
The community health nurse...
a. Participates in surveillance, recognizes trends in epidemiology data, and utilizes this data through population level actions such as health education, screening, immunizations, and communicable disease control, and management.
b. Uses prevention and protection approaches with the patient to identify risk factors and to address issues such as communicable disease, injury, chronic disease, and the physical environment.
c. Applies the appropriate level of prevention (primordial, primary, secondary, tertiary, and quaternary) to improve health.
d. Facilitates informed decision making with the patient for protective and preventive measures.

Source: Adapted with permission from Community Health Nurses of Canada. (2019). *Canadian Community Health Nursing Professional Practice Model & Standards of Practice* (p. 19). Retrieved from https://www.chnc.ca/standards-of-practice.

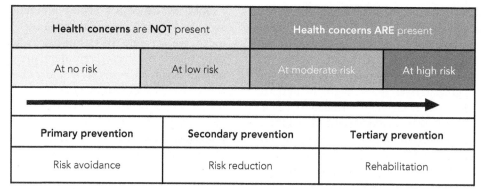

Health concerns are **NOT** present		Health concerns **ARE** present	
At no risk	At low risk	At moderate risk	At high risk

Primary prevention	Secondary prevention	Tertiary prevention
Risk avoidance	Risk reduction	Rehabilitation

Fig. 4.1 Levels of Disease Prevention on the Risk Continuum.

relationship to health promotion, disease prevention, and treatment. The figure shows the relationship between the three levels of disease prevention and risk. As discussed in Chapter 1, activities and programs at the primary-prevention level are initiated when patients are at no risk to low risk and have the goal of risk avoidance. In primary prevention, prevention activities strive to prevent movement toward disability and death. Early treatment and intervention programs at the secondary-prevention level are initiated when patients are at moderate risk and have the goal of risk reduction. Treatment programs at the tertiary-prevention level (health recovery) are initiated when patients are at a high risk and have the goal of rehabilitation. Health enhancement, a health promotion strategy, is used to develop or enhance the health and well-being of patients at any point on the risk continuum.

While disease prevention measures can contribute to improved population health, individuals may make choices contrary to the interventions proposed by the CHN based on considerations such as culture, religion, or health beliefs. For example, a family in the community might refuse to have its preschool child immunized. In such a situation, the CHN needs to be respectful and nonjudgemental, weigh the risks and benefits to the population, and assess and educate the family appropriately to ensure that the patient has made an informed choice.

Community health nursing interventions aimed at health promotion encourage the enhancement of the well-being of patients. In Canada, many community health nursing strategies are directed at populations and aggregates and emphasize the determinants of health and the use of the health promotion strategies outlined in the Ottawa Charter. Refer to Box 4.2 for excerpts from Standard 1, which provides direction for the CHN working on health promotion.

Harm reduction is a set of strategies and ideas aimed at reducing harm to an individual or society by modifying harmful or hazardous behaviours that are difficult and, in some cases, impossible to prevent. It is a movement for social justice built on a belief in and respect for the rights of people who engage in harmful or hazardous behaviours such as drug use (Harm Reduction Coalition, 2014). It is accomplished through strategies such as the implementation of policies or programs (often not requiring

---

BOX 4.2   Canadian Community Health Nursing Standards of Practice

Standard 1: Health Promotion
The community health nurse …
a. Applies health promotion theories and models in practice.
b. Collaborates with patient to do a comprehensive, evidenced informed, and strength-based holistic health assessment using multiple sources and methods to identify needs, assets, inequities, and resources.
c. Seeks to identify and assess the root and historical causes of illness, disease, and inequities in health, acknowledge diversity and the adverse effects of colonialism on Indigenous people, and when appropriate, incorporate Indigenous ways of knowing, including connectedness and reciprocity to the land and all life in health promotion.

Source: Community Health Nurses of Canada. (2019). *Canadian Community Health Nursing Professional Practice Model & Standards of Practice* (p. 18). Retrieved from https://www.chnc.ca/standards-of-practice.

---

abstinence) to decrease the adverse health consequences of substance use (Centre for Addiction and Mental Health, 2010; Davis, 2006; Health Canada, 2005b). Harm reduction strategies focus on the eventual goal of abstinence as opposed to abstinence as a prerequisite for program participation (Davis, 2006).

Examples of harm reduction strategies include needle-exchange programs, supervised injection facilities, methadone maintenance programs, and smokeless tobacco programs. Although provincial and territorial research findings on the patterns of substance use vary, commonalities exist in its prevalence. The Canadian Centre on Substance Use and Addiction (2017) recently identified priority needs for action, including the need for more evidence to inform decisions about cannabis, and the mobilization of resources to address the death toll from opioid abuse in Canada. These priority needs could be addressed through harm-reduction strategies, such as providing free access to naloxone kits and educating youth about the legalization of cannabis. Harm-reduction strategies are one of the foundational concepts of health promotion and CHNs play an important role in promoting harm reduction programs in the community.

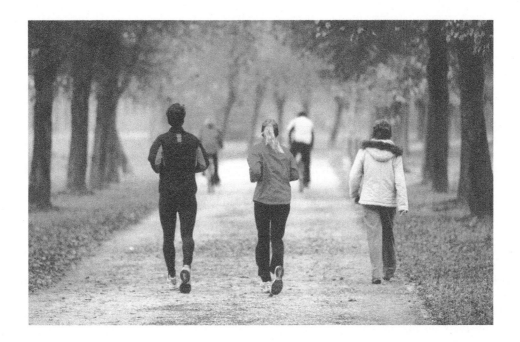

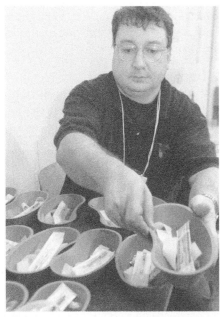

Community nurses may participate in health promotion and harm reduction programs. Health promotion may be aimed at enhancing the well-being of patients, for example, by encouraging participation in exercise programs (top). On the bottom a nurse prepares injection kits for Vancouver's needle-exchange program, an example of a harm reduction program. (© iStockphoto/Gartner [top]; THE CANADIAN PRESS/Richard Lam [bottom])

Despite Canada having a wide variety of harm-reduction policies in place, some areas of the country have few or no policies. For example, access to harm-reduction interventions among substance users is highly variable across the country, with policies and programs to address low-threshold opioid substitution, and safer inhalation kits being almost nonexistent (Wild, Pauly, Belle-Isle, et al., 2017). Vancouver is well known for an established harm reduction infrastructure with harm reduction programs. However, street-involved young people who use drugs continue to be vulnerable to overdose, death, hepatitis, and high rates of syringe sharing. Interviews with at-risk youth in Vancouver identified limitations of current risk-reduction programs, including offering little support to improve their life chances, and distance from services (Bozinoff, Small, Long, DeBeck & Fast 2017). CHNs working with these populations need to consider current research when developing harm reduction programs to address their needs. Harm reduction is discussed further in Chapter 15.

Closely associated with the concept of harm reduction is the concept of resiliency. **Resiliency** is the capacity of patients (individuals, families, groups, communities) to cope effectively when faced with considerable adversity or risk (University of Calgary, 2007). Resiliency develops and changes over time, depending on changes in risk and protective factors. **Risk factors** are variables that create stress and therefore challenge the patient's health status. For example, hypertension is a risk factor for a CVA, poverty is a risk factor for certain infectious diseases, and a community disaster is a risk factor for increased community crime rates. **Protective factors** are variables that assist in managing the stressors associated with being at risk. Examples of protective factors include literacy, social support networks, family support systems, and community empowerment through public participation. If stress outweighs one's protective factors and creates an imbalance, a previously resilient patient may become incapable of usual functioning. The following are examples of risk factors and associated protective factors:

- Risk factor—inaccessibility to family doctors; protective factor—the provision of local walk-in clinics
- Risk factor—domestic violence; protective factor—extended family support
- Risk factor—gang violence in a community neighbourhood; protective factor—an established community

coalition of concerned citizens, the police force, and health care providers
- Risk factor—bullying in schools; protective factors—antibullying campaigns (e.g., Pink Shirt Day, https://www.pinkshirtday.ca/)

EVOLUTION OF HEALTH PROMOTION

Canada has been at the forefront in the evolution of health promotion. Health promotion extends beyond individuals to families, aggregates, populations, and communities. A review of the key developments of health promotion in Canada will help identify other aspects of health promotion to be considered by CHNs.

The evolution of community health nursing and health care (see Chapter 2) and the discussion earlier in this chapter on the definitions of *health* reveal that when the medical approach prevailed, health care's focus was on illness and that *health* was defined as the absence of disease. Developmentally and historically, the emphasis was on the control of infectious and communicable diseases. In the mid-1900s, the advent of antibiotics and vaccinations generally brought these diseases under control. Box 4.3 lists landmark health promotion initiatives that have affected health promotion. Fig. 4.2 presents information on key documents and initiatives that have shaped perspectives on health and health policies in Canada.

Lalonde Report

In 1974 Marc Lalonde, then minister of Health and Welfare Canada, introduced the notion of health promotion nationally and internationally in the report titled *A New Perspective on the Health of Canadians*. The Lalonde Report initiated a shift, especially in Canada, from a primarily biomedical view of disease and health to a consideration of certain aspects of health promotion. It also increased the awareness of human biology, environment, and lifestyle as determinants of health and, therefore, as influencers of health (Lalonde, 1974; Vollman et al., 2017). Lalonde (1974) proposed the need for a more comprehensive approach to health care. He urged improvements to the environment, increased knowledge in human biology, and modifications of self-imposed risks due to individual health choices to increase the population health status of Canadians (Lalonde, 1974; Vollman et al., 2017). The report raised policymakers' awareness of health promotion, not only in Canada but also in the United States and Europe. The Lalonde Report and its focus on health promotion resulted in health promotion research, healthy public policy, and interventions directed toward lifestyle changes. Health promotion research identified associations between personal risk factors and health status. Healthy public policy focused on areas such as smoking and drinking and driving. Health promotion interventions have included the implementation of health education and mass media campaigns to dissuade unhealthy behaviours such as smoking and sedentary lifestyles (Health Canada, 2005c).

Alma-Ata Declaration

In 1978, the Alma-Ata Declaration, which focuses on primary health care, was presented at the WHO International

BOX 4.3   Landmark Health Promotion Initiatives

1974 *A New Perspective on the Health of Canadians* (the Lalonde Report) is released.
1978 Alma-Ata Declaration is adopted (at WHO International Conference on Primary Health Care in Alma-Ata, USSR [Kazakhstan]).
1984 WHO Working Group develops concepts, principles, priorities, and dilemmas of health promotion.
1986 Ottawa Charter for Health Promotion is adopted (at WHO First Global Conference on Health Promotion in Ottawa, Canada).
1986 *Achieving Health for All: A Framework for Health Promotion* (the Epp Report) is released.
1988 Adelaide Recommendations on Healthy Public Policy were adopted (at WHO Second Global Conference on Health Promotion in Adelaide, Australia).
1991 Sundsvall Statement on Supportive Environments for Health is released (at WHO Third Global Conference on Health Promotion in Sundsvall, Sweden).
1996 *Population Health Promotion: An Integrated Model of Population Health and Health Promotion* (by Hamilton and Bhatti) is released.
1997 Jakarta Declaration on Leading Health Promotion Into the 21st Century is adopted (at WHO Fourth Global Conference on Health Promotion in Jakarta, Indonesia).

2000 Health Promotion: Bridging the Equity Gap is adopted (at WHO Fifth Global Conference on Health Promotion in Mexico City, Mexico).
2002 The conference "Strengthening the Social Determinants of Health: The Toronto Charter for a Healthy Canada" is held in Toronto, Canada.
2005 The Bangkok Charter for Health Promotion in a Globalized World is adopted (at the WHO Sixth Global Conference on Health Promotion, in Bangkok, Thailand).
2007 World Conference on Health Promotion and Health Education by the International Union for Health Promotion and Education is held in Vancouver, Canada.
2008 WHO's Commission on Social Determinants of Health (established in 2005) releases its final report on the social determinants of health, titled *Closing the Gap in a Generation: Health Equity Through Action on the Social Determinants of Health*.
2009 The conference "Promoting Health and Development: Closing the Implementation Gap" closes with the adoption of the Nairobi Call to Action (at the WHO Seventh Global Conference on Health Promotion in Nairobi, Kenya).
2011 The Rio Political Declaration on Social Determinants of Health is adopted (at the WHO Eighth World Conference on Social Determinants of Health in Rio de Janeiro, Brazil).
2016 The Shanghai Declaration on Promoting Health is adopted (at the WHO Ninth Global Conference on Health Promotion in Shanghai, China).

Illness focused

←

- Provider centred
- Limited community participation
- Public policies based on assumptions that medical technology alone can improve health status

Document	The Lalonde Report: A New Perspective on the Health of Canadians	The Alma-Ata Declaration on PHC	The Black Report	The Healthy Communities Initiative: Toronto 2000	The Ottawa Charter: A Framework for Health Promotion	Review of PHC and HFA by 2000
Author(s)	(Marc Lalonde) Health and Welfare Canada	WHO and UNICEF	Sir Douglas Black	Dr. Trevor Hancock	(Jake Epp) Health and Welfare Canada	WHO
Place	Ottawa, Ont.	Alma-Ata, Kazakhstan, USSR	United Kingdom	Toronto, Ont.	Ottawa, Ont.	Riga, Latvia
Year	1974	1978	1980	1984	1986	1988
Main ideas	Introduction of the "health field concept" (4 domains): • Human biology • Lifestyle • Environment • Health care system as determinant of health Focused on lifestyle modification Approaches seen by some as blaming the victim	5 principles: 1. Accessibility 2. Emphasis on health promotion 3. Intersectoral collaboration 4. Appropriate technology 5. Community participation Plus 8 essential elements	Study of British civil servants—showed that class was associated with mortality outcomes	Began to examine the socioenvironmental determinants of health Multisectoral health policies and health planning emerged Community visioning and empowerment seen as a health-promoting process	Challenges outlined: • Reducing health inequities • Increasing disease prevention Health promotion seen as enabling people to increase control over their health and lives	Renewed commitment to principles of PHC Some disappointment with progress in some areas and locations Health still a highly centralized approach in many parts of the world

→ **Improved well-being?**

- Better community participation, dialogue, and collaboration

CNA position paper on PHC	RNABC position paper on PHC	ANAC submission to the Royal Commission on Aboriginal Peoples	Community Action Program for Children (CAPC)	Royal Commission on the Future of Health in Canada (the Romanow Report)	The Chief Public Health Officer's Report on the State of Public Health in Canada 2008: Addressing Health Inequalities	A Life Course Approach to the Social Determinants of Health for Aboriginal Peoples
CNA	RNABC	ANAC	Health Canada	Roy J. Romanow	Public Health Agency of Canada (Dr. David Butler Jones)	Jeff Reading
Ottawa, Ont.	Vancouver, BC	Ottawa, Ont.	Ottawa, Ont.	Saskatoon, Sask.	Ottawa, Ont.	Ottawa, Ont.
1989	1991	1993	1994	2002	2008	2009
		Established a need for dialogue and collaboration and for community-based approaches, including the use of traditional healers	Community-based information gathering for health planning and implementation	Limits of the role of the health care system: • Definition of PHC is reduced to "health care for individuals" and "services to communities" • Intersectoral collaboration is reduced to "interdisciplinary teamwork" • Prevention is reduced to "early detection and action"	Reports on the health trends in Canada such as the growing prevalence of obesity and diabetes. Includes discussion of the determinants of health and their impact on the health of Canadians and the inequalities that develop because of the determinants of health.	In-depth examination of the social determinants of health, specifically related to the unique context of Indigenous peoples' health

Fig. 4.2 A Conceptual Evolution of "Health": National and International Perspectives on Health and Health Policies From 1974 to 2009. (Adapted from Ehrlich, A., & Ladouceur, M. G. (2002). *A conceptual evolution of "health": National and international perspectives on health and health policies from 1974 to the present.* Hamilton, ON: School of Nursing, McMaster University.)

Conference in Alma-Ata, USSR (Kazakhstan) to address the unacceptable inequalities in the health status between developed and developing countries (see Appendix 3). From this conference came an awareness and acknowledgement that to improve health, more had to be done beyond funding health services such as hospitals (Catford, 2004, 2014). This shift in thinking made primary health care the chosen strategy for health care delivery to achieve the goal of "health for all by the year 2000." Primary health care identified social and environmental conditions as determinants of health outside of the health care sector and helped make evident the need for intersectoral cooperation, if the population's health status was to improve. The result was a shift in power from health care providers to communities and the consumers of health care services (Catford, 2004).

World Health Organization Principles of Health Promotion

In 1984, a WHO working group was charged with "reorienting health services" and prepared a report on health promotion that identified principles as well as subject areas, priorities, and dilemmas (Catford, 2004). Table 4.1 presents the principles of health promotion proposed by the WHO working group with associated implications. In 2014, Catford stated, "very encouraging strides have been made with Ottawa's four challenges to build health public policy, create supportive environments, develop personal skills and support community action."

Ottawa Charter for Health Promotion

The Ottawa Charter for Health Promotion (WHO, 1986) defined and developed the concept and components of health promotion (see Appendix 4). The Ottawa Charter increased awareness of and expanded upon the determinants of health in its discussions of the prerequisites for health, such as peace, shelter, education, food, income, a stable ecosystem, sustainable resources, social justice, and equity (Vollman et al., 2017).

The Ottawa Charter identified several health promotion strategies for practice—advocating, enabling, and mediating—as necessary to help communities, groups, and individuals to reach their optimal levels of health. The new perspective on health promotion included in the Ottawa Charter contributed to a change in the roles assumed by health care providers, who moved from the expert "in control" role to the roles of advocate, facilitator, supporter, and mediator (Young & Hayes, 2002). The advocacy role is discussed in further detail

TABLE 4.1   Principles of Health Promotion and Their Implications

Principles of Health Promotion	Discussion	Implications
1. Health promotion involves the population as a whole in the context of their everyday life, rather than focusing on people at risk for specific diseases.	This principle recognizes the need to enable people to take charge of and responsibility for their health. It identifies population health as a major part of health promotion.	• Health care providers need to empower and promote self-care with patients. • Populations require access to information about health. • Health care providers need to use a variety of dissemination methods.
2. Health promotion is directed toward action on the determinants or causes of health.	The intersectoral aspects of health promotion are evident. Intergovernmental responsibility exists for the "total" environment, which is outside of individual and group influence.	• All levels of government are responsible for ensuring that all environments support and promote health by implementing appropriate and timely interventions. • Health care providers should assume an advocacy role and be involved in intersectoral collaboration to influence the development of healthy public policy.
3. Health promotion combines diverse, but complementary, methods or approaches.	Diverse strategies and approaches could include communication, education, legislation, organizational change, community development, and health hazard management.	• Health care providers need to carefully plan and be selective in choosing appropriate and mixed strategies and approaches.
4. Health promotion aims particularly at effective and concrete public participation.	Public participation collectively and individually requires further development of problem definition and decision-making life skills.	• Health care providers need to be flexible, innovative, and transparent to facilitate individual, group, and community involvement in decision making. • Health care providers need to build on and support individual, group, and community strengths.
5. Health professionals—particularly in primary health care—have an important role in nurturing and enabling health promotion.	Health promotion is not a medical service; it is an activity mainly used in the health and social fields.	• Health care providers need to develop skills in health promotion, such as empowerment, health education, and advocacy.

Source: Adapted from Catford, J. (2014). Turn, turn, turn: Time to reorient health services. Health Promotion International, 29(1), 1–4.

later in this chapter and in several other chapters throughout this text.

Also, at this time Canada experienced a shift from an individual-based health promotion approach toward a population health promotion approach that integrated the Ottawa Charter. The five major actions (referred to as "action means" in the Ottawa Charter) for promoting health are:

- Build healthy public policy (e.g., mandatory seatbelt use in automobiles)
- Create supportive environments (e.g., smoke-free workplaces)
- Strengthen community action (e.g., funding for heart health initiatives such as healthy food choices in restaurants)
- Develop personal skills (e.g., through community literacy programs)
- Reorient health services (e.g., interprofessional community health centres)

These five action means shifted the health promotion emphasis to include communities and shifted the responsibility for health primarily to governments, communities, and individuals (Young & Hayes, 2002). Note that the five action means are referred to as *health promotion strategies* in this text; recent Canadian literature has also called them *health promotion strategies* (Canadian Public Health Association, 1996; Community Health Nurses Association of Canada, 2019; Health Canada, 2005a; Ministry of Health Promotion, 2008; Reutter & Eastlick Kushner, 2009). Health promotion strategies make up the "how" component of a plan to meet specified goals. Therefore, the population health promotion model (see Fig. 1.1 on page 7) considers the question "*How* should we take action?" in light of the five action means.

The Ottawa Charter was created primarily in response to the need for action on the social and economic determinants of health. Although the Ottawa Charter has become the foundation for health promotion strategies in Canada and around the world, it has not been beyond criticism. McPhail-Bell, Fredericks, and Brough (2013) used critical discourse to examine how the Ottawa Charter was created in 1987 and concluded that it was a WHO-dominated process that focused primarily on industrialized countries. The authors also concluded that the process was informed by Western-centric world views and that non-Western voices were silent. The Australian authors were particularly concerned about the "invisibility" of input from Indigenous peoples and developing countries. They challenged health care providers to use the Ottawa Charter as it was originally intended, to promote health through participation, empowerment, and social justice for *all* people.

Epp Report: A Canadian Framework for Health Promotion

In 1986 Jake Epp, as the minister of Health and Welfare Canada, proposed a national framework for health promotion as a strategy to achieve the goal of "health for all." In his framework, the following three national health challenges

were identified as requiring particular focus: (1) reducing health inequities between low- and high-income groups; (2) increasing prevention efforts by reducing or eliminating risks to decrease injuries, diseases, chronic illnesses, and related disabilities; and (3) enhancing coping abilities, especially helping people to manage chronic conditions, mental health problems, and disabilities (Epp, 1986).

The Epp framework (Epp, 1986) identified the following mechanisms as necessary for health promotion and for meeting the identified health challenges:

- Self-care as related to healthy personal decisions and actions regarding an individual's own health (e.g., an individual deciding to become physically active)
- Mutual aid associated with individuals helping and supporting other individuals to deal with health concerns (e.g., bereavement groups)
- The creation of healthy environments to enhance health (e.g., smoke-free spaces)

Epp's framework further supported a community and policy focus in health promotion through the actions of fostering public participation (e.g., encouraging physical activity for heart health), strengthening community health services (e.g., increasing community mental health services), and coordinating healthy public policy (e.g., affordable, accessible housing).

Both the Epp Report and the Ottawa Charter take a socioenvironmental approach to health promotion. In both documents, "health is seen as more than just the absence of disease and engaging in healthy behaviours; rather, this approach emphasizes connectedness, self-efficacy, and capacity to engage in meaningful activities" (Reutter & Eastlick Kushner, 2009, p. 4).

Developments in Health Promotion

The identification of the determinants of health within the framework of health promotion introduced by Lalonde (1974), Epp (1986), and the Ottawa Charter (WHO, 1986) demonstrated progressive thinking in health care. As noted in Chapter 1, research has shown that many of the 12 determinants, specifically economic and social inequities, influence the health status of Canadians. Of note is the influence of chronic childhood poverty on long-term health status. Lethbridge and Phipps (2005) concluded that there is an important pathway between poverty, low birthweight, and high prevalence of rates of asthma for Maritime children. For further discussion of each of the determinants of health, including policy implications, refer to Mikkonen and Raphael's report *Social Determinants of Health: The Canadian Facts*, which is available on the authors' website (see the link on the Evolve website). The document provides a succinct review of the determinants of health from a Canadian perspective.

The WHO Second Global Conference on Health Promotion was held in Adelaide, Australia, in 1988. It focused on the importance of healthy public policy and the re-establishment of commitment to the Ottawa Charter (Wass, 2000). Industrial countries were urged to establish policies to reduce inequities between rich and poor countries. Other priorities identified for action included the health of women, the elimination of malnutrition and hunger, a decrease in the availability of alcohol and tobacco, and the provision of increased supportive environments through alliance formations (Vollman et al., 2017).

The WHO Third Global Conference on Health Promotion was held in Sundsvall, Sweden, in 1991. It had as its main focus the provision of supportive environments to promote health at a community level. The four key actions to promote the creation of these supportive environments were as follows:

(1) strengthening advocacy through community action, particularly through groups organized by women; (2) enabling communities and individuals to take control over their health and environment through education and empowerment; (3) building alliances for health and supportive environments in order to strengthen the co-operation between health and environmental campaigns and strategies; and (4) mediating between conflicting interests in society in order to ensure equitable access to supportive environments for health. (WHO, 1991, pp. 3–4)

Population Health Promotion Model, Revisited

CHNs use the population health model to facilitate planned change with individuals, families, groups, and communities. In 1994, a document titled *Strategies for Population Health: Investing in the Health of Canadians,* prepared by a federal, provincial, and territorial advisory committee, endorsed a population health approach (as cited in Public Health Agency of Canada [PHAC], 1994). The population health approach had originally been introduced in 1989 by the Canadian Institute for Advanced Research (CIFAR). CIFAR had started the discussion on population health as a new concept to aid in understanding the determinants of health and the interplay among them (Evans, Barer, & Marmor, 1994). The population health approach created much debate about how it related to or was different from health promotion, especially since it also focused on the determinants of health (Young & Hayes, 2002). Many health promotion leaders in Canada expressed concerns about the population health approach and its possible negative influence on the integration of health promotion into public health practice in Canada (Bhatti, 1996; Labonte, 1995; Raphael & Bryant, 2002; Robertson, 1998).

A few years later, Hamilton and Bhatti (1996) introduced the population health promotion (PHP) model. This model builds on the Ottawa Charter: it incorporates the Ottawa Charter's five action means, the determinants of health, and health promotion strategies. It integrates the challenge of reducing inequities in the population as outlined by both the Epp Report (Health Canada, 2005a,) and the CIFAR population health model (Young & Hayes, 2002). This PHP model clarifies the relationship between health promotion and population health. In support of the model, Health Canada (2005a) identifies the two theories as "synergistic" rather than contrasting concepts, and the PHAC (2001) describes the PHP model as showing "how a population health approach can be

implemented through action on the full range of health determinants by means of health promotion strategies."

Fig. 1.1 in Chapter 1 presents the three-dimensional diagram of the PHP model. The interrelating parts of the model that guide actions to improve health are (1) On "what" should we take action? (referring to the determinants of health); (2) With "whom" should we act? (referring to the patient); and (3) "How" should we take action? (referring to the health promotion strategies of the Ottawa Charter). The foundations of the model are evidence-informed decision making; sources for evidence-informed decision making, which include research, experiential learning, and evaluation; and values and assumptions. With this model, any of the five health promotion strategies can be developed and implemented at various levels, from the individual to society. The choice of health promotion strategy depends on factors such as the values and assumptions held about the determinants of health, desired outcomes, and available evidence. The model can be used from a variety of entrance points (PHAC, 2001). For example, the determinants of health to be influenced or a health issue for a particular aggregate can be entrance points, and one or more of the determinants can be addressed simultaneously. Fig. 4.3 demonstrates the application of the PHP model to an

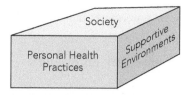

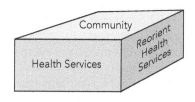

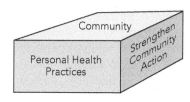

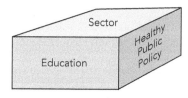

e.g.: Support community action to obtain available HPV vaccine and establish an HPV program.

e.g.: Boards of Education can ensure that HPV vaccine information is included in the school curriculum.

e.g.: Communities can provide opportunities for HPV testing, HPV counselling, and administration of the HPV vaccine and ensure that all opportunities are available and accessible.

e.g.: Social marketing campaigns can heighten public awareness of the importance and availability of the HPV vaccine.

Fig. 4.3 The Population Health Promotion Model Applied to a Female Aggregate. From Public Health Agency of Canada. [2001]. *An Integrated Model of Population Health and Health Promotion.* (Adapted and reproduced with permission from the Minister of Health, 2016.)

at-risk aggregate—girls and young women (9 to 26 years of age) who are at risk for a specific sexually transmitted infection. This infection is caused by exposure to the human papillomavirus (HPV) and can be prevented by the administration of an HPV vaccine. Health promotion programs have been shown to increase HPV vaccine uptake by creating realistic perceptions about the vaccine (Vanderpool, Casey, & Crosby, 2011).

The PHAC has identified eight key elements that need to be addressed in the population health approach model. These elements, presented in Figure 4.4, are as follows (PHAC, 2008a):

1. *Focus on the health of populations.* A population health approach assesses health status and disparities in health status through the lifespan at the population level.
2. *Address the determinants of health and their interactions.* A population health approach appraises the determinants of health and their interrelationships.
3. *Base decisions on evidence.* A population health approach uses evidence in assessment, planning, and development of interventions in health promotion.
4. *Increase upstream investments.* A population health approach capitalizes on its potential by focusing its energy and interventions to deal with foundational contributors to health and wellness.
5. *Apply multiple interventions and strategies.* A population health approach uses a variety of interventions and strategies to address the health concerns of patient as individual, family, group or aggregate, community, population, or society.
6. *Collaborate across sectors and levels.* A population health approach includes horizontal and vertical intersectoral collaboration to affect health.
7. *Employ mechanisms for public involvement.* A population health approach partners with the community in planning, implementing, and evaluating health promotion programs.
8. *Demonstrate accountability for health outcomes.* A population health approach focuses on the extent of change in health outcomes that result from interventions.

Although CHNs may work in health promotion with individuals and families, many work with populations and aggregates in their communities. CHNs need to always assess the determinants of health; consider social and economic inequalities; consider interventions needed to affect the determinants of health, such as empowering communities; advocate for healthy public policy; and establish and promote partnerships that contribute to the highest level of health for the patient. This integration of the determinants of health is complex. A document that can assist CHNs with the development of health promotion activities to effect change in population health determinants is *How Our Programs Affect Population Health Determinants: A Workbook for Better Planning and Accountability* (Labonte, 2003). (See the link on the Evolve website.)

International Health Promotion Conferences

The WHO Fourth Global Conference on Health Promotion took place in Jakarta, Indonesia, in 1997. The conference produced the Jakarta Declaration on Leading Health Promotion Into the 21st Century (WHO, 2001). This was the first health promotion conference held in a developing country and the first to involve the private sector. To the prerequisites for health introduced in the Ottawa Charter, the Jakarta conference added social security, social relations, empowerment of women, and respect for human rights. Poverty (income) was identified as the social determinant that influences health the most. In addition, the declaration expanded on the Ottawa Charter strategies. The five priorities identified for the twenty-first century were (1) to promote social responsibility for health; (2) to increase investments for health development; (3) to consolidate and expand partnerships for health; (4) to increase community capacity and empower the individual; and (5) to secure an infrastructure for health promotion. The WHO link on the Evolve website offers further information.

The WHO Sixth Global Conference on Health Promotion took place in Bangkok, Thailand, in 2005 and produced the Bangkok Charter for Health Promotion in a Globalized World (WHO, 2005). The Bangkok Charter addresses the need for global governance of health as affected by all the determinants of health, especially the health gaps between the rich and the poor. The Bangkok Charter made four global health promotion commitments. It would make health promotion "central to the global development agenda; a core responsibility for all of government; a key focus of communities and civil society; a requirement for good corporate practice" (WHO, 2005). The following five action areas were identified for all sectors and

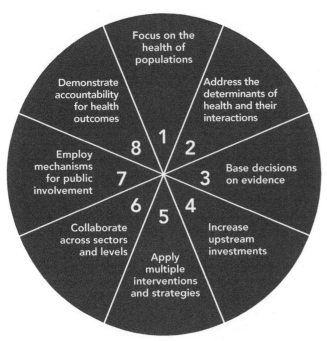

Fig. 4.4 Population Health Approach: The Organizing Framework. From Public Health Agency of Canada. [2013]. *Canadian best practices portal: Population health approach: The organizing framework.* (Adapted and reproduced with permission from the Minister of Health, 2016.)

settings to narrow the inequalities in the social determinants that affect health: (1) advocacy for health for all; (2) investment in sustainable policies, actions, and infrastructure; (3) capacity building in policy development, leadership, health promotion practice, knowledge transfer and research, and health literacy; (4) regulation and legislation that provides an optimal level of security from harm to provide opportunity for health and well-being for all that is equal; and (5) partnerships and alliances among public, private, nongovernmental, and international organizations to create measures that are sustainable (WHO, 2006).

The WHO Seventh Global Conference on Health Promotion took place in Nairobi, Kenya, in 2009, and followed up on the work done at the Bangkok conference. WHO member states were encouraged to work toward meeting the four global health promotion commitments established in the Bangkok Charter. Support was provided to member states to develop and implement pilot projects to address the social determinants of health to reduce the gap between the rich and the poor (WHO, 2010). (See the WHO Overview link on the Evolve website.)

In 2011, the Government of Canada participated in the WHO World Conference on Social Determinants of Health in Rio de Janeiro, Brazil. The conference produced the Rio Political Declaration on Social Determinants of Health. It was authored by representatives of all the heads of government, ministers, and government representatives at the conference (WHO, 2011). The document's main ideas are as follows: that health equity is a shared responsibility and requires the engagement of all sectors of government, society, and all members of the international community; and that the promotion of health equity is essential for a better quality of life and well-being for all. The document acknowledges that there is a need to adopt better governance for health and development (e.g., give a voice to all groups and sectors), and to promote participation in policymaking and implementation (e.g., use participatory processes).

In 2016, leaders from around the world endorsed the Shanghai Declaration on Health Promotion, which stressed the links between health and well-being and highlighted the need for people to be able to control their own health. The Declaration highlighted the role of good governance and health literacy in improving health and called on governments to introduce universal health coverage as an efficient way to promote health. Leaders committed to considering the growing importance and value of traditional medicine as well as implementing fiscal policies as a powerful tool to enable new investments in health and well-being (Kickbusch & Nutbeam, 2017).

Summary of the Evolution of Health Promotion

Catford (2004) captures the development of health promotion during the past several decades by categorizing health promotion dimensions related to its main focuses. According to Catford, in the 1970s, the first dimension of health promotion focused on managing preventable diseases and risk behaviours (e.g., heart disease, tobacco use). The health promotion strategy most countries adopted was providing health information and "simple" education. In the 1980s, the emphasis shifted to the importance of complementary intervention approaches as outlined in the Ottawa Charter, such as building healthy public policy and strengthening community action. In the 1990s, the focus was on providing health promotion to individuals and groups in their communities (e.g., cities, neighbourhoods, workplaces, schools, health care settings).

Catford (2004) suggests that in the 2000s, a fourth dimension of health promotion is evident in the inclusion of the social determinants of health (see Chapter 1), which provide a much broader focus than disease control and prevention. Leadership is essential to ensuring that health promotion continues to be a primary focus; therefore, CHNs actively promoting health in their nursing practice need to continue demonstrating their leadership role in influencing healthy public policy, creating supportive environments, and strengthening community-based action. In addition, CHNs need to take action on the social environments that contribute to risk, the socioeconomic determinants of health as well as health inequities (CPHA, 2010).

Canadian community health nursing practice incorporates strategies from primary health care, the Ottawa Charter, the Epp framework, the population health model, and the determinants of health. For a synopsis of the reports and initiatives that contributed to the shift from an illness-focused perspective to a population- and health-promotion focus in primary health care in Canada, refer to Ehrlich and Ladouceur (2002).

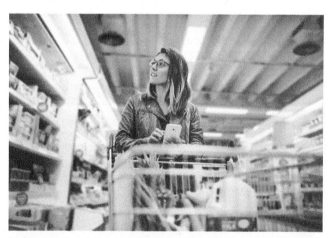

Making healthy choices when grocery shopping is one way in which a person practises self-efficacy. (iStockphoto/PeopleImages)

HEALTH PROMOTION MODELS, THEORIES, AND FRAMEWORKS

Models, theories, and frameworks provide different ways of looking at health and health promotion. Several models, theories, and frameworks have been developed in an attempt to explain health behaviour and health behavioural change (Clark, 2008; Heiss, 2009). They may focus on behavioural change in individuals, health changes in communities and organizations, healthy public policy, broader contextual factors that influence health, or human caring.

Individual-Focused Perspectives

Individual-focused models mainly consider health promotion interventions that shape individuals' or groups' health behaviours (Sallis, Cervero, Ascher, et al., 2006; Young & Hayes, 2002). These models tend to encourage individual responsibility for health, and when people do not change their health behaviour, poor health is viewed as their fault. The advantage of these models for CHNs is that they facilitate the exploration of the reasons for individual health-related behaviours (Meade, 2007). The theory and model most widely associated with individual-focused health promotion and used in community health nursing are the theory of planned behaviour and the transtheoretical model (also called the stages of change model). Both focus on explaining an individual's behavioural health change and help explain and facilitate personal health practices, which is one of the determinants of health.

Theory of Planned Behaviour

In 1980, Ajzen and Fishbein developed the theory of reasoned action (renamed the "theory of planned behaviour") to understand and predict individual changes to health behaviour (Clark, 2008). The theory assumes that a relationship exists among attitudes, beliefs, intention, and behaviour (McKenzie, Neiger, & Thackeray et al., 2009; Park & Lee,

2012). Another underlying assumption of this theory is that the most influential factor in behavioural change is the intent to act. The theory postulates that beliefs, attitudes, and perceived behavioural control influence individual, group, and aggregate intention and thus behaviour (McKenzie et al., 2009). Therefore, to develop interventions and programs that will meet patient needs, the CHN needs to assess these three factors in all patient situations. In addition, the CHN needs to identify the patient's intention for behavioural change.

Transtheoretical Model (or Stages of Change Model)

The transtheoretical model, often referred to as the *stages of change model,* was first introduced in the early 1980s by Prochaska and DiClemente (1983) and continues to be used today (Lam, Wiley, Siu, et al., 2010). The model proposes that the process of intentional behavioural change usually proceeds through five stages: precontemplation, contemplation, preparation, action, and maintenance. A sixth stage, termination, was later added, and it is most often associated with changing addictive behaviours such as substance use. Table 4.2 applies the transtheoretical model to the process of smoking cessation.

The transtheoretical model includes stages, challenges (e.g., consciousness raising, recognition of the benefits of change), constructs (e.g., situational self-efficacy), temptations (e.g., coping with a situation with confidence without reverting to previous unhealthy behaviours), and decisional balance (e.g., consideration of the pros and cons of changing behaviour) (Cancer Prevention Research Center, n.d.).

TABLE 4.2 Application of the Transtheoretical Model to Promoting Smoking Cessation

Stages of Change	Patient Behaviour	Challenge	Suggested Actions for the Community Health Nurse
Precontemplation	Patient has no intention to change behaviour within the next 6 months (no readiness for change)	Consciousness raising	• Assess patient interest in quitting smoking • Provide information to the patient on the health risks associated with smoking • Explore with the patient the feasibility of smoking cessation
Contemplation	Patient thinking of changing behaviour within the next 6 months	Recognition of the benefits of change	• Discuss information on the potential benefits of quitting smoking
Preparation	Patient has serious intention to change behaviour within the next 30 days (readiness for change)	Support to overcome barriers to quitting smoking	• Assist patient to identify potential barriers • Explore with the patient how to overcome the barriers
Action	Patient has initiated behavioural change within past 6 months (behavioural change)	Program of change	• Develop a smoking cessation plan with the patient • Monitor patient progress
Maintenance	Patient has changed behaviour for longer than 6 months (behavioural change)	Follow-up with continued support	• Plan routine follow-up contacts with the patient • Prepare a plan to prevent relapse
Termination	Patient is no longer tempted to re-establish the unhealthy behaviour (permanent behavioural change)	No need for follow-up	• Capacity building by identifying strengths • Supporting changed behaviour

Source: Adapted from Nutbeam, D., & Harris, E. (2004). *Theory in a nutshell: A practical guide to health promotion theories.* Sydney: McGraw Hill (based on Prochaska, J. O., & DiClemente, C. C. [1983]. Stages and processes of self-change of smoking: Toward an integrative model of change. *Journal of Consulting and Clinical Psychology, 51*[3], 390–395).

For a more comprehensive discussion of this model (and other models), see the *Theory at a Glance: A Guide for Health Promotion Practice* and the Cancer Prevention Research Center links on the Evolve website.

Many research studies have used this model with aggregates such as smokers in smoking cessation programs (Callaghan & Herzog, 2006; Spencer, Pagell, Hallion, et al., 2002); obese individuals in weight-loss programs (Beresford, Curry, Kristal, et al., 1996; Glanz, Patterson, Kristal, et al., 1998); and persons and aggregates with sedentary lifestyles trying to increase their physical activity behaviours (Riebe, Blissmer, Greene, et al., 2005; Spencer, Adams, Malone, et al., 2006).

Critics have raised several issues with the transtheoretical model and have challenged its scientific merit, despite the finding that more than 500 published studies have used this model for smoking cessation (see Herzog [2005] and West [2005] for specifics on the debate).

For CHNs working with patients or developing individual-focused health promotion programs, this model of change provides direction regarding what to assess, which processes to use, and what nursing actions to take when patients are at different stages of change. This model encourages CHNs to become familiar with community resources that would benefit patients going through specific stages of change for a particular behaviour.

Community-Focused Perspectives

We now turn to perspectives that consider health as more than just an individual responsibility. Two of the most common theories and frameworks that attempt to explain changes in communities are the diffusion of innovation theory and the community mobilization framework.

Diffusion of Innovation Theory

The diffusion of innovation theory provides guidance on effective ways to encourage patients to adopt ideas, practices, programs, or products that are considered "new" or innovative. *Innovation* is any new idea, practice, or product, and *diffusion* is the process for gaining acceptance of that innovation in the community or throughout society (Nutbeam & Harris, 2004). This theory shows that individuals adopt innovations at different rates. Patients exposed to an innovation are classified in one of the following five categories: innovators (quick adopters), early adopters (keeners), early majority, late majority, and laggards. Although the innovators hastily adopt the innovation, these people are often viewed as impulsive. The early adopters are willing to change and have the resources to adopt the innovation. The early majority usually comprise 30 to 35% of the general population, and they are open to change and recognize the benefits of change. The late majority usually comprise 30 to 35% of the general population and are doubtful about adopting the innovation. The laggards are resistant to adopting the innovation (Nutbeam & Harris, 2004). In general, patients are more likely to adopt innovative health-related practices if the following six conditions exist: compatibility, flexibility, reversibility, simplicity, advantageousness, and cost-efficiency.

Dearing (2009) indicates that a potential adopter's perception of the attributes of an innovation affect his or her adoption decision. A potential adopter assesses the following:
- The relative advantage of the innovation in terms of effectiveness and cost-efficiency in relation to the alternatives
- The simplicity of the innovation (i.e., how easy it is to understand)
- The compatibility of the innovation (i.e., its similarity with established ways of achieving the same goal)
- The observability of the innovation (i.e., the degree to which results can be observed)
- The trialability of the innovation (i.e., the degree of commitment for full adoption)

To be effective, CHNs involved in the development and implementation of innovative health promotion ideas and practices need to consider the types of adopters for an innovation and the six conditions that influence adoption of the innovation. Social marketing strategies, which are discussed later in the chapter, can be used to disseminate and cultivate acceptance of innovative ideas and practices.

The theoretical components of diffusion need to be considered to make health promotion programs sustainable in communities, organizations, and individuals. When innovations are introduced in a community, diffusion can include implementing new initiatives, advancing policies, and using mass media (National Cancer Institute, 2005). When innovations are introduced in an organization, diffusion can include initiating programs, modifying regulations, and adjusting worker roles. When innovations are introduced to individuals, diffusion includes adopting a health behaviour and requires lifestyle changes.

CHNs must know the community they work with and be able to anticipate what would most likely influence the community's response to new health promotion ideas, practices, and programs. Also, CHNs can identify community leaders as role models for change, which can speed up the adoption of the innovation. See Table 4.3 for the top 10 misconceptions that can happen in practice to work against diffusion. CHNs need to be aware of these mistakes to avoid them.

Community Mobilization Framework

Health promotion involves working with communities that can be defined as a geographical community (e.g., neighbourhood, town) or a community of interest (e.g., older adults, disabled group with diabetes, obese children, transgendered persons). Rothman's community mobilization framework identifies the following three health promotion community mobilization approaches to bring about community change: (1) social planning (i.e., problem solving at the community level to deal with community physical, mental, and social health concerns), which is described as a task-oriented strategy with a health care provider as expert "leader"; (2) locality development (i.e., community participation and cooperation to deal with community health concerns with a focus on process, consensus, and community self-help with a health care provider as facilitator); and (3) social action (i.e., a process with the focus on shifting power relationships and resources

TABLE 4.3 Top 10 Misconceptions That Can Happen in Practice to Work Against Diffusion

1. *Evidence matters the most in the decision making of potential adopters.*
   Interventions of unknown effectiveness and of known ineffectiveness often spread while effective interventions do not.
   Evidence is most important to only a subset of early adopters and is most often used by them to reject interventions (e.g., HPV is linked to cancer, yet many young women are still not vaccinated against it).
   Solution: Emphasize other variables in the communication of innovations such as compatibility, cost, and simplicity.

2. *Our perceptions are the same as those of potential adopters.*
   Potential adopters do not always have the same evidence that we have about prototype interventions. This can contribute to inaccurate perceptions of a particular program because the evidence needed by the potential adopters has not been disseminated (e.g., research on the lack of adverse effects of the HPV vaccine may not be readily available to potential adopters).
   Solution: Seek out and listen to representative potential adopters to learn wants, information sources, advice-seeking behaviours, and reactions to prototype interventions.

3. *Intervention creators are effective intervention communicators.*
   While the creators of interventions are sometimes effective communicators, the opposite is much more common.
   Solution: Use information from the experts but rely on others who you know will elicit attention and information-seeking by potential adopters (e.g., public health campaigns by experts should be designed in consultation with parents of school-aged females) when planning communication.

4. *Interventions should be introduced as soon as they are ready.*
   Interventions are often publicized as soon as they are created or tested. However, if the results of the interventions are uncertain or complex, they can be confusing for potential adopters (e.g., if HPV vaccination clinics are introduced before adequate dissemination of new research on the effectiveness of HPV vaccines).
   Solution: Publicize interventions only after clear results and prepare messages that report on those results to elicit positive reactions from potential adopters.

5. *Information will influence the decision making of all adopters.*
   Information is necessary and can be sufficient for adoption decisions about inconsequential innovations, but for consequential interventions that imply changes in organizational routines or individual behaviours, information alone may not be enough.
   Solution: Pair information resources with social influence in an overall dissemination strategy (e.g., invite a well-known student to attend an HPV clinic and to participate in educational events).

6. *Authority and influence are the same.*
   People who have high positional or formal authority are sometimes influential, but often this is not the case.
   Solution: Determine who potential adopters seek out for advice and ask those influencers for their help in propelling diffusion (e.g., female community leaders who have already received the HPV vaccine).

7. *Innovators should select future health care strategies.*
   The first to adopt often do so for counter-normative reasons, so they may not represent the majority of potential adopters. Although an innovator's opinions are important, the opinions of others must also be obtained when selecting future health care strategies (e.g., females who attended the day-time HPV vaccination clinic may be satisfied, but there may be a need to offer evening clinics to reach all of the female target population).
   Solution: Identify the opinions of all of the potential adopters when selecting future health care strategies.

8. *Change agents, authority figures, opinion leaders, and innovation champions all have the same influence on health promotion.*
   It is unusual for people to have the same influence in communities and complex organizations.
   Solution: Use formative evaluation to determine the functions that different persons are able to fulfill in diffusion.

9. *Demonstration sites should be selected based on the criteria of motivation and capacity.*
   Criteria of motivation and capacity make sense when effective implementation is the only objective, but spread also relies on the perceptions by others of the initial adopters (e.g., a demonstration site at a small youth group centre may not have the capacity to service large numbers of students, but it may have a more positive influence on potential adopters than a larger HPV vaccine clinic at a community health centre).
   Solution: Consider motivation and capacity as well as which demonstration sites could have a positive influence on potential adopters.

10. *Single interventions are the best solution to a health problem.*
    Potential adopters differ according to a variety of factors, so a single intervention is unlikely to fit all populations (e.g., HPV education in schools and with community groups such as Girl Guides).
    Solution: Communicate a cluster of evidence-informed practices so that potential adopters can get closer to a best fit of intervention to organization prior to adoption.

Source: Dearing, J. W. (2009). Applying diffusion of innovation theory to intervention development. *Research on Social Work Practice, 19*(5), 503–518.

so that change occurs to the benefit of the disadvantaged in the community) (Nutbeam & Harris, 2004). (See the Ontario Health Promotion Resource System link on the Evolve website.)

The distinction between "working with," "working for," and "working on" communities is important as one examines the perspective of community-level work (Wass, 2000). When "working with" the community, health care providers form partnerships with community members as community development and capacity building occur. Thereby, communities incorporate health promotion approaches to bring about needed changes. When "working for" the community, health care providers are recognized as experts who lead the planning and implementation of health promotion approaches, with some involvement of community members as required to bring about the needed changes. When "working on" the community, health care providers, using health promotion approaches, are viewed as experts and assume complete planning and decision-making responsibilities with little or no input from the community to bring about the needed changes. "Working with" the community is the approach CHNs prefer for fostering community engagement and mobilization.

Public Policy–Focused Perspectives

CHNs consider the sociopolitical issues that may underlie individual, family, group, community, population, or system problems (Community Health Nurses of Canada [CHNC], 2019). Sociopolitical issues are influenced by the public policies created by municipal (local), provincial or territorial, and federal governments. Therefore, CHNs need to be familiar with and knowledgeable about the available models for healthy public policy development, the policies and legislation that mandate their professional practice roles and responsibilities, and the healthy public policies mandated within their community programs and service delivery. It is also important for CHNs to recognize the need for intersectoral collaboration in relation to healthy public policy development. Within a population health focus with an emphasis on the determinants of health, policy development is broader than just health care. Therefore, depending on the issue, other societal sectors may need to be involved (e.g., agriculture, justice, and transportation) in the building of healthy public policy.

The CHN's role in building health public policy is strongly supported by the Canadian Nurses Association (CNA). In 2012, the CNA presented evidence to the federal government from its National Expert Commission report that indicated health inequities in Canada are directly related to income, housing, nutrition, and social support (CNA, 2012). In response to that report, CNA engaged in efforts to promote healthy public policy, including supporting Bill C-32 *Cracking Down on Tobacco Monitoring Aimed at Youth Act* (Government of Canada, 2009) and Bill C-304 *Secure Adequate Accessible and Affordable Housing Act* (Government of Canada, 2010). CNA is also involved annually in prebudget consultations with the federal government to identify priority foci for health funding, including supporting the need for innovative and cost-effective ways to support working family caregivers, First

Nations people, Inuit, Métis, and older persons (CNA, 2015). These actions by CNA show support for the CHN's role as an advocate in creating healthy public policy.

Three frameworks are available to help in building healthy public policy: Milio's framework for the development of healthy public policy, Weiss's framework on the relationships between evidence and policy, and the health impact assessment on policy development and implementation.

Milio's Framework

In 1987, Milio coined the term *healthy public policy* and identified that policy development proceeds through initiation, action, implementation, evaluation, and reformulation stages (as cited in Nutbeam & Harris, 2004). These stages are cyclical and dynamic rather than linear as policy moves through the social and political processes. In Milio's framework, *policyholders* (i.e., politicians, bureaucrats), *policy influencers* (i.e., aggregates inside and outside of governments), the *public* (i.e., individuals who influence policy adoption, such as taxpayers and voters), and the *media* (i.e., print and electronic, affecting policymakers and public knowledge and perceptions about the issue) are foundational to healthy policy development. Milio maintained that the community or organization must become a key stakeholder, even though most policy development is initiated by only a few individuals. The four elements that affect policy development as identified by Milio are *social climate* (i.e., social, economic, and political context when the policy is introduced), *influence* (best if the policy is associated with committed groups who have the most power on the issue), *interests* (i.e., what could be gained, lost, or compromised), and *capacity* (i.e., ability to affect the issue). Social climate is the most powerful of these elements.

The CHN's roles as an advocate in creating public policy, as a support for community action to influence public policy, and as an advocate for societal change are identified in the CCHN Standards. In community health nursing, with its health promotion focus, development of healthy public policy is often directed at particular aggregate groups based on age, health challenges, lifestyle, and healthy choice issues. Examples include crib safety for infants and young children, restraint use in long-term care institutions, seatbelt use for populations, and a tobacco ban in communities. An understanding of Milio's framework would, for example, help the CHN identify the main players and key elements to consider in strategy development when proposing a health issue for healthy policy development.

Weiss's Models of Policy Development

Weiss developed knowledge-driven, problem-solving, interactive, political, and tactical models to provide clarification of the different ways that evidence has guided healthy policy development (as cited in Nutbeam & Harris, 2004). Box 4.4 provides a synopsis of each of these models.

Ecological Models

Ecological models in health promotion address broad contextual factors that influence health (Green & Kreuter, 1999;

BOX 4.4 Weiss's Models of Policy Development

Model	Key Considerations
Knowledge driven	• New research knowledge immediately influences healthy public policy. • New knowledge is rapidly accepted into policy development.
Problem solving	• Mechanisms during the decision-making process related to policy development include collection and consideration of the evidence.
Interactive	• The evidence is collected from a variety of sources. • During policy development, knowledge from research is one consideration. • Other considerations include social pressures, experience, and political situation.
Political	• "Evidence is used to justify a predetermined position."*
Tactical	• Preferable data are used. • Evidence is used to support an unpopular decision or to explain and avoid an unpopular decision. • Unsubstantiated research findings are used to delay decision making.

Source: Adapted from Nutbeam, D., & Harris, E. (2004). Theory in a nutshell: A practical guide to health promotion theories. Sydney: McGraw Hill.
*Nutbeam & Harris, 2004, p. 65.

Lyons & Langille, 2000). These models have a system-level focus and explore the relationships between individuals and communities and between sociocultural and environmental factors that influence health (McLaren & Hawe, 2005). Therefore, when using an ecological perspective, the health promotion strategies target multiple levels, such as healthy public policy, community, organization, and intrapersonal and interpersonal factors that affect health (Green & Kreuter, 1999; McLaren & Hawe, 2005; Sallis et al., 2006). One example of an ecological model is the PRECEDE–PROCEED model developed by Green and Kreuter (1999). Sallis et al. (2006) describe a more recent example of the application of the ecological model to change population health in communities through improving physical activity. The researchers explored the ecological model and its influence on the four domains of active living: recreation, transport, occupation, and household. (See the article by Sallis et al. [2006] for further detail on the approach used.) The PRECEDE–PROCEED model is discussed in depth in Chapter 10.

Existential and Humanistic Theoretical Perspectives

In recent literature, existential and humanistic theoretical perspectives have emerged as orientations that inform nursing practice. Within these orientations, the classic and evolving theoretical work of Watson (1979, 1999) emphasizes caring for humankind as foundational to nursing as a profession and, more specifically, the therapeutic interpersonal relationship between the nurse and the patient. Watson's description of caring as the moral imperative to act justly and ethically to effect a positive change in the welfare of others aligns well with health promotion initiatives for community patients. Watson's emphasis on holistic health identifies that all human beings have "carative" needs that can be met through individualized nursing interventions focused on a human care process involving mutual participation of both the nurse and the patient (Watson, 1999). Although not widely acknowledged as a health promotion model, Watson's theory of human caring, when applied in health promotion initiatives within the community context, provides a holistic and progressive patient-inclusive approach.

HEALTH PROMOTION APPROACHES

The following three approaches provide different ways of viewing health and of promoting optimal health and well-being: (1) biomedical, (2) behavioural, and (3) socioenvironmental. These approaches were originally referred to as *models*. Table 4.4 describes the components of each of these approaches.

Biomedical Approach

The biomedical approach was introduced in the eighteenth century with the discovery of disease pathogens and has continued to develop to the present. "Health promotion began with a medical approach focusing on immunization and screening for existing diseases, then shifted to a focus on changing individual risk behaviours" (Clark, 2008). This approach focuses on the treatment and prevention of disease, especially on the biological and physiological risk factors associated with disease and ill health. The prevention of disease includes the three levels of prevention. For example, hypertension is a risk factor for cardiovascular events such as a CVA. Finding hypertension in patients early and counselling about dietary changes, especially fat and salt intake, are important preventive strategies.

Behavioural Approach

The behavioural approach was first introduced with the Lalonde Report (1974) and has been further developed since then. This approach focuses on using lifestyle changes, especially behavioural risk factors, to promote health. For example, obesity is a risk factor for hypertension, and obesity and smoking are risk factors for cardiovascular disease. Health communication activities in this example would focus on quit-smoking campaigns and physical activity and nutritional messages for weight loss. Social marketing, the use of mass media, or both could be used to support the adoption of a healthy lifestyle.

Socioenvironmental Approach

The socioenvironmental approach started with the Alma-Ata Conference on Primary Health Care in 1978, when community participation and intersectoral collaboration were identified as necessary for dealing with social and environmental

TABLE 4.4 Three Approaches Used in Health Promotion

Approach	Perception of Health	Examples of Leading Health Problems	Examples of Strategies to Manage Health Problems
Biomedical	Health is the absence of diseases, conditions, and disorders	• Hypertension • Cardiovascular diseases • Diabetes • Obesity • Human immunodeficiency virus/ acquired immunodeficiency syndrome	• Medical and pharmacological treatments specific to health problem • Primary prevention (e.g., immunization) • Secondary prevention, e.g., early case finding through screening programs • Tertiary prevention (e.g., cardiovascular rehabilitation programs)
Behavioural	Health is the result of lifestyle choices, specifically healthy ones	• Poor stress management • Smoking • Sedentary lifestyle • Poor eating habits • Substance abuse	• Health communication • Health education • Self-help or mutual aid • Advocacy for healthy public policies to change behaviours and promote healthy lifestyle choices (e.g., smoking bans)
Socioenvironmental	Health is the result of the determinants of health, specifically social, economic, and environmental, that provide benefits and barriers to individual and community health	• Unemployment • Poverty • Lack of social support and isolation • Environmental pollution	• Building healthy public policy • Creating supportive environments • Strengthening community action • Developing personal skills • Reorienting health services

Source: Adapted from Hershfield, L., & Hyndman, B. (2004). *HP-101: Health promotion on-line course, module 4*, Ontario Health Promotion Resource System. Retrieved from https://www.publichealthontario.ca/en/education-and-events/online-learning/health-promotion-courses

determinants of health. This approach focuses on health as a resource and considers the psychosocial and environmental risk factors related to the determinants of health in relation to health and health promotion. For example, the risk condition associated with the social determinant of health of poverty in the community affects people's ability to purchase healthy foods and, thereby, affects their cardiovascular health. Community policy development pertaining to "food security" would address this social determinant of health. The importance of the socioenvironmental approach in health promotion can be summarizes as:

> Lack of health care is not the cause of the huge global burden of illness; water-borne diseases are not caused by lack of antibiotics but by dirty water, and by political, social and economic forces that fail to make clean water available to all; heart disease is not caused by a lack of coronary care units but by the lives people lead; which are shaped by the environments in which they live; obesity is not caused by moral failure on the part of individuals but by the excess availability of high-fat and high-sugar foods. The main action on the social determinants of health must come from outside the health sector. (WHO, 2008, p. 43)

The Senate Subcommittee on Population Health (2009) recommends that priority be given to the following determinants of health: clean water; food security; parenting and early childhood learning; violence against Indigenous women, children, and elders; education; housing; economic development; and health care. The report also addresses health disparities, promotes the well-being of all Canadians, and recommends a whole-government approach to address health issues of Canadians. Health care providers usually subscribe to one or all of these approaches, influencing their view of health and health promotion, their definitions of *health,* and their decisions about which health promotion strategies and activities to use to deal with patient health challenges. CHNs often subscribe to all three approaches, depending on the setting in which they work.

HEALTH PROMOTION STRATEGIES

Several strategies are used to promote population, community, group, family, and individual health. As noted earlier, the Ottawa Charter identified five areas requiring action in health promotion practice: building healthy public policy, creating supportive environments, strengthening community action, developing personal skills, and reorienting health services. Because of the complexity of health issues, addressing them is best done using a combination of strategies to achieve an identified goal or goals. The Ottawa Charter shifted the health promotion approach from an individual level with a focus on behavioural and disease orientation to a population health level with a focus on the determinants of health and a health orientation (Tang et al., 2005). Each of the Ottawa Charter strategies is discussed next.

Strengthening Community Action

The strategy of strengthening community action, as outlined in the Ottawa Charter, refers to empowering communities. It involves engaging communities from the grassroots, or "bottom up" (referred to as "locality development" by Rothman, as cited in Nutbeam & Harris, 2004), so as to involve community members in identifying health issues and planning and initiating interventions specific to their communities. Thereby, communities take ownership and have control over health issues affecting them and the health of their members. The term most frequently used for this strategy in Canada (as well as Australia and the United Kingdom) is *community development;* in the United States, this strategy is most often referred to as *community organizing* or *community building* (Labonte, 1997). **Community development** is the process of involving the community in identifying and strengthening the daily, cultural, and political aspects of life that promote and support health (CPHA, 2010). Partnerships are essential in community development. The goal is a secure and healthy community with buy-in from all community members.

The resources or assets and possible contributions of the partners are identified and "mapped" to build a capacity list rather than a deficiency list. *Asset mapping* with a capacity-building focus serves as the starting point for determining the resources and assets available in the community, identifying further community resources to be developed. The asset-mapping approach usually shows the connections between and among community assets because communities are built on these types of connections and supports. A community working on capacity building would focus on establishing green space, sponsoring numerous support groups, and working toward low crime rates.

The information gained from asset mapping should be used to promote community development. Often, a coalition of community partners is engaged with this goal of effecting positive community change. The Health Data Research Network Canada serves as an example of a capacity-building project using partnerships. This multilevel-strategy project links local, provincial, and national health departments by producing widespread partnerships as a way of developing and distributing knowledge about health and social challenges in Canada (Health Data Research Network Canada, 2021).

The Canadian Healthy Communities project, developed and launched by Health Canada in 1987 (active until 1992), is an example of community development. (WHO established its Healthy Communities program shortly afterward.) Currently, provincial Healthy Communities networks are found in British Columbia, Ontario, Quebec, and New Brunswick. The Healthy Communities process includes an intersectoral approach, with health being the major focus for policymaking and citizen engagement at the municipal level. The project includes the following components: wide community participation (communities identify their own health issues), involvement of all sectors of the community, local government commitment, and creation of healthy public policies (Ontario Healthy Communities Coalition, 2019). These components relate directly to the Ottawa Charter health promotion strategies.

The significance of the Healthy Communities process to CHNs is that it deals with many of the determinants of health that fall outside the scope of the health care system. For example, implementing policies to provide better access to nutritious food would have a significant positive impact on patients' health status. CHNs in several Canadian communities have contributed to building healthy communities by identifying health issues in the community, assisting community members to explore health issues, advocating for identified issues, and establishing coalitions with other organizations and sectors such as education and housing (CNA, 2005). The CNA backgrounder titled *Healthy Communities and Nursing: A Summary of the Issues* provides information on why the issue of healthy communities is important to nurses and offers some suggestions as to what nurses can do about this issue, for example, becoming informed about community health issues and working with others in the community to advocate for healthier communities (CNA, 2005).

The PHAC has a Healthy Communities Division within the Centre for Health Promotion, which addresses the issues of family violence, rural health, mental health, injury prevention, and physical activity and also provides consultation with regard to community capacity building with the goal of improving Canadians' health (PHAC, 2008b). The use of community capacity to bring about change through an action plan, usually developed and implemented with community partners, is known as **community mobilization**. *Community mobilization* involves individuals in a community working together as a group to influence healthy public policy and to bring about change regarding a health issue. The reduction in tobacco use is an example of community mobilization. The healthy public policy around smoking developed from the grassroots, meaning that it was initiated by individuals in the community who were concerned about the effects of smoking. They formed community groups, which partnered with community agencies and organizations, to advocate for policy changes on smoking at the municipal, provincial, and federal levels. Usually, these groups included CHNs, either as representatives of their local health agency or as fellow concerned citizens. As a result of the community mobilization around tobacco use, municipal, provincial, and federal governments in Canada have developed and implemented policies to restrict tobacco use.

Community-based strategies and community development strategies are distinct (Boutilier, Cleverly, & Labonte, 2000; Labonte, 1997; Hershfield & Hyndman, 2004). Usually defined by an outside organization or professional, *community-based strategies* connect programs and services to community groups. The decision-making power is most often with the sponsoring organization or professional and not with the community participants. By contrast, *community development strategies* involve a health concern or issue as defined and raised by community residents rather than a sponsoring organization or a health care provider such as a physician or CHN. When community development strategies are used, the decision-making power rests primarily with community residents. In community development strategies, the CHN may fulfill a liaison role.

Having gained recognition in the 1990s (Ontario Prevention Clearinghouse, 2002), the term **capacity building** refers to the process of actively involving communities, individuals, or organizations in all phases of planned change to deal with their health issues and increase their skills, knowledge, and willingness to take action. Capacity building focuses on community strengths but also acknowledges deficits. Capacity building requires a strong foundation that can support and sustain what the community needs to address its health concerns or issues, often through the establishment and maintenance of partnerships. A project led by the Canadian Public Health Association (CPHA) serves as an example of capacity building. Voluntary Organizations Involved in Collaborative Engagement (VOICE) in Health Policy was a national project with the goal of enhancing the policy capacity of volunteer health organizations. The project was divided into three phases and concluded in 2004 with an action plan to continue enhancing policy collaboration (Stanhope and Lancaster, 2011). Health Canada's Community Action Program for Children and Canada Prenatal Nutrition Program provide two other examples of capacity building.

Community capacity includes the identification of resources, commitment, and time required to ensure the success of the health project or program. As well, capacity building at the community level involves community members' taking action to deal with their needs as well as the social and political support required for successful implementation of programs (Smith, Tang, & Nutbeam, 2006).

To build community capacity, CHNs need to work collaboratively with the community. When working with the community, the CHN begins with an assessment to (1) determine what stage the community is at, (2) assist the community to identify health concerns and strengths, (3) assist the community to identify how to use its strengths to deal with the identified health challenges, and (4) explore how the community feels it can best manage its health challenges. Following assessment and planning, the CHN works with the community to develop strategies. See Standard 5 ("Capacity Building") of the CCHN Standards in Appendix 1.

Empowerment, a key concept in health promotion, refers to a process that is used to actively engage the patient to gain greater control and involves political efficacy, improved quality of community life, and social justice. Community empowerment results from collective individual efforts to influence and manage the effects of the determinants of health. Patient empowerment is a key component of health promotion (Uys, Majumdar, & Gwele, 2004).

Community inclusion and engagement are aspects of health promotion and part of the dialogue within the field of population health. People need to experience a sense of belonging if they are to feel comfortable actively participating in decisions that will affect the health of their community. Social networks and supports contribute to the development of this sense of belonging. Social and political actions that influence policy are also needed to ensure equity and social justice and that the determinants of health are addressed. For further information about inclusion, see the links for Health Canada's *An Inclusion Lens* (a workbook developed in Atlantic Canada) and Health Nexus (previously known as the Ontario Prevention Clearinghouse) on the Evolve website. Table 4.5 provides examples of inclusion and exclusion

TABLE 4.5 **Examples of Inclusion and Exclusion in Relation to the Eight Dimensions of An Inclusion Lens**		
Dimension	**Examples of Inclusion**	**Examples of Exclusion**
Cultural	• Valuing of contributions • Acknowledgement of differences and diversity	• Intolerance • Gender stereotyping
Economic	• Fewer disparities • Personal security	• Unemployment • Stigma • Inequality
Functional	• Ability to be involved • Valuing of social roles	• Inability to function • Overextended
Participatory	• Ability to make choices • Accessibility of programs	• Lack of encouragement to participate in decision making • Blockage of communication
Physical	• Friendly environment • Access to community services	• Unfriendly environment • Unsustainable environments
Political	• Social protection of vulnerable groups • Active participation by citizens in the community	• Victim blaming • Restrictive policies
Relational	• Belonging • Supportive family	• Isolation • Family violence
Structural	• Community capacity building • Two-way communication	• Withholding of information • Restrictive boundaries

Source: Adapted from Health Canada. (2002). *An inclusion lens: Workbook for looking at social and economic exclusion and inclusion.* Halifax: Minister of Health. Retrieved from https://www.allianceon.org/sites/default/files/documents/Workbook%20for%20looking%20at%20Social_and_Economic_Inclusion_Lens%202002.pdf

in relation to the eight dimensions of inclusion identified in *An Inclusion Lens*.

The community health action model, a new model currently in development, considers many of the concepts that have been discussed in this section. The model does the following:

- Serves as a model for community health promotion
- Incorporates community development and community health assessment
- Incorporates a population health approach
- Empowers the community
- Views health care providers as resources for the community versus experts
- Considers community assets and strengths
- Considers community resiliency and community capacity (Racher & Annis, 2007)

CHNs value and believe in the concepts of partnerships and empowerment, which are supported in the CCHN Standards. They build partnerships derived from the concepts of primary health care, caring, and empowerment (CHNC, 2019). In the standards of practice, the two primary health care principles directly related to partnerships and empowerment are that individuals and communities should actively participate in decisions affecting their health and life and that partnerships should be established between disciplines, communities, and all health sectors (CHNC, 2019). See the "Cultural Considerations: Community Inclusion" box.

Building Healthy Public Policy

Building healthy public policy, as outlined in the Ottawa Charter, refers to creating environments that support health and reduce inequities in health and social policies. It requires coordinated action by federal, provincial, and municipal government levels, and specific areas of governments such as agriculture and health, to identify and develop public policies that affect health. Healthy public policy development is the process of "putting health issues on decision makers' agendas" (CPHA, 2010, p. 35). An example of healthy public policy is the ban on the use of cellphones and other handheld devices while driving. That policy was developed to reduce the risk of motor vehicle–related injuries. A focus on the concept of health, rather than illness, has engaged policy discussions over the past two decades regarding the relationship between health and social and economic conditions such as education, housing, employment, and the environment. A shift from institution-based care to community-based care has presented the opportunity for individuals to participate in health decisions with health care providers. This empowerment of individuals and communities has resulted in the development of healthy public policy such as bylaws that restrict smoking in public places, environmental protection legislation prohibiting the use of leaded gasoline in motor vehicles, and laws requiring seatbelt use. Policies can be developed from the top down (i.e., originating from the government) or from the bottom up (i.e., originating from the community).

🌐 CULTURAL CONSIDERATIONS

Community Inclusion

One of the basic elements of a CHN's capacity for health promotion is knowledge of the community's cultural values and influences. Cultural values can have an impact on participation rates, recruitment, and the effectiveness of a population health strategy. For example, in some Middle Eastern, African, and Asian countries, conservative social norms have been shown to influence women's participation in regular physical activity. Milligan identified some of the cultural considerations that can influence participation in health promotion programs, such as family composition, social, economic, and environmental factors.* In some cultures, it is customary for women to be accompanied by a male relative to public gatherings. Therefore, health promotion strategies to increase physical activity in this population may need to focus on family-centred interventions and education through social media modalities. Simpler interventions to address conservative social norms may also include culturally appropriate sportswear and swimwear or women-only exercise classes. Riggs, van Gemert, Gussy, et al. (2012) proposed planning culturally appropriate strategies that consider local, vernacular, and experiential knowledge.† What works

for one group may not work for another due to cultural diversity. For example, "*miswak*" is a teeth-cleaning twig that is commonly used for dental hygiene in developing countries. If CHNs understand that *miswak* is a culturally acceptable practice, they could incorporate *miswak* into their oral health education interventions, along with the use of toothbrushes. Accepting the practice shows that CHNs understand and respect the population that uses the practice, which could result in better participation rates and recruitment in oral education interventions with this population. Recognizing traditional cultural values and influences and incorporating them into health promotion strategies can help increase the CHN's capacity for effective health promotion interventions in culturally diverse populations.

Questions to Consider

1. What strategies could the CHN use to increase participation rates for a physical activity program for Asian women?
2. How could the CHN incorporate assessment of cultural influences into everyday practice?

Sources: *Milligan, F. (2014). Cultural influences on healthy lifestyle behaviours. *British Journal of Cardiac Nursing, 9*(4), 202–203. †Riggs, E., van Gemert, C., Gussy, M., et al. (2012). Reflections on cultural diversity in oral health promotion and prevention. *Global Health Promotion, 19*(1), 60–63.

In 2004, Canada's first ministers committed to a collaborative process to set health goals and targets for Canada. In 2005, provincial, territorial, and federal ministers of health outlined health goals for Canada based on the following four areas: basic needs (social and physical environments); belonging and engagement; healthy living; and a system for health (Keon & Pepin, 2008). These health goals were developed using an extensive consultation, confirmation, and approval process involving experts and grassroots representatives from all provinces and territories and formed the basis for future policy development. For further reading on the historical efforts of the federal, provincial, and territorial governments to develop and implement healthy public policy in Canada, refer to the Senate of Canada report *Population Health Policy: Federal, Provincial, and Territorial Perspectives* (see the link on the Evolve website).

Current health policy development challenges in Canada pertain to the constraints of changing social, economic, and political climates. The 2011 Rio Political Declaration on Social Determinants of Health acknowledges that there is a need to adopt better governance for health and development (e.g., give a voice to all groups and sectors) and to promote participation in policymaking and implementation (e.g., use participatory processes) in relation to social and economic determinants of health (WHO, 2011). CHNs can play a pivotal role in advocating at the community, provincial, and federal levels for healthy public policy to address the socioeconomic determinants of health. CHNs collaborate with the community to identify areas in need of policy development and then participate in implementing and evaluating that policy. The CHN uses excellent communication skills to help set clear policies with measurable outcomes (CPHA, 2010). Healthy public policy development and implementation is a strategy that CHNs can use to support health and reduce inequities in health, but policy development can be a complex and lengthy process.

Creating Supportive Environments

Creating supportive environments, as outlined in the Ottawa Charter, refers to providing environments in all settings—home, work, and play—that are safe, satisfying, stimulating, and enjoyable. Health equality and the social determinants of health contribute to the creation of supportive environments for health promotion. Environment is a determinant of health and is, therefore, interconnected with health. This interconnectedness leads to improved population health if improvements have been made in the environment. Butler-Jones (2009) stated that "people's actions are very much shaped by the social and environmental conditions in which they live and work" (p. 47). For example, poor communities often experience population health disparities. These populations live in environments that lack material and social supports and tend to experience poorer health as compared to the general Canadian population. A large body of evidence links poverty to poor health (Auger & Alix, 2016). Approximately 10% of health outcomes are influenced by the physical environment, and 50% of the health of a population is explained by socioeconomic factors (Senate Subcommittee on Population Health, 2009). The environment as a determinant of health is discussed in Chapter 17. Despite Canada's reputation

as a leader in health promotion and population health, health disparities in the population continue to exist (Raphael, 2016). Child poverty has persisted as a major Canadian issue, with income disparity among families with children continuing to create a bigger gap (Lethbridge & Phipps, 2005).

As an example of the CHN role in creating a supportive environment, consider the case of a CHN working in a rural agricultural community. This CHN works with this community to plan and implement a program pertaining to farm safety. A farm is more than an industrial worksite, it is also a home. The CHN uses strategies such as providing education about farm safety by working with parent–school councils, local youth groups such as 4-H clubs, school staff, and organizations such as the Canadian Agricultural Safety Association, an association that works to improve farm safety practices in Canada.

Another example of the creation of a supportive environment is the Baby-Friendly Hospital Initiative. This initiative was developed by WHO and UNICEF in 1991 (UNICEF, 2009). This program, known in Canada as the Baby Friendly Initiative (BFI) and available at six designated sites across the country (Alberta Breastfeeding Committee, 2015), integrates both hospital and community care for breastfeeding mothers and infants. Breastfeeding protects the health of babies, mothers, and families and supports the environment (Horta, Bahl, Martines, et al., 2007). Quebec and New Brunswick have mandated the implementation of BFI (Alberta Breastfeeding Committee, 2015). Refer to the Alberta Breastfeeding Committee and UNICEF links on the Evolve website for further information.

Creating a supportive environment, within the Ottawa Charter, includes social marketing, advocacy, health communication, and mutual aid, which are discussed later in this chapter. See the link for WHO's report on addressing health inequalities on the Evolve website. For further information on how to address the multiple determinants of health, see the Senate of Canada report link on the Evolve website.

Developing Personal Skills

Developing personal skills, as outlined in the Ottawa Charter, refers to building individual capacity so that persons will make lifestyle choices that promote health. One aspect of this strategy is the provision of health education to empower patients as individuals and to promote patient involvement in health care decisions. This strategy also includes the adoption of healthier behaviours, such as stress management, healthy eating, and physical activity. Moving toward the adoption of healthier lifestyles through behavioural change is difficult even for motivated patients.

When developing health education, CHNs assess learner needs and consider the economic factors that can influence learning, such as access to a computer. CHNs use their content expertise to offer formal and informal teaching to community groups, families, and individuals (CPHA, 2010). Health education can occur in public places or through social media strategies such as Facebook and Twitter. Health education with community groups may occur in various setting such as homes, clinics, schools, workplaces, and churches, on a range of issues, such as the hazards of vaping or elder abuse. CHNs also educate groups of learners who then become educators for other groups in the community. This activity is usually referred to as "train the trainer" sessions. One example is a CHN who educates a select community group to teach about healthy food choices to promote a healthy lifestyle. These trainees then individually teach nutrition information to community groups in various settings.

Several teaching methods are appropriate for health education, including lectures, demonstrations, small groups, and health fairs. Health fairs are commonly used with populations to disseminate information and to determine population interest and further learning needs. One example of a program for developing personal skills is Aboriginal Head Start in Urban and Northern Communities (AHSUNC), a national program provided in urban and northern settings to Indigenous preschool children and their families. AHSUNC aims to promote the development of a positive sense of self to encourage learning. CHNs in their communities could facilitate community development through the administration of this type of program for children and their parents. (See the Tool Box on the Evolve website for links to resources for planning general and workplace health fairs.)

Health Literacy

The effectiveness of health education and health promotion interventions is directly influenced by the patient's health literacy. **Health literacy** is defined as "the ability to access, understand, evaluate, and communicate information as a way to promote, maintain, and improve health in a variety of settings across the lifespan" (Rootman & Gordon-El-Bihbety, 2008, p. 11). Low literacy has been identified as a barrier to accessing health services and understanding health information (Ronson & Rootman, 2009; Rootman & Gordon-El-Bihbety, 2008); and it may prevent people from seeking health care. In ethnocultural communities, a low level of health literacy can create a barrier to accessing health services because of limited language abilities resulting in a lack of information on available health services (Zanchetta & Poureslami, 2006). Persons with lower levels of literacy are inclined to live and work in less healthy environments (Ronson & Rootman, 2009).

DETERMINANTS OF HEALTH

Literacy
- Low literacy and low health literacy contribute to lower incomes and decreased community engagement, which are related to poorer health.
- Approximately 55% of working-aged Canadian adults have less than adequate health literacy skills.
- Approximately 88% of older adults (65 years of age and older) have less than adequate health literacy skills.
- Approximately 10% of Canadians live with a learning disability, approximately 80% of whom experience difficulty learning to read.
- Canadians with the lowest health literacy scores are 2.5 times more likely than Canadians with high health literacy scores to report their health status as "fair" to "poor."

source: Rootman, I., & Gordon-El-Bihbety, D. (2017). *A vision for a health literate Canada*. Ottawa: Canadian Public Health Association. Retrieved from https://www.cpha.ca/vision-health-literate-canada-report-expert-panel-health-literacy

Health literacy has been an issue in health promotion for many years. In 1986, literacy was identified as a national priority; in 1994, the CPHA initiated a national literacy and health program; in 2000, Ottawa hosted the first Canadian conference on literacy and health; in 2005, British Columbia created the Health and Learning Knowledge Centre, which is focused on research; in 2007, the results of the International Adult Literacy and Skills Survey, which included thousands of Canadians and resulted in the development of a health literacy measurement tool, were published; and in 2008, a report titled *A Vision for a Health Literate Canada: Report of the Expert Panel on Health Literacy* was released by CPHA, providing information on the extent of the literacy problem in Canada and proposing a national strategy for health literacy. This report includes definitions, concepts, an assessment of the scope of the problem, a discussion of the barriers to literacy and the effectiveness of interventions, and the panel's recommendations.

Ronson and Rootman (2009) suggested that literacy is related to the following:
- Overall health status
- Comorbidity burden
- Life expectancy
- Lifestyle practices
- Culture
- Income and socioeconomic status
- Living and working conditions
- Educational attainment
- Gender
- Early life

Literacy, therefore, is linked to some of the determinants of health (e.g., income and education). In addition, the data suggest that literacy is associated with health status, community involvement, and health literacy. The CHN needs to be constantly aware of the challenges that health literacy presents in many patient situations. The CHN works with patients to develop personal skills and partners with others to create supportive environments, strengthen community action on literacy, and build healthy public policy to address health literacy issues.

Other common activities used to further the Ottawa Charter strategy of developing personal skills include health communication and social marketing, mutual aid, and advocacy directed at the individual. These activities are discussed later in this chapter.

LEVELS OF PREVENTION

Related to Community Health Education
Primary Prevention
A CHN provides education at a health fair regarding healthy eating using *Eating Well With Canada's Food Guide*.

Secondary Prevention
A CHN provides education at a health fair about the need for blood pressure screening for early diagnosis and treatment of hypertension.

Tertiary Prevention
A CHN provides education to a community group of individuals and their families coping with the effects of brain injury.

Reorienting Health Services

Reorienting health services, as outlined in the Ottawa Charter, refers to reforming health services and the health sector so that they include a health promotion focus. This change requires movement beyond the focus on cure and clinical services. Health care reform would need to consider areas such as the link between the determinants of health and population health; social justice; the individual as a holistic being; community-based care that is accessible, affordable, acceptable, and appropriate for the patients; a greater focus on population health and on health research; and modifications to professional education (Vollman et al., 2017). In contributing toward achieving this goal, a CHN may, for example, work with community partners to reorient mental health services from a hospital to a community location that is accessible, available, and appropriate to meet specific community mental health promotion needs. One of the most common activities used to further the Ottawa Charter strategy of reorienting health services are health communication and social marketing.

Activities to Facilitate Health Promotion Strategies

Health Communication and Social Marketing Activities

Used in the delivery of health promotion messages to various targeted populations, health communication and social marketing activities are designed to inform individuals so that they can make decisions related to maintaining and improving their health and well-being and those of their families and communities. In 1971, ParticipACTION became the first Canadian government program that incorporated health communication and social marketing strategies with a mandate to improve the health of Canadians (Bauman, Madil, Craig, et al., 2004). ParticipACTION is directed at positively influencing attitudes, beliefs, values, and behaviours to increase physical activity in the general population as well as specific aggregates such as youth, older adults, and workers. In February 2007, ParticipACTION was officially renewed, with funding from sources such as government, labour, education, and business (ParticipACTION, 2010).

Health communication involves disseminating information to promote knowledge, distributing health risk information, demonstrating how to access health care programs, and creating awareness of health issues using various forms of mass and social media. Examples include television, radio, flyers, newspapers, magazines, Facebook, Instagram, Pinterest, YouTube, and Twitter. ParticipACTION initially used television, radio, and print to get out its messages and, at a national level, a document titled *Canada's Physical Activity Guide to Healthy Active Living*. More recently, ParticipACTION programs have expanded to include a social media campaign using blogs, Twitter, and Facebook to reach a larger audience (see http://www.participaction.com).

The CHN needs to plan health communication messages that are inclusive and considerate of the patient's ability to access and understand health information. For example, not all patients use the Internet, and some have low literacy levels. When developing health communication messages, it is important to evaluate the message to ensure that it is at an appropriate reading level for the patient population. One common method for establishing the reading level of education materials is the Simple Measure of Gobbledygook, which utilizes a hand-scoring method to determine the grade level of patient education material (Grabeel, Russomanno, Oelschlegel, Tester, & Heidel, 2018).

Communicating health messages through social marketing focuses on specific populations and uses structured messages to effect positive behavioural change in lifestyle areas such as diet and substance use to improve health and decrease health inequities (French, Blair-Stevens, McVey, et al., 2009). The four *P*s of marketing, also known as the marketing mix, are the key elements of social marketing: *product* (benefits), *price* (costs such as physical, psychological, social, and financial for the target audience related to the benefits), *place* (convenient access), and *promotion* (using the most appropriate media form to convey the messages to the target audience) (Grier & Bryant, 2005). ParticipACTION demonstrated use of the four *P*s of social marketing in the following ways:

- *Product*: benefits through physical activity such as improved health and well-being
- *Price*: physical activity was inexpensive, easy to do, and readily available
- *Place*: physical activity could be carried out in the home, school, or workplace or outdoors in the community
- *Promotion*: various communication approaches were used (e.g., television and radio advertisements and social media campaigns)

Weinreich (2006) added the following four additional *P*s to social marketing: *publics, partnership, policy,* and *purse strings. Publics* includes external groups, such as policymakers and the target audience, and internal groups, such as organizational managers. *Partnership* refers to teaming up with relevant agencies and organizations in the community that have similar goals. *Policy* refers to creating a supportive environment by introducing and supporting policies that fit with the social marketing program for sustainability. *Purse strings* refers to the identification and use of funding from sources such as grants or donations that will assist with creating and operating the program. Social marketing activities target specific audiences and are based on audience research that is used to understand the target audience, identify barriers, and monitor interventions. The main focus is to develop attractive and motivational interactions with the target audience, using the four *P*s or marketing (Andreasen, 2002).

Social marketing campaigns via the Internet are becoming one of the preferred methods of communicating health messages to the public. For example, in 2018 Health Canada implemented the social media campaign titled "End Stigma Campaign" to address the opioid crisis in Canada (https://www.canada.ca/en/services/health/campaigns/drug-prevention.html). That campaign is designed to increase awareness of the health risks of opioids and end stigma surrounding substance use. It provides access to a variety of resources including printed materials, a link to a YouTube video and resources to learn how to end stigma and increase awareness of the opioid crisis in Canada. CHNs can promote and use these existing social marketing strategies to communicate health messages to a variety of patient populations.

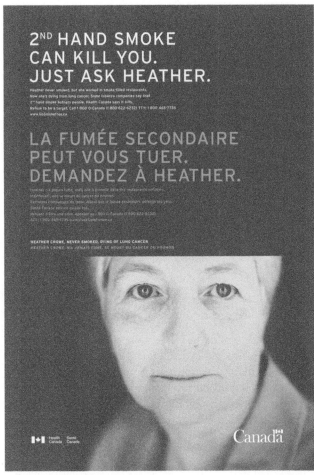

Heather Crowe developed lung cancer after years of exposure to second-hand smoke in her work environment. The antismoking campaign based on her experience provides an example of a social marketing strategy aimed at educating the public about the risks of tobacco use. From 2nd Hand Smoke Can Kill You. Just Ask Heather. (Health Canada. Adapted and reproduced with permission from the Minister of Health, 2016.)

Mutual Aid

In *A Framework for Health Promotion,* Jake Epp identified mutual aid as a health promotion mechanism (Epp, 1986). *Mutual aid,* most commonly referred to as *self-help,* is defined as a process whereby persons share common experiences, situations, or problems with others and view one another as equals (Self-Help Resource Centre, n.d.; Young & Hayes, 2002). Self-help groups are used for individual support usually when access to persons who have gone through

a similar problem is viewed as helpful. Self-help groups provide individuals with emotional and practical support, information exchange, and, often, assistance with problem solving (Self-Help Resource Centre, n.d.). Some self-help groups, such as breast cancer support groups, Alcoholics Anonymous, and Mothers Against Drunk Driving also engage in community education and advocacy. CHNs can promote self-help groups as a health promotion mechanism where individuals share their common experiences and support each other.

One example of a mutual aid service for youth and adults experiencing mental health issues is the Alberta Health Services "Community Helpers" program (https://www.albertahealthservices.ca/findhealth/service.aspx?id=1073813). This is a suicide prevention program that takes place in community-based settings and works with existing community strengths to find community members to act as "natural helpers" to work with youth and adults with mental health problems. In contrast to traditional models of help, these natural helpers already have a youth connection and are persons whom youth have related to in the past when they have encountered problems and need extra support.

CHNs can support mutual aid by promoting the use of self-help groups by discussing with patients (individuals and families) appropriate and available self-help groups and the assistance they provide; referring patients to self-help groups as appropriate; and assisting in the establishment of self-help groups as needed in the community.

Advocacy

Advocacy is defined as "interventions such as speaking, writing or acting in favour of a particular issue or cause, policy or group of people" (PHAC, 2008d). Advocacy enhances the power of patients by involving them in the identification of their health concerns or issues and encouraging them to participate in developing solutions, including policy-related solutions. Advocacy involves taking action to influence decision makers in communities and governments to support a policy or cause that promotes health. Advocacy often involves promoting the health of disadvantaged groups, such as people living in poverty (CPHA, 2010).

Advocacy for health includes looking after those who are helpless or have been discriminated against and empowering patients to raise awareness of their health issues, such as concerns about traffic patterns in a school area. Regardless of the need for advocacy, CHNs need to work *with* the patient rather than do *for* the patient. Advocacy is discussed throughout this text.

HEALTH PROMOTION SKILLS

CHNs need to be familiar with resources that are available to facilitate and enhance their health promotion skills. Often, CHNs have the theoretical knowledge of *what* needs to happen to effect change to improve patient

A qualitative study by Cusack, Hall, Scruby, et al., (2008) worked with focus groups of CHNs to explore perceptions of early postpartum discharge (EPD) and its effect on CHNs' practice in Winnipeg, Manitoba. The study identified three main themes: passion for the CHN role, the influence of EPD on CHN practice, and building a CHN future. It also identified 9 subthemes: valuing public health nursing, building capacity and developing relationships, changes in practice, erosion of health promotion, a new role for CHNs, proper tools, continuity of care, relationships with community partners, and resources to support public health programs. The CHNs perceived that the introduction of EPD affected their role in community-level interventions and health promotion activities, thus altering their scope of practice. Although the CHNs in this study valued their new role in EPD, they identified a need for more resources and funding to be directed to the public health system to support CHNs' increased responsibilities and to continue support of their traditional health promotion roles with all patients.

Application for CHNs

It is important to understand the impact new programs such as the EPD have on the roles of CHNs. The introduction of EPD added new responsibilities for CHNs, but additional resources and staffing were not provided, putting at risk CHNs' other program commitments. CHNs perceived that they were being forced to give up their established community commitments and involvement. Time normally allocated for population health approach activities, including health promotion activities, had to be directed to EPD care in the community. Organizations need to consider and plan for the introduction of new programs for health care delivery, and CHNs need to be involved in this planning process to ensure the availability of sufficient resources and staffing. CHNs' involvement would contribute to making sure that the established population health programs would not be compromised with the introduction of new program delivery modes.

Questions for Reflection and Discussion

1. What health promotion activities could a CHN implement with early discharge patients (mothers, neonates, postoperative) in their homes?
2. What questions would be important to ask CHNs when a new program of delivery in the community is being considered?

Source: Cusack, C., Hall, W., Scruby, L., et al. (2008). Public health nurses' (PHNs) perceptions of their role in early postpartum discharge. *Canadian Journal of Public Health, 99*(3), 206–211.

health. The necessary "how to" information on the skills needed to promote health in the community is available through many resources including online websites. Two health promotion skills, working with focus groups and preparing funding proposal applications, are briefly introduced here.

Working With Focus Groups

Focus groups in health promotion are informal sessions using an interactive strategy to gain insight into the perceptions, beliefs, and opinions of generally 6 to 12 representatives (or stakeholders) of the target population. These representatives may include patients, caregivers, municipal council members, professionals (e.g., lawyers, dentists, engineers), and volunteers. Focus groups are used in assessment, particularly social assessment, and serve as "pretests" in health promotion program development and evaluation. In most cases, focus groups are led by skilled moderators who create supportive environments so that group members can speak liberally and instinctively about the issues, programs, or services. The leader usually follows a structured interview format in a 60- to 90-minute facilitated and recorded discussion. Several web-based resources further elaborate on the "how to" of this skill (see the Tool Box on the Evolve website).

Preparing Funding Applications

The survival of a health program may be challenged due to fiscal constraints and, therefore, is dependent on government funding. This funding involves the submission of an application for funding to various government organizations. Stiff competition for available funds often exists. Therefore, succinct and skilled completion of funding proposals is critical. CHNs need to become familiar with how to write funding proposals so that they can apply directly or assist a program in the community to apply directly for funding. Several web-based tools provide guidance on the "how to" of the skill of writing a funding proposal (see the Health Communication Unit online proposal writing course link on the Evolve website).

Developing Health Promotion Capacity

In summary, health promotion practice has undergone a shift from a primary focus on the individual to include a focus on families, groups, communities, populations, and systems. However, health promotion strategies often address individuals as patients. CHNs need to develop many skills applicable to working with patients. Table 4.6 summarizes the knowledge, skills, commitment, and resources that health care providers, including CHNs, require. Table 4.7 presents the organizational elements necessary to support CHNs as they function within their health promotion practice.

TABLE 4.6 The Basic Elements of Practitioners' Health Promotion Capacity

Category	Basic Elements of Capacity
Knowledge	• A holistic understanding of health and its determinants • An awareness of population health promotion principles • An understanding of a variety of strategies and processes through which effective health promotion interventions can be undertaken • A recognition of the contextual specificity of the strengths and weaknesses of different health promotion strategies and processes • A familiarity with the conditions, aspirations, and culture of the population(s) with which one works
Skills	• Program planning (needs assessment, design, implementation, and evaluation) • Communication across sectors, disciplines, and socioeconomic or community boundaries • Working with others (e.g., nurturing relationships, participation, and intersectoral partnerships; facilitation; conflict mediation) • Integrating research and practice (both in the program planning cycle and as a means of critically reflective practice) • Capacity building (both within one's own organization and with the external communities and organizations with which one works) • Being strategic and selective in making decisions about what to do and how to do it
Commitment	• Personal energy, enthusiasm, patience, and persistence • Values of population health promotion • Willingness to be flexible, to innovate, and to take thoughtful risks • Learning from experience of oneself and others • Self-confidence and credibility • Believing in and advocating for health promotion
Resources	• Time to engage in health promotion practice and in personal and professional development that enhances such practice • Tools for more efficient and effective practice, including resource inventories and repertoires of good ideas and best practices • Infrastructure, including office space, capital equipment, and effective means of communication • Supportive managers, colleagues, and allies with whom to work and learn • Access to adequate funding for health promotion activities

Source: Reprinted with permission from *Building Health Promotion Capacity* by Scott McLean, Joan Feather, and David Butler-Jones © University of British Columbia Press (2005). All rights reserved by the Publisher.

TABLE 4.7 The Basic Elements of Organizational Health Promotion Capacity

Category	Basic Elements of Capacity
Commitment	• Health promotion is valued at all levels of the organization • There are a shared vision, a mission, and strategies for engaging in population health promotion to address the determinants of health • Policies, programs, and practices are consistent with the organization's vision, mission, and strategies ("walking the talk") • Partnerships are valued and nurtured both across the organization and with diverse external organizations and communities
Culture	• Styles of leadership and management empower health promotion practice, foster lifelong learning, and support healthy working environments • Positive and nurturing relationships are fostered among employees • Communication is open and timely, enabling employees to solve problems, learn from mistakes, and share successes • Critical reflection, innovation, and learning are fostered
Structures	• Health promotion is a shared responsibility, being an integral part of job titles, job descriptions, and performance evaluations among at least several employees • There are effective policies and practices of human resource recruitment, retention, and professional development • There are participatory, empowering, and evidence-informed practices for strategic planning, needs assessment, program planning, and evaluation • Employees are organized into work teams that promote intra-institutional collaboration
Resources	• A significant number of employees in key positions and units have high levels of individual capacity for health promotion • Adequate funding is provided for the programmatic and infrastructural costs of engaging in health promotion activities • Appropriate infrastructure exists, including office space, capital equipment, technology, and effective means of communication • Active engagement with communities brings additional resources

Source: Reprinted with permission of the Publisher from McLean, S., Feather, J., & Butler-Jones, D. (2005). *Building Health Promotion Capacity*. UBC Press.

STUDENT EXPERIENCE

Working alone or with a student study group, identify a health promotion program or healthy public policy relevant to your community. Search local newspaper websites for relevant programs or policies. Create your own inclusion and exclusion lens by responding to the following key questions about any policy, program, or practice.

Questions About Exclusion:
1. Who is being excluded from this policy, program, or practice?
2. What are the reasons for this exclusion?
3. Does anyone benefit from this exclusion?

Questions About Inclusion:
1. Who will be included in this policy, program, or practice?
2. What are the reasons for this inclusion?
3. Does being included benefit those people?
Bring your completed work to class for discussion.

CHAPTER SUMMARY

4.1 Various definitions of *health* have developed over time and have influenced the development of health promotion. CHNs should be aware of the distinctions between the following foundational concepts in health promotion: injury prevention, disease, disease course, illness, illness trajectory, disease prevention, health protection, risk avoidance, risk reduction, health enhancement, and harm reduction.

4.2 The concept of health has evolved from a medical approach to a population health promotion model designed to enable patients to increase control over and improve their health. Significant milestones in the development of health promotion in Canada include the Lalonde Report, the Ottawa Charter for Health Promotion, and the Epp Report.

4.3 Health promotion models, theories, and frameworks include the theory of planned behaviour and the

transtheoretical model (individual focused); the diffusion of innovation theory and the community mobilization framework (community focused); and Milio's framework and Weiss's framework (public policy–oriented).

4.4 Three approaches used in health promotion are the biomedical (absence of disease), behavioural (lifestyle choices), and socioenvironmental (determinants of health) approaches.

4.5 Health promotion strategies include strengthening community action, building healthy public policy, creating supportive environments, developing personal skills, and reorienting health services. They are based on the Ottawa Charter and are fundamental to community health nursing practice in Canada.

4.6 CHNs require many skills to develop their health promotion practice, including working with focus groups and preparing funding proposal applications.

CHN IN PRACTICE: A CASE STUDY

Health Promotion Strategies

Tim is a CHN who lives and works in a large urban centre. He has been teaching prenatal classes to high school students in his assigned district for a couple of years. It his first time teaching at a particular high school. The students at this high school comprise a multicultural population consisting mainly of second-generation immigrants from Asia and Africa. Ten pregnant girls have signed up for the prenatal class, eight of whom are from ethnocultural communities. Tim usually incorporates various teaching methods such as lecture, videos, and the dissemination of print materials.

Think About It

1. If you were the CHN, what would you include in your assessment as you prepare to teach this particular aggregate?
2. Locate a pamphlet (online, from a pharmacy, or from a local health unit) on a topic related to pregnancy and prenatal care. Using a tool to assess readability (see the resources on plain language and readability in the Tool Box on the Evolve website), evaluate the pamphlet for readability and usability for this aggregate. Identify whether you would use this pamphlet and provide a rationale. Bring your pamphlet and results to class.

TOOL BOX

The Tool Box contains useful resources that can be applied to community health nursing practice. These related resources are found either in the appendices at the back of this text or on the Evolve website at http://evolve.elsevier.com/Canada/Stanhope/community/.

Appendices
- Appendix 1: Canadian Community Health Nursing Professional Practice Model and Standards of Practice
- Appendix 3: Declaration of Alma-Ata
- Appendix 4: The Ottawa Charter for Health Promotion

Tools

Basics of Conducting Focus Groups. (http://managementhelp.org/businessresearch/focus-groups.htm)

This is an excellent resource for anyone planning to conduct or learn about focus groups. It provides a step-by-step guide for the novice.

Community Tool Box. (http://ctb.ku.edu/en)

This resource acts as a support for nurses in the community who strive to promote health. The resource is organized as a tool box and provides practical skills-building information on more than 250 topics as well as examples, checklists, and resources relating to community health.

How to Organize a Workplace Health Fair. (https://www.2020onsite.com/blog/13-tips-for-throwing-an-awesome-health-fair)

This step-by-step guide includes the phases from planning to evaluation of a workplace health fair.

Literacy and Essential Skills Toolkit. (http://www12.esdc.gc.ca/sgpe-pmps/p.5bd.2t.1.3ls@-eng.jsp?pid=2688)

This Human Resources and Skills Development Canada tool kit is a series of user-friendly tools that offer support in the following areas: assessment, learning, and training applicable to employees and learners; community groups; and employers and practitioners. The tool kit also offers many tip sheets and resources on how to take action on literacy.

Plain Language Services. (http://www12.esdc.gc.ca/sgpe-pmps/p.5bd.2t.1.3ls@-eng.jsp?pid=2688)

This site provides the reader with information and tools to assist in the preparation of plain-language documents.

The Readability Test Tool. (https://readability-score.com/)

This site provides an explanation of readability and provides tools on how to measure written materials for readability such as the Gunning Fog score and the Flesch-Kincaid grade level score.

Rural Communities Impacting Policy: Rural Tackle Box. (http://www.predc.ca/rural-tackle-box.html)

This site provides tools on how to influence policy to maintain healthy communities.

10 Tips for Running Successful Focus Groups. (http://www.groupsplus.com/pages/mn091498.htm)

This site provides tips that can help CHNs conduct more effective focus groups.

REFERENCES

Adams, C., Drake, C., Dang, M., et al. (2014). Optimization of injury prevention outreach for helmet safety. *Journal of Trauma Nursing, 21*(2), 133–138. https://doi.org/10.1097/JTN.0000000000000047.

Alberta Breastfeeding Committee. (2015). *BFI in Canada.* http://www.breastfeedingalberta.ca.

Andreasen, A. R. (2002). Marketing social marketing in the social change marketplace. *Journal of Public Policy and Marketing, 21*(1), 3–13.

Auger, N., & Alix, A. (2016). Income, income distribution, and health in Canada. In D. Raphael (Ed.), *Social determinants of health* (3rd ed.) (pp. 90–102). Canadian Scholars' Press.

Bauman, A., Madil, J., Craig, C. L., et al. (2004). ParticipACTION: This mouse roared, but did it get the cheese? *Canadian Journal of Public Health, 96*(Suppl. 2), S14S19.

Beresford, S. A., Curry, S. J., Kristal, A. R., et al. (1996). *Report of the roundtable on population health and health promotion.* Health Canada, Health Promotion Development Division.

Bhatti, T. (1996). *Report of the roundtable on population health and health promotion.* Health Canada, Health Promotion Development Division.

Boutilier, M., Cleverly, S., & Labonte, R. (2000). Community as a setting for health promotion. In B. D. Poland, L. W. Green, & I. Rootman (Eds.), *Settings for health promotion: Linking theory and practice* (pp. 250–307). Sage.

Bozinoff, N., Small, W., Long, C., et al. (2017). Still "at risk": An examination of how street-involved young people understand, experience, and engage with "harm reduction" in Vancouver's inner city. *International Journal of Drug Policy, 45*, 33–39. https://doi.org/10.1016/j.drugpo.2017.05.006.

Butler-Jones, D. (2009). The role of public health in the health of Canada's children. *Chronic Diseases in Canada, 29*(2), 47.

Callaghan, R. C., & Herzog, T. A. (2006). The relation between processes-of-change and stage-transition in smoking behavior: A two-year longitudinal test of the transtheoretical model. *Addictive Behaviors, 31*(8), 1331–1345.

Canadian Centre on Substance Use and Addiction (CCSA). (2017). *Annual Report 2016–2017: Real need, real action.* Retrieved from https://www.ccsa.ca/real-need-real-action-ccsa-annual-report-2016-2017.

Canadian Nurses Association. (2005). *CNA backgrounder: Healthy communities and nursing: A summary of the issues.* https://www.cna-aiic.ca/~/media/cna/page-content/pdf-en/bg5_healthy_communities_e.pdf?la=en.

Canadian Nurses Association. (2012). *A nursing call to action.* https://www.cna-aiic.ca/~/media/cna/files/en/nec_report_e.pdf.

Canadian Nurses Association. (2015). *Submission to the Standing Committee on Finance 2015 pre-budget consultations: Healthier Canadians and communities.* http://cna-aiic.ca/~/media/cna/page-content/pdf-en/cna-2015-pre-budget-submission_e.pdf.

Canadian Public Health Association. (1996). *Action statement for health promotion in Canada.* https://www.cpha.ca/action-statement-health-promotion-canada.

Canadian Public Health Association (CPHA). (2010). *Public health—community health nursing practice in Canada: Roles and activities* (4th ed.).

Cancer Prevention Research Center. (n.d.). *Detailed overview of the transtheoretical model of change.* http://web.uri.edu/cprc/detailed-overview/.

Catford, J. (2004). Health promotion's record card: How principled are we 20 years on? *Health Promotion International, 19*(1), 1–4.

Catford, J. (2014). Turn, turn, turn: Time to reorient health services. *Health Promotion International, 29*(1), 1–4.

Centre for Addiction and Mental Health. (2010). *Health promotion resources.* https://www.camh.ca/-/media/files/guides-and-publications/addiction-guide-en.pdf.

Clark, M. J. (2008). *Community health nursing: Advocacy for population health* (5th ed.). Pearson Prentice Hall.

Community Health Nurses of Canada. (2019). *Canadian community health nursing: Professional practice model and standards of practice.* https://www.chnc.ca/standards-of-practice.

Cusack, C., Hall, W., Scruby, L., et al. (2008). Public health nurses' (PHNs) perceptions of their role in early postpartum discharge. *Canadian Journal of Public Health, 99*(3), 206–211.

Davis, S. (2006). *Community mental health in Canada: Theory, policy, and practice*. UBC Press.

Dearing, J. W. (2009). Applying diffusion of innovation theory to intervention development. *Research on Social Work Practice, 19*(5), 503–518.

Dewey, J. (1963). *Experience and education*. Collier Books.

Dunn, H. L. (1959). High-level wellness for man and society. *American Journal of Public Health, 49*(6), 786–792. http://www.pubmedcentral.nih.gov/picrender.fcgi?artid=1372807&blobtype=pdf.

Ehrlich, A., & Ladouceur, M. G. (2002). *A conceptual evolution of "health": National and international perspectives on health and health policies from 1974 to the present*. School of Nursing, McMaster University.

Epp, J. (1986). *Achieving health for all: A framework for health promotion*. Ottawa: Minister of Supply and Services.

Erikson, E. H. (1963). *Childhood and society* (2nd ed.). Norton.

Evans, R. G., Barer, M. L., & Marmor, T. R. (Eds.). (1994). *Why are some people healthy and some people not?* Aldine de Gruyter.

French, J., Blair-Stevens, C., McVey, D., et al. (2009). *Social marketing and public health: Theory & practice*. Elsevier.

Glanz, K., Patterson, R. E., Kristal, A. R., et al. (1998). Impact of worksite health promotion on stages of dietary change: The working well trial. *Health Education and Behavior, 25*(4), 448–463.

Government of Canada. (2009). *Bill C-32: Cracking down on tobacco monitoring aimed at youth*. Parliament of Canada.

Government of Canada. (2010). *Bill C-304 secure adequate accessible and affordable housing act*. Parliament of Canada.

Grabeel, K. L., Russomanno, J., Oelschlegel, S., et al. (2018). Computerized versus hand-scored health literacy tools: A comparison of Simple Measure of Gobbledygook (SMOG) and Flesch-Kincaid in printed patient education materials. *Journal of the Medical Library Association, 106*(1), 38–45. https://doi.org/10.5195/jmla.2018.262.

Green, L. W., & Kreuter, M. W. (1999). *Health promotion planning: An educational and ecological approach* (3rd ed.). Mayfield.

Grier, S., & Bryant, C. (2005). Social marketing in public health. *Annual Review of Public Health, 26*, 319–339.

Hamilton, N., & Bhatti, T. (1996). *Population health promotion: An integrated model of population health and health promotion*. Health Promotion Development Division, Health Canada.

Harm Reduction Coalition. (2014). *Principles of harm reduction*. https://harmreduction.org/about-us/principles-of-harm-reduction.

Health Data Research Network Canada (2021). For the Public. https://www.hdrn.ca/en/public.

Health Canada. (2002). *An inclusion lens: Workbook for looking at social and economic exclusion and inclusion*. Minister of Health. https://www.allianceon.org/sites/default/files/documents/Workbook%20for%20looking%20at%20Social_and_Economic_Inclusion_Lens%202002.pdf.

Health Canada. (2004). *Canadian addiction survey: A national survey of Canadians' use of alcohol and other drugs*. http://www.ccsa.ca/Resource%20Library/ccsa-004804-2004.pdf.

Health Canada. (2005a). *Health promotion: Does it work?* http://publications.gc.ca/collections/Collection/H12-36-03-2002E.pdf.

Health Canada. (2005b). *National framework for action to reduce the harms associated with alcohol and other drugs and substances in Canada*. https://www.ccsa.ca/national-framework-action-reduce-harms-associated-alcohol-and-other-drugs-and-substances-canada-0.

Health Canada. (2005c). *Social marketing*. http://www.hc-sc.gc.ca.

Heiss, G. L. (2009). Health promotion and risk reduction in the community. In F. A. Maurer, & C. M. Smith (Eds.), *Community/public health nursing practice: Health for families and populations* (4th ed., pp. 472–490). Saunders/Elsevier.

Hershfield, L., & Hyndman, B. (2004). *HP-101: Health promotion on-line course, module 4*. Ontario Health Promotion Resource System. Retrieved from a web page formerly available at https://www.publichealthontario.ca/en/education-and-events/online-learning/health-promotion-courses.

Herzog, T. A. (2005). When popularity outstrips the evidence: Comment on West. *Addiction, 100*(8), 1040–1041.

Horta, B., Bahl, R., Martines, J., et al. (2007). *Evidence on the long-term effects of breastfeeding*. World Health Organization.

Keon, W., & Pepin, L, (2008) Population heath policy: Federal, provincial and territorial perspectives. Retrieved from https://sencanada.ca/Content/SEN/Committee/392/soci/rep/rep09apr08-e.htm#_ftn14.

Kickbusch, I., & Nutbeam, D. (2017). A watershed for health promotion. The shanghai conference 2016. (Editorial). *Health Promotion International* (32), 2–6. https://doi.org/10.1093/heapro/daw112.

Kumar, S., & Preetha, G. (2012). Health promotion: An effective tool for global health. *Indian Journal of Community Medicine, 37*(1), 5–12. https://doi.org/10.4103/0970-0218.94009.

Labonte, R. (1995). Population health and health promotion: What do they have to say to each other? *Canadian Journal of Public Health, 86*(3), 165–168.

Labonte, R. (1997). Community, community development, and the forming of authentic partnerships: Some critical reflections. In M. Minkler (Ed.), *Community organizing and community building for health* (pp. 88–102). Rutgers University Press.

Labonte, R. (2003). *How our programs affect population health determinants: A workbook for better planning and accountability*. Health Canada, Population and Public Health Branch. http://www.sparc.bc.ca/how-our-programs-affect-population-health-determinants.

Lalonde, M. (1974). *A new perspective on the health of Canadians: A working document*. Government of Canada.

Lam, C., Wiley, A., Siu, A., et al. (2010). Assessing readiness to work from a stages of change perspective: Implications for return to work. *Work, 37*(3), 321–329.

Lethbridge, L., & Phipps, S. (2005). Chronic poverty and childhood asthma in the Maritimes versus the rest of Canada. *Canadian Journal of Public Health, 96*(1), 18–23. https://www.ncbi.nlm.nih.gov/pmc/articles/PMC6975801/pdf/41997_2005_Article_BF03404007.pdf.

Lubkin, I. M., & Larsen, P. D. (2009). *Chronic illness: Impact and interventions* (7th ed.). Jones & Bartlett.

Lyons, R., & Langille, L. (2000). *Healthy lifestyle: Strengthening the effectiveness of lifestyle approaches to improve health*. Public Health Agency of Canada.

Maville, J. A., & Huerta, C. G. (2008). *Health promotion in nursing* (2nd ed.). Delmar, Cengage Learning.

McKenzie, J. F., Neiger, B. L., & Thackeray, R. (2009). *Planning, implementing, and evaluating health promotion programs: A primer* (5th ed.). Pearson Education.

McLaren, L., & Hawe, P. (2005). Ecological perspectives in health research. *Journal of Epidemiology and Community Health, 59*, 6–14.

McLean, S., Feather, J., & Butler-Jones, D. (2005). *Building health promotion capacity: Action for learning, learning from action*. UBC Press.

McPhail-Bell, K., Fredericks, B., & Brough, M. (2013). Beyond the accolades: A postcolonial critique of the foundations of the Ottawa Charter. *Global Health Promotion, 20*(2), 22–29.

Meade, C. D. (2007). Community health education. In M. A. Nies, & M. McEwan (Eds.), *Community/public health nursing: Promoting the health of populations* (4th ed., pp. 104–134). Saunders Elsevier.

Milligan, F. (2014). Cultural influences on healthy lifestyle behaviours. *British Journal of Cardiac Nursing, 9*(4), 202–203.

Ministry of Health Promotion. (2008). *Ontario public health standards*. Government of Ontario. http://www.health.gov. on.ca/en/pro/programs/publichealth/oph_standards/.

Morrison, V., Gagnon, F., Morestin, F., & Keeling, M. (2014). *Keywords in healthy public policy*. National Collaborating Center for Healthy Public Policy. https://www.ncchpp.ca/docs/ Keywords_EN_Gabarit.pdf.

National Cancer Institute. (2005). *Theory at a glance: A guide for health promotion practice* (2nd ed.). U.S. Department of Health and Human Services, National Institutes of Health, National Cancer Institute. http://sbccimplementationkits.org/ demandrmnch/ikitresources/theory-at-a-glance-a-guide-for-health-promotion-practice-second-edition/.

Nutbeam, D., & Harris, E. (2004). *Theory in a nutshell: A practical guide to health promotion theories*. McGraw Hill.

Ontario Healthy Communities Coalition. (2019). *Our legacy*. https://greencommunitiescanada.org/wp-content/ uploads/2019/11/Legacy-Report-web.pdf.

Ontario Prevention Clearinghouse. (2002). Capacity building for health promotion: More than bricks and mortar. *OHPE Bulletin, 308*(308), 2003. http://www.mentalhealthpromotion.net/ resources/capacity-building-for-health-promotion.pdf.

Park, C., & Lee, J. (2012). Choice intention regarding hospice care based on the theory of reasoned action. *Journal of Hospice & Palliative Nursing, 14*(1), 34–44. https://doi.org/10.1097/ NJH.0b013e3182331002.

ParticipACTION. (2010). *About ParticipACTION*. https://www. participaction.com/en-ca/about.

Piaget, J. (1963). *The origins of intelligence in children*. Norton.

Prochaska, J. O., & DiClemente, C. C. (1983). Stages and processes of self-change of smoking: Toward an integrative model of change. *Journal of Consulting and Clinical Psychology, 51*(3), 390–395.

Public Health Agency of Canada (PHAC). (1994). *Strategies for population health: Investing in the health of Canadians*. http:// publications.gc.ca/collections/Collection/H88-3-30-2001/pdfs/ other/strat_e.pdf.

Public Health Agency of Canada (PHAC). (2001). *Population health promotion: An integrated model of population health and health promotion*. http://www.phac-aspc.gc.ca/ph-sp/php-psp/php3-eng.php#Developing.

Public Health Agency of Canada (PHAC). (2008a). *Centre for health promotion: Healthy communities division*. http://www. phac-aspc.gc.ca/chhd-sdsh/index-eng.php.

Public Health Agency of Canada (PHAC). (2008b). *Glossary of terms relevant to the core competencies for public health, A–D*. http://www.phac-aspc.gc.ca/php-psp/ccph-cesp/glos-eng.php.

Public Health Agency of Canada (PHAC). (2008d). *Population health approach: The organizing framework*. http://cbpp-pcpe. phac-aspc.gc.ca/population-health-approach-organizing-framework/.

Public Health Agency of Canada (PHAC). (2010). *Creating a healthier Canada: Making prevention a priority. A declaration on prevention and promotion from Canada's Ministers of Health and Health Promotion*. https://www.canada.ca/en/public-health/ services/health-promotion/healthy-living/creating-a-healthier-canada-making-prevention-a-priority.html.

Racher, F. E., & Annis, R. C. (2007). *The community health action model: Health promotion by the community*. https://pubmed. ncbi.nlm.nih.gov/18763474/.

Raphael, D. (2016). *Social determinants of health: Canadian perspectives* (3rd ed.). Canadian Scholars' Press.

Raphael, D., & Bryant, T. (2002). The limitations of population health as a model for a new public health. *Health Promotion International, 17*(2), 189–199.

Reutter, L., & Eastlick Kushner, K. (2009). Health and wellness. In P. A. Potter, A. G. Perry, J. C. Ross-Kerr, et al. (Eds.), *Canadian fundamentals of nursing* (4th ed., pp. 1–13). Elsevier Canada.

Riebe, D., Blissmer, B., Greene, G., et al. (2005). Long-term maintenance of exercise and healthy eating behaviors in overweight adults. *Preventive Medicine, 40*(6), 769–778.

Riggs, E., van Gemert, C., Gussy, M., et al. (2012). Reflections on cultural diversity in oral health promotion and prevention. *Global Health Promotion, 19*(1), 60–63. https://doi. org/10.1177/1757975911429872.

Robertson, A. (1998). Shifting discourses on health in Canada. From health promotion to population health. *Health Promotion International, 13*(2), 155–166.

Ronson, B., & Rootman, I. (2009). Literacy and health literacy: New understandings about their impact on health. In D. Raphael (Ed.), *Social determinants of health* (2nd ed., pp. 171–185). Canadian Scholars' Press.

Rootman, I., & Gordon-El-Bihbety, D. (2017). *A vision for a health literate Canada*. Canadian Public Health Association. https:// www.cpha.ca/vision-health-literate-canada-report-expert-panel-health-literacy.

Sallis, J. F., Cervero, R. B., Ascher, W., et al. (2006). An ecological approach to creating active living communities. *Annual Review of Public Health, 27*, 297–322.

Self-Help Resource Centre. (n.d.). *Self-help and health promotion*. http://www.selfhelp.on.ca/resource/health_promo_factsheet.pdf.

Senate Subcommittee on Population Health. (2009). *A healthy productive Canada: A determinant of health approach*. http:// www.parl.gc.ca/content/sen/committee/402/popu/rep/ rephealth1jun09-e.pdf.

Sheinfeld Gorin, S., & Arnold, J. (1998). *Health promotion handbook*. Mosby.

Singh-Grewal, D., Schneider, R., Bayer, N., et al. (2006). Predictors of disease course and remission in systemic juvenile idiopathic arthritis: Significance of early clinical and laboratory features. *Arthritis & Rheumatism, 54*(5), 1595–1601.

Smith, B. J., Tang, K. C., & Nutbeam, D. (2006). WHO health promotion glossary: New terms. *Health Promotion International, 21*(4), 340–345.

Spencer, L., Adams, T. B., Malone, S., et al. (2006). Applying the transtheoretical model to exercise: A systematic and comprehensive review of the literature. *Health Promotion Practice, 7*(4), 428–443.

Spencer, L. S., Pagell, F., Hallion, M. E., et al. (2002). Applying the transtheoretical model to tobacco cessation: A review of the literature. *American Journal of Health Promotion, 17*(1), 7–71.

Stanhope, J., & Lancaster, J. (2011). Environmental health in Canada. In M. Stanhope, J. Lancaster, H. Jessup-Falcioni, et al. (Eds.), *Community health nursing in Canada* (3rd ed.) (pp. 474–476). Toronto, ON: Mosby Elsevier.

Tang, K., Beaglehole, R., & O'Byrne, D. (2005). Policy and partnership for health promotion: Addressing the determinants of health. *Bulletin of the World Health Organization, 83*(12), 884–885.

UNICEF. (2009). *The baby-friendly hospital initiative.* http://www.unicef.org/nutrition/files/BFHI_2009_s1.pdf.

University of Calgary. (2007). *Introduction to children's mental health.* https://socialwork.ucalgary.ca/sites/default/files/Course_Outlines/Spring_2020/SOWK_555.03_1_Matheson_P20.pdf.

Uys, L. R., Majumdar, B., & Gwele, N. (2004). The Kwazulu-Natal health promotion model. *Journal of Nursing Scholarship, 36*(3), 192–196.

Vanderpool, R., Casey, B., & Crosby, R. (2011). HPV-related risk perceptions and HPV vaccine uptake among a sample of young rural women. *Journal of Community Health, 36*(6), 903–909. https://doi.org/10.1007/s10900-010-9345-3.

Vollman, A. R., Anderson, E. T., & McFarlane, J. (2017). *Canadian community as partner: Theory & multidisciplinary practice* (4th ed.). Lippincott Williams & Wilkins.

Wass, A. (2000). *Promoting health: The primary health care approach* (2nd ed.). Harcourt Saunders.

Watson, J. (1979). *Nursing: The philosophy and science of caring.* Little, Brown and Company.

Watson, J. (1999). *Human science and human care: A theory of nursing.* Jones & Bartlett.

Weinreich, N. K. (2006). *What is social marketing?.* http://www.social-marketing.com/Whatis.html.

West, R. (2005). Time for a change: Putting the transtheoretical (stages of change) model to rest. *Addiction (Abingdon, England), 100*(8), 1036–1039.

Wild, T. C., Pauly, B., Belle-Isle, L., et al. (2017). Canadian harm reduction policies: A comparative content analysis of provincial and territorial documents, 2000–2015. *International Journal of Drug Policy, 45*, 9–17. https://doi.org/10.1016/j.drugpo.2017.03.014.

World Health Organization (WHO). (1947). *World Health Organization Act 1947. Constitution of the world health organization: section 3.* http://www5.austlii.edu.au/au/legis/cth/consol_act/whoa1947273/s3.html.

World Health Organization (WHO). (1986). *The ottawa charter for health promotion.* http://www.who.int/healthpromotion/conferences/previous/ottawa/en/.

World Health Organization (WHO). (1991). *Health promotion: Sundsvall statement on supportive environments for health.* http://www.who.int/healthpromotion/conferences/previous/sundsvall/en/.

World Health Organization (WHO). (2001). *Health promotion: Jakarta declaration on leading health promotion Into the 21st century.* http://www.who.int/healthpromotion/conferences/previous/jakarta/declaration/en/.

World Health Organization (WHO). (2005). *Health promotion: The Bangkok charter for health promotion in a globalized world.* http://www.who.int/healthpromotion/conferences/6gchp/bangkok_charter/en/.

World Health Organization (WHO). (2006). *Health promotion in a globalized world.* http://apps.who.int/iris/bitstream/10665/21113/1/A59_21-en.pdf.

World Health Organization (WHO). (2008). *Closing the gap in a generation: Health equity through action on the social determinants of health.* http://apps.who.int/iris/bitstream/10665/43943/1/9789241563703_eng.pdf.

World Health Organization (WHO). (2010). *Overview: 7th global conference on health promotion.* http://www.who.int/healthpromotion/conferences/7gchp/overview/en/index.html.

World Health Organization (WHO). (2011). *Rio political declaration on social determinants of health.* https://www.who.int/sdhconference/declaration/Rio_political_declaration.pdf?ua=1.

Young, L. E., & Hayes, V. E. (2002). *Transforming health promotion practice: Concepts, issues, and applications.* F. A. Davis.

Zanchetta, M. S., & Poureslami, I. M. (2006). Health literacy within the reality of immigrants' culture and language. *Canadian Journal of Public Health, 97*(Suppl. 2), 526–530.

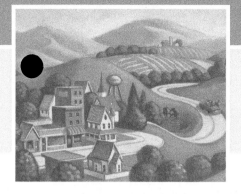

Evidence-Informed Practice in Community Health Nursing

OUTLINE

Evidence-Informed Practice, 117
The Evidence-Informed Practice Process, 118
    Formulating the Clinical Question, 119

Gathering and Assessing Evidence, 121
Determining Which Evidence Is Best to Inform
    Practice, 125

OBJECTIVES

After reading this chapter, you should be able to:
5.1 Explain evidence-informed practice.

5.2 Discuss the evidence-informed practice process.

KEY TERMS*

action research, 124
best practice guidelines, 118
ethnography, 124
evidence-informed practice, 118
grounded theory, 124
knowledge exchange, 125
meta-analysis, 122

participatory action research (PAR), 124
phenomenology, 124
qualitative research, 120
quantitative research, 120
randomized controlled trials (RCTs), 123
systematic review, 122

* See the Glossary on page 468 for definitions.

In this chapter, the basic principles of evidence-informed practice are described as they apply to nursing in general and community health nursing in particular. The process of evidence-informed decision making is also discussed, from formulating the clinical question to gathering and assessing evidence to determining which practice to apply. This chapter emphasizes the importance of integrating evidence-informed decisions in community health nursing practice. It also notes additional resources that provide more information on evidence-informed practice.

EVIDENCE-INFORMED PRACTICE

Evidence-informed practice has become central to daily nursing practice (Canadian Nurses Association [CNA], 2018). It provides nurses with guidance in current nursing practice to help make the most relevant and individualized nursing care decisions in their practice (DiCenso, Guyatt, & Ciliska, 2005; Melnyk & Fineout-Overholt, 2011). Consequently, CHNs need to acquire the skills for evidence-informed practice, including the ability to develop clinical questions, access available evidence to answer these questions, interpret the information correctly, and apply the evidence appropriately in their nursing practice to deliver the highest-quality care to patients (CNA,

2018; Community Health Nurses of Canada, 2019; Kirkpatrick et al., 2012). CHNs support knowledge development, generation, and translation (CPHA, 2010). In addition, CHNs need to stay current in the knowledge related to their area of practice and to appropriately apply this knowledge to patient situations to be competent practitioners and to be able to validate decisions made in their daily nursing practice.

To promote the use of knowledge and evidence by public health practitioners and policy makers, the PHAC has funded the following six National Collaborating Centres for Public Health (NCCPH) to synthesize, translate and share knowledge: Aboriginal Health, Determinants of Health, Environmental Health, Infectious Diseases, Health Public Policy, and Methods and Tools. One of those centres, the National Collaborating Centre for Methods and Tools (2012) supports public health professionals to find and use innovative high-quality methods and tools to build capacity for evidence informed public health. Evidence-informed health care involves the process of critiquing and disseminating the best evidence available from research, context, and experiences, and using that evidence to improve practice and policy (Thomas, Ciliska, Dobbins, et al., 2004). Many factors influence clinical decisions, including science-based interventions and community preferences (Melnyk & Fineout-Overholt, 2011;

Thomas et al., 2004). The application of scientific evidence in nursing is not new. For example, infection-control measures, such as handwashing, are based on sound scientific knowledge. However, it is important to underline that evidence-informed practice includes more than the use of scientific evidence, as will be discussed in this chapter. Although this chapter provides an overview of research as it relates to community health nursing, students will need to review details of the research process using additional resources.

Evidence-informed practice entails combining the best evidence derived from research, clinical practice, knowledge, and expertise, and unique patient experiences, values, preferences, and choices when making clinical decisions (Kirkpatrick et al., 2012; Straus, Richardson, Glasziou, et al., 2005). It is critical to the caring context in community health nursing. Evidence-informed practice is a continuous interactive process that involves explicit, conscientious, and judicious consideration of the best available evidence to provide care (CNA, 2018). The CNA position statement on evidence-informed decision making and nursing practice (see the link on the Evolve website) outlines the responsibilities of individual nurses; professional and nursing specialty associations; nursing regulatory authorities; researchers; educators and educational institutions; health service delivery organizations; governments; and national and provincial or territorial health information institutions (CNA, 2018). The Sigma Theta Tau International Honour Society of Nursing (2005) defines *evidence-informed nursing* as "an integration of the best evidence available, nursing expertise, and the values and preferences of the individuals, families and communities who are served" (p. 1). CHNs use the best evidence available and nursing expertise to create best practice guidelines. **Best practice guidelines** are recommendations pertaining to specific health issues or practice areas based on the most recent research evidence and key expert experiences and judgements (Health Canada, 2007). The Registered Nurses Association of Ontario (RNAO) has published over 50 best practice guidelines as well as toolkits and educator's resources to support their implementation on such topics as smoking cessation and enhancing health adolescent development (https://www.rnao.ca/bpg). By using best practice guidelines, health care providers consider global concepts such as health promotion as a framework for implementing standard decisions and rules about care (see the links for the Institute for Clinical Evaluative Sciences and the Public Health Agency of Canada on the Evolve website for several sources on best practices).

THE EVIDENCE-INFORMED PRACTICE PROCESS

The evidence-informed practice process is a problem-solving strategy based on sound evidence from various sources. The following sources of evidence are key to community health nursing practice:

- The CHN's professional knowledge and clinical experience
- Scientific knowledge—high-quality quantitative and qualitative research from a variety of disciplines; population

health status statistics such as surveillance data, community health status, frequency, causes, and modifying factors
- People in the community—their beliefs, preferences, and concerns
- Knowledge of the community milieu, such as resource availability and accessibility

In community health nursing practice, assumptions are made every day about patient health situations. These assumptions need to be challenged. Doing so entails accessing, interpreting, and appropriately applying the most appropriate evidence. CHNs also need to use the best available evidence to make policy recommendations.

Historically, nurses have used multiple sources of evidence or knowledge in their practice. Unsystematic clinical observations by a CHN can lead to the development of hypotheses (hunches) of what might be happening. However, alone they may not accurately reflect the real problem or concern of the population. The model for evidence-informed practice and decision making (Fig. 5.1) is based on a systematic approach. Using this model, the CHN develops a clinical or community question and answers that question by taking into consideration the best available evidence from the key sources of evidence.

The evidence-informed practice puzzle in Fig. 5.2 presents the questions CHNs ask when they follow evidence-informed practice to provide the highest-quality care to their patients. As previously mentioned, the term *patient* is used in the broadest sense; that is, a patient can be the individual, family, aggregate or group, population, community, or society. Every piece of the puzzle calls for reflection and decision making in each unique patient situation.

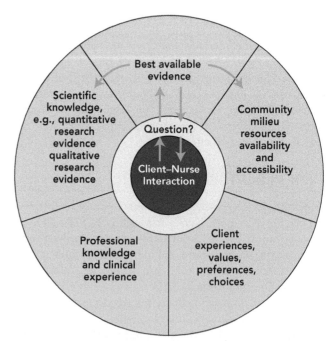

Fig. 5.1 Model for Evidence-Informed Practice and Decision Making in Community Health Nursing.

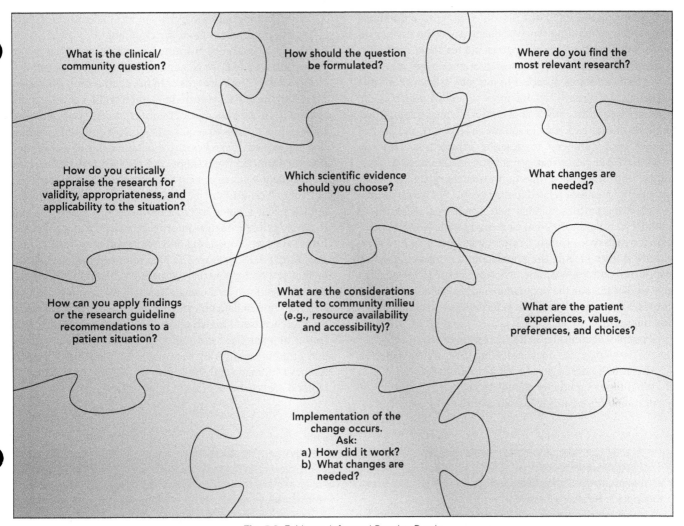

Fig. 5.2 Evidence-Informed Practice Puzzle.

Formulating the Clinical Question

The first step in the evidence-informed practice process is to produce a sound, researchable clinical question. Doing so involves beginning with a clear idea of the question, then defining and refining it so that it has a clear focus and is answerable. Various methods are available to help clearly define a clinical question. One is the PICO approach, in which P = population, I = intervention, C = comparison of evidence, and O = outcome (Wakefield, 2014).

Major, Clarke, Cardenas, et al. (2006) sought to understand key barriers to providing asthma care to elementary school children in an effort to determine best practices for delivering quality care. Using the PICO approach, they defined the component parts of the clinical question as follows:

- P—elementary school-aged children living with asthma
- I—elementary school health education, interventions, and barriers
- C—literature and focus groups with CHNs caring for children in schools
- O—best practices and collaborative strategies with schools, families, health care providers, and the community

With these component parts in mind, the clinical question became "What is the best community health promotion strategy for elementary school-aged children with asthma?" Current practices and interventions were examined in the literature, and current best practices were explored with focus groups of CHNs currently caring for this population. Major et al. (2006) recommended that programs and strategies for this population should be collaborative in nature with teachers, CHNs, families, and patients. The study authors also recommended that all of these groups be involved in planning, implementing, and evaluating asthma care programs and strategies. The PICO approach can help CHNs define a clinical question that has a clear focus for the research needed to determine best practices.

The clinical question directs the search for relevant research evidence in the literature. A well-formulated question provides the keywords to search the literature in order to retrieve relevant research evidence. At first glance, creating a clinical question may seem easy. However, the CHN needs to formulate the clinical question in such a way that it is answerable and searchable if the literature searches are to be effective and provide relevant information.

DiCenso et al. (2005) describe different types of questions and the corresponding types of quantitative and qualitative studies that would be most appropriate for those questions. **Quantitative research** is a research methodology that tests hypotheses and uses numbers to describe relationships, differences, and cause–effect interactions among variables. By contrast, **qualitative research** is a research methodology that explores human experiences and uses words, text, and themes (rather than numbers) to describe experiences. DiCenso et al. (2005) indicate that quantitative studies answer "how many" and "how much" questions, whereas qualitative studies answer questions related to how people feel about or how people experience situations and conditions. Also, these authors identify the different elements to include in the question for each type of study. For example, questions for quantitative studies include the population, the interventions or exposures, and the outcome, whereas questions for qualitative studies include the population and the situation. Box 5.1 provides two examples of how to formulate a structured clinical question.

Examples of clinical questions are as follows:

1. For new parents, does providing free smoke detector alarms to homes help reduce injuries from fires?
2. What type of guidance should be provided to a group of new mothers regarding infant car seats?
3. Which community programs are most effective in reducing obesity among school-age children?
4. Should a policy be instituted requiring vaccination for hepatitis A and B for all adults travelling out of Canada?

Remember: The keywords used in your question will determine how successful you are in extracting the relevant information from the available literature related to your question. Information on how to acquire the skills of question formulation and keyword searches can be obtained through evidence-informed practice workshops and relevant texts. Librarians are excellent sources of help in conducting library searches, but your question must be clearly stated to locate the information needed. Some Internet resources that CHNs can use to develop their evidence-informed practice are listed on the Evolve website. Depending on your community health nursing practice setting, as well as your roles and responsibilities, certain Internet resources will be more helpful than others. Exercise caution when using information from websites that claim to contain data on evidence-informed practice. Ensure the evidence from the website is credible by examining such factors as references and the qualifications of the organization or group sponsoring the website (e.g., the Public Health Agency of Canada and the Registered Nurses' Association of Ontario are reliable sources of information).

BOX 5.1   Examples of Transforming Unstructured Clinical Questions into Structured Clinical Questions

Example 1: Smoking Cessation

You are a school nurse at a large high school in your community. You have just completed a day of information sessions with students on the harmful effects of smoking and have offered to meet with whomever is interested in quitting smoking. The next day, an 18-year-old girl, who has been smoking half a pack of cigarettes a day for the past year, drops in at your office. She has tried to quit smoking a number of times but with no success. She asks you whether "the patch" is an effective aid to quit smoking.

Type of Study: Quantitative

Initial Question: Is the nicotine patch effective?

Digging Deeper: One limitation of this type of question is that it does not specify the population. The effectiveness of the nicotine patch may differ in adolescents versus adults, in women versus men, in heavy smokers versus light smokers, as well as in those who have smoked for many years versus those who have smoked only for a few years. Another limitation of this question is that it does not include an outcome, which we know is smoking cessation.

Improved (Searchable) Question: A searchable question would specify the relevant patient population, the management strategy, and the patient-relevant consequences of that intervention, as follows:

Population: Young women who are moderate smokers
Intervention: Nicotine replacement therapy
Outcome: Smoking cessation

Formulated Question: Among young women who are moderate smokers, does nicotine replacement therapy increase the probability of smoking cessation?

Example 2: Caregiver Stress

You are a public health nurse who has been visiting an elderly man with Alzheimer's disease. His daughter is his primary caregiver. As his condition deteriorates, she is increasingly worried about his safety and finds the situation physically and emotionally draining. She is experiencing anguish and guilt as she realizes that her father will soon need to be placed in a special care unit. She asks you whether others in this situation have similar feelings and what she can expect to feel once he is placed in the special care unit.

Type of Study: Qualitative

Initial Question: What is it like to place a relative in special care?

Digging Deeper: Limitations of this formulation of the question include failure to specify the population and insufficient details about the situation.

Improved (Searchable) Question: A searchable question would specify the relevant patient population and situation:
Population: Caregivers
Situation: Placing a relative with Alzheimer's disease in a special care unit

Formulated Question: How do caregivers describe their experiences of deciding to place a relative with Alzheimer's disease in a special care unit?

Source: DiCenso, A., Guyatt, G., & Ciliska, D. (2005). *Evidence-based nursing: A guide to clinical practice* (pp. 24–27). Mosby.

Gathering and Assessing Evidence

To effectively answer the formulated clinical question, CHNs access a variety of sources, such as their professional knowledge and experience; scientific knowledge; patient experiences, values, preferences, and choices; and knowledge of the community milieu and its available and accessible resources.

Community Health Nurses' Professional Knowledge and Experience

CHNs' professional knowledge, clinical experience in the community, and clinical-reasoning skills will help in (1) identifying patient issues for study and anticipating possible patient responses to proposed strategies; (2) integrating all available evidence into nursing practice decisions; and (3) evaluating community health nursing practice decisions. When CHNs access scientific knowledge of all types, they need to choose the most relevant information for each patient's clinical situation. Asking the right questions will help determine what acceptable evidence is. As well, CHNs need to have the skills to critically appraise the available evidence, including the research methods of quantitative and qualitative studies. The choice of research methodology is dependent on the nature of the patient's health concern.

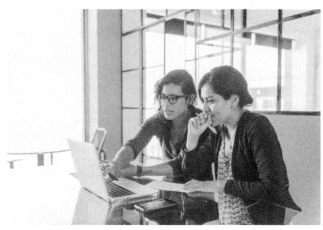

Although it might sometimes be easier to rely on past experience and knowledge, CHNs strive to use the most recent evidence-informed data as one of their primary sources of decision making. This type of data can be found in peer-reviewed, published research articles that are usually free and accessible online. (iStockphoto/ferrantraite)

Clinical Practice Guidelines

Clinical practice guidelines are systematically developed recommendations or statements that facilitate nursing decision making and provide the most suitable clinical interventions for particular patients (CNA, 2004). These statements provide nurses with the most current, reliable information about a particular problem. The most rigorous research available is used to develop clinical practice guidelines. However, when research evidence is found to be weak, these guidelines are developed using expert opinion and consensus (CNA, 2004; DiCenso et al., 2005). Examples of clinical practice guidelines in nursing are as follows: Adult Asthma Care Guidelines for Nurses: Promoting Control of Asthma; Assessment and Care of Adults at Risk for Suicidal Ideation and Behaviour; Assessment and Device Selection for Vascular Access; Assessment and Management of Foot Ulcers

for People With Diabetes; Assessment and Management of Pain. All are available through the Registered Nurses' Association of Ontario website (see the link on the Evolve website). The "Ethical Considerations" box relates to the application of clinical practice guidelines to public health emergencies.

ETHICAL CONSIDERATIONS

Public health emergencies present unique ethical challenges because health care workers are often at increased personal risk when caring for patients experiencing emergencies such as environmental disasters and life-threatening communicable diseases. One example of a recent communicable disease outbreak is the enterovirus D68, one of more than 100 nonpolio enteroviruses that causes respiratory illness and is spread by coughing, sneezing, or touching a surface that has been touched by an infected person. Symptoms range from mild cold symptoms to paralysis and severe respiratory illness requiring hospitalization. In October 2014, four Canadian deaths and numerous clinical cases were attributed to D68; a total of 75 specimens tested positive for the virus. Communicable diseases can cause disproportionate damage or harm to vulnerable populations and increase personal risk to CHNs. When this happens, CHNs need to identify and address ethical issues and evidence-informed guidelines to deliver the highest-quality care to patients. Evidence-informed guidelines for the care of these patients could include policies and procedures related to infection-control practices and personal protective equipment.

Ethical principles that apply to the above situation include (see Box 6.4):

- *Nonmaleficence.* The CHN acts according to the standards of due care, always seeking to do no harm (e.g., ensuring informed consent).
- *Beneficence.* This principle is complementary to nonmaleficence and requires that the CHN do good (e.g., provide competent care).

CHNs have an ethical obligation to perform actions that are in keeping with the principles of nonmaleficence and beneficence as long as those actions do not place health care providers at high risk for personal harm.

The CNA *Code of Ethics for Registered Nurses* also provides criteria to consider when contemplating the CHN duty to provide care during a public health emergency such as a communicable disease outbreak, including:

- The significance of the risk to vulnerable populations if the CHN does not assist.
- Whether care is directly relevant to preventing harm to the population.
- Whether the benefits of providing care outweigh the harm that a CHN may incur.

Questions to Consider

You are the CHN working with a vulnerable population of middle-aged diabetic patients.

1. How would you prevent the spread of the enterovirus D68 among this vulnerable population?
2. What is the significance of the risk to this vulnerable population if the spread of enterovirus D68 is not controlled? Are there any best practice guidelines to prevent the spread of the enterovirus D68 in your province?

Scientific Knowledge

CHNs need to determine the scientific evidence that is best suited to answering their clinical question. The following questions can help CHNs evaluate the quality and acceptability of a source to their clinical question:

1. Does the information come from a reliable source (e.g., a peer-reviewed journal)?
2. Is the author a credible source?
3. What is the research sample, and how was it selected? Is it representative of the population?
4. What research method was used, and was it appropriate?
5. How were the data analyzed?
6. What are the findings? Are they valid? Are they realistic and based on the data?
7. Can this research evidence be applied to my patient population?
8. What are the implications of this research evidence for my patient population? (Wakefield, 2014)

The most common types of research CHNs will use to answer their clinical question are systematic reviews, randomized controlled trials, and participatory action research. You may want to refer to textbooks on research to review study designs and the research process in depth.

A **systematic review**, or an *overview*, is a summary or synthesis of the research evidence that relates to a specific question and to the effects of an intervention. According to Im and Chang (2012), a systematic review in nursing includes:

- A systematic approach in the methods used to retrieve, sort, and analyze the literature on a particular topic
- Explicit step-by-step descriptions of the procedures used to analyze the literature
- Comprehensive covering of all available sources of the literature
- The ability to be reproduced by peers or the discipline

The "Evidence-Informed Practice" box provides one example of a systematic review found in the Cochrane Library (a collection of high-quality, independent evidence to inform health care decisions). Systematic reviews can involve a rigorous process with several steps and several evaluators to analyze all available resources of the literature that relate to the same question or the effects of an intervention.

The abundance of research information available on a topic can be overwhelming. Systematic reviews help CHNs manage this information overload and provide a grading of the quality of the available information. In addition, systematic reviews are useful knowledge sources, providing quick and easy access to large amounts of available research information that has been reviewed and summarized.

A meta-analysis is sometimes used in a systematic review. A **meta-analysis** systematically analyzes the results of multiple studies that are comparable to produce a summary of those results (Ciliska, Cullum, & Marks, 2001; Munn, Tufanaru, & Aromataris, 2014). A systematic review can include several meta-analyses, depending on the outcomes that were identified. For example, Ruppar, Conn, Chase, et al. (2014) conducted a meta-analysis with data from 344 studies testing

EVIDENCE-INFORMED PRACTICE

Nurses and other health care providers often advise or counsel patients regarding smoking cessation. Rice and Stead (2006) questioned whether this health promotion activity is effective. As a result, they conducted a systematic review to determine the effectiveness of nursing interventions in smoking cessation. The authors, using an evidence-informed approach, searched the resources of the Cumulative Index to Nursing and Allied Health Literature (CINAHL) and the Cochrane Tobacco Addiction Group to identify randomized trials exploring nursing interventions for smoking cessation. Twenty of the 29 studies identified that smoking cessation interventions significantly increased the odds of the patient quitting smoking, particularly when the activity was provided during hospitalization. Smoking cessation interventions for nonhospitalized patients showed that the advice and support of nurses provided some benefit. Overall, the systematic review indicated reasonable evidence that smoking cessation interventions by nurses could be effective.

Application for CHNs

The review of the trials indicated that the health promotion activity of advising and counselling smokers had some benefit and, therefore, should be used as a community health nursing intervention for encouraging smoking cessation. As well, the review showed the benefit of follow-up care for patients discharged from hospital who require continued support and counselling for smoking cessation.

Questions for Reflection and Discussion

1. State one clinical question raised by the systematic review described above.
2. What evidence-informed practice sources would you use to obtain answers to this clinical question? Elaborate on why you have chosen these evidence-informed practice sources.

Source: Rice, V. H., & Stead, L. F. (2006). Nursing interventions for smoking cessation. *Cochrane Database of Systematic Reviews.* ISSN: 1464–780X. http://www.cochrane.org

the impact of supervised exercise interventions on lipid outcomes. They concluded that there was a greater effect on lipid outcomes with interventions that used low-intensity exercise. One of the limitations of a meta-analysis is that only studies that have similar data collection methods and analysis can be combined, which limits the number and type of studies that can be pooled (Munn et al., 2014). Past and current systematic reviews and meta-analyses that are relevant to CHNs in their nursing practice are available from the Effective Public Health Practice Project (EPHPP) website (see the Tool Box on the Evolve website).

Ciliska et al. (2001) developed three basic appraisal questions to ask when evaluating systematic reviews:

1. Are the results of this systematic review valid?
   Ask yourself:
   - Is this a systematic review of similar studies?
   - Does the systematic review include a description of the strategies used to find all relevant trials?

A Systematic Review of Motor Vehicle Crashes in Indigenous Populations in Canada

Motor vehicle crashes (MVCs) represent one of the causes of unintentional death among Indigenous populations in Canada. In 2013, Short, Mushquash, and Bédard conducted a systematic review of the published and grey literature* on MCVs involving Indigenous people in Canada. They used the literature search approach outlined by Cochrane, including use of the Haddon matrix of injury epidemiology and prevention to identify trends in MVC-related risk factors. Examples of phrases used to search the literature included the terms "pre crash," "crash," and "post crash." The risk factors identified were human, vehicle/equipment, physical environment, and social environment variables. The initial search revealed 223 studies, but that number was narrowed down by focusing on studies published after 1980, with at least one of the objectives identified as well as measurable outcomes. As a result, 20 studies were reviewed: 17 were in peer-reviewed journals and seven were grey literature. The authors found higher rates of injury and death from MCVs among Indigenous populations in Canada than non-Indigenous populations, particularly in western Canada. Review of pre crash and crash factors indicated several relevant risk factors for this population, including adult males, seat belt nonadherence, alcohol misuse, road surface (e.g., loose gravel, muddy roads), interactions with wild animals, vehicle type (e.g., trucks heavier than 4.5 tons), and vehicle year (e.g., older than 1990). This systematic review of the literature revealed that Indigenous populations in Canada are at twice the risk for death, hospitalizations, and injury related to MVCs than non-Indigenous populations in Canada. This evidence can assist CHNs in planning health promotion strategies for Indigenous populations in Canada by targeting the risk factors identified in the review and evaluating strategies based on those indicators.

Questions to Consider

1. Formulate a researchable, clinical question on the issue of motor vehicle crashes among Indigenous people in Canada.
2. How could you use this systematic review to develop an injury prevention program for this population?
3. What sources of evidence could you obtain from the community to help you plan an intervention?

* *Grey literature* is literature that is produced by organizations outside of commercial or academic research (e.g., annual reports, minutes of meetings).
Source: Short, M., Mushquash, C. J., & Bédard, M. (2013). Motor vehicle crashes among Canadian Aboriginal people: A review of the literature. *Canadian Journal of Rural Medicine, 18*(3), 86–98.

- Does the systematic review include a description of how the validity of the individual studies was assessed?
- Were the results consistent from study to study?
- Were individual or aggregate data used in the analysis?
2. What were the results?
   Ask yourself:
   - How large was the treatment effect?

- Were the results statistically significant?
3. Will the results help me in caring for my patients?
   Ask yourself:
   - Are my patients so different from those in the study that the results do not apply?
   - Is the intervention/treatment feasible in my setting?
   - Were all clinically important outcomes (harms as well as benefits) considered?

The "Cultural Considerations" box discusses a systematic review of research on motor vehicle crashes in Indigenous populations in Canada.

Im and Chang (2012) propose the following guidelines for CHNs who conduct their own systematic integrated literature review:

1. Use multiple sources for article retrieval (e.g., select databases that are specific to your question, such as CINAHL, PubMed, CNA Nurse One, Cochrane Library).
2. Adopt a framework that will guide the analysis of each article (e.g., feminist perspective, the Roy adaptation model of nursing).
3. Determine the evaluation criteria that will be used to analyze the articles (e.g., *Cochrane Handbook for Systematic Review of Interventions*).
4. Use specific quantitative or qualitative methods to analyze the articles.

One consideration with systematic reviews is the possible problem of bias, particularly publication bias. The reviewer(s) who develop the systematic review may select only published studies that have significant results. However, other unpublished studies (e.g., academic research that has not been published in a peer-reviewed journal) may confirm or contradict the reported results (DiCenso et al., 2005; Melnyk & Fineout-Overholt, 2011).

Systematic reviews can overestimate the effectiveness of an intervention, especially if unpublished studies are not included in the review. In the systematic review, the reviewer needs to be transparent about the efforts made to access unpublished studies as well as the process used for obtaining published studies. Cochrane (formerly the Cochrane Collaboration) websites listed on the Evolve website provide guidance on conducting a systematic review and searching the health promotion and public health literature. The quality of the research studies included in systematic reviews will, in turn, influence the quality of the systematic reviews themselves. The Evidence for Policy and Practice Information Coordinating Centre (EPPI-Centre) has developed guidelines for the systematic review of empirical research studies in education (see the Tool Box on the Evolve website). This site provides questions to consider when appraising research studies (e.g., health promotion intervention studies). The EPHPP also provides examples of systematic reviews and summary statements of relevance to CHNs.

Randomized controlled trials (RCTs) are the gold standard of evidence gathering in evidence-informed practice. RCTs are one of the best sources of research on the efficacy and safety of clinical practices and interventions, and medications (Beam, Aliaga, Ahlfeld, et al., 2014; DiCenso et al., 2005; Melnyk & Fineout-Overholt, 2011). RCTs are often considered the strongest evidence because the people being studied are randomly assigned to either the control group or the experimental group. Random assignment controls for biases and differences that can occur due to the intervention. You may refer to research textbooks for details on random assignment (also called *random allocation*), blinding, and loss to follow-up, which can affect bias in a study.

RCTs are as applicable to nursing practice in communities as they are to other areas of health care. RCTs can inform CHN practice and help address population health concerns. For example, Sichieri, Paula Trotte, de Souze et al. (2009) conducted a clustered RCT to determine whether an education program aimed at discouraging students from drinking sugar-sweetened beverages could prevent excessive weight gain. They concluded that participation in a program designed to decrease sugar-sweetened beverage intake significantly reduced body mass index among overweight children as compared with those children who did not participate in the program. These findings could have implications for CHNs trying to develop programs and policies to address childhood obesity in their patient populations.

The reason for the limited number of community health nursing RCT studies is often related to ethical issues. It is considered unethical to withhold an intervention from the control group—for example, withholding administration of the human papillomavirus (HPV) vaccine from a group of teens to determine the psychological effects of HPV infection. However, this ethical issue could be addressed by offering the intervention to the control group after the research study has been completed. It would also be unethical to assign individuals to an experimental group when harm could occur; for example, assigning pregnant women to a smoking group (experimental group) to determine the effects of smoking on the fetus (this type of study would not receive ethical approval).

Regardless of the type of study design, the quality of a study must always be established before a decision is made to use the study's findings. Several tools are available to evaluate the quality of a quantitative study. Refer to the EPHPP quality assessment tool listed in the Tool Box on the Evolve website. This tool can help CHNs determine whether the findings of a study can be used in their community health nursing practice.

Qualitative research has gained importance because it allows exploration of the "meaning" of situations to patients. Qualitative research has contributed to the development of theories relevant to nursing practice. A system for rating the strength of qualitative evidence has yet to be developed. However, meta-synthesis—the summarizing of results from multiple qualitative studies—is increasingly being used and likely will lead to the development of a rating system. Qualitative research, with its interpretive perspective, assigns meaning to experiences. The

types of qualitative approaches most familiar to CHNs are **phenomenology** (to understand the meaning of the lived experience); **grounded theory** (for theory development); **ethnography** (to understand a culture from the emic [insider] perspective); and **action research** (a systematic study of practice interventions) (Melnyk & Fineout-Overholt, 2011).

Participatory action research (PAR), a form of qualitative research, is widely used in community health nursing practice to identify health needs and guide practice (Cusack, Cohen, Mignone, et. al., 2018; Nadin, Crow, Prince & Kelley, 2018). PAR is a subcategory of action research that assists participants in articulating needs and developing strategies to address those needs. Nadin and colleagues (2018) used PAR to develop the Wiisokotaatiwin Palliative Care Program in the community of Naotkamegwanning First Nation, Ontario. The researchers engaged the community through conducting a needs assessment and establishing a leadership team with elders and band members. The project resulted in the development of a palliative care program influenced by local cultural protocols (Cultural Considerations box).

🌐 CULTURAL CONSIDERATIONS

Using Participatory Action Research

Participatory action research (PAR) can assist CHNs to make decisions for program development in culturally diverse populations. Nadin and colleagues (2018) used PAR in the design, implementation, and evaluation of an innovative, palliative care program for the First Nations rural community of Naotkamegwanning in Ontario. That program was developed within the context of the Improving End-of-Life-Care in First Nations Communities project, a 5-year PAR project where researchers partnered with First Nations communities to develop local palliative care programs. The Naotkamegwanning program was embedded in and influenced by local cultural protocols, values, and beliefs. For example, there is no word for "palliative care" in the Anishinaabe language, so with direction from the elders and the leadership team, the program was called Wiisokotaatiwin, which translates as "taking care of each other or supporting each other". The vision of the program was to have coordinated, comprehensive community services available for those who wish to return home to journey, and to maintain the use of traditions and spiritual beliefs.

PAR can be an integral part of implementing a community development process and building community capacity to guide program development in culturally diverse populations.

Source: Nadin, S., Crow, M., Prince, H., & Kelley, M. L. (2018). Wiisokotaatiwin: development and evaluation of a community-based palliative care program in Naotkamegwanning First Nation. *Rural & Remote Health, 18*(2), 41–58. https://doi.org/10.22605/RRH4317.

The partnership between the CHN and the patient also involves determining how the research will be used to create or support the change. PAR is often conducted to (1) resolve health service delivery issues and problems and (2) empower individuals, populations, and communities with the motivation to promote social action (Melnyk & Fineout-Overholt, 2011). Janzen, Ochocka, Jacobson, et al. (2010) used PAR to develop a framework for providing community-based mental health supports to people from diverse backgrounds. The researchers engaged key stakeholders in the community—including representatives from five cultural groups, service providers, and mental health organizations—to help develop the framework. The framework synthesized previous culture-oriented and power-oriented models for community mental health practice and had three components: *values* that guided *actions* that produced desired *outcomes.*

It is critical that CHNs recognize that both quantitative and qualitative studies contribute to nursing knowledge. DiCenso et al. (2005) assert that these two paradigms are complementary. In the qualitative paradigm, meanings of phenomena are explored, theories are generated, and "relationships between identified concepts" are identified. In the quantitative paradigm, hypotheses are tested, and numbers are used in data analysis and in presenting study findings to make generalizations about aggregates and populations and to make predictions. In addition, this paradigm tests the theories developed in qualitative studies (DiCenso et al., 2005). Fade (2003) also posited the need for both types of study to achieve a complete understanding of an issue.

Patient Experiences, Values, Preferences, and Choices

CHNs who value evidence-informed practice take into consideration patient experiences, values, preferences, and choices about care and services. Since the goal in nursing is to deliver the best possible care to patients and to have the best possible patient outcomes, the evidence can also be based on unsystematic clinical observations by the CHN and discussions with the patient (DiCenso et al., 2005).

CHNs need to evaluate patient openness and readiness to implement the change recommended by the research (DiCenso et al., 2005). In this process, it is important to assess patient experiences, values, preferences, and choices because they will influence patient willingness to implement the change or intervention.

Sometimes, a patient may request a particular intervention, but the CHN may have determined, based on the critical appraisal of the available evidence, that the intervention would not be a wise choice. The CHN would then need to explain to the patient the evidence presented by the research and help the patient make an informed decision.

Community Milieu

In partnership with the patient, the CHN must consider the community milieu to determine which interventions would most likely be of benefit to the patient. Community milieu includes such factors as expertise available in the community, urban or rural setting, social and physical environments, and resource availability and accessibility. For example, adequate fiscal and human resources should be available in the community to support selected programs.

BOX 5.2 Questions on the Appropriateness and Applicability of an Evidence-Informed Practice

1. How will the results of the study direct my patient care practice?
   a. What is the fit between the characteristics of the study participants and my patients? Can the study results be applied to my patients?
   b. What is the feasibility of applying the treatment or intervention in our setting?
   c. How were the clinically relevant outcomes—that is, harms and benefits—considered?
   d. What are my patient's experiences, values, preferences, and choices for prevention of the outcome and the potential adverse effects?
   e. What community milieu resources (including their availability and accessibility) need to be considered?
2. How can the study findings be applied to the care of my patient?
   a. What is the meaning and relevance of the study to my practice?
   b. How does the study facilitate my understanding of the context of my practice?
   c. How does the study enhance my knowledge about my practice?

Source: Adapted from Ciliska, D., & Thomas, H. (2008). Research. In J. L. Leeseberg Stamler & L. Yiu (Eds.), *Community health nursing: A Canadian perspective* (2nd ed., pp. 227–244). Pearson Education Canada.

Determining Which Evidence Is Best to Inform Practice

CHNs have access to a vast amount of evidence that can be used to inform practice. However, not all evidence is appropriate or applicable. It is important to use appropriate criteria to determine which evidence is the best to inform practice. Box 5.2 presents questions to consider regarding the appropriateness and applicability of an evidence-informed practice to a patient situation.

Mowinski Jennings and Loan (2001) have noted that when selecting the appropriate evidence to apply to practice in partnership with the patient, it is important to support the patient in the decision-making process. CHNs must ensure that the evidence is presented at an appropriate literacy level for each patient, advise the patient of the benefits and risks of an intervention, and consider patient preferences and values in relation to the practice. CHNs use evidence-informed practice as a process to improve practice and patient outcomes, and to influence policies that will improve the health of the patient (DiCenso et al., 2005).

Knowledge exchange is a collaborative, problem-solving process in which researchers and decision makers exchange knowledge to solve problems. It involves mutual learning through the process of collaboratively planning, producing, developing, disseminating, and applying knowledge to decision making (Canadian Foundation for Healthcare Improvement, 2016). It is a continuous process that involves complex and unpredictable settings that are influenced by a variety of factors such as political, cultural, historical, and organizational factors. Knowledge exchange involves working in collaboration with key stakeholders at every stage of the process (Hunter, Rushmer, & Best, 2014). Through knowledge exchange, CHNs, in their roles as researchers and in working collaboratively with other researchers and health care decision makers, can influence health care policy, and the ensuing health care policy changes and application of research evidence can positively affect community health. The access and use of evidence-informed practice encourage CHNs to be professional, to provide care in a safe manner, and to be accountable for their community health nursing practice.

Evidence-informed practice skills can help CHNs deal with these uncertainties as they occur in nursing practice. The application of evidence-informed practice can also help CHNs explain and justify the decisions they make on a daily basis in their community health nursing practice.

STUDENT EXPERIENCE

Patient situation: A 24-year-old paraplegic patient who is bedridden has developed reddened broken skin in the coccyx area. This patient became paraplegic due to a motorcycle accident and has just been discharged home, where he will be living with his recently separated mother. Use the approach to clearly identify the clinical question.
1. P = Identify the target population
2. I = Identify appropriate interventions for this population
3. C = Compare the evidence
4. O = Identify appropriate outcomes for this patient

Questions
1. What have you learned from this evidence-informed practice exercise?
2. How has this exercise changed your thoughts and feelings about evidence-informed practice?

CHAPTER SUMMARY

5.1 Evidence-informed practice combines the best evidence derived from research, clinical practice, knowledge and expertise, and unique patient experiences, values, preferences, and choices when making clinical decisions.

5.2 The evidence-informed practice process starts with defining a researchable clinical question. The PICO approach can help clearly define the clinical question (P = population; I = intervention; C = comparison of evidence, and O = outcome). The process then moves into gathering and assessing evidence from a variety of sources to answer the clinical question. The best available evidence comprises the CHN's professional knowledge and clinical experience; scientific knowledge—high-quality quantitative and qualitative research from a variety of disciplines; patient experiences, values, preferences, and choices; and knowledge of the community milieu, such as resource availability and accessibility.

CHN IN PRACTICE: A CASE STUDY

Expanding Clinic Services

The director of a part-time, nurse-managed community health clinic is in the process of determining how best to expand services to operate as a full-time clinic in the most cost-effective as well as clinically effective manner. The nurse, who is the director, gathers evidence on nurse-managed community clinics in other rural settings to evaluate cost-effectiveness and clinical effectiveness of various models. The nurse also considers evidence from the following sources in the decision-making process: patient satisfaction research data, knowledge of clinic staff, expert opinion of community advisory board members, evidence from community partners, and data on service needs in the province. Having examined the evidence, the nurse decides that incremental (step-by-step) growth toward full-time status is warranted. Evidence of needs in the community and analysis of statistical data indicate that adding services for children is a priority. As the first step, a CHN with a pediatric clinical background is hired, while planning for full-time status continues.

Think About It
1. Which of the following is demonstrated by the evaluation of the evidence gathered?
   a. Effectiveness of the intervention in communities
   b. Application of the data to populations and communities
   c. Economic consequences of the intervention
   d. Barriers to implementation of the interventions in communities
2. Explain how this example applies principles of evidence-informed practice.

📶 TOOL BOX

The Tool Box contains useful resources that can be applied to community health nursing practice. These related resources are found on the Evolve website at http://evolve.elsevier.com/Canada/Stanhope/community/.

Tools

Canadian Task Force on Preventive Health Care. (https://www.canadiantaskforce.ca/)

This website provides screening guidelines for depression, cervical cancer, hypertension, diabetes, and breast cancer.

Cochrane. (https://www.cochrane.org/)

This website (formerly the Cochrane Collaboration) provides reviews from A to Z on such topics as cardiovascular health, medications and alcohol, infectious diseases, sexual health, human immunodeficiency virus/acquired immunodeficiency syndrome (HIV/AIDS), various types of injuries, mental and social health, nutrition, overweight and obesity, physical activity, occupational health and safety, population screening and population group, and tobacco control.

Effective Public Health Practice Project. Quality Assessment Tool for Quantitative Studies. (https://www.ncbi.nlm.nih.gov/books/NBK38243/)

This website includes the tool and a dictionary for tool use. It also includes links to systematic literature reviews.

Evidence for Policy and Practice Information and Coordinating Centre (EPPI-Centre). (http://eppi.ioe.ac.uk/cms/Portals/0/PDF%20reviews%20and%20summaries/EPPI%20REPOSE%20Guidelines%20A4%202.1.pdf)

This website includes guidelines for the reporting of primary empirical research studies in education (the REPOSE guidelines). It also provides a variety of links to references on research methods (e.g., on appraising and synthesizing research and using research evidence).

REFERENCES

Beam, K., Aliaga, S., Ahlfeld, S., et al. (2014). A systematic review of randomized controlled trials for the prevention of bronchopulmonary dysplasia in infants. *Journal of Perinatology*, 34(9), 705–710. https://doi.org/10.1038/jp.2014.126

Canadian Foundation for Healthcare Improvement. (2016). *Glossary of knowledge exchange terms.* http://www.cfhi-fcass.ca/PublicationsAndResources/ResourcesAndTools/GlossaryKnowledgeExchange.aspx.

Canadian Nurses Association (CNA). (2004). Making best practice guidelines a reality. *Nursing Now* (Vol. 17). https://www.cna-aiic.ca/~/media/cna/page-content/pdf-en/nn_best_practice_ejan_2005_e.pdf?la=en.

Canadian Nurses Association (CNA). (2018). *Position statement: Evidence-informed decision-making and nursing practice.* https://www.cna-aiic.ca/-/media/cna/page-content/pdf-en/evidence-informed-decision-making-and-nursing-practice-position-statement_dec-2018.pdf.

Canadian Public Health Association (CPHA). (2010). *Public health—community health nursing practice in Canada: Roles and activities* (4th ed.).

Ciliska, D., Cullum, N., & Marks, S. (2001). Evaluation of systematic reviews of treatment of prevention interventions. *Evidence-Based Nursing*, 4(4), 100–105.

Ciliska, D., & Thomas, H. (2008). Research. In J. L. Leeseberg Stamler, & L. Yiu (Eds.), *Community health nursing: A Canadian perspective* (2nd ed.) (pp. 227–244). Pearson Education Canada.

Community Health Nurses of Canada (CHNC). (2019). *Canadian community health nursing: Professional practice model and standards of practice.* https://www.chnc.ca/standards-of-practice.

Cusack, C., Cohen, B., Mignone, J., et al. (2018). Participatory action as a research method with public health nurses. *Journal of Advanced Nursing*, 74(7), 1544–1553. https://doi.org/10.1111/jan.13555

DiCenso, A., Guyatt, G., & Ciliska, D. (2005). *Evidence-based nursing: A guide to clinical practice.* Mosby.

Fade, S. A. (2003). Communicating and judging the quality of qualitative research: The need for a new language. *Journal of Human Nutrition and Dietetics*, 16(3), 139–149.

Health Canada. (2007). *Best practices: Treatment and rehabilitation for seniors with substance use problems.* http://www.hc-sc.gc.ca/hc-ps/pubs/adp-apd/treat_senior-trait_ainee/index-eng.php.

Hunter, D. J., Rushmer, R. R., & Best, A. A. (2014). Knowledge exchange in public health. *Public Health (Elsevier)*, 128(6), 495–496. https://doi.org/10.1016/j.puhe.2014.04.011

Im, E.-O., & Chang, S. J. (2012). A systematic integrated literature review of systematic integrated literature reviews in nursing. *Journal of Nursing Education*, 51(11), 632–640. https://doi.org/10.3928/01484834-20120914-02

Janzen, R., Ochocka, J., Jacobson, N., et al. (2010). Synthesizing culture and power in community mental health: An emerging framework. *Canadian Journal of Community Mental Health*, 29(1), 51–67.

Kirkpatrick, P., Wilson, E., & Wimpenny, P. (2012). Research to support evidence-based practice in COPD community nursing. *British Journal of Community Nursing*, 17(10), 486–492.

Major, D. A., Clarke, S. M., Cardenas, R. A., et al. (2006). Providing asthma care in elementary schools: Understanding barriers to determine best practices. *Family & Community Health*, 29(4), 256–265.

Melnyk, B. M., & Fineout-Overholt, E. (2011). *Evidence-based practice in nursing and healthcare: A guide to best practice.* Lippincott, Williams & Wilkins.

Mowinski Jennings, B., & Loan, L. A. (2001). Misconceptions among nurses about evidence-based practice. *Journal of Nursing Scholarship*, 33(2), 121–127.

Munn, Z., Tufanaru, C., & Aromataris, E. (2014). Data extraction and synthesis. *American Journal of Nursing*, 114(7), 49–54.

Nadin, S., Crow, M., Prince, H., et al. (2018). Wiisokotaatiwin: Development and evaluation of a community-based palliative care program in Naotkamegwanning first nation. *Rural and Remote Health*, 18(2), 41–58. https://doi.org/10.22605/RRH4317

National Collaborating Centre for Methods and Tools. (2012). *A model for evidence-informed decision-making in public health [Fact Sheet].* http://www.nccmt.ca/uploads/media/media/0001/01/9e2175871f00e790a936193e98f4607313a58c84.pdf.

Rice, V. H., & Stead, L. F. (2006). Nursing interventions for smoking cessation. *Cochrane Database of Systematic Reviews.* ISSN: 1464–780X. http://www.cochrane.org.

Ruppar, T. M., Conn, V. S., Chase, J. D., et al. (2014). Lipid outcomes from supervised exercise interventions in healthy adults. *American Journal of Health Behavior*, 38(6), 823–830. https://doi.org/10.5993/AJHB.38.6.4

Short, M., Mushquash, C. J., & Bédard, M. (2013). Motor vehicle crashes among Canadian Aboriginal people: A review of the literature. *Canadian Journal of Rural Medicine*, 18(3), 86–98.

Sichieri, R., Paula Trotte, A., de Souza, R., et al. (2009). School randomised trial on prevention of excessive weight gain by discouraging students from drinking sodas. *Public Health Nutrition*, 12(2), 197–202. https://doi.org/10.1017/S1368980008002644

Sigma Theta Tau International Honour Society of Nursing. (2005). *Evidence-based nursing position statement.* http://www.nursingsociety.org/about-stti/position-statements-and-resource-papers/evidence-based-nursing-position-statement.

Straus, S. E., Richardson, W. S., Glasziou, P., et al. (2005). *Evidence-based medicine: How to practice and teach EBM.* London: Elsevier/Churchill Livingstone.

Thomas, B., Ciliska, D., Dobbins, M., et al. (2004). A process for systematically reviewing the literature: Providing the research evidence for public health nursing interventions. *Worldviews on Evidence-Based Nursing*, 1(3), 176–184.

Wakefield, A. (2014). Searching and critiquing the research literature. *Nursing Standard*, 28(39), 49–57.

6

Ethics in Community Health Nursing Practice

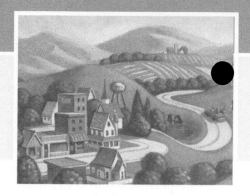

OUTLINE

History of Nursing and Ethics, 129
Ethical Decision Making, 129
Ethics, 130
    Definitions, Theories, and Principles, 130
    Rule Ethics, 131
    Ethical Principles, 132
    Virtue Ethics, 135
    Relational Ethics, 136
    Ethics of Care, 136

Nursing Code of Ethics, 137
Nursing Code of Ethics and Community Health Nursing, 138
Advocacy and Ethics, 139
    Definitions, Codes, and Standards, 139
    Conceptual Framework for Advocacy, 140
    Practical Framework for Advocacy, 140
Principles for the Justification of Public Health Interventions, 140

OBJECTIVES

After reading this chapter, you should be able to:

6.1 Describe the history of the ethics of nursing.
6.2 Apply the steps of the ethical decision-making framework in community health nursing practice.
6.3 Distinguish among rule ethics, ethical principles, virtue ethics, relational ethics, and the ethics of care.
6.4 Identify the main code of ethics adopted in community health nursing.

6.5 Understand how the code of ethics is applied in community health nursing.
6.6 Apply the ethical principles for effective advocacy to community health nursing.
6.7 List the ethical principles that can help determine whether a public health intervention is justified.

KEY TERMS*

accountability, 138
autonomy, 133
beneficence, 133
bioethics, 131
code of ethics, 129
communitarianism, 134
confidentiality, 138
consequentialism, 131
deontology, 131
distributive justice, 133
equality, 135
equity, 135
ethical (moral) distress, 130
ethical courage, 130
ethical decision making, 129
ethical dilemmas, 130
ethical disengagement, 130
ethical issues, 129

ethical problems, 130
ethical uncertainty, 130
ethical violations, 130
ethics, 130
feminist ethic, 137
morality, 130
morals, 131
nonmaleficence, 133
principlism, 132
relational ethics, 136
social justice, 135
teleology, 131
utilitarianism, 131
values, 131
veracity, 132
virtue ethics, 135
virtues, 135

*See the Glossary on page 468 for definitions.

The work of community health nurses (CHNs) involves ethical decision making and practice. CHNs focus on protecting, promoting, preserving, and maintaining health while preventing disease. These goals reflect the ethical principles of beneficence or promoting good and nonmaleficence or preventing harm. CHNs struggle with ethical decision making that can have an impact on the rights of individuals and families versus the rights of groups, communities, and society. These struggles reflect the tension between individual rights–based ethical theories and communitarianism or global rights–based theories.

In addition, CHNs use consequence-based ethical theory and obligation-based ethical theory to guide their ethical decision making. They apply ethical principles to their practice, including the principles of autonomy, beneficence, nonmaleficence, and distributive justice. They are guided by codes of ethics and ethical decision-making frameworks. Ethics is a body of knowledge and, as such, is more than "being a good person." Ethical decision making is a part of clinical decision making and clinical practice (Bernheim & Melnick, 2008). This chapter applies the core knowledge of ethics to ethical decision making in community health nursing.

HISTORY OF NURSING AND ETHICS

Modern nursing has a rich heritage of ethical practice, beginning with Florence Nightingale (1820–1910). Nightingale proposed that the practice of nursing is based on ethical values and principles. These values and principles have endured and are reflected in the Canadian Nurses Association *Code of Ethics for Registered Nurses* (Canadian Nurses Association [CNA], 2017). Nightingale saw nursing as a call to service, and she thought that those who became nurses should be people of good moral character. She was passionate about the need to provide care to vulnerable people and about the importance of a sanitary environment, as seen in her work with soldiers in the Crimean War (1854–1856). Because of her commitment to vulnerable individuals in communities, her championing of primary prevention, and the work she did to show that healthy environments save soldiers' lives, Nightingale is considered nursing's first moral leader and first community health nurse.

Nurses' codes of ethics are important in the history of all areas of nursing practice, including community health nursing. A nursing **code of ethics** is a framework that nurses use to guide their ethical obligations and actions within the profession. Nurses' codes of ethics clarify the values and guidelines of ethical conduct in nursing practice. The Nightingale Pledge written in 1863 (Box 6.1) is generally considered to be one of the earliest nursing codes of ethics (American Nurses Association [ANA], 2014a). Modelled on the Hippocratic Oath, it was composed as a tribute to Florence Nightingale. The ANA House of Delegates formally adopted the first *American Code of Ethics for Professional Nurses* in 1950. It was amended and revised five more times until, in 2001, after 5 years of work, the ANA House of Delegates adopted the *Code of Ethics for Nurses with Interpretive Statements*.

BOX 6.1 The Nightingale Pledge

The Nightingale Pledge was written by Lystra Gretter in 1893. It states:

I solemnly pledge myself before God and in the presence of this assembly, to pass my life in purity and to practice my profession faithfully. I will abstain from whatever is deleterious and mischievous, and will not take or knowingly administer any harmful drug. I will do all in my power to maintain and elevate the standard of my profession, and will hold in confidence all personal matters committed to my keeping and all family affairs coming to my knowledge in the practice of my calling. With loyalty will I endeavor to aid the physician in his work, and devote myself to the welfare of those committed to my care.

Source: American Nurses Association (ANA). (2014b). *Florence Nightingale Pledge*. https://www.nursingworld.org/ana/about-ana/

Shortly after the first ANA code of ethics was adopted in the United States, the first known international code of ethics for nursing was developed by the International Council of Nurses (ICN) in 1953 and was adopted in Canada in 1954 (CNA, 2017). Since that time, the *ICN Code of Ethics for Nurses* has undergone various reviews with the most recent revisions made in 2012 (International Council of Nurses [ICN], 2012). The *ICN Code of Ethics for Nurses* has four principal elements that outline the standards of ethical conduct for nurses. The four elements and examples of nursing responsibilities in relation to each are shown in Box 6.2.

In 1980, CNA developed its own code entitled *CNA Code of Ethics: An Ethical Basis for Nursing in Canada*. It was revised and updated five more times by 2017 and was retitled *Code of Ethics for Registered Nurses* (CNA, 2017). The CNA code of ethics is not based on any particular ethical theory but arises from principle-based ethics, the ethics of care, virtue ethics, and values. The CNA code of ethics outlines seven nursing values and ethical responsibilities for registered nurses: (1) providing safe, compassionate, competent, and ethical care; (2) honouring health and well-being; (3) promoting informed decision-making; (4) preserving dignity; (5) maintaining privacy and confidentiality; (6) promoting justice; and (7) being accountable. New and updated content in the 2017 edition reflects contemporary practice in Canada, including medical assistance in dying, workplace bullying, job action, and advanced health care planning.

ETHICAL DECISION MAKING

Ethical decision making is the component of ethical thought that focuses on the process of how ethical decisions are made. It involves making decisions in an orderly process that considers ethical principles, patient values and abilities, and professional obligations, and it occurs when health care providers make decisions about ethical issues and concerns in practice. **Ethical issues** are moral challenges facing the nursing

BOX 6.2 **ICN Code of Ethics for Nurses**

1. Nurses and people
   a. Respect patients' rights, values, customs, and spiritual beliefs.
   b. Hold all patient information confidential.
   c. Share responsibility for the care of vulnerable populations.
   d. Advocate for equity and social justice for all.
   e. Demonstrate professional values (e.g., respect, compassion, competence).
2. Nurses and practice
   a. Maintain lifelong professional learning.
   b. Maintain personal health and well-being.
   c. Safeguard patients' dignity and rights when using technology.
3. Nurses and the profession
   a. Implement accepted standards of nursing practice.
   b. Use evidence-informed practice.
   c. Create a positive practice environment.
   d. Practise to sustain and protect the natural environment.
   e. Challenge unethical practices and settings.
4. Nurses and coworkers
   a. Sustain collaborative and respectful relationships at work.
   b. Safeguard the patient when their care is endangered by health care personnel.
   c. Advance ethical conduct in practice.

Source: Adapted from International Council of Nurses. (2012). *ICN code of ethics for nurses.* https://www.icn.ch/sites/default/files/inline-files/2012_ICN_Codeofethicsfornurses_%20eng.pdf

BOX 6.3 **Types of Ethical Experiences and Situations**

- **Ethical problems** are conflicts between one or more values and include uncertainty about the right course of action (e.g., a CHN notices that a colleague never washes her hands prior to or after patient care).
- **Ethical uncertainty** is a feeling of indecision or a lack of clarity about a matter, accompanied by a sense of unease or discomfort (e.g., a patient asks a CHN for more pain medication but is at the maximum dosage for that prescription).
- **Ethical dilemmas** involve equally compelling reasons for and against two or more possible courses of action (e.g., a palliative care patient wants to stop eating, but the family does not want the CHN to withhold food and fluids).
- **Ethical (moral) distress** involves knowing the right thing to do but—for various reasons—being unable to take the right action or prevent potential harm (e.g., a patient cannot afford a new baby seat, but the old one is unsafe).
- **Ethical disengagement** can arise if the disregard of ethical commitments is seen as normal (e.g., a CHN discusses confidential patient information over lunch in a public place because others have done so).
- **Ethical violations** are actions or failures to act that breach fundamental duties to others, such as patients and coworkers (e.g., a CHN observes another CHN verbally abusing a patient and does nothing).
- **Ethical courage** is shown when a nurse stands firm on a point of moral principle in the face of fear or threat to oneself (e.g., a CHN provides care to a patient with an infectious disease such as the Ebola virus).

Source: Adapted from Canadian Nurses Association (CNA). (2017). *Code of ethics for registered nurses,* 2017 edition. https://www.cna-aiic.ca/~/media/cna/page-content/pdf-en/code-of-ethics-2017-edition-secure-interactive

profession. In community health nursing, one such challenge is how to prepare an ethical and competent workforce for the future. In contrast, *ethical dilemmas* are puzzling moral problems in which a person, group, or community can envision morally justified reasons for both taking and not taking a certain course of action. In community health nursing, an example of an ethical dilemma is how to allocate resources to two equally needy populations when the resources are sufficient to serve only one. Ethical decision-making frameworks help nurses think through how to respond to these and other types of ethical experiences.

The other types of ethical experiences and situations CHNs may encounter are ethical uncertainty, ethical questions, ethical distress, ethical disengagement, and ethical violations. When CHNs can name the type of ethical experience or situation they are facing, they are better able to discuss it with colleagues and managers. Box 6.3 defines various types of ethical experiences and situations and provides examples of each from the perspective of a CHN.

CHNs often experience ethical situations that require them to make decisions about their practice. Ethical decision-making frameworks can help because they provide a method for making sound ethical decisions that can be morally justified. A few of these frameworks are discussed in this chapter.

One ethical model that can help CHNs engage in ethical decision-making is the Oberle and Raffin model (CNA, 2017). That model promotes reflection on the ethical issue

and offers a nursing model for considering ethical issues in practice. It can be applied to many types of clinical situations. The model outlines a process that begins with assessing the situation and ends with reflecting and reviewing the ethical actions. Table 6.1 outlines the Oberle and Raffin model as applied to the ethical dilemma of a mother who is refusing to vaccinate her child.

ETHICS

Definitions, Theories, and Principles

Ethics is a branch of moral philosophy that includes both a body of knowledge about the moral life and a process of reflection for determining what persons ought to do or be in this life. It involves consideration of moral practices, beliefs, and standards of individuals or groups (Fry & Johnstone, 2002). The study of ethics refers to the study of human actions and whether they are "good" or bad," "desirable" or "undesirable" (Ivanov & Oden, 2013). Ethics refers to the Aristotelian approach to practical reasoning based on virtue, whereas **morality** refers to values of duty, obligations, and conduct. Personal, cultural, and professional values are all aspects of morality. These values often provide the morals or guidelines needed to address the ethical questions of How should

TABLE 6.1   Ethical Reflection on Refusal to Vaccinate

Steps	Questions for Ethical Reflection	Answers
1. Assess the ethics of the situation including the relationships, goals, beliefs, and values	Which ethical principles are involved?	The ethical principle of autonomy is involved and the right to refuse or withdraw consent for treatment
	What relationships are involved?	Parental consent is required for treatment
	Does the CNA *Code of Ethics* address the issue?	
	What are my values and beliefs on the issue?	
	What is the goal of action?	Goal is to promote and respect informed decision making (CNA, 2017)
2. Reflect on and review potential actions	What actions will produce the most good?	Educating patient on pros and cons of vaccination will produce the most good and cause the least harm
	What actions will cause the least harm?	
	What are the patient's expectations for action?	Patient is strongly refusing vaccination
3. Select an ethical action	What do I believe is the best action?	Educate patient and family on pros and cons of childhood vaccination
	Can I support the patient's choice for action?	
	Do I have the knowledge and skills required for action?	CHNs have the required knowledge and skills to educate patients, families, and communities
4. Engage in the ethical action	Did I apply the *Code* to my actions?	Respect for patient's autonomy was maintained and informed decision making was promoted
	Am I acting as any reasonable and prudent nurse would act in this situation?	
5. Reflect on and review the action	Did I achieve the desired goal?	Yes, the desired goal was achieved
	Were harms minimized and good maximized?	
	What could have been done differently?	

I behave? What action should I take? What kind of person should I be? What are my obligations to myself and to fellow humans? **Morals** are shared generational societal norms about what constitutes right or wrong conduct (e.g., thou shalt not kill). **Values** are standards or qualities that are esteemed, desired, considered important, or have worth or merit (e.g., competent, compassionate care) (Fry & Johnstone, 2002; Racher, 2007).

The study of ethics is divided into three main branches: (1) meta-ethics, (2) normative ethics, and (3) applied ethics. The branch of *meta-ethics* seeks to understand the nature of morality and how human values are developed and maintained. The branch of *normative ethics* is concerned with the general principles or obligations that guide human actions. General obligations that humans have as members of society include the following:

- To not harm others
- To respect others
- To tell the truth
- To keep promises

Finally, the branch of *applied ethics* relates to the application of ethical principles to situations people face in everyday life (e.g., human ethics review for research). **Bioethics,** a branch of applied ethics, is concerned about life issues in relation to the principles of autonomy, beneficence, nonmaleficence, and distributive justice (Dunbar, 2003). Bioethics first became an important consideration in research and clinical practice in the 1960s as society struggled with human rights, antiracism, and new technologies that made clinical decisions controlling life and death more complex and problematic.

Today the study of bioethics continues to be concerned with preventing the abuse of the rights of individuals. However, Sherwin (2011) suggests that bioethics ought to also be concerned with questions relating to critically evaluating institutional and organizational polices that influence the ways in which societies seek to promote and protect the health of populations. CHNs consider morals, values, and ethical principles when making decisions about individual patient situations and the health of populations.

Rule Ethics

CHNs have an ethical duty to follow the rules and principles, or policies and procedures set out by the profession and the organizations in which they work. This ethical duty is supported by the theory of rule ethics. Two theories form the foundation of rule ethics: **teleology** (Greek for "logic of ends" or consequences) and **deontology** (Greek for "what is due" or "duty"). The goal of rule ethics is to outline moral duties and obligations by setting out rules or principles (Racher, 2007).

Consequentialism, a type of teleology, holds that the morality of an action is dependent on the outcome of that action. **Utilitarianism,** a well-known form of consequentialism, holds that a morally right action is one that produces the greatest amount of good or the least amount of harm in a given situation. In utilitarianism, "the moral value of an action is determined by its overall benefit" (Chaloner, 2007, p. 43). A utilitarian approach involves deciding on a course of action based on an anticipated favourable outcome. It is the outcome or consequence of the action that is important and not the action itself.

CHNs are often faced with making decisions that challenge fundamental beliefs, such as having to decide on the allocation of scarce resources for community health promotion strategies. In such circumstances, CHNs may conclude that the decision they must make is right or wrong in itself, regardless of the amount of good that might come from it. This thinking typifies a deontological approach, which focuses on whether an action or decision is right or wrong rather than on whether the outcome of an action or decision is right or wrong. In a deontological approach, the outcome of an action or decision is not the primary reason for acting in a certain way. For example, a CHN decides to allocate her time to a harm reduction strategy for 10 patients with substance use issues instead of a smoking cessation program for 100 patients. Some would say that the decision is based on deontological ethics because it is focused on the rightness of the decision to help a small group of patients who are more vulnerable than the larger group of patients. If the CHN decided to allocate her time to the 100 patients instead of the 10 patients, this decision could be justified based on a utilitarian perspective that the greatest number of patients would be served, which would create the greatest good. Either way, the CHN could justify her actions and decisions based on one of these two ethical theories.

Utilitarianism and deontology emerged from the Enlightenment's focus on universals, rationality, and isolated individuals. Both ethical theories maintain that there is a universal first principle (the principle of utility for utilitarianism, and the principle of duty for deontology) that serves as a rational norm for our behaviour and allows us to calculate the rightness or wrongness of each individual action. According to both utilitarianism and deontology, as in classic liberalism, the individual is the special centre of moral concern. Giving priority to the individual means that the rights of the individual should never (or rarely) be sacrificed for the rights of the larger society (Steinbock, London, & Arras, 2008).

✳ HOW TO …

Apply the Utilitarian Ethics Decision Process

1. Determine the outcome or consequence of the action that is important to society and derived from the principle of utility.*
2. Identify the communities or populations that are affected or most affected by the moral rules.
3. Analyze viable alternatives for each proposed action based on the moral rules.
4. Determine the outcome or consequence of each viable alternative on the communities or populations most affected by the decision.
5. Select the action on the basis of the rules that produce the greatest amount of good or the least amount of harm for the communities or populations that are affected by the action.

---

* Moral rules of action that produce the greatest good for the greatest number of communities or populations affected by or most affected by the rules.

✳ HOW TO …

Apply the Deontological Ethics Decision Process

1. Determine the action (e.g., tell the truth) that serves as a standard by which you can perform your moral obligations.
2. Examine personal motives for the proposed action to ensure that they are based on good intentions in accord with moral rules.
3. Determine whether the proposed action can be generalized so that all persons in like situations are treated similarly.
4. Select the action that treats persons as ends in themselves and never as mere means to the ends of others.

Ethical Principles

A primary ethical principle that applies to community health nursing practice is veracity. **Veracity** means telling the truth, and it is a CHN's duty to tell the truth. Veracity promotes trust in the nurse–patient therapeutic relationship. Sometimes, however, a situation arises in which it is difficult to tell the truth because the consequences of telling the truth may bring about more harm than good (utilitarianism). For example, a junior high school student asks the CHN not to tell her parents that she smokes. When the parent asks the CHN if her child smokes, the CHN is morally justified in telling the truth, but she may jeopardize her relationship with the student if she does tell the truth. This example illustrates the following about ethical thinking:

- Ethical judgements or decisions can be based on ethical principles. The goal of an ethical judgement is to choose that action or state of affairs that is good or right in the circumstances.
- Ethical judgements generally do not have the certainty of scientific judgements. For example, a CHN accepts a parent's refusal to vaccinate her child, despite the scientific proof that vaccines can prevent diseases such as measles.

Principlism, an approach to problem solving in bioethics, can help guide a CHN's practice. The four ethical principles that form the foundation of principlism are autonomy, nonmaleficence, beneficence, and distributive justice (Box 6.4). These principles are compatible with teleological and deontological theories.

Health care providers have specific ethical obligations because of the ethical rules and principles that guide the practices and goals of the profession. The principles of autonomy, beneficence, nonmaleficence, and distributive justice have dominated the development of the field of bioethics. One of the best descriptions and fullest articulations of principlism in bioethics appears in the seventh edition of Beauchamp and Childress's *Principles of Biomedical Ethics* (2012). The principlism approach to ethical decision making in health care arose in response to life-and-death decision making in acute care settings, where the question to be resolved tended to concern a single localized issue such as the withdrawing or withholding of treatment (Holstein, 2001). In these circumstances, preserving and respecting a patient's autonomy became the dominant issue.

BOX 6.4   Ethical Principles

- **Autonomy.** This principle is derived from the Greek words *autos* (self) and *nomos* (rule), which means to self-rule. Autonomy means the ability to self-govern and be one's own person. It is based on human dignity and respect for the individual. Autonomy requires that individuals be permitted to choose those actions and goals that fulfill their life plans unless those choices result in harm to themselves or others. The need for informed consent is based on this principle.
- **Nonmaleficence.** According to ancient writings from Hippocrates, nonmaleficence requires that we "do no harm." It is impossible to avoid harm entirely, but this principle requires that health care providers act according to the standards of due care, always seeking to produce the least amount of harm possible, e.g., prevent injury by conducting a home safety assessment.
- **Beneficence.** This principle is complementary to nonmaleficence and requires that we "do good," which is reflected in the provision of high-quality nursing care based in competent, compassionate practice. Health care providers have special obligations of beneficence to patients, but we are often limited by time, place, and talents in the amount of good we can do. We have general obligations to perform those actions that maintain or enhance the dignity of other persons whenever those actions do not place an undue burden on health care providers.
- **Distributive justice.** This principle requires that there be a fair distribution of the benefits and burdens in society based on the needs and contributions of its members. *Benefits* in this context refers to basic needs, including material and social goods, liberties, rights, and entitlements. Distributive justice focuses on the position of one social group in relationship to others and encourages nurses to explore the root causes of disparities and what can be done to eliminate them.* Consistent with the dignity and worth of its members and within the limits imposed by its resources, this principle requires that a society determine a minimal level of goods and services be available to its members. For CHNs, this principle takes on considerable importance, especially when caring for vulnerable populations (e.g., in harm reduction strategies).

* Myllykoski, H. (2011). Social justice: Who cares? *Alberta RN, 67*(4), 28–29; Peter, E. (2011). Fostering social justice: The possibilities of a socially connected model of moral agency. *Canadian Journal of Nursing Research, 43*(2), 11–17; Woods, M. (2012). Exploring the relevance of social justice within a relational nursing ethic. *Nursing Philosophy, 13*(1), 56–65.

Despite its success as a basis for analysis in bioethics, principlism has come under attack from a variety of quarters (e.g., Boylan, 2000; Callahan, 2000; Clouser & Gert, 1990; Walker, 2009), and there are grounds for this criticism. The primary critiques are as follows: (1) the principles are too abstract to serve as guides for action; (2) the principles can conflict in a given situation, and there is no independent basis for resolving the conflict; (3) effective ethical problem solving must be rooted in concrete, individual experiences; (4) ethical judgements may depend more on the judgement of a sensitive person than on the application of abstract principles; and

(5) principlism's view of morality is narrowly constrained. Nonetheless, the four principles remain a popular guide for ethical decision making in health care.

Autonomy involves respect for the patient's right to make informed decisions about his or her own health care. However, in community health, this may involve restricting patients' rights where individual choice may negatively impact on the rights or well-being of others. For example, usually a patient has the right to refuse treatment, but in the case of a contagious disease such as tuberculosis, a patient who is noncompliant with his or her medications may be isolated or quarantined until treatment is complete. This example shows that there are exceptions to this rule.

Nonmaleficence and *beneficence* represent the two ends of the spectrum of "do no harm" and "do good." Doing good means CHNs provide high-quality, competent, compassionate care through evidenced-informed practice and by following organizational policies and procedures. Doing no harm means CHNs act according to the standards of care and avoid harming their patients (e.g., using handwashing to prevent the spread of infection). Avoiding harm can also include preventing harm (e.g., conducting a fall risk assessment). CHNs base their professional practice on these two fundamental ethical principles of nonmaleficence and beneficence.

Distributive justice refers to the allocation of benefits and burdens to members of society. Some benefits of society are wealth, education, and public services. Among the burdens to be shared are things such as taxes, poverty, pollution, and homelessness. Justice requires that the distribution of benefits and burdens in a society be fair or equal. It is widely agreed that the distribution should be based on what one needs and deserves, but there is considerable disagreement on how these terms should be defined.

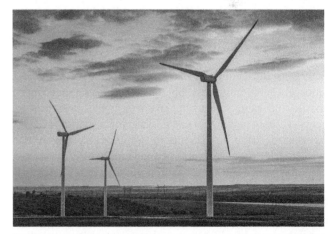

Distributive justice means that as a society, we share both benefits and burdens. Among the burdens to be shared are the location of garbage incinerators, windmills, and power plants and their impact on greenhouse gas emissions. (iStockphoto/VR_Studio)

How is it possible to apply the principle of distributive justice to prenatal services? A CHN can face this interesting question when the target group is women with low educational levels who cannot afford the cost of travelling to health care visits or the time to attend them. This is a challenging issue considering that quality prenatal care can potentially reduce the rates of incidence of maternal mortality and morbidity (U.S. Department of Health and Social Services and Centers for Disease Control and Prevention, 2008). Phillippi (2009) identified societal, maternal, and structural barriers for this population in accessing prenatal care, including inadequate space in waiting rooms. Maternal and societal barriers include a lack of education, which could be addressed through targeted population health strategies. Applying the principles of distributive justice for this issue means the CHN is justified in using scarce resources to create more child-friendly waiting and examining rooms. The CHN could seize this opportunity to minimize the barriers for this population by using the principle of distributive justice to allocate resources to education and improving clinic space.

The three primary theories of distributive justice are egalitarianism, libertarian theory, and liberal democratic theory. *Egalitarianism* is the view that everyone is entitled to equal rights and equal treatment in society. Ideally, each individual has an equal share of the goods of society, and it is the role of government to ensure that this happens. The government has the authority to redistribute wealth if necessary to ensure equal treatment. Thus, egalitarians are supportive of *welfare rights*—that is, the right to receive certain social goods necessary to satisfy basic needs. These include adequate food, housing, education, and police and fire protection (Anderson, Rodney, Reimer-Kirkham, et al., 2009), and the opportunity to acquire basic needs (Kayman & Ablorh-Odjidja, 2006). Egalitarianism has practical and theoretical weaknesses. For example, it would be almost impossible to ensure the equal distribution of goods and services in any moderately complex society. But the distribution of material resources must be sufficient to ensure participants' independence and "voice" (Kirkham & Browne, 2006). Also, egalitarianism cannot provide an incentive for each of us to do our best because there is no promise of our merit being rewarded.

Libertarian theory holds that the right to private property is the most important right. Libertarians recognize only *liberty rights*, the right to be left alone to accomplish our goals. Stubager (2008) notes that "libertarians ... loathe social hierarchies and value instead the free and equal interaction of people without regard to social positions of any kind" (p. 329). Libertarians see a limited role for government, namely the protection of property rights of individual citizens through providing police and fire protection. Although they agree that there is a need for jointly shared, publicly owned facilities such as roads, they reject the idea of welfare rights and view taxes to support the needs of others as the coercive taking of their property. In addition, the libertarian position entails a basic respect for and tolerance of other people—including those who deviate from one's own norms or the norms of the society (Stubager, 2008).

Rawls (2001) developed a version of *liberal democratic theory* that attempted to reconcile the potentially competing values of liberty and equality. He acknowledged that inequities are inevitable in society, but he tried to establish an approach in which everyone benefits, especially the least advantaged. Rawls developed basic principles of justice that he believed "free and rational individuals would agree to in a hypothetical situation of pure equality" (Duignan, 2014). When he developed his principles, Rawls (2001) imagined a group of people who had no awareness of their particular socioeconomic and historical circumstances or personal goals. Behind a "veil of ignorance," Rawls (2001) maintained that all individuals are rational and would agree on the following two principles:

(a) Each person has the same indefeasible claim to a fully adequate scheme of equal basic liberties, which scheme is compatible with the same scheme of liberties for all; and (b) Social and economic inequalities are to satisfy two conditions: first, they are to be attached to offices and positions open to all under conditions of fair equality of opportunity; and second, they are to be to the greatest benefit of the least-advantaged members of society (the difference principle). (Rawls, 2001, pp. 42–43).

> ✳ **HOW TO ...**
>
> **Apply the Principlism Ethics to the Decision Process**
> 1. Determine the ethical principles (autonomy, nonmaleficence, beneficence, distributive justice) that are relevant to an ethical issue or dilemma.
> 2. Analyze the relevant principles within a meaningful context of accurate facts and other pertinent circumstances.
> 3. Act on the principle that provides, within the meaningful context, the strongest guide to action that can be morally justified by the tenets foundational to the principle.

As the veil-of-ignorance device and the justice principles indicate, Rawls (and other justice theorists) assumed the Enlightenment concept of isolated individuals in competition for scarce resources. In this view, justice is about ensuring fairness to individuals. Moreover, violating the principles of distributive justice is an offence to the dignity of the collective preferences of autonomous, rational moral agents. The interests of the community may be in conflict with the interests of individuals; yet, confined to the Enlightenment ideal, the needs of society are not directly addressed, nor is society given any priority. This Enlightenment assumption has been challenged recently by a number of ethical theories loosely grouped together under the heading *communitarianism*. **Communitarianism** maintains that abstract, universal principles are not an adequate basis for moral decision-making; instead, these theorists argue, history, tradition, institutions, cultural heritage, global values and responsibilities, and concrete moral communities should be the basis of moral thinking and action (Solomon, 1993; Ten Have, 2011). Virtue ethics and the ethics of care, discussed later in the chapter, have a communitarianism focus.

Justice considerations play a prominent role in community health nursing. According to CNA (2010), "justice includes respecting the rights of others, distributing resources fairly, and preserving and promoting the common good (the good of the community)" (p. 26). Kass (2005), while describing principles of public health, highlights the importance of fairness in decision procedures and in balancing benefits and burdens. Stone and Parham (2007) describe the principle of justice as building on and functioning with the principle of equal and substantial respect. "Justice informs how to show such respect and how to respond when people are disrespected" (Stone & Parham, 2007, p. 356). For example, the issue of justice arises regarding the equitable or fair treatment or equitable opportunity for patient participation and input.

To effect equity, CHNs need to ensure equity in access to health care and equity in health outcomes (Pauly, MacKinnon, & Varcoe, 2009). For example, people who are street involved, either homeless or drug users, often delay or do not access health care for a variety of complex and multifaceted reasons, including concerns about stigma related to drug use and homelessness. In this case, attention is required to address the stigma and discrimination experienced by those who are disadvantaged.

It is important to be clear on the definition of two sometimes confused concepts: *equity* and *equality*. In health care, **equity** refers to "the fulfillment of each individual's needs as well as the individual's opportunity to reach full potential as a human being" (CNA, 2006, p. 14). **Equality** is also an important ethical concept and refers to the right for equal treatment in society, including under the law, such as security, voting rights, freedom of speech and assembly, and the extent of property rights. However, it also refers to the right to equal access to education, health care, and other social goods such as economic good and fundamental political rights (Easley & Allen, 2007). It includes equal opportunities and obligations and involves the whole society. *Egalitarianism* is closely related to the concept of equality as it favours the right of all people to be equal in worth, social status, and politics. In order to respect the elements of equity and equality, it becomes important for CHNs to ensure that their assessment of needs leads to the fair distribution of resources without compromising the access and opportunities for the targeted group to benefit from those resources.

Social justice is an area of particular concern for community health. **Social justice** refers to "the fair distribution of society's benefits and responsibilities and their consequences. It focuses on the relative position of one social group in relation to others in society as well as on the root causes of disparities and what can be done to eliminate them" (CNA, 2006, p. 7). A social justice framework can be useful in addressing the vulnerabilities of people; this framework has the potential to engage all community players. The Federal Initiative to Address HIV/AIDS in Canada is based on the belief that the principles of social justice should guide the development of all Canadian public policy across all jurisdictions—equity, fairness, and inclusion of all Canadians—reflecting broad determinants of health and the broadest definition of health. The initiative focuses on ensuring that people living with and vulnerable to HIV/AIDS are partners in shaping policies

and practices that affect their lives (Public Health Agency of Canada [PHAC], 2014). The guiding principles for a social justice approach are (1) an integrative approach; (2) an approach that operates across the determinants of health; (3) a rights-based approach that respects, promotes, and fulfills rights; and (4) an approach that presents a lens of social inclusion for policy design, program development, and evaluation (PHAC, 2006).

Virtue Ethics

Virtue ethics, one of the oldest ethical theories, dates back to the ancient Greek philosophers Plato and Aristotle. Rather than being concerned with rules or actions, as utilitarianism and deontology are, virtue ethics focuses on the character of the moral agent. Virtue ethics asks, What kind of person should I be? The goal of virtue ethics is to enable persons to flourish as human beings. It involves the integration of seeing, feeling, and acting (Racher, 2007). According to Aristotle, **virtues** are acquired, excellent traits of character that dispose humans to act in accord with their natural good. During the seventeenth and eighteenth centuries, the Greek concept of the "good" as a principle of explanation of actions went out of favour. Because virtue ethics was closely tied to the concept of the good, interest in virtues as an element of normative ethics also declined. Examples of virtues include benevolence, compassion, discernment, trustworthiness, integrity, and conscientiousness (Beauchamp & Childress, 2012). The appeal to virtues results in a significantly different approach to moral decision making in health care (Fletcher, 1999). Rather than focusing on moral justification by relying on theories and principles, virtue ethics emphasizes practical reasoning applied to character development. The following values identified in the CNA code of ethics would be considered virtues: dignity, confidentiality, and accountability. CHNs are responsible not only for their own good character but also for the kind of communities they collectively develop (Racher, 2007).

✳ HOW TO ...

Apply the Virtue Ethics Decision Process
1. Identify the virtues that are relevant to the ethical dilemmas or issues.
2. Identify moral considerations that arise from a communal perspective and apply the considerations to specific communities.
3. Identify and apply virtues that facilitate a communal perspective.
4. Modify moral considerations as needed to apply to the specific ethical dilemmas or issues.
5. Seek ethical community support to enhance character development.
6. Evaluate and modify the individual or community character traits that impede communal living.

Source: Modified from Volbrecht, R. M. (2002). *Nursing ethics: Communities in dialogue* (p. 138). Prentice Hall.

Relational Ethics

Relational ethics refers to the relational context of practice and asks, "What should I be doing for others?" Relational-based ethics approaches would argue that when considering how to act and think, CHNs must consider the relationships they have with their patients and how those relationships are influenced by their thoughts and actions (Evans, Bergum, Bamforth, et al., 2004; Leung & Esplen, 2010; Olmstead, Scott, & Austin, 2010; Wright & Brajtman, 2011). Relationships would be the starting point of ethical inquiry.

The core elements of relational ethics are engaged interaction, mutual respect, embodied knowledge, uncertainty and vulnerability, and an interdependent environment (Austin, 2001; Austin, Goble, & Kelecevic, 2009; Shaw, 2011). *Engaged interaction* means that the patient's own stories form the basis for ethical decision making. *Mutual respect* is inherent in patient relationships, and CHNs have *embodied knowledge* that influences care. The *uncertainty and vulnerability* of patients in the community make relational ethics especially important for CHNs. Nurses have an ethical obligation to be aware of the vulnerable status of their patients and adjust care accordingly to prevent harm. Canada has a wide range of harm-reduction strategies in place, including a well-established harm-reduction infrastructure in British Colombia (Wild et al., 2017). However, many parts of the country have few or no policies, and access to harm-reduction strategies is variable and, in some cases, nonexistent. One population of particular concern is substance users because access to low-threshold opioid substitution and safe inhalation kits is almost nonexistent in some communities (Wild et al., 2017). The Canadian Centre on Substance Use and Addiction (2020) has identified the death toll from opioid abuse as a priority for action, thus supporting the need for CHNs to be aware of the vulnerable status of their patients and adjust care accordingly to prevent harm.

The *interdependent environment* refers to the relationships that exist between nurses and patients, groups, communities, society, and the world (e.g., the *ICN Code of Ethics for Nurses*). The concept of interdependent environment challenges nurses to recognize the social and political nature of individuals.

The relational ethics approach suggests that individuals often apply their personal values within their social world (Kenny, Sherwin, & Baylis, 2010). This concept has implications for CHNs in the development of healthy public policy: patients are social, independent beings who have a unique perspective and should be encouraged to apply their personal values to the development of policy. A relational ethics approach to making decisions helps CHNs reflect on how they ought to act and think in relation to others, and to consider the relationships they have with their patients in an effort to provide ethically sound nursing care and make ethical decisions in the community setting. Table 6.2 presents the core elements of relational ethics and how CHNs can use them when making decisions.

Ethics of Care

The central focus of ethics of care theory is the relationship that exists between those who care for others and those who rely on that care (Rowa-Dewar & Ritchie, 2014). Nurses have written about caring as the essence or moral ideal of nursing (Leininger, 1984; Watson, 1985). This view was partly in response to the technological advances in health care science and to the desire of nurses to differentiate nursing practice from medical practice. The ethics of care is a core value of community health nursing.

Carol Gilligan and Nel Noddings are two of the most influential authors on the ethics of care (Volbrecht, 2002). Gilligan's moral orientation toward care and responsibility distinguishes the moral agency of nurses for leadership and practice, and it also distinguishes between the moral judgement of women and

TABLE 6.2 Core Elements of Relational Ethics Applied to Community Health Nursing

Core Elements	CHN's Role	CHN's Actions
Engaged interactions	Communicator	Provides education on wound care
	Counsellor	Conducts a nursing assessment
	Teacher	Develops plan of care using mutual goals
	Decision maker	Discusses options for palliative care
Mutual respect	Negotiator	Readjusts care based on patient's schedule
	Team building	Meets with social worker
	Patient advocate	Arranges family meeting
Embodied knowledge	Researcher	Participates in research (e.g., assesses community health needs)
	Coordinator of care	
	Professional development supporter	Attends conferences
	Policy/procedure administrator	Is a member of the policy and procedure committee
	Expert clinician	Reads appropriate literature
Interdependent environment	Team leader	Applies code of ethics to practice
	Advocate for social justice	Is active in professional associations
		Is active in healthy public policy development
Vulnerability, uncertainty	Advocate	Advocates for quality care
	Consultant	Is a member of the ethics committee
	Risk manager	Develops policies and procedures

men (Storch, Rodney, & Starzomski, 2004). In fact, Gilligan (1982) describes a personal journey where, by listening and talking to people, she began to notice two distinct voices about morality and two ways of describing the interpersonal relationships between self and others—male and female. This insight was the beginning of a feminist ethics approach to caring.

> *The different voice I describe is characterized not by gender [emphasis added] but theme. Its association with women is an empirical observation, and it is primarily through women's voices that I trace its development. But this association is not absolute, and the contrasts between male and female voices are presented here to highlight a distinction between two modes of thought and to focus [on] a problem of interpretation rather than to represent a generalization about either sex. (Gilligan, 1982, p. 2)*

Gilligan's 1982 book is based on three qualitative studies about conceptions of morality and self, and about experiences of conflict and choice. From these studies, she formulated three basic premises about responsibility, care, and relationships:

1. Being sensitive to the needs of others and assuming responsibility for taking care of others will lead people to listen to voices other than their own.
2. People not only define themselves in a context of human relationships but also judge themselves in terms of their ability to care for others.
3. Self and others are interdependent, and life can only be sustained by the care in relationships.

Noddings's (1984) personal journey started at a point different from that of Gilligan. Noddings noticed that ethics was described in the literature primarily using principles and logic. The goal for Noddings's book, therefore, was to express a feminist view that could be accepted or rejected by women *and* men.

✳ HOW TO …

Apply the Ethics of Care Decision Process
1. Recognize the caring relationships that exist between a CHN and patients.
2. Identify the caring experiences that form the basis for relating to self and patients.
3. Assume responsibility for promoting and enhancing caring in relationships with patients.

The basic premises of Noddings's (1984) book, in her own voice, are as follows:

1. "The essential elements of caring are located in the relation between the one caring and the cared-for." (p. 9)
2. "Caring requires me to respond … with an act of commitment: I commit myself either to overt action on behalf of the cared-for or I commit myself to thinking about what I might do." (p. 81)

3. "We are not 'justified'—we are *obligated*—to do what is required to maintain and enhance caring." (p. 95)
4. "Caring itself and the ethical ideal that strives to maintain and enhance it guide us in moral decisions and conduct." (p. 105)

What both Gilligan and Noddings have in common is a **feminist ethic of care,** which advocates for inclusive morality that strengthens relationships and solves problems without the need for specific rules and principles. Feminism involves political positioning to promote social and individual change to address inequalities that are assigned as masculine and feminine. A feminist ethic of care is also concerned with eliminating racism and classism (Green, 2012). CHNs can apply a feminist ethic of care by recognizing their obligation to maintain and enhance caring for all patients and families through social and individual change, regardless of sex, race, or class.

CHNs can use a variety of ethical decision-making frameworks to reflect on what they ought to do in practice. Ethical decision making requires consideration of personal and professional moral practices, beliefs, and standards. CHNs care for patients regardless of sex, race, or class and are guided by the CNA (2017) *Code of Ethics for Registered Nurses.* The preceding ethical decision-making theories can provide useful frameworks to help CHNs address the ethical challenges they face every day while caring for diverse and challenging patient populations in the community.

NURSING CODE OF ETHICS

Canadian nurses have adopted the CNA *Code of Ethics for Registered Nurses* (CNA, 2017). CNA, a national nursing body, links with all provincial and territorial associations representing nurses. This national organization works with these affiliated associations in developing standards of nursing practice, education, and ethical conduct (Keatings & Smith, 2010). The CNA code of ethics "can assist nurses in practicing ethically and working through ethical challenges that arise in their practice with individuals, families, communities and public health systems" (p. 1). The purpose of the CNA code of ethics is as follows (CNA, 2017):

- To provide guidance for ethical relationships, responsibilities, behaviours, and decision making in conjunction with standards, best practices, research, laws, and regulations.
- To provide guidance for nurses during ethical challenges that arise in practice.
- To serve as an ethical basis from which nurses can advocate for quality practice environments that support the delivery of safe, compassionate, competent, and ethical care.

The purpose of the code is reflected in its seven primary values. Each primary value is accompanied by responsibility statements that are intended to help nurses work through ethical experiences.

NURSING CODE OF ETHICS AND COMMUNITY HEALTH NURSING

In nursing practice, CHNs are required to uphold the values identified in the CNA *Code of Ethics for Registered Nurses.* CHNs are often faced with unique situations of ethical conflict that challenge CNA code of ethics nursing values such as **confidentiality**, which is the duty to not disclose a patient's personal and private information (CNA, 2017); and **accountability**, which means being answerable to oneself and others (patient, profession, society) for one's own actions. Oberle and Tenove (2000) explored the ethical problems faced by Canadian public health nurses (PHNs) working in rural and urban settings and identified some strategies to support ethical nursing practice. The "Evidence-Informed Practice" box provides further information on this study.

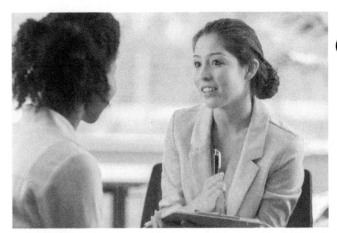

Maintaining privacy and confidentiality is one of the nursing values and ethical responsibilities identified in the CNA Code of Ethics. (iStockphoto/SDI Productions)

EVIDENCE-INFORMED PRACTICE

Oberle and Tenove (2000) undertook a study to identify recurring ethical problems faced by PHNs in Canada. The exploratory qualitative study comprised interviews with 22 PHNs who were deemed by supervisors to be reflective and articulate regarding ethical problems. Eleven PHNs worked in urban settings, and 11 worked in rural settings. The interviews, which were basically unstructured, were tape-recorded and lasted from 30 minutes to 2 hours. The tape recordings were transcribed and then analyzed.

The analyses resulted in five interrelated themes: "relationships with health care professionals; systems issues; character of relationships; respect for persons; and putting self at risk" (p. 425). Each of the five themes had two or three subthemes related to ethical problems in public health nursing. Examples of subtheme ethical problems were perceived inequities in power, unacceptable practice, inequitable resource allocation, conflict between ethics and law, inadequate systems support for nursing, conflicts between individual and community rights, conflicts between nurses' and patients' values, and conflicts between service to patients and physical danger to self.

Application for CHNs
This study concluded that ethics permeates every aspect of public health nursing.

Questions for Reflection and Discussion
1. Are more ethical concerns likely to arise for PHNs working in rural versus urban communities? Support your thinking with an example.
2. Have you observed or experienced any of the subtheme ethical problems outlined in the study findings? Explain.

Source: Oberle, K., & Tenove, S. (2000). Ethical issues in public health nursing. *Nursing Ethics, 7*(5), 425–439.

The *Canadian Community Health Nursing Standards of Practice* (CCHN Standards) discussed in Chapter 1 and found in Appendix 1, must also be followed in ethical, legal, and professional nursing practice situations. The CCHN Standards outline the expectations of CHNs in relation to the knowledge, skills, values, and decision making required in community health nursing practice. In addition, they indicate that CHNs need to consider factors that affect the health status of patients, such as the determinants of health as outlined in Chapter 1.

The CNA code of ethics and the CCHN Standards help CHNs identify ethical problems, issues, and dilemmas; provide CHNs with guidance on responding to ethical experiences; and provide CHNs with rules for professional conduct. Should the code and standards not be followed, ethical distress, professional misconduct, or legal ramifications would likely result. As the "Levels of Prevention" box indicates, ethical decision making is necessary at the three levels of community health prevention.

LEVELS OF PREVENTION

Related to Ethical Decision Making

Primary Prevention
A CHN struggles with providing influenza vaccines to only those who can afford to pay for the vaccine.

Secondary Prevention
A CHN recognizes that a group of low-income lone parents do not have adequate income to provide a healthy diet for their children.

Tertiary Prevention
Due to time restraints and lack of resources, a CHN can only provide diabetic screening clinics to a small group of older-person patients.

EVIDENCE-INFORMED PRACTICE

Flicker and Guta (2008) used a case study analysis to explore ethical issues related to adolescent participation in sexual health research. The study also identified access barriers and facilitators to adolescents' use of community services health resources. One of the ethical issues was whether parental consent should be required for adolescent participation in sexual health research. The authors raised the following concerns about parental consent: that it was unwarranted, unjust, and confusing and could silence those voices that most need to be heard. Other ethical issues concerned safeguarding youth by paying more attention to issues of confidentiality and anonymity and ensuring youth-friendly processes, protocols, and consent procedures. In addition to suggesting that institutional review boards should be encouraged to adopt context-dependent strategies that address the unique vulnerabilities of the adolescent, the authors state that "attention to flexibility, vulnerability, and community-specific needs is necessary to ensure appropriate ethical research practices that attend to the health and well-being of young people" (p. 3).

Application for CHNs

CHNs need to be sensitive to ethical issues related to adolescent health research to avoid inadvertent harm. This case study analysis provides some strategies for CHNs to use to encourage adolescent participation in sexual research. It also highlights legal and ethical areas in public health that CHNs may find useful in evidence-informed clinical practice.

Questions for Reflection and Discussion

1. What are some examples of ethical situations with which CHNs, specifically those involved with a research team, might be confronted?
2. See the link for the CNA *Code of Ethics for Registered Nurses* on the Evolve website. Based on the primary nursing values, outline the CHN's responsibilities in relation to conducting research projects with adolescents.

Source: Flicker, S., & Guta, A. (2008). Ethical approaches to adolescent participation in sexual health research. *Journal of Adolescent Health, 42*, 3–10.

ADVOCACY AND ETHICS

Definitions, Codes, and Standards

Advocacy is a powerful ethical concept in community health nursing. But what does *advocacy* mean? Christoffel (2000) offers two definitions that are useful, since they seem to differentiate between community health nursing and public health nursing. The following definition relates to community health nursing: "*Advocacy* is the application of information and resources (including finances, effort, and votes) to effect systemic changes that shape the way people in a community live" (p. 722). In contrast, "*public health advocacy* is advocacy that is intended to reduce death or disability in groups of people.... Such advocacy involves the use of information and resources

to reduce the occurrence or severity of public health problems" (pp. 722–723). The former definition is intended to address the quality of life of individuals in a community, whereas the latter is intended to address the quality of life for aggregates or populations. Thus, both definitions have an ethical basis grounded in quality of life. Advocacy is addressed in the CNA *Code of Ethics for Registered Nurses* (CNA, 2017) as well as in the CCHN Standards (Community Health Nurses of Canada [CHNC], 2019).

The CNA code of ethics indicates that advocacy is a nursing responsibility. According to Hogan (2008), a body of literature emphasizes the importance of advocacy ethics in informing public health nursing practice (Cohen & Reutter, 2007). The importance of the advocacy ethic is reflected in the responsibility statements that accompany the following primary nursing values: promoting health and well-being, promoting and respecting informed decision making, preserving dignity, maintaining privacy and confidentiality, and promoting justice (see the CNA link on the Evolve website).

Under the nursing value of promoting health and well-being, the code states that when an intervention interferes with an individual's rights, "nurses use and advocate for the use of the least restrictive measures possible for those in their care" (CNA, 2017, p. 10). Under the nursing value of promoting and respecting informed decision making, the code states, "nurses advocate for persons in their care if they believe that the health of those persons is being compromised by factors beyond their control, including the decision-making of others" (p. 11). Under the nursing value of preserving dignity, the CNA code of ethics states, "When a person receiving care is terminally ill or dying, nurses foster comfort, alleviate suffering, advocate for adequate relief of discomfort and pain and support a dignified and peaceful death" (p. 14). Under the nursing value of maintaining privacy and confidentiality, the code states, "Nurses advocate for persons in their care to receive access to their own health-care records through a timely and affordable process when such access is requested" (p. 15). Moreover, "Nurses respect policies that protect and preserve people's privacy, including safeguards in information technology" (p. 15). Under the nursing value of promoting justice, the code states that nurses "advocate for fair treatment and for fair distribution of resources for those in their care" (p. 17).

Similarly, the CCHN Standards document lists advocacy as part of the CHN's role. It also states that CHNs need to advocate "for and with the patient to act for themselves" and "for healthy public policy and social justice by participating in legislative and policymaking activities that influence the health determinants and access to services" (p. 19).

See the CNA and ICN links on the Evolve website for further information on codes of ethics, and the CHNC website for information on incorporating the standards into community health nursing practice. For an example of a code of ethics developed by a health care agency, see the VON Canada link on the Evolve website.

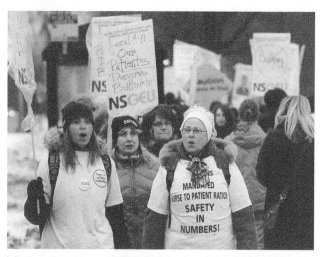

Advocacy is a responsibility of all nurses. Nova Scotia nurses are shown here picketing in favour of mandated nurse-to-patient ratios. (THE CANADIAN PRESS/Andrew Vaughan)

Conceptual Framework for Advocacy

Hogan (2008) noted that PHNs need to know their ethical responsibilities related to advocacy. She stated that "advocacy ethics … needs to be considered and emphasized when examining public health nursing training and education including familiarity with frameworks for advocacy such as the practical approach to advocacy suggested by Bateman (2000) or the conceptual framework for advocacy identified by Christoffel (2000)" (p. 36).

The conceptual framework for public health advocacy proposed by Christoffel (2000) has three stages:

1. *Information stage,* which focuses on gathering data about public health problems, including such factors as extent of the problem, patterns of frequency, and effectiveness of and barriers to public health programs;
2. *Strategy stage,* which focuses on tactics such as disseminating the gathered information and policy statements to lay and professional audiences, identifying objectives, building and funding coalitions, and working with legislators;
3. *Action stage,* which focuses on implementing the strategies through tactics such as lobbying, testifying, issuing press releases, passing laws, and voting.

Some of the principles that underlie this framework include scientific integrity in data gathering and dissemination, respect for persons (i.e., lay and professional people), honesty regarding fundraising, truthfulness in lobbying and testifying, and justice in passing laws.

Practical Framework for Advocacy

Bateman (2000) takes a practical approach to advocacy. He places the advocate's core skills (i.e., interviewing, assertiveness and force, negotiation, self-management, legal knowledge and research, and litigation) within the context of six ethical principles for effective advocacy, as shown in Box 6.5. Although his focus is on the individual, it can also apply to groups and communities.

Regarding the first ethical principle, Bateman (2000) is sensitive to the ethical conflict between patients' best interests

---

BOX 6.5   Ethical Principles for Effective Advocacy

1. Act in the patient's (group's, community's) best interests.
2. Act in accordance with the patient's (group's, community's) wishes and instructions.
3. Keep the patient (group, community) properly informed.
4. Carry out instructions with diligence and competence.
5. Act impartially and offer frank, independent advice.
6. Maintain patient confidentiality.

Source: Adapted from Bateman, N. (2000). *Advocacy skills for health and social care professionals* (p. 63). Jessica Kingsley.

and the best interests of groups, communities, and societies but does not elaborate on this conflict. The second ethical principle works in tandem with the first principle and puts the patient in charge. For example, the CHN might say to the patient, "This is what I think we can do. What do you want me to do?" (Bateman, 2000, p. 51). Of course, the advocate can refuse the request if oneself or others may be harmed. By following the third ethical principle, the patient is empowered to make knowledgeable decisions. The fourth ethical principle addresses standards of practice. The fifth addresses fairness and respect for persons (nursing in community health is more collaborative than independent in nature). The last ethical principle, confidentiality, ensures that information will be shared only on a need-to-know basis.

PRINCIPLES FOR THE JUSTIFICATION OF PUBLIC HEALTH INTERVENTIONS

CHNs are often challenged to answer the question of whether a public health intervention or action is justified. There are ethical aspects to this kind of question, and Upshur (2002) outlines four ethical principles that can help answer it: the harm principle, the principle of least restrictive means, the reciprocity principle, and the transparency principle.

The harm principle is a foundational principle for justifying public health actions. It sets out the justification to take action to restrict the liberty of an individual or a group in order to prevent harm to others (e.g., a TB patient is living in a crowded shelter and placing others at risk).

The ethical principle of using the least restrictive means recognizes that a variety of means exist to achieve public health needs, but the full authority and power of public health officials should be used only in exceptional circumstances; education, facilitation, and discussion should precede any restriction or coercive measures (e.g., educate the patient regarding risk for transmission and compliance with treatment).

The reciprocity principle holds that once a public health action is warranted, society is obligated to support individuals and communities in their efforts to comply with that public health intervention. Complying with public health requests can place an added burden on individuals or communities. Therefore, resources must also be put in place to support the action (e.g., provide a TB patient with an alternative housing arrangement and enroll him in a directly observed therapy program).

The transparency principle refers to the manner and context in which decisions are made. All key stakeholders, especially patients, should be involved in the decision, and clear communication should be provided about the action to be taken. CHNs can answer the question of whether the need for a public health intervention exists by applying Upshur's (2002) ethical principles to the decision-making process.

👤 STUDENT EXPERIENCE

1. Access the CNA's *Code of Ethics for Registered Nurses* (2017) and *Social Justice* (2010) documents (see the links on the Evolve website).
2. Read through the documents and familiarize yourself with the nursing values and ethical responsibilities as well as the attributes and framework of social justice in the respective documents.
3. Read this scenario and answer the questions that follow:
   Mr. Smith is an 85-year-old man who resides on the eighth floor in an older-persons' apartment building. His spouse passed away 4 months ago, and he has no other family. He has had many falls over the last 3 weeks, resulting in severe leg and hip pain that has prevented him from attending church or socializing with his friends. He is experiencing urinary incontinence and is having difficulty managing his own personal care. He is unable to complete household tasks and has lost over 5 kg since his spouse died. He has a diagnosis of chronic obstructive pulmonary disease (COPD) and hypertension and is having difficulty taking his medications on schedule. You are the CHN assigned to Mr. Smith.
   a. Choose one of the ethical models presented in the CNA *Code of Ethics for Registered Nurses* document and apply it to Mr. Smith's situation. What ethical action would you take?
   b. How would you apply the *Social Justice* document's decision tree model in Mr. Smith's situation?

CHAPTER SUMMARY

6.1 Nursing's first code of ethics was the Nightingale Pledge of 1893, which outlined the ethical values and principles that guide nursing practice. In 1950, the ANA adopted its Code for Professional Nurses based on that pledge, and in 1953 the ICN developed an international code of ethics for nurses. Canada adopted the ICN code in 1954. CNA developed its own Canadian code of ethics in 1980, which has gone through four updates to its current version, which was revised in 2017.

6.2 Oberle and Raffin's model for ethical reflection includes: (1) assessing the ethics of the situation, (2) reflecting on and reviewing potential actions, (3) selecting an ethical action, (4) engaging in the ethical action, and (5) reflecting on and reviewing the action.

6.3 Ethical theories include utilitarianism, deontology, virtue ethics, relational ethics, and the ethics of care. Ethical principles that guide CHN's practice include autonomy, nonmaleficence, beneficence, and distributive justice.

6.4 CHNs in Canada are required to uphold the values identified in the CNA *Code of Ethics for Registered Nurses* as well as the *ICN Code of Ethics for Registered Nurses*.

6.5 The CNA code of ethics applies to all registered nurses and contains the ethical principles that guide practice. CHNs are also guided by the CCHN Standards, which also address ethical principles such as advocacy.

6.6 Ethical principles for effective advocacy are as follows: act in the patient's best interests; act in accordance with the patient's wishes and instructions; keep the patient properly informed; carry out instructions with diligence and competence; act impartially and offer frank, independent advice; and maintain patient confidentiality. CHNs also apply the principles of advocacy by participating in legislative and policymaking activities that influence the determinants of health and access to services in the community and by CHNs supporting individuals, families, communities, and populations to develop the skills necessary to advocate for themselves and change policies to improve community health.

6.7 Principles relevant to ethical deliberation in public health practice include the harm principle, the principle of least restrictive means, the reciprocity principle, and the transparency principle.

📋 CHN IN PRACTICE: A CASE STUDY

Ethical Considerations in Planning Care

In October 2005, the news media in Canada focused on the evacuation of Indigenous people from the community of Kashechewan, a Cree First Nation community of about 1900 people located near the western shore of James Bay on the Albany River in Northern Ontario. The measure was essential because the community's water supply was tainted and had become a serious health threat. Prior to the evacuation, high levels of *Escherichia coli* were found in the reserve's drinking water, requiring that chlorine levels be increased to "shock" levels, which, in turn, caused an increase in common skin problems such as scabies and impetigo. Part of the problem was that an intake pipe for the community's water treatment plant was downstream from the sewage lagoon. This resulted in many boil-water orders and, eventually, the evacuation.

This community was not just facing problems with water quality, however. The tainted water drew attention to the living conditions on the reserve: deteriorating and inadequate housing and community services, as well as repeated spring flooding requiring multiple evacuations since 2004 at the public's

Continued

CHN IN PRACTICE: A CASE STUDY—Cont'd

expense. The conditions inspired public debate over the quality of life for the members of the Kashechewan First Nation community and the need to relocate to a safer location.

An Ontario agency organizing the October 2005 evacuation from the Cree reserve searched for communities to take in the displaced people. Many people went to surrounding northern communities such as Sudbury, Cochrane, and Timmins. Another 250 were flown to Ottawa. The Kashechewan people remained away for a month while the Canadian military installed water purification systems that supplied up to 50 000 L of clean water per day; also, building materials were shipped in for housing reconstruction. However, spring flooding in April 2006 necessitated yet another evacuation. As part of a longer-term solution, the federal government offered to move the community to a better area a short distance from its current location. However, the Kashechewan people wished to relocate within their traditional lands. The government signed an agreement with the First Nation on July 30, 2007, giving the reserve $200 million to improve and repair the infrastructure of the existing community, including housing and flood-control services.

This scenario is an example of a situation that CHNs might face while working in remote communities.

Think About It

1. Identify two ethical dilemmas presented by this population health crisis and describe the potential involvement of CHNs in this situation.
2. What do you think of the quality of life of residents who were evacuated and relocated in different communities? (Reflect on the residents' beliefs and values that make up their personal value system.)
3. How should the Indigenous culture have been considered in relocating the residents from the community of Kashechewan?
4. Which aspects of the CNA code of ethics might apply to this situation, especially considering the health concerns of the Indigenous population (e.g., diseases of the respiratory system, which accounted for 18.8% and 11.6% of all hospital separations for First Nations males and females, respectively, in 1997, and injuries and poisonings, which accounted for 17.7% and 9.3% of all hospital separations for First Nations males and females, respectively, in 1997*)?
5. Which CHNC Standards could be employed to help empower the community of Kashechewan to deal with this crisis?

*Health Canada, 2014.

Sources: Brennan, R. (2007). Ottawa to rebuild troubled reserve. *Toronto Star,* July 30; CBC News. (2006). *Kashechewan: Water crisis in Northern Ontario,* November 9. Retrieved from http://www.cbc.ca/news2/background/aboriginals/kashechewan.html; Government of Canada. (2005). *Progress on Kashechewan action plan* [Press release], November 3; Health Canada. (2014). *A statistical profile on the health of First Nations in Canada: Determinants of health, 2006 to 2010.* Retrieved from http://publications.gc.ca/collections/collection_2014/sc-hc/H34-193-1-2014-eng.pdf; McGuire, A. (2006). Flooding forces evacuation of Kashechewan First Nation. *Ottawa Citizen,* April 24, A1.

 TOOL BOX

The Tool Box contains useful resources that can be applied to community health nursing practice. These related resources are found either in the appendices at the back of this text or on the Evolve website at https://evolve.elsevier.com/Canada/Stanhope/community/.

Appendix

- Appendix 1: Canadian Community Health Nursing Standards of Practice

Tools

Toronto Central Community Care Access Centre (2008). *Community Ethics Toolkit.* (https://www.suncountry.sk.ca/gsCMSDisplayPluginFile/show/id/598/menu_id/88/lang_type/en_US/page_type/service/page_id/175)

The *Community Ethics Toolkit* was created to facilitate the broader implementation of a common approach for ethical decision making across the community health and support sector. It consists of a code of ethics for the community health and support sector; a decision-making worksheet; guidelines for using the decision-making worksheet; guidelines for conducting case reviews; and additional resources.

REFERENCES

American Nurses Association (ANA). (2014a). *Code of ethics for nurses with interpretive statements.* American Nurses.

American Nurses Association (ANA). (2014b). *Florence nightingale pledge.* https://www.nursingworld.org/ana/about-ana/.

Anderson, J. M., Rodney, P., Reimer-Kirkham, S., et al. (2009). Inequities in health and healthcare viewed through the ethical lens of critical social justice: Contextual knowledge for the global priorities ahead. *Advances in Nursing Science, 32*(4), 282–294.

Austin, W. (2001). Relational ethics in forensic psychiatric settings. *Journal of Psychosocial Nursing and Mental Health Services, 39*(9), 12–19.

Austin, W., Goble, E., & Kelecevic, J. (2009). The ethics of forensic psychiatry: Moving beyond principles to a relational ethics approach. *Journal of Forensic Psychiatry and Psychology, 20*(6), 835–850.

Bateman, N. (2000). *Advocacy skills for health and social care professionals.* Jessica Kingsley.

Beauchamp, T. L., & Childress, J. F. (2012). *Principles of biomedical ethics* (7th ed.). Oxford University Press.

Bernheim, R. G., & Melnick, A. (2008). Principled leadership in public health: Integrating ethics into practice and management. *Journal of Public Health Management and Practice, 14*(4), 348–366.

Boylan, M. (2000). Interview with Edmund D. Pellegrino. In M. Boylan (Ed.), *Medical ethics: Basic ethics in action.* Prentice Hall.

Brennan, R. (2007). *Ottawa to rebuild troubled reserve.* Toronto Star. July 30.

Callahan, D. (2000). Universalism and particularism fighting to a draw. *The Hastings Center Report, 30*(1), 37.

Canadian Centre on Substance Use and Addiction. (2020). *Focused on the future: Strategic plan 2021-2026.* https://www.ccsa.ca/focused-future-strategic-plan-2021-2026.

Canadian Nurses Association (CNA). (2006). *Social justice.* Author.

Canadian Nurses Association (CNA). (2010). *Social justice* (2nd ed.). https://www.cna-aiic.ca/~/media/cna/page-content/pdf-en/social_justice_2010_e.pdf.

Canadian Nurses Association (CNA). (2017). *Code of ethics for registered nurses, 2017 edition.* https://www.cna-aiic.ca/~/media/cna/page-content/pdf-en/code-of-ethics-2017-edition-secure-interactive.

CBC News. (2006). *Kashechewan: Water crisis in northern Ontario.* November 9. http://www.cbc.ca/news2/background/aboriginals/kashechewan.html.

Chaloner, C. (2007). An introduction to ethics in nursing. *Nursing Standard, 21*(32), 42–45.

Christoffel, K. K. (2000). Public health advocacy: Process and product. *American Journal of Public Health, 90*(5), 722–723.

Clouser, K. D., & Gert, B. (1990). A critique of principlism. *Journal of Medicine and Philosophy, 15*, 219.

Cohen, B. E., & Reutter, L. (2007). Development of the role of public health nurses in addressing child and family poverty: A framework for action. *Journal of Advanced Nursing, 60*(1), 96–107.

Community Health Nurses of Canada. (2019). *Canadian community health nursing: Professional practice model and standards of practice.* https://www.chnc.ca/standards-of-practice.

Duignan, B. (2014). *John Rawls. Encyclopedia britannica.* http://www.britannica.com/biography/John-Rawls.

Dunbar, T. (2003). Autonomy versus beneficence: An ethical dilemma. *Primary Health Care, 13*(1), 38–41.

Easley, C. E., & Allen, C. A. (2007). A critical intersection: Human rights, public health nursing, and nursing ethics. *Advances in Nursing Science, 30*(4), 367–382.

Evans, M., Bergum, V., Bamforth, S., et al. (2004). Relational ethics and genetic counseling. *Nursing Ethics, 11*(5), 459–471.

Fletcher, J. J. (1999). Virtues, moral decisions, and healthcare. *NursingConnections, 12*(4), 26–32.

Flicker, S., & Guta, A. (2008). Ethical approaches to adolescent participation in sexual health research. *Journal of Adolescent Health, 42*, 3–10.

Fry, S., & Johnstone, M.-J. (2002). *Ethics in nursing practice: A guide to ethical decision-making* (2nd ed.). Blackwell: International Council of Nurses.

Gilligan, C. (1982). *A different voice: Psychological theory and women's development.* Harvard University Press.

Government of Canada. (2005). *Progress on Kashechewan action plan [Press release].* November 3.

Green, B. (2012). Applying feminism ethics of care to nursing practice. *Journal of Nursing Care, 1*(3), 1–4. https://doi.org/10.4172/2167-1168.1000111.

Health Canada. (2014). *A statistical profile on the health of First Nations in Canada: Determinants of health, 2006 to 2010.* http://publications.gc.ca/collections/collection_2014/sc-hc/H34-193-1-2014-eng.pdf.

Hogan, M. (2008). *Public health nursing practice in Canada: A review of the literature for the Community Health Nurses Association of Canada.* (Available from infor@chnac.ca).

Holstein, M. B. (2001). Bringing ethics home: A new look at ethics in the home and the community. In M. B. Holstein, & P. B. Mitzen (Eds.), *Ethics in community-based elder care.* Springer.

International Council of Nurses. (2012). *ICN code of ethics for nurses.* https://www.icn.ch/sites/default/files/inline-files/2012_ICN_Codeofethicsfornurses_%20eng.pdf.

Ivanov, L., & Oden, T. (2013). Public health nursing, ethics and human rights. *Public Health Nursing, 30*(3), 231–238.

Kass, N. E. (2005). An ethics framework for public health and avian influenza pandemic preparedness. *Yale Journal of Biology & Medicine, 78*, 235–250.

Kayman, H., & Ablorh-Odjidja, A. (2006). Revisiting public health preparedness: Incorporating social justice principles into pandemic preparedness planning for influenza. *Journal of Public Health Management and Practice, 12*(4), 373–380.

Keatings, M., & Smith, O. B. (2010). *Ethical and legal issues in Canadian nursing* (3rd ed.). Mosby.

Kenny, N., Sherwin, S., & Baylis, F. (2010). Re-visioning public health ethics: A relational perspective. *Canadian Journal of Public Health, 101*(1), 9–11.

Kirkham, S. R., & Browne, A. (2006). Toward a critical theoretical interpretation of social justice discourses in nursing. *Advances in Nursing Science, 29*(4), 324–339.

Leininger, M. (Ed.). (1984). *Care: The essence of nursing and health.* Slack.

Leung, D., & Esplen, M. (2010). Alleviating existential distress of cancer patients: Can relational ethics guide clinicians? *European Journal of Cancer Care, 19*(1), 30–38.

McGuire, A. (2006). *Flooding forces evacuation of Kashechewan first nation.* Ottawa Citizen, A1, April 24.

Meagher-Stewart, D., Aston, M. L., Edwards, N. C., et al. (2007). Managements' perspective on Canadian public health nurses' primary health care practice. *Primary Health Care Research & Development, 8*, 170–182.

Myllykoski, H. (2011). Social justice: Who cares? *Alberta RN, 67*(4), 28–29.

Noddings, N. (1984). *Caring: A feminine approach to ethics and moral education.* University of California Press.

Oberle, K., & Tenove, S. (2000). Ethical issues in public health nursing. *Nursing Ethics, 7*(5), 425–439.

Olmstead, D., Scott, S., & Austin, W. (2010). Unresolved pain in children: A relational ethics perspective. *Nursing Ethics, 17*(6), 695–704.

Pauly, B. M., MacKinnon, K., & Varcoe, C. (2009). Revisiting "who gets care?" Health equity as an arena for nursing action. *Advances in Nursing Science, 32*(2), 118–127.

Peter, E. (2011). Fostering social justice: The possibilities of a socially connected model of moral agency. *Canadian Journal of Nursing Research, 43*(2), 11–17.

Phillippi, J. C. (2009). Women's perceptions of access to prenatal care in the United States: A literature review. *Journal of Midwifery & Women's Health, 54*(3), 219–225.

Public Health Agency of Canada (PHAC). (2006). *Direction #9: Move to a social justice framework.* Author.

Public Health Agency of Canada (PHAC). (2014). *Strengthening federal action in the Canadian response to HIV/AIDS.* http://www.phac-aspc.gc.ca/aids-sida/fi-if/fa-if/2-eng.php.

Racher, F. (2007). The evolution of ethics for community practice. *Journal of Community Health Nursing, 24*(1), 65–76.

Rawls, J. (2001). In E. Kelly (Ed.), *Justice as fairness: A restatement.* Harvard University Press.

Rowa-Dewar, N., & Ritchie, D. (2014). Protecting children from smoking in the home: An ethics of care perspective. *British Journal of Community Nursing, 19*(5), 214–218.

Shaw, E. (2011). Relational ethics and moral imagination in contemporary systemic practice. *Australian and New Zealand Journal of Family Therapy, 32*(1), 1–14.

Sherwin, S. (2011). Looking backwards, looking forward: Hopes for bioethics' next twenty-five years. *Bioethics, 25*(2), 75–82. https://doi.org/10.1111/j.1467-8519.2010.01866.x.

Solomon, R. C. (1993). *Ethics: A short introduction.* Dubuque, IA: Brown & Benchmark.

Steinbock, B., London, J., & Arras, A. J. (2008). *Ethical issues in modern medicine.* McGraw-Hill.

Stone, J. R., & Parham, G. P. (2007). An ethical framework for community health workers and related institutions. *Family & Community Health, 30*(4), 351–363.

Storch, J. L., Rodney, P., & Starzomski, R. (2004). *Toward a moral horizon: Nursing ethics for leadership and practice.* Pearson Education Canada.

Stubager, R. (2008). Education effects on authoritarian-libertarian values: A question of socialization. *British Journal of Sociology, 59*(2), 327–350.

Ten Have, H. (2011). Global bioethics and communitarianism. *Theoretical Medicine and Bioethics, 32*(5), 315–326.

Upshur, R. E. G. (2002). Principles of the justification of public health intervention. *Canadian Journal of Public Health, 93*(2), 101–103.

U.S. Department of Health and Social Services and Centers for Disease Control and Prevention. (2008). *Safe motherhood: Promoting health for women before, during, and after pregnancy.* Atlanta. CDC.

Volbrecht, R. M. (2002). *Nursing ethics: Communities in dialogue.* Prentice Hall.

Walker, T. (2009). What principlism misses. *Journal of Medical Ethics, 35,* 229–231.

Watson, J. (1985). *Nursing: Human science and human care.* Appleton-Century-Crofts.

Wild, T. C., Pauly, B., Belle-Isle, L., et al. (2017). Canadian harm reduction policies: A comparative content analysis of provincial and territorial documents, 2000–2015. *International Journal of Drug Policy, 45,* 9–17. https://doi.org/10.1016/j.drugpo.2017.03.014.

Woods, M. (2012). Exploring the relevance of social justice within a relational nursing ethic. *Nursing Philosophy, 13*(1), 56–65.

Wright, D., & Brajtman, S. (2011). Relational and embodied knowing: Nursing ethics within the interprofessional team. *Nursing Ethics, 18*(1), 20–30.

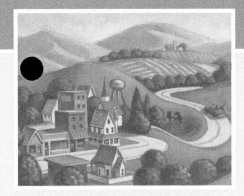

7

Diversity and Relational Practice in Community Health Nursing

R. Lisa Bourque Bearskin, Sonya L. Jakubec

OUTLINE

Diversity, Culture, Race, and Ethnicity, 146
Key Demographic Groups for Community Health Nursing in Canada, 147
  An Aging Population, 147
  Indigenous Peoples, 148
  Immigrant Population, 148
Types of Diversity, 149
  Ethnic Diversity, 149
  Multiculturalism, 152
  Linguistic Diversity, 152
  Religious Diversity, 153
  Sexual Diversity, 153
  Disability/Diverse Abilities, 154
Diversity, Inequities, and the Determinants of Health, 156

Approaches to Diversity in Community Health Nursing Practice, 157
Cultural Competence, 159
  Developing Culturally Responsive Care, 160
  Inhibitors to Culturally Responsive Care, 160
Cultural Safety, 163
  Cultural Humility, 164
Cultural Nursing Assessment, 165
  Relational Practice: Assessment and Intervening Processes, 165
Applying Cultural Skills in Community Health Practice, 167
  Working With Immigrant and Refugee Populations, 167
  Using an Interpreter, 168

OBJECTIVES

After reading this chapter, you should be able to:

7.1 Define *diversity, culture, race,* and *ethnicity.*
7.2 Describe key demographic groups that have implications for community health nursing in Canada.
7.3 Understand the different types of diversity in Canada: ethnic, linguistic, religious, sexual, and physical abilities.
7.4 Describe the determinants of health that affect the health of Canadians.
7.5 Discuss the approaches to diversity in community health nursing practice.

7.6 Explain cultural competence and its application to community health nursing.
7.7 Explain the concept of cultural safety and its application to community health nursing.
7.8 Conduct a cultural nursing assessment and describe relational practice and its application to community health nursing.
7.9 Discuss some important skills and tools required for a diverse community health practice.

KEY TERMS*

allophones, 152
anti-oppressive practice, 146
bias, 160
cisgender, 154
cultural awareness, 161
cultural blindness, 160
cultural competence, 159
cultural interaction, 161
cultural interpretation, 168
cultural knowledge, 161
cultural nursing assessment, 165
cultural pluralism, 146
cultural proficiency, 162
cultural safety, 163
cultural sensitivity, 161

cultural skill, 162
cultural understanding, 161
culture, 147
culture shock, 160
diversity, 146
ethnicity, 147
ethnocentrism, 160
gender, 154
gender identity, 154
heterosexual, 153
homosexual, 153
immigrant, 167
interpretation, 168
linguistic interpretation, 168
microaggressions, 152

multiculturalism, 152
newcomer, 167
prejudice, 162
queer or questioning, 153
race, 147
racializing, 146
racially visible, 146
racism, 162
refugee, 167

relational practice, 165
sexual orientation, 153
sexuality, 153
stereotyping, 162
structural racism, 163
transgender, 154
translation, 168
visible minority, 146

*See the Glossary on page 468 for definitions.

Canada is a rich tapestry of diverse people. Indigenous peoples represent Canada's original inhabitants, and over time the country's cultural landscape has been transformed by settler colonialism and immigration patterns (Dickason & Newbigging, 2019). Canada is a multicultural nation that values **cultural pluralism,** or the right of groups to maintain their cultural identity (UNESCO, 2001). The diversity of the country's people, culture, and languages shapes how differences in individual and community health are understood and approached. Understanding how oppression operates to advantage and disadvantage people from diverse groups is central to the community health nurse's advocacy role, and to creating conditions for community health.

Community health nurses (CHNs) are responsible for ensuring that nursing practice addresses these issues of oppression, discrimination, and equity, and for providing care that is culturally congruent with and culturally responsive to the beliefs of the individuals, families, groups, and communities they serve. CHNs provide care for diverse patients, and CHNs themselves are culturally and socially diverse.

This chapter focuses on Canada's culture, ethnic mix, and various areas of diversity, as well as strategies for providing anti-oppressive care that is equity-informed and results in culturally safe service to patients. To develop CHN practice in a way that supports care to all patients, as well as professional and social change, diversity must be understood with a view towards developing anti-oppressive practice as a professional value. **Anti-oppressive practice** involves not only accepting and valuing people of different cultures, ages, genders, sexual orientation, abilities, and all lifestyles, beliefs, and practices, but also seeking to dismantle the forces and contexts of oppression and colonization. This chapter introduces relational practice and describes how it establishes a path towards awareness and anti-oppressive practices.

DIVERSITY, CULTURE, RACE, AND ETHNICITY

CHNs who work with people from a variety of backgrounds benefit from understanding the concepts of diversity, culture, race, and ethnicity in their nursing practice. **Diversity** in a cultural context considers similarities, differences, and power relations across age, gender, race, religion, occupation, sexual orientation, and poverty (Campinha-Bacote,

2018; Lowe & Archibald, 2009; Racine & Petrucka, 2011; Spector, 2017). More broadly and beyond culture, diversity focuses on unique patient assets that build capacity. The two types of diversity are visible and invisible (Clair, Beatty, & MacLean, 2005). *Visible diversity* includes attributes such as age, physical appearance, and gender (Clair et al., 2005). People who are visibly diverse have a greater risk of experiencing discrimination, stereotyping, and marginalization (Srivastava, 2007). Invisible diversity includes attributes that are not readily seen, such as religion, national origin, occupation, sexual orientation, and illness. Consideration must also be given to people who are *invisibly diverse* because their inconspicuous attributes may not be acknowledged (Srivastava, 2007).

Throughout this chapter, the two terms *visible minority* and *racially visible* will be used, as they are the terms used by Statistics Canada under the *Employment Equity Act*. According to Statistics Canada (2020b), the term **visible minority** is used to describe people of colour; that is, people who are neither Indigenous nor White. However, the term **racially visible** is more accurate in describing diverse aggregates and indicates visible diversity by way of colour. Srivastava (2007) and Nestel (2012) identify limitations that occur when the terms *visible minority* or *people of colour* are used: heterogeneous groups of non-White people are slotted into one category, which ignores class and ethnic differences. In health care, this practice, known as **racializing,** has many of the pitfalls of categorization, including bias, discrimination, and limiting opportunities for diversity (Varcoe, Browne, Wong, et al., 2009). Being able to identify the limitations of these terms and their implications for health care enables CHNs to relate more openly and relationally with patients.

The concepts of culture, race, and ethnicity also influence our understanding of human beliefs, perceptions, and behaviour as well as actions in health care practice (Napier, Arcano, Butler, et al., 2014). Culture provides direction on the appropriate behaviours for situations in everyday life. It also provides cues to nurses on how individuals may interact. The terms *race* and *ethnicity* are used to identify distinguishable groups within cultures. However, the imprecise use of these terms is problematic and can cause misidentification of various populations (Bourque Bearskin, 2014; Nestel, 2012).

Although there are many definitions of **culture,** Srivastava (2007) defines it as "a term that applies to all groups of people where there are common values and ways of thinking and acting that differ from those of another group" (p. 15). Srivastava also describes culture using the acronym CULTURE: C = commonly, U = understood, L = learned, T = traditions, U = unconscious, R = rules of, E = engagement.

Culture has six distinguishing features:

1. *Culture is learned.* It is based on the events and experiences that we internalize as we grow and develop from infancy onward. We are not born with culture.
2. *Culture is adaptive.* It adjusts to environmental and technological changes that occur over time.
3. *Culture is dynamic.* It is not static and responds to changes created by new situations and demands.
4. *Culture is invisible.* It is something one experiences. It is apparent through rituals, language, celebrations, and dress.
5. *Culture is shared.* Persons from the same culture identify with the same values, beliefs, and patterns of behaviour, yet maintain individuality. Everyone is unique.
6. *Culture is selective.* It differentiates between outsiders and insiders through boundaries for desirable, acceptable, or unacceptable behaviour. It also influences how people view and respond to situations and issues. (Srivastava, 2007, p. 15)

Race is primarily a social classification based on an imagined hierarchy of human value that relies on phenotypes, skin colour, and other expressions of group superiority and inferiority to identify group membership (Nestel, 2012). Individuals may be of the same race but of different ethnicities and cultures. For example, Black people—who may have been born in Africa, the Caribbean, North America, or elsewhere—are a heterogeneous group, but they are often (wrongly) viewed as culturally and racially homogeneous.

Racism and other forms of oppression (for example, through social exclusion or medicalizing social issues) operate to produce health inequities and limit professional knowledge and agency (Ford, 2019; McGibbon, 2012; Raphael, 2017). McGibbon and Etowa (2009) promote antiracist frameworks to guide the profession, and to prevent the many forms of racism that often become invisible to nurses. For example, individual racism, internalized racism, systemic racism, environmental racism, and cultural racism negatively affect health status. Awareness and understanding of the different varieties of racism enables nurses to be more culturally sensitive and to adopt aspects of cultural safety, which will be discussed later in this chapter.

Ethnicity is the state of belonging to a social group that shares common cultural patterns (e.g., beliefs, values, customs, behaviours, traditions). It is influenced by education, income level, geographical location, and association with individuals from ethnic groups other than one's own. Therefore, a reciprocal relationship exists between the individual and society. Some examples of ethnicity are African, Chinese, Greek, Irish, Italian, Ukrainian, and Vietnamese. *Ethnicity* is used more often than *race* to identify and categorize individuals (Srivastava, 2007).

KEY DEMOGRAPHIC GROUPS FOR COMMUNITY HEALTH NURSING IN CANADA

In Canada, key demographic groups that have implications for anti-oppressive and equity-informed practice are the aging older population and people with disabilities, Indigenous peoples, and immigrant communities. Demographic trends are important for the profession in many ways, including professional position statements and advocacy for city or municipal design, as well as social, health, and community services planning. For example, the rapidly growing aging and immigrant populations will affect planning for translators/interpreters, adapted/accessible/universal design, and the location of health care services. Awareness of diverse needs can support CHN practice, and advocacy for supports and resources that may be otherwise outside of the dominant, privileged view. For instance, awareness of the experiences of a demographic group in an area could alert CHNs to inequitable access to transportation, or to additional sexual health support services that may be required in a community.

Diversity and diverse groups' concerns are highlighted, with a specific emphasis on the concerns of Indigenous people, and expanded upon in Chapter 14. Health inequity among Indigenous populations continues to widen, despite advances in Indigenous health research (Allan & Smylie, 2015; Greenwood, De Leeuw, & Lindsay, 2018); community health approaches for equity-informed practice more broadly are discussed in Chapter 15.

While professional nursing codes and CHN standards provide guidance, acknowledging, confronting, and transforming oppressive practices is the work of everyone within the profession (Lancellotti, 2008). All nurses, for example, are responsible for ensuring that nursing practice is culturally congruent with and culturally responsive to the beliefs of the individuals, families, groups, organizations, and communities they serve. At times, these very codes and norms require scrutiny for their taken-for-granted assumptions that perpetuate oppression and racism (Smith, 2019).

An Aging Population

Demographic trends around age, such as an aging population, an increase in older persons living in suburban neighbourhoods, and the overall declining birth rate highlight the diversity of community health needs and concerns. A key contributor to the changing demographic landscape in Canada is the growing population of older persons. This trend has emerged both due to the immigration of older persons and because people are living longer. At this time, about 3 in 10 Canadians are aged 65 years of age and older, and this proportion is steadily increasing (Statistics Canada, 2019c). In 2019, more people were aged 55 to 64 than those aged 15 to 24, and older persons represented 17.5% of the population; this percentage is projected to rise to 22.7% by 2031. The largest proportion of older persons lives in the Atlantic provinces, while the western provinces and northern territories have the youngest populations (Statistics Canada, 2019c). A growing number of older persons is living in Canadian suburbs, which has important implications for older-person belonging, community connection, and health and well-being in those locations (Jakubec, Olfert, Choi, et al., 2019).

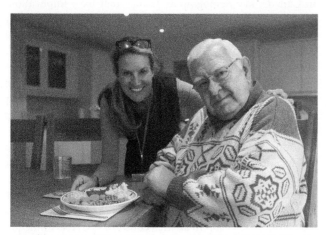

An older person enjoys a meal and a visit. (iStockphoto/SolStock)

Indigenous Peoples

Prior to European contact, an estimated 500 000 Indigenous people lived in what is now known as Canada. By 1871, this number was reduced to 102 000 as a result of infectious diseases such as influenza, smallpox, measles, and tuberculosis, to which Indigenous peoples had no immunity (Indian and Northern Affairs Canada, 1996). The word *Indigenous* often refers to the original inhabitants of a country who identify with a particular heritage based on their home nation or linguistic family. Early European immigrants forced Indigenous communities to relocate while claiming the land and resources as their own. This displacement has caused First Nations people, Inuit, and Métis to become resistant to the government's agenda to control and monopolize Canadian resources through its numerous assimilation policies (Indian and Northern Affairs Canada, 1996). For more information about First Nations people, Inuit, and Métis and community health nursing practice, see Chapter 14.

In Canada, First Nations people, Inuit, and Métis are now the fastest-growing populations in the country. In 2016, 2.1 million people, or 6.2% of the total Canadian population, reported Indigenous ancestry. Of the three main Indigenous groups, the largest was First Nations, with 1.5 million people. Within this group, Cree (356 660), Mi'kmaq (168 480), and Ojibway (125 725) were the most common ancestries. Métis ancestry was reported by 600 000 people, and Inuit ancestry was reported by 79 125 (Statistics Canada, 2017).

First Nations People

Canada has more than 600 different First Nations communities (Statistics Canada, 2013a), each with its own unique history, language, traditions, and ceremonies. It is important to note that some First Nations people identify themselves with their linguistic group (e.g., Cree, Blackfoot, Dene, or Chipewyan), whereas others identify themselves with their community of origin (e.g., Blood Tribe or Beaver Lake Cree Nation) or treaty area (e.g., Treaty 6 or Treaty 7).

The most important means of Canadian control over First Nations communities was and still is the *Indian Act,* which consolidated the various laws relating to Indigenous peoples that had been passed by the Canadian government in the years since Confederation and by the British colonial authorities before them.

Inuit

Three quarters of Inuit in Canada reside in 53 communities spread across the Northwest Territories, Yukon, Nunavut, Northern Quebec, and Labrador (Indigenous and Northern Affairs Canada, 2015). Over 90% of these communities are accessible by air only. Inuit communities are located in four land-claim regions: Nunatsiavut (Labrador), Nunavik (Northern Quebec), Nunavut Territory, and Inuvialuit Settlement Region (Northwest Territories and Yukon). Of the Inuit who live in southern Canada, about half live in cities. The largest populations are in Edmonton, Montreal, Ottawa, Yellowknife, and St. John's (Indigenous and Northern Affairs Canada, 2014).

Métis

The Métis National Council (n.d.) defines a Métis person as "*a person who self-identifies as Métis, is distinct from other Aboriginal peoples, is of historic Métis Nation Ancestry and who is accepted by the Métis Nation.*" The "historic Métis Nation" refers to the Indigenous people historically known as Métis or mixed blood (with parents of Indigenous and European ancestry) who resided in the "historic Métis Nation Homeland," which refers to the area of land in west central North America used and occupied as the traditional territory of the Métis. "Métis Nation" refers to the Indigenous people descended from the historic Métis Nation, which now comprises all Métis Nation citizens. Métis are members of the Aboriginal peoples of Canada per section 35 of the Constitution Act of 1982. They have their own distinct dialect (called the Michif language), but Métis are diverse linguistically, depending on the combination of ancestry (e.g., Cree, Dene, English, French).

Immigrant Population

With the development and colonization of Canada came an influx of immigrants into the country. Historically, the patterns of immigration to Canada have varied, with a mix of places of origin represented. Many immigrants have come from Europe, Asia, the United States, Africa, and the Caribbean. Often, the reasons for leaving the country of origin have included lack of economic prosperity, persecution, and war.

Canada's ethnocultural composition has changed over time. While in the past, immigrants came mainly from European countries, between 2006 and 2011 the largest source of immigrants was Asia (Astle, Barton, Johnson, et al., 2019; Statistics Canada, 2013c). According to the 2011 National Household Survey (NHS), Canada reported the second-highest proportion of foreign-born individuals, which is about one in five people and represents about 21%

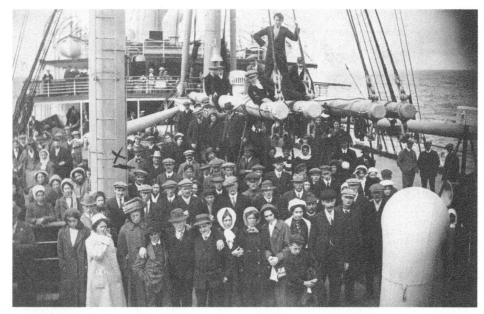

In the early 1900s, immigrants to Canada were mainly European in origin, as with the group shown here setting sail on the Empress of Ireland in 1910. Today, however, most immigrants coming to Canada are from other parts of the world, especially Asia and Africa. (Glenbow Archives, NA-1960-1)

of the overall population. During the past 5 years, there has been a slight increase in the number of immigrants coming from Africa, Caribbean, and Central and South America. The majority of immigrants move to urban centres in Ontario, British Columbia, Quebec, and Alberta (Statistics Canada, 2013c).

Citizenship and Immigration Canada (2016a) and the *Immigration and Refugee Protection Act* outline permanent resident status categories such as economic classes (e.g., federal skilled trades class, live-in caregivers) and noneconomic classes (e.g., family members, people seeking humanitarian and compassionate consideration). In addition, this classification also outlines the temporary status of residents as temporary workers, students, and visitors (Citizenship and Immigration Canada, 2016b). The top source countries for new people arriving in Canada are the Philippines (13.1%), China (10.5%), and India (10.4%) (Statistics Canada, 2013c).

New immigrants are showing a preference to live in metropolitan areas such as Toronto, Vancouver, and Montreal (Statistics Canada, 2011b). These three cities are the most racially and culturally diverse in Canada. Canada has a history of admitting large numbers of immigrants of various ethnic origins. In 2015, Canada planned to welcome 260 000 to 285 000 new permanent residents, 65% of which would be economic immigrants (Citizenship and Immigration Canada, 2015). Changes to the *Citizenship Act* in 2015 require immigrants to prove that they have an attachment to Canada and are contributing to the economy. These changes will impact where new immigrants choose to take up residence. For evidence-informed resources on health care for immigrant and refugee children, youth, and families, see the Caring for Kids New to Canada link on the Evolve website.

TYPES OF DIVERSITY

In Canada, diversity is experienced in a number of important ways: ethnic, religious, linguistic, sexual, and based on physical abilities (that also relate to age). Understanding that diversity is expressed and experienced uniquely, but with shared concerns and issues of social determinants of health (discussed later in this chapter), is essential to advocacy and supporting patient strengths in an asset-based approach to CHN practice.

Ethnic Diversity

Over 200 ethnic groups live in Canada, and 13 of these groups have populations of over 1 million people. In 2011, visible minorities represented 19.1% of the total population, of which 30.9% were born in Canada and 65.1% were born outside of Canada. The median age of the visible minority population was about 7 years younger than that of the overall total population (Statistics Canada, 2013c). In all, 4% of the visible minority population were nonpermanent residents (Statistics Canada, 2013c).

The influx of visible minorities is projected to continue to rise. For example, in 2031, it is estimated that 55% of foreign-born people in the population may be born in Asia, and 20% could be born in Europe (Statistics Canada 2010b). The projected (2011–2031) distribution of the immigrant population by continent of birth appears in Fig. 7.1. The population of selected prominent cultural groups across Canada appears in Fig. 7.2.

The ethnocultural population varies according to generations. The 2011 census indicated that 22% of the overall Canadian population were first-generation Canadians (born outside of Canada). Second-generation Canadians accounted for 17.4% of the overall population and were defined as individuals born in Canada but with one or both parents born

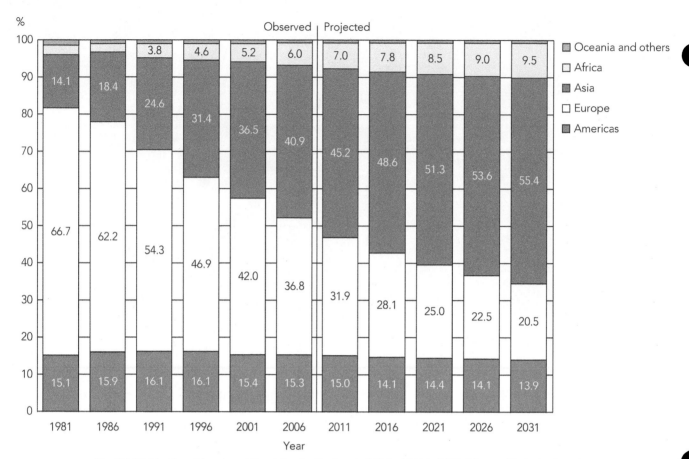

Fig. 7.1 Distribution of Immigrant Population by Continent of Birth, 1981 to 2031. (*Source:* Statistics Canada. (2010b). *Projections of the diversity of the Canadian population: 2006–2031,* Figure 2. http://www.statcan. gc.ca/pub/91-551-x/91-551-x2010001-eng.pdf.)

outside of Canada. Third-generation Canadians accounted for 60.7% of the overall population and were defined as individuals born in Canada with parents who were also born in Canada. Three out of 10 second-generation Canadians were visible minorities. The median age of all second-generation visible minorities was 13.6 years, whereas the median age of the second generation who are not visible minorities was 43.4 years (Statistics Canada, 2013c).

Canada's ethnic mix is changing rapidly, particularly in urban areas, mainly because of increased rates of non-European immigration in recent decades. Immigrants are making up an increasingly large proportion of the general population. This means that a growing number of Canadians do not speak English or French and have a religion that is non-Christian. These facts affect how health care is delivered to large segments of the community and the ability of this population to access health care.

Population projections are estimates of how a population will grow and change in the future. Statistics Canada data indicate important trends in Canadian demographics by the year 2031:

- Three in 10 (between 29% and 32%) of Canadians could be a visible minority (i.e., belonging to the South Asian, Chinese, Arabic, West Asian, Black, Filipino, Latin American, Japanese, or Korean groups) (Statistics Canada, 2010b).
- The population that is not from a visible minority group is also projected to grow between 2001 and 2017—but at a slower rate of only 1% to 7% (Statistics Canada, 2010a).

- Visible minorities will continue to live in urban centres. Almost 96% of the racially visible population will live in census metropolitan areas—with more than 71% residing in Toronto, Vancouver, and Montreal, alone (Statistics Canada, 2010b).

In 2011, South Asians, Chinese, and Blacks formed the largest racially visible groups in Canada, representing 61.3% of the overall visible minority population, with Arabic and West Asian being the fastest-growing populations (Statistics Canada, 2013c). Projections for 2031 indicate that approximately 36% of the visible minority group will be under 15 years of age and 18% will be over 65 years of age (Statistics Canada, 2010b). The population projections in Table 7.1 have implications for policy development and health care service delivery. CHNs need to be aware of changing demographic patterns in their communities so that they can be proactive in their program planning. For example, if the community's growth reflects an increase in a cultural group that is susceptible to certain diseases, then the CHN would assess current services offered and work with the community to identify and fulfill program and service needs.

Table 7.2 presents projections for 2031 on the median age of different groups in Canada. These statistical projections also have implications for policy development and health care service delivery. For example, First Nations people, Inuit, and Métis and visible minorities will be, on average, much

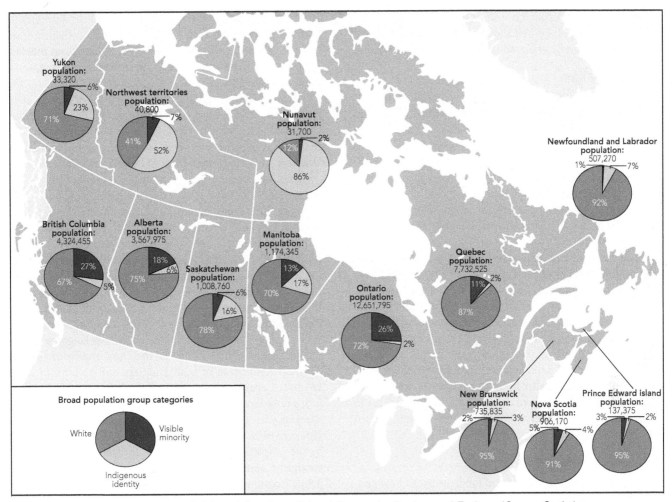

Fig. 7.2 Population of Selected Prominent Cultural Groups, by Province and Territory. (*Source:* Statistics Canada. (2011a). *2011 National Household Survey*. https://www12.statcan.gc.ca/nhs-enm/2011/dp-pd/prof/index.cfm?Lang=E.)

TABLE 7.1 Racially Visible, Indigenous, and Immigrant Populations as a Percentage of the Total Canadian Population

Group	2011 Census Data (% of General Population)	Projections for 2031 (% of General Population)	Increase (%)
Racially visible*	19.1	29–32	10–13
Indigenous people	4.3	5.3	1–2
Immigrants	20.6	22.2	4.2

*Refers to Chinese, South Asian, Black, Filipino, Latin American, Southeast Asian, Arabic, West Asian, Japanese, and Korean groups, and excludes Indigenous people.
Source: Statistics Canada. (2010b). *Projections of the diversity of the Canadian population: 2006–2031.* http://www.statcan.gc.ca/pub/91-551-x/91-551-x2010001-eng.pdf

TABLE 7.2 Projections for 2031: Median Age of Racially Visible and Indigenous Groups and the Rest of Canada

Group	2031 Projections (Median Age in Years)
Racially visible*	35.5
Canadian born	16.6
Born outside Canada	44.3
Rest of Canada†	43.3
Indigenous people	26.6
Rest of Canada‡	43.1

*Refers to Chinese, South Asian, Black, Filipino, Latin American, Southeast Asian, Arabic, West Asian, Japanese, and Korean groups, and excludes Indigenous people.
†Refers to all persons, including Indigenous people, but not persons included under "racially visible."
‡Refers to all persons, including racially visible, but not Indigenous people.
Sources: Statistics Canada. (2010b). *Projections of the diversity of the Canadian population: 2006–2031.* http://www.statcan.gc.ca/pub/91-551-x/91-551-x2010001-eng.pdf; Statistics Canada. (2015). *Population projections by Aboriginal identity in Canada, 2006 to 2031.* http://www.statcan.gc.ca/pub/91-552-x/2011001/hl-fs-eng.htm

younger than the rest of the population. These age projections might be used to advocate for health equity and social justice, to lend support for the continuation or expansion of existing programs or the development of new programs that better respond to age-based patient health concerns.

For further information on Canada's ethnocultural makeup, see the link for Statistics Canada's *Immigration and Ethnocultural Diversity in Canada* report on the Evolve website.

Multiculturalism

In 1971, Canada was the first country to adopt multiculturalism as an official policy. **Multiculturalism** recognizes the diverse ancestry of citizens and supports the ideals of equality and mutual respect among the population's ethnic and cultural groups (Jedwab, 2020). In some cases, multiculturalism is seen as a protective wellness factor within diverse populations. School policies on multiculturalism were found to be a protective factor for students who experience interpersonal violence in school environments (Le & Johansen, 2011).

Some critics of multiculturalism argue that it downplays the special status of Indigenous peoples and French Canadians (Library of Parliament, 2018). Others suggest that multiculturalism could be viewed as another form of assimilation and colonialism that further marginalizes diverse populations, in particular, racialized women (Pillay, 2015). Multiculturalism is less popular in Quebec than other provinces because of the belief that the federal government's multicultural policy minimizes Quebec's nationalist aspirations. Quebec emphasizes a multiethnic policy—a form of interculturalism that aims to preserve historical identity and achieve sovereignty within the Canadian state (Library of Parliament, 2018).

Linguistic Diversity

Language is the basis of culture and fundamental to how people make sense of their everyday lives. Language is a universal tool for translating information and knowledge within cultural groups, and each language has its own nuances, meanings, rules, and symbols (Hoffman-Goetz, Donelle, & Ahmed, 2014). The National Collaborating Centre for Indigenous Health (2016) considers language to be a social determinant of health that is essential to improving the health outcomes of Indigenous people.

More than 200 languages are spoken in Canada. In 2016, 21% of Canadians were **allophones,** or people whose mother tongue is a language other than French or English. At the same time, two-thirds of the population who speak a nonofficial language at home also speak English or French (Statistics Canada, 2017). Between 2011 and 2016, more than 1.2 million immigrants, or about 250 000 people per year, settled in Canada. In 2016, 21.9% of the Canadian population was born outside Canada. In recent decades, the countries of origin of people immigrating to Canada have become increasingly diverse. Until the 1970s, immigrants came mainly from Western countries and Eastern Europe. Since then, growing numbers of people from Asia, the Middle East, Latin America, the Caribbean, and Africa have settled in Canada. With this increasingly diversified pattern of immigration, Canada's linguistic landscape has altered considerably. An increasing share of immigrants report a language other than English or French as their mother tongue or language spoken most often at home (Statistics Canada, 2019a).

In 2016, nearly three-quarters (72.5%) of immigrants had a language other than English or French as their mother tongue, compared with 50.7% in 1971. Similarly, an increasing proportion of immigrants speak an "other" language most often at home. There is diversity across the country of the top immigrant languages spoken, with Tagalog predominant in the prairie provinces and territories, Punjabi in British Columbia, Mandarin in Ontario, Arabic in Quebec and the maritime provinces, with Mandarin being the top immigrant language in Prince Edward Island (Statistics Canada, 2017).

Among the over 60 Indigenous languages in Canada, the largest language family is Algonquian, which includes Cree, Ojibway, Innu/Montagnais, and Oji-Cree. Those whose mother tongue is Algonquian live mainly in Saskatchewan, Manitoba, Alberta, Quebec, Nova Scotia, and New Brunswick (Statistics Canada, 2018). Not all people who reported speaking an Indigenous language at home reported it at as their mother tongue; that is, they reported another language (e.g., English or French) as their mother tongue but may be learning the Indigenous language as a second language at school.

Trends are on the increase for Indigenous language speaking and learning across Canada; this is an encouraging trend for the transmission of both language and culture. In 2016, 263 840 Canadians reported that they could speak an Indigenous language. The proportion of Indigenous-language speakers who acquired it as a second language increased from 18% in 1996 to 26% in 2016. From 1996 to 2016, the total number of people who could speak an Indigenous language well enough to conduct a conversation rose by 8%. First Nations people accounted for 79% of all Indigenous-language speakers, Inuit for 16%, and Métis for 4%. By comparison, the proportions of the entire population with an Indigenous identity were First Nations at 58%, Métis at 35%, and Inuit at 4%. The extent to which Indigenous languages are spoken depends on a number of personal, family, and geographical factors. For instance, families where at least one parent had an Indigenous language as their mother tongue were more likely to have children who could speak an Indigenous language (Statistics Canada, 2018).

Language is obviously an important part of the everyday expression of a profession's work. Language strongly impacts relationships with patients and other members of the health care team, as well as the reputation of the profession. Respectful, relational nursing care requires a deep commitment to developing therapeutic communication and requires attention to what is not spoken as well as to what is spoken. Individuals and the profession must be aware of language that enacts disrespect, racism, and discrimination—including **microaggressions,** the subtle, often automatic and unconscious, verbal and nonverbal slights, insults, and disparaging messages directed toward people in relation to their gender, age, disability, and cultural or racial group membership. These expressions are perceived as racist by racialized targets; and while they rarely reflect vindictive intent, they inadvertently inflict insult and create unsafe environments for work, services, or care and, if they remain unchecked in our institutions and professions, they contribute to systemic racism

(Grullon, Hunnicutt, Morrison, et al, 2018). Particularly well-hidden in the CHN discourse are these unchecked patterns of microaggressions. The terminology used, the subtle comments, hidden normalization, and practices of oppression are upheld by a long history of racism within professional nursing and community health. The extent to which white privilege and colonialism are embedded in the language of science, medicine, nursing, and health contributes to the subtle and not-so-subtle forms of racism in nursing and the health of communities (Smith, 2019).

Religious Diversity

According to the 2011 NHS, 67.3% of Canadians reported that they were affiliated with a Christian religion. In addition, 7.2% of Canadians reported that they were affiliated with one of the following religions: Muslim, Hindu, Sikh, and Buddhist. The proportion of the population that reported having no religious affiliation was 23.9% (an increase of about 7% from 10 years earlier). Roman Catholics comprise the largest Christian religious group in Canada, and the largest number live in Quebec and Ontario. In all, 4.5% of the Indigenous population reported an affiliation to traditional Indigenous spirituality, representing 0.2% of the overall Canadian population (Statistics Canada, 2013c). Census data projections suggest that the number of people with a non-Christian religion will more than double by 2031 (Statistics Canada, 2010b).

Sexual Diversity

Sexuality is another way in which people differ from one another. Around the world, sexual orientation and gender identity diversity can and does contribute to discrimination, marginalization, harassment in housing, the workplace, or classroom, as well as contributing to increased risks of violence (such as physical attacks, arbitrary arrest, torture, sexual assault, suicide, and murder) (Government of Canada, 2020). Canadians have become much more accepting of sexual diversity; however, this acceptance is evolving and still relatively new. It was only in 2005, after a long series of court battles over same-sex marriage, that Canada became the fourth country in the world to develop a *Civil Marriage Act*. In 2015, a landmark ruling in the United States made same-sex marriage a legal right nationwide in that country. According to the 2016 census, the number of same-sex marriages has more than tripled since 2005, whereas the number of same-sex common-law couples has risen by 28.0%. In 2016, married spouses represented one third (33.4%) of all same-sex couples in Canada (Statistics Canada, 2019b).

CHNs should understand sexual diversity to be able to support diverse patients in a nondiscriminatory manner, and to stand with patients to address discrimination and oppression. Practice and policy in community health have begun consider the sexual diversity of patients, including different sexual orientations and gender identities, same-sex families, and gender transitions from female to male and male to female. Understanding the language of sexual diversity is important in building knowledge and sensitivity that informs community health practices and policies. The acronym LGBTQ2 encompasses both sexual orientation and gender identity and stands for lesbian, gay, bisexual, transgender, queer or questioning, and two spirited. Within an Indigenous context, individuals who feel that their body has both a masculine and feminine spirit may refer to themselves as "two spirited" (Wilson, 1996).

Sources vary considerably in their conception of sexual diversity because few data have been collected on this topic and because sexual orientation and gender identity are generally underreported. Limited research exists on sexual diversity because people do not always feel safe to publicly report their gender identity or sexual orientation; some fear discrimination, prejudice, physical harm, or other expressions of hatred and intolerance (Ziegler, 2019). An understanding of sexual diversity is important to be able to expose intolerance and oppression, which is apparent in the increased rates of hate crimes in relation to sexual orientation (Statistics Canada, 2020a). Consider that 28% of lesbian, gay, and bisexual youth are at higher risk for suicide versus 4% of heterosexual youth (Centre for Suicide Prevention, 2018). In Ontario alone, 1 in 10 youth identify as LGBTQ2. Nurses who are open to discussing gender and sexuality in relation to health care can reduce these risk factors for sexually diverse patients in the community.

CHNs must face health concerns regarding gender and sexuality with awareness and sensitivity. Most home health care providers have not felt comfortable asking specific questions about sexuality and gender because of a lack of knowledge regarding the appropriate terminology to use (Daley & MacDonnell, 2015). This is why the CHN must become familiar, comfortable, accepting, and aware of sexuality, sexual orientation, and gender identities in relation to community health and well-being.

Sexuality is the way that people experience and express themselves as sexual beings. **Sexual orientation** is a person's sexual identity in relation to the gender to which they are attracted. An individual's sexual orientation can be said to be heterosexual, homosexual, or bisexual. Sexual orientation is biological: people are born heterosexual, homosexual, or bisexual. People who identify as **heterosexual** are sexually attracted to people of the opposite sex. Those who identify as **homosexual** are sexually attracted to people of the same sex. Homosexuality can be further classified as *gay* and *lesbian*. Men who are sexually attracted to men often use the term gay to describe their sexual orientation, whereas women who are sexually attracted to women may use the term lesbian. The word *gay* may be used interchangeably by both men and women to describe their sexual orientation. People who are attracted to both men and women use the term *bisexual* to describe their sexual orientation. **Queer or questioning** is the umbrella term for individuals who do not identify as heterosexual (Ziegler, 2019). In 2015, Statistics Canada reported that 1.7% of Canadians between the ages of 18–59 identified as gay or lesbian, whereas 1.3% of Canadians in the same age group identified as bisexual.

Gender refers to a person's identity and social classifications, often based on masculine or feminine qualities and traits (Zunner & Grace, 2012). **Gender identity** refers to one's personal sense of gender and can be classified as cisgender or transgender. **Cisgender** refers to one's gender identity being aligned with their gender assigned at birth. A cisgender female is a person who was born female, identifies as female, and uses feminine pronouns such as she and her. **Transgender** refers to an incongruence in a person's gender identity with the gender assigned at birth. A transgender male is a person who was born female, identifies as male, and may use male pronouns such as him and he (LGBT Health Program, 2015). The sexual orientation of transgender individuals can be heterosexual, lesbian, gay, bisexual, or queer. As with cisgender people, sexual orientation should never be assumed. When asking a patient about their sexual activities, avoid asking questions such as "Do you have a girlfriend?" or "In the last 6 months how many men have you had sex with?" Such questions assume heterosexuality. For patients who do not identify as heterosexual, these types of questions may cause the patient to not fully disclose or discuss anything further as they may feel that you are not open or may pass judgement. Instead, when asking about sexual activity or sexuality, make general statements such as "Do you have sex with men, women, or both?" By asking this question, the CHN is opening the door for further discussion and letting the patient know that their sexuality is not a barrier and that they can feel comfortable having these conversations (Ziegler, 2019).

Very little information exists regarding diversity within LGBTQ2 communities (Scheim & Bauer, 2015). Recent statistics suggest that perhaps 0.5% of the adult population identifies as a trans person, broadly defined. In Ontario, an estimated 23% of trans people completed social and medical gender transition. It is important to note that some trans people live in their felt gender either full-time or part-time, and that trans populations are heterogeneous. Scheim and Bauer (2015) undertook a research study on transgender persons in Ontario that provides insight into the sex, gender, and transition-related characteristics of this population and their implications for policy, practice, and research. There is much to learn in order for community health and well-being to be supported for all people who have been marginalized because of their gender or sexuality in any way.

The Registered Nurses' Association of Ontario (RNAO, 2007) recommends that nurses receive education and training on human rights and health equity that address LGBTQ2 health issues. Cultivating an atmosphere of acceptance and understanding of LGBTQ2 individuals' identities requires people to change the belief that sexual identity is a private matter, when in fact it is a community health concern that requires public attention (Canadian Centre for Diversity and Inclusion, 2020.). The Canadian Centre for Diversity and Inclusion provides a variety of tools for practice issues regarding assessment and self-awareness, which are available on the Evolve website. Keeping abreast of best practices for this population will help CHNs be able to distinguish a person's

biological sex, gender identity, gender expression, and sexual orientation. An understanding of gender fluidity will help CHNs avoid stereotyping women and men into the confines of labels and boundaries of traditional gender roles. CHNs can also support families with transgender children to help them through the stages of gender identity development and the various cultural, legal, and ethnic considerations.

CHNs follow the nursing process and ask questions in a comprehensive assessment, which includes a health history, not to pathologize sexuality or gender identities, but to address needs and facilitate supports and to teach or advocate where there are barriers. When assessing a patient, it is important to ask questions about gender and sexuality as a general part of their health history. With some patients, a sexual or gender history may come up as part of the discussion initiated by the patient. However, the more likely scenario will be that the nurse needs to start the conversation. Before bringing up the topic of sex, sexuality, or gender, it is extremely important to explain to the patient why you are asking these questions, and that you ask all your patients these questions. Patients may ask why the CHN is asking these questions, so it is important to provide them with answers that will further facilitate discussion. For example, if a patient asks why you are asking about their sexuality, the CHN could say "Your sexuality and sexual health are important aspects of your overall health and important to discuss."

When talking to patients about gender and sexuality, it is extremely important to avoid making assumptions. Making heterosexist and gender assumptions could jeopardize the helping relationship. For example, when taking a health history, if the CHN asks a female patient "Do you have a boyfriend?" they are assuming that this patient identifies as heterosexual. If the patient identifies as lesbian, she may answer "no." Not only could this affect the relationship with patients, but it could also cause the CHN to miss key points from the health history. Instead, the CHN can ask "Do you have a partner?" Partner is a gender-neutral term and is appropriate to use when questioning all patients, in order to avoid assumptions. Similarly, to avoid assumption when asking about sexual activity, the CHN should ask "Do you have sex with men, women, or both?" CHNs can effectively obtain a complete sexual history using the algorithm presented in Box 7.1. Assessing gender can be approached along the same open, supportive, and nondiscriminatory lines. When meeting a new patient, ask which gender pronoun they prefer you use. Depending on the circumstance, the CHN can use their preferred pronouns or list those pronouns on their nametag. By creating an open and neutral environment in your assessment and clinical practice, and by routinely asking these questions, CHNs will be able to effectively communicate with patients without making assumptions, and with the potential to break down possible barriers to health and health care.

Disability/Diverse Abilities

Disability is a narrow term used to describe an impairment that restricts activities and participation. It is estimated that

BOX 7.1   Algorithm For Taking A Sexual History

Set the Stage
- Bring up the sexual history as part of the overall history.
- Explain that you ask these questions of all patients.
- Ensure confidentially.

Begin with Three Screening Questions
- Have you been sexually active in the last year?
- Do you have sex with men, women, or both?
- How many people have you had sex with in the last year?

Multiple Partners, New Partners
- Ask about:
  - Partners
  - STI/HIV protection
  - Substance abuse
  - Sexual functioning and satisfaction
  - History of STIs
  - Other concerns

Long-Term Monogamous Partner
- Ask about:
  - Pregnancy plans/protection
  - Trauma/violence
  - Sexual function and satisfaction
  - Other concerns

Not Sexually Active
- Ask about:
  - Past partners
  - Any questions or concerns

Follow Up as Appropriate
- Counselling and education
- Referral
- STI or HIV testing

Source: Adapted from Makadon, H. & Goldhammer, H. (2015). Taking a sexual history and creating affirming environments for lesbian, gay, bisexual, and transgender people. *Journal of the Mississippi State Medical Association, 56*(12), 358–362.

22% or over 6.2 million Canadians over age 15 live with at least one type of disability (Fig. 7.3). The most common disability types are pain, flexibility, mobility, and mental health, with over one-quarter of persons living with a disability reporting a severe disability, and more than 8 out of 10 people using aids or assistive devices (Statistics Canada, 2018).

The stereotypical view that people with a disability live with a specific injury or genetic predisposition such as deafness or blindness does not capture the full meaning of the concept. A nurse may encounter people with chronic or progressive mobility disorders; visual, hearing, or other sensory impairment; chronic illness; mental illness or problematic substance use; or cognitive or intellectual disabilities. Often a disability is an underlying reality, but serious consideration must be given to access to care or adaptive

services when a person is seeking other health and support (e.g., immunization, postpartum care, trauma-informed care, or sexual health support). Access to social care and supports (e.g., housing, education, employment, recreation, and socialization activities) must also be considered for health and well-being of people who experience the diversity of disabilities.

According to World Health Organization (WHO, 2018), disability rates are increasing due to population aging and a rise in chronic health conditions. Chronic diseases are the largest cause of death worldwide (WHO, 2020). In Canada, 65% of all deaths per year are caused by four major chronic conditions: cancer, diabetes, and cardiovascular and chronic respiratory diseases. As seen during the COVID-19 pandemic in 2020, people living with chronic diseases are also at greater risk of influenza and other communicable diseases. In this double-risk scenario, the burden of chronic diseases in terms of morbidity and mortality is great. It is estimated that these diseases cost the Canadian economy $190 billion each year, with $68 billion going to treatment and the rest to lost productivity (Public Health Agency of Canada, 2016).

Patterns of disability involve a range of personal factors (e.g., self-confidence, self-efficacy, and social supports) and environmental factors (e.g., accessible housing, transit, and walkways, and supported employment programs) as well as health conditions (e.g., psychological health, and physical injuries or illnesses). Individuals, families, and communities living with disabilities continue to have poorer health outcomes, lower educational achievements, and high rates of poverty and social isolation. Historically, people with disabilities have been provided services that have led to segregation in institutions or hospital-type settings. However, many individuals have not let their disability define who they are and lead productive and fulfilling lives. Understanding disability through a human rights lens requires nurses to think differently and become aware of issues that prevent differently abled persons from reaching their full potential when addressing activities of daily living.

In 2010, Canada ratified the UN Convention on the Rights of Persons with Disabilities. Outlined in the Convention's articles are strategies that, alongside the *Canadian Human Rights Act*, promote inclusion, awareness, collaboration, and engagement with all stakeholders from a human rights perspective. Every four years, Canada must report to the UN on progress, and it is acknowledged that while there has been advancement, people with disabilities continue to face numerous challenges and barriers that include language and communication, learning and training, and safety and security (Government of Canada, 2018).

Awareness of the demographics and statistics around disability is just one area of concern for CHNs. Awareness of the structural inequities and systematic oppression of people with disabilities is also essential to supporting health and well-being for all people. These inequities are discussed in the following section.

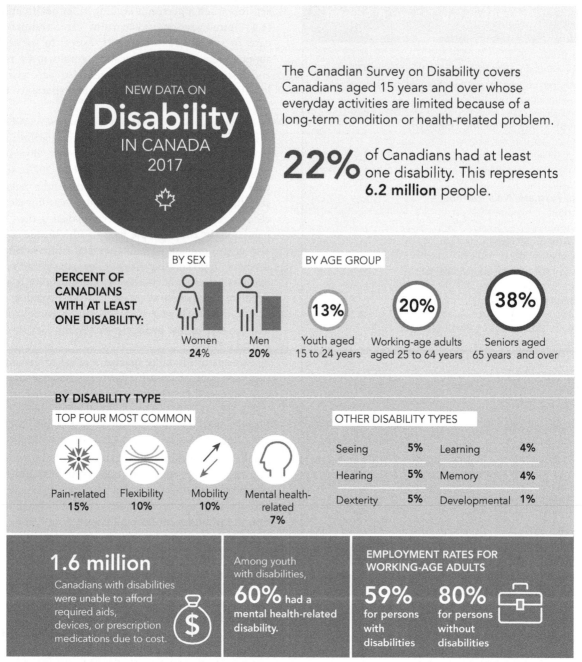

NEW DATA ON
Disability
IN CANADA
2017

The Canadian Survey on Disability covers Canadians aged 15 years and over whose everyday activities are limited because of a long-term condition or health-related problem.

22% of Canadians had at least one disability. This represents **6.2 million** people.

BY SEX

BY AGE GROUP

PERCENT OF CANADIANS WITH AT LEAST ONE DISABILITY:

Women 24%   Men 20%

13% Youth aged 15 to 24 years

20% Working-age adults aged 25 to 64 years

38% Seniors aged 65 years and over

BY DISABILITY TYPE

TOP FOUR MOST COMMON

Pain-related 15%   Flexibility 10%   Mobility 10%   Mental health-related 7%

OTHER DISABILITY TYPES

Seeing   5%   Learning   4%
Hearing   5%   Memory   4%
Dexterity   5%   Developmental   1%

1.6 million Canadians with disabilities were unable to afford required aids, devices, or prescription medications due to cost.

Among youth with disabilities, **60%** had a mental health-related disability.

EMPLOYMENT RATES FOR WORKING-AGE ADULTS

59% for persons with disabilities   **80%** for persons without disabilities

Fig. 7.3 New Data on Disability in Canada, 2017. (*Source:* Statistics Canada. [2017]. *Canadian survey on disability, 2017.* https://www150.statcan.gc.ca/n1/en/pub/11-627-m/11-627-m2018035-eng.pdf?st=jDFl7_N_.)

DIVERSITY, INEQUITIES, AND THE DETERMINANTS OF HEALTH

The circumstances in our daily lives are shaped by the distribution of money, power, and resources at global, national, and local levels, as well as public policy decisions (Ford, 2019). "The social determinants of health are mostly responsible for health inequities—the unfair and avoidable differences in health status seen within and between countries" (WHO, n.d.). The "Determinants of Health" box presents data that indicates how diversity—including race, immigrant or refugee status, access to health care,

sexual diversity, ethnicity, gender, and disability—impact the health of Canadians.

From an equity perspective, the WHO recommends that actions on the social determinants of health occur across sectors. Action across sectors has proved to be an effective way to address community health issues, most notably for tobacco control and in combating global epidemics and pandemics, for instance HIV/AIDS. They are also highly effective in health-emergency situations, which usually require the rapid participation and cooperation of various sectors (e.g., health, security and emergency responders, trade and industry, education, housing, environment, and travel) (WHO, 2015, p. 7).

DETERMINANTS OF HEALTH

Diversity

- One in 6 Canadian adults has experienced racism.*
- Racism is a form of social exclusion, one of the social determinants of health,[†‡] and it contributes to lower income and social status, a determinant of health.[‡]
- Racism not only has a direct effect on a person's health but also influences how health practitioners provide care.[§]
- People who have immigrant or refugee status are more likely to be refused health care and, therefore, less likely to use preventive health care services.[‖]
- The use of health care services among visible minorities varies. For example, Japanese and Korean people tend to visit family physicians less often than South Asians.[#]
- Over 34% of LGBTQ2 individuals self-reported living with extreme levels of stress, whereas almost 23% of the general Canadian population live with high levels of stress.[**]
- Indigenous workers earn between 30% to 40% less than non-Indigenous workers with the same level of education.[††]
- In 2005, recent-immigrant men earned 63 cents for every dollar earned by Canadian-born men, and recent-immigrant women earned 56 cents for every dollar earned by Canadian-born women,[‡‡] thereby contributing to lower socioeconomic status.
- Full-time working women make 20% less on average than full-time working males, which represents less than a 2% reduction in the gender gap over the last 20 years.[††]
- Visible minority workers with a high school diploma working full-time in the private sector earn 27% less than their nonvisible minority counterparts. This gap decreases by about 12% in the public sector.[††]
- Almost 66% of Indigenous children take part in sports regularly (about the same as Canadian children in general); with Métis and Inuit children being most involved in sports. First Nations children living off-reserve have higher rates of sports participation than those living on reserve, and parents of Indigenous children participating in sports generally have higher levels of education and income than parents of nonparticipating children.[§§]
- In 2006, 7.3% of the visible minority population in Canada was over 65 years of age, compared with 13% of the total population,[‡‡] which indicates that as a whole, the visible minority population is younger than the overall Canadian population.
- In 2012, 13.7% of the Canadian adult population reported limited daily activities due to a disability.[‖‖]

* Ipsos-Reid, 2005.
[†‡] Allan & Smylie, 2015; Cameron, Carmargo Plazas, Santos Salas, et al., 2014.
[‡] Mikkonen & Raphael, 2010.
[§] Williams & Mohammed, 2013.
[‖] Pollock, Newbold, Lafrenière, et al., 2012.
[#] Quan, Fong, DeCoster, et al., 2006.
[**] Mental Health Commission of Canada, 2015.
[††] McInturrff & Tulloch, 2014.
[‡‡] Statistics Canada, 2009.
[§§] Statistics Canada, 2007.
[‖‖] Statistics Canada, 2013b.

APPROACHES TO DIVERSITY IN COMMUNITY HEALTH NURSING PRACTICE

The diversity of community health nursing practice settings is as wide-ranging as the Canadian landscape. CHNs have an obligation to contribute to a community's health by delivering services that engage and respond to diverse communities and their needs. The Canadian Nurses Association position statement on promoting cultural competence in nursing states that nurses require "knowledge, skills, attitudes or personal attributes to maximize respectful relationships with diverse populations" (Canadian Nurses Association, 2018, p. 1) (see the CNA links on the Evolve website).

Each of the seven standards of the Canadian Community Health Nursing Professional Practice Model and Standards of Practice addresses diversity and cultural practice standards:

- *Standard 1: Health Promotion*—requires the CHN to recognize the impact of specific issues (including culture) on health.
- *Standard 2: Prevention and Health Protection*—requires the CHN to apply a wide array of local knowledge and cultural activities focused on minimizing incidents of disease and injuries.
- *Standard 3: Health Maintenance, Restoration and Palliation*—requires the CHN to acknowledge diversity, respect the population's specific requests, and provide culturally relevant teaching, counselling, and coordination of health care supports.
- *Standard 4: Professional Relationships*—requires the CHN to connect with patients in culturally meaningful ways and to interact with patients based on respect and acceptance of cultural diversity.
- *Standard 5: Capacity Building*—requires the CHN to collaborate with individuals, families, groups, and communities in culturally congruent ways that build on existing strengths.
- *Standard 6: Access and Equity*—requires the CHN to provide culturally sensitive care and facilitate inclusive, equitable access to services in the community.
- *Standard 7: Evidence Informed Practice*—requires the CHN to read, understand, synthesize, adapt, and implement the evidence in areas related to practice with diverse populations.
- *Professional Responsibility and Accountability*—requires the CHN to embrace self-awareness and recognize how cultural biases influence nursing practice (Community Health Nurses of Canada, 2019).*

Numerous approaches, models, strategies, and skills exist to guide the CHN in working with diverse populations. At the core of all of them is an intention to listen to the unique experience of others. Understanding that every person has a story and that their experience is invaluable is essential to nursing in communities (Spadoni, Hartrick Doane, Sevean, et al., 2015). Ultimately, the art of asking questions is one of the most important skills a CHN has to elicit accurate and pertinent

*Adapted with permission from *Canadian Community Health Nursing, Professional Practice Model & Standards of Practice* (p. 8), Community Health Nurses of Canada. Reprinted with permission.

information from diverse patients. That art also applies to the questions CHNs should ask themselves to ensure they are providing culturally responsive care to patients. Campinha-Bacote (2002) developed the mnemonic "ASKED," which represents key questions CHNs should reflect on:

- *Awareness:* Am I aware of my personal biases and prejudices toward cultural groups?
- *Skills:* Do I have the skills to perform a culturally based assessment?
- *Knowledge:* Do I understand the patient's world view and the field of biocultural ecology?
- *Encounters:* How many encounters have I had with patients from different backgrounds?
- *Desire:* Why do I want to be culturally competent?

These questions can help CHNs incorporate notions of diversity and culture into their way of thinking and ongoing reflexive practice (Campinha-Bacote, 2002). They can also help CHNs provide safe, competent, and ethical care based on patients' cultural values and beliefs.

Other interactional strategies for establishing relationships with structurally vulnerable or stigmatized patients have been developed. For example, Porr and colleagues (Porr, 2015; Porr, Drummond, & Olson, 2012) looked at the relational tools that could be used to build relationships with single mothers living on public assistance. They proposed that establishing a therapeutic relationship with this patient group entails six interdependent stages: (1) projecting optimism, (2) focusing on child as mediating presence, (3) ascertaining motives, (4) exercising social facility, (5) engaging in concerted intentionality, and (6) redrawing professional boundaries. This model requires the nurse to always be present (face to face), be aware of stressors from a social-context lens, take the time to listen, maintain a caseload of patients over an extended period of time, and build a mentorship or support network with colleagues for debriefing and exploring alternative strategies to connect individuals and families with community agency services (Bourque Bearskin, 2014).

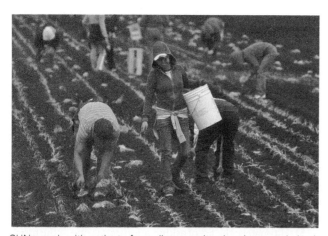

CHNs work with patients from diverse cultural and economic backgrounds. One such group is migrant workers, who often have high occupational mobility and who may seek health care only when they are too ill to work. It is important for a CHN to support these patients regarding disease prevention, health maintenance, health protection, and health promotion activities before the patient moves. (iStockphoto/Joseph Sorrentino)

When CHNs approach patients equitably, they practise nursing with awareness and an underlying respect for diversity (see the "Evidence-Informed Practice" box). *Enhancing Cultural Competency: A Resource Kit for Health Care Professionals* (Alberta Health Services, 2009) provides general information on topics such as barriers to health care, diverse world views, language, literacy, health practices, communication, prevalent diseases, and political and acculturation issues.

EVIDENCE-INFORMED PRACTICE

A critical ethnographic research study by McCabe and Holmes (2014) explored the experience of nurses who provided sexual health care to adolescents with physical and/or developmental disabilities. Participants were selected using a purposive sampling technique. The study was conducted in an urban pediatric rehabilitation facility that provides services to youth who have congenital and acquired disabilities. One of the aims of the study was to understand the institutional and social discourses that informed nurses' interactions.

Participants helped identify factors that inform nursing action and inaction. They reported that therapeutic relationship training, combined with a broader understanding of social and health determinants, prepared nurses well to engage with patients and families regarding the sexuality and gender of youth with disabilities. Nurses also considered themselves to be well positioned and knowledgeable on ways to engage patients and families on this sensitive topic. As well, because nurses occupy the role of "caring agent," they are well positioned to build family-oriented and strengths-based approaches to promoting sexual health. However, nurses found that providing care was complicated by the limited time and space they had to interact with patients. Institutional-level barriers were identified as scheduling and pre-established priorities as well as social barriers of stigma attached to the sexuality of youth with disabilities. In addition, attempts by nurses to normalize the issues of sexuality in disabled youth were found to cause more harm than good; instead, acknowledgement of the differences and support for alternatives was helpful to patients.

Application for CHNs
- Recognize that everyone, including disabled youth, has a gender identity and sexuality interests.
- Be aware of your own personal beliefs about sexuality and gender fluidity.
- Be ready to assert your own personal privacy boundaries.
- Include sexuality and sexual preferences as part of your regular assessments.
- Use accurate language to reference body parts, processes, and functions.
- Consider the contextual reality of disability and consider the differences as well as the universal interests.

Questions for Reflection and Discussion
1. Why would attempts to normalize sexuality in particular populations be found unhelpful?
2. What options does the CHN have to promote healthy sexuality and experiences?
3. How can diversity be approached as a strength and from an asset-based perspective?

Source: McCabe, J., & Holmes, D. (2014). Nursing, sexual health and youth with disabilities: A critical ethnography. *Journal of Advanced Nursing, 70*(1), 77–86. https://doi.org/10.1111/jan.12167.

CULTURAL COMPETENCE

In response to Canada's diverse cultural landscape, the demand has grown for CHNs to provide high-quality, effective, culturally sensitive, respectful, and culturally agile care (Government of British Columbia, 2020). Many definitions of *cultural competence* exist, and many are contested for their essentialist views of culture that suggest there are some natural and unchanging characteristics of people from cultural groups, making claims of defined categorization (Powell, 2016; Wesp, Scheer, Ruiz, et al., 2018). **Cultural competence** is an ongoing process, rather than an outcome, and the process is thought to fit within other practices and ways of being, such as cultural agility and humility. A culturally competent health care provider is aware of his or her own cultural identity and views on different cultures and is sensitive to and accepting of patients' differing views (Srivastava, 2007). In order to address unique individuals in their specific contexts and environments, nurses need to move beyond essentialist perspectives of cultural competence that provide a checklist of attributes (Greene-Moton & Minkler, 2020; Gregory, Harrowing, Lee, et al., 2010). A more emancipatory view of cultural competence draws on the intersectional, feminist, postcolonial, and critical race theories (Wesp et al., 2018).

The cultural competence process helps nurses understand culture as socially constructed within a historical context that reflects the values and assumptions of the society at a particular time (Campinha-Bacote, 1999, 2018). According to this view, culture is not to be thought of in terms of race or bloodline, but rather as "everyday experiences of marginalization" (Kirkham & Anderson, 2002, p. 2). Cultural competence begins by acknowledging experiences and the fundamental variations in the ways patients respond to health care challenges. A nurse can begin by asking patients questions about health inequities, poverty, and policies and practices that may include or exclude access to appropriate services (Rowan, Rukholm, Bourque-Bearskin, et al., 2013). At the same time, the nurse would seek to understand the patient's health promotion activities; social connections; ability to cope with pain; grieving practices; and culturally specific beliefs, values, and practices (which are individually expressed and also socially or culturally informed).

The Nova Scotia Department of Health produced a *Cultural Competence Guide for Primary Health Care Professionals in Nova Scotia* that comprises tools and resources that can assist health care providers in administering culturally competent health care (see the link on the Evolve website). This document addresses key concepts that impact the health status of Nova Scotia's diverse communities, such as power, privilege, equity, racism, and oppression (Nova Scotia Department of Health, 2005). It also includes a discussion on the eight steps to developing cultural competence (Box 7.2), consideration of the determinants of health such as equity and access, and inequitable access to primary health care.

An example of cultural competence with a community-level focus was the establishment of a coalition between two Saskatchewan Indigenous communities, a health region,

---

BOX 7.2 Eight Steps to Developing Cultural Competence

1. Know yourself by analyzing your values, behaviours, views, and assumptions.
2. Be aware of racism and the systems or behaviours that foster racism.
3. Reframe your thinking by engaging in activities that encourage others' views and perspectives.
4. Become familiar with the core cultural aspects of your community.
5. Partner with patients to facilitate a comparison of their perceptions and your findings of the core cultural aspects of the community.
6. Familiarize yourself with different cultures and their perceptions and practices for health and illness, and explore with patients their cultural uniqueness (diversity) regarding health and illness.
7. Establish rapport, respect, and trust with patients and co-workers by being open, understanding, and willing to accept varying perceptions.
8. Establish an environment that is welcoming for the diverse cultures within your community.

Source: Nova Scotia Department of Health. (2005). *A cultural competence guide for primary health care professionals in Nova Scotia* (p. 13, Section 2). https://www.mycna.ca/~/media/nurseone/page-content/pdf-en/cultural_competence_guide_for_primary_health_care_professionals.pdf.

---

and three tertiary educational institutions. The objective was to determine cultural elements that demonstrated respect in the delivery of direct health care and ways to deliver health education programs for Indigenous peoples that were respectful of their cultural diversity. Another example is the decades-long recognition of diversity within the Canadian Institutes of Health Research. The refocus on diversity and Indigenous knowledge-making resulted in an action plan for research and knowledge mobilization to strengthen First Nation, Inuit, and Metis peoples' health (Canadian Institutes of Health Research, 2016). The approach used by these communities demonstrates cultural competence through collaboration, respect, and trust, building system-wide integration of Indigenous knowledge. Effectively addressing structural racism and discrimination requires this level of systemic change.

An example of cultural competence with an individual-level focus involves a recent Chinese immigrant who speaks little English and goes to an urban community health centre because of a urinary tract infection. The culturally competent CHN understands the need to use strategies that allow the CHN to communicate effectively with the patient. The CHN also understands that the patient has the right to effective care, to judge whether she has received the care she wants, and to follow up with appropriate action if she does not receive the expected care. In this interaction, the CHN demonstrates cultural competence by being sensitive to the patient's modesty by using a female interpreter to explain the physical examination procedures. The CHN also explores with this patient the use of traditional medicines and practices for pain and infections.

CHNs working with Indigenous people in Canada need to understand that this population has specific health care beliefs and care practices. They may have healers, often called *medicine healers, traditional knowledge holders,* or *shamans,* who provide service to people in their communities. Some of the traditions found in First Nations communities are smudging with sage or sweetgrass and gifting of tobacco; using sweat lodges, which are associated with spirituality; using the medicine wheel to represent a holistic balance; and connecting with the circle of life to reach balance and harmony. CHNs need to be aware of their own values, beliefs, and biases toward healing and health care practices that may differ from their own.

Developing Culturally Responsive Care

The values of inclusivity, respect, valuing differences, equity, and commitment underlie culturally competent care for individuals, families, groups, and communities. These values should be embedded in all processes, policies, and practices of nurses and health care organizations (RNAO, 2007). Culturally competent care is provided not only to individuals of racial or ethnic groups but also to individuals belonging to groups based on factors such as age, religion, sexual orientation, and socioeconomic status. Nurses need to be culturally competent to provide nursing care that meets the needs of these persons. Cultural nursing assessment is discussed later in this chapter.

Developing cultural competence is an ongoing life process that involves every aspect of patient care. It is challenging and at times painful as nurses struggle to adopt new ways of thinking and performing. Core principles of developing cultural competence are highlighted by McFarland and Wehebe-Alama (2018), who draw from the origins of culture care principles and suggest the following two principles as a starting point:

1. Maintain a broad, objective, and open attitude toward individuals and their cultures.
2. Avoid seeing all individuals as alike.

Nurses develop cultural competence in different ways, but the key elements are having direct experience with patients of other cultures, reflecting on this experience, and promoting mutual respect for differences. Burchum (2002) identified five attributes of cultural competence: (1) cultural awareness, (2) cultural knowledge, (3) cultural understanding, (4) cultural sensitivity, and (5) cultural skill. Two other attributes of cultural competence are cultural interaction and cultural proficiency. Table 7.3 presents these seven attributes, their dimensions, and considerations for CHNs.

CHNs can help culturally diverse patients in relation to their health literacy and self-management. Educational or self-help groups facilitated by the CHN or others can help patients from different cultures learn new adaptation strategies and ways to relate to other families, the community, schools, and workplaces. An important role of the CHN working with diverse populations is that of advocate. CHNs have an obligation to support access to health care for diverse groups who may not have that access. CHNs also

advocate at the local, provincial, and federal levels for policies that support adaptation of diverse groups, for example, assisting patients from different countries to adjust in their new or unfamiliar environment. For example, a policy change that was initiated by a municipality to assist a culturally diverse group of wheelchair users involved the requirement that all local public buildings have ramps to accommodate wheelchairs. As a result of this change, all public buildings in the community now have wheelchair access. CHNs can use an environmental scan to assess communities to ensure that issues affecting diverse groups are addressed.

To provide culturally competent care, CHNs need to appreciate and understand the diversity issues experienced by and the cultural backgrounds of their patients. Although research has identified certain health beliefs and practices within First Nations, Inuit, francophone, Black, and Chinese cultures, CHNs need to remember that those beliefs and practices differ among regions of the country, within communities, and among individuals.

Inhibitors to Culturally Responsive Care

When CHNs fail to provide culturally competent care, it may be because they do not understand relational practice, are pressured by supervisors to improve productivity by increasing their caseloads, or are pressured by colleagues who are not knowledgeable about other cultures. These and similar forces inhibit the delivery of culturally responsive care and may result in some of the following CHN behaviours:

- **Ethnocentrism.** Ethnocentrism is a type of cultural prejudice in which one believes that his or her "own cultural values, beliefs, and behaviours are the best, preferred, and the most superior ways" (Srivastava, 2007, p. 5). For example, CHNs who assume that their way of providing nursing care is the only right way are ethnocentric.
- **Cultural blindness.** Cultural blindness is a denial of diversity and inability to recognize the uniqueness of individual patients. For example, a CHN, attempting to be culturally unbiased, treats all patients in the same manner, conducts nursing assessments with the same questions, and consequently fails to gain an understanding of each patient's culture and diversity. Hilario, Browne, and McFadden (2018) show how nurses have perpetuated systemic racism through practices of cultural blindness in research as well as community practice.
- **Bias.** Bias is "the negative evaluation of one group and its members relative to another" (Choi & Jakubec, 2017). Bias may be intentional or unconscious. For example, a CHN who is biased implements nursing care based on personal attitudes, cognitive errors, prejudices, and stereotypes.
- **Culture shock.** Culture shock is a condition that involves feelings of anxiety because of exposure to unfamiliar environments and culture. The person feels threatened and helpless while trying to adapt to the unfamiliar culture with its different practices, values, and beliefs. For example, a person from Somalia arrives in Canada and finds the unfamiliar environment and culture overwhelming.

TABLE 7.3   Attributes and Dimensions of Cultural Competence

Attributes and Definitions	Dimensions	CHN Considerations
Cultural awareness is self-examination and in-depth exploration of one's own beliefs and values as they influence behaviour*,†	• Understand your own culture • Know your ethnocentric views, biases, and prejudices • Be aware of similarities and differences between and among cultures	CHNs who have developed cultural awareness are: • Receptive to learning about the cultural dimensions of the patient • Able to understand their own cultural beliefs and behaviour and how these can influence the delivery of competent care to persons from cultures other than their own‡ • Able to recognize that health is expressed differently across cultures and that culture influences an individual's responses to health, illness, disease, and death
Cultural knowledge is information about organizational elements of diverse cultures and ethnic groups. Emphasis is on learning about the patient's world view from an emic (native) perspective. An understanding of the patient's culture decreases misinterpretations and the misapplication of scientific knowledge and facilitates the patient's cooperation with the health care regimen.*,‖	• Know about cultures other than your own • Be able to recognize differences in communication styles between and within cultures • Become familiar with conceptual and theoretical frameworks	Cultural competence is knowledge-based care.§ McFarland and Wehebe-Alama‖ point out that nurses who lack cultural knowledge may develop feelings of inadequacy and helplessness if they are unable to effectively help their patients. Although it is unrealistic to expect that nurses will have knowledge of all cultures, they need to be aware of and know how to obtain the knowledge of cultural influences that affect groups with whom they most frequently interact
Cultural understanding refers to continuous reflections on the effects of culture (values, beliefs, and behaviours) for diverse patients#	• Understand that "Western medicine" does not have all the answers • Recognize how culture shapes your beliefs, values, and behaviours • To avoid stereotyping, be aware that there are racial, ethnic, and cultural variations • Understand the concerns and issues that occur when your values, beliefs, and practices differ from those of the dominant culture • Know that marginalization influences patterns of seeking care	CHNs who achieve cultural understanding practise with patients in a manner that demonstrates recognition of a variety of ways of knowing. CHNs also recognize and accept that patients from various cultures use alternative and complementary therapies. CHNs also deal with problems such as marginalization that result from differing beliefs and values
Cultural sensitivity is "knowing how."§ Cultural sensitivity refers to being able to reflect on the influence of one's own culture on practice, and to appreciate, "respect, and value cultural diversity"#	• Appreciate and respect your individual patient's beliefs and values • Appreciate and value diversity • Appreciate and genuinely care about those of other cultures • Recognize how your own cultural background may influence professional practice	In all patient interactions, CHNs are aware of and respect patient cultural diversity. CHNs also consider how personal and professional identity influence nursing practice. CHNs' verbal and nonverbal behaviours are polite and respectful**
Cultural interaction refers to the verbal and nonverbal communication between persons of different cultures	• Interact with those of other cultures • Engage in practice with those of other cultures	CHNs engage in effective communication, use the appropriate language and literacy level, and learn directly from patients about their life experiences and the significance of these experiences for health‖

Continued

TABLE 7.3 Attributes and Dimensions of Cultural Competence—cont'd

Attributes and Definitions	Dimensions	CHN Considerations
Cultural skill refers to the effective integration of cultural awareness and cultural knowledge to obtain relevant cultural data and meet the needs of culturally diverse patients.[††]	• Perform cultural assessments that consider beliefs and values, family roles, health practices, and the meanings of health and illness • Perform physical assessments that incorporate knowledge of racial variations • Be sure to communicate, either personally or through appropriate use of interpreters and other resources, in a manner that is understood and is responsive to those who speak other languages • Make sure your nonverbal communication techniques take into consideration the patient's use of eye contact, facial expressions, body language, touch, and space • Know how to provide care that incorporates the development of a respectful and therapeutic alliance with the patient • Provide care that overcomes biases and is modified to respect and accommodate the values, beliefs, and practices of the patient without compromising your own values • Provide care that is beneficial, safe, and satisfying to your patient • Know how to provide care that elicits a feeling by the patient of being welcome, understood, important, and comfortable • Provide care that addresses disadvantages arising from the patient's position in relation to networks • Use self-empowerment strategies in your patient care	CHNs use appropriate touch during conversation, modify the physical distance between themselves and others, and use strategies to avoid cultural misunderstandings while meeting mutually agreed-upon goals[††]
Cultural proficiency refers to the demonstration of new knowledge and cultural skills, including the communication of this information	• Add new knowledge by conducting research, by developing new culturally sensitive therapeutic approaches, and by delivering this information to others • Demonstrate a commitment to change though ongoing reflective practice	CHNs participate in and use research in nursing practice with culturally diverse patients

Source: Adapted from Burchum, J. L. (2002). Cultural competence: an evolutionary perspective. *Nursing Forum, 37*(4), 5–15.
*Campinha-Bacote, 2002.
[†]Misener, Sowell, Phillips, et al., 1997.
[‡]Pottinger, Perivolaris, & Howes, 2007.
[§]Srivastava, 2007.
[||]McFarland & Wehebe-Alama, 2018.
[#]Burchum, 2002.
[**]Giger, Davidhizar, Purnell, et al., 2007.
[††]Stanhope & Lancaster, 2018.

- **Stereotyping.** Stereotyping occurs when generalizations are applied to an individual without exploring individual values, beliefs, and behaviours. For example, a CHN decides that an Italian patient with diabetes eats too much pasta and therefore cannot control blood sugar levels. As a result, the CHN does not ask the patient about the kinds of foods he eats on a regular basis.
- **Prejudice.** Prejudice is a negative attitude about a person or group without factual data (Srivastava, 2007). For example, "older persons do not have sex."
- **Racism.** Racism is a form of prejudice in which members of one cultural group perceive themselves to be superior

to another cultural group (Canadian Public Health Association, 2018). For example, "White people in Canada are superior to other racial groups."

Being aware of patients' cultural beliefs and knowing about other cultures may help CHNs to be less judgmental, more accepting of cultural variations, and less likely to engage in the behaviours previously listed, which inhibit cultural competence.

Racism

Racism is most frequently thought of in terms of a response to skin colour, ethnic origin, or religion; however, it can be directed at other aspects of culture such as cultural celebrations, traditional dress, and traditional food. The most common types of racism cited in the literature are overt and systemic. *Overt racism* is an open demonstration by attitudes, actions, policies, and practices of a feeling of superiority over individuals or groups with the intent of harming or damaging (Government of Canada, 2019a). Hate crimes, for example, are considered as one example of overt racism. *Systemic racism* can be identified by *institutional racism,* which involves policies within organizations, corporations, and institutions that are not equally applied to all individuals and groups, producing inequitable opportunities and impacts based on race (Bourque Bearskin, 2014; Bourque Bearskin et al., 2016; RNAO, 2007). An example would be when a job position is available only to persons who are Canadian born. Founded on the ideology of white supremacy, another form of systemic racism is **structural racism,** the normalization and legitimization of an interplay of historical, cultural, institutional, and interpersonal dynamics that routinely advantages White people while producing cumulative and chronic adverse outcomes for people of colour. While there are numerous examples of this, educational requirements and admissions policies, or policing and incarceration patterns are just two examples. Because of the layered dynamics, it is difficult to specifically identify where and how structural racism occurs. The results of structural racism are apparent in inequalities in power, access, opportunities, treatment, and policy impacts and outcomes, whether they are intentional or not (Alberta Civil Liberties Research Centre, 2020). The Black Lives Matter movement is calling on all people to investigate the systemic racism within our communities and society as a whole, including within the institutions of health care and nursing.

Racism *will* be encountered in institutions and it grossly impacts community health nursing practice (RNAO, 2007). The CHN may experience racism in patient interactions, collegial nursing interactions, workplace organizational systems, and community systems. Racism in CHN practice (whether toward a patient or toward the CHN) needs to be labelled and addressed when it occurs, or it can lead to oppression. It may also be detrimental to patient health and access to health care services. The Canadian Public Health Association recognizes that we are all either overtly or inadvertently racist and that the influence of this racism affects the health of individuals and populations (Canadian Public Health Association, 2018). The CHN needs to consider the culture, beliefs, and values of patients, as well as the role of power imbalances, oppression, and racism that occurs within each nurse–patient interaction.

CULTURAL SAFETY

Cultural safety is defined by the patient in nurse–patient interactions (De & Richardson, 2008). **Cultural safety** refers to gaining an understanding of others' health beliefs and practices so that health care actions work toward equity and avoid discrimination. There is recognition of and respect for cultural identity so that power balance exists between the health care provider and the patient (Anderson, Perry, Blue,

et al., 2003; Racine, 2014; Ramsden, 2002; Srivastava, 2007). The recognition of kinship and love in an ethical, relational practice have been more recently emphasized as a vehicle for enacting cultural safety (Sheppard, 2020).

The term *cultural safety* was first coined by Irihapeti Ramsden, a Maori nurse in New Zealand. She identified the need to address cultural issues in relation to health care interactions between Maori patients and non-Maori health care providers. Ramsden asserted that cultural safety extends beyond the concept of cultural competence and that nurses need to be self-aware, be conscious of their own culture, and understand theories of power relations. In this context, cultural safety is an outcome of nursing care that enables those who receive the service to define safe service. Ramsden's research offers insight into the historical and political issues surrounding the delivery of health care services to the Maori population (Ramsden, 2002).

The National Aboriginal Health Organization (2006) asserted that cultural safety is built on the principle of biculturalism, which differs from transcultural nursing concepts in that transcultural nursing care develops from the dominant culture. Gray and Thomas (2006) support the view of culture as relational, and as a sociopolitical construct it involves power relationships in nurse–patient interactions. Therefore, when CHNs use a cultural safety lens, they involve the patient in addressing health inequities and striving for social justice. Cultural safety is about fostering an understanding of the relationship between minority status and health status so that practices and systems of health care that do not support the health of minority groups are identified and addressed (Arieli, Friedman, & Hirschfeld, 2012).

According to De and Richardson (2008), cultural safety is based on:

- The health care provider's analysis of his or her cultural self and its influence on patient interactions
- Acknowledgement of the power imbalance between the health care provider and the patient
- The health care provider learning and applying basic skills.

For the CHN to work effectively with patients from various cultural backgrounds and to provide culturally responsive health care, cultural safety and cultural competence need to be addressed and implemented in patient interactions (Bourque Bearskin, 2014; Bourque Bearskin et al., 2016; De & Richardson, 2008; Dion Stout & Downey, 2006).

The concept of cultural safety has become widely applied by organizations working with First Nations, Inuit, and Métis people. The Canadian Indigenous Nurses Association (CINA), Indigenous Physicians Association of Canada, the former National Aboriginal Health Organization (Saint Elizabeth Health, 2020), and the National Collaborating Centre for Aboriginal Health have all identified Indigenous peoples as a key group requiring culturally safe practice.

According to the Truth and Reconciliation Commission of Canada (2015), colonization continues to affect the traditional values and social structures of Indigenous people in Canada. It also contributes to inequities in the health status of Indigenous people in Canada. The context of colonialism encouraged the development of dominant systems of care that resulted in discrimination against and disempowerment of Indigenous peoples. Some of these influences have carried over to postcolonial times, sparking a desire for improved cultural competence and safety (National Aboriginal Health Organization, 2006; Saint Elizabeth Health, 2020).

Cultural safety requires a set of basic skills that can be learned through cultural sensitivity and cultural competence training. A culturally safe nurse–patient relationship requires that nurses understand the need for: Indigenous peoples' access to traditional health care practices and ceremonies; engagement, dialogue, and consultations with health care administrators and providers; health administrators' and providers' respect for the rights of diverse knowledge; and the enactment of ethical commitments, culturally safe practices, and collective thinking. All of these elements can lead to a holistic understanding of culture and a sense of humility to raise the nurse's consciousness of cultural safety.

The Canadian Indigenous Nurses Association website (https://indigenousnurses.ca/) provides further information on its cultural competence and cultural safety initiative (see the link on the Evolve website).

Cultural Humility

The concept of cultural humility encompasses a process that requires CHNs to continually engage in self-reflection and self-critique as lifelong learners and reflective practitioners.

Cultural humility also brings into check the power imbalances that exist in the dynamics of the health care setting (Tervalon & Murray-Garcia, 1998). CHNs will be better prepared for culturally safe practice by learning cultural humility (Levi, 2009). Approaching health care with cultural humility goes beyond the concept of cultural safety to encourage individuals to identify and acknowledge their own biases. Cultural humility acknowledges that it is impossible to be adequately knowledgeable about cultures other than one's own and requires that we take responsibility for our interactions with others beyond acknowledging or being sensitive to our differences (Greene-Moton & Minkler, 2020). Having a sense of humility is being comfortable with a position of not knowing and not being the expert. The "Evidence-Informed Practice" box considers how CHNs can apply cultural humility with patients who experience diversities of abilities, language, culture, and who are seeking community support.

Cultural humility is not an end in itself; rather, it is a commitment to a way of being and an active process of relating to one another (Hoskins, 1999; Racher & Annis, 2007). Hoskins (1999) outlined five major processes that can help people work toward cultural humility: (1) acknowledging the pain of oppression, (2) engaging in acts of humility, (3) acting with reverence, (4) engaging in mutuality, and (5) maintaining a position of not knowing.

⚄ EVIDENCE-INFORMED PRACTICE

A qualitative research study by Khanlou, Haque, Mustafa, et al. (2017) focused on the lived experiences of new immigrant Canadian mothers of children with autism spectrum disorder. Equal access for autism services remains suboptimal for diverse groups. In Canada, little is known about the barriers that immigrant mothers face in accessing services and support for their children with developmental disabilities.

In this qualitative study, 21 immigrant mothers of children with autism, from diverse ethnocultural backgrounds, were interviewed. Structural support challenges, such as delays in diagnosis, impacted available financial and community health support featured for these family caregivers. Fragmented and dispersed services were common. Barriers to instrumental support (the tangible support that mothers can get from formal networks such as family and friends, and from informal networks, such as social institutions and compassionate service providers) as a result of loss of social ties and stigma were routinely experienced. Lack of expected support from partners and negative perceptions of services were identified as emotional and perceptive challenges. Attention at all these sites to support by community health practitioners and decision makers will be important to address intersecting inequalities and the unique circumstances of family caregivers.

Application for CHNs

Research on the lived experiences of others helps CHNs understand how individuals define and live with experiences in their own ways. Although research informs CHNs about the

lived experiences of particular groups, it does not define those groups. Rather, it enhances CHNs' understanding that certain commonalities and individual differences exist within groups. CHNs who communicate verbally with ease can never truly understand what it is like to learn a new language as an adult, or to have autism spectrum disorder with restricted social and communication abilities. However, they are responsible for meeting the needs and respecting the rights of patients with diverse neuro-developmental circumstances. That may entail changing the way they communicate and interrelate with this group and their caregivers.

Questions for Reflection and Discussion

1. You are going to make a home visit with a family caregiver who is a recent immigrant with limited English language abilities and who is the primary support person for a child with a neuro-developmental disability who uses an electronic communication device but otherwise is nonverbal. What might you consider related to communication strategies and practice possibilities prior to the visit? What questions might you ask during the visit?
2. You are going to be presenting a paper of a relevant community health topic at the local chapter of the Canadian Autism Spectrum Disorders Alliance. What factors do you need to consider when making this presentation?
3. Which components of the model for evidence-informed practice and decision making discussed in Chapter 5 would be applicable to Khanlou et al.'s research study?

Source: Khanlou, N., Haque, N., Mustafa, N., Vazquez, L., Mantini, A., & Weiss, J. (2017). Access barriers to services by immigrant mothers of children with autism in Canada. *International Journal of Mental Health and Addiction, 15*(2), 239–259.

CULTURAL NURSING ASSESSMENT

Culturally competent and safe care requires culturally responsive attitudes, knowledge, and skills, which are developed and enhanced through cultural nursing assessments. A **cultural nursing assessment** is a systematic way of identifying the beliefs, values, meanings, and behaviours of people while considering their history, life experiences, and the social and physical environments in which they live.

CHNs need to conduct a cultural nursing assessment for all patients. It is important that CHNs be aware that some patients might be reluctant to openly acknowledge cultural identity, such as racial background, religion, age, and sexual orientation. This reluctance to disclose information may be due to a fear of prejudice or discrimination, commitment to assimilation as a Canadian, mistrust of authority, or discomfort with direct questioning and other forms of nonverbal communication such as direct eye contact. CHNs need to seek information from sources such as family members, interpreters, traditional cultural health practitioners, and educational resources on how to integrate cultural concepts into patient care to meet their patients' total health care needs. In addition, they need to be able to distinguish between cultural and socioeconomic class issues so as not to misinterpret behaviour as having a cultural origin when, in fact, it should be attributed to socioeconomic class.

Many factors need to be considered when conducting a cultural nursing assessment, such as communication, space, social organization, time, environmental control, and biological variations (Giger, 2016). The Giger and Davidhizar Transcultural Assessment Model can assist CHNs in bringing together the variety of factors and dimensions in an assessment. A synopsis of the model is provided in Appendix 5. Key areas of competency for cultural assessment are awareness of population demographic changes; general information about cultural groups; how and when to use a focused assessment; how to use an interpreter; and how to assess and consider the social, political, and economic factors in the community (Astle et al., 2019).

When using Giger and Davidhizar's Transcultural Assessment Model, CHNs must recognize that it does little to address power and privilege, but it does provide a way to begin a cultural assessment. The model includes the following categories:

1. *Culturally unique individual.* The CHN needs to elicit patient cultural data as outlined in the "Culturally Unique Individual" section (see Appendix 5).
2. *Communication.* An understanding by the CHN of differences in communication patterns can help overcome communication barriers due to culture; therefore, the quality of patient care will be improved. Some patients from diverse cultural backgrounds may be reluctant to speak to a traditional CHN about nontraditional health care beliefs and practices. The use of therapeutic communication skills such as conveying respect, warmth, and genuineness is necessary. The CHN should assess the patient's need for an interpreter.
3. *Space.* The physical distance between the patient and the CHN is an important consideration in promoting the comfort level of the patient during interactions. The CHN should take the cue from the patient and inquire about appropriate physical distance in interviews.
4. *Social organization.* There are various types of families, such as traditional nuclear, lone-parent, blended, same-sex, and communal families. CHNs need to incorporate the family cultural beliefs and concerns into a patient care plan (see Chapter 12).
5. *Time.* It is important for the CHN to recognize that patients from different cultures may view time differently. The CHN may become quite frustrated when many members arrive approximately 30 minutes past the scheduled start time of the group meeting. A culturally sensitive CHN will be aware that this lateness is not an avoidance of the topic but rather reflects the group's cultural view of time.
6. *Biological variations.* To provide culturally competent and safe nursing care, CHNs need to be familiar with the biological variations associated with racial groups and to consider the uniqueness of cultural groups and individuals. This awareness also needs to incorporate the fact that biological parameters are usually based on White standards and that these norms may not be applicable to non-White patients. Use extreme caution with guidelines that suggest White-centred norms.

Skills such as listening, explaining, acknowledging, recommending, understanding, and negotiating help the CHN to be nonjudgmental with patients. It is vital that CHNs listen to patients' perceptions of their health concerns and, in turn, that CHNs explain to patients their perceptions of their concerns. To develop recommendations for managing health concerns, CHNs and patients need to acknowledge and discuss similarities and variations between their perceptions. CHNs also negotiate with patients on nursing care actions to meet patients' needs.

Relational Practice: Assessment and Intervening Processes

Relational practice "is guided by conscious participation with patients using a number of relational skills including listening, questioning, empathy, mutuality, reciprocity, self-observation, reflection and a sensitivity to emotional contexts" (College of Nurses of Ontario, 2018, p. 11). It helps CHNs make better-informed, culturally competent decisions about the best care for diverse patients (e.g., patients of different gender identities, sexual orientation, abilities, spirituality, income, language, and geographical locations) (RNAO, 2006). Relational practice places CHN care within the context of relationships (Bergum & Dossetor, 2005; Pollard, 2015). It asks CHNs to look beyond the restrictive labels of ethnicity, visible minority, age, and so on to see patients as individuals with their own history and identity (Hartrick Doane & Varcoe, 2015). Relational practice has been shown to improve health outcomes for patients and the job satisfaction of nurses (Andersen & Havaei, 2015; Johannessen, Werner, & Steihaug, 2013).

In their practice, CHNs will engage with individuals, families, groups, and communities that have varying degrees of "differences." CHNs must listen to and care for all patients, regardless of their personal views on those differences. It is in these "hard spots" of nursing where holistic relational views can provide a basis for understanding culture and diversity and help nurses to ensure they are providing safe, competent, and ethical nursing care (Hartrick Doane & Varcoe, 2006).

Relational practice requires a deep-seated commitment to respect, which means different things to different people. At the heart of relational practice is the recognition that individuals are diverse in terms of personal characteristics as well as how they perceive the world and react to others. CHNs who seek to understand diversity through a cultural safety lens become more aware of their personal views of ethnicity and recognize that ethnicity is intersected by other markers that are socially and culturally constructed—these are often difficult conversations to have in nursing (Arieli et al., 2012; Greenwood, Wright, & Nielsen, 2006). Nursing is not as culturally diverse as the general Canadian population, as the poor representation of minorities in nursing demonstrates (Lowe & Archibald, 2009).

The hallmark of professional nursing practice within these systems of care is safe, patient-focused care founded on trusting therapeutic relationships. There are many examples of how trusting therapeutic relationships have been severed in clinical practice. For example, cultural safety studies have noted the prevalence of stereotyping, perceived discrimination, and derogatory comments by health care providers (Allan & Smylie, 2015; Martin & Kipling, 2006). Hartrick Doane & Varcoe (2005) explain that relational practice builds on the strengths of individuals and recognizes differences without bias, keeping in mind the power dynamics involved in delivering health care services to patients. Relational practice helps nurses work with differences, thereby neutralizing the power dynamic. Key concepts in relational practice are a heightened sense of self-awareness, self-reflexivity in relation to others, a holistic perspective of the context and culture, and relational capacities. *Relational capacities* are ways of being in a relationship; that is, being able and willing to understand others and express or share your own personal meaning. CHNs who engage in relational practice are fully present with patients and demonstrate mindfulness, mutuality, intentionality, genuineness, warmth, respect, care, knowledge of boundaries, the ability to provide and receive constructive feedback, assertiveness, conflict-resolution skills, and a willingness to share information in meaningful ways (Hartrick Doane & Varcoe, 2005).

Relational practice requires good communication skills. Active listening skills, nonverbal communication skills, and compassion increase the CHN's ability to develop effective therapeutic relationships with patients. They also provide CHNs with greater self-awareness and awareness of patients' cues that can reveal the root causes of pain, suffering, or challenging behaviours (Hartrick Doane & Varcoe, 2005). This expanded awareness is necessary to address multiple levels (e.g., individual, group, policy) of community health intervention. The "How to" box provides guidelines for relational practice.

✳ HOW TO …

Apply the Process of Relational Practice to Working With Patients

1. *Enter into relation.*
   - Participate consciously and intentionally.
   - Stop to look and listen.
   - Show unconditional positive regard for the patient.
   - Get "in sync" with the patient.
   - Walk alongside the patient.
2. *Be in collaborative relation.*
   - Understand that the patient collaborates with the nurse.
   - Understand that the patient and nurse work together to assess and intervene.
3. *Inquire into the health and healing experience.*
   - Ask the patient what is meaningful and significant with regard to their circumstances.
   - Keep the patient (individual, family, group, or community) as the central focus.
4. *Follow the lead of the patient.*
   - Take cues from the patient.
   - Take a stance of unknowing and uncertainty.
   - Use theoretical knowledge to enhance sensitivity to patient experience.
   - Scrutinize theoretical knowledge against patient experience.
5. *Listen.*
   - Listen through phenomenological, critical, and spiritual lenses.
   - Listen through a socioenvironmental health promotion lens.
6. *Engage in self-observation.*
   - Be self-aware.
7. *Practice letting be and support change.*
   - Get to know who patients are and what is happening without imposing your views.
   - Create the opportunity for patients to learn more about their own experience, patterns, capacities, challenges, and contextual constraints.
8. *Engage in collaborative knowledge development.*
   - Draw on patient knowledge (experiential, historical, sociocultural) to build understanding and plan interventions (scientific, theoretical, biomedical, political, practical).
9. *Recognize patterns.*
   - Identify underlying patterns of experience.
   - Identify patient responses.
   - Identify patterns of capacity.
   - Identify capacity–adversity patterns.
10. *Name and support patient capacity.*
    - Recognize the patient's capacity.
    - Look beyond the surface.
    - Honour the patient's version of the story.
    - Work with the patient (at an individual and community level) to enhance capacity and address adversity.
11. *Engage in emancipatory action.*
    - Recognize and name inequities.
    - Recognize and name structural conditions.
    - Draw on and share contextual knowledge.
    - Introduce alternative discourses.
    - Devote energy to remedying structural inequities.
    - Create coalitions.

Source: Hartrick Doane, G. & Varcoe, C. (2005). *Family nursing as relational inquiry. Developing health promoting practice.* Lippincott, Williams & Wilkins.

APPLYING CULTURAL SKILLS IN COMMUNITY HEALTH PRACTICE

Culture is a key determinant of health. When CHNs come in contact with patients who are culturally different from themselves, they need to adapt general cultural concepts to the situation until they are able to learn directly from the patients about their culture. CHNs can further develop cultural competence through self-reflection as well as by reading about, taking courses on, and learning about cultures from multicultural people and groups.

CHNs need to know whether specific risk factors exist for a given cultural population. For example, Southeast Asians are often at risk for hepatitis B (with its attendant effects on the liver), tuberculosis, intestinal parasites, and visual, hearing, and dental problems; the incidence of hypertension in Black populations is higher and more severe and occurs earlier in life than in White populations (Arcangelo & Peterson, 2011); and the incidence of type 2 diabetes in Indigenous peoples is considerably higher than in the general population. However, it is important to note that some health concerns that appear to be linked to culture may in fact be more closely linked to other determinants of health. For example, the higher incidence of type 2 diabetes among Indigenous peoples is linked to determinants of health such as low income, unemployment, lower educational levels, poor social conditions, and difficulty accessing health care (Statistics Canada, 2007). These links mean that CHNs must consider the socioeconomic factors (e.g., poverty, employment, housing, and violence) that influence health rather than focus solely on race and ethnicity (Beckmann Murray, Proctor Zentner, Pangman, et al., 2009). Only then can CHNs focus on levels of prevention that relate to the broader determinants of health.

LEVELS OF PREVENTION

Related to Culture and Literacy

Primary Prevention

A CHN determines that the health information on immunization requirements is culturally appropriate and at a suitable health literacy level for each patient.

Secondary Prevention

A CHN screens the health literacy level of a patient so that programs are developed and provided at the appropriate health literacy level.

Tertiary Prevention

A CHN, through intersectoral partnerships, establishes literacy community programs and services to meet the needs of patients requiring culturally appropriate teaching about health during cardiac rehabilitation.

In addition to the broader determinants of health, CHNs need to understand the variety of nontraditional healing practices that their patients may use. Many of these treatments have proved effective and can be blended with traditional Western medicine. The key is to know which practices are being used so that the blending can be done knowledgeably.

For example, Chinese patients may use traditional practices such as acupuncture or massage therapy, and Indigenous peoples may wish to consult community elders, including a shaman (Srivastava, 2007).

An awareness of cultural values, beliefs, and practices will guide the nurse in planning and delivering culturally appropriate, holistic care (Giger, 2016). A patient's cultural values, beliefs, and practices need to be considered and respected by the CHN when planning health care for the patient. However, to plan appropriate nursing interventions with patients, CHNs need to explore individual patients' cultural values, beliefs, and practices rather than just rely on a list of expected cultural practices.

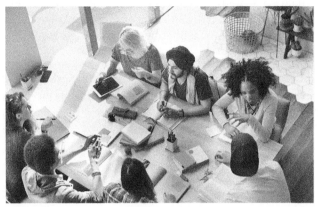

CHNs working with patients who are culturally different from themselves need to adapt general cultural concepts to the situation until they are able to learn directly from patients about their culture. Similarly, working with diverse patients requires attention, listening, and adaptation. (iStockphoto/Rawpixel)

Working With Immigrant and Refugee Populations

An **immigrant** is a person who has moved from their country of origin (their homeland) and is choosing to settle permanently in another country to become a citizen of that country. A **refugee** is a person who needs protection and is escaping being persecuted in their homeland. If they stay or return to their homeland, they will risk being tortured or killed (Government of Canada, 2019b). Refugees often seek protection in safe countries like Canada. A **newcomer** is an immigrant or refugee who has been in a country for a short time, usually less than 5 years.

Newcomers may have limited access to health care if they lack health care benefits, financial and social resources, English or French language abilities, and transportation. CHNs need to consider the background of newcomer patients. Often, the community and the family (if available) must be relied on to provide information, support, and other aid. CHNs also need to know the major health concerns and risk factors for the cultural groups they work with, such as vulnerability to specific diseases, and consider related social determinants of health.

Regardless of the approach to assessment, CHNs must consider multiple factors that influence the health of individuals, families, groups, and the community:

- Language barriers
- Low literacy levels

- Financial constraints
- Differences in social, religious, and cultural backgrounds between the newcomer and the health care provider
- Health care providers' lack of knowledge about high-risk diseases in the newcomer groups they care for
- Reliance by many newcomers on traditional healing or folk health care practices that may be unfamiliar to their Canadian health care providers
- The fact that refugees experience more physical and mental health problems and greater poverty than immigrants (Beckmann Murray et al., 2009)

In late 2015, Canada announced that it would resettle 25 000 Syrian refugees who were forced to flee their war-torn country. The "Cultural Considerations" box looks at providing mental health promotion and support for this group.

🌐 CULTURAL CONSIDERATIONS

Layers of Mental Health Promotion and Support for Syrian Refugees

Syria's civil war has caused the largest refugee displacement crisis of our time. Nearly half of the population has been forced to leave the country since 2011; the population comprises almost 8 million people inside Syria and more than 4 million registered refugees who have fled to neighbouring countries in the Middle East as well as Europe. In 2015, several thousand refugees began the process of migration to Canada. The psychological and social stresses from extreme loss and grief often experienced by refugees can double the prevalence of severe disorders (e.g., psychosis, severe depression, and disabling anxiety) and increase mild to moderate mental health disorders from 10% to 20%. Four layers of mental health promotion and support are recommended for Syrian refugees: (1) ensuring social consideration in basic services and security—providing basic needs in ways that protect the dignity of all people; (2) strengthening community and family support; (3) providing focused psychosocial support—nonspecialized workers in health, education, or community services can deliver such interventions, after training, within the community; and (4) delivering clinical services to those who need it (i.e., people with pre-existing mental health disorders and emergency-induced problems such as psychosis, drug abuse, severe depression, disabling anxiety symptoms, severe post-traumatic stress symptoms as well as those who are at risk for harming themselves or others).

Questions to Consider

1. How might CHNs promote mental health care, psychosocial support, and access to services in nonstigmatizing ways?
2. Consider some of the different approaches for distinct refugee groups (e.g., children, men, women, older persons, those who have experienced torture).

Sources: Hassan, G., Kirmayer, L. J., Mekki-Berrada, A., et al. (2015). *Culture, context and the mental health and psychosocial wellbeing of Syrians: A review for mental health and psychosocial support staff working with Syrians affected by armed conflict.*; World Health Organization & United Nations High Commissioner for Refugees. (2012). *Assessing mental health and psychosocial needs and resources: Toolkit for major humanitarian settings.* http://www.who.int/mental_health/resources/toolkit_mh_emergencies/en/.

When working with newcomer populations, CHNs need to recognize that their own background, beliefs, and knowledge may be significantly different from those of the people receiving their care. CHNs can assess their cultural beliefs and practices by using cultural competence checklists (see the "Tool Box" at the end of this chapter).

CHNs need to be aware of the importance of the family to newcomer patients. Often, children and adolescents adjust to the new culture more easily than older family members—something that can lead to family conflict. Family members can help translate their culture, religion, beliefs, practices, support systems, and risk factors for the health care provider. They can also assist with decision making and provide support to enable the person or group seeking care to change behaviours to become more health conscious. CHNs need to strive to understand the role of the family for newcomer populations and to treat individuals in the context of their families.

Similarly, the role of the community in the care of newcomers is important. Communities can help patients with communication, explanation, crisis intervention, emotional and other forms of support, and housing. CHNs need to assess the community carefully and learn what strengths, resources, and talents are available. For further information about newcomers, see the Ontario Council of Agencies Serving Immigrants (OCASI) link on the Evolve website.

Using an Interpreter

Clear communication between nurses and patients and their families is vital. Communication is often a complex area of CHN practice. Language barriers may interfere with CHNs' efforts to provide assistance or undertake an assessment. When CHNs do not speak or understand the patient's language, they need to obtain an interpreter (Ku & Flores, 2005). **Interpretation** is the process by which a spoken or signed message in one language is relayed, with the same meaning, in another language. Srivastava (2007) distinguishes **linguistic interpretation** as interpretation of spoken words only from **cultural interpretation,** which is the interpretation of spoken words but with additional information about the culture. **Translation** is the written conversion of one language into another (Bowen, 2015). It is best not to use community members as interpreters, although it may be necessary to do so if no other interpreters are available. Regardless, the need for confidentiality must be addressed with the interpreter. Strategies to help CHNs select and use an interpreter effectively are listed in the "How to" box. Where interpreters are not available, the CHN could use interpreters by telephone or video conferencing and provide paper-based information in a variety of languages that would meet the needs of the diverse population in the community. The "CHN in Practice: A Case Study, Interpretation in the Home Visit" box considers a situation in which an interpreter would be involved in a CHN visit with a patient.

✦ HOW TO ...

Select and Use an Interpreter

1. Select an interpreter who has knowledge of health-related terminology when feasible.
2. Use family members with caution because of the patient's need for privacy; family members may lack the ability to communicate effectively in both languages, and family members may exhibit biases that influence the patient's decisions.
3. Be aware that the gender of the interpreter may be of concern; in some cultures, women may prefer a female interpreter and men may prefer a male.
4. Be aware that the age of the interpreter may also be of concern. For example, older patients may want a more mature interpreter. Children may have limited comprehension and language skills and may have difficulty interpreting complex information.
5. Understand that differences in socioeconomic status, religious affiliation, and educational level between the patient and the interpreter may lead to problems in interpreting information.
6. Identify the patient's origin of birth and spoken language or dialect before selecting the interpreter. For example,

Chinese patients speak different dialects, depending on the region in which they were born.

7. Avoid using an interpreter from the same community as the patient to avoid a possible breach of confidentiality.
8. Avoid using professional jargon, colloquialisms, abstractions, idiomatic expressions, slang, similes, and metaphors. Speak slowly and use plain language.
9. Clarify roles with the interpreter.
10. Introduce the interpreter to the patient and explain to the patient what the interpreter will be doing.
11. Observe the patient for nonverbal messages such as facial expressions, gestures, and other forms of body language. If the patient's responses do not fit with the question, the nurse needs to check that the interpreter understood the question.
12. Increase accuracy in transmission of information by asking the interpreter to translate the patient's own words and ask the patient to repeat the information communicated by the interpreter.
13. Review the material with the patient at the end of the interview to ensure the patient's understanding.

Sources: Giger, J. N. (2016). *Transcultural nursing: Assessment and intervention* (7th ed.). Mosby/Elsevier; Randall-David, E. (1994). *Culturally competent HIV counseling and education.* Maternal and Child Health Clearinghouse.

📋 CHN IN PRACTICE: A CASE STUDY

Interpretation in the Home Visit

Mr. Ping's health has been deteriorating. He was recently discharged from Vancouver General Hospital, and Mary has been assigned as his CHN. Mr. Ping is an older person who speaks Cantonese and little English. He has one daughter, Shu, who lives in Toronto. Shu contacted her friend, Sally Wong, a grade-school teacher in Vancouver, to ask if Sally could act as an interpreter when Mary visited her father. On the first visit, Sally was able to establish a close enough relationship with Mr. Ping to engage him in a discussion about his health. He confided to Sally that he had been diagnosed with cancer of the small intestine, and he feared he was dying. Through Sally, Mr. Ping stated that he did not want Mary or Sally to discuss his diagnosis with his daughter. He refused treatment because he believed that people never got better after they were diagnosed with cancer; he believed that they always died.

Think About It

1. What knowledge and skills should Mary have and what actions should she take to demonstrate her ability to provide culturally competent care to the Ping family?
2. Since Sally volunteered to be an interpreter for Mr. Ping, what are some of the possible limitations of this interaction that Mary would need to consider?
3. Identify how Mary would apply the Giger and Davidhizar Transcultural Assessment Model to the Ping family situation.

Answers are on the Evolve website at http://evolve.elsevier.com/ Canada/Stanhope/community/.

Be aware that interpreters may not understand medical language, which can influence the accuracy of the interpretation. As well, interpreters may emphasize their personal preferences by influencing both the nurse's and the patient's decisions to select and participate in treatment modalities. CHNs may minimize the risk of interpretation errors by learning basic words and sentences of the most commonly spoken languages in the community and by having key written materials translated into the language of sizable patient populations.

Five steps that will help CHNs work effectively with interpreters are:

1. Identify when the need for an interpreter exists.
2. Use an appropriate interpreter.
3. Explain the role of the interpreter and the health professional.
4. Verbally engage the patient in conversation.
5. Monitor for interpretation errors (Srivastava, 2007).

Box 7.3 presents guidelines the CHN can use when conducting an interpretation session.

As in all areas of health care, resources for interpretation are finite, and choices must be made about how best to serve the needs of the whole community. The degree of accommodation depends on the proportion of patients in the community who speak a language other than French or English. If there is a large volume of a particular cultural or linguistic group, health care agencies may be required to provide translations of all their written materials and to use interpreters regularly. If the volume of patients is not sufficiently large, perhaps only portions of the written materials will be translated and no interpreter provided.

BOX 7.3   Working With Interpreters: Guidelines for the Interpretation Session

- Face the patient directly.
- Always speak in the first person as if talking directly to the patient.
- Introduce yourself (and the interpreter) to the patient(s).
- Describe your role and the purpose of the session.
- Speak slowly, clearly, in simple language and directly to the patient, not the interpreter.
- While the interpreter is speaking, observe the patient's nonverbal communication.
- Verify interpretations of any nonverbal behaviour ("I notice you are tapping your foot—is this something you do when you are nervous or is there something else ...?").

- Be patient; remember that the interpreter may require much more time to interpret something than you needed in English.
- Ask open-ended questions as needed to clarify what the patient says or to hear what the patient may wish to convey.
- Observe and evaluate what is going on before interrupting the interpreter.
- Always ask that the patient repeat instructions.
- Provide written information (preferably in the patient's language) for instructions, appointments, and contact information.
- Provide information as to how the patient may access an interpreter (preferably the same interpreter) in the future.

Source: Srivastava, R. H. (2007). *The health care professional's guide to clinical cultural competence* (p. 140). Elsevier Canada. Reprinted with permission.

STUDENT EXPERIENCE

Storytelling can help students develop ways of knowing and explore issues (Lordly, 2007). Through the exchange of experiences through storytelling, you will be able to identify similarities in experiences and enhance your knowledge of culturally competent care.

Activity

1. Journal and reflect on one experience that you have had with a specific cultural group such as an ethnic group, a group of older persons, members of a homeless shelter, a deaf individual, or members of a criminal or gang culture. What did you learn about that cultural group from this experience?
2. Choose a culture that you are unfamiliar with and write, using storytelling, about
   a. Your attitudes, beliefs, values, and experiences as a member of that culture; and
   b. Your difficulties in accessing health care services.

CHAPTER SUMMARY

7.1 Diversity is an element of Canadian society and all aspects of CHN practice. *Diversity* in a cultural context includes consideration of similarities, differences, and power relations across age, gender, race, religion, occupation, sexual orientation, and poverty. *Culture* refers to common values and ways of thinking and acting that differ from those of another group. Culture is learned, adaptive, dynamic, invisible, shared, and selective. *Race* is a social classification based on an imagined hierarchy of human value that relies on phenotypes, skin colour, and other expressions of group superiority and inferiority to identify group membership. *Ethnicity* is the state of belonging to a social group that shares common cultural patterns (e.g., beliefs, values, customs, behaviours, traditions).

7.2 Key demographic groups for community health nursing in Canada are older persons, Indigenous peoples, and immigrants.

7.3 The population of Canada is diverse in terms of ethnicity, language, religion, sexuality, and abilities. Canada is a multicultural society that recognizes its citizens' diverse ancestry and values cultural pluralism. CHNs need to perform a broad assessment on every patient with whom they interact. Considering the aging population and other determinants, disability and adaptations are increasingly community health interests.

7.4 The circumstances in our day-to-day life related to gender, culture, age, ability, and social status are shaped by the distribution of money, power, resources, and decision making at global, national, and local levels. Issues and concerns related to diversity can be seen as determinants of health.

7.5 Diversity in CHN practice should be considered from an asset-based perspective; that is, that while the conditions of diversity may be determined by power relations, people who experience diverse cultures, ages, abilities, and all ways of being have strengths as a result of their differences.

7.6 Cultural competence is an ongoing process rather than an outcome. In order to practice with cultural competence, CHNs apply cultural knowledge and skills appropriate to patient interactions without personal biases.

7.7 When CHNs use a cultural safety lens, they reflect an understanding of others' health beliefs and practices so that health care actions work toward equity and avoid discrimination. Culturally safe CHN care incorporates the patient's beliefs, values, attitudes, and behaviours and is provided with sensitivity. A CHN who works toward cultural safety has a keen sense of his or her own cultural values and beliefs and uses cultural knowledge as well as specific skills—such as intracultural communication and cultural assessment—to evaluate and select interventions for patient care.

7.8 CHNs need to perform a cultural nursing assessment on every patient with whom they interact. Relational practice is an approach to assessment and interventions that addresses the imbalance of power between

CHNs and patients. At the heart of relational practice is the recognition of diversity and how each individual perceives the world they live in and how they react to others.

7.9 In addition to relational practice, a number of skills and tools support culturally competent and safe practice. For example, when CHNs do not speak or understand the patient's language, they need to use an interpreter or, in the case of written materials, a translator.

CHN IN PRACTICE: A CASE STUDY

Cultural Competence and the Home Visit

Carolyn, a CHN for the Bigstone Cree Nation (in northern Alberta), received a referral for follow-up for Marie, a 59-year-old Cree-speaking woman. The CHN calls Marie to set up a home visit and Marie immediately reports that she was recently diagnosed with cervical cancer, which she says is at stage III and moving into stage IV. On Carolyn's first home visit, she observes Marie to be upset and distressed. Marie explains to Carolyn that her mother died of stage IV cervical cancer 10 years ago and that her mother delayed diagnosis and refused treatment. In conversation, Carolyn learns that the cancer diagnosis and pending treatment is being overshadowed by the sudden death of her son, Lionel, in a car collision. Losing Lionel at this crucial time is causing Marie to consider refusing treatment. However, Marie's relatives are trying to convince her that her other children and grandchildren still need her and that she should seek medical treatment. Marie also mentions that she heard that cervical cancer has a genetic predisposition.

During another home visit, Carolyn meets Marie's sister Cora, who has come to help Marie physically, spiritually, and emotionally. Cora is a retired registered nurse with 35 years of nursing experience in Indigenous communities. During the

visit, Marie begins to talk to Carolyn about traditional medicine and approaches to treatment. She tells Carolyn that she recalls a medicine man who claims to know of over 100 herbs used to treat cancer. Marie also talks about a relative who was recently diagnosed with prostate cancer and tells Carolyn that his treatment from a traditional healer is reported to have cured the prostate cancer. Marie tells Carolyn, "It was just gone—without any treatment." Cora, Marie's sister responds, "But he was treated. It was just a different kind of treatment." There are many medicines to treat all kinds of illnesses and there are many ways to get well.

Think About It

1. What are some of the issues surrounding Marie's decision to not seek immediate medical attention?
2. How could Carolyn gain cultural competence to best support Marie?
3. Imagine that you are the CHN working on this case. How would you implement the health promotion strategies of strengthening community action; building healthy public policy; creating supportive environments; developing personal skills; and reorienting health services (see Chapter 4)?

 TOOL BOX

The Tool Box contains useful resources that can be applied in community health nursing practice. These related resources are found either in the appendices at the back of this text or on the text's website at https://evolve.elsevier.com/Canada/Stanhope/community/.

Appendices

- Appendix 1: Canadian Community Health Nursing Standards of Practice
- Appendix 5: The Giger and Davidhizar Transcultural Assessment Model

Tools

Better Communication, Better Care: A Provider Toolkit for Serving Diverse Populations. (http://www.lacare.org/sites/default/files/la0784_provider_toolkit_201902.pdf)

This tool kit was prepared for health care providers and contains information on how to interact and communicate with patients from diverse cultures.

Canadian Ethnocultural Council. (https://www.ethno-cultural.ca/canadian-ethnocultural-council-1)

The Canadian Ethnocultural Council (CEC) is a nonprofit, nonpartisan coalition of national ethnocultural umbrella

organizations which, in turn, represent a cross-section of ethnocultural groups across Canada. The CEC's objectives are to ensure the preservation, enhancement, and sharing of the cultural heritage of Canadians; the removal of barriers that prevent some Canadians from participating fully and equally in society; the elimination of racism; and the preservation of a united Canada. One of its key initiatives is "Hepatitis C and Other Related Communicable Diseases in High-Risk Immigrant Ethnic Communities."

Cultural Competence Checklist: Personal Reflection. (https://www.asha.org/siteassets/uploadedFiles/Cultural-Competence-Checklist-Personal-Reflection.pdf)

This web-based tool is a one-page cultural competence checklist to increase awareness of how patients from different cultures are viewed.

Cultural Competence Checklist: Service Delivery. (https://www.asha.org/siteassets/uploadedfiles/cultural-competence-checklist-service-delivery.pdf)

This web-based tool is a one-page cultural competence checklist to assess how to improve service delivery to culturally diverse patients.

REFERENCES

Alberta Civil Liberties Research Centre. (2020). *Forms of racism.* http://www.aclrc.com/forms-of-racism.

Alberta Health Services. (2009). *Enhancing cultural competency: A resource kit for health care professionals.* [Seminal Reference] http://fcrc.albertahealthservices.ca/pdfs/Enhancing_Cultural_Competency_Resource_Kit.pdf.

Allan, B., & Smylie, J. (2015). *First peoples, second class treatment: The role of racism in the health and well-being of Indigenous peoples in Canada.* Wellesley Institute.

Andersen, E., & Havaei, F. (2015). Measuring relational care in nursing homes: Psychometric evaluation of the relational care scale. *Journal of Nursing Measurement, 23*, 82–92.

Anderson, J., Perry, J., Blue, C., et al. (2003). Rewriting cultural safety within the postcolonial and postnational feminist project: Towards new epistemologies of healing. *Advances in Nursing Science, 26*(3), 196–214 [Seminal Reference].

Arcangelo, V., & Peterson, A. M. (2011). *Pharmacotherapeutics for advanced practice: A practical approach* (3rd ed.). Lippincott, Williams & Wilkins.

Arieli, D., Friedman, V. J., & Hirschfeld, M. J. (2012). Challenges on the path to cultural safety in nursing education. *International Nursing Review, 59*(2), 187–193.

Astle, B. J., Barton, S. S., Johnson, L., et al. (2019). Global health. In B. J. Astle, & W. Duggleby (Eds.), *Canadian fundamentals of nursing* (6th ed.) (pp. 115–132). Elsevier Canada.

Beckmann Murray, R., Proctor Zentner, J., Pangman, V., et al. (2009). *Health promotion strategies through the life span* (2nd Cdn ed.). Pearson Prentice Hall.

Bergum, V., & Dossetor, J. (2005). *Creating environment. Relational ethics: The full meaning of respect.* University Publishing Group. [Seminal Reference].

Bourque Bearskin, R. L. (2014). *Mâmawoh kamâtowin: Coming together to help each other: Honouring indigenous nursing knowledge. PhD Dissertation.* Edmonton, Canada: University of Alberta.

Bourque Bearskin, R. L., Cameron, B. L., King, M., et al. (2016). Mâmawoh kamâtowin "coming together to help each other in wellness": Honouring indigenous nursing knowledge. *International Journal of Indigenous Health, 11*(1), 18–33.

Bowen, S. (2015). *The impact of language barriers on patient safety and quality of care: Final report prepared for the Société Santé en Français.* https://www.reseausantene.ca/wp-content/uploads/2018/05/Impact-language-barrier-qualitysafety.pdf.

Burchum, J. L. (2002). Cultural competence: An evolutionary perspective. *Nursing Forum, 37*(4), 5–15 [Seminal Reference].

Cameron, B., Carmargo Plazas, P., Santos Salas, A., et al. (2014). Understanding inequalities in access to healthcare services for Aboriginal people: A call for nursing action. *Advances in Nursing Science, 37*(3), E1–E16. https://doi.org/10.1097/ANS.0000000000000039.

Campinha-Bacote, J. (1999). A model and instrument for addressing cultural competence in health care. *Journal of Nursing Education, 38*(5), 204–207 [Seminal Reference].

Campinha-Bacote, J. (2002). The process of cultural competence in the delivery of healthcare services: A model of care. *Journal of Transcultural Nursing, 13*(3), 181–184 [Seminal Reference].

Campinha-Bacote, J. (2018). Cultural competemility: A paradigm shift in the cultural competence versus cultural humility debate—Part I. *OJIN: Online Journal of Issues in Nursing, 24*(1). https://ojin.nursingworld.org/MainMenuCategories/ANAMarketplace/ANAPeriodicals/OJIN/TableofContents/Vol-24-2019/No1-Jan-2019/Articles-Previous-Topics/Cultural-Competemility-A-Paradigm-Shift.html.

Canadian Centre for Diversity and Inclusion. (2020). *Research and tool kits.* https://ccdi.ca/toolkits/.

Canadian Institutes of Health Research. (2016). *Action plan: Building a healthier future for first nations, Inuit and Metis peoples.* https://cihr-irsc.gc.ca/e/50372.html.

Canadian Nurses Association. (2018). *Position statement: Promoting cultural competence in nursing.* https://www.cna-aiic.ca/-/media/cna/page-content/pdf-en/position_statement_promoting_cultural_competence_in_nursing.pdf?la=en&hash=4B394DAE5C2138E7F6134D59E505DCB059754BA9.

Canadian Public Health Association. (2018). *Position statement on racism and health.* https://www.cpha.ca/racism-and-public-health.

Centre for Suicide Prevention. (2018). *Sexual minorities and suicide prevention.* https://www.suicideinfo.ca/resource/sexual-minorities-suicide-prevention/.

Choi, L., & Jakubec, S. L. (2017). An on-line learning journey of diversity and bias. In D. K. Deardorff, & L. A. Arasaratnam-Smith (Eds.), *Intercultural competence in higher education: International approaches, assessment and application* (pp. 169–173). Routledge.

Citizenship and Immigration Canada. (2015). *Report on plans and priorities 2015–2016.* https://www.canada.ca/en/immigration-refugees-citizenship/corporate/publications-manuals/report-plans-priorities/2015-2016.html.

Citizenship and Immigration Canada. (2016a). *Permanent resident program.* http://www.cic.gc.ca/english/resources/tools/perm/index.asp.

Citizenship and Immigration Canada. (2016b). *Temporary residents.* http://www.cic.gc.ca/english/resources/tools/temp/index.asp.

Clair, J., Beatty, J., & MacLean, T. (2005). Out of sight but not out of mind: Managing invisible social identities in the workplace. *Academy of Management Review, 30*(1), 78–95 [Seminal Reference].

College of Nurses of Ontario. (2018). *Competencies for entry-level registered nurse practice.* https://www.cno.org/globalassets/docs/reg/41037-entry-to-practice-competencies-2020.pdf.

Community Health Nurses of Canada. (2019). *Canadian community health nursing professional practice model and standards of practice.* https://www.chnc.ca/standards-of-practice.

Daley, A. E., & MacDonnell, J. A. (2015). "That would have been beneficial": LGBTQ education for home-care service providers. *Health and Social Care in the Community, 23*(3), 282–291. https://doi.org/10.1111/hsc.12141.

De, D., & Richardson, J. (2008). Cultural safety: An introduction. *Pediatric Nursing, 20*(2), 39–43.

Dickason, O. P., & Newbigging, W. (2019). *Indigenous peoples within Canada: A concise history* (4th ed.). Oxford University Press.

Dion Stout, M., & Downey, B. (2006). Nursing, indigenous peoples and cultural safety: So what? Now what? *Contemporary Nurse, 22*, 327–332.

Ford, C. (2019). *Racism: Science & tools for the public health professional.* American Public Health Association.

Giger, J. N. (2016). *Transcultural nursing: Assessment and intervention* (7th ed.). Mosby/Elsevier.

Giger, J., Davidhizar, R., Purnell, L., et al. (2007). American academy of nursing expert panel report: Developing cultural competence to eliminate health disparities in ethnic minorities and other visible populations. *Journal of Transcultural Nursing*, *18*(2), 95–102.

Government of British Columbia. (2020). Cultural agility. https://www2.gov.bc.ca/gov/content/careers-myhr/job-seekers/about-competencies/indigenous-relations/cultural-agility.

Government of Canada. (2018). *Rights of people with disabilities*. https://www.canada.ca/en/canadian-heritage/services/rights-people-disabilities.html.

Government of Canada. (2019a). *Canada's anti-racism strategy*. https://www.canada.ca/en/canadian-heritage/campaigns/anti-racism-engagement.html.

Government of Canada. (2019b). *How Canada's refugee system works*. https://www.canada.ca/en/immigration-refugees-citizenship/services/refugees/canada-role.html.

Government of Canada. (2020). *Canada and the world: The human rights of lesbian, gay, bisexual, transgender, queer, 2 spirit and intersex persons*. https://www.international.gc.ca/world-monde/issues_development-enjeux_developpement/human_rights-droits_homme/rights_lgbti-droits_lgbti.aspx?lang=eng.

Gray, P. D., & Thomas, D. J. (2006). Critical reflections on culture in nursing. *Journal of Cultural Diversity*, *13*(2), 76–82.

Greene-Moton, E., & Minkler, M. (2020). Cultural competence or cultural humility? Moving beyond the debate. *Health Promotion Practice*, *21*(1), 142–145.

Greenwood, M., de Leeuw, S., & Lindsay, N. (2018). Challenges in health equity for Indigenous peoples in Canada. *The Lancet*, *391*(10131), 1645–1648. https://doi.org/10.1016/S0140-6736(18)30177-6.

Greenwood, S., Wright, T., & Nielsen, H. (2006). Conversations in context: Cultural safety and reflexivity in child and family health nursing. *Journal of Family Nursing*, *12*(2), 201–224 [Seminal Reference].

Gregory, D., Harrowing, J., Lee, B., et al. (2010). Pedagogy as influencing nursing students' essentialized understanding of culture. *International Journal of Nursing Education Scholarship*, *7*(1), 1–17.

Grullon, E., Hunnicutt, C., Morrison, M., et al. (2018). A need for occupational justice: The impact of racial microaggression on occupations, wellness, and health promotion. Occupation: A Medium of inquiry for students. *Faculty & Other Practitioners Advocating for Health through Occupational Studies*, *3*(1), Article 4. https://nsuworks.nova.edu/occupation/vol3/iss1/4.

Hartrick Doane, G., & Varcoe, C. (2005). *Family nursing as relational inquiry: Developing health-promoting practice*. Lippincott, Williams & Wilkins. [Seminal Reference].

Hartrick Doane, G., & Varcoe, C. (2006). The "hard spots" of family nursing: Connecting across difference and diversity. *Journal of Family Nursing*, *12*(1), 7–21.

Hartrick Doane, G., & Varcoe, C. (2015). *How to nurse? Relational inquiry with individuals and families in changing health and healthcare contexts*. Lippincott, Williams & Wilkins.

Hassan, G., Kirmayer, L. J., Mekki-Berrada, A., et al. (2015). *Culture, context and the mental health and psychosocial wellbeing of Syrians: A review for mental health and psychosocial support staff working with Syrians affected by armed conflict*. UNHCR.

Hilario, C., Browne, A., & McFadden, A. (2018). The influence of democratic racism in nursing inquiry. *Nursing Inquiry*, *25*(1)e12213 -n/a. https://doi.org/10.1111/nin.12213.

Hoffman-Goetz, L., Donelle, L., & Ahmed, R. (2014). *Health literacy in Canada: A primer for students*. Canadian Scholars' Press.

Hoskins, M. L. (1999). Worlds apart and lives together: Developing cultural attunement. *Child and Youth Care Forum*, *28*(2), 73–85 [Seminal Reference].

Indian and Northern Affairs Canada. (1996). *Report of the Royal Commission on Aboriginal peoples (RCAP)*. [Seminal Reference] https://www.bac-lac.gc.ca/eng/discover/aboriginal-heritage/royal-commission-aboriginal-peoples/Pages/final-report.aspx.

Indigenous and Northern Affairs Canada. (2014). *Urban Aboriginal peoples*. https://www.canada.ca/en/indigenous-services-canada.html.

Indigenous and Northern Affairs Canada. (2015). *Inuit*. https://www.canada.ca/en/indigenous-services-canada.html.

Ipsos-Reid. (2005). *March 21st, international day for the elimination of racial discrimination: One in six Canadians say they have been the victim of racism*. https://www.ipsos.com/en-ca/march-21st-international-day-elimination-racial-discrimination.

Jakubec, S. L., Olfert, M., Choi, L., et al. (2019). Understanding belonging and community connection for seniors living in the suburbs. *Urban Planning*, *4*(2), 43–52. https://doi.org/10.17645/up.v4i2.1896.

Jedwab, J. (2020). Multiculturalism. *Canadian Encyclopedia*. https://www.thecanadianencyclopedia.ca/en/article/multiculturalism.

Johannessen, A.-K., Werner, A., & Steihaug, S. (2013). Work in an intermediate unit: Balancing between relational, practical and more care. *Journal of Clinical Nursing*, *23*, 586–595. https://doi.org/10.1111/jocn.12213.

Khanlou, N., Haque, N., Mustafa, N., et al. (2017). Access barriers to services by immigrant mothers of children with autism in Canada. *International Journal of Mental Health and Addiction*, *15*(2), 239–259.

Kirkham, S., & Anderson, J. M. (2002). Postcolonial nursing scholarship: From epistemology to method. *Advances in Nursing Science*, *25*(1), 1–17 [Seminal Reference].

Ku, L., & Flores, G. (2005). Pay now or pay later: Providing interpreter services in health care. *Health Affairs*, *24*(2), 435–444 [Seminal Reference].

Lancellotti, K. (2008). Culture care theory: A framework for expanding awareness of diversity and racism in nursing education. *Journal of Professional Nursing*, *24*(3), 179–183. https://doi.org/10.1016/j.profnurs.2007.10.007.

Le, T. N., & Johansen, S. (2011). The relationship between perceived school multiculturalism and interpersonal violence: An exploratory study. *Journal of School Health*, *81*(11), 688–695.

Levi, A. (2009). The ethics of nursing student international clinical experiences. *Journal of Obstetric, Gynecologic, and Neonatal Nursing*, *28*(1), 94–99. https://doi.org/10.1111/j.1552-6909.2008.00314.x.

LGBT Health Program. (2015). *Guidelines and protocols for hormone therapy and primary health care for trans clients*. Sherbourne Health Centre.

Library of Parliament. (2018). *Canadian multiculturalism*. https://lop.parl.ca/sites/PublicWebsite/default/en_CA/ResearchPublications/200920E.

Lordly, D. (2007). Once upon a time. … Storytelling to enhance teaching and learning. *Canadian Journal of Dietetic Practice and Research*, *68*(1), 30–35.

Lowe, J., & Archibald, C. (2009). Cultural diversity: The intention of nursing. *Nursing Forum*, *44*(1), 11–18. https://doi.org/10.1111/j.1744-6198.2009.00122.x.

Martin, D., & Kipling, A. (2006). Factors shaping Aboriginal nursing students' experiences. *Nurse Education Today, 26*(8), 688–696.

McCabe, J., & Holmes, D. (2014). Nursing, sexual health and youth with disabilities: A critical ethnography. *Journal of Advanced Nursing, 70*(1), 77–86. https://doi.org/10.1111/jan.12167.

McFarland, M., & Wehebe-Alama, H. B. (2018). *Leininger's transcultural nursing: Concepts, theories, research, and practices* (4th ed.). McGraw-Hill.

McGibbon, E. (Ed.). (2012). *Oppression: A social determinant of health.* Fernwood Publishing.

McGibbon, E., & Etowa, J. (2009). *Anti-racist health care practice.* Canadian Scholars' Press.

McInturrff, K., & Tulloch, P. (2014). *Narrowing the gap: The difference that public sector wages make.* https://www.policyalternatives.ca/publications/reports/narrowing-gap.

Mental Health Commission of Canada. (2015). *Informing the future: Mental health indicators for Canada.* http://www.mentalhealthcommission.ca/English/document/68796/informing-future-mental-health-indicators-canada.

Métis National Council (n.d.). Métis nation citizenship. http://www.metisnation.ca/index.php/who-are-the-metis/citizenship.

Mikkonen, J., & Raphael, D. (2010). *Social determinants of health: The Canadian facts.* York University School of Health Policy and Management. http://www.thecanadianfacts.org.

Misener, T. R., Sowell, R. L., Phillips, K. D., et al. (1997). Sexual orientation: A cultural diversity issue for nursing. *Nursing Outlook, 45*(4), 178–181 [Seminal Reference].

Napier, A. D., Arcano, C., Butler, B., et al. (2014). Culture and health. *The Lancet, 384*(9954), 1607–1639.

National Aboriginal Health Organization. (2006). *Discussion paper series in Aboriginal health: Legal issues—first Nations, Métis, and Inuit women's health.* https://www.deslibris.ca/ID/203529.

National Collaborating Centre for Aboriginal Health (NCCAH). (2016). *Infographic: Culture and language as social determinants of first nations, Inuit and Metis health.* https://www.nccih.ca/495/Infographic__Culture_and_language_as_social_determinants_of_First_Nations,_Inuit,_and_M%C3%A9tis_health.nccih?id=172.

Nestel, S. (2012). *Colour coded health care: The impact of race and racism on Canadians' health.* Wellesley Institute.

Nova Scotia Department of Health. (2005). *A cultural competence guide for primary health care professionals in Nova Scotia.* https://www.mycna.ca/~/media/nurseone/page-content/pdf-en/cultural_competence_guide_for_primary_health_care_professionals.pdf.

Pillay, T. (2015). Decentring the myth of Canadian multiculturalism. In A. A. Abdi, L. Shultz, & T. Pillay (Eds.), *Decolonizing global citizenship education* (pp. 69–80). SensePublishers.

Pollard, C. L. (2015). What is the right thing to do: Use of a relational ethic framework to guide clinical decision-making. *International Journal of Caring Sciences, 8*(2), 362–368.

Pollock, G., Newbold, K. B., Lafranière, G., et al. (2012). Discrimination in the doctor's office: Immigrants and refugee experiences. *Critical Social Work, 13*(2), 60–79.

Porr, C. J. (2015). Important interactional strategies for everyday public health nursing practice. *Public Health Nursing, 32*, 43–49. https://doi.org/10.1111/phn.12097.

Porr, C., Drummond, J., & Olson, K. (2012). Establishing therapeutic relationships with vulnerable and potentially stigmatized patients. *Qualitative Health Research, 22*, 384–396.

Pottinger, A., Perivolaris, A., & Howes, D. (2007). The end of life. In R. H. Srivastava (Ed.), *The health care professional's guide to clinical cultural competence* (pp. 227–246). Elsevier Canada.

Powell, D. (2016). Social determinants of health: Cultural competence is not enough. *Creative Nursing, 22*(1), 5–10.

Public Health Agency of Canada. (2016). *How healthy are Canadians? A trend analysis of the health of Canadians from a healthy living and chronic disease perspective.* https://www.canada.ca/content/dam/phac-aspc/documents/services/publications/healthy-living/how-healthy-canadians/pub1-eng.pdf.

Quan, H., Fong, A., DeCoster, C., et al. (2006). Variation in health services utilization among ethnic populations. *Canadian Medical Association Journal, 174*(6), 787–791.

Racher, F. E., & Annis, R. C. (2007). Respecting culture and honoring diversity in community practice. *Research and Theory for Nursing Practice, 21*(4), 255–270.

Racine, L. (2014). The enduring challenge of cultural safety in nursing. *The Canadian Journal of Nursing Research/Revue Canadienne de Recherche en Sciences Infirmieres, 46*(2), 6–9.

Racine, L., & Petrucka, P. (2011). Enhancing decolonization and knowledge transfer in nursing research with non-Western populations: Examining the congruence between primary healthcare and postcolonial feminist approaches. *Nursing Inquiry, 18*(1), 12–20.

Ramsden, I. (2002). *Cultural safety and nursing education in Aotearoa and Te Waipounamu.* Victoria University. [Seminal Reference].

Randall-David, E. (1994). *Culturally competent HIV counseling and education. Maternal and child health Clearinghouse.* [Seminal Reference].

Raphael, D. (2017). Implications of inequities in health for health promotion practice. In I. Rootman, A. Pederson, K. L. Frohlich, et al. (Eds.), *Health promotion in Canada: New perspectives on theory, practice, policy, and research* (4th ed.) (pp. 167–183). Canadian Scholars' Press.

Registered Nurses' Association of Ontario. (2006). *Establishing therapeutic relationships—best practice guideline.* http://rnao.ca/bpg/guidelines/establishing-therapeutic-relationships.

Registered Nurses' Association of Ontario. (2007). *Embracing cultural diversity in health care: Developing cultural competence.* http://rnao.ca/bpg/guidelines/embracing-cultural-diversity-health-care-developing-cultural-competence.

Rowan, M. S., Rukholm, E., Bourque-Bearskin, R. L., et al. (2013). Cultural competence and cultural safety in Canadian schools of nursing: A mixed methods study. *International Journal of Nursing Education Scholarship, 10*(1), 1–10. https://doi.org/10.1515/ijnes-2012-0043.

Saint Elizabeth Health. (2020). *First nations, Inuit and Metis program: NAHO publications and resources.* https://fnim.sehc.com/se-learning/naho-publications-and-resources.

Scheim, A. E., & Bauer, G. R. (2015). Sex and gender diversity among transgender persons in Ontario, Canada: Results from a respondent-driven sampling survey. *The Journal of Sex Research, 52*(1), 1–14.

Sheppard, D. M. (2020). Getting to the heart of cultural safety in Unama'ki: Considering kesultulinej (love). *Witness: The Canadian Journal of Critical Nursing Discourse, 2*(1), 51–65.

Smith, K. (2019). Facing history for the future of nursing. *Journal of Clinical Nursing, 29*(9–10), 1429–1431. https://doi.org/10.1111/jocn.15065.

Spadoni, M., Hartrick Doane, G., Sevean, P., et al. (2015). First-year nursing students—developing relational caring practice through inquiry. *Journal of Nursing Education, 54*(5), 270–275.

Spector, R. (2017). *Cultural diversity in health and illness* (9th ed.). Pearson Prentice Hall.

Srivastava, R. H. (2007). *The health care professional's guide to clinical cultural competence*. Elsevier Canada.

Stanhope, M., & Lancaster, J. (2018). *Foundations for population health in community/public health nursing* (5th ed.). Elsevier Inc.

Statistics Canada. (2007). *Study: Sports participation among Aboriginal children*. http://www.statcan.gc.ca/daily-quotidien/070710/dq070710b-eng.htm.

Statistics Canada. (2009). *Earnings and incomes of Canadians over the past quarter century, 2006 census: Findings (Cat. No. 97-563-XIE2006001)*. http://www12.statcan.ca/census-recensement/2006/as-sa/97-563/index-eng.cfm.

Statistics Canada. (2010a). *Canada's ethnocultural mosaic, 2006 census: National picture*. http://www12.statcan.ca/census-recensement/2006/as-sa/97-562/p2-eng.cfm.

Statistics Canada. (2010b). *Projections of the diversity of the Canadian population: 2006–2031*. http://www.statcan.gc.ca/pub/91-551-x/91-551-x2010001-eng.pdf.

Statistics Canada. (2011a). *2011 national household survey*. https://www12.statcan.gc.ca/nhs-enm/2011/dp-pd/dt-td/Index-eng.cfm.

Statistics Canada. (2011b). *The Canadian population in 2011: Population counts and growth*. https://www12.statcan.gc.ca/census-recensement/2011/as-sa/98-310-x/98-310-x2011001-eng.cfm.

Statistics Canada. (2013a). *Aboriginal peoples in Canada: First nations people, Métis and Inuit*. http://www12.statcan.gc.ca/nhs-enm/2011/as-sa/99-011-x/99-011-x2011001-eng.pdf.

Statistics Canada. (2013b). *Disability in Canada: Initial findings from the Canadian survey on disability*. http://www.statcan.gc.ca/pub/89-654-x/89-654-x2013002-eng.pdf.

Statistics Canada. (2013c). *Immigration and ethnocultural diversity in Canada: National household survey, 2011*. http://www12.statcan.gc.ca/nhs-enm/2011/as-sa/99-010-x/99-010-x2011001-eng.pdf.

Statistics Canada. (2015). *Population projections by Aboriginal identity in Canada, 2006 to 2031*. http://www.statcan.gc.ca/pub/91-552-x/2011001/hl-fs-eng.htm.

Statistics Canada. (2017). *Census in brief: Ethnic and cultural origins of Canadians: Portrait of a rich heritage*. https://www12.statcan.gc.ca/census-recensement/2016/as-sa/98-200-x/2016016/98-200-x2016016-eng.cfm.

Statistics Canada. (2018). *Insights on Canadian society—results of the 2016 Census. Aboriginal languages and the role of second language acquisition*. https://www150.statcan.gc.ca/n1/pub/75-006-x/2018001/article/54981-eng.htm.

Statistics Canada. (2019a). *Immigration and language in Canada*. https://www150.statcan.gc.ca/n1/pub/89-657-x/89-657-x2019001-eng.htm.

Statistics Canada. (2019b). *Census in brief: Same-sex couples in Canada 2016*. https://www12.statcan.gc.ca/census-recensement/2016/as-sa/98-200-x/2016007/98-200-x2016007-eng.cfm.

Statistics Canada. (2019c). *Canada's population estimates: July 1, 2019*. https://www150.statcan.gc.ca/n1/daily-quotidien/190930/dq190930a-eng.htm.

Statistics Canada. (2020a). *Police-reported hate crime in Canada, 2018*. https://www150.statcan.gc.ca/n1/pub/85-002-x/2020001/article/00003-eng.htm.

Statistics Canada. (2020b). *Visible minority of person*. https://www23.statcan.gc.ca/imdb/p3Var.pl?Function=DEC&Id=45152.

Tervalon, M., & Murray-Garcia, J. (1998). Cultural humility versus cultural competence: A critical distinction in defining physician training outcomes in multicultural education. *Journal of Health Care for the Poor and Underserved, 9*(2), 117–125 [Seminal Reference].

Truth and Reconciliation Commission of Canada. (2015). *Honouring the truth, reconciling for the future: Summary of the final report of the Truth and Reconciliation Commission of Canada*. http://www.trc.ca/websites/trcinstitution/index.php?p=890.

UNESCO. (2001). *Universal declaration on cultural diversity*. [Seminal Reference] http://www.unesco.org/new/fileadmin/MULTIMEDIA/HQ/CLT/pdf/5_Cultural_Diversity_EN.pdf.

Varcoe, C., Browne, A. J., Wong, S., et al. (2009). Harms and benefits: Collecting ethnicity data in a clinical context. *Social Science & Medicine, 68*, 1659–1666.

Wesp, M., Scheer, M., Ruiz, M., et al. (2018). An emancipatory approach to cultural competency: The application of critical race, postcolonial, and intersectionality theories. *Advances in Nursing Science, 41*(4), 316–326. https://doi.org/10.1097/ANS.0000000000000230.

Williams, D. R., & Mohammed, S. A. (2013). Racism and health I: Pathways and scientific evidence. *American Behavioral Scientist, 57*(8), 1152–1173.

Wilson, A. (1996). How we find ourselves: Identity development and two-spirit people. *Harvard Educational Review, 66*, 303–317 [Seminal Reference].

World Health Organization. (2015). *First draft of the framework for country action across sectors for health and health equity*. https://www.who.int/nmh/events/action-framework/en/.

World Health Organization. (2018). *Disability and health*. https://www.who.int/news-room/fact-sheets/detail/disability-and-health.

World Health Organization. (2020). *Chronic diseases and health promotion*. https://www.who.int/chp/about/integrated_cd/en/.

World Health Organization. (n.d.). *Social determinants of health*. http://www.who.int/social_determinants/sdh_definition/en/.

World Health Organization & United Nations High Commissioner for Refugees. (2012). *Assessing mental health and psychosocial needs and resources: Toolkit for major humanitarian settings*. http://www.who.int/mental_health/resources/toolkit_mh_emergencies/en/.

Ziegler, E. (2019). Sexuality and gender. In C. Pollard, & S. Jakubec (Eds.), *Varcarolis's Canadian psychiatric mental health nursing* (2nd Cdn ed.). Elsevier Canada.

Zunner, B., & Grace, P. (2012). The ethical nursing care of transgender patients: An exploration of bias in health care and how it affects this population. *American Journal of Nursing, 112*(12), 61–64.

8

Epidemiological Applications

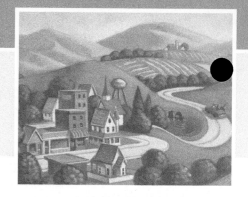

OUTLINE

Epidemiology: An Overview, 177
History of Epidemiology, 178
Common Epidemiological Measures in Community
  Health Nursing, 180
  Measures of Morbidity and Mortality, 180
Epidemiological Models and Approaches, 185
  The Epidemiological Triangle, 185
  The Web of Causation, 186
  The Life Course Approach, 188
Levels of Prevention, 189
  Primary Prevention, 189
  Secondary Prevention, 189

Tertiary Prevention, 189
The Natural History of Disease Related to Levels of
  Prevention, 189
Screening, 189
  Reliability and Validity, 191
The Basics of Epidemiological Research, 192
  Types of Epidemiological Studies, 192
  Sources of Data, 195
  Age-Adjusted Death Rates, 196
  Comparison Groups, 196
How Community Health Nurses use Epidemiology, 196

OBJECTIVES

After reading this chapter, you should be able to:

8.1 Define the types of epidemiology and discuss the steps
     in the epidemiological process.
8.2 List some of the important milestones in the history of
     epidemiology.
8.3 Describe the common epidemiological measures used in
     community health nursing.
8.4 Explain the epidemiological triangle, the web of
     causation, and the life course approach.

8.5 Describe the three levels of prevention and how they
     relate to the natural history of disease.
8.6 Describe the characteristics of a successful screening
     program in epidemiology.
8.7 Describe the types of studies used in epidemiology.
8.8 Explain how community health nurses use epidemiology
     in nursing practice.

KEY TERMS*

agent, 185
analytical epidemiology, 177
case fatality rate (CFR), 183
descriptive epidemiology, 177
distribution, 177
ecological study, 192
endemic, 182
environment, 185
epidemic, 182
epidemiological triangle, 185
epidemiology, 177
experimental or intervention studies, 193
host, 185
incidence rate, 180
morbidity, 180
mortality, 180
natural history of disease, 189
negative predictive value, 192

pandemic, 182
point epidemic, 182
positive predictive value, 192
prevalence rate, 182
primary prevention, 189
proportion, 180
proportionate mortality ratio (PMR), 184
public health surveillance, 195
rate, 180
reliability, 191
screening, 189
secondary prevention, 189
sensitivity, 191
specificity, 191
surveillance, 195
tertiary prevention, 189
validity, 191
web of causation, 186

*See the Glossary on page 468 for definitions.

Epidemiology is the study of the distribution of factors that determine health-related states or events in a population, and the use of this information to control health problems. The term originally applied to infectious epidemics, such as cholera and tuberculosis (TB). It now applies to infectious diseases; chronic diseases such as cancer; cardiovascular disease; mental health–related events; other health-related events, including accidents, injuries, and violence; occupational and environmental exposures and their effects; health status and outcomes; determinants of health; and health system performance.

As the basic science of public health, epidemiology has made major contributions to (1) our understanding of the factors that contribute to health and disease; (2) the development of health promotion and disease prevention measures; (3) the detection and characterization of emerging infectious agents; (4) the evaluation of health services and policies; and (5) the practice of nursing in community health. This chapter examines key epidemiological concepts and processes. Community health nurses (CHNs) need to be able to understand and use epidemiological data. Readers are encouraged to consult resources that provide detailed information on epidemiology.

EPIDEMIOLOGY: AN OVERVIEW

Epidemiology is classified as either descriptive or analytical. **Descriptive epidemiology** examines health outcomes in terms of what, who, where, and when. It asks questions such as, What is the disease? Who is affected? Where are they? When do these events occur? Thus, descriptive epidemiology discusses a disease in terms of person, place, and time. By contrast, **analytical epidemiology** examines the etiology (origins or causes) of a disease and associated determinants of health. It asks questions such as, How does the disease occur? Why are some people affected more than others? Determinants of health may be individual, relational, social, communal, or environmental.

Epidemiology, like both the research process and community health nursing process, consists of a set of steps that help investigate a health pattern. Step one of the epidemiological process is to define the health pattern and explore current statistics related to that health pattern. The health pattern can refer to an outbreak of disease (e.g., measles), or it can refer to injuries (e.g., needle stick injuries), accidents, or even wellness (e.g., normal blood pressure). Step two involves using epidemiological methods to describe the distribution—who, where, and when—of a disease, event, or injury (e.g., mortality, morbidity, incidence). Step three involves searching for factors that explain the pattern or risk of occurrence (e.g., poor handwashing protocols). Step four involves determining what has influenced the occurrence of a particular disease or injury or why and how events occurred as they did (e.g., low level of measles vaccinations).

CHNs are often involved in investigating the **distribution**, or the pattern of, a health outcome in a population and determining the factors that influence those patterns, especially

---

BOX 8.1 Steps in Investigating a Disease Outbreak

- Research the most recent statistics on the rate of the disease in the community (e.g., the current rate of measles in the community).
- Establish that an outbreak exists by verifying the diagnosis and comparing previous rates of the disease with the current rate of the disease (chart audits, trends in rates).
- Establish a working case definition using laboratory data, and clinical symptoms (chart audit)
- Find cases systematically and collect data on those cases (contact tracing).
- Conduct descriptive epidemiology. Characterize the outbreak in terms of "person, place, and time" to determine the personal characteristics of the cases, changes in disease frequency over time, and differences in disease frequency based on location.
- Develop hypotheses about the cause or source of the disease outbreak (e.g., an outbreak of measles occurred at elementary schools in a community).
- Evaluate the hypotheses and refine them if necessary. Conduct additional studies if necessary (e.g., the outbreak occurred in one elementary school after an unvaccinated child returned to school after experiencing flu-like symptoms).
- Implement control and prevention measures (check all children and teachers' vaccination records and vaccinate as needed).
- Communicate findings to local health authorities (report case of measles immediately to nursing supervisor).

Source: Adapted from Centers for Disease Control and Prevention. (2015). *Investigating an outbreak*. https://www.cdc.gov/csels/dsepd/ss1978/lesson6/section2.html

---

if that health pattern involves the outbreak of disease in the community. Box 8.1 outlines the steps a CHN can use in consultation with the health care team to investigate a disease outbreak (Centers for Disease Control and Prevention, 2015). Although the steps are ordered here, several of these steps may occur at the same time.

Like nursing, epidemiology builds on and draws from other disciplines and methods, including clinical medicine, laboratory sciences, social sciences, quantitative methods (especially biostatistics), and public health policy and goals. It is important to note that epidemiology focuses on *populations*, whereas clinical medicine focuses on *individuals*. Moreover, epidemiology studies populations to determine the causes of health and disease in communities and to investigate and evaluate interventions that will prevent disease and maintain or restore health.

Epidemiology differs from clinical medicine in that it studies populations to (1) monitor their health, (2) identify the determinants of health and disease in communities, and (3) investigate and evaluate interventions to prevent disease and maintain or restore health. A CHN uses epidemiology to assess the complex interplay of social and environmental factors that affect the client's well-being and understand the broader context in which the client lives.

Specifically, CHNs use epidemiological methods and findings to determine the needs of a population and then work with the health care team and the clients to develop community health programs and implement preventive measures. In this way, community health nursing practice connects the disciplines of nursing, epidemiology, and medicine.

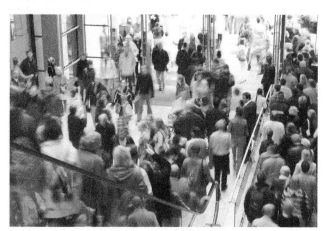

Epidemiology is the study of the health of populations. (iStockphoto/sculpies)

HISTORY OF EPIDEMIOLOGY

Hippocrates (c. 460–375 BCE) was first to use the ideas that are now part of epidemiology (Merril & Timmreck, 2006). He examined health and disease in a community by looking at geography, climate, the seasons of the year, the food and water consumed, and the habits and behaviours of the people. His approach, like descriptive epidemiology, looked at how health is influenced by personal characteristics, place, and time. Louis Pasteur (1822–1895) developed the germ theory of disease as well as pasteurization. Pasteur also recognized the role of personal factors, such as immunity and host resistance, when he saw that only certain people were susceptible to disease (Vandenbroucke, 1990). Joseph Lister (1827–1912), a British surgeon, developed antiseptic surgery, and Robert Koch (1843–1910), a German scientist, developed pure-culture techniques and identified the organisms that cause such diseases as TB, anthrax, and cholera.

In the eighteenth and nineteenth centuries, comparison groups began to be used to measure change in and the effects of some experimental action or treatment. Also at this time, quantitative methods (numerical measurements or counts) came into use. One of the most famous studies using a comparison group is the mid-nineteenth-century investigation of cholera by John Snow (1813–1858), whom some call the "father of epidemiology" (Merril & Timmreck, 2006). Snow drew a map of the areas of cholera occurrence in London and found that the cases were clustered around a single public water pump. He was thus able to show that the contaminated water supply was related to the outbreak of cholera. He later observed that cholera rates were higher among households whose water intake was downstream from the city than among households whose water came from farther upstream, where there was less contamination. However,

TABLE 8.1   Cholera Death Rates per Household by Source of Water Supply in John Snow's 1853 Investigation

Company	Number of Houses	Death From Cholera	Deaths per 10 000 Households
Southwark and Vauxhall	40 046	1 263	315
Lambeth	26 107	98	37
Rest of London	256 423	1 422	59

Source: Adapted from Snow, J. (1855). On the mode of communication of cholera. In Snow on cholera. The Commonwealth Fund.

when households in the same area had different sources of water, differences observed in rates of cholera could not be attributed to location or economic status. Snow showed that households receiving water from the Lambeth Company, which moved its water intake away from sewage contamination, had cholera rates considerably lower than those supplied by Southwark and Vauxhall, a company that still drew water from a contaminated section of the river. Snow conducted a "natural experiment" in London (Table 8.1) and was able to document that foul water was the vehicle of transmission of the agent that caused cholera (Rothman, 2002).

In the field of nursing, Florence Nightingale (1820–1910) made a major contribution to the development of epidemiology in her work with British soldiers during the Crimean War (1854–1856). At this time, sick and injured soldiers were cared for in cramped quarters that had poor sanitation and were infested by lice and rats. They also had access to insufficient food and medical supplies. Nightingale looked at the relationship between the environmental conditions and the recovery of the soldiers. Using simple epidemiological measures, such as rate of illness per 1 000 soldiers, she was able to show that improving environmental conditions and providing additional nursing care decreased the mortality rate among the soldiers (Cohen, 1984; Palmer, 1983).

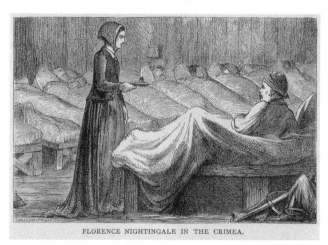

FLORENCE NIGHTINGALE IN THE CRIMEA.

Florence Nightingale, a skilled statistician for her time, had a significant influence on the study of epidemiology. (iStockphoto/whitemay)

Several changes followed and influenced the development of epidemiology. Before the twentieth century, the epidemiological focus was on the elimination of infectious diseases, such as cholera and bubonic plague (Naidoo & Wills, 2005). Improvements in sanitation, water, and housing were considered most essential to improve health. During the twentieth century, prevention and treatment of many infectious and communicable diseases were made possible, and the study of the causes of death shifted to chronic conditions, such as heart disease and cancer. Negative lifestyle factors have been shown to contribute to many of the chronic conditions that lead to death. Highly effective vaccinations, immunizations, and mass health screening programs contributed to the downward shift in disease (morbidity) and death (mortality) statistics.

Table 8.2 shows the leading causes of death in Canada from 2013 to 2017 (Statistics Canada, 2018a). Many of these deaths were due to chronic illnesses. Within a biomedical approach, cardiovascular diseases are often associated with negative lifestyle behaviours, such as smoking, unhealthy diets, and physical inactivity (Spenceley, 2007). According to Raphael (2009), the social determinants of health, specifically those that affect socioeconomic conditions for the client, contribute to chronic disease and other negative health outcomes. The Health Nexus and the Ontario Chronic Disease Prevention Alliance document titled *Primer to Action: Social Determinants of Health* (see the link on the Evolve website) provides information on the relationship between the social determinants of health and chronic disease and suggests actions to be taken.

Over the past 20 years, the development of genetic and molecular techniques has increased the epidemiologist's ability to classify persons in terms of exposures or inherent susceptibility to disease. Examples included the identification of genetic traits that indicate an increased risk for breast cancer and markers that identify exposure to environmental toxins, such as lead or pesticides. These developments are of particular interest to CHNs who deal with people in their living and work environments and have to understand the effects of environment(s) on health and well-being. CHNs are able to assess a broad range of health outcomes as well as factors that contribute to wellness and illness.

Unfortunately, in recent years, new infectious diseases (e.g., COVID-19, Lyme disease, legionnaires' disease, hantavirus, Ebola virus, severe acute respiratory syndrome [SARS], HIV/AIDS, avian influenza), as well as new forms of old diseases (e.g., drug-resistant strains of TB, new forms of *Escherichia coli* [*E. coli*]), have emphasized that potential dangers continue to exist to community health. Also, possible threats from terrorist attacks with infectious agents (e.g., anthrax, smallpox) have once again brought infectious disease epidemiology to the spotlight. Knowledge of epidemiological tools is vital to safeguarding the community and to improving health care management. As mentioned earlier, epidemiological methods are applied to a broader spectrum of health-related outcomes, including accidents, injuries, and violence, and occupational and environmental exposures. They are also applied to psychiatric and sociological phenomena; health-related behaviours; and health services research.

In the United States, following the terrorist attacks of September 11, 2001, and the apparently unrelated appearances of "anthrax letters," public health acquired a broader significance and heightened public awareness. Letters containing finely milled anthrax were sent to US senators and prominent

TABLE 8.2 Age-Standardized Mortality Rates in Canada by Selected Causes (Both Sexes), 2013 to 2016

	RATE PER 100 000 POPULATION			
	2013	2014	2015	2016
All causes of death (per 1 000)	717.8	728.3	737.7	736.8
Sepsis	6.5	6.6	6.9	5.3
Viral hepatitis	1.5	1.6	1.5	1.2
HIV	0.7	0.6	0.5	0.5
Malignant neoplasms (colon, rectum, anus, pancreas, trachea, bronchus, lung, breast)	213.7	216.9	215.0	218.1
Diabetes mellitus	20.0	19.9	20.0	18.9
Alzheimer's disease	18.0	18.0	18.4	18.0
Major cardiovascular diseases	193.6	194.9	195.5	191.9
Influenza and pneumonia	16.4	18.6	18.6	21.3
Chronic lower respiratory diseases	32.9	34.1	33.4	35.1
Chronic liver disease and cirrhosis	8.3	8.4	8.8	8.9
Nephritis, nephrotic syndrome, and nephrosis	9.6	8.5	8.7	8.7
Certain conditions originating in the perinatal period	3.1	3.2	3.1	3.0
Congenital malformations, deformations, and chromosomal abnormalities	2.8	2.8	2.8	2.8
Accidents (unintentional injuries)	32.5	32.6	33.0	33.0
Intentional self-harm (suicide)	11.3	11.5	12.0	12.3
Assault (homicide)	1.4	1.3	1.2	1.3

Source: Adapted from Statistics Canada. (2018a). *Death and age-specific mortality rates, by selected grouped causes* (Table 13-10-0392-01). https://www150.statcan.gc.ca/t1/tbl1/en/tv.action?pid=1310039201

news anchors, postal workers, and others. Five people died after becoming infected with anthrax and 17 contracted anthrax but survived. Those anthrax letters caused heightened public awareness of the role of the epidemiologist in tracing the origins of infectious diseases, which in that case was linked to the letters and not an outbreak. In Canada, in 2004, the Public Health Agency of Canada (PHAC) was established in response to the SARS outbreak, with additional responsibilities for chronic disease prevention, injury prevention, and emergency preparedness (Issa, 2008; PHAC, 2006). In the United States and especially in Canada, there is renewed awareness of the importance of a sound public health infrastructure, particularly with regard to disease surveillance and outbreak investigations. This infrastructure can carry on critical day-to-day public health functions while also monitoring, anticipating, and responding to events. Epidemiologists were among the first to respond to events such as the 9/11 terrorist attacks, anthrax letters, SARS, and Ebola. Subsequently, numerous epidemiological studies were designed and initiated to understand the impact of a range of exposures related to those events. Epidemiological methods and epidemiologists play a key role in public health planning and emergency preparedness.

Epidemiology looks at the distribution of health states and events in the community. Individuals differ in their probability or risk of disease, so the primary concern is to identify how they differ. Mapping cases of a disease in an area—as John Snow mapped cholera cases in London, and as many epidemiologists currently map various health-related events—can be instructive, even though it is limited in what it can reveal. A higher number of cases may simply be the result of a larger population with more potential cases or the result of a longer period of observation. Any description of disease patterns should take into account the size of the population at risk for the disease. That is, we should look not only at the numerator (the number of cases) but also at the denominator (the number of people in the population at risk) and at the amount of time each was observed. For example, 50 cases of influenza might be seen as a serious epidemic (outbreak of influenza) in a population of 250, over a period of 10 days, but it would be a low rate in a population of 250 000. Using proportions (ratio) and rates (measures of frequency) instead of simple counts of cases correctly identifies a population at risk.

COMMON EPIDEMIOLOGICAL MEASURES IN COMMUNITY HEALTH NURSING

Measures of Morbidity and Mortality

CHNs must be familiar with epidemiological measures to be able to describe the distribution of disease and health outcomes within populations. **Morbidity** refers to the occurrence of disease in a population—for example, the number of reported cases of coronary artery disease in males between the ages of 40 and 60. Measurements of morbidity include **incidence rate** and prevalence rate. By contrast, **mortality** refers to the number of deaths in a population—for example, the number of deaths from coronary artery disease among men between the ages of 40 and 60. Mortality rates include case fatality rate, infant mortality rate, and proportionate mortality rate.

Table 8.3 presents definitions, examples, and formulas for the basic epidemiological measures that CHNs need to be familiar with. These measures help CHNs identify and understand health issues present in a community, populations most at risk, and the health services needed in the community.

Proportion

A *proportion* is a type of ratio in which the numerator is part of the denominator. Because the numerator is included in the denominator, a proportion can range from 0 to 1. Proportions are often multiplied by 100 and expressed as a percentage, which literally means a rate or proportion "per 100." In public health statistics, however, if the proportion is very small, a larger multiplier is used to avoid small fractions. Thus, the proportion may be expressed as a number per 1 000 or per 100 000.

Rate

A *rate* is a ratio, but it is not a proportion because the denominator is a function of both the population size and the dimension of time, whereas the numerator is the number of events. Furthermore, depending on the units of time and the frequency of events, a rate may exceed 1. As its name suggests, a rate is a measure of how quickly something is happening—how rapidly a disease is developing in a population or how rapidly people are dying. Rates deal with change over time; that is, they express movement from one state of being to another (e.g., from well to ill, alive to dead, or ill to cured). A population must be monitored over time to observe the changes in state, and, typically, those persons who have already experienced the event are excluded from the population that is monitored.

Population at Risk

A *population at risk* comprises those for whom there is some finite probability (even if small) of experiencing an event. For example, although the risk of breast cancer in men is small, a few men do develop breast cancer and therefore are part of the population at risk. There are some outcomes for which certain people would never be at risk (e.g., men can never be at risk for ovarian cancer, nor can women be at risk for testicular cancer). A high-risk population, on the other hand, would include those persons who, because of exposure, lifestyle, family history, or other factors, are at greater risk for a disease than the population at large. It seems that all persons are susceptible to HIV infection, although the degree of susceptibility may vary. Persons who have multiple sexual partners without adequate protection or intravenous drug users are in the high-risk population for HIV infection. However, others who do not fit these categories may unknowingly be at high risk—for example, individuals who are in monogamous relationships but are unaware that their partners have multiple sexual relationships. Similar to proportions, risk estimates also have no dimensions, but they are a function of the length of time of observation. Given a continuous rate, increasing exposure time will mean that a larger proportion of the population will eventually become ill.

Ratio

A *ratio* can be used to calculate an approximation of a risk. For example, the infant mortality "rate" is the number of

TABLE 8.3   Basic Epidemiology Measures

Measure	Definition	Examples and Formulas
Proportion	Proportion is a type of ratio that shows the relationship between the total number and the frequency of occurrence in the case of a particular health event	In 2016, a total of 2 404 624 deaths were recorded in country X, of which 709 894 were reported as caused by cardiovascular diseases. Therefore, the proportion of deaths caused by heart disease in 2016 was $$\frac{709894}{2404624} = 0.295, \text{ or } 29.5\%$$
Rate	Rate is a measure of the frequency of a health event in a specific population in a defined time period	The formula for calculating rate is $$\frac{\text{\# of events in a time period}}{\text{Total population at risk during the same time period}} \times 1000 \text{ (10 000 or 100 000)}$$ For example, in country X, the birth rate for a given year would be calculated as follows: $$\frac{\text{\# of births in (year)}}{\text{Total population in (year)}}$$ $$\frac{37\ 850\,(2015)}{3\ 970\ 000\,(2015)} = 0.0095 \times 1\ 000 = 9.5$$ Therefore, in country X, 9.5 births per 1 000 population occurred in the year 2015
Risk	Refer to Table 8.6	Refer to Table 8.6
Ratio	Refer to Table 8.6	Refer to Table 8.6
Incidence rate	Incidence rate is a measure of the number of new cases of a disease or an event in a population at risk over a defined period	The formula for calculating incidence rate is $$\frac{\text{\# of new cases in a time period}}{\text{Total population at risk during the same time period}}$$ For example, 80 new cases of breast cancer were found in 2016 within a population of 8 000 women aged 50 to 75, so the incidence rate for this population in 2016 was $$\frac{80}{8\ 000} = 0.01$$
Prevalence rate	Prevalence rate identifies the number of persons in a population who have a disease or experience a health event in a specific time period (old and new cases included)	The formula for calculating the prevalence rate is $$\frac{\text{\# of people in a population with the disease in a time period}}{\text{Total population at risk during the same time period}}$$ For example, 8 000 women were screened for breast cancer from January 1, 2015, to December 31, 2015. 35 of them had previously been diagnosed with a cancer event and 20 were newly diagnosed with a cancer event; the prevalence rate in this group for 2015 is as follows: $$\frac{55}{8\ 000} = 0.006875, \text{ or } 687.5 \text{ per 100 000}$$

Note: Country X could be Canada; note, however, that these numbers are fictitious.
Source: The definitions are adapted from Greenberg, Daniels, Flanders, et al., 2005.

infant deaths in a given year divided by the number of live births in that same year (*infants* are defined as being younger than 1 year). It approximates the risk of death in the first year of life for infants born in a specific year. It is important to note that in a particular year, some of the infants who die before their first birthday would have been born in the previous year, and some of the infants born that year may die in the following year. However, because about two-thirds of infant deaths occur within the first 28 days of life, the number of infants in the numerator (deaths in a given year) will be smaller than the denominator (live births in that same year). One of the assumptions used in the calculation of infant mortality is that the current-year deaths among the previous year's

cohort (group of individuals with similar characteristics) will approximate the following year's deaths among the current year's cohort. Although technically a ratio, infant mortality rate is an approximation of the true proportion and, therefore, an estimate of the risk. Infant mortality rate is calculated using the following formula:

$$\frac{\text{Number of infant deaths under 1 year of age during a given year}}{\text{Number of live infant births under 1 year during the same year}} \times 1\ 000$$

For example, in city X in Canada, which has a population of 200 000, there were 200 infant deaths and 20 000 live births in 2015. Therefore, the infant mortality rate for 2015 would be as follows:

$$\frac{200}{20\ 000} \times 1\ 000$$

Therefore, there have been 10 infant deaths per 1 000 live births during 2015 in city X.

Measures of Incidence

Measures of *incidence* reflect the number of new cases or events. The population at risk is considered to be individuals who have not experienced the event or outcome of interest but who are at risk of experiencing it. Note that for this calculation, existing (or prevalent) cases are excluded from the population at risk because they already have the condition and are no longer at risk of developing it.

In community health nursing practice, CHNs need to be familiar with the concepts of *epidemic, endemic,* and *pandemic* because diseases tend to occur at specific times in specific geographical locations and affect specific populations. People who are exposed to specific agents or pathogens are more likely to develop a disease or a condition that may spread to others in their community. In some situations, the disease or condition may also spread to other communities and geographical locations, as in the case of the global spread of SARS, which will be discussed in a later chapter.

An **epidemic** is the occurrence of a greater number of cases of a disease, an injury, or other condition than expected in a particular area or group. Therefore, it describes a situation in which the incidence of a disease has increased (has new cases). For example, with the global eradication of smallpox, any occurrence of smallpox anywhere might be considered an epidemic. A **point epidemic** is a time-and-space–related pattern that is particularly important in infectious disease investigations. It is also a significant indicator for toxic exposures in environmental epidemiology. A point epidemic is most clearly visible when the frequency of cases is graphed against time. The sharp peak that is characteristic of such graphs indicates a concentration of cases over a short interval of time. The peak often indicates a population's response to a simultaneous exposure to a common source of infection or contamination. Knowledge of the incubation or latency period (the time between exposure and development of signs and symptoms) for the specific disease entity can help determine the probable time of exposure. A common point epidemic is an outbreak of gastrointestinal illness caused by a foodborne pathogen. CHNs need to be alert for a sudden increase in the number of cases of a disease and then need to chart the outbreak, determine the probable time of exposure, and, by careful investigation, isolate the probable source of the agent.

An **endemic** disease is a disease with a constant presence in a particular population or geographical area. For example, community-acquired pneumonia is usually present in a particular population within a region. By contrast, a **pandemic** is an epidemic occurring in a geographically widespread area or in a large population. For example, the Ebola virus outbreak in 2014 in West Africa would be considered a pandemic.

Prevalence Rate

The *prevalence rate* is a measure of existing disease in a population at a particular time (i.e., the number of existing cases divided by the current population). The prevalence of a specific risk factor or exposure can also be calculated. For example, if a breast cancer screening program reveals that 35 of the 8 000 women screened have a previous diagnosis of breast cancer and 20 with no previous history of breast cancer are diagnosed as having breast cancer, then the prevalence rate would be calculated as shown in Table 8.3. The "Evidence-Informed Practice" box discusses a study focused on identifying the prevalence and incidence of a disease.

ⓢ EVIDENCE-INFORMED PRACTICE

Issekutz, Graham, Prasad, et al. (2005) undertook a national epidemiological study of CHARGE syndrome over 3 years, which was coordinated by the Canadian Pediatric Surveillance Program (CPSP). In the study, physicians provided information on a monthly basis to the CPSP on clients with CHARGE syndrome. The study population comprised clients with select conditions grouped as CHARGE syndrome (coloboma, heart defects, atresia choanae, retarded growth and development, genital hypoplasia, and ear abnormalities). The prevalence of CHARGE in births was calculated on the basis of national and provincial birth rates obtained from Statistics Canada.

The main objective of the study was to estimate the birth prevalence of CHARGE syndrome in Canada between January 1, 1999, and December 31, 2002. The national birth incidence of those with CHARGE syndrome was 3.5 per 100 000 live births. No cases of this syndrome were reported in Alberta. In Newfoundland and Labrador, and the Maritime provinces (Nova Scotia, New Brunswick, and Prince Edward Island) the birth incidence was 10.66 per 100 000, and 12.84 per 100 000, respectively. This translates into a CHARGE occurrence of 1 in every 8 500 live births in the Atlantic provinces. Provincial and regional variations in the birth

rate of those with this syndrome were identified to be higher than previously reported in the literature. The findings of this study are consistent with previous reports, in that patients who survive infancy are more likely to survive through childhood.

Application for CHNs
Epidemiological measures, such as the prevalence and incidence of disease, are important for CHNs when planning community health nursing care for aggregates in their geographical area.

Questions for Reflection and Discussion
1. Explain the difference between the terms *prevalence* and *incidence.*
2. How would knowledge of change in the occurrence of CHARGE syndrome over time contribute to the assessment and planning role of a CHN?
3. A higher incidence of CHARGE syndrome exists in the Maritime provinces and Newfoundland and Labrador. What could CHNs explore about client experiences, values, preferences, or choices when conducting home visits with families caring for children with CHARGE syndrome?

Source: Issekutz, Graham, Prasad, et al., 2005.

TABLE 8.4   Common Mortality Rates

Rate/Ratio	Definition and Example*
Crude mortality rate	An estimate of the risk of death for a person in a given population at a specified time. *Example:* In year X, there were 2 304 500 deaths in a total population of 295 364 888, or 780.2 per 100 000
Age-specific mortality rate	The number of deaths among persons of a given age group divided by the total number of deaths in the population of that age group at a specified time. *Example:* In year X, the age-specific mortality rate for 40- to 60-year-olds was 240 per 100 000
Cause-specific mortality rate	The number of deaths from a specific cause in a population at a specified time. *Example:* In year X, the cause-specific rate for accidents was 42.6 per 100 000
Case fatality rate	The proportion of persons diagnosed with a particular disease (i.e., cases) who die within a specified period. *Example:* If 15 of every 100 males diagnosed with prostate cancer dies within 5 years, the 5-year case fatality rate is 15%. The 5-year survival rate is 85%
Proportionate mortality ratio	The proportion of all deaths that are the result of a specific cause who die within a specified period. *Example:* In year X, there were 650 670 deaths from cardiovascular diseases and 2 506 451 deaths from all causes, or 26% of all deaths were due to heart disease
Infant mortality rate	The number of infant deaths before 1 year of age in a year divided by the number of live births in the same year. *Example:* In year X, there were 29 200 infant deaths and 3 068 715 live births, or 9.5 per 1 000 live births
Neonatal mortality rate	The number of infant deaths under 28 days of age in a year divided by the number of live births in the same year. *Example:* In year X, there were 17 886 neonatal deaths and 4 068 914 live births, or 4.4 per 1 000 live births
Postneonatal mortality rate	The number of infant deaths from 28 days to 1 year of age in a year divided by the number of live births in the same year. *Example:* In year X, there were 8 489 postneonatal deaths and 4 068 914 live births, or 2.1 per 1 000 live births

*Examples are not based on actual data. Refer to the chapter discussion for calculation formulas.

Mortality Rates

Mortality rates reflect both the incidence and prevalence of death rates. Table 8.4 provides examples of common mortality rates. Many mortality rates are not true rates but proportions. Although measures of mortality reflect serious health problems and changing patterns of disease, they have limited usefulness. They provide information only about fatal diseases and do not provide direct information about either the level of an existing disease in the population or the risk of getting a particular disease. Also, a person may have one disease (e.g., prostate cancer) and yet die from a different cause (e.g., cerebrovascular accident).

Because of population changes during the course of a year, the usual practice is to estimate the population at mid-year as the denominator for annual rates. The *crude annual mortality rate* is an estimate of the risk of death for a person in a given population for that year. These rates are multiplied by a scaling factor, usually 100 000, to avoid small fractions. The result is then expressed as the number of deaths per 100 000 persons. Although the crude mortality rate is calculated easily and represents the actual death rate for the total population, it has certain limitations. It does not reveal specific causes of death, which change in relative importance over time. Also, the mortality rate is affected by the population's age distribution, since older adults are at much greater risk of death than are younger people.

Mortality rates are also calculated for specific groups (e.g., age-specific, gender-specific, or race-specific mortality rates). To determine the *age-specific mortality rate*, the number of deaths occurring in the specified group is divided by the population at risk at a specific time. This rate is then considered the risk of death for persons in the specified group during the period of observation. Differences in the age distribution between two populations can lead to bias. Standardized mortality rates build on age-specific mortality rates and correct for age distribution differences and therefore control for bias.

The *cause-specific mortality rate* is an estimate of the risk of death from a specific disease in a population. It is the number of deaths from a specific cause divided by the total population at risk, usually multiplied by 100 000. Two related measures should be distinguished from the cause-specific mortality rate. The **case fatality rate (CFR)** is the proportion of persons diagnosed with a particular disease (i.e., cases) who die within a specified period. The CFR is considered an estimate of the risk of death within that period for a person newly diagnosed with the disease (e.g., the proportion of persons globally with cases of avian influenza A(H5N1) who die within 5 years). Since the CFR is the proportion of diagnosed individuals who die within the period, 100 minus the CFR yields the survival rate. For example, if 433 cases of H5N1 were diagnosed over a 5-year period and 262 deaths occurred, the CFR would be 60.5%, and the 5-year survival rate would be 39.5% (Proteus, 2009). To review further information on CFRs and on the avian influenza, see the Proteus link on the Evolve website. Persons diagnosed with a particular disease often want to know the probability of their survival. Case fatality rates provide that information.

The second measure to be distinguished from the cause-specific mortality rate is the **proportionate mortality ratio (PMR)**, which is the proportion of all deaths for a specific population, that are the result of a specific cause within a specified period. The denominator is not the population at risk of death but the total number of deaths in the population; therefore, the PMR is not a rate, nor does it estimate the risk of death. The magnitude of the PMR is a function of both the number of deaths from the cause of interest and the number of deaths from other causes. The formula for calculating the PMR, usually expressed as a percentage, is as follows:

$$\frac{\text{Total number of deaths due to a specific cause}}{\text{Total number of deaths from all causes}} \times 100$$

If rates of death from certain causes decline over time, rates of death from other causes that remain fairly constant may have increasing PMRs. For example, in Canada in 2017, intentional self-harm (suicide) accounted for a total of 223 deaths with an age-specific mortality rate of 10.9 per 100 000 for persons 15 to 19 years of age. The total number of deaths from all causes in this age group was reported as 732 with an age-specific mortality rate at 35.9 per 100 000 persons (Statistics Canada, 2018a). Using the formula for calculating the PMR, the proportion of deaths from self-harm (suicide) for this age group was 30.5%. By comparison, suicide accounted for 36 or 1.9 deaths per 100 000 persons 10–14 years of age, with the total number of deaths from all causes in this age group reported as 198 (Statistics Canada, 2018a). The PMR for suicide for the 10–14 years age group was calculated as 18.2%. This example demonstrates that the risk of death from suicide in the age group 15 to 19 years was higher than that of risk for the age group of 10–14 years (based on the rates) and that suicide accounted for a far greater proportion of all deaths in this older age group (based on the PMR).

The infant mortality rate is used all over the world as an indicator of overall health and availability of health care services. The risk of death declines considerably during the first year of life, so neonatal (i.e., newborn) and postneonatal mortality rates are of significance. In Canada, in 2014, infant mortality rates were 4.7 per 1 000 live births, compared with 4.5 per 1 000 live births in 2017 (Statistics Canada, 2018b). Table 8.5 presents Canadian infant mortality rates from 2014 to 2017. Some provinces and territories (Nova Scotia, Manitoba, Saskatchewan, Northwest Territories, and Nunavut) have reported an increase in infant mortality rates per 1 000 live births in 2014 compared with 2017.

Measures of Association

Measures of association indicate the strength of the relationship between the variables being studied. The most frequently used measures of association in epidemiology are risk, relative risk, attributable risk, ratio, odds ratio, and potential years of life lost (Table 8.6). Of note, attributable risk and relative risk are used by epidemiologists to compare rates of exposure between those exposed to a risk and those not exposed to a risk.

Epidemiological concepts and data are used in ongoing assessments of client health concerns. As will be discussed in Chapter 9, an initial component of a community health assessment is the collection of vital statistics such as incidence, prevalence, morbidity, and mortality rates for specific diseases and other data such as patterns of the use of health services and immunization rates.

The clinical epidemiology glossary in the Tool Box on the Evolve website includes additional terms CHNs will find useful in their practice.

TABLE 8.5	Infant Mortality Rates by Province and Territory (Both Sexes), 2014 to 2017			
	2014	**2015**	**2016**	**2017**
Canada	4.7	4.5	4.5	4.5
Newfoundland and Labrador	6.1	4.7	4.5	4.4
Prince Edward Island	1.4	2.2	7.1	3.0
Nova Scotia	4.4	4.1	5.1	4.1
New Brunswick	4.0	4.1	5.1	2.8
Quebec	4.4	4.8	4.3	4.0
Ontario	4.6	4.4	4.7	4.7
Manitoba	6.2	6.4	5.5	7.2
Saskatchewan	5.7	5.3	5.8	6.6
Alberta	4.9	4.6	4.4	4.9
British Columbia	4.2	3.3	3.4	3.1
Yukon	2.5	6.9	6.7	*
Northwest Territories	6.0	5.9	6.2	4.9
Nunavut	16.7	12.8	17.7	11.1

NOTE: The infant mortality rate is calculated as the number of deaths of children less than 1 year of age per 1 000 live births.
*Data not available for specific reference period.
Source: Statistics Canada. (2018a). *Death and age-specific mortality rates, by selected grouped causes* (Table 13-10-0392-01). https://www150.statcan.gc.ca/t1/tbl1/en/tv.action?pid=1310039201

TABLE 8.6 Analytical Measures of Association in Epidemiology

Measure	Description	Formula
Risk	*Risk* refers to the probability that an event will occur within a specified period	Different measures of risk (e.g., absolute risk, attributable risk, and relative risk) are considered in determining the morbidity and mortality of a disease. The formulas associated with each measure can be found in epidemiological texts
Relative risk (RR)	A measure of the probability of the occurrence of a disease for persons who are exposed and persons who are not exposed to the risk factor	$\dfrac{\text{Incidence in exposed group}}{\text{Incidence in unexposed group}}$
Attributable risk (AR)	A measure of the incidence of a disease in individuals who have been exposed to the risk factor, expressed as a percentage	$\dfrac{\text{Incidence in exposed group} - \text{Incidence in unexposed group}}{\text{Incidence in exposed group}}$
Ratio	A measure of the relationship between two numbers expressed as the quotient of one divided by the other	$\dfrac{\text{Number X}}{\text{Number Y}}$
Odds ratio (OR)	A measure of the odds/probability that an event is the same for two groups. OR is used when incidence rates are not available	$\dfrac{\text{Odds of exposure for cases}}{\text{Odds of exposure for controls}}$ The OR is calculated by using contingency tables (refer to epidemiology text for specifics)
Potential years of life lost (PYLL)*	A ratio for a specific period of the total years of life lost before the age of 75 to the total population under 75. It is an indicator of premature mortality	$\dfrac{\text{Sum of differences between age at death and 75 for all deaths in a given year}}{\text{Total population aged 0 - 75 estimated in that year}} \times 1000$

Source: *Association of Public Health Epidemiologists in Ontario. (2006). *Calculating potential years of life lost (PYLL).* http://core.apheo.ca/index.php?pid=190

CHN IN PRACTICE: A CASE STUDY

Epidemiology

CHNs can use epidemiological data to assess individual and community-based health needs and evaluate the impact of interventions designed to meet those needs. The First Nations and Inuit Health Branch of Indigenous Services Canada Health have summarized epidemiological data specific to First Nations and Inuit populations in a "Quick Stats" sheet that can be useful when planning interventions. Summarized data include health and wellness indicators such as infant mortality, average number of decayed, missing, and filled teeth rates of TB, hospital rates for intentional harm, percentage living in crowded homes, and access to health services.

Health Indicators	First Nations	Inuit
Infant Mortality	9.2/1 000	12.2/1 000
Decayed, Missing, Filled Teeth (3–5 years)	7.6	8.2
TB	26.6/ 100 000	189.3/100 000
Intentional Harm	146/100 000	226/100 000
Living in Crowded Homes	36.8%	51.7%

Think About it

1. How could the CHN use these data to develop, implement, and evaluate harm reduction and health promotion programs for this population?
2. First Nations and Inuit populations have less favourable results across many health outcomes as compared to the rest of Canada. Why is this so, and what can be done about it?

Source: First Nations and Inuit Health Branch, Indigenous Services Canada. (2018). *First Nations in Canada Health and Wellness Indicators, Quick Stats, 2018 Edition.* https://health-infobase.canada.ca/fnih/doc/first_nations.pdf

EPIDEMIOLOGICAL MODELS AND APPROACHES

Several models and approaches can help CHNs identify and explore connections among the various factors and causes that contribute to specific health challenges. A few are discussed here.

The Epidemiological Triangle

Epidemiologists understand that disease results from complex relationships among causal agents, susceptible persons, and environmental factors. These three elements—agent, host, and environment—are referred to as the **epidemiological triangle** (Fig. 8.1A). Changes in one of the elements of the triangle can influence the occurrence of disease by increasing or decreasing a client's risk for disease. Often, the patient is an individual; however, a patient can be a group. For example, a group of miners (host) were diagnosed with pneumoconiosis as a result of their working conditions in an underground mine (environment) and their exposure to coal dust (agent). Fig. 8.1B shows that interactions between agent and host are influenced by the environmental context in which they exist. Alternatively, agent and host may in turn influence the environment. These three elements, or variables, are defined as follows:

1. **Agent:** an animate or inanimate factor that must be present or lacking for a disease or condition to develop.
2. **Host:** a living species (human or animal) capable of being infected or affected by an agent.
3. **Environment:** all that is internal or external to a given host or agent and that is influenced by and influences the host and the agent. Environment also includes social and physical factors.

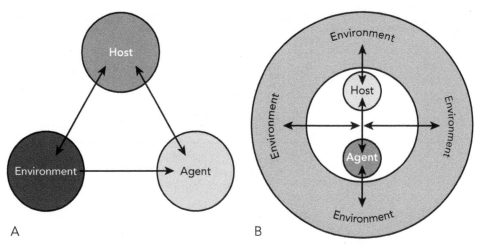

Fig. 8.1 The Epidemiological Triangle and Agent–Host–Environment Interactions.

BOX 8.2   Examples of Agent, Host, and Environmental Factors in the Epidemiological Triangle

Agent
- Infectious agents (e.g., bacteria, viruses, fungi, parasites)
- Chemical agents (e.g., heavy metals, toxic chemicals, pesticides)
- Physical agents (e.g., radiation, heat, cold, machinery)

Host
- Genetic susceptibility
- Immutable characteristics (e.g., age, sex)
- Acquired characteristics (e.g., immunological status)
- Lifestyle factors (e.g., diet, exercise)

Environment
- Climate (e.g., temperature, rainfall)
- Plant and animal life (e.g., agents or reservoirs or habitats for agents)
- Human population distribution (e.g., crowding, social support)
- Socioeconomic factors (e.g., education, resources, access to care)
- Working conditions (e.g., levels of stress, noise, satisfaction)

Examples of these three components are listed in Box 8.2. Fig. 8.2 provides examples of client situations using the epidemiological triangle for the events of TB, MVA, family violence, and homelessness. In the TB example, the host is a new immigrant with poor nutritional status; the agent is the mycobacterium tuberculosis organism; and the environment is the crowded housing in which the host lives, and the fact that the host has poor hygiene and has been in contact with a person infected with TB.

The Web of Causation

A causal relationship (one thing or event causing another) is often more complex than the epidemiological triangle conveys. The term **web of causation,** also referred to as *web of*

causality, recognizes the complex interrelationships among many factors, sometimes interacting in subtle ways to increase (or decrease) the risk of disease. Also, associations are sometimes mutual, with lines of causality going in both directions. Refer to Fig. 8.3 for an example of the application of the web of causation for the causal variables for cardiovascular disease, a medical event. In this web diagram, the contributing factor identified as "social pressures" would include the social and economic determinants of health. A growing body of evidence shows that poverty, social exclusion, and unavailability of health and social services are major factors contributing to the incidence of cardiovascular disease in populations (Raphael, 2004). As well, gender, especially being female, contributes to differences in causes, risk factors, processes, and treatment of cardiovascular disease (Armstrong, 2010).

In this web of causality, the linked factors illustrate relationships among the data. For example, such factors as heredity, diet, and exercise can contribute to prevention or development of myocardial infarction. To explore the relationships in the web of causality, Edwards and Moyer (2000) suggest asking the following two questions: (1) "What factors are contributing to the problem?" and (2) "What issues does each problem cause?" (p. 432). The CHN can use the web of causation for assessment purposes and to identify prevention intervention strategies.

Fig. 8.4 presents an example of the web of causation applied to homelessness, which is a social problem. In this figure, it is evident that homelessness is a complex social problem, and the multiple factors that contribute to it do not act in isolation of one another. Some of the key interrelated factors that contribute to homelessness are income, social support networks, education, the physical environment, employment and working conditions, health services, and culture. Conditions such as lack of affordable housing and lack of community supports and services can lead to an inability to manage other aspects of living, such as maintenance of relationships with family and friends and as well as employment status, and these conditions may also enhance health risks such as malnutrition.

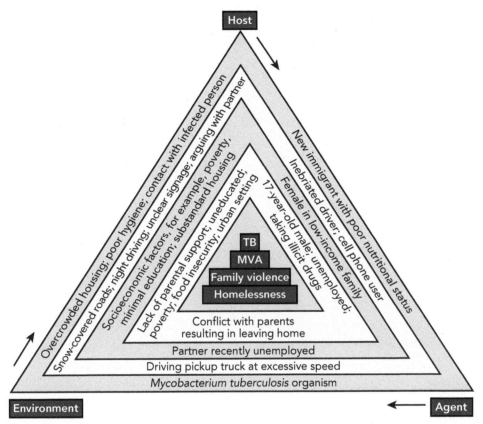

TB, Tuberculosis; MVA, motor vehicle accident

Fig. 8.2 Examples of Client Situations Using the Epidemiological Triangle.

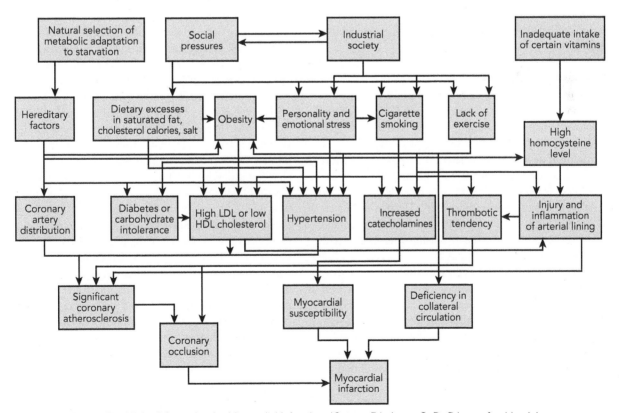

Fig. 8.3 The Web of Causation for Myocardial Infarction. (*Source*: Friedman, G. D. *Primer of epidemiology*. McGraw-Hill. Reproduced with permission.)

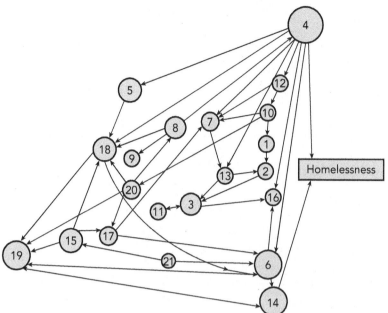

1. Changed economic factors
2. Decreased job market
3. Loss of employment
4. Poverty
5. Decreased food security
6. Lack of affordable housing
7. Access to health care
8. Cuts to social programs
9. Domestic violence
10. Physical chronic diseases
11. Educational level
12. Stress
13. Occupation
14. Poor hygiene
15. Loss of friends
16. Loss of family support
17. Addiction problems
18. Criminalization
19. Mental illness
20. Lack of available community services
21. Culture (e.g., Indigenous)

Fig. 8.4 The Web of Causation for Homelessness. *Note*: These are some possibilities and are not to be considered all-inclusive.

It needs to be noted that the relationship between mental health, substance abuse, and homelessness is multidirectional. The questions this point raises are: Does homelessness lead to mental illness and abuse of alcohol and drugs? Does mental illness lead to homelessness? Does substance abuse lead to homelessness? For further information on homelessness, see HeretoHelp, a project of the BC Partners for Mental Health and Addictions Information (the link is on the Evolve website).

The Life Course Approach

A life course approach attempts to understand how early life factors influence health or disease risk in adulthood (Kuh, Ben-Shlomo, Lynch, et al., 2003). A life course approach involves an exploration of how the social determinants of health influence development across the lifespan in relation to immediate as well as long-term health and illness status (Ben-Schlomo & Kuh, 2002; Braveman & Gottlieb, 2014; Evans-Polce, Doherty, & Ensminger, 2014; Hertzman, Power, Matthews, et al., 2001; Raphael, 2009; Senate Subcommittee on Population Health, 2009). The increasing interest in recent years in conceptualizing health and disease risk using a life course approach has led to a paradigm shift in the understanding of disease; disease prevention, especially in relation to chronic illness; and health and wellness (Ben-Schlomo & Kuh, 2002; Senate Subcommittee on Population Health, 2009). The life course approach to epidemiology includes an analysis of biological, psychosocial, and behavioural data collected from longitudinal studies that cover childhood to adulthood.

Over the life course, three types of effects influence a person's health in adulthood: latent, pathway, and cumulative effects. *Latent effects* relate to biological and developmental events that take place during the fetal or infancy stage that

influence a person's health later in life. *Pathway effects* relate to early life events and environments, especially the social environment, that place an individual on a particular life path that influences their childhood and adult health. *Cumulative effects* refer to the multiple environmental risks experienced at different ages that together increase the risk of disease in adulthood (Hertzman et al., 2001; PHAC, 2009). Many studies have been conducted to explore each of these effects and the link between early life factors and diseases in adulthood (Ben-Schlomo & Kuh, 2002; Evans-Polce et al., 2014; Hertzman et al., 2001; PHAC, 2009). However, life course research studies are difficult to conduct due to the complexity of this type of cohort study (Ben-Schlomo & Kuh, 2002).

Canadian researcher Clyde Hertzman was influential in creating a framework that "connects population health to human development, highlighting the unique role of early childhood development as a determinant of health" (World Health Organization [WHO], 2006). The linkage of population health to early child development has helped establish the connection between the effects of the environment in early life on a person's health in adulthood. The Centre of Excellence for Early Childhood Development is one organization that fosters the dissemination of scientific knowledge on the development of young children and works in partnership with several community groups, such as Canadian universities, First Nations communities, and professional associations. The centre has as its mandate to identify and synthesize scientific research on early childhood development and disseminate that knowledge to decision makers and practitioners. Another source of scientific knowledge on early childhood development is the Encyclopedia on Early Childhood Development (see the link on the Evolve website), which is produced by the Centre of Excellence for Early Childhood Development and the Strategic Knowledge

Cluster on Early Child Development at the Université de Montréal and Université Laval (Quebec, Canada).

LEVELS OF PREVENTION

In their daily practice, CHNs are often involved in activities related to all three levels of prevention. Consider, for example, how the three levels of prevention apply to TB infection control. In the prepathogenesis period, primary prevention activities include health promotion programs with both the general population and specific vulnerable groups (e.g., the homeless, HIV-positive persons, certain vulnerable immigrant groups) to reduce the incidence of TB. In the early period of pathogenesis, secondary prevention activities include routine Mantoux screening tests of specific groups (e.g., health care providers, childcare workers) and identifying and screening people who have had contact with a client known to have active TB. The use of directly observed therapy for the treatment of clients with TB in the community falls within the realm of tertiary prevention, which focuses on restoring client health. Given the emergence of new drug-resistant strains of TB, CHNs face the challenge of designing and implementing programs to increase long-term adherence and providing aftercare for clients in a variety of community settings.

Primary Prevention

Primary prevention refers to activities that seek to prevent the occurrence of a disease (based on the natural history of a disease) or an injury. Interventions at this level of prevention are aimed at individuals, groups, and populations who are susceptible to disease but have no discernible pathology (i.e., they are in a state of prepathogenesis). This first level of prevention includes broad efforts, such as:

1. *Environmental protection,* which includes basic sanitation, food safety, home and workplace safety, and air quality control. An example is a CHN working proactively to develop and advocate for policies and legislation that lead to the prevention of environmental hazards. Another example is a CHN consulting with industries, local governments, and groups of concerned citizens and public educators about preventable environmental health problems.
2. *Specific protection against disease or injury,* which includes immunizations, proper use of seat belts and infant car seats, preconception folic acid supplementation to prevent neural tube defects, fluoridation of the water supply to prevent dental caries, and actions taken to reduce exposure to cancer-causing agents.

Many CHNs are actively involved in primary prevention activities in homes, in community settings, and at the primary level of health care (e.g., in public health clinics, physicians' offices, community health centres, and rural health clinics).

Secondary Prevention

Secondary prevention refers to activities that seek to detect disease early in its progression (early pathogenesis), before clinical signs and symptoms become apparent, to make a diagnosis and begin treatment. Health screening programs are the mainstay of secondary prevention. Early and periodic screenings are critical for diseases, such as breast cancer, for which there are few specific primary prevention strategies.

Interventions at the secondary level of prevention may occur in community settings as well as at primary and secondary levels of health care. In developing countries, wherever safe water can be made available, oral rehydration therapy (ORT) is an inexpensive and effective way to treat infant diarrheal disease. For example, a CHN can teach mothers to recognize the early signs of infant dehydration and administer a homemade ORT solution made with water, sugar, and salt. In another example of secondary prevention, a CHN obtains a family history of cancer, heart disease, diabetes, or mental illness as part of a client's health history and then follows up with education about appropriate screening procedures. Other secondary prevention interventions include a mammography to detect breast cancer, a Papanicolaou (Pap) test to detect cervical cancer, a colonoscopy for early detection of colon cancer, and screening of pregnant women for gestational diabetes.

Tertiary Prevention

Tertiary prevention refers to activities that take place during the middle and later periods of pathogenesis; the goals are to interrupt the course of the disease, reduce the amount of disability that might occur, and begin rehabilitation. Tertiary prevention interventions occur most often at secondary and tertiary levels of health care (e.g., in specialized clinics, hospitals, rehabilitation centres) but may also occur in community and primary care settings. Examples of tertiary prevention are medical treatment, physical and occupational therapy, and rehabilitation.

The Natural History of Disease Related to Levels of Prevention

The goal of epidemiology is to identify and understand the causal factors and mechanisms of disease, injuries, and disability so that effective interventions can be implemented to prevent the occurrence of these adverse processes before they begin or before they progress. The **natural history of disease** refers to the progression of the disease process from onset to resolution. Leavell and Clark (1965) provide a classic description of two distinct periods in the natural history of the disease process: prepathogenesis (the period when no disease is present but susceptibility to disease exists) and pathogenesis (the period from early pathogenesis to convalescence). These two periods in the natural history of a disease are related to the three levels of prevention of communicable and noncommunicable diseases commonly used in community health nursing practice. Leavell and Clark's depiction of the natural history of a disease appears in Fig. 8.5. This figure illustrates the relationship between the natural history of a disease and the three levels of prevention.

SCREENING

Screening, a key component of many secondary prevention interventions, involves the testing of groups of individuals

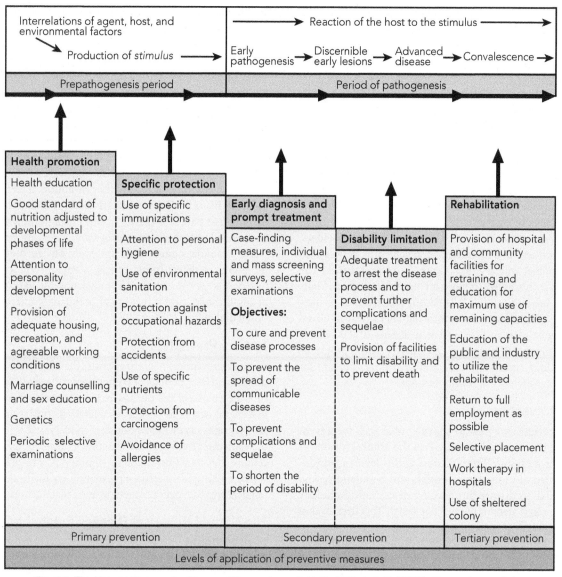

Fig. 8.5 The Natural History of a Disease. (*Source*: Leavell, H. R., & Clark, I. G. (1965). *Preventive medicine for the doctor in his community: An epidemiological approach.* McGraw-Hill. Reproduced with permission.)

who are at risk for a certain condition but do not manifest any symptoms. The goal is to determine the likelihood that these individuals will develop the disease. From a clinical perspective, the aim of screening is early detection and treatment when these are likely to result in a more favourable prognosis. From a public health perspective, the objective is to sort out, efficiently and effectively, those who probably have the disease from those who probably do not, again to detect early cases for treatment or begin prevention and control programs. A screening test is *not* a diagnostic test. Effective screening programs must include referrals for diagnostic evaluation for those who have positive results for the disease to confirm whether they do have the disease and need treatment.

CHNs need to stay current on screening guidelines, since they are regularly reviewed and revised on the basis of epidemiological research results. In Canada, these screening guidelines are referred to as Clinical Practice Guidelines, which recommend routine screening for such conditions as dyslipidemia,

diabetes mellitus, hypertension, women's health, and men's health. As community health advocates, CHNs are responsible for planning and implementing screening and prevention programs aimed at high-risk populations. Box 8.3 outlines criteria for planning a successful screening program. Box 8.4 presents Wilson and Jungner's (1968) classic screening criteria for the early detection of disease. Box 8.4 also includes a synthesis of the screening criteria up to the present time. Andermann, Blancquaert, Beauchamp, et al. (2008) report that the Wilson and Jungner screening criteria are still the "gold standard of screening assessment" (p. 18). A synthesis of emerging screening criteria over the past 40 years shows that Wilson and Jungner's screening criteria remain undisputed. However, newer policy tools are available that take into consideration the growing interest in genetic screening, increased consumerism, a focus on evidence-informed care, and the need for cost effectiveness. Criteria for screening programs and policies should also include a response to a recognized need, a targeted

BOX 8.3 Characteristics of a Successful Screening Program.

- *Valid (accurate):* The program has a high probability of correct classification of persons tested.
- *Reliable (precise):* Results are consistent from place to place, time to time, and person to person.
- *Facility for large group administration:* The program is (a) fast both in administration of the test and in obtaining results; and (b) inexpensive in both personnel required and the materials and procedures used.
- *Innocuous:* The test has few, if any, adverse effects, and it is minimally invasive.
- *High yield:* The program can detect enough new cases to justify the effort and expense (*yield* defined as the amount of previously unrecognized disease that is diagnosed and treated as a result of screening).

BOX 8.4 Screening Criteria for the Early Detection of Disease.

Wilson and Jungner's classic screening criteria:
- The condition sought should be an important health problem.
- There should be an accepted treatment for patients with recognized disease.
- Facilities for diagnosis and treatment should be available.
- There should be a recognizable latent or early symptomatic stage.
- There should be a suitable test or examination.
- The test should be acceptable to the population.
- The natural history of the condition, including development from latent to declared disease, should be adequately understood.
- There should be an agreed policy on whom to treat as patients.
- The cost of case-finding (including diagnosis and treatment of patients diagnosed) should be economically balanced in relation to possible expenditure on medical care as a whole.
- Case-finding should be a continuing process and not a "once and for all" project.*

Synthesis of emerging screening criteria proposed over the past 40 years:
- The screening program should respond to a recognized need.
- The objectives of screening should be defined at the outset.
- There should be a defined target population.
- There should be scientific evidence of screening program effectiveness.
- The program should integrate education, testing, clinical services, and program management.
- There should be quality assurance, with mechanisms to minimize potential risks of screening.
- The program should ensure informed choice, confidentiality, and respect for autonomy.
- The program should promote equity and access to screening for the entire target population.
- Program evaluation should be planned from the outset.
- The overall benefits of screening should outweigh the harm.

* Reprinted with permission from Andermann, A., Blancquaert, I., Beauchamp, S., & Dery, V. (2008). Revisiting Wilson & Jungner in the genomic age: A review of the screening criteria over the past 40 years. *Bulletin of the World Health Organization, 86*(4), 317–319. http://www.who.int/bulletin/volumes/86/4/07-050112/en/

population, scientific evidence of effectiveness, and the integration of education, testing, clinical services, and program management (Andermann et al., 2008).

Reliability and Validity

For a measure to be accepted as scientific proof, it must be both reliable and valid.

Reliability

The **reliability** of a measure refers to its consistency or repeatability. Consider the example of a blood pressure screening that is being carried out in a community. A large number of people are being screened, and follow-up or repeat measurements are taken for some individuals with higher blood pressure. If the sphygmomanometer used for the screening shows extremely varying measures on two consecutive readings for the same person, then the sphygmomanometer lacks reliability. The instrument would be unreliable even if the overall mean of repeated measurements was close to the true overall mean for the persons measured. The problem would be that the readings would not be reliable for any individual, and reliability is what a screening program requires.

On the other hand, suppose the readings on a particular sphygmomanometer are reliably reproducible but tend to be about 10-mm Hg too high. This instrument is producing consistent readings, but the uncorrected (or uncalibrated) instrument lacks accuracy. In short, a measure can be reliable but not provide usable or sound results.

The following three major sources of error can affect the reliability of tests:
1. Variation inherent in the trait being measured (e.g., blood pressure changes with time of day, activity, level of stress, and other factors)
2. Observer variation, which can be divided into intraobserver reliability (consistency by the same observer) and interobserver reliability (consistency from one observer to another)
3. Inconsistency in the instrument, which includes the internal consistency of the instrument (e.g., whether all items in a questionnaire measure the same thing) and the stability (or test–retest reliability) of the instrument over time

Validity

Validity refers to whether a measure really measures what we intend it to measure, and how accurately it does so. The validity of a screening test is measured by sensitivity and specificity. **Sensitivity** quantifies how accurately the test identifies those with the condition or trait. It represents the proportion of persons with the disease whom the test correctly identifies as positive (true positives). High sensitivity is needed when early treatment is crucial and when identification of all cases is important.

Specificity indicates how accurately the test identifies those without the condition or trait (i.e., the proportion of persons whom the test correctly identifies as negative for the disease [true negatives]). High specificity is needed when rescreening is impractical and when reducing false positives is important.

The sensitivity and specificity of a test are determined by comparing the results from a particular test with results from a definitive diagnostic procedure (sometimes called the *gold standard*). For example, the Pap test is used frequently to screen for cervical dysplasia and carcinoma. The definitive diagnosis of cervical cancer requires a biopsy and histological confirmation of malignant cells.

The ideal for a screening test is 100% sensitivity and 100% specificity. That is, the test is positive for 100% of those who actually have the disease and is negative for 100% of those who do not have the disease. In practice, sensitivity and specificity are often inversely related. That is, if the test results are such that one can choose a particular point beyond which a person is considered positive (a "cut point")—as in a blood pressure reading to screen for hypertension or a serum glucose reading to screen for diabetes—then moving that critical point to improve the sensitivity of the test will result in a decrease in specificity; in other words, an improvement in specificity can be made only at the expense of sensitivity.

Associated with sensitivity and specificity is the predictive value of a screening test. The **positive predictive value** (also called *predictive value positive*) is the proportion of persons with a positive screening test who actually have the disease; it is interpreted as the probability that an individual with a positive test has the disease. The **negative predictive value** (or *predictive value negative*) is the proportion of persons with a negative screening test who do not have the disease; it is interpreted as the probability that an individual with a negative screening test actually does not have the disease. Although sensitivity and specificity are relatively independent of the prevalence of disease, predictive values are affected by the level of disease in the screened population and by the sensitivity and specificity of the test. When the prevalence is very low, the positive predictive value will be low, even with tests that are sensitive and specific. In addition, lower specificity produces lower positive predictive values because of the increase in the proportion of false-positive results.

Table 8.7 presents a description of each of these measurement terms with an accompanying formula. Screening tests are related to the period of pathogenesis in the natural history of disease as part of secondary prevention during early diagnosis, specifically early case-finding. Refer again to Fig. 8.5 for an illustration of the natural history of disease to see the relationship between screening and secondary prevention.

Two or more tests can be combined, in a series or in parallel, to enhance sensitivity or specificity. In *series testing*, the final result is considered positive only if *all* the tests in the series were positive, and it is considered negative if *any* test was negative. For example, if a blood sample were screened for HIV, a positive enzyme-linked immunosorbent assay (ELISA) might be followed up with a Western blot, and the sample would be considered positive only if both tests were positive. Series testing enhances specificity, which produces fewer false positives, but sensitivity will be lower. In series testing, sequence is important; a very sensitive test is often used first to pick up all cases, including false positives, and then a second, very specific test is used to eliminate the false positives.

In *parallel testing*, the final result is considered positive if *any* test was positive, and it is considered negative only if *all* tests were negative. To return to the example of a blood sample being tested for HIV, a blood bank might consider a sample positive if a positive result were found on either the ELISA or the Western blot. Parallel testing enhances sensitivity, which produces fewer false negatives, but specificity will be lower.

THE BASICS OF EPIDEMIOLOGICAL RESEARCH

Types of Epidemiological Studies

The four main types of studies used by epidemiologists to explore health and illness in populations are (1) descriptive, (2) analytical, (3) ecological, and (4) experimental or intervention studies. Descriptive and analytical studies are observational. In these studies, the investigator observes events as they are or have been and does not intervene to change anything or to introduce a new factor. An **ecological**

TABLE 8.7	Screening Tests: Sensitivity, Specificity, and Predictive Values	
Measurement	**Description**	**Formula**
Sensitivity	A measurement (expressed as a percentage) that identifies a test's ability to identify those persons with the disease	$\dfrac{\text{Number of persons with a positive test}}{\text{Total number of persons with the disease}} \times 100$
Specificity	A measurement (expressed as a percentage) that identifies a test's ability to identify those persons who do not have the disease	$\dfrac{\text{Number of persons with a negative test}}{\text{Total number of persons without the disease}} \times 100$
Positive predictive value	The probability (expressed as a percentage) that persons with a positive screening test have the disease	$\dfrac{\text{Number of persons with a positive test who have the disease}}{\text{Total number of persons with a positive test}} \times 100$
Negative predictive value	The probability (expressed as a percentage) that persons with a negative screening test do *not* have the disease	$\dfrac{\text{Number of persons with a negative test who do not have the disease}}{\text{Total number of persons with a negative test}} \times 100$

Sources: Adapted from Fletcher & Fletcher, 2004; Gordis, 2008.

study bridges both descriptive and analytical epidemiology. **Experimental or intervention studies** include interventions to test preventive or treatment measures, techniques, materials, policies, or medications.

Descriptive Studies

Descriptive studies describe the distribution of disease, death, and other health outcomes in a population according to person, place, and time. They provide a picture of how things are or have been—the who, where, and when of disease patterns. In a descriptive study, common measurements of disease occurrence are frequency, incidence rates, morbidity and mortality rates, and prevalence. Populations based on certain factors, such as age, socioeconomic status, and gender, that are at high or low risk for diseases can be identified using descriptive measurements. Also, in descriptive epidemiology, trends for specific diseases can be observed over time. Descriptive epidemiology generates hypotheses, and analytical epidemiology tests the hypotheses (Cassells, 2007). A descriptive epidemiological study was conducted using the Canadian Community Health Survey (CCHS) data to describe the epidemiology of major depression in Canadians (Patten, Wang, Williams, et al., 2006). The study participants were 15 years of age or older and lived in family homes. Households were randomly selected, and one study participant 15 years of age or older from the household was interviewed (based on willingness to participate). The Statistics Canada national survey data that were reviewed had been collected between May and December 2002. As expected in descriptive epidemiology, the findings included annual and lifetime prevalence rates based on characteristics such as gender, age group, marital status, socioeconomic status, urban and rural status, and presence or absence of one or more chronic medical conditions. One of the rationales for conducting this descriptive epidemiology was to generate etiological hypotheses.

Analytical Studies

Analytical studies search for the determinants of the patterns observed—the how and why. Epidemiological concepts and methods are used to identify what factors, characteristics, exposures, or behaviours might account for differences in the observed patterns of disease occurrence. Analytical epidemiology includes study designs such as cross-sectional (prevalence survey), case-control (retrospective, case comparison), prospective cohort (concurrent cohort, longitudinal, follow-up), and retrospective cohort (nonconcurrent cohort). Surveys and polls are examples of cross-sectional studies. Two well-known and influential longitudinal studies conducted in the United States on heart disease and other common health conditions are the Framingham Heart Study and the Nurses' Health Study. A recent example of a Canadian cohort study is the National Longitudinal Survey of Children and Youth (NLSCY), a long-term study that follows the development and well-being of persons from birth to adulthood. The NLSCY is designed to collect information on the factors influencing a child's social, emotional, and behavioural development and to monitor the impact of those factors over

time (Statistics Canada, 2010). Some of the findings were as follows: (1) children were more aggressive in their behaviour when parenting practices were more punitive; (2) children experienced higher levels of anxiety when parental practices were punitive; (3) children became less aggressive in their behaviour over an 8-year span of time when parental practices had changed from punitive to nonpunitive practices; (4) children became less anxious when parental practices had changed from punitive to nonpunitive practices; and (5) children from low-income homes, when tested 8 years later, had higher scores in aggressive behaviour than children from higher-income homes (Statistics Canada, 2010).

The advantages and disadvantages of analytical study designs are summarized in Table 8.8.

Ecological Studies

The identifying characteristic of *ecological studies* is that only aggregate data, such as population rates, are used rather than data on individuals' exposures, characteristics, and outcomes. In ecological studies, the descriptive component considers variations in disease rates by person, place, or time. The analytical component in ecological studies tries to determine whether a relationship exists between disease rates and variations in rates for possible risk (or protective) factors or characteristics.

Experimental or Intervention Studies

Experimental or intervention studies, such as clinical trials and community trials, have particular significance for CHNs. The goal of a clinical trial is generally to evaluate the effectiveness of an intervention, such as a medical treatment for disease, a new drug or an existing drug used in a new or different way, a surgical technique, or other treatment. Randomized clinical trials are used to test hypotheses about specific interventions. In clinical trials, the sample should be randomly assigned to two treatments, that is, the new treatment and the currently used treatment. In randomization, treatments are assigned to patients (subjects) so that all possible treatment assignments have a predetermined probability; however, neither the subject nor the investigator determines the actual assignment of any participant. Randomization avoids the bias that may result if subjects choose to be in one group or the other or if the investigator or clinician chooses particular subjects for each group.

Masking or "blinding" treatment assignments is a second kind of treatment allocation. Generally, it is best to use the double-blinded study method, in which neither the subject nor the investigator knows who is getting which treatment. Clinical trials usually are the best way to show causality because of the objective way in which subjects are assigned and the greater control over other factors that could influence outcome. Like cohort studies, they are prospective and provide the clearest evidence using a time sequence.

Clinical trials tend to be conducted in a contrived (versus natural) situation, under controlled conditions, and with specific client populations. That means that treatment may

TABLE 8.8   Comparison of Analytical Study Designs

Study Design	Advantages	Disadvantages
Ecological	• Is a quick, easy, and inexpensive first study • Uses readily available existing data • May prompt further investigation or suggest other/new hypotheses • May provide information about contextual factors not accounted for by individual characteristics	• Ecological fallacy: the associations observed may not hold true for individuals • Problems in interpreting temporal sequence (cause and effect) • Is more difficult to control for confounding and "mixed" models (ecological and individual data); more complex statistically
Cross-sectional (prevalence survey)	• Gives general description of scope of problem; provides prevalence estimates • Is often based on a population (or community) sample, not just those who sought care • Is useful in health care evaluation and planning • Obtains data at once; less expensive and quicker than cohort because there is no follow-up • Provides baseline for prospective study or to identify cases and controls for case-control study • Correlational cross-sectional studies identify relationships (associations)	• Does not include calculation of risk; prevalence, not incidence • Has an unclear temporal sequence • Is not good for rare diseases or rare exposures unless large sample size or stratified sampling • Can result in selective survival, which can be major source of selection bias; surviving subjects may differ from those who are not included (e.g., death, institutionalization) • Can result in selective recall or lack of past exposure information, which can create bias
Case-control (retrospective, case comparison)	• Is less expensive than cohort; smaller sample required • Is quicker than cohort; no follow-up • Can investigate more than one exposure • Is best design for rare diseases • Can be important tool for etiological investigation, if well designed • Is best suited to disease with relatively clear onset (timing of onset can be established so that incident cases can be included)	• Is more susceptible than cohort studies to various types of bias (selective survival, recall bias, selection bias in choice of both cases and controls) • May result in confounding if information on other risk factors is not available • Antecedent consequence (temporal sequence) not as certain as in cohort; not well suited to rare exposures • Gives only an indirect estimate of risk • Is limited to a single outcome because of sampling effect on disease status
Prospective cohort (concurrent cohort, longitudinal, follow-up)	• Is best estimate of disease incidence • Is best estimate of risk • Involves fewer problems with selective survival and selective recall • Establishes temporal sequence more clearly • Provides broader range of options for exposure assessment	• Is expensive in time and money • Is more difficult to organize • Is not good for rare diseases • Can result in a biased estimate due to attrition of participants • May have a very long latency period; may miss cases • May be difficult to examine several exposures
Retrospective cohort (nonconcurrent cohort)	• Combines advantages of both prospective cohort and case-control • Takes less time (even if follow-up into future) than prospective cohort • Is less expensive than prospective cohort because relies on existing data • Entails a temporal sequence that may be clearer than that of case-control	• Shares some disadvantages with both prospective cohort and case-control • Is subject to attrition (less to follow-up) • Relies on existing records that may result in misclassification of both exposure and outcome • May have to rely on surrogate measurement of exposure (e.g., job title) and vital records information on cause of death

not be as effective when applied in more realistic clinical or community conditions in a more diverse patient population. There are also more ethical considerations in experimental studies than in observational studies. For example, the question arises as to whether it is fair to withhold a treatment if the treatment truly appears to have the potential to cure a disease or alleviate suffering in order to systematically evaluate the treatment using experimental and control groups. Finally, clinical trials are expensive with regard to time, personnel, facilities, and, in some cases, supplies.

Community trials are similar to clinical trials in that an investigator determines what the exposure or intervention will be. However, community trials often deal with health promotion and disease prevention rather than treatment of an existing disease. The intervention is usually undertaken on a large scale, and the unit of treatment is a community, region, or group rather than individuals. Although a pharmaceutical process, such as fluoridation of water or mass immunizations, may be involved in a community trial, these trials often involve educational, programmatic, or policy interventions. Examples of community interventions would be measuring the rate of diabetes or cardiovascular disease in a community after increasing the availability of exercise programs and facilities or where a much larger supply of healthful fresh foods has been made available.

Although community trials provide the best means of testing whether changes in knowledge or behaviour, policy, programs, or other mass interventions are effective, they do present some problems. For many interventions, it may take years for the effectiveness to become evident—for example, the effect of exercise programs and healthful food on the rates of either diabetes or heart disease. While the study is being carried out over time, other factors can influence the outcome either positively (making the intervention look more effective than it really is) or negatively (making the intervention look less effective than it really is). Comparable community populations without similar interventions for comparative analysis are often difficult to find. Even when comparable communities are available—especially when the intervention is improved knowledge or changed behaviour—it is difficult and unethical to prevent the control communities from making use of generally available information, thereby making them less different from the intervention communities. Finally, because community trials are often undertaken on a large scale and over long periods, they can be expensive, require a large staff, have complicated logistics, and need extensive communication about the study.

Sources of Data

The following three major categories of data sources are commonly used in epidemiological investigations:

1. *Routinely collected data:* census data, vital records (birth and death certificates), and **surveillance** data (systematic collection of data related to disease occurrence)
2. *Data collected for other purposes but useful for epidemiological research:* medical, health department, and insurance records
3. *Original data collected for specific epidemiological studies.*

Routinely Collected Data

The Canadian census is conducted every 5 years by Statistics Canada and collects population data, including demographic (age, race, and sex) and geographical distribution, and information about economic status, housing, and education. These data provide denominators for various rates, such as CFR, infant mortality rate, and maternal mortality rate.

Vital records—collected by provincial and territorial governments in Canada—are the primary source of birth and mortality statistics. Registration of births and deaths, mandated in most countries, serves as one of the most complete sources of health-related data. However, the quality of specific information varies. For example, on birth information forms, sex and date of birth are fairly reliable, whereas information such as gestational age, level of prenatal care, and the mother's smoking during pregnancy is less reliable. On death certificates, the quality of the cause-of-death information varies due to the differing history forms used. It also varies from place to place, depending on the location's diagnostic capabilities and local practice. Vital records are readily available in most parts

of the world; they are an inexpensive and convenient resource and allow the study of long-term trends. Mortality data, however, are informative only in the case of fatal diseases.

Public health surveillance is defined by WHO (2014) as the "continuous, systematic collection, analysis and interpretation of health-related data needed for the planning, implementation, and evaluation of public health practice." Surveillance can serve as an early warning system for public health emergencies, document the impact of programs and strategies, and monitor the epidemiology of public health problems so that decisions can be made on the allocation of resources. The federal government provided funding in 2004 to support the development and implementation of the pan-Canadian Health Surveillance System—an electronic information system for collecting health data that would guide public health actions in areas such as communicable diseases and population health issues, as well as the management of infectious diseases (KPMG, 2009). One resulting initiative was the "Skills Online" continuing education program, which offered Internet-based training to build the skills and knowledge needed to meet the core competencies for public health. This initiative, through self-study modules, provided health care providers opportunities to enhance their skills in epidemiology, surveillance, and information management. Although the "Skills Online" is no longer supported by PHAC, many online courses are now available to public health professionals. (PHAC, 2014).

Data Collected for Other Purposes

Hospital, physician, health department, and insurance records provide information on morbidity, as do surveillance systems such as cancer registries and health-department reporting systems, which solicit reports of all cases of a particular disease within a geographical region. Other information, such as occupational exposures, may be available from employer records.

Original Data Collected for Specific Epidemiological Studies

Statistics Canada and the Canadian Institute for Health Information support and carry out surveys that provide information on the health of Canadians, such as lifestyle behaviours. For example, the CCHS is a cross-sectional survey that collects information on health status, health care utilization risk factors, and determinants of health for the Canadian population. It relies on a representative sample of respondents and is designed to provide reliable estimates at the health region level. Provincial governments also carry out surveys to collect data on the health of the population in their provinces. Since 1999, various health units in Ontario have conducted an ongoing monthly telephone provincial survey as part of program planning. In this study, a random sample of 100 adults, 18 years and older, are interviewed about risky behaviours that have an impact on public health—for example, excessive sun exposure, failure to use a seat belt, and smoking. This survey conducted on behalf of the participating health units, in partnership with the Institute for Social

Research at York University, is called the Rapid Risk Factor Surveillance System (2009).

Age-Adjusted Death Rates

Rates, which are key to epidemiological studies, can be misleading when compared across different populations of different ages. Therefore, it is necessary to consider adjusting rates based on the age of the population. For example, the risk of death increases considerably after 40 years of age, so a higher crude death rate is expected in a population of older people compared with a population of younger people (Gordis, 2008). Comparing the overall mortality rate of an area that has a large population of older adults with that of an area that has a predominately younger population would be misleading. Methods that adjust for differences in populations can be used to make fairer comparisons between groups.

Age adjustment is based on the assumption that a population's overall mortality rate is a function of the age distribution of the population and age-specific mortality rates. Age adjustment, or the standardization of rates, reduces bias when the populations to be compared comprise different age groups (Cassells, 2007). Age adjustment can be performed by direct or indirect methods. Both methods require *a standard population,* which can be an external population, such as the Canadian population in a given year; a combined population of the groups under study; or some other standard chosen for relevance or convenience.

In the direct method of age adjustment, the age-specific death rates of the study population are applied to the age distribution of a standard population to determine the expected death rate. The (hypothetical) expected death rate is the number of deaths the study population would have if it had the same age distribution as the standard population. The CHN can then compare the two populations, which are now similar in age distribution. The indirect age-adjusted method, as the name suggests, is more complicated. The age-specific death rates of the standard population, when applied to the study population's age distribution, produce an index rate that is used with the crude rates of both the study population and the standard population to produce the final indirect adjusted rate, which is also hypothetical.

The indirect method may be required when the age-specific death rates of the study population are unknown or unstable (e.g., when based on relatively small numbers). Often, instead of an indirect adjusted rate, a standardized mortality ratio is calculated. That is, the number of observed deaths in the study population is divided by the number of deaths expected on the basis of the age-specific rates in the standard population and the age distribution of the study population (Gordis, 2008; Greenberg, Daniels, Flanders, et al., 2005).

Comparison Groups

Comparison groups are often used in epidemiology. To determine the rate of disease based on a suspected risk factor, the exposed group would be compared with a group of unexposed persons. For example, to investigate the effect of smoking during pregnancy on the rate of low birth weight,

calculate the rate of low-birth-weight infants born to women who smoked during their pregnancy and the (lower) rate of low-birth-weight infants born to nonsmoking women. Ideally, you want to compare one group of people who all have a certain characteristic, exposure, or behaviour with a group of people who are like them in all ways except that characteristic, exposure, or behaviour. In the absence of that ideal, you can either randomize people to exposure or treatment groups in experimental studies or select comparison groups that are comparable in observational studies.

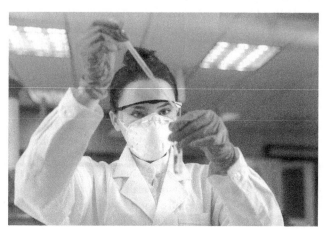

Epidemiological methods and epidemiologists are at the very centre of public health planning and response to diseases and pandemics. (iStockphoto/Eugeneonline)

HOW COMMUNITY HEALTH NURSES USE EPIDEMIOLOGY

CHNs use the epidemiological results of various databases (e.g., databases on morbidity and mortality rates) when planning and conducting a community health assessment. In their community practice, CHNs use epidemiology to identify the extent of the health concern; health threats or unhealthy behaviours occurring in their practice community; and populations at risk in their practice community (case-finding). For example, analyzing the leading cause of death in a community could help the CHN to target strategies toward specific populations and behaviours, such as adolescents at risk for motor vehicle accidents.

CHNs are often members of interprofessional teams (which consist of epidemiologists, researchers, policymakers, and others) that analyze health and disease causation in the community in order to develop and initiate appropriate prevention programs using the most relevant and up-to-date evidence-informed community interventions. CHNs may identify client health concerns and work with nurse researchers and other discipline-specific researchers to explore options that would improve patients' quality of life. Based on epidemiological data, policymakers at various levels of government make health care spending decisions such as the amount and type of financial support (e.g., grants) to make available and the allocation of resources (e.g., health care providers, community programs, and material resources).

CHNs are a key part of interprofessional teams that analyze the causes of health and disease in the community and are responsible for both preventing and treating illnesses. CHNs often use epidemiological principles and techniques to deal with the factors that affect individuals, families, and populations that cannot be as easily controlled in the community as might be the case in acute care settings. For example, in the community it is difficult to control water and food supplies; air quality conditions, including pollutants; the disposal of garbage; and the use of lead-free paint.

CHNs are involved in the surveillance and monitoring of disease trends. Those working in homes, clinics, schools, occupational health, and public health often can identify patterns of disease in a group. For example, if several children in a school experience abdominal problems within a short period (e.g., a 24-hour period), the CHN would try to trace the common source of contamination. Did they eat the same food, drink water from the same source, or swim in the same pool? Similarly, if workers in a factory all displayed similar symptoms, the occupational health nurse (OHN) would look for causative factors in the workplace such as the preparation of cafeteria food.

CHNs incorporate epidemiology into their daily practice and function in a variety of ways. In many settings, CHNs collect, report, analyze, interpret, and communicate epidemiological data. CHNs involved in the care of individuals with communicable diseases, such as TB, gonorrhea, and gastroenteritis, practise epidemiology when they identify, report, treat, and provide follow-up on cases and contacts. Those working in schools collect data on the incidence and prevalence of accidents, injuries, and illnesses in the school population. CHNs are also key players in the detection and control of local epidemics, such as outbreaks of mumps. CHNs practise in a variety of settings and are actively involved in primary, secondary, and tertiary prevention (see "The Natural History of Disease Related to Levels of Prevention" on page 189 and the "Levels of Prevention" box that follows).

LEVELS OF PREVENTION

Related to Cardiovascular Disease

Primary Prevention

At a large competitive industrial facility, an OHN discusses strategies to manage various psychosocial stresses with a group of high-level management personnel who have no diagnosed medical conditions.

Secondary Prevention

An OHN implements blood pressure screening for all workers at the worksite in an industrial facility.

Tertiary Prevention

In an industrial facility, an OHN holds monthly group meetings with personnel diagnosed with cardiovascular disease to discuss reducing the impact of personal risk factors on cardiovascular health.

Nursing documentation on client records is an important source of data for epidemiological reviews. For example, client demographics (quantifiable statistics of a given population) and health histories are often collected or verified by nurses. As nurses collect and document client information, they might not be thinking about the epidemiological connection. However, the reliability and validity of such data can be key factors in determining the quality of future epidemiological studies and how CHNS apply those findings in practice.

CHNs critique the findings from epidemiological research studies, particularly population studies, to determine whether they can be applied to their community health nursing practice. Consider, for example, how normal growth is categorized in children based on epidemiological studies of growth patterns and body size, but there are difficulties in the definitions of "normal" growth. Unfortunately, epidemiological data may not take into consideration other factors such as cultural values and childrearing practices when determining normal growth and growth standards (Ruben, 2009). When children are categorized at either end of the weight range in a manner that does not fit with the clinical findings, CHNS must re-examine the implications of using labels such as "underweight" or "failure to thrive" and consider other factors before intervening. For example, infants can be labelled as underweight with a poor negative outcome, but they are clinically well nourished (Ruben, 2009).

The problem of defining normal growth is compounded in the Indigenous population due to interfering factors such as sociodemographic and economic determinants of health. There are few published reviews of undernutrition and obesity among Indigenous children of Canada, but those that do exist report concerns with the availability of high-quality data and underrepresentation of the population in collected data. Indigenous sample sizes are generally too small in national surveys to determine adequate Indigenous rates to be estimated (Ruben, 2009). To help address this concern, the First Nations and Inuit Health Branch of Indigenous Services Canada has compiled a "Quick Stats" sheet on First Nations and Inuit health and wellness indicators in Canada (First Nations and Inuit Health Branch, 2018). That sheet summarizes data from several sources, including Statistics Canada, Canadian HIV/AIDS Reporting System, and the First Nations Oral Health Survey. It includes population data on demographics, health status and outcomes, determinants of health, and health system performance. CHNs can use that information to develop, implement, and evaluate community health strategies for Indigenous populations.

CHNs use epidemiological data along with clinical assessment to help individuals and populations address health issues and concerns. CHNs working with Indigenous populations would need to discuss with the community elders the relevance of epidemiological data to the population. The CHN would work with the elders and the community to identify and develop a community action plan that would involve the establishment of community partnerships to address community needs and develop appropriate interventions. In summary, CHNs use epidemiology data to assist them in explaining the multiplicity of factors that influence population health and illness (Clark, 2008).

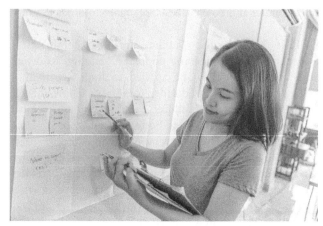

Community health nurses use epidemiological data along with clinical assessment to help individuals and populations address health issues and concerns. (iStockphoto/SamuelBrownNG)

In the late 1990s, chronic disease epidemiology was an area of research focus by epidemiologists (Susser & Susser, 1996), and this focus continues today. However, epidemiologists continue to struggle with the best approach to understanding causation (Barreto, 2005). The different approaches taken in the study of causation include those that focus on individual-level risk factors, population health, and the life course (Evans-Polce et al., 2014; Krieger, 2001; McMichael, 1999; Susser, 2004). The risk factor approach looks at relationships between individual-level risk factors that cause disease in populations. Debate has arisen over the use of this approach in epidemiology. Supporters argue that identifying risk factors is crucial in public health research and that risk factor studies need to continue with a greater focus on validity and precision (McMichael, 1999; Susser, 2004). Critics argue that this approach takes a narrow view and limits findings by studying individuals as the locus of disease at the expense of environment and societal influences, where risks often begin (Stanley, 2002). McMichael (1999) maintained that a social-ecological systems perspective with a focus on population health and upstream thinking is needed to gain an understanding of the determinants of health, disease causation, and well-being. Susser and Susser (1996) proposed a paradigm shift referred to as *eco-epidemiology*, which takes a multidimensional focus that integrates molecular, societal, individual, and population levels. Susser (2004) proposes that "an integrated approach to

investigating disease and its prevention will necessarily subsume levels of causation, life course trajectories, kinds of causes, and types of disease" and calls on epidemiologists to unite and adapt the eco-epidemiology framework (p. 520). As noted earlier in the chapter, the life course approach considers how early life factors influence health or disease risk in adulthood. It challenges the traditional view that contemporary risk factors affect the health of adults and recognizes the importance of adopting healthy lifestyles over the lifespan to prevent chronic diseases, such as cardiovascular disease and diabetes (PHAC, 2009; Raphael, 2004; Senate Subcommittee on Population Health, 2009). See the "Evidence-Informed Practice" box for a discussion on the importance of using epidemiological data to make decisions in CHN practice.

EVIDENCE-INFORMED PRACTICE

A quantitative study by Fantus, Shah, Qiu, et al. (2009) analyzed the incidence of all-cause injury and specific injury categories reported for 2004 in Indigenous communities in Ontario (N=28 816). The research study compared the rate and categories of injuries leading to hospitalization for First Nations peoples with residents living in small non-Indigenous northern (N=211 834) and southern (N=650 002) communities. Hospital discharge data were used to determine the incidence rate for all-cause injury and specific injury type. In the First Nations communities, the relative risk for injury was 3.0 relative to the southern communities and 2.5 relative to the northern communities. The study findings indicated that the most likely reasons for hospitalization of residents in First Nations communities compared with those in non-Indigenous communities was accidental poisoning, assault, and intentional self-harm, with females in First Nations communities being most vulnerable to these injuries.

Injuries that required hospital admission were higher in First Nations communities in northern Ontario relative to those in northern and southern Ontario communities. This interesting finding underscores the importance of using a geographical comparison group when doing research.

Application for CHNs
Geographical information is a useful way for CHNs to identify population priorities. By knowing which aggregate or population locations have the greatest risk of disease or injury, CHNs can focus on programs that will more effectively fit the needs of the communities they serve.

Questions for Reflection and Discussion
1. Which determinants of health are evident in this study?
2. Explain the relevance of each of the determinants of health identified.
3. What primary care interventions could a CHN implement that would address injury prevention?

Source: Fantus, D., Shah, B. R., Qiu, F., et al. (2009). Injury in First Nations communities in Ontario. *Canadian Journal of Public Health*, 100(4), 258–262.

STUDENT EXPERIENCE

Complete the following chart by exploring websites such as the PHAC's Infectious Diseases site at https://www.canada.ca/en/public-health/services/infectious-diseases.html.

Prevalence Rate	Location	Reasons for Prevalence Rate
Infectious Diseases Currently Prevalent in Canada		

Prevalence Rate	Location	Reasons for Prevalence Rate
Infectious Diseases Prevalent in Canada in the Early 1900s		
Infectious Diseases Currently Prevalent in Developing Countries		

CHAPTER SUMMARY

8.1 *Epidemiology* is the study of the distribution of factors that determine health-related states or events in a population, and the use of this information to control health problems. The steps in the epidemiological process are (1) define the health pattern and explore current statistics related to the health pattern; (2) use epidemiological methods to describe the distribution of a disease, event, or injury; (3) search for factors that explain the pattern or risk of occurrence; and (4) determine what has influenced the occurrence of a particular disease or injury or why and how events occurred as they did.

8.2 The nineteenth century saw many milestones in the evolution of epidemiology, including the development of the germ theory, the identification of the microorganisms that cause disease, and the use of epidemiology to show that environmental conditions could contribute to death. During the twentieth century, prevention and treatment of many infectious and communicable diseases were made possible, due to highly effective vaccinations, immunizations, and mass health screening programs. In addition, the development of genetic and molecular techniques increased the epidemiologist's ability to classify persons in terms of exposures or inherent susceptibility to disease.

8.3 Common epidemiological measures in community health nursing include proportion, rate, incidence rate, prevalence rate, mortality rate, risk, relative risk (RR), attributable risk (AR), ratio, odds ratio (OR), and potential years of life lost (PYLL).

8.4 The epidemiological triangle involves an interrelationship between agent, host, and environment. The interactions of factors, exposures, and characteristics form the web of causation that affects the risk for contracting a disease. The life course approach includes biological, psychosocial, and behavioural data collected from longitudinal studies starting from childhood and through to adulthood. The life course approach attempts to link early life factors with diseases that occur in adulthood.

8.5 The two distinct periods in the natural history of a disease are the prepathogenesis period and the period of pathogenesis. During the prepathogenesis period, CHNs use primary prevention activities, including health promotion programs, with both the general population and specific vulnerable groups to reduce the incidence of a disease. In the early period of pathogenesis, secondary prevention activities include routine screening tests of specific groups. In the later stages of pathogenesis, tertiary prevention is used to restore the client's health.

8.6 Screening is a key component of secondary prevention. It involves the testing of groups of individuals who are at risk for certain conditions but do not manifest any symptoms. The goal is to determine the likelihood that these individuals will develop the disease of concern. A screening test is not a diagnostic test. Screening tests used in epidemiology should be acceptable to the population being screened and should respond to a recognized need. They should be for a defined target population, and the screening program should include education, testing, clinical services, and program management. The overall benefits of screening should outweigh any harm to the client.

8.7 The four main types of epidemiological studies are descriptive, analytical, ecological, and experimental or intervention studies. Sources of data for epidemiological studies include public health surveillance data, medical and health records, and original data collected for specific epidemiological studies.

8.8 CHNs use the epidemiological results of various databases (e.g., databases on morbidity and mortality rates) when planning and conducting community health assessments. CHNs use epidemiology to identify the extent of health concerns, health threats or unhealthy behaviours, and populations at risk. CHNs are also involved in the surveillance and monitoring of disease trends.

CHN IN PRACTICE: A CASE STUDY

Foodborne Illness

Marnie, a public health nurse (PHN) is employed by the Warren Public Health Unit. She was contacted by a local church after several church members became sick following its annual picnic. Of the 200 people who attended the picnic, 100 were ill with diarrhea, nausea, and vomiting. Ten people required emergency medical treatment or hospitalization. Incubation periods ranged from 1.5 to 30 hours, with a mean of 6 hours and a median of 3.5 hours. The duration of the illness ranged from 1 to 80 hours, with a mean of 30 hours and a median of 15 hours.

The annual church picnic was a potluck lunch buffet. The menu included macaroni casserole (brought by the Carusos), turkey with gravy and stuffing (brought by the Smiths), potato salad (brought by the Changs), green bean casserole (brought by the Champs), chili (brought by the Turners), homemade bread (brought by Grand-Maman Rivest), chocolate cake (brought by the Bushes), and cookies (brought by the Beckmans). Marnie interviewed the church members who were ill and discovered that three specific food items were clearly associated with the illness: turkey, gravy, and stuffing.

Marnie interviewed the Smiths, who brought the turkey, gravy, and stuffing to the picnic. A review of their food-handling procedures showed that after the turkey had been cooked, it had been left out for 4 hours to come to room temperature—a time and temperature sufficient for bacterial growth and toxin production. Furthermore, the same dishes were used for cooking the turkey and the other foods.

Marnie educated the Smiths on proper food-handling practices, emphasizing handwashing, proper cooling and preserving methods, and better sanitation of dishes. Marnie also offered a similar educational session to the entire church congregation.

Think About It

1. What agent do you think was responsible for this foodborne illness?
2. How can you apply the data in this situation to the epidemiological triangle?

TOOL BOX

The Tool Box contains useful resources that can be applied in community health nursing practice. These related resources are found on the Evolve website at http://evolve.elsevier.com/Canada/Stanhope/community.

Tools

Clinical Epidemiology Glossary. (http://www.ebm.med.ualberta.ca/Glossary.html)

This website provides common terms used in epidemiology and their definitions. For some of the terms, such as *odds ratio, relative risk,* and *specificity (of a diagnostic test)*, calculation links are also provided.

REFERENCES

Andermann, A., Blancquaert, I., Beauchamp, S., et al. (2008). Revisiting Wilson and Jungner in the genomic age: A review of screening criteria over the past 40 years. *Bulletin of the World Health Organization, 86*(4), 317–319. http://www.who.int/bulletin/volumes/86/4/07-050112/en/.

Armstrong, E. (2010). Gender, health, and care. In T. Bryant, D. Raphael, & M. Rioux (Eds.), *Staying alive: Critical perspectives on health, illness, and health care* (pp. 331–346). Canadian Scholars' Press.

Association of Public Health Epidemiologists in Ontario. (2006). *Calculating potential years of life lost (PYLL).* http://core.apheo.ca/index.php?pid=190.

Barreto, M. L. (2005). Commentary: Epidemiologists and causation in an intricate world. *Emerging Themes in Epidemiology, 2*(3), 1–2.

Ben-Schlomo, Y., & Kuh, D. (2002). A life course approach to chronic disease epidemiology: Conceptual models, empirical challenges and interdisciplinary perspectives. *International Epidemiological Association, 31*, 285–293.

Braveman, P., & Gottlieb, L. (2014). The social determinants of health: It's time to consider the causes of the causes. *Public Health Reports, 129*, 19–31.

Cassells, H. (2007). Epidemiology. In M. A. Nies, & M. McEwen (Eds.), *Community/public health nursing: Promoting the health of populations* (4th ed., pp. 50–73). Saunders.

Centers for Disease Control and Prevention. (2015). *Investigating an outbreak.* https://www.cdc.gov/csels/dsepd/ss1978/lesson6/section2.html

Clark, M. J. (2008). *Community health nursing: Advocacy for population health* (5th ed.). Pearson Prentice Hall.

Cohen, I. B. (1984). Florence Nightingale. *Scientific American, 250*(3), 128–137.

Edwards, N. C., & Moyer, A. (2000). Community needs and capacity assessment: Critical component of program planning. In M. J. Stewart (Ed.), *Community nursing: Promoting Canadians' health* (pp. 420–442). Harcourt Canada.

Evans-Polce, R. J., Doherty, E. E., & Ensminger, M. E. (2014). Taking a life course approach to studying substance use treatment among a community cohort of African American substance users. *Drug and Alcohol Dependence, 142*, 216–223. https://doi.org/10.1016/j.drugalcdep.2014.06.025.

Fantus, D., Shah, B. R., Qiu, F., et al. (2009). Injury in First Nations communities in Ontario. *Canadian Journal of Public Health, 100*(4), 258–262.

First Nations and Inuit Health Branch, Indigenous Services Canada. (2018). *First Nations in Canada health and wellness*

indicators, Quick Stats, 2018 edition. https://health-infobase.
canada.ca/fnih/doc/first_nations.pdf.

Fletcher, R. W., & Fletcher, S. W. (2004). *Clinical epidemiology: The essentials.* Lippincott, Williams & Wilkins.

Gordis, L. (2008). *Epidemiology* (4th ed.). Elsevier/Saunders.

Greenberg, R. S., Daniels, S. R., Flanders, W. D., et al. (2005). *Medical epidemiology* (4th ed.). McGraw-Hill.

Hertzman, C., Power, C., Matthews, S., et al. (2001). Using an interactive framework of society and life course to explain self-rated health in early adulthood. *Social Science & Medicine, 53*(12), 1575–1585.

Issa, J. (2008). Revisiting SARS, five years later: Public health chief David Butler-Jones on warding off the next one. *National Review of Medicine, 5*(4). http://www.nationalreviewofmedicine.com/issue/2008/04/5_policy_politics04_4.html.

Issekutz, K. A., Graham, J. M., Prasad, C., et al. (2005). An epidemiological analysis of CHARGE syndrome: Preliminary results from a Canadian study. *American Journal of Medical Genetics, 133A,* 309–317.

KPMG. (2009). *2009 performance evaluation of the Canada Health Infoway public health surveillance program.* https://www.infoway-inforoute.ca/en/component/edocman/56-infoway-phs-evaluation-report-march-2009/view-document.

Krieger, N. (2001). Theories of social epidemiology in the 21st century: An ecosocial perspective. *International Journal of Epidemiology, 30*(4), 668–677.

Kuh, D., Ben-Shlomo, J., Lynch, J., et al. (2003). Life course epidemiology. *Journal of Epidemiology & Community Health, 57,* 778–783.

Leavell, H. R., & Clark, I. G. (1965). *Preventive medicine for the doctor in his community: An epidemiological approach.* McGraw-Hill.

McMichael, A. J. (1999). Prisoners of the proximate: Loosening the constraints on epidemiology in an age of change. *American Journal of Epidemiology, 149*(10), 887–897.

Merril, R., & Timmreck, T. C. (2006). *Introduction to epidemiology* (4th ed.). Jones and Bartlett.

Naidoo, J., & Wills, J. (2005). *Public health and health promotion: Developing practice* (2nd ed.). Baillière-Tindall.

Palmer, I. S. (1983). *Florence Nightingale and the first organized delivery of nursing services.* American Association of Colleges of Nursing.

Patten, S. B., Wang, J. L., Williams, J. V. A., et al. (2006). Descriptive epidemiology of major depression in Canada. *Canadian Journal of Psychiatry, 51*(2), 84–90.

Proteus. (2009). *Avian influenza information page.* http://www.ryerson.ca/~tsly/avian_flu_page.htm.

Public Health Agency of Canada. (2006). *Centre for infectious disease and emergency preparedness branch (IDEP).* http://www.phac-aspc.gc.ca.

Public Health Agency of Canada. (2009). *The chief public health officer's report on the state of public health in Canada 2009:*

Growing up well—Priorities for a healthy future. http://www.phac-aspc.gc.ca/cphorsphc-respcacsp/2009/fr-rc/index-eng.php.

Public Health Agency of Canada. (2014). *Skills online.* http://www.phac-aspc.gc.ca/php-psp/ccph-cesp/index-eng.php.

Raphael, D. (2004). *Social determinants of health: Canadian perspectives.* Canadian Scholars' Press.

Raphael, D. (2009). *Social determinants of health* (2nd ed.). Canadian Scholars' Press.

Rapid Risk Factor Surveillance System. (2009). *History.* https://www.rrfss.ca/history

Rothman, K. J. (2002). *Epidemiology: An introduction.* Oxford University Press.

Ruben, A. (2009). Undernutrition and obesity in Indigenous children: Epidemiology, prevention and treatment. *Pediatric Clinics of North America, 56*(6), 1285–1302.

Senate Subcommittee on Population Health. (2009). *A healthy, productive Canada: A determinant of health approach.* http://www.parl.gc.ca/content/sen/committee/402/popu/rep/rephealth1jun09-e.pdf.

Snow, J. (1855). On the mode of communication of cholera. In *Snow on cholera.* The Commonwealth Fund.

Spenceley, S. (2007). Chronic illness. In R. Day, P. Paul, B. Williams, et al. (Eds.), *Brunner and Suddarth's textbook of medical-surgical nursing* (1st Cdn ed., pp. 148–159). Lippincott, Williams & Wilkins.

Stanley, F. (2002). From Susser's causal paradigms to social justice in Australia. *International Journal of Epidemiology, 31*(1), 40–45.

Statistics Canada. (2010). *National longitudinal survey of children and Youth (NLSCY).* http://www23.statcan.gc.ca/imdb/p2SV.pl?Function=getSurvey&SDDS=4450.

Statistics Canada. (2018a). *Death and age-specific mortality rates, by selected grouped causes (Table 13-10-0392-01).* https://www150.statcan.gc.ca/t1/tbl1/en/tv.action?pid=1310039201.

Statistics Canada. (2018b). *Infant mortality rates, by province and territory (Table 13-10-0368-01).* https://www150.statcan.gc.ca/t1/tbl1/en/tv.action?pid=1310036801.

Susser, E. (2004). Eco-epidemiology: Thinking outside the black box. *Epidemiology, 15*(5), 19–520.

Susser, M., & Susser, E. (1996). Choosing a future for epidemiology: II. From black box to Chinese boxes and ecoepidemiology. *American Journal of Public Health, 86*(5), 674–677.

Vandenbroucke, J. P. (1990). Epidemiology in transition: A historical hypothesis. *Epidemiology, 1*(2), 164.

Wilson, J. M. G., & Jungner, G. (1968). *Principles and practice of screening for disease.* World Health Organization. http://apps.who.int/iris/bitstream/10665/37650/1/WHO_PHP_34.pdf.

World Health Organization (WHO). (2006). *Socio-economic determinants of health.* http://www.who.int.

World Health Organization (WHO). (2014). *Public health surveillance.* http://www.who.int/topics/public_health_surveillance/en/.

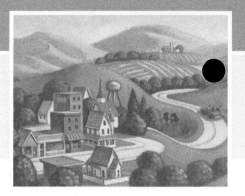

9

Working With the Community

OUTLINE

What Is a Community?, 203
The Community As Partner, 204
  Community and the Determinants of Health, 206
Characteristics of Community Health Nursing Practice, 207
  Community Health, 207
  Strategies to Improve Community Health, 209
  Healthy Communities, 209
  Community Partnerships and Coalitions, 210
Community Development, 211
  Community Capacity Building, 211
  Outcomes of Community Development, 212
Assessing Community Health, 213
  Data Collection and Interpretation, 213
  Data-Collection Methods, 214
  Identifying Community Health Concerns, 218

Planning for Community Health, 218
  Analyzing Health Concerns, 218
  Identifying Health Concern Priorities, 219
  Establishing Goals and Objectives, 220
  Identifying and Prioritizing Intervention Activities, 221
Implementation in the Community, 221
  The Community Health Nurse's Role, 221
  The Community Health Concern and the Community
    Health Nurse's Role, 222
  The Social Change Process and the Community Health
    Nurse's Role, 222
Evaluating the Intervention for Community
  Health, 222

OBJECTIVES

After reading this chapter, you should be able to:

9.1 Define *community*.
9.2 Discuss the process of working with the community as partner.
9.3 Identify the characteristics of community health nursing practice.
9.4 Describe the community development process.

9.5 Explain the three steps used to assess community health.
9.6 Discuss the main activities involved in planning for community health initiatives.
9.7 Understand the factors that shape the implementation of community health initiatives.
9.8 Explain how to evaluate interventions for community health.

KEY TERMS*

asset mapping, 212
change agent, 222
change partner, 222
coalition, 210
community capacity building, 211
community competence, 213
community forum, 217
community health, 208
community health assessment, 213
community health concerns, 214
community health strengths, 214
community partnerships, 210
data collection, 213
data gathering, 214
data generation, 214
database, 214

evaluation, 222
focus group, 215
goals, 220
healthy community, 209
implementation, 221
informant interviews, 214
interdependent, 204
intervention activities, 221
objectives, 220
participant observation, 215
partnership, 210
secondary analysis, 217
survey, 217
sustainability, 213
windshield survey, 206

*See the Glossary on page 468 for definitions.

When Florence Nightingale was stationed at Scutari (now Üsküdar, a municipality of Istanbul), she defined her community as war-torn Crimea. There, she discovered that the lack of fresh air, sanitation, and hygiene was contributing to the death of wounded soldiers. Lillian Wald found that the New York neighbourhoods in her community were impoverished, with poor housing conditions and sanitation, improper nutrition, and crowding that contributed to the problems of new mothers and children. Both women became political activists, worked with the leaders in their communities, and even solicited help from their respective governments to help change the conditions for the individuals and families in their communities. Community health nurses (CHNs) need to know how to assess a community and work with the community as partner to maximize community health.

This chapter clarifies community concepts and provides a guideline for community health nursing practice with the community as the unit of care. The Canadian Community Health Nursing Standards of Practice (CCHN Standards) includes expectations for assessment, planning, intervention, and evaluation when working with the community (Community Health Nurses of Canada [CHNC], 2019). Some examples of working with the community are listed in Box 9.1. For the complete CCHN Standards, refer to Appendix 1.

Working with the community as the unit of care and as partner may be a new experience for some CHNs, as many are accustomed to working with individuals, groups, and families as patients. The term *community health nursing process,* coined in the CCHN Standards (CHNC, 2019), refers to the process by which CHNs make their community health nursing decisions. This process involves a comprehensive health community assessment, planning, implementation, and evaluation. Recall from Chapter 1 that the patient refers to the individual, family, group or aggregate, community, population, or society. CHN professional practice involves working with the community to collect data and to draw conclusions about the community's strengths and assets, resources, and health concerns (assessment) and includes further decision making during planning, implementation, and evaluation. This chapter provides CHNs with the knowledge necessary to conduct a community health assessment and to complete the community health nursing process with the community as the unit of care and as partner. Completing a community health assessment will assist the CHN in identifying community strengths and assets and community health concerns (actual and potential).

WHAT IS A COMMUNITY?

The concept of community varies widely, but in the context of community health nursing, it refers to people and the relationships that emerge among them as they develop and commonly

BOX 9.1 Examples of Working With the Community as the Unit of Care

The following examples of activities, excerpted and adapted from the CCHN Standards, provide direction for CHNs when working with the community as the unit of care. The relevant CCHN standard of practice is noted at the end of each example.

Standard 1: Health Promotion
- Develop a cardiovascular health promotion program for adults. (a)
- Collaborate with the community to conduct an assessment of assets and needs. (b)
- Incorporate healing circles into practice. (c)
- Consider overcrowding as a contributing factor to community health problems. (d)
- Provide Indigenous-specific resources, including presentations and education materials. (g)
- Evaluate and modify smoking cessation programs, in partnership with the teens. (h)

Standard 2: Prevention and Health Protection
- Recognize the differences between the levels of prevention (primary, secondary, tertiary, and quaternary) and select the appropriate level of preventive intervention. (c)
- Help communities create an emergency preparedness plan. (e)
- Advocate for safe injection sites. (f)

Standard 3: Prevention and Health Protection
- Maintains accurate records of COVID-19 immunizations.

Standard 4: Professional Relationships
- Conduct a windshield survey to assess the need for health education on vaping. (b)
- Collaborate with community elders to translate health education material. (e)
- Invite family members to childhood vaccinations. (f)
- Consult with social work regarding the need for home care services. (k)

Standard 5: Capacity Building
- Provide public health education to combat vaccine hesitancy. (c)
- Join a high school health committee. (i)

Standard 6: Health Equity
- Explore options to fund health services for uninsured families. (m)
- Implement a healthy baby club for at-risk teenage mothers. (a)

Standard 7: Evidence-Informed Practice
- Attend the Community Health Nurses annual conference. (b)
- Refer to agency policies and procedures to guide care. (a)

Standard 8: Professional Responsibility and Accountability
- Apply the ethical principle of autonomy when obtaining informed consent. (b)
- Document care in a timely and thorough manner. (j)

Source: Adapted with permission from Community Health Nurses of Canada. (2019). *Canadian Community Health Nursing Professional Practice Model & Standards of Practice* (pp. 18–26). https://www.chnc.ca/standards-of-practice. Community Health Nurses of Canada. Reprinted with permission.

share agencies, institutions, and a physical environment; members may be defined in terms of geography or a common interest or focus. When community agencies such as schools, social services, and government interact, solutions to health concerns are more probable. CHNs quickly learn that society consists of many different kinds of communities, such as a community of interest (e.g., a group of individuals who want to cut hiking and walking trails in their community or a group of older persons who support affordable healthy food options in their community); a community of concern (e.g., a local group that is concerned about low literacy levels in their community or a group of older persons that is concerned about the limited lighting of city sidewalks in some areas); a neighbourhood community (e.g., neighbours in a specific geographical area who meet to set up a neighbourhood watch program); and communities of practice (e.g., practitioners sharing knowledge and learning).

CHNs also may work in partnership with political communities, such as school districts, municipalities, or counties, to develop a health promotion policy pertaining to a widespread health concern (e.g., bullying). Because each community is unique and its defining characteristics will affect the nature of the partnership, CHNs planning an intervention with a community must take into account its specific characteristics.

In most definitions, the concept of community includes three dimensions—*people*, *place*, and *function*—which are described as follows:

1. The *people* are the community residents.
2. *Place* refers to both geographical and time dimensions.
3. *Function* refers to the aims and activities of the community.

CHNs regularly need to examine how the personal, geographical, and functional dimensions of community shape their nursing practice with individuals, families, groups, and populations. They can use both a conceptual definition and a set of indicators for the concept of community in their practice.

In this chapter, the components of community are considered to be **interdependent** (they are mutually reliant upon each other), and their function is to meet a wide variety of collective needs. This definition of community includes personal, geographical, and functional dimensions and recognizes the interaction among the systems within a community. Indicators of the three dimensions appear in Table 9.1.

THE COMMUNITY AS PARTNER

The community is the primary setting for practice for CHNs providing health promotion and disease prevention interventions using a population health approach. Community health nursing has often been considered unique because its focus of care is the community. The idea of health-related care being provided within the community is not new. In the nineteenth

TABLE 9.1 Concepts of Community Specified

Dimension	Measures	Examples of Data Sources
People or person	Population: number and density	Statistics Canada
	Demographic structure of population, such as age, sex, socioeconomic and racial distributions, rural and urban character, and dependency ratio	Statistics Canada
	Informal groups such as block clubs, service clubs, and friendship networks	Churches, older persons' centres Civic groups Local newspaper
	Formal groups such as schools, churches, businesses, industries, governmental bodies, unions, and health and welfare agencies	Telephone directory United Way Social service agencies Chamber of Commerce Regional health units/health authority
	Linking structures (intercommunity and intracommunity contacts among organizations)	Tourist bureau Local and government offices
Place	Geopolitical boundaries	Maps
	Local or folk name for area	Local newspaper
	Size in kilometres, acres, blocks, or census tracts	Census data
	Transportation avenues, such as rivers, highways, railroads, and sidewalks	Chamber of Commerce Municipal offices
	History	Library archives and local histories
	Physical environment such as land-use patterns and condition of housing	Local housing office
Function	Production, distribution, and consumption of goods and services	Provincial or territorial offices Business and labour Local library
	Socialization of new members	Social and local research reports
	Maintenance of social control	Police station
	Adaptation to ongoing and expected change	Social and local research reports
	Provision of mutual aid	Churches and religious organizations

century, most people stayed at home during an illness and were cared for by laypersons and members of religious orders. In the mid-1800s, the Nightingale model of nursing training emerged, but the practice environment for most nurses continued to be in the home rather than the hospital.

As the range of community health nursing services continued to expand in the nineteenth century, many health organizations (e.g., the Canadian Red Cross Society and the Victorian Order of Nurses [VON]) started up, but their services often overlapped. For instance, both the VON nurses and government health agency home health nurses visited mothers with newborn babies or patients with tuberculosis. These CHNs practised in patients' homes, not in the hospital. Early textbooks on public health nursing included lengthy descriptions of the home environment and tools for assessing the extent to which that environment promoted the health of family members. Health education about the domestic environment was often a major part of home nursing care.

By the 1950s, schools, prisons, industries, and neighbourhood health centres, as well as homes, had all become areas of practice for nurses in community health. CHNs in these settings focused on the individual patient or family seeking care and were referred to as providing community-based nursing (Kushner, 2006; Zotti, Brown, & Stotts, 1996). Nurses practising in the community (location of practice) and caring for the individual, family, or group living in the community (unit of care) were not necessarily focusing on the community itself as the unit of care.

For CHNs, embracing the idea of community as partner involves developing partnerships with the community as a means of community practice. The "Ethical Considerations" box discusses a situation in which the CHN and the community are partners in health.

Conceptualizing the community as patient is different from conceptualizing the community as partner. A CHN who conceptualizes the community as patient provides prevention and early intervention programs for the total population, such as offering mass health screening and immunization programs in the community; the CHN is often viewed as the expert. In the community-as-patient approach, a community assessment emphasizes the use of epidemiological data and disease occurrences with a focus that is needs defined. The interventions used by the CHN are often directed by government policy and legislation or regulations with an expectation of patient adherence.

By contrast, when a CHN approaches the community as partner, everyone in a defined community (total population) or aggregate (preschool, teachers) represents the person. The core of the assessment includes demographics of the population and values, beliefs, and history. The emphasis is on identifying community strengths or assets to address community-identified health concerns and to further develop community capacity in a collaborative milieu that is supportive to and meaningful for community members. The CHN partners with community groups such as other health care providers, community stakeholders, and

ETHICAL CONSIDERATIONS

Working with a CHN, a group of women who live in a low-income neighbourhood have identified food security as a major issue for many of the children in their community. They proposed to the local government that programs could be developed by community members. Those programs included a breakfast program for school children, food banks for individuals and families, a community kitchen program, and a community garden if start-up funding and support by the local government could be provided. This is the first time that community members have worked together to address some of their community's health concerns. The response of the local government was to zone for a grocery store chain in the neighbourhood that provides bulk discount food, a change that would also provide increased tax revenue for the city.

The ethical principles that apply to the preceding case are as follows:

- *Beneficence:* Patients are most empowered and their dignity most respected if their own input is recognized. In this case, the community members' suggestions were ignored.
- *Distributive justice:* The bulk discount food store does not solve all of the community's food security problems. Many people may still not be able to afford or access the food there.
- *Autonomy:* CHNs recognize the importance of patient autonomy when working with the community as partner. The community members were trying to achieve autonomy by having their own garden so that they did not have to depend fully on external sources.
- *Promoting health and well-being:* Promoting the health and well-being of vulnerable populations is a primary ethical value for CHNs.

Questions to Consider

1. What are the CHN's responsibilities in promoting social justice in this situation?
2. What are some actions the CHN could take to promote social justice in this situation?

nonprofit agencies. The CHN blends professional knowledge with knowledge of the specific community to use and work with community resources for planning and implementation purposes. During this partnership, epidemiological data and disease and injury prevention data are also considered by the CHN.

Vollman, Anderson, and McFarlane (2017) proposed a community health action model with a community-as-partner focus. A partnership conveys an egalitarian relationship between the CHN and the community. This egalitarian relationship encourages community involvement, autonomy, and empowerment. According to Vollman et al. (2017), the people in your community are your partners, and these partners need to be included during the entire community health nursing process. To facilitate the community partnership, the CHN may work with a community agency, perhaps directly with someone in that agency with ties to the particular community health issue (Jessup-Falcioni & Viverais-Dresler, 2005).

Community partners can facilitate the development of community rapport and trust that are necessary for the CHN to gain access to and information from the community. The "Cultural Considerations: Community Wisdom" box outlines the importance of developing community rapport and trust when forming partnerships.

🌐 CULTURAL CONSIDERATIONS

Community Wisdom

Viewing the community as partner is not a new concept for CHNs who care for Indigenous populations. The importance of using community wisdom to identify root causes of illness, disease, and health inequities has been well recognized as an effective approach to discussing community health programs and policies with First Nations populations. For example, in an effort to address the health problem of early childhood caries, Cidro and colleagues partnered with the elders in the community to identify traditional and culturally based infant oral health practices in one remote Canadian Cree Nation community.* A participatory research approach was used to conduct 20 interviews and four focus groups with grandmothers in the community. Respondents discussed the importance of traditional foods and medicines to address oral health issues. The authors concluded that local health knowledge keepers should be a part of the discussions around community health programs and policies and are essential to building community partnerships to address health issues. Bingham and colleagues also recognized the importance of creating a partnership between the target population of at-risk Indigenous women and the community to explore the impact of high HIV infection rates.† The authors concluded that policy reforms and community-based culturally safe initiatives are needed for this population and that reforms must be conducted in partnership with the community.

Questions to Consider

1. What impact could traditional foods have on the oral health of First Nations children?
2. How can CHNs create strong partnerships with at-risk Indigenous women?

Sources: * Cidro, J., Zahayko, L., Lawrence, H., et al. (2014). Traditional and cultural approaches to childrearing: Preventing early childhood caries in Norway House Cree Nation, Manitoba. *Rural and Remote Health, 14*(4), 1–11. † Bingham, B., Leo, D., Zhang, R., et al. (2014). Generational sex work and HIV risk among Indigenous women in a street-based urban Canadian setting. *Culture, Health & Sexuality, 16*(4), 440–452. https://doi.org/10.1080/13691058.2014.8 88480

Considerations for providing care to an aggregate or entire community are the same as those for providing care to an individual or a family patient. For example, the community must perceive that a health concern exists; believe that the CHN can assist in addressing this health concern; perceive that its contributions are valued; be assured of confidentiality for nonpublic information; and be involved from the beginning in the partnership. Role negotiation (who will do what) and role separation (CHN as data collector and CHN

as facilitator) are other important aspects of partnership and trust. For example, a school principal speaks to a CHN regarding concerns about the number of overweight and obese children in the school and requests assistance to deal with this health concern. The community of interest in this situation is the schoolchildren. The CHN has a role as data collector—examining the pediatric literature to determine the incidence and prevalence of childhood obesity in the community. As well, the CHN has a role as facilitator—partnering with the school principal and school community to conduct a "windshield survey" of the school and the surrounding school catchment area to determine factors such as nutrition policies and practices, food costs, and food security. The CHN then negotiates the "educator" role in partnership with the school health education teachers and conducts a nutrition education session during the school's health education classes. A **windshield survey** is an observational method used as part of a community assessment that scans the community's physical environment. A windshield survey is discussed in more detail later in this chapter. The CHN decides to interview certain members individually and conduct focus groups with students, teachers, parents, lunch monitors, and physical activity coordinators. School community strengths and assets are identified and strategies for implementation are determined by all stakeholders.

The community-as-partner model, based on Betty Neuman's system model, is a nursing framework for community health assessment that incorporates two central components: the nursing process and the community as partner (see Appendix 6). The community in this community-as-partner model is composed of a central population and eight subsystems depicted diagrammatically as a wheel with people as the hub surrounded by the subsystems. Working as partners, the CHN and the community plan, implement, and evaluate strategies to reduce stressors, restore stability, and avert future health concerns. (A comprehensive discussion of the community-as-partner model is presented in Vollman et al. [2017].)

Other community health assessment models that are sometimes used in community health are the general systems model for community and population assessment, comprehensive health assessment (it looks for all relevant community health information), familiarization assessment (the windshield survey), problem-oriented assessment (it assesses the community with regard to one problem), subsystem or population-oriented assessment (it assesses a single aspect of community such as schools or resources for older adults), and assets assessment (it focuses on strengths and capacities rather than on health concerns alone) (Maurer & Smith, 2013).

Community and the Determinants of Health

The "Determinants of Health" box provides examples of social and economic determinants of health that relate to community-oriented practice and that influence the health of populations. Health status variations exist between populations residing in urban and rural communities, which suggests that the determinants of health need to be addressed, especially to deal with the health disparities that exist in rural communities. CHNs need to consider other determinants of health that might exist in their community, such as social and physical environments, including rural versus urban living (e.g., farm accidents versus motor vehicle accidents), income, geography, and culture. Dunn (2002) stated that "social and economic factors strongly influence the health of Canadians and such factors can be modified by social and economic policy" (p. ii).

DETERMINANTS OF HEALTH

Community-Level Determinants of Health

- Rural Canadians, compared with their urban counterparts, have completed a lower level of education; live in poorer socioeconomic conditions; demonstrate less healthy behaviours; and have more chronic illnesses, lower life expectancy, higher mortality rates, and a stronger sense of community belonging.[*]
- Rural Canadians face greater economic difficulties than their urban counterparts.[†]
- Rural Canadians have higher smoking rates (especially men), greater exposure to second-hand smoke, and lower likelihood of eating the recommended five daily servings of fruit and vegetables (especially men).[‡]
- The most common causes of mortality due to injury in rural communities are due to motor-vehicle and farm accidents, and injuries.[‡]
- In Canadian people aged 6 to 79 years, the number of decayed teeth, missing teeth, and oral pain decreases with increasing income, whereas the number of filled teeth increases with income.[§]

Obesity is more prevalent among economically disadvantaged women in Canada and is mainly concentrated among the poor in the Atlantic provinces.[I]

- Four in ten Indigenous children in Canada live in poverty[#]
- In Canada, the gap between the poor and rich families remains very wide.[#]
- In 2011–2012, 8.3% of Canadian households, or almost 1.1 million households, experienced food insecurity. Of that amount, 5.8% was reported as moderate and 2.5% was severe.[**]

Sources: [*] Canadian Institute for Health Information (CIHI). (2006). *How healthy are rural Canadians? An assessment of their health status and health determinants.* https://secure.cihi.ca/free_products/rural_canadians_2006_report_e.pdf
[†] Pong, 2007.
[‡] DesMeules, Luo, Wang, et al., 2007.
[§] Ravaghi, Quiñonez, & Allison, 2013.
[I] Hajizadeh, Campbell, & Sarma, 2014.
[#] Campaign 2000, 2014.
[**] Statistics Canada, 2012.

CHARACTERISTICS OF COMMUNITY HEALTH NURSING PRACTICE

The most effective way for CHNs to achieve healthy changes is in partnership with the community. In community-oriented practice, the CHN and the community seek to achieve changes together. Community-oriented practice includes considering the dimensions of community health that are unique to each community, and then involving the community in maintaining, improving, promoting, and protecting its own health and well-being. Fundamental to community-oriented practice are the concept of Healthy Communities and the need to develop community partnerships. The common goal of community-oriented practice is an ongoing series of health-promoting changes developed in partnership with the community.

Community Health

Community health has three dimensions: status, structure, and process. Each dimension has a unique effect on a community's health.

Status

The status of community health is often measured by traditional morbidity and mortality rates, life expectancy indices, and risk-factor profiles. This information for all regions in Canada is currently available on the Statistics Canada website through census data (see the link on the Evolve website). Canadian census data include profiles of individual communities and detailed data for small groups (such as lone-parent families, ethnic groups, occupational groups, and immigrants). The Canadian census is conducted every 5 years and aims to include every Canadian living in and outside of the country. Individuals without an address, such as the homeless, are not likely to be included and therefore are invisible aggregates. The census also includes those who are residing in Canada with a permit (e.g., a study, work, or temporary resident permit) and their dependents. The questions used every 5 years are similar, so comparisons can be made to determine changes that have occurred in Canada's population over time. The Government of Canada's decision in the summer of 2010 to make the previously mandatory long-form census voluntary (which it was for the 2011 census) has research and evaluation implications. According to Collier (2010), "The population data obtained from a voluntary survey will be biased, researchers say, and will inhibit research into the social determinants of health" (p. E563). That may well be the case for the 2011 census data. However, the mandatory long-form census was reinstated by the federal government at the end of 2015 so that it would be used in the 2016 census.

Data to assess the status of a community is also available through the Canadian Institute for Health Information (CIHI), a nonprofit autonomous organization that provides data and analysis on the health of Canadians and Canada's health system. The CIHI, along with Statistics Canada, reports on the health indicators that reflect and affect the health of Canadians and the performance of the Canadian health care system. Another source of data is the Canadian Community Health Survey (CCHS), which was initiated in 2000 (Statistics Canada, 2016). The CCHS closely examines health determinants and, since 2007, collects data on an annual basis. The CCHS is conducted by Statistics Canada to provide cross-sectional estimates of health determinants, health status, and health system use for 133 health regions across Canada as well as the territories. The primary use of the CCHS is for health surveillance and population health research. Health indicators provide information on the health of the population, health services, and community characteristics.

Other Canadian health surveys include the Canadian Health Measures Survey (Statistics Canada, 2015), and the National Longitudinal Survey of Children and Youth (Statistics Canada, 2010). These health surveys provide prevalence rates for risk factors, disease, disability, and the use of health services, and they are used to look at associations among risk factors. In 2011, Health Canada published *Healthy Canadians: A Federal Report on Comparable Health Indicators 2010* (see the link on the Evolve website). The report includes statistics on findings such as smoking among teenagers, diabetes, and perceived health (Health Canada, 2011).

Structure

Community health, when viewed from the structure of the community, is usually defined in terms of *services, resources,* and the *characteristics of the community structure itself.* Measures of community health services and resources include service-use patterns, treatment data from various health agencies, and provider-to-patient ratios. These data provide information such as the number of available hospital beds or the number of emergency department visits to a particular hospital.

Characteristics of the community structure are commonly identified as social indicators, or correlates, of health. Measures of community structure include demographic data such as socioeconomic and racial distributions, age, gender, and educational levels. Their relationships to health status have been thoroughly documented (Fournier & Karachiwalla, 2020).

Recent evidence has shown that the social determinants of health are key factors that influence the health of populations (Raphael, 2016). The social determinants of health include gender, housing, income and income distribution, and educational levels (Mikkonen & Raphael, 2010). Some studies have found that certain social determinants of health have more impact on health and the incidence of illness than traditional biomedical and behavioural risk factors (Raphael, 2016).

Process

The view of community health as the process of effective community functioning or problem solving is well established. However, it is especially appropriate to community health nursing because it directs the study of community health to promote effective community action for health promotion, which is an important goal of CHNs.

Community health typically refers to the process of involving the community in maintaining, improving, promoting, and protecting its own health and well-being. This definition emphasizes the process dimension but also includes the dimensions of status and structure. Indicators for the dimensions of community health (status, structure, and process) are listed with measures and examples of data sources in Table 9.2.

TABLE 9.2   Concept of Community Health Specified

Dimension	Measures	Examples of Data Sources
Status	Vital statistics (live births, neonatal deaths, infant deaths, maternal deaths)	Census data District health unit annual vital statistics
	Incidence and prevalence of leading causes of mortality and morbidity	Census data District health unit/health authority
	Health-risk profiles of selected aggregates	District health unit Support groups Local nonprofit organizations
	Functional ability levels	Census data
Structure	Health facilities such as hospitals, long-term care facilities, industrial and school health services, health units, voluntary health associations	Local Chamber of Commerce United Way
	Health-related planning groups	Local newspapers Local magazines Local government
	Health personnel resources, such as physicians, dentists, and nurses	Telephone directory Provincial and labour statistics Professional licensing boards
	Health-resource use patterns, such as bed-occupancy days and patient or provider visits	Statistics Canada District health units and hospital annual reports
Process	Commitment to community health	Local government
	Awareness of self and others and clarity of situational definitions	Local history Neighbourhood help organizations Local or neighbourhood newspapers and radio programs Local government
	Conflict containment and accommodation	Social services department
	Participation	Existence of and participation in local organizations
	Management of relationships with society	Windshield survey—observation of interactions
	Machinery for facilitating participant interaction and decision making	Notices for community organizations and meetings in public places (e.g., supermarkets, newspapers, radio)

The use of status, structure, and process dimensions to define community health is an effort to develop a broad definition of community health, involving indicators that often are not included when discussions focus only on individual and family risk factors as the basis for community health.

Strategies to Improve Community Health

Although several strategies to community disease prevention and health promotion exist, the strategy chosen often depends on whether the status, structure, or process dimension of community health is being emphasized. Consider the following examples:

- If the emphasis is on the *status dimension,* the best strategies are usually primary or secondary prevention activities because the objective is either to prevent a disease or to treat it in its early stages. An immunization program is an example of a community health nursing intervention at the primary prevention level when contracting the disease will likely occur if the immunization is not received. A breast cancer–screening program is an example of secondary prevention because the focus is on detecting and treating disease in the early stages, as well as determining the incidence and prevalence of breast cancer in the identified population.
- If the emphasis is on the *structural dimension,* the best strategies are usually interventions directed at health services or based on population demographic characteristics. Interventions directed at health services might include developing a new program in occupational health nursing at a workplace where recurring illnesses and injuries have been identified through an assessment. Interventions based on demographic characteristics may include community development. For example, a group of community leaders may come together because they have recognized that school-age children do not have easy access to recreational opportunities after school. The leaders, in partnership with the health units or authorities and the school board, may be able to plan for after-school recreational activities.
- If the emphasis is on the *process dimension*—usually the level of intervention of the CHN—the best strategy is usually health promotion. For example, if family-life education is lacking in a community because of ineffective communication among families, children, school board members, religious leaders, and health care providers, the most effective CHN strategy may be to open discussion among these groups and help community members develop education programs and advocate for programs.

Healthy Communities

In the late 1980s, World Health Organization (WHO) developed an international healthy cities movement promoting healthy communities. The term *Healthy Cities movement* is used interchangeably with *Healthy Communities movement.* This movement, also discussed in Chapter 4, incorporates the primary health care principles of health promotion to achieve "health for all." "A **'healthy community'** is one where people, organizations and local institutions work together to improve the social, economic and environmental conditions that make people healthy—the determinants of health" (British Colombia Healthy Communities, 2021).

The health of a community includes the health care system and involves policies that affect social, economic, and environmental life, and the activities of individuals, groups, and corporations (Capital Regional District, 2008). A healthy community has the following characteristics:
- "Clean and safe physical environments
- Peace, equity, and social justice
- Adequate access to food, clean water, shelter, income, safety, work and recreation for all
- Strong, mutually-supportive relationships and networks
- Wide participation of residents in decision-making
- Strong cultural and spiritual heritage
- Diverse and robust economy
- Opportunities for learning and skill development
- Access to health services, including public health and preventive programs" (Vancouver Coastal Health, 2009).

The Healthy Communities movement emphasizes the determinants of health, which include social determinants (e.g., healthy public policy), environmental determinants (e.g., green space), economic determinants (e.g., stable employment), physical determinants (e.g., physical activity), psychological and spiritual determinants (e.g., sense of belonging), and cultural determinants (e.g., community identity) (BC Healthy Communities, 2009). (For further information on Healthy Communities, see the Healthy Cities/Healthy Communities link on the Evolve website.) Many communities across Canada have adopted the movement, including Victoria in British Columbia, Buffalo Narrows in Saskatchewan, Brandon in Manitoba, Waterloo in Ontario, Trois-Rivières in Quebec, and Bathurst in New Brunswick. For additional information on other Canadian communities engaged in the Healthy Communities movement, see pp. 32–38 of the Senate Subcommittee on Population Health (link is on the Evolve website).

Canadian Nurses Association (CNA, 2005) summarizes the issues pertaining to healthy communities and nursing in a backgrounder (see the link on the Evolve website). The CNA backgrounder provides information on the Healthy Communities process and, in particular, the range of policies at the community level that can affect health—for example, a policy for sidewalk snow removal that should result in fewer falls and injuries. The process of Healthy Communities development is important to CHNs because it deals with several of the determinants of health as well as policy development to improve on these determinants, which is a strategy that CHNs can support. Additionally, CHNs can apply for funding where available for community projects that support Healthy Communities initiatives (BC Healthy Communities, 2009). Some of the ways that CHNs have been involved in the Healthy Communities movement are: identifying community health issues; supporting community members in the research, organization, and presentation of the issues; and establishing coalitions with others such as the educational sector.

Community Partnerships and Coalitions

A **partnership** is a relationship between individuals, groups, organizations, or governments, in which the parties actively work together at all stages of assessment planning, implementation, and evaluation. In the community context, the term *partnership* is often used synonymously with *coalition* and *alliance,* ideally with power shared among all participants in the processes of change for improved community health. **Community partnerships** involve collaborative decision-making efforts in health planning, with the goal of reducing health inequities and improving community health. Consequently, successful strategies for improving community health must include collaborative partnerships in the community for greater health impact. Vollman et al. (2017) use the community-as-partner model to emphasize the fundamental thinking of interprofessional primary health care and the developing reverence for public involvement in health decision making.

Partnership is a concept that is essential for CHNs to know and use, as are the concepts of community, community as partner, and community health. Experienced CHNs know that partnership is important because health is generated through new and increasingly effective means of lay and professional collaboration at the individual, family, group, or community level. This collaboration can also be referred to as *intersectoral collaboration* when there is joint action and a shared responsibility among groups, professionals, the community, and other groups not normally associated with health. For example, air pollution is an issue for many urban neighbourhoods. An example of an intersectoral collaboration is one that developed among parents of asthmatic children, local politicians, industry, and other citizens to create a policy about leaf burning in the township. Another is the spring cleanup organized in several communities, whereby citizens volunteer to pick up garbage along roadways on a selected activity day, sponsored by a local business such as Tim Hortons in partnership with the local government, with the intention of promoting exercise and cleaner neighbourhoods. An example of a formal partnership is the Peace Works Community Partnerships Project, which took place in the late 1990s in the eastern part of Prince Edward Island. Partnerships were established between families, youth groups, schools, police, and local businesses to address the issue of increased community violence, with the goal of more peaceful schools and communities.

Effective partnerships usually have the following characteristics:
- Equality in decision making
- A shared vision
- Integrity
- Agreement on specific goals
- A plan of action to meet the goals.

A growing body of literature supports the significance and effectiveness of partnerships in improving community health. One Government of Canada partnership initiative that is having an impact on the physical environment as a determinant of health is the Homeless Partnering Strategy (HPS), a community-based program designed to prevent and reduce homelessness by providing direct support and funding to 61 communities across Canada. The HPS has a housing-first approach that involves moving homeless individuals from the streets or shelters into permanent housing, while also providing services to assist individuals to sustain their housing. (Employment and Social Development Canada, 2016b). Another program that emphasizes the importance of partnerships is the New Horizons for Seniors Program, which partners with seniors to make a difference in their communities by promoting volunteerism and education on topics such as elder abuse (Employment and Social Development Canada, 2021).

In international health, the goal of partnership models is generally to empower people, through their lay leaders, to control their own health destinies and lives. Partnerships can also be established between nurses. CNA supports the idea that nurses and the nursing profession in Canada must contribute to the advancement of global health and equity and that one way this can be achieved is by establishing partnerships with nurses and nursing associations around the world, especially in developing countries. The CNA (2012) position statement "International Health Partnerships" shows that CNA has been establishing partnerships with national nursing associations in developing countries for more than 30 years with the goal of increasing the ability of these nursing associations to fortify the nursing profession as well as the quality of nursing and health services provided to their populations (see the link on the Evolve website).

Many activities in the Healthy Communities movement are conducted by coalitions. A **coalition** refers to two or more groups that share a mutual issue or concern and join forces, thereby increasing their influence in achieving a common goal. Most often, the groups are representative of organizations and agencies that have an assigned interest (mandate) in the issue and citizens who have come together to form a "community of interest." These community coalitions usually continue for a long period of time. Members come to a coalition as representatives of their own organization or as community members; however, the expectation is that members will advocate on behalf of the coalition to advance their shared interests in health promotion and not their own self-interest (Moyer, 2005; Nies & McEwen, 2019). Coalitions can have many purposes, and many coalitions are not just locally based but have provincial and national affiliates. For example, Heart Health coalitions exist in at least 10 provinces and territories and in more than 50 Canadian communities (Health Canada, 2004). As well, Healthy Communities coalitions are located in several provinces, with four provincial organizations forming the Canadian Healthy Communities Network in 2009. Coalitions often add credibility to the health community because they have broad community support and present a united front with a coordinated, consistent message. However, conflict may at times arise among groups due to the variety of groups in a coalition, their varying strengths and weaknesses, and the personalities that they bring to the coalition. Conflict-management and team-building skills are necessary to deal with issues that arise in coalitions. Working with groups is discussed further in Chapter 13.

TABLE 9.3 Components of the Community Development Process

Components	Concepts	Elements	Indicators
Capacity building	Strengthens and enables the knowledge, skills, commitment, and resources needed at individual and organization level	Education Organizational development Resource building	Positive leadership Stakeholder involvement Support for volunteers
Intersectoral networking	Provides resources for network development and building alliances	Sectors work together to solve health problems and achieve goals	Coalitions Alliances Partnerships
Local area development	Provides access to human and financial resources for action	Human resources Financial resources Volunteer support Shared experiences	Support groups Local leadership Funding sources Assets identified

Source: Based on Winnipeg Regional Health Authority. (2017). *Community development framework.* https://wrha.mb.ca/files/community-development-framework.pdf

COMMUNITY DEVELOPMENT

Kretzmann and McKnight (1993) defined *community development* as "building communities from the inside out." Community development occurs when a community is engaged in a dynamic, continuous process of social change that can lead to permanent enhancements in people's lives; it can include a broad range of strategies such as capacity building and empowerment (Winnipeg Regional Health Authority (WRHA), 2017). The process of community development involves working with the community as the unit of care. It implies that the CHN and other health care providers partner with community members to involve them in making decisions to improve their health. A community development approach involves people in determining what health services are needed, which is in keeping with the principles of primary health care. The WRHA (2017) identifies three components of the community development process: capacity building, intersectoral networking, and local area development (Table 9.3). Table 9.3 outlines the components of the community development process.

Community Capacity Building

Community capacity building involves identifying and working with existing community strengths to promote a positive view of the community; therefore, it is focused on helping communities become stronger based on their strengths rather than letting their weaknesses define them (McKnight & Kretzmann, 2005). The process of capacity building relies heavily on collaboration and partnerships. It ensures that partners develop the skills and resources required to hold programs together, thereby increasing their chances for long-term success. CHNs work with communities to build capacity by actively involving the community in decisions about programs and initiatives that are based on the specific needs and resources of the community and then building partnerships and identifying resources to address those needs. The "Evidence-Informed Practice" box shows the importance of engaging community partners in capacity building.

EVIDENCE-INFORMED PRACTICE

Horton and MacLeod (2008) undertook a qualitative study to explore the experience of capacity building among health education workers in the Yukon. The study used interpretive descriptive analysis and was undertaken through individual and small-group interviews with 21 Yukon health education workers. Themes that emerged included the ways in which participants build on their own and community members' strengths; participants' focus on achieving outcomes that are immediately important and relevant to the community; and how they live and work in the community while undertaking capacity building. The health education workers asked learners to share practical skills and knowledge and used these in their teaching to build on strengths. This strategy engaged the learners. It is very important to understand that health education workers who live in their communities can make a difference in capacity building. The findings indicated the spaces in which policy and organizational practices can support communities to enhance capacity building.

Application for CHNs

The findings support the importance of recognizing the knowledge and experiences of community members and involving community members in capacity building. CHNs need to work with community strengths and assets and build on these to promote capacity building. Engaging a community in capacity building is often related to a CHNs' engagement in a community at a relationship level ("living in relationship with the community") and at a working level ("working in interactive relationships with community members") (p. 71). *Relationship level* refers to the personal level of residing in a community, whereas the *working level* refers to the professional aspect of working with the community while residing in that community.

Questions for Reflection and Discussion

1. Why is it important to promote community capacity building?
2. Do you think that living in and knowing the community would be a disadvantage to a CHN who also works in that community? Support your viewpoint.
3. Based on the study findings, what is one clinical question that you would ask in order to search the literature?

Source: Horton, J., & MacLeod, M. (2008). The experience of capacity building among health education workers in the Yukon. *Canadian Journal of Public Health, 99*(1), 69–72.

TABLE 9.4 Features of Community Capacity

Feature	Description
Participation	The active involvement of people in improving their own and their community's health and well-being. Participating in a project means the target population, community members, and other stakeholders are involved in project activities such as making decisions and evaluation.
Leadership	Developing and nurturing both formal and informal local leaders during a project. Effective leaders support and direct, deal with conflict, acknowledge and encourage community members' voices, share leadership, and facilitate networks to build on community resources. Leaders bring people with diverse skill sets together and may have both interpersonal and technical skills. Finally, effective leaders have a strategic vision for the future.
Community structures	Smaller or less formal community groups and committees that foster belonging and give the community a chance to express views and exchange information. Examples are church groups, youth groups, and self-help groups.
External supports	Funding bodies such as government departments, foundations, and regional health authorities that can link communities and external resources. At the beginning of a project, early external support may nurture community momentum.
Asking why	A community process that uncovers the root causes of community health issues and promotes solutions. The community comes together to critically assess the social, political, and economic influences that result in differing health standards and conditions. Exploration through "asking why" helps refine a project to reflect the community needs.
Obtaining resources	Finding time, money (other than from funding bodies), leadership, volunteers, information, and facilities from both inside and outside the community.
Skills, knowledge, and learning	The qualities in the project team, the target population, and the community that the project team uses and develops.
Linking with others	Linking your project with individuals and organizations. These project links help the community deal with its issues. Examples are creating partnerships or linking with networks and coalitions.
Sense of community	A feeling fostered by building trust with others. Community projects can strengthen a sense of community when people come together to work on shared community problems. Collaborations give community members confidence to act and courage to feel hopeful about change.

Source: Public Health Agency of Canada. (2008). *The community capacity building tool.* http://www.phac-aspc.gc.ca/canada/regions/ab-nwt-tno/downloads-eng.php

Table 9.4 describes nine features of community capacity (Public Health Agency of Canada, 2008).

McKnight and Kretzmann (2005) held that greater success in community capacity building comes from focusing on a community's capacities, skills, and assets rather than its deficiencies, needs, and problems. Asset mapping is one of the skills required of CHNs when working in community development. **Asset mapping** involves identifying community-based assets such as individuals, local associations, businesses, public institutions (e.g., schools, libraries, fire stations), non-profit organizations, and the community's physical characteristics (Briggs & Huang, 2017; Kretzmann & McKnight, 1993). The three approaches to asset mapping are as follows: (1) the whole-assets approach (which is comprehensive and provides a complete map of the community and its support systems); (2) the storytelling approach (a social history that reveals assets in the community); and (3) the heritage approach (a picture, map, or list of anything that is part of a community's heritage) (Government of Canada, 2009). Resources on asset mapping include *Asset Mapping: A Handbook* (Canadian Community Economic Development [CED] Network, 2016) and *Canadian Asset Map for Stem Cell and Regenerative Medicine* (International Biopharma Solutions, 2012) (see the links on the Evolve website). The CED handbook provides extensive guidelines on and examples for using mapping as a tool.

The use of community capacity to bring about change through an action plan (usually developed and implemented with community partners) is known as *community mobilization*. Community mobilization seeks to influence healthy public policy and may include individuals residing in the community joining together to bring about change in reference to a health issue. For example, Fighting for a Supervised Injection Site in Vancouver is a group of citizens who mobilized over the issue of safe drug use in Downtown Eastside Vancouver; and Building a Gay, Lesbian, Bisexual and Transgendered (GLBT) Community Organization in Nova Scotia is a group of citizens who mobilized to create a safe community for its GLBT community members. For further information on these examples of community mobilization and others, see the Canadian HIV/AIDS Legal Network link on the Evolve website.

Outcomes of Community Development

When community members are involved as partners in community development, outcomes such as empowerment, sustainability, and community competence are most likely to occur. By using partnership in the community development process, community members and the community overall should gain control over the issues that affect them and thereby become empowered. Participation that encourages empowerment is crucial in promoting community health and sustainability (Diem, 2005). **Sustainability** refers to the maintenance and continuation of established community programs and is more likely to occur when members of the community are involved as partners in the community development process. **Community competence** has been linked to community empowerment; a competent community is able to use its problem-solving abilities to identify and deal with community health issues (Minkler & Wallerstein, 2005). By identifying and managing their own issues, communities are more likely to experience feelings of empowerment.

CHNs are in an ideal position to be involved in community development because they possess the knowledge required to work with the community and nursing practice skills in community development. As mentioned in Chapter 1, CHNs take the approach of *working with* rather than *working for* the community, which demonstrates the forward thinking needed in community development. They have an established rapport with members in their communities and can therefore mobilize the community in meeting its health needs through the community health nursing process.

ASSESSING COMMUNITY HEALTH

Assessment is the first phase of the community health nursing process. There are many approaches to assessing a community. According to Maurer and Smith (2013), they include a comprehensive needs assessment approach, which tries to determine what the particular problems or needs are within a community using an extensive systematic process to assess all community aspects; a problem-oriented approach, which assesses a community based on a specific health concern; a single-population approach, which is an assessment of one population group in a community such as older adults or men; and the familiarization approach, which uses existing data on a community such as census data, surveys, or health reports. In Canada, one widely used comprehensive community health needs assessment model is the community-as-partner model (Vollman et al., 2017). In that model, there is a focus on the nursing process and partnering with the community to identify priority issues and concerns. CHNs engage the community in the assessment process from the beginning, and key stakeholders assist with the planning and implementation of the community assessment process. Another community health needs-assessment model is the community health assessment process, which takes into account the determinants of health in the planning process and is endorsed by the Community Health Assessment Network of Manitoba. The associated *Community Health Assessment Guidelines, 2009* are available through the link on the Evolve website, under the Manitoba Health and Healthy Living Accountability Support Branch.

Community health assessment is the process of thinking critically about the community and involves getting to know and understand the community as partner. This process helps the CHN to understand the patient health concerns and to know what community strengths and resources are available

to the CHN to partner with the patient to address the patient's concerns. The community health assessment phase involves a logical, systematic approach. Community health assessment helps (1) identify community strengths, resources, assets, capacities, and opportunities; (2) clarify health concerns; (3) identify community constraints; (4) identify the economic, political, and social factors affecting the community; and (5) identify the determinants of health affecting community health.

Community health assessments can be extensive, such as the comprehensive needs assessment approach, or shorter, such as the single-population approach. Either way, the necessary initial assessment phase of the community health nursing process with the community as partner is applied. CHNs undertake a community health assessment for many reasons that direct the type of data collected, the emphasis on different clusters of data, the sources of data, and the data-collection methods. One reason to conduct a community health assessment is to validate the existence of a suspected or identified health concern, determine the extent of the health concern, and generate some possible resolutions. Another reason is to identify community assets and gaps in resources so that alternative solutions can be developed to address the identified gaps. Yet another reason is to determine the actual health status of the community; in doing so, the CHN may focus on a particular population group (aggregate) within the community or the entire community.

A couple of examples will help to clarify these differing purposes. For instance, a CHN concerned about an apparent increase in the incidence of rubella in a community might conduct a community health assessment to verify the existence and extent of the health concern within a susceptible population, such as females of child-bearing years, and their level of immunity. This action might enable the CHN to prevent fetal deformities either by increasing immunization levels among the target group or by promoting contraceptive use by those who are not immune. Another example is a CHN who has been recently assigned to a new or rapidly expanding town. A comprehensive needs assessment is conducted to establish baseline information on the health status of a community and the capacity of the community to meet its health concerns. Before a community health assessment is started, certain planning considerations must be addressed. For a discussion on planning considerations, see the *Community Health Assessment Guidelines, 2009* link on the Evolve website (under the Manitoba Health and Healthy Living Accountability Support Branch), specifically pp. 6–22.

Assessing community health requires:

1. Gathering relevant existing data and generating missing data.
2. Developing a composite database.
3. Interpreting the composite database to identify community strengths and health concerns.

Data Collection and Interpretation

Data collection is the process of acquiring existing, readily available information or developing new information about the community and its health. The systematic collection of data about community health requires:

- Gathering or compiling existing data
- Generating missing data
- Interpreting data
- Identifying community abilities and health concerns

For key considerations on data gathering and analysis for community health assessments, see the *Community Health Assessment Guidelines, 2009* link on the Evolve website (under the Manitoba Health and Healthy Living Accountability Support Branch), especially pp. 23–26.

A multitude of data must be collected to complete a comprehensive health assessment of a community as patient. An assessment model or framework identifies the various categories of data to be collected and assists in organizing the data collected. No sole instrument provides all the information needed; therefore, CHNs often select parts of various assessment instruments that meet their needs and address concerns of relevance to the community. Even though an assessment model or framework assists with data gathering and generation, in a comprehensive assessment of a community, the amount of community information can become overwhelming. Therefore, CHNs need to decide what information is most important to collect, the data sources most appropriate to use, and the data-collection methods deemed most effective. Most often, CHNs will conduct smaller and more focused assessments. These small, focused community assessments could be done using the windshield survey method to gain initial insights about the community (Escoffery, Miner, & Trowbridge, 2004). Depending on factors such as health concern, purpose, and resource availability, CHNs may conduct either a comprehensive community health needs assessment or a condensed community health needs assessment.

Data Gathering

Data gathering is the process of obtaining existing, readily available data. The following data usually describe the demography of a community:

- Age of residents
- Gender distribution of residents
- Socioeconomic characteristics
- Racial distributions
- Vital statistics, including selected mortality and morbidity data
- Community institutions, including health care organizations and the services they provide
- Health personnel characteristics

Often these data have been collected by others via structured interviews, questionnaires, or surveys and are available in published research reports online, by searching for the topic or specific government department website. These data give CHNs a snapshot of how the patients receiving services fit into the community.

Data Generation

Data generation is the process of developing data that do not already exist, through interaction with community members.

This type of information is more difficult to obtain and is generally not statistical. Data that often must be generated include:

- Knowledge and beliefs
- Values and sentiments
- Goals and perceived concerns
- Norms
- Problem-solving processes
- Power
- Leadership
- Influence structures

These data are more likely to be collected by interviews and observation.

Composite Database Analysis

Combining the gathered and generated data creates a composite **database.** Data analysis seeks to make sense of the data, as follows:

1. First, data are analyzed and synthesized, and themes are noted.
2. **Community health concerns**—actual, possible, or potential community health challenges with identifiable contributing factors in the environment—are determined.
3. **Community health strengths**—community resources available to meet community health concerns—are identified.
4. The resources available to meet the health concerns are identified.

Data collection and interpretation (diagnostic reasoning) are critical aspects of the community health nursing process.

Data-Collection Methods

Several methods to collect data are needed. Methods that encourage the CHN to consider the community's perception of its health concerns and abilities are as important as methods structured to identify knowledge that the CHN considers essential.

Seven methods of collecting data are:

1. Informant interviews
2. Focus groups
3. Participant observation
4. Windshield surveys
5. Community forums
6. Secondary analysis of existing data
7. Surveys

These methods can be grouped into two distinct but complementary categories: methods that rely on what is directly observed by the data collector and methods that rely on what is reported to the data collector.

Collection of Direct Data

Informant interviews, focus groups, participant observation, windshield surveys, and *community forums* are five methods of directly collecting data. All five methods require sensitivity; openness; curiosity; the ability to listen, taste, touch, and smell; and the ability to see life as it is lived in a community.

Informant interviews, which consist of directed talks with selected members of a community about community members or groups and events, are basic to effective data collection. Talking to key informants is a critical part of the community assessment. Key informants are not always people who have a formal title or position—they often have an informal role within the community. Examples are a member of a minority group who is listened to by other members of the group, a church deacon, and a parent who is active and vocal about the school health curriculum. When selecting key informants, it is critical to choose people whose views represent those of the community.

Key informant interviews can provide data that describe a community that has well-defined clusters of individuals with similar concerns, such as persons of low income, those with concerns about adolescent pregnancy, and those with worries about the health of babies. These data could be difficult to acquire without interviews, but interviews can be time consuming.

HOW TO …

Identify a Key Informant for Interviews
The following people may be key informants:
- Health care providers such as social workers
- Church leaders
- Community members recommended by CHNs
- A president of the school council organization
- The mayor or other local politicians
- Informal leaders, such as a mother who organized the local chapter of Mothers Against Drunk Driving

In community health assessment, a **focus group** is a small group of individuals residing in the community who are brought together to share their beliefs, opinions, and experiences about a selected discussion topic. In focus groups, participants are able to interact with one another and build on one another's ideas. During the community health assessment process, focus groups are used throughout the assessment phase. A focus group may be conducted to explore high-risk behaviour in specific aggregate groups; for example, to try to determine factors that contribute to smoking behaviour in youth. Also, a focus group might be conducted to explore possible alternative interventions for identified health concerns in youth who smoke to determine youth perceptions of actions that promote smoking cessation. Moreover, a focus group might be conducted to evaluate the effectiveness of a smoking cessation program that has been implemented among youth.

Participant observation is the deliberate sharing, if conditions permit, in the life of a community. For example, if the CHN lives in the community, participating in activities such as clinical organizations and church life and reading the newspaper provides the CHN with "observations" of the community's life. Informant interviews and participant observation are good ways to generate information about community beliefs, norms, values, power and influence structures, and problem-solving processes. Such data can

seldom be reported in numbers, so often they are not collected. One limitation of participant observation is that conclusions may be based on one person's opinion or intuition and are therefore unchecked. Any conclusions drawn by the CHN from participant observation should be confirmed with the participants.

A windshield survey or walking survey can be easily conducted by a CHN driving or walking through a community. It involves collecting data on the community based on observations made through a car windshield, while riding public transportation, or during a walk. A survey can facilitate an understanding of the geographical features of the community and "the location of agencies, services, businesses, and industries and location of possible areas of environmental concern through 'sight, sense, and sound'" (Cassells, 2019, p. 96).

While driving a car, riding public transportation, or walking, the CHN can observe many dimensions of a community's life and environment, such as:
- Common characteristics of people on the street
- Accessibility, such as access to buildings and sidewalk design
- Neighbourhood gathering places
- The rhythm of community life
- Housing quality and alternatives
- Recreational opportunities
- Geographical boundaries

CHNs can use windshield surveys for short and rapid community health assessments. See the "How to …" box below. A CHN doing such a survey as part of a community health assessment should go out twice: once during the day when people are at work and children are at school, and a second time in the evening after work is done and school is out. This survey can be completed on foot to provide the opportunity for interaction and a "feel" for the community, or by driving slowly through the community if it covers a large geographical area. Figure 9.1 is an example of a walking or windshield survey.

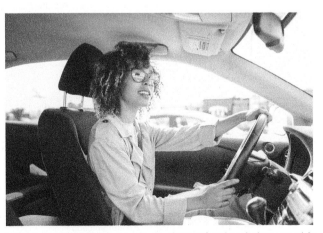

A windshield/walking survey is an observational technique used in community health assessment that offers the community health nurse some early insights about the community in which he or she is working. iStockphoto/kate_sept2004

I. Community Core (Elements)	Observations	Data
1. *History.* What can you glean by looking (e.g., old, established neighbourhoods; new subdivision)? Ask people willing to talk: How long have you lived here? Has the area changed? As you talk, ask if there is an "old-timer" who knows the history of the area.		
2. *Demographics.* What sorts of people do you see? Young? Old? Homeless? Alone? Families? Is the population homogeneous?		
3. *Ethnicity.* Do you note indicators of different ethnic groups (e.g., restaurants, festivals)? What signs do you see of different cultural groups?		
4. *Values and beliefs.* Are there churches, mosques, temples? Does it appear homogeneous? Are the lawns cared for? With flowers? Gardens? Signs of art? Culture? Heritage? Historical markers?		

II. Subsystems	Observations	Data
1. *Physical environment.* How does the community look? What do you note about air quality, flora, housing, zoning, space, green areas, animals, people, human-made structures, natural beauty, water, climate? Can you find or develop a map of the area? What is the size (e.g., kilometres, blocks)?		
2. *Health and social services.* Is there evidence of acute or chronic conditions? Shelters? Alternative therapists or healers? Are there clinics, hospitals, practitioners' offices, public health services, home health agencies, emergency centres, nursing homes, social service facilities, mental health services? Are there resources outside the community but readily accessible to residents?		
3. *Economy.* Is it a "thriving" community, or does it feel "seedy"? Are there industries, stores, places of employment? Where do people shop? Are there signs that people can find employment (e.g., Help Wanted signs, classified ads)? Are there signs of thrift stores, pawn shops, and other services for people with money issues? How active is the food bank?		
4. *Transportation and safety.* How do people get around? What types of private and public transportation are available? Do you see buses, bicycles, taxis? Are there sidewalks, bike trails? Is getting around in the community possible for people with disabilities? What types of protective services are there (e.g., fire, police, sanitation)? Is air quality monitored? What types of crimes are committed? Do people feel safe? Are there signs of racism or intolerance?		
5. *Politics and government.* Are there signs of political activity (e.g., posters, meetings)? What party affiliation predominates? What is the governmental jurisdiction of the community (e.g., elected mayor, city council with single-member districts)? Are people involved in decision making in their local governmental unit?		
6. *Communication.* Are there "common areas" where people gather? What newspapers do you see in the stands? Do people have TVs, mobile music devices, cell phones? What do they watch and listen to? What are the formal and informal means of communication?		

Fig. 9.1 Windshield/Walking Survey. (From Vollman, A. R., Anderson, E. T., & McFarlane, J. M. [2017]. *Canadian community as partner: Theory and multidisciplinary practice in nursing* [4th ed., p. 177]. Lippincott, Williams & Wilkins. Reproduced with permission.)

Continued

	Observations	Data
7. *Education.* Are there schools in the area? How do they look? How does it function? What is the reputation of the school(s)? What are major educational issues? What are the dropout rates? Are extracurricular activities available? Are they used? Is there a school health service? A school nurse? Are there adult education and second-language programs readily available?		
8. *Recreation.* Where do children play? What are the major forms of recreation? Who participates? What facilities for recreation do you see? Are they in good order or disrepair? Are there signs that pets are welcome? What about the performing arts and social and other leisure activities (e.g., festivals, zoo, museum, sports teams)?		
III. Perceptions	**Observations**	**Data**
1. *The residents.* How do people feel about the community? What do they identify as its strengths? Problems? Ask several people from different groups (e.g., old, young, unskilled/skilled workers, service worker, professional, clergy, stay-at-home parent, lone parent) and keep track of who gives what answer.		
2. *Your perceptions.* What are your general statements about the "health" of this community? What are its strengths? What concerns or potential concerns can you identify? Who are the gatekeepers to the community and/or population of interest? Who are the champions that might support your work? Who in the community might become a partner in the process? Where will resistance be found?		

Fig. 9.1, cont'd

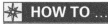

HOW TO …

Obtain a Quick Assessment of a Community
- One way to get a quick, initial sense of the community is to do a windshield assessment using a format like the one provided in Fig. 9.1.
- CHNs interested in doing a windshield assessment need to take public transportation, have someone else drive while they take notes, or stop frequently to write down what they see.
- The windshield survey example is organized into 14 elements with specific questions to answer that are related to each element. Some of the questions need to be answered by visiting the library to get secondary data.
- CHNs who use this approach will have an initial descriptive assessment of the community when they are finished.
- Interventions are planned based on the windshield survey findings.

A **community forum** is a meeting in which involved parties can gain an understanding of a particular issue of concern to them. For a community forum to be effective, it is important for the discussion leader to build a trusting, open relationship with participants. Community forums do not involve decision making. Examples of community forums are town hall meetings where members of the public meet face to face in a community centre to discuss a community issue; community-to-community forums where members from neighbouring communities such as a First Nations reserve and a local community meet face to face to discuss issues of mutual interest; and Internet forums that provide the opportunity for a discussion to occur using online technology. For information on developing a community forum, see the *Guide to Community to Community Forums in British Columbia* link on the Evolve website.

Collection of Reported Data

Secondary analysis and surveys are two methods of collecting reported data. In **secondary analysis**, the CHN uses previously gathered data, such as minutes from community meetings and available epidemiological data. This type of analysis is extremely valuable because it saves time and effort. Many sources of data are readily available and useful for secondary analysis, including:
- Public documents
- Census data
- Health surveys
- Health surveillance
- Minutes from meetings
- Statistical data
- Internet sites and informatics
- Health records

A **survey** is a method of assessment in which data from a sample of persons are reported to a data collector. A health survey can be cross-sectional (provided to participants once only) or longitudinal (provided to the same participants at different times) (Fournier & Karachiwalla, 2020). Surveys can be conducted by interview, telephone, mail, or the Internet. The use of computers for linking databases and for conducting surveys has created ethical and social issues (Fournier & Karchiwalla, 2020). Health surveys most often are used for surveillance of health behaviour, illness levels, and health consequences (Fournier & Karchiwalla, 2020). They are as useful as observational methods and secondary analyses but require time-consuming and costly data collection as the reliability and validity of the questions need to be determined. Thus, the CHN does not often use the survey method. There are many population health surveys conducted in Canada, including the Canadian Health Measures Survey, the National Longitudinal Survey of Children and Youth, the Canadian Community Health Survey, the National Population Health Survey, and the Participation and Activity Limitation Survey (Statistics Canada, 2012).

Assessment Issues

Gaining entry or acceptance into the community is perhaps the biggest challenge in assessment. If the CHN does not live in the community, he or she is most likely to be considered an outsider. The CHN is often seen to represent an established health care system that is neither known nor trusted by community members, who may therefore react with indifference or even active hostility to the CHN. In addition, CHNs may feel insecure about their skills as a community worker, and the community may refuse to acknowledge its need for those skills. Because the CHN's success depends largely on the way he or she is viewed, entry into the community is critical. It takes time to establish trust and rapport. It is crucial that ethical principles such as autonomy, beneficence, nonmaleficence, and distributive justice are followed and that the possibility for bias is minimized by upholding professional standards and being aware of the influence of one's own values and beliefs and how these may affect the establishment of trust with community patients. Often the CHN can gain trust and entry into the community in the following ways:

- Taking part in community events
- Being present and listening with interest
- Visiting people in formal leadership positions
- Using an assessment guide
- Using a peer group for support
- Keeping appointments
- Clarifying community members' perceptions of health needs
- Respecting an individual's right to choose whether he or she will work with the CHN

If the CHN lives in the community, establishing and maintaining professional boundaries may be problematic. In small communities, patients may also be very familiar to the CHN in that they could be relatives or friends. CHNs may have to set boundaries between their personal and professional lives in order to find a balance that is respected by patients and the CHN. For example, if the CHN is well known in the community, some community members may solicit, in a public place, the CHN's advice, or the CHN may inadvertently ask a patient about his or her progress in a public place.

Maintaining *confidentiality* is important. CHNs need to protect the identity of community members who provide sensitive or controversial data. In some cases, the CHN may consider withholding data; in other situations, the CHN may be legally required to disclose data. For example, CHNs are required by law to report child abuse.

Identifying Community Health Concerns

The data collected from the various sources and the creation of a composite database will result in a wealth of information on health concerns and the community strengths that can support health promotion for the health concern. To organize this information into a manageable list of community health needs, develop a profile of each health concern with the following elements: the identified health concern, clearly stated; the health risk to the community; the persons affected; and the community factors that led to the health concern(s). This process is an important first step for planning. In the planning phase, priorities are established and interventions are identified.

Consider the example of the community health concern of infant malnutrition. The community health assessment data on infant malnutrition would be organized as follows:

1. Infant malnutrition health concern: infants younger than 1 year
2. Risk to community: because of children in poor health, may need to provide new services
3. Persons affected: some families in the community
4. Community factors that led to the health concern:
   - Lack of regular developmental screening for infants in the community
   - No outreach program to identify at-risk infants
   - Families' lack of knowledge about the community nutrition program
   - Confusion among families in the community about criteria for enrollment in the nutrition health program
   - Community families' lack of infant-related nutritional knowledge
5. Community strengths:
   - Healthy Baby clubs that address healthy nutrition and screening for health concerns in infants

For more information on analyzing data to identify needs and assets in the community, see the *Community Health Assessment Guidelines, 2009* link on the Evolve website (under the Manitoba Health and Healthy Living Accountability Support Branch), specifically pp. 25–26.

PLANNING FOR COMMUNITY HEALTH

The planning phase, the second phase of the community health nursing process, includes:

- Analyzing the community health data to identify the community health concerns
- Establishing priorities among the identified community health concerns
- Establishing goals and objectives
- Identifying intervention activities that will accomplish the objectives

Analyzing Health Concerns

When analyzing health concerns, the CHN seeks to clarify the nature of the concern. Therefore, the CHN identifies the following:

- The origins and effects of the health concern
- The points at which intervention might be undertaken

TABLE 9.5 Health Concern Analysis: Infant Malnutrition

Community: Stanfield Township
Health concern: Infant malnutrition

Factors Contributing to the Health Concern and Outcomes	Relationship of Factors	Data Supportive to Relationships
1. Inadequate diet	Diets lacking in required nutrients contribute to malnutrition.	All township infants and their mothers seen by public health nurses in 2019 were referred to dietitians because of poor diets.
2. Community norms	Bottle-fed babies are less apt to receive adequate amounts of safe milk containing necessary nutrients.	Area general practitioners and CHNs agree that 90% of mothers in the township bottle-feed.
3. Poverty	Infant formulas are expensive.	Of new mothers in the township, 60% are receiving social assistance.
4. Disturbed mother–child relationship	Poor mother–child relationship may result in infant's failure to thrive.	Data from charts of 43 nursing mothers show infants diagnosed with failure to thrive.
5. Teenage pregnancy	Teenage mothers are most apt to have inadequate diets prenatally, to bottle-feed, to be poor, to lack parenting skills, and to have low literacy skills.	Of births in 2019, 90% were to women 19 years of age or younger.

- The parties that have an interest in the health concern and its solution
- The direct and indirect factors that contribute to the health concern
- The outcomes of the health concern
- Relationships among health concerns (whether one health concern contributes to or is affected by other health concerns)

This analysis is important because the CHN can anticipate that several of the same factors that contribute to a health concern and affect its outcomes also contribute to many other health concerns.

Analysis should be undertaken for each identified health concern. It often requires organizing a special group composed of the CHN and persons whose areas of expertise relate to the health concern, individuals whose organizations are capable of intervening, and representatives of the community experiencing the health concern—the patient. Together, they can identify the contributing factors and explain the relationships between each factor and the health concern.

This process is shown in Table 9.5, in an example of a health concern analysis for infant malnutrition. All the tables pertaining to the health concern for Stanfield Township are based on fictitious data. Factors that contribute to the health concern of infant malnutrition and its outcomes are listed in the first column. These factors are from all areas of community life. Social and environmental factors are as appropriate as those oriented to the individual. For example, teenage pregnancy is a social factor, and high unemployment is an environmental factor; both are related to infant malnutrition. In the second column of Table 9.5, the relationship between each factor and the health concern are noted. The third column contains data from the community and the literature that support the relationship, using the example of suspected infant malnutrition. From the best evidence available, infant malnutrition is thought to be related to inadequate diet,

community norms, poverty, disturbed mother–child relationships, and teenage pregnancy. This example demonstrates how some of the determinants of health can affect a patient situation.

Identifying Health Concern Priorities

Infant malnutrition represents only one of several community health concerns identified by the assessment of the fictitious Stanfield Township (Table 9.6). In reality, a CHN in partnership with the community will likely identify several community health concerns and rank those concerns together with the community. Health concerns may include a lack of clinics, poor housing conditions, a mortality rate from cardiovascular disease that is higher than the national norm, and—as expressed by many residents—a desire to be smoke-free.

The CHN and the community partners rank each health concern that is identified as part of the assessment process and determine its importance to resolving the concern. The criteria, rationale for ranking, and the priority of the health concern are identified in an effort to focus on the top priority for the community. In this fictitious case, the top-ranked criterion related to resolving the concern of infant malnutrition is the availability of nutritionists and dieticians, whereas the lowest-ranked criterion is the quickness of resolving the problem. The act of ranking criteria is known as *prioritizing*. By prioritizing, CHNs and the community can focus and agree on the most important criterion to address the health concern. For more information on selecting priorities from identified needs, see the *Community Health Assessment Guidelines, 2009* link on the Evolve website (under the Manitoba Health and Healthy Living Accountability Support Branch), specifically pp. 27–28.

Community Health Concern Priority Criteria

Answers to the following questions have been helpful in ranking identified health concerns:

1. How aware is the community of the health concern?

TABLE 9.6   Health Concern Priority: Infant Malnutrition in Stanfield Township

Criterion	Rationale for Ranking	Health Concern Priority
1. Community awareness of the health concern	Health service providers, teachers, and a variety of leaders have mentioned the health concern	2
2. Community motivation to resolve the health concern	Most believe that this health concern is not solvable because most of those affected are poor	4
3. CHN's ability to influence health concern resolution	CHNs are skilled at raising consciousness and mobilizing support	3
4. Ready availability of expertise relevant to health concern resolution	Public health unit/regional health authority nutrition program and nutritionists and dietitians are available	1
5. Severity of outcomes if health concern is left unresolved	The effects of marginal health services are not well documented	5
6. Quickness with which health concern resolution can be achieved	The time taken to mobilize a rural community with no history of social action is lengthy	6

TABLE 9.7   Community Health Concern Priority: All Identified Community Health Concerns in Stanfield Township

Criteria	Health Concern	Rationale for Rating	Health Concern Priority
1. Community awareness of the health concern	Community's desire to be smoke-free	Health service providers, teachers, and a variety of leaders have mentioned the health concern	2
2. Community motivation to resolve the health concern	Poor housing standards	Most believe that this health concern is not solvable because most of those affected are poor	4
3. CHN's ability to influence health concern resolution	Mortality rate from cardiovascular disease	CHNs are skilled at raising consciousness and mobilizing support	3
4. Ready availability of expertise relevant to health concern resolution	Infant malnutrition	Public health unit/regional health authority nutrition program and nutritionists and dietitians are available	1
5. Severity of outcomes if health concern is left unresolved	Lack of primary health care clinics	The effects of marginal health services are not well documented	5
6. Quickness with which health concern resolution can be achieved	Teen pregnancy	The time taken to mobilize a rural community with no history of social action is lengthy	6

2. Is the community motivated to resolve or better manage the health concern?
3. Is the CHN able to influence a solution for the health concern?
4. Are experts available to resolve the health concern?
5. How severe are the outcomes if the health concern is unresolved?
6. How quickly can the health concern be resolved?

Using the example of infant malnutrition again, the criteria are listed in the first column of Table 9.6. Note that this one health concern is only an example to show how to evaluate each health concern using the six criteria.

The members of the partnership answer questions related to their ability to influence or change the situation, and the CHN and the community agree on the ability to resolve the health concern. One example of the difference between the perceptions of the CHN and community members is smoking in public buildings; the CHN might identify smoking as a public health concern, but community members might view smoking as an issue of individual choice and personal freedom. For

example, recently, a mid-sized community, through the local municipal government and the health unit, passed a regulation to forbid smoking in all public places, including restaurants and bars. The outcry from the community residents has been loud. Many residents believe their individual rights and freedoms have been taken away by government regulations. It does not matter to them that lung cancer rates are high.

This process is repeated separately for each identified health concern, and all of the health concerns are compared. Priorities among the identified health concerns are established. The health concerns with the highest priority are the ones selected as the focus for intervention. Table 9.7 shows how all health concerns in Stanfield Township community example were prioritized after each one was separately evaluated.

Establishing Goals and Objectives

Once high-priority health concerns are identified, relevant goals and objectives are developed. **Goals** are generally broad statements of desired outcomes. **Objectives** are the precise statements indicating the means of achieving the desired

TABLE 9.8   Goals and Objectives: Infant Malnutrition in Stanfield Township

Community: Stanfield Township
Health concern: Infant malnutrition
Goal statement: To reduce the incidence and prevalence of infant malnutrition

Present Date	Objectives	Completion Date
Sept. 2021	1. Developmental levels will be assessed for 80% of the infants seen by the health unit, neighbourhood health centre, and private physicians	Sept. 2023
Sept. 2021	2. Nutrition program eligibility will be determined for 80% of infants seen by the health unit, neighbourhood health centre, and private physicians	Oct. 2023
Sept. 2021	3. An outreach program will be implemented to identify at-risk infants not now known to health care providers	Dec. 2023
Sept. 2021	4. Nutrition program eligibility will be determined for 25% of at-risk infants	Dec. 2023
Sept. 2021	5. Of all infants eligible for nutrition program food supplements, 75% will be enrolled in the program	Jan. 2023
Sept. 2021	6. Of the mothers of infants enrolled in the nutrition program, 50% will demonstrate three ways of incorporating nutrition program supplements into their infants' diets	Jan. 2023

outcomes. Table 9.8 provides an example of one of the goals and the specific objectives associated with it for the infant malnutrition health concern in Stanfield Township. The goal is to reduce the incidence and prevalence of infant malnutrition. Using a humanistic caring model, the broadly stated goal is used to measure the desired patient outcomes. However, when using behavioural models, the objectives are *precise, behaviourally stated,* and *measurable* and can be reached in a series of steps implemented over time rather than all at once. In this Stanfield Township example, the specific objectives pertain to (1) assessing infant developmental levels, (2) determining nutrition program eligibility, (3) implementing an outreach program, (4) enrolling infants in the nutrition program, and (5) providing supplemental foods in existing diets. Writing goals and objectives will be covered in more detail in Chapter 10.

As noted, establishing goals and objectives involves collaboration between the CHN and representatives of the community groups affected by both the health concern and the proposed intervention. This often requires a great deal of negotiation among everyone taking part in the planning process. One important advantage offered by the continuous active involvement of people affected by the outcomes is that they have a vested interest in those outcomes and are therefore supportive of and committed to the success of the intervention. Once goals and objectives are chosen, intervention activities to accomplish the objectives can be identified.

Identifying and Prioritizing Intervention Activities

Intervention activities are the means or strategies used to meet objectives, effect change, and break the health concern cycle. Because alternative intervention activities do exist, they must be identified and evaluated. An example of how intervention activities are identified then prioritized for infant developmental levels for Stanfield Township is illustrated in Table 9.9.

To achieve the objective related to the assessment of infant developmental levels for Stanfield Township (see Table 9.8, objective 1), five intervention activities are listed in the second column of Table 9.9. Each is relevant to the first objective. The first two activities involve nutrition program personnel as the principal change agents. The last three involve the CHN as

the principal change agent but also include the nutrition program personnel, the staff of the health unit, the neighbourhood health centre, and physicians as the change partners.

The expected effect of each of the activities is considered in the second column of Table 9.9. The resources that will be needed to implement the intervention are noted in the third column, and the priority of the intervention for the best outcome to meet the objective and resolve the health concern is noted in the fourth column. It is more valuable in the long term to educate others on how to assess infant development (activity 4) than to do it for them (activity 1). It is also necessary to analyze the change process needed to complete the objective (activity 5). Activity 5 must be done before any other interventions can be considered.

IMPLEMENTATION IN THE COMMUNITY

Implementation, the third phase of the community health nursing process, involves the work and activities aimed at achieving the goals and objectives. Implementation efforts may be made by the person or group that established the goals and objectives, or they may be shared with or even delegated to others.

Implementation is shaped by the CHN's chosen roles, the type of health concern selected as the focus for intervention, the community's readiness to take part in resolving the health concern, and the social change process. The CHN taking part in community intervention has knowledge and skills, but the question for the CHN is how to use that knowledge and those skills to benefit the implementation for community health.

The Community Health Nurse's Role

CHNs can act as content experts, helping communities select and attain task-related goals. In the Stanfield Township example of infant malnutrition, the CHN can use epidemiological skills to determine the incidence and prevalence of malnutrition. The CHN can serve as a process expert by increasing the community's ability to document the health concern rather than by providing help only as an expert in the area.

Content-focused roles often are considered change agent roles, whereas process roles are considered change partner

TABLE 9.9   Plan: Intervention Activities to Assess Infant Developmental Levels in Stanfield Township

Community: Stanfield Township
Objective 1: Developmental levels will be assessed for 80% of the infants seen by the health unit, neighbourhood health centre, and private physicians.

Date	Possible Interventions	Resources for the Intervention	Priority of Intervention for Best Outcome
Sept. 2021	1. The nutrition program supplies personnel to assess infant developmental levels	Personnel and time are insufficient; existing community resources (potential) are ignored	5
Sept. 2021	2. The nutrition program provides in-service education to staff on the assessment of infant development	Not enough personnel in the nutrition program to provide education. The need for education must be assessed	4
Sept. 2021	3. The CHN provides in-service education to staff in assessment of infant development	Not enough CHNs to provide education. More resources are needed	3
Sept. 2021	4. The CHN helps the nutrition program personnel identify in-service educational needs of area health care providers regarding the assessment of infant development	This activity is most likely to build on existing community strengths; a CHN skilled in needs assessment and interpersonal techniques is needed	2
Sept. 2021	5. The CHN helps the nutrition program personnel, the staff of the health unit, the neighbourhood health centre, and physicians to identify driving and restraining forces relative to implementation of the objective	This is the first step in the change process and is necessary for lasting change to occur	1

roles. **Change agent** roles stress gathering and analyzing facts and implementing programs, whereas **change partner** roles include those of enabler-catalyst, teacher of problem-solving skills, and activist-advocate.

The Community Health Concern and the Community Health Nurse's Role

The role the CHN chooses depends on the nature of the health concern, the community's decision-making ability, and professional and personal choices. Some health concerns clearly require certain intervention roles:

- If a community lacks democratic problem-solving abilities, the CHN may select educator, facilitator, and advocate roles. Problem-solving skills must be explained, and the CHN becomes a role model.
- A difficulty with determining the health status of the community, on the other hand, usually requires fact-gatherer and analyst roles.
- Some health concerns require multiple roles. Managing conflict among the involved health care providers demands process skills.
- Collecting and interpreting the data necessary to document a health concern requires both interpersonal and analytical skills.
- The community's history of taking part in decision making is a critical factor. In a community skilled in identifying and successfully managing its health concerns, the CHN may best serve as technical expert or advisor.

Different roles may be required if the community lacks problem-solving skills or has a history of unsuccessful change efforts. The CHN may need to focus on developing problem-solving capabilities or on making one successful change so that the community becomes empowered to take on the job of promoting change on its own behalf.

The Social Change Process and the Community Health Nurse's Role

The CHN's role also depends on the social change process. Not all communities are open to change. Ability to change is often related to the extent to which a community focuses on traditional norms. The more traditional the community, the less likely it is to change. Other barriers such as lack of human and fiscal resources and accessibility to health services in the community may also hinder change; the CHN needs to determine what these are so that appropriate interventions can be initiated.

The CHN, as a change agent, needs to be familiar with the principles of change and the types of community organizations that support change (Maurer & Smith, 2013). The Rothman model of community organization is most commonly used to initiate community change. Rothman identified three models of community organization: locality development, social planning, and social action (Maurer & Smith, 2013). In practice, Rothman's three models are often used in combination.

EVALUATING THE INTERVENTION FOR COMMUNITY HEALTH

Simply defined, **evaluation** is the appraisal of the effects of some organized activity or program. Evaluation, the final phase of the community health nursing process, may involve designing and conducting evaluation research or the more elementary process of assessing progress by contrasting the objectives and the results. For key considerations on the evaluation of a community health assessment, see the *Community Health Assessment Guidelines, 2009* link on the Evolve website (under the Manitoba Health and Healthy Living Accountability Support Branch), specifically pp. 32–33.

Evaluation begins in the planning phase, when goals and measurable objectives are established, and goal-attaining activities are identified. After implementing the intervention, the extent of the accomplishment of objectives, and the effects of intervention activities have to be assessed and documented in the progress notes. Community health nursing progress notes direct CHNs to perform such evaluations concurrently with implementation. In assessing the data recorded there, the CHN is requested to evaluate whether the objectives were met and the extent to which these were met or unmet and whether the intervention activities used were effective. Such a process is oriented toward evaluating the effectiveness of the intervention based on the goals and objectives developed by the CHN and the community.

The measurement of outcomes is a particularly important part of the evaluation process. Evaluation needs to be ongoing—that is, before and during the implementation process (formative evaluation) and after the outcome (summative evaluation). This is one reason for placing emphasis on measurable goals and objectives, since the focus will be on measuring the extent to which they have been met and about the effectiveness or ineffectiveness of community interventions. Questions raised with the community to determine whether a health concern has been resolved or the risk reduced are as follows: To what extent have the goals and measurable objectives been met? What changes, if any, are needed in the goals and objectives? Outcome measures also answer questions about the results of the intervention, such as the following: Which interventions have been effective, and why? Which interventions have been ineffective, and why? Has the health concern been resolved or the risk reduced? What lessons have been learned? What changes are needed? Process and outcome evaluation are discussed in greater detail in Chapter 10.

Often, data collected over time can provide important outcomes information about health trends within the community. Epidemiological data and trends do not provide the only measure of success, but they do provide important information about the intervention. CHNs need to consider the collection of this type of outcomes data for use as part of the evaluation phase. Outcomes can be measured by looking at changes from before and after the intervention to resolve the health concerns.

In the example of infant malnutrition in Stanfield Township, one would consider the number of cases of infant malnutrition in the community before providing education to other health providers about the assessment of infant development. A time period for evaluation would be chosen, perhaps 1 year after completion of the intervention. The number of cases of infant malnutrition would be measured to see if a change had occurred and there were fewer cases.

👤 STUDENT EXPERIENCE

1. Find community health assessment data on your community or another community.
2. See *A Picture of Our Health: Community Health Assessment, 2014*, which covers southern Manitoba, at https://www.southernhealth.ca/public/assets/AnnualReports/9f0c298e22/Community-Health-Assessment-2014.pdf
3. Compare the key data findings for your selected community with those of *A Picture of Our Health*. What were the similarities and differences?
4. Identify the sources of data and methods of data collection that were used for the community health assessment of your selected community. Were similar sources used in your community compared with what was used for southern Manitoba?
5. Using an online search, identify and record contact information for the major community health agencies as well as other community resources and assets in your selected community.

CHAPTER SUMMARY

9.1 A *community* refers to people and the relationships that emerge among them as they develop and commonly share agencies, institutions, and a physical environment; members may be defined in terms of geography or a common interest or focus.

9.2 The concept of *community as partner* means that the CHN emphasizes community strengths or assets to deal with community-identified health concerns and develop community capacity. The CHN works in partnership with the community in an approach that is supportive to and meaningful for community members. A *partnership* is a relationship between individuals, groups, organizations, or governments, in which the parties actively work together in all stages of assessment planning, implementation, and evaluation. In the community context, *partnership* is often used synonymously with *coalition* and *alliance*.

9.3 The most effective way for CHNs to achieve healthy changes is through partnership with the community. CHNs work with the community to achieve community health, engage in Healthy Communities development, and build effective partnerships that address health issues together.

9.4 The steps in the community development process are defining the issue; initiating the process; planning community conversations; talking, discovering, and connecting; creating an asset map; mobilizing the community; taking action; and planning and implementing.

9.5 Assessing community health requires gathering existing data, generating missing data, and interpreting the composite database to identify strengths and health concerns. Seven methods of collecting data are as follows: informant interviews, focus groups, participant observation, windshield surveys, community forums, secondary analysis of existing data, and surveys.

9.6 Planning for community health includes analyzing the community health data to identify community health concerns, establishing priorities among the identified community health concerns, establishing goals and objectives, and identifying intervention activities that will accomplish the objectives.

9.7 Implementation, the third phase of the community health nursing process, involves transforming a plan for improved community health into the achievement of goals and objectives. Implementation is shaped by the CHN's chosen roles, the type of health concern selected as the focus for intervention, the community's readiness to take part in resolving the health concern, and the characteristics of the social change process.

9.8 Evaluation begins in the planning phase and must involve developing measurable goals and objectives. It is the appraisal of the effects of a program and the extent to which the community health concerns have been resolved. Measurement of outcomes is a particularly important part of the evaluation process. Evaluation needs to occur before and during the implementation process (formative evaluation) and after the outcome (summative).

 CHN IN PRACTICE: A CASE STUDY

Caring for Older Persons in the Community

Alan is a CHN and a member of a committee assigned to assess the health care needs of the aging baby boomers in Woodsbury, a small northern community. The community is located in a scenic area near a large freshwater lake. The winter temperatures can vary from −15° to −40°C. The average annual snowfall has been declining but is usually around 80 cm. The summers are dry and warm. The major industries in the community are mining and forestry. The unemployment rate has been low, but due to declining demand for some resources, the unemployment rate has been steadily increasing.

Alan and the committee are aware that as the baby-boomer population ages, health care providers need to prepare for a rapid increase in the number of people older than 65 years. The committee's purpose is to make suggestions to the district health unit or regional health authority and municipal officials about how to prepare for the increase in health services that will be needed for the older adults in the area.

The ethnic composition of this community is 80% White (consisting of French Canadians and those of British, Finnish, German, and Dutch descent) and 20% Indigenous. Currently, 25%

of the population in Woodsbury is older than 65 years. However, in 25 years, this percentage is expected to increase to more than 50%. Many of these older adults have practised a lifestyle that included a high-fat diet, smoking, and frequent alcohol use. Consequently, many have heart disease or chronic obstructive pulmonary disease. Currently, five primary health care providers are in the community. Waiting times to see these health providers range from 1 to 3 weeks. Only one of these providers specializes in geriatric care. One 54-bed long-term care facility is in the most northern location of the district, located 50 km from Woodsbury. Because of the rural location, there is no public transit system. The long-term-care residents are dependent on family or friends for transportation to appointments in Woodsbury.

Think About It
1. Define the community.
2. Outline the data-collection methods that Alan might decide to use to assess the community.
3. Present the available data on this community.
4. Identify potential community partners that Alan and the committee might consider working with.

 CHN IN PRACTICE: A CASE STUDY

Community Asset Mapping

Community asset mapping is based on the assumption that all individuals, physical structures, natural resources, institutions, businesses, or informal organizations play a role in strengthening community capacity. Traditional assets are those assets that clearly support community health (e.g., health services). Nontraditional assets are those assets that may be overlooked but are important to support health (e.g., the location of ATM machines) (Briggs & Huang, 2017).

Think About It
1. Break into small groups and locate a map of your school's campus.
2. Using the "Campus Community Asset Inventory" document the special features of the physical assets of your campus and how they relate to and support student health (e.g., Student Wellness Centre; located in the nursing building; two private offices; two RNs and one physician provide health promotion, screening, and diagnostic tests; excellent support for student health).
3. Identify both traditional and nontraditional assets that support student health.

4. If possible, working in small groups of 4–6, walk around your campus for 20–30 minutes and identify the assets that support student health.

Campus Community Asset Inventory

Physical Asset (Traditional or Nontraditional)	Specific Features	How They Relate to Student Health

5. After returning to the classroom, discuss the following questions:
   a. Why is community asset mapping important for CHNs?
   b. How do nontraditional assets influence student health?
   c. How could CHNs use community mapping to help plan, implement, and evaluate interventions for student health on your campus?

🛜 TOOL BOX

The Tool Box contains useful resources that can be applied in community health nursing practice. These related resources are found either in the appendices at the back of this text or on the Evolve website at http://evolve.elsevier.com/Canada/Stanhope/community/.

Appendices

- Appendix 1: Canadian Community Health Nursing Standards of Practice
- Appendix 6: Community-as-Partner Model

Tools

The Community Development Facilitator's Guide. (http://publications.gc.ca/site/eng/9.647495/publication.html)

This resource is used to facilitate use of *The Community Development Handbook* so that CHNs are able to facilitate workshops in the community.

The Community Development Handbook. (http://publications.gc.ca/site/eng/245322/publication.html)

This introductory guide to community development provides information to deepen the CHN's interest in and understanding of community development.

Public Health Agency of Canada. The Community Capacity Building Tool. (http://www.phac-aspc.gc.ca/canada/regions/ab-nwt-tno/downloads-eng.php)

This planning tool document assists communities to build community capacity in health promotion projects.

REFERENCES

BC Healthy Communities. (2009). *Funding.* http://bchealthycommunities.ca.

Bingham, B., Leo, D., Zhang, R., et al. (2014). Generational sex work and HIV risk among indigenous women in a street-based urban Canadian setting. *Culture, Health and Sexuality, 16*(4), 440–452. https://doi.org/10.1080/13691058.2014.888480.

Briggs, L., & Huang, Y. (2017). Asset-based community maps: A tool for expanding resources in community health programs. *Pedagogy in Health Promotion, 3*(3), 195–201. https://doi.org/10.1177/2373379916664736.

British Colombia Healthy Communities (2021). What is a healthy community? https://planh.ca/big-picture/what-healthy-community.

Campaign 2000. (2014). *2014 report card on child and family poverty in Canada.* Retrieved from a website no longer accessible. http://www.campaign2000.ca/anniversaryreport/CanadaRC2014EN.pdf.

Canadian Community Economic Development (CED) Network. (2016). *Asset mapping: A handbook.* https://ccednet-rdec.ca/en/toolbox/asset-mapping-handbook.

Canadian Institute for Health Information (CIHI). (2006). *How healthy are rural Canadians? An assessment of their health status and health determinants.* https://secure.cihi.ca/free_products/rural_canadians_2006_report_e.pdf.

Canadian Nurses Association (CNA). (2005). *CNA backgrounder: Healthy communities and nursing: A summary of the issues.* https://www.cna-aiic.ca/~/media/cna/page-content/pdf-en/bg5_healthy_communities_e.pdf?la=en.

Canadian Nurses Association (CNA). (2012). *Position statement: International health partnerships.* https://www.cna-aiic.ca/~/media/cna/page-content/pdf-en/ps82_intl_health_partnerships_e.pdf.

Capital Regional District (2016). Setting our table. https://www.crd.bc.ca/docs/default-source/crd-document-library/plans-reports/planning-development/draft-regional-food-agriculture-strategy-web.pdf?sfvrsn=77e42cca_6.

Cassells, H. (2019). 6: Community assessment. In M. A. Nies, & M. McEwen (Eds.), *Community/public health nursing: Promoting the health of populations* (7th ed.) (pp. 92–106). Saunders.

Cidro, J., Zahayko, L., Lawrence, H., et al. (2014). Traditional and cultural approaches to childrearing: Preventing early childhood caries in Norway House Cree Nation, Manitoba. *Rural and Remote Health, 14*(4), 1–11.

Collier, C. (2010). Long form census change worries researchers. *Canadian Medical Association Journal: Canadian Medical Association Journal, 182*(12), E563–E564.

Community Health Nurses of Canada (CHNC). (2019). *Canadian community health nursing: Professional practice model and standards of practice.* https://www.chnc.ca/standards-of-practice.

DesMeules, M., Luo, W., Wang, F., et al. (2007). Rural places: Variations in health. *Health Policy Research Bulletin, 14*, 19–22. http://www.hc-sc.gc.ca/sr-sr/alt_formats/hpb-dgps/pdf/pubs/hpr-rps/bull/2007-people-place-gens-lieux/2007-people-place-gens-lieux-eng.pdf.

Diem, E. (2005). Collaborative assessment. In E. Diem, & A. Moyer (Eds.), *Community health nursing projects: Making a difference* (pp. 83–121). Lippincott, Williams & Wilkins.

Dunn, J. R. (2002). *Are widening inequalities making Canada less healthy? The health determinants partnership.* http://en.healthnexus.ca/sites/en.healthnexus.ca/files/resources/widening_income_equalities.pdf.

Employment and Social Development Canada. (2021). About the new horizons for seniors program. https://www.canada.ca/en/employment-social-development/programs/new-horizons-seniors.html.

Employment and Social Development Canada. (2016b). *Homelessness strategy.* http://www.edsc.gc.ca/eng/communities/homelessness/indexs.html.

Escoffery, C., Miner, K. R., & Trowbridge, J. (2004). Conducting small-scale community assessments. *American Journal of Health Education, 35*(4), 237–241.

Fournier, B., & Karachiwalla, F. (2020). *Shah's public health and preventive health care in Canada* (6th ed.). Elsevier Inc.

Government of Canada. (2009). *Canadian rural partnership asset mapping: A handbook.* https://ccednet-rdec.ca/en/toolbox/asset-mapping-handbook.

Hajizadeh, M., Campbell, M. K., & Sarma, S. (2014). Socioeconomic inequalities in adult obesity risk in Canada: Trends and decomposition analyses. *The European Journal of Health Economics, 15*(2), 203–221. https://doi.org/10.1007/s10198-013-0469-0.

Health Canada. (2004). *The Canadian heart health initiative: A policy in action.*

Health Canada. (2011). *Healthy Canadians. A federal report on comparable health indicators 2010.* http://publications.gc.ca/collections/collection_2011/sc-hc/H21-206-2010-eng.pdf.

Horton, J., & MacLeod, M. (2008). The experience of capacity building among health education workers in the Yukon. *Canadian Journal of Public Health, 99*(1), 69–72.

International Biopharma Solutions. (2012). *Canadian asset map for stem cell and regenerative medicine.* https://www.ic.gc.ca/eic/site/lsg-pdsv.nsf/vwapj/camscrmr_crcdcsmr_eng.pdf/$file/camscrmr_crcdcsmr_eng.pdf.

Jessup-Falcioni, H., & Viverais-Dresler, G. (2005). *Community health nursing (NURS 2296 EL). Online course. Envision.* Laurentian University.

Kretzmann, J. P., & McKnight, J. L. (1993). *Building communities from the inside out: A path toward finding and mobilizing assets.* Institute for Policy Research. https://ccednet-rcdec.ca/en/toolbox/building-communities-inside-out-path-toward-finding-and.

Kushner, K. E. (2006). Community-based nursing practice. In J. C. Ross-Kerr, & M. J. Wood (Eds.), *Canadian fundamentals of nursing* (3rd ed.) (pp. 51–65). Elsevier Canada.

Maurer, F. A., & Smith, C. M. (2013). *Community/public health nursing practice: Health for families and populations* (5th ed.). Elsevier.

McKnight, J. L., & Kretzmann, J. P. (2005). Mapping community capacity. In M. Minkler (Ed.), *Community organizing and community building for health* (2nd ed.) (pp. 158–172). Rutgers University Press.

Mikkonen, J., & Raphael, D. (2010). *Social determinants of health: The Canadian facts.* York University School of Health Policy and Management. http://www.thecanadianfacts.org.

Minkler, M., & Wallerstein, N. (2005). Improving health through community organization and community building. In M. Minkler (Ed.), *Community organizing and community building for health* (2nd ed.) (pp. 26–50). Rutgers University Press.

Moyer, A. (2005). Building coalitions. In A. Diem, & A. Moyer (Eds.), *Community health nursing projects: Making a difference* (pp. 297–323). Lippincott, Williams & Wilkins.

Nies, M., & McEwen, M. (2019). *Community/public health nursing: Promoting the health of populations* (7th ed.). Elsevier.

Pong, R. W. (2007). *Rural poverty and health: What do we know?* http://documents.cranhr.ca/pdf/Presentation_Senate_Committee_on_rural_poverty_-_May_2007.pdf.

Public Health Agency of Canada. (2008). *The community capacity building tool.* http://www.phac-aspc.gc.ca/canada/regions/ab-nwt-tno/downloads-eng.php.

Raphael, D. (Ed.). (2016). *Social determinants of health: Canadian perspectives* (3rd ed.) Canadian Scholars' Press.

Ravaghi, V., Quiñonez, C., & Allison, P. J. (2013). The magnitude of oral health inequalities in Canada: Findings of the Canadian Health Measures Survey. *Community Dentistry and Oral Epidemiology, 41*(6), 490–498. https://doi.org/10.1111/cdoe.12043

Statistics Canada. (2010). *National longitudinal survey of children and youth (NLSCY).* http://www23.statcan.gc.ca/imdb/p2SV.pl?Function=getSurvey&SDDS=4450.

Statistics Canada. (2012). *Health facts sheets 82-625-X.* http://www.statcan.gc.ca/pub/82-625-x/2013001/article/11889-eng.htm.

Statistics Canada. (2015). *Canadian health measures survey.* http://www.statcan.gc.ca/eng/survey/household/5071.

Statistics Canada. (2016). *Canadian community health survey: Annual component.* http://www23.statcan.gc.ca/imdb/p2SV.pl?Function=getSurvey&Id=164081.

Vancouver Coastal Health. (2009). *Healthy communities.* http://www.vch.ca/about-us/accountability/healthy-communities/.

Vollman, A. R., Anderson, E. T., & McFarlane, J. (2017). *Canadian community as partner: Theory and multidisciplinary practice in nursing* (4th ed.). Lippincott, Williams & Wilkins.

Winnipeg Regional Health Authority. (2017). *Community development framework.* https://wrha.mb.ca/community-development/.

Zotti, M. E., Brown, P., & Stotts, R. C. (1996). Community based nursing versus community health nursing: What does it all mean? *Nursing Outlook, 44*(5), 211–217.

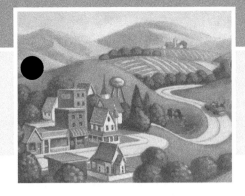

10

Health Program Planning and Evaluation

OUTLINE

The Health Program Management Process, 227
Health Program Planning for Community Health
  Nursing, 228
Health Program Planning Models, 229
  Program Logic Model, 229
  PRECEDE-PROCEED Model, 230
The Health Program Planning Process, 232
  Assessing and Defining the Patient Health Concern, 233

Identifying Health Program Goals and Objectives, 234
Planning for Implementation, 236
Weighing Health Concern Solution Options, 237
Choosing the Best Solution, 237
The Health Program Evaluation Process, 237
  Health Program Evaluation Sources, 238
  Health Program Evaluation Criteria, 239

OBJECTIVES

After reading this chapter, you should be able to:

10.1 Compare the health program management process
  with the community health nursing process.
10.2 Explain the application of the health program planning
  process to nursing in the community.

10.3 Identify the limitations and advantages of the program
  logic model and the PRECEDE-PROCEED model in
  health program planning.
10.4 Describe the steps in the health program planning process.
10.5 Describe the health program evaluation process as well
  as evaluation sources and criteria.

KEY TERMS*

assessment, 233
goals, 234
health program, 228
health program evaluation process, 228
health program implementation process, 228
health program management process, 227
health program planning process, 228

objectives, 234
operational health planning, 228
outcome evaluation, 233
outcomes, 234
process evaluation, 233
strategic health planning, 228

*See the Glossary on page 468 for definitions.

Health program management is an area in which community health nurses (CHNs) are often integral members of an interprofessional team focused on improving the health of communities. Therefore, it is critical that CHNs become familiar with health program management, from health program assessment to evaluation. This chapter focuses primarily on health program planning and evaluation. Although presented in separate discussions, these factors are related and interdependent processes that work together to bring about a successful program. Other chapters in this text provide examples of implementation.

THE HEALTH PROGRAM MANAGEMENT PROCESS

The **health program management process** addresses health issues of populations and consists of four steps: assessing,

planning, implementing, and evaluating a health program, in partnership with the patient. As interprofessional team members, CHNs are often most heavily involved in health program planning, implementation, and evaluation. It is important to note, however, that single interventions or programs may not adequately address complex health issues, and an integrated approach may be needed to effectively target multiple risk and protective factors in populations (Domitrovich, Bradshaw, Greenberg, et al., 2010).

The health program management process is similar to the community health nursing process in that both involve community assessment, planning, implementation, and evaluation. Like the community health nursing process, the health program management process consists of a rational decision-making system designed to help CHNs determine:
- When to make a decision to develop a health program
- Where they want to be at the end of the health program

- What to do to have a successful health program
- How to develop a plan to go from where they are to where they want to be
- How to know that they are getting where they want to go
- How to implement the health program plan
- What to measure to know whether what they are doing is appropriate
- Whether to modify or terminate existing health programs (based on evaluation findings).

Health programs may be implemented with a variety of patients, including individuals, families, groups or aggregates, communities, and populations. Health programs in the community need to be planned based on the findings of a community health assessment. The community health assessment process was discussed in Chapter 9 and will be discussed briefly later in this chapter under "The Health Program Planning Process."

A **health program** consists of a variety of planned activities to address the assessed health concerns of patients and builds on patient strengths to meet specific goals and objectives. The following are examples of health programs in the community that CHNs are involved with:

- Immunization programs for school-aged children
- Hearing screening programs for locomotive engineers
- Family-planning programs for teenagers
- Smoking-cessation programs for women
- Heart health programs for post–myocardial infarction patients.

The following are more broadly based aggregate and population health programs:

- Community school health programs
- Home health care programs
- Disaster management programs
- Occupational health and safety programs
- Environmental health programs
- Community health programs directed at specific health concerns through special interest groups (e.g., Canadian Heart and Stroke Association, Canadian Cancer Society, Canadian Diabetic Association)
- Community wellness programs
- Stress-management programs.

The first step in the health program management process is a community health assessment, which involves identifying the need for specific health programs. The second step is the **health program planning process,** which is an organized approach to identifying and choosing interventions to meet specified goals and objectives that address patient health concerns. The overarching goal of planning is to ensure that health care services are acceptable, equitable, efficient, and effective. As outlined in *Canadian Community Health Nursing Professional Practice Model and Standards of Practice* (Community Health Nurses of Canada [CHNC], 2019), CHNs are expected to plan health programs using a variety of sources, including high-quality data and community wisdom (Appendix 1). The third step, the **health program implementation process,** is the systematic process of putting the health program's planned activities into action.

The last step, the **health program evaluation process,** is the systematic process of appraising all aspects of a program to determine their impact; this process is undertaken in partnership with the individual, family, group, community, population, or system in partnership with individuals, employers, and policymakers (Appendix 1). The evaluation process of a health program needs to start early and, therefore, should be designed during the health program planning process.

HEALTH PROGRAM PLANNING FOR COMMUNITY HEALTH NURSING

Health program planning involves systematic decision making on broad goals and specific objectives on the basis of various types of information. Health program planning facilitates how resources (time, money, and people) are used so that they will have the utmost impact, particularly in times of fiscal restraint and limited resources when efficiency is critical. In planning a health promotion program, the CHN needs to ensure that there are opportunities for the continuing participation of key stakeholders in program decision making and that the process has flexibility to accommodate contextual changes as the program evolves. The intent of health promotion programs is to have a positive impact on the knowledge, attitudes, and behaviours of patients.

Health program planning can:

- Benefit patients, CHNs, and the community
- Focus attention on what the CHN and other community partners are attempting to do with the patient to address the health concern
- Assist in identifying the community resources and activities that are required to meet the health program objectives
- Reduce role ambiguity (uncertainty) by giving responsibility to the patient, the CHN, and other partners to meet health program objectives
- Reduce uncertainty within the health care program environment
- Increase the abilities of the CHN and others involved in the health program to cope with the external environment
- Help the CHN and health program participants (patients) anticipate activities
- Allow for quality decision making and better control over the actual health program results.

Strategic health planning involves matching patient health needs, patient and provider strengths and competencies, and resources. Strategic health planning would focus on a question such as, How can we attract health care providers and retain them in rural practice settings? **Operational health planning** is used on a smaller scale and starts with a specific objective in relation to health program planning. For example, the operational health planning objective could be "to increase the number of family physicians and CHNs by 20% in the rural primary health care practice setting." Everyone involved with health program planning can anticipate the following areas for discussion:

- What will be required to implement the health program?
- What will occur during implementation?
- What will be the health program outcomes?

Health program planning should involve an assessment of the situation (issue), which should include any literature pertaining to the issue and evaluations of similar proposed program interventions. It should also consider socioenvironmental and other determinants of health. The Public Health Ontario website includes an "Online Health Program Planner" that has interactive worksheets to help make evidence-informed decisions when planning health programs. This planner also includes a six-step process that can be used for planning a health promotion program (see the Tool Box on the Evolve website). One example of a program in Ontario that has implemented this six-step planning process is the NutriSTEP program for preschoolers and toddlers.

HEALTH PROGRAM PLANNING MODELS

Population-based program health planning began with the need for mass immunizations, such as the program to administer the first polio vaccine (Barreto, Van Exan, & Rutty, 2006). Planning models include steps for planning a program that, if used, will likely increase its success. As well, they provide structure and organization to the planning process. There are many different planning models to choose from. Some models are more applicable to health planning than others.

A few models that have been used by CHNs and multidisciplinary teams for health program planning are the Planned Approach to Community Health Model, or PATCH (McKenzie, Neiger, & Thackeray, 2016); the 4-Step Planning Process (Finnegan & Ervin, 1989); Mobilizing for Action Through Planning and Partnership, or MAPP (McKenzie et al., 2016); and Targeting Outcomes of Programs (Bennet & Rockwell, 2005). These models are described briefly in Table 10.1. One element common to each of these models is the health program management approach of mobilizing the community for the assessing, planning, implementing, and evaluating health promotion programs.

When choosing a model, CHNs need to evaluate which is most useful to their health program and community health planning. Questions to determine a model's usefulness include, Are the steps or elements sequential? Does the model adapt to stakeholder needs? Will the model support improving health conditions?

Although a number of health program planning models exist, the two most commonly used in community health are the program logic model and the PRECEDE-PROCEED model.

Program Logic Model

The program logic model (PLM) is used in health care as a health program planning, implementation and evaluation model that describes the effectiveness of programs. It depicts the components of a health program from start to finish as a diagram. This model is useful because it clarifies the logical linkages between program inputs (resources and activities), outputs (products, program deliverables, and audiences or targets), and program outcomes related to a specific health concern. It involves stakeholders such as CHNs who are familiar with the health program and program patients (Vollman, Anderson, & McFarlane, 2017). A PLM depicts a cause-and-effect sequence or path toward a stated outcome by identifying the links between the health concern, inputs, and outputs.

The first element of the PLM (the "situation element") is a statement on the health concern and its causes; who is affected by the health concern and where; and who is interested in the health concern, such as the stakeholders and other projects that might focus on the stated health concern. The second element (the "input element") is the resources essential to support the program are identified. Resources can include a combination of human (including partners who might be involved in program planning, delivery, and evaluation), financial, organizational, and community resources. The third element (the "output element") is the outputs of the program—what specific activities will be undertaken during the program. Program outputs should provide quantitative or qualitative information on the people who were affected: such as their numbers, their characteristics, and how they participated in the program. The fourth element of the PLM (the "outcomes element") is the program's short-term, intermediate, and long-term outcomes. Outcomes need to communicate the impacts of the program; they usually include changes in knowledge, skills, and behaviour.

A sample schematic diagram using the elements of the PLM is displayed in Fig. 10.1. This figure was developed based on Statistics Canada data that showed the number of falls by older persons residing in the community of Pine Ridge (a pseudonym) was higher than the provincial average. Pine Ridge is a small rural retirement community with a population consisting mainly of older persons. The CHN conducted a community health assessment and determined that there were no educational health programs on the prevention of falls for persons 65 years of age or older who were residing in their own homes. Based on these findings, the CHN conducted focus groups with older persons residing in Pine Ridge and determined that they also identified concerns about the occurrence of falls and the lack of information on prevention of falls. In collaboration with other community health team members, including older person representatives, it was decided that a health program for this population should be delivered by the CHN and the community occupational health therapist. A PLM was the chosen planning model for the educational intervention health program. Fig. 10.1 identifies the basic elements of this educational intervention health program using the PLM. For other examples and more detailed information on logic models, see the University of Wisconsin Program Development and Evaluation link on the Evolve website and the Innovation Network's *Logic Model Workbook* listed in the Tool Box on the Evolve website.

TABLE 10.1   Health Program Planning Models

Model and Description	Phases or Steps
The PATCH (Planned Approach to Community Health) model: It increases the capacity of members of the community and empowers them to participate, and thus provides the community with a sense of program ownership. The PATCH model is applicable in addressing specific health issues of populations	The five phases are: 1. *Mobilizing the community.* The identified community is organized with community representatives and working and steering groups providing program information 2. *Collecting and organizing data.* Working and steering groups analyze quantitative and qualitative data to identify community health concerns 3. *Choosing health priorities.* Further data are collected, such as the determinants of health, to assist in stating and selecting health priorities 4. *Developing a comprehensive intervention plan.* A plan is developed based on the available resources that includes strategies, timelines, and a task list for various activities such as publicizing, recruitment, and program evaluation 5. *Evaluation.* This should be ongoing to assess the progress of the program at each stage as well as the program activities, with feedback of the results directed to the community*[†]
4-Step Planning Process: It is an organized response to opportunities and challenges for the patient as individual, organization, and community	The four steps are: 1. *Defining.* Outcome goals are developed based on community desires 2. *Analyzing.* Critical evaluation of multiple data sources to identify need/challenge 3. *Choosing.* Selection of activities to most likely yield desired outcomes 4. *Mapping.* Each implementation step is mapped out with identification of resources and evaluation[‡]
Mobilizing for Action through Planning and Partnerships (MAPP): It is a community-driven strategic planning tool for improving community health and quality of life	The six phases are: 1. *Organizing for success.* Organizing the planning process and developing the planning partnership 2. *Visioning.* Guiding the community through a collaborative, creative process that leads to a shared community vision and common values 3. *Assessments.* Identifying important information for improving community health 4. *Strategic issues.* Participants develop an ordered list of the most important issues facing the community 5. *Goals/strategies.* Formulated as statements related to identified issues with broad strategies for addressing issues and achieving goals identified 6. *Action cycle.* Links planning, implementation, and evaluation[†]
Targeting Outcomes of Planning (TOP): It focuses on outcomes in planning, implementing, and evaluating programs. TOP assesses needs, targets outcomes, assesses program opportunities, designs programs to achieve stated outcomes, tracks program outcomes, and evaluates outcome achieved	There are seven levels working downward for the proposal. The downward levels starting with level 7 are resources, activities, participants, reactions, KASA (knowledge, attitudes, skills, aspirations), practices, and SEE (social, economic, and environmental conditions and outcomes).[§] The seven levels working upward for the results start with level 1, which is SEE. TOP assists with answering the following four questions: 1. Why have a program? 2. How should the program be conducted? 3. Is the program design implemented? 4. What benefits does the program deliver?

Sources: *Issel, L. M. (2008). *Health program planning and evaluation: A practical systematic approach for community health* (2nd ed.). Jones & Bartlett.
[†]McKenzie, Neiger, & Thackeray, 2016.
[‡]Finnegan & Ervin, 1989.
[§]Bennett & Rockwell, 2005.

PRECEDE-PROCEED Model

The Green and Kreuter (1999) PRECEDE-PROCEED model is widely used for planning due to its comprehensiveness; however, for some it can be a complex planning model. It is founded on the disciplines of epidemiology; the social, behavioural, and educational sciences; and health administration. Many researchers have used this model, including Ezeonwu and Berkowitz (2014), who described the model as a guiding framework when they developed and implemented a collaborative community-wide health fair and assessed its impact on underserved populations. Ranjbaran, Dehdari, & Sadeghniiat-Haghighi (2015) used the model to design interventions for patients experiencing poor sleep quality after coronary artery bypass graft surgery and measured predisposing, reinforcing, and enabling factors before and after the intervention. They concluded that an intervention based on the PRECEDE-PROCEED model could further improve the sleep quality of this population.

Fig. 10.2 illustrates the nine phases of the PRECEDE-PROCEED model. PRECEDE stands for Predisposing,

Inputs Resources	Activities	Outputs	Outcomes—Impact		
			Short-term	Intermediate	Long-term
• Have CHN and OT as program lead (in-kind service). • Gain financial support from provincial ministry ($10 000). • Make fall prevention a priority of the provincial/territorial health program mandate. • Have as guest speakers community health professionals with expertise in older person health. • Ensure access to health professionals such as geriatrician, family physician; CHNs (e.g., nurse practitioners, public health nurses, home health nurses) with assessment skills. • Utilize home workers such as Red Cross homemakers. • Utilize community resources such as the older person centre; clergy; older person. • Print out resources such as handouts ($2 000). • Engage in social marketing (community flyers, radio and paper ads) ($2 000 allocated). • Allocate space for educational sessions. • Provide transportation services ($1 000 for volunteers' gas allowance). • Provide refreshments for educational session breaks ($300). • Pay part-time student salary ($4 000).	• Recruit older person as target audience participants. • Recruit older person as peer educators. • Hire students (part-time) to assist with fall educational program. • Develop age-appropriate fall prevention promotion material for handouts. • Launch marketing program: dissemination of flyers, bulletin board postings, public service announcements, print media. • Inform older person about fall prevention through dissemination of print materials by health care professionals and clergy. • Educate older person about fall prevention through 6 education classes/sessions, including group discussions. • Offer 6 classes/sessions on fall prevention led by CHN and OT at donated space located at older adult centre. • Prepare for some older person who may request one 6-week session to be held in the evening.	• 200 community flyers distributed • 10 daily radio public service announcements ×1 week • 1 newspaper announcement • # of older person enrolled (50) • # of older person who completed the program (40) • 6 educational classes held per session with one session held in the evenings • 5 sessions held • 5 program participants became peer educators in the community	• By the end of the third class, 80% of Pine Ridge older person in the fall prevention education program can identify at least two environmental hazards in their home. • By the last class, 90% of Pine Ridge older person in the fall prevention education program will verbalize appreciation of the safety issues pertaining to their homes.	• By the end of the fall prevention educational program, 90% of Pine Ridge older person who completed the fall prevention educational program will report having made environmental changes to reduce the risk of the number of falls. • By the end of the fall prevention educational program, 95% of the Pine Ridge older person who completed the fall prevention program will report more confidence in their mobility in their homes.	• The number of reported falls by Pine Ridge older person who participated in the fall prevention educational program will be decreased by 80% after 1 year of completion of the fall prevention educational program.

CHN, community health nurse; OT, occupational therapist.

Fig. 10.1 Program Logic Model for Fall Prevention for Older Persons of Pine Ridge.

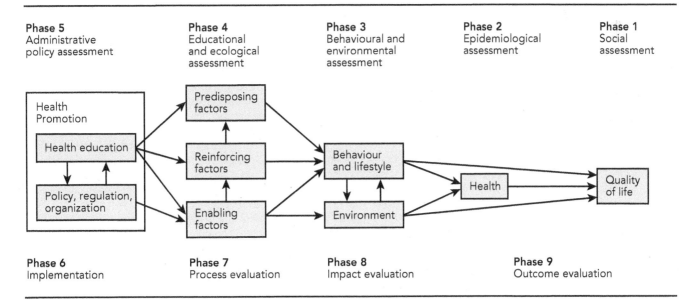

PRECEDE

Phase 5
Administrative
policy assessment

Phase 4
Educational
and ecological
assessment

Phase 3
Behavioural and
environmental
assessment

Phase 2
Epidemiological
assessment

Phase 1
Social
assessment

Phase 6
Implementation

Phase 7
Process evaluation

Phase 8
Impact evaluation

Phase 9
Outcome evaluation

PROCEED

Fig. 10.2 The PRECEDE-PROCEED Model. (From Green et al., *Health Program Planning, Implementation, and Evaluation.* Baltimore: Johns Hopkins University Press, 2022. Reproduced with permission.)

Reinforcing, and Enabling Constructs in Ecosystem Diagnosis and Evaluation (factors that occur before program implementation). PRECEDE is the process of systematic planning and evaluation of health education programs (Green & Kreuter, 2005). PROCEED is the acronym for Policy, Regulatory and Organizational Constructs in Educational and Environmental Development (factors that support program implementation). PROCEED involves implementing and evaluating the program. Originally, there were eight phases in the PRECEDE-PROCEED model. Currently, there are nine phases, with the PRECEDE phases being phases 1 to 5 and the PROCEED phases being phases 6 to 9. The PRECEDE phases set the direction and objectives for the ensuing phases of PROCEED to address the need for health promotion interventions and additionally the traditional educational approaches used to change unhealthy behaviours. These interventions include, for example, political and economic interventions that affect the social environment and its support for healthy lifestyles. Alternatively stated, this model's continuum of phases centre on planning, implementation, and evaluation of a health promotion program plan.

Throughout the PRECEDE-PROCEED model, two basic assumptions are emphasized: (1) health and health risks are caused by multiple factors (determinants of health), and (2) efforts to effect behavioural, environmental, and social change must be multidimensional or multisectoral, and participatory in that the target audience is actively involved in the change process (Green & Kreuter, 2005). Using the model starts with a vision of the desired goal or outcome and then works back to identify what is influencing the achievement of that goal (causes) and what precedes the desired outcome. Using the data from the Pine Ridge Older Persons Fall-Prevention Program, the nine phases of the PRECEDE-PROCEED model are identified and explained in Table 10.2.

THE HEALTH PROGRAM PLANNING PROCESS

Planning health programs and planning for the evaluation of health programs are two important activities, whether the health program being planned is a national health program such as seat belt use, a provincial health care program such as immunizations, a local health program such as heart health initiatives for elementary schoolchildren, or a health education program on diet and exercise for a group of obese patients. Regardless of the type of health program, the planning process is the same.

TABLE 10.2 The PRECEDE-PROCEED Model and Its Application to the Pine Ridge Older Persons Fall-Prevention Program

Phase	Description	Pine Ridge Fall-Prevention Program Data
Phase 1: Social assessment	Identification of the social challenges affecting target populations using a variety of methods, such as focus groups, surveys, and community forums. The aim is to engage the target population in the identification of their specific needs and aspirations to facilitate their achievement of the best quality of life	• A community health assessment determined that there were no educational programs on the prevention of falls for persons 65 years of age or older who were residing in their own home • Focus groups were conducted with older adults residing in Pine Ridge, and they identified concerns about the occurrence of falls and the lack of information on prevention of falls • In collaboration with other community health team members, including older adult representatives, it was decided that a program for this population should be delivered by the CHN and the community occupational health therapist
Phase 2: Epidemiological assessment	Determination of health concerns, ranking, and development of objectives using data such as vital statistics, morbidity, and mortality	• Statistics Canada data showed an above-average number of falls by older persons (residing in the pseudo-community of Pine Ridge) when compared to the provincial average
Phase 3: Behavioural and environmental assessment	Assessment of personal and environmental factors contributing to health challenge(s) for the target population	• Behavioural and lifestyle risk factors included wearing inappropriate footwear, not using mobility aids appropriately, and a fear of falling • Environmental risk factors included inadequate lighting and obstacles such as scatter rugs, too much clutter, and pets
Phase 4: Educational and ecological assessment	Examination of the causes of health behaviour according to three kinds of factors: predisposing (knowledge, attitudes, values, beliefs, perceptions); enabling (barriers that help or hinder behavioural and environmental changes); and reinforcing (rewards and feedback that support changes)	• Predisposing: value safety in the home by preventing falls in order to prevent injury such as fractures • Enabling: availability of health care providers, community willingness to provide an educational program • Reinforcing: professional, peer support to modify the environment

TABLE 10.2   **The PRECEDE-PROCEED Model and Its Application to the Pine Ridge Older Persons Fall-Prevention Program—cont'd**

Phase	Description	Pine Ridge Fall-Prevention Program Data
Phase 5: Administrative policy assessment	Assessment of administrative and policy concerns that need to be addressed prior to program implementation include assessment of capabilities and resources that can be used to develop and implement the program, budget allocation, implementation schedule, compatibility of program with organizational objectives, etc.	• $10 000 in government funding is needed • A variety of health care providers are needed to collaborate to deliver the program • Community resources must be organized to support the program • An older persons centre would need to donate space for educational program delivery
Phase 6: Implementation	Implementation of the planned activities	• Fall-prevention program flyers were developed and 200 were disseminated • Fifty participants enrolled • A fall-prevention program was conducted with 10 older persons per educational session. Each session was made up of 6 weekly classes. Five fall-prevention educational sessions were held • Five program participants became peer educators in the community • Some older persons requested a 6-week session of evening classes
Phase 7: **Process evaluation**	Evaluation of implementation process	• Ten older persons dropped out (five due to changes in their health and living arrangements; five due to inability to attend the scheduled evening classes they had originally requested) • The location used provided comfort and accessibility • Guest speakers were well received
Phase 8: Impact evaluation	Evaluation of changes in predisposing, enabling, and reinforcing factors, and program effectiveness	**Short-Term Impact Outcomes** • By the end of the third class, 80% of the Pine Ridge older persons in the fall-prevention program will identify two or more environmental hazards in their home • By the last class, 90% of the Pine Ridge older persons in the fall-prevention program will verbalize an understanding of the safety issues pertaining to their homes **Intermediate Impact Outcomes** • At the end of the fall-prevention program, 90% of Pine Ridge older persons will report having made environmental changes to reduce the risk of the number of falls • At the end of the fall-prevention program, 95% of Pine Ridge older persons who completed the fall-prevention program will report more confidence in their mobility in their homes
Phase 9: **Outcome evaluation**	Measurement of overall changes in achieving program objectives	**Long-Term Outcome Evaluation** • The number of reported falls by Pine Ridge older persons who participated in the fall-prevention program will decrease by 80% after 1 year of completion of program

Assessing and Defining the Patient Health Concern

The initial and most critical step in health program planning is assessing and defining the patient health concern. The target population or patient to be served by any health program, often referred to as *key stakeholders,* must be identified and involved in designing the health program to be developed. The interprofessional planning team needs to verify that a current health concern exists and is being ignored or unsuccessfully treated in a patient group. **Assessment** is defined as a systematic appraisal of the type, depth, and scope of health concerns and strengths as perceived by patients, health care providers, or both (Box 10.1).

- *Preactive:* projecting future health concerns
- *Reactive:* defining the health concern based on past health concerns identified by the patient or the agency
- *Inactive:* defining the health concern based on the existing health status of the population to be served
- *Interactive:* describing the health concern using past and present data to project future population needs

The term *patient,* as used throughout this text, refers to the individual, family, group or aggregate, community, population, or society. The patient should also be defined by biological and psychosocial characteristics, by geographical location, and by the concerns to be addressed. For example, in a community with a large number of preschool children who require immunizations to enter school, the patient population may be described as all children between 4 and 6 years of age residing in the local district who have not had up-to-date immunizations. This example identifies for the CHN who the patient is, what the health concern is, how large the population is, and where the patient is located.

A health education program may be necessary to alert the population to the existing health concern. In the example of the immunization of preschool children, public service announcements on television and radio and in newspapers may be used to alert parents to laws requiring immunizations, to the health concerns of communicable diseases, and to which communicable diseases (e.g., smallpox) have been successfully eradicated by immunization programs. Health concerns to be met for the patient population must be identified collaboratively by the patient, the CHN, or the interprofessional team. If the patient does not recognize the health concern or is not involved in the planning, the program usually fails.

Determining the *size and location of a patient population* for a health program involves more than counting the number of persons in the community who may be eligible for the health program. More specifically, it involves defining the number of persons with the health concern who are underserved by existing health programs and the number of eligible persons who have and have not taken advantage of existing services. For example, consider again the community need for a preschool immunization program. In planning the health program, the estimates of numbers of preschool children in the district may be obtained from census data or birth certificates. The CHN then needs to determine the number of children underserved and the number of children who have not used services for which they are eligible.

Boundaries for the patient population are established by defining the size and location of the patient population. The boundaries stipulate who is included in or excluded from the health program. If the fictional immunization program were designed to serve only preschool children of low-income families, all other preschool children would be excluded.

What people think about the need for a health program, or *program feasibility,* might differ among health care providers, agency administrators, policymakers, and potential patients. Collecting data on the opinions and attitudes of all persons directly and indirectly involved with the health program's success is necessary to determine the program's feasibility and the need to redefine the health concern, and to decide to develop a new health program or expand an existing one. Before implementing a health program, CHNs need to *identify available resources.* Health program resources include personnel, facilities, equipment, and financing. If any one of the four categories of health program resources is unavailable, the health program is likely to be inadequate to meet the health concerns of the patient population.

A number of assessment data sources exist to assist the CHN in the assessment process, as discussed in Chapter 9. Some of the major data sources used for assessment, summarized in Table 10.3, are key informants, statistical indicators, community forums, a survey of existing community agencies with similar health programs, and a survey of residents of the community to be served (patient population) (Rossi, Lipsey, & Henry, 2018).

The demand for a health program is determined by working with the patient. This stage of planning creates options for solving the health concern and considers several solutions. Each option for a health program solution is examined for its uncertainties (risks) and consequences, leading to a set of **outcomes** (the results or impact of health program interventions).

Some alternative solutions to the health concern will present more risks or uncertainties than others, prompting the following considerations:

- The CHN needs to decide between the solution that involves more risk and the solution that is free of risk.
- A "do nothing" decision is always one with the least risk to the provider.
- When choosing a solution, the CHN looks at whether the desired outcome can be achieved.
- After careful consideration, the CHN rethinks the solutions.
- Information collected with the data source is used to develop these alternative solutions.
- Decision trees are useful graphic aids that give a picture of the solutions and the consequences and risks of each solution.

Identifying Health Program Goals and Objectives

Goals are defined as broad statements that identify the main purpose(s) for the health program. For example, the goal of an exercise program for middle-aged adults is to help participants be healthy and participate in regular exercise. **Objectives** are defined as specific measurable statements that identify the steps planned to reach the overall health program goal. For example, in an exercise program for middle-aged adults, a learning objective is that each program participant will increase his or her daily walking by 15 minutes during the first week of the exercise program. Therefore, several

TABLE 10.3 Summary of Community Health Assessment Data Sources

Name	Definition	Advantages	Disadvantages
Community forum	Community, group, organization, open meeting	• Low cost • Learn perspectives of large number of persons	• Limited data • Limited expression of views • Discourages less powerful • Becomes arena to discuss political issues
Focus groups	Open discussion with small representative groups	• Low cost • Patients participate in identification of health concern • Initiates community support for the program	• Time consuming • Allows focus on irrelevant or political issues
Key informants	Identify, select, and question knowledgeable leaders	• Provides picture of services required	• Bias of leaders • Community characteristics may be incorrectly perceived by informants
Statistical indicators approach (e.g., census data)	Existing data used to determine health concern	• Excellent data on health concerns and characteristics of patient groups	• Growth and change in population may make data outdated
Survey of existing community agencies	Estimates of patient populations via services used at similar community agencies	• Easy method to estimate size of patient group • Know extent of services offered in existing programs	• All cases of health concern may not be reported • Exaggeration of services may occur
Survey of residents of the community to be served	Measurement of total or sample patient population by interview or questionnaire	• Direct and accurate data on patient population and their health concerns	• Expensive • Technically demanding • Need many interviews or observations • Interviews may be biased

objectives (short term, intermediate, and long term) are stated to meet each program goal. Action-oriented verbs are used to specify the change expected. Some examples of action verbs are *identify, define, compare, contrast, apply, decrease, increase, demonstrate,* and *state.*

If the objectives are too general, health program evaluation becomes impossible. The objectives must be specific and stated so that anyone reading them could conduct the health program without further instruction. To be truly effective, the health program plan should begin with a general health program goal and move on to specific objectives. For example, a health program goal might be to reduce communicable diseases in the District of Wakefield (a fictitious location). Table 10.4 provides one example of an objective to meet this goal. The stated objective is this: The Wakefield District immunization program will decrease the incidence rates of vaccine-preventable illnesses by 10 to 25% by providing immunization clinics in all schools in the district by December 2022. Other objectives would also need to be developed to meet this goal. The objective that follows is developed using the SMART acronym (Specific, Measurable, Attainable, Realistic, Timely) to assist in meeting the criteria necessary to write a "good" objective. Websites available to help CHNs develop skill in writing objectives using the SMART tool are listed in the links on the Evolve website: *A Guide to Writing Learning Objectives* and "Bloom's Taxonomy Action Verbs."

The purpose of a goal is to focus on the major reason for the health program. A general health program goal may be to reduce the incidence of low-birth-weight babies in Wakefield

District in 2022 by improving access to prenatal care. Each specific health program objective includes the following:
- A measurable behaviour
- The circumstances under which the behaviour is observed
- The minimal acceptable standard for the performance of the behaviour.

A specific objective for this Wakefield District health program may be to open a prenatal clinic in each health unit or regional health authority within the district by January 2022 to serve the population within each census tract of the district. This specific objective is an action-oriented approach to meeting the goal.

Specific health program activities are then planned to meet each specific objective, and resources, such as the number of CHNs, equipment, supplies, and location, are planned for each of the objectives. It is assumed that as each specific objective is met, the general program goal will also be partly achieved. Remember that several specific objectives are required to meet a general health program goal.

It is important for the CHN and other members of the health program planning team to track activities planned and the team member who will work on the various activities. A Gantt chart is a useful tool for visually tracking the activities pertaining to the achievement of the health program objectives and, therefore, toward meeting the identified health program goal. The chart indicates the health program activities with the time frame for accomplishment. A Gantt chart is useful to depict the order of tasks, health program progress, and possible dependencies between tasks. A Gantt chart considers the concepts of

TABLE 10.4 Using the SMART Acronym to Develop an Objective to Meet the Program Goal "To Reduce Communicable Diseases in the District of Wakefield"

Objectives Using SMART	Criteria	Example Program Objective Using Wakefield District Data
S = specific	The objective must be specific and stated using an action-oriented verb to determine the behaviour expected.	The Wakefield District Immunization program...
M = measurable	Change must be measurable to know when the objective has been met.	will decrease the incidence rates of vaccine-preventable illnesses by 10 to 25%...
A = achievable/attainable	The objective can be accomplished by the patient or organization.	by providing immunization clinics...
R = realistic	For the situation, the objective can be achieved given the resources.	in all schools in the district...
T = time frame	The target time or date for accomplishing the objective must be stated.	by December 2022

Fall Prevention Program for Pine Ridge Older Persons

Objective 1:

To increase awareness of the fall prevention program by at least 75% of the older Persons of Pine Ridge within 3 months

	January	February	March	April
Develop print resources to be distributed to the local papers	CHN and OT			
Contact local clergy by telephone	CHN			
Develop posters to be displayed at older Person centres and other organizations		CHN		
Prepare newsletter to distribute to the community home care agencies			CHN and volunteers	CHN and volunteers

CHN, Community health nurse; OT, occupational therapist.

Fig. 10.3 Gantt Chart for the First Objective of the Fall-Prevention Program for Older Persons of Pine Ridge.

events and time, with events listed on the left side of the chart and time indicated horizontally at the top of the chart showing the planned start and completion dates for health program activities. Time is represented on the chart lines (duration of activity) by horizontal colour bars to show the start and completion of an activity. Because changes in the health program necessitate redrawing the chart, the CHN needs to consider using a computer-generated chart program such as Microsoft Project or Excel. Fig. 10.3 is a Gantt chart for the first objective of the fall-prevention program for older persons of Pine Ridge.

Planning for Implementation

In this planning phase, the CHN, working with the patient, considers the possibilities of solving a health concern using one of the solutions identified. The CHN considers the costs, resources, and program activities required for each of the solutions. To illustrate, consider again the immunization scenario. If the proposed solution is to encourage parents to obtain the immunizations for their children (the best consequence), examples of activities include developing a script for a health education program and implementing a television program to encourage parents to take children to their health care provider. If one of the other alternatives, such as providing community health nursing clinics at daycare centres (the worst possible consequence) or providing community health nursing clinics at the health unit or health authority for all ages of children were chosen, offering a clinic 8 hours per day at the health unit or health authority and providing a mobile clinic to each daycare centre for 4 hours per day to provide the immunizations would be possible activities.

For each alternative, the CHN lists the resources required to implement the activity. In the example, personnel could include CHNs, volunteers, and clerks; supplies might include handouts, adhesive bandages, medications, records, and consent forms; equipment might include syringes, needles, stethoscopes, and blood pressure cuffs; and facilities might include a television studio for a media blitz on the education program, a room with chairs, and emergency carts. The costs of personnel, supplies, equipment, and facilities for each solution should be listed and considered. As indicated, patients need to review each solution for acceptance.

Weighing Health Concern Solution Options

Each alternative is weighed to judge the costs, benefits, and acceptability of the idea to the patient, community, and CHN. The solution that would provide the desired outcomes needs to be considered. Looking at available information through literature reviews or interviews might show whether someone else has tried any of the options in another place or with another population. The results from other sources would be helpful in deciding whether a chosen solution would be useful.

Choosing the Best Solution

Patients, CHNs, and the interprofessional health planning team in consultation with the sponsoring agency select the best solution. Working with patients throughout the health planning process helps to promote acceptance of the plan; solutions that are derived from key stakeholders meeting to explore, decide, and commit to possible options that address particular health program needs are more likely to be successful. One type of meeting that could be used is a *charette*. A charette is a workshop-like public meeting that brings people of similar interests together to explore creative ways of designing a program or addressing an issue. Traditionally, charettes have been used in the arts to capture a visual portrayal of ideas. Charettes are becoming more popular in other fields, such as business, urban planning to promote health, and government (see the link to the Health Canada website in the Tool Box on the Evolve website for more information on charettes.) Providing a rationale for recommending particular solutions helps the CHN to get support (i.e., agency and community support) for the plan to be implemented.

THE HEALTH PROGRAM EVALUATION PROCESS

Health program evaluation is a systematic process that examines the intended and unintended impacts of a health program. An evaluation produces data to inform decision making about ways to support health programs and best use resources.

The five steps identified by the Public Health Agency of Canada (PHAC, 2008) for evaluating public health programs are:
1. Focus on determining exactly what needs to be known about the health program.
2. Choose suitable strategies to answer the evaluation questions.
3. Design or revise data-collection tools.
4. Collect and analyze the data.
5. Make decisions about the health program based on responses to the evaluation questions.

See the link to Public Health Ontario's 10 steps for conducting an evaluation on the Evolve website.

The major benefit of a health program evaluation is that it shows whether a program is meeting its purpose. It should answer the following questions:
- Are the health needs for which the program was designed being met?
- Are the health concerns it was designed to resolve being resolved?

Health program justification and continued funding for programs are a result of demonstration through evaluation that the program is meeting its goals. Evaluation is important for health program continuance and improvement. CHNs at all levels of education and preparation can participate in the planning and evaluation of a health program.

The "Ethical Considerations" box presents an example of a program evaluation and considers how ethical principles apply to it.

ETHICAL CONSIDERATIONS

A CHN working as a member of an interprofessional team is involved in the evaluation of the human papillomavirus (HPV) immunization program, which is offered free of charge to Grade 8 girls by the Ontario Ministry of Health. The program takes place at school-based clinics administered by registered nurses from Ontario's Public Health Units. Childhood immunizations require the explicit consent of parents and, despite the known benefits of vaccines, some parents have refused to provide consent for their children's immunization due to concerns over adverse effects. The team is evaluating the program and is using the Canadian Nursing Coalition for Immunization Program Evaluation Toolkit (see the link on the Evolve website).

Ethical principles that apply to this program are as follows:
- *Autonomy:* When a community health intervention interferes with the individual rights of persons receiving care, CHNs use and advocate for the use of the least restrictive measures possible for those in their care. CHNs recognize and support a capable person's right to refuse or withdraw consent for care or treatment at any time. CHNs also recognize and support a parent's right to refuse consent for care for their child.
- *Distributive justice:* CHNs ensure that health care is provided with the person's informed consent.

Questions to Consider
1. During planning for the HPV immunization program, what steps should health care providers have taken to ensure that participants gave their consent freely and provided informed consent?
2. What are the elements to consider in the refusal of parental consent for the vaccine?

Quality assurance audits are prime examples of formative health program evaluation in health care delivery. Evaluation data are used to justify continuing programs in community health. Health program records—including patient evaluations and community indexes—serve as the major source of information for health program evaluation. Surveys, interviews, observations, and diagnostic tests are ways to assess consumer and patient responses to health programs. When the planning process begins, health program evaluation starts with assessment—that is, process evaluation. The types of evaluation are process or formative and outcome or summative, and these are described in Table 10.5.

Health Program Evaluation Sources

Major sources of information for health program evaluation are health program patients, program records, and community indicators. The program participants, or patients, of the service have a unique and valuable role in program evaluation. Whether the patients for whom the program was designed accept the services determines to a large extent whether the program achieves its purpose. Thus, their reactions, feelings, and judgements about the program are important to the evaluation.

To assess the response of participants in a health program, the CHN as evaluator may use a written survey in the form of a questionnaire, an attitude scale, interviews, and observations. *Attitude scales* are probably used most often, and they are usually phrased in terms that will ascertain whether the health program has met its objectives. The patient satisfaction survey is an example of an attitude scale often used in the health care delivery system to evaluate the health program objectives. The "Evidence-Informed Practice" box discusses

TABLE 10.5   Types of Health Program Evaluation

Type of Evaluation	Definition and Purpose	Examples of Questions Connected to This Type of Evaluation	Practice Example
Process/Formative	Process evaluation entails making a judgement about program delivery while the program is in development. It begins with an assessment of the need for the program. It focuses on what the program does and for whom. The purpose is to improve the program	Was the target group reached? Was the target group satisfied with the program? What is working in the program? Why? What is not working in the program and why not? Were the resources used suitable? Which program objectives have not been met and why? What in the program needs to be changed if it is to be implemented elsewhere?	In a weight-loss program for older persons, 20 persons signed up for the program, which was more than the targeted number of 15. Verbal feedback from the group members indicated that 95% were very satisfied with the program and the other 5% were satisfied. Responses showed satisfaction with the time of day, location, program content such as menu preparation, physical activity, and group support. Areas requiring change were the need for more individualized exercises based on individual participant ability, especially for participants over 75 years of age. One consideration for future program delivery would be to conduct a preassessment of the older persons' physical activity level and abilities
Outcome/ Summative	Outcome evaluation examines the results of a program—that is, the effects of the program. It also provides information to use in order to decide whether to continue, adjust, or terminate the program. Its purpose is to examine the changes that occurred as a result of the program and to determine whether the program is having the intended effect	To what extent have the short-term objectives been met? To what extent have the intermediate objectives been met? To what extent have the long-term objectives been met? What changes have occurred due to program delivery?	Short-term objectives were fully met—e.g., all participants were able to gradually increase their weekly activity and to follow the recommended total caloric intake and all participants lost at least 3 pounds within the first 3 weeks of the program. The immediate objectives were that all participants indicated that they followed the recommended food preparation and meal plans; however, those over 75 years of age were not able to increase their physical activity. Within 2 months, the participants had each lost a minimum of 10 pounds. The long-term objectives were partially met as 80% of the participants continued with the healthy eating and exercise program, except for those over 75 years of age who continued to be challenged with the physical activity component

Source: Adapted from Clark, M. J. (2008). *Community health nursing: Advocacy for population health* (5th ed.). Pearson Prentice Hall.

a program evaluation by Campbell, Patterson, Adams, et al. (2008) that is based on a survey of patients and nurses.

The second major source of information for health program evaluation is *program records,* especially clinical records. Clinical records provide the CHN evaluator with information about the care given to the patient and the results of that care. To determine whether a health program goal has been met, one might summarize the data from a group of records. For example, if one overall goal is to reduce the incidence of low-birth-weight babies through prenatal care, records would be reviewed to obtain the number of mothers who received prenatal care and the number of low-birth-weight babies born to them.

The third major source of health program evaluation is a *community health index.* Health and illness indicators, such as mortality and morbidity data, are probably cited more frequently than any other single index for health program evaluation. Incidence and prevalence are valuable indexes used to measure program effectiveness and impact (see Chapter 8 for further discussion on rates and ratios).

Health Program Evaluation Criteria

The following criteria are used in health program evaluation: relevance, adequacy, progress, efficiency, effectiveness, impact, and sustainability (Veney & Kaluzny, 2005). These criteria are related to the type of evaluation that is conducted in regard to health program evaluations. To conduct a health program evaluation, the first step is to choose the type of evaluation required. The second step is to identify the goal and objectives for evaluation. The third step is to decide who will be involved in the evaluation. The final step is to answer the questions found in Table 10.6. Depending on the answers to those questions, the health program will be found to be successful or not.

In summary, health program planning is evolving as new program planning models are introduced. Furthermore, CHNs need to monitor the quality and necessity of health programs in order to justify existing and proposed program delivery within the current fiscal environment.

EVIDENCE-INFORMED PRACTICE

Campbell et al. (2008) undertook a participatory evaluation project with researcher evaluators and sexual assault nurse examiners (SANEs) to develop an evaluation survey of SANE nursing practice and patient psychological well-being. The project was developed to determine whether the nursing care provided by SANEs was consistent with a logic model of "empowering care." In this project, *empowering care* was defined as providing health care, support, and resources; treating patients with dignity and respect; believing patients' stories; helping patients regain control and choice; and respecting patients' decisions. An evaluation survey was developed and tested with 52 sexual assault victims in one SANE program. According to the findings, SANE nursing actions included all aspects of the definition of *empowering care.* As well, the majority of sexual assault victims described having positive psychological well-being outcomes. The established partnership in this project led to further collaborative endeavours. The program evaluation process contributed to SANEs' capacity building and the sustainability of the SANE program.

Application for CHNs
The logic model and other program planning models are tools that the CHN needs to be familiar with. Models are necessary for CHNs so that an organized approach is used in program planning and program evaluation. Program evaluation offers opportunities for CHNs to communicate and work with patients to further improve community health.

Questions for Reflection and Discussion
1. What aspects of the logic model of "empowering care" do you feel would be appropriate in your own nursing care?
2. As the CHN working on this collaborative team, what process evaluation questions could you ask?
3. Related to evidence-informed practice, locate the most recent evidence on SANEs and their use of the logic model of care.

Source: Campbell, R., Patterson, D., Adams, A. E., et al. (2008). A participatory evaluation project to measure SANE nursing practice and adult sexual assault patients' psychological well-being. *Journal of Forensic Nursing, 4*(1), 19–28.

TABLE 10.6 Health Program Evaluation Considerations

Criterion	Explanation	Type of Evaluation	Questions to Consider	CHN Implications
Relevance	It is an important component of the initial planning phase. It considers whether the program is suitable to meet the needs of the target group	Process evaluation	1. Did the community health needs assessment determine that the program is necessary?	As money, health care providers, facilities, and supplies for delivering health care services are monitored more and more closely, the assessment conducted by the CHN will be used to determine whether the program is required

Continued

TABLE 10.6   Health Program Evaluation Considerations—cont'd

Criterion	Explanation	Type of Evaluation	Questions to Consider	CHN Implications
Adequacy	It looks at the extent to which the program addresses the entire health concern defined in the assessment. The magnitude of the health concern is determined by vital statistics, incidence, prevalence, and expert opinion	Process evaluation	1. Does the program have the capacity to positively influence the health concern? 2. Are there clearly identified parameters of the services required to address the target group health concerns?	The CHN will need access to a variety of data sources
Progress	It involves monitoring program activities—such as hours of service, number of health care providers used, number of referrals made, and amount of money spent to meet program objectives. It provides an evaluation of the progress of the program. Progress *evaluation* occurs primarily while implementing the program	Process evaluation	1. How frequently would activities be monitored? 2. What aspects of the activities would be monitored (e.g., hours of service, patients served, types of health care providers available)? 3. What is the fit between the program plan and implementation regarding budgeting?	The CHN who completes a daily or weekly log of clinical activities (e.g., the number of patients seen in a clinic or visited at home, number of phone contacts, number of referrals made, number of community health promotion activities such as mass media campaigns) is contributing to the progress evaluation of the community health nursing intervention
Efficiency	It is the relationship between the program outcomes and the resources spent	Process evaluation (ongoing) and outcome (end result of the program)	1. Are the costs of this program similar to other programs with the same goal? 2. If the program costs are greater or less than what is planned, is the program needed? 3. Is the program needed if the productivity level is high or low compared with similar programs? 4. What are benefits of the program to the target group and to the community? 5. What are benefits of the program to the target group and to the community?	The CHN as evaluator may be able to determine whether the program provides better benefits at a lower cost than a similar program or whether the benefits to the patients or number of patients served justify the costs of the program
Effectiveness	It is an evaluation of program effectiveness that may help the CHN determine both patient and provider satisfaction with the program activities as well as whether the program met its stated objectives	Outcome evaluation	1. How satisfied are the health care providers, target group, and community with the program outcomes? 2. Are the health concerns of the target group being addressed?	The CHN determines both patient and provider satisfaction with the program activities, as well as whether the program met its stated objectives
Impact	If an evaluation of impact is the goal, long-term effects such as changes in morbidity and mortality must be investigated	Outcome evaluation	1. To what extent has (have) the overall goal(s) been met? 2. What changed as a result of the program for the target population?	The CHN determines both the short- and long-term impact of the program on the target population
Sustainability	The program can be continued if the resources and the program effects can be sustained over time	Outcome evaluation	1. Did the program receive external funding? 2. What new resources are available to support the program once the initial funding is exhausted?	When program evaluation is completed, dissemination of the results is required to be communicated to any funding bodies, appropriate community agencies, stakeholders, and the public. The CHN may be involved with this process

Source: Based on Veney, A., & Kaluzny, J. (2005). *Evaluation and decision making for health services* (4th ed.). Health Administration Press.

LEVELS OF PREVENTION

Related to Health Program Planning and Evaluation

Primary Prevention

A CHN plans a community-wide cancer prevention program with the local government and health department to make women aware of the health risks associated with cervical cancer.

Secondary Prevention

An occupational health nurse (OHN) develops a screening program for women aged 35 to 65 to determine the incidence and prevalence of cervical cancer before implementing a health promotion program to educate women about the importance of regular screening.

Tertiary Prevention

An OHN evaluates the incidence and prevalence of cervical cancer among the target population of women aged 35 to 65 after the implementation of a cervical cancer screening program and provides health promotion programs to educate women about the importance of regular screening.

STUDENT EXPERIENCE

Explore the *Logic Model Workbook* and the "How to Make a Gantt Chart Using Microsoft Excel" website (the links are on the Evolve website).

Program development using the program logic model (PLM) usually involves a team approach. Your team consists of a CHN (who will take the role of coordinator), a health promotion consultant, a public health nutritionist, and two community key informants (a parent, and a teacher). Analysis by the team of the community health assessment data has identified that childhood obesity is a health concern in community X. The team is in the initial stages of planning a health program to address this health concern.

The CHN, in consultation with the team, will coordinate preparation of a two-page draft health program plan using the PLM and a one-page Gantt chart. The program goal is to reduce the incidence of childhood obesity in community X. Together, the team will prepare at least three SMART objectives for this goal that will be discussed and prioritized by the team. Share your PLM and the Gantt chart for your community with your classmates.

CHAPTER SUMMARY

10.1 The health program management process addresses health issues of populations and consists of four steps: assessing, planning, implementing, and evaluating a health program, in partnership with the patient. The community health nursing process also consists of assessing, planning, implementing, and evaluating nursing care in partnership with the patient.

10.2 Health program planning involves systematic decision making on broad goals and specific objectives on the basis of various types of information. *Strategic health planning* involves matching patient health needs, patient and provider strengths and competencies, and resources. *Operational health planning* is used on a smaller scale and starts with a specific objective in relation to health program planning.

10.3 The two most commonly used models for health program planning are the program logic model (PLM) and the PRECEDE-PROCEED model. PLM clarifies the logical linkages of program inputs (resources and activities), outputs (products, program deliverables, and audiences or targets), and program outcomes related to a specific health concern. The PRECEDE-PROCEED model is founded on the disciplines of epidemiology; the social, behavioural, and educational sciences; and health administration. Two assumptions are emphasized: health and health risks are caused by multiple factors (determinants of health), and efforts to effect behavioural, environmental, and social change must be multidimensional or multisectoral, and participatory.

10.4 The steps in the health program planning process are (1) assessing and defining the patient health concern; (2) identifying health program goals (broad statements that identify main purpose) and objectives (specific measurable statements); (3) planning for implementation (consider costs, resources, and program activities for each possible solution); (4) weighing health concern solution options; and (5) choosing the best solution to the health concern in consultation with patients, the interprofessional planning team, and the organization.

10.5 The health program evaluation process is a systematic process that examines the intended and unintended impacts of a health program. Evaluation of a program entails (1) focusing on what needs to be known about the health program, (2) choosing suitable strategies to answer the evaluation questions, (3) designing or revising data-collection tools, (4) collecting and analyzing data, and (5) making decisions about the health program based on responses to the evaluation questions. Sources of data for program evaluation include: the patients, program records, and community health indices. The main criteria for a program evaluation are whether the program met the health needs for which the program was designed and resolved the health concern identified.

CHN IN PRACTICE: A CASE STUDY

Health Promotion Program for Mill Employees

Jean is the occupational health nurse at the lumber mill in Pine Ridge. She noticed that many of the workers exhibit poor health habits, such as smoking and eating high-fat foods. Through talking with workers who visited the occupational health office, Jean learned that many of them wanted to take better care of themselves but believed they could not because of the long hours they worked and the high stress of their jobs. She decided to investigate whether poor health habits were a problem for everyone working in the mill or if they were common only to those who visited the occupational health office.

Jean sent surveys to all 800 employees at the mill and received responses from 40%. From the surveys, Jean learned that 30% of employees worked 10 to 12 hours each work day, 40% smoked one-half to two packs of cigarettes a day, and the most recent meal consumed by 85% of the workers did not include any fruits or vegetables.

Jean went to the president of the mill, shared this information with him, and discussed how poor health could decrease productivity. The president supported her suggestion to implement a health promotion program for the mill employees and offered to provide the required space and office materials for the program. Jean is now planning to develop a health education program that will focus on helping the employees to adopt healthy lifestyle behaviours. One of the health program objectives is to have the employees engage in healthy eating behaviours.

Think About It

1. Using the four elements of the program logic model, write up a health program plan for the healthy eating program objective for the mill employees.
2. Develop a Gantt chart to monitor the accomplishment of the activities.

TOOL BOX

The Tool Box contains useful resources that can be applied in community health nursing practice. These related resources are found either in the appendices at the back of this text or on the Evolve website at http://evolve.elsevier.com/Canada/Stanhope/community/.

Appendix

- Appendix 1: Canadian Community Health Nursing Standards of Practice

Tools

The Health Canada Policy Toolkit for Public Involvement in Decision Making (http://www.hc-sc.gc.ca/ahc-asc/pubs/_public-consult/2000decision/index-eng.php)

This site provides information on a charette, how it works, and its logistics.

Public Health Ontario. Online Health Program Planner (http://www.publichealthontario.ca/en/ServicesAndTools/ohpp/Pages/default.aspx)

Links are provided on this site to tools such as webinars, workbooks, and worksheets on a variety of topics pertaining to health program planning, such as situational assessment, program logic models, and objective writing.

How to Make a Gantt Chart Using Microsoft Excel (https://www.ablebits.com/office-addins-blog/2014/05/23/make-gantt-chart-excel/)

This site provides the "how to" for preparing a Gantt chart using Microsoft Excel.

The Health Planner's Toolkit. The Planning Process (https://cdn2.hubspot.net/hubfs/316071/Resources/Article/A_CE_Health_Care_Guide.pdf)

This resource includes everything required to carry out a program planning process as well as a health impact assessment.

At a Glance: The Ten Steps for Conducting an Evaluation (http://www.publichealthontario.ca/en/eRepository/At_A_Glance_Evaluation_2015.pdf)

This document outlines 10 steps for conducting a program evaluation.

Innovation Network. Logic Model Workbook (http://www.innonet.org/client_docs/File/logic_model_workbook.pdf)

This site provides the step-by-step process for creating and using the program logic model.

REFERENCES

Barreto, L., Van Exan, R., & Rutty, C. (2006). Polio vaccine development in Canada: Contributions to global polio eradication. *Biologicals, 34,* 91–101.

Bennett, C., & Rockwell, K. (2005). *Targeting outcomes of programs (TOP).* http://citnews.unl.edu.

Campbell, R., Patterson, D., Adams, A. E., et al. (2008). A participatory evaluation project to measure SANE nursing practice and adult sexual assault patients' psychological well-being. *Journal of Forensic Nursing, 4*(1), 19–28.

Clark, M. J. (2008). *Community health nursing: Advocacy for population health* (5th ed.). Pearson Prentice Hall.

Community Health Nurses of Canada (CHNC). (2019). *Canadian community health nursing: Professional practice model and standards of practice.* https://www.chnc.ca/standards-of-practice.

Domitrovich, C., Bradshaw, C., Greenberg, M., et al. (2010). Integrated models of school-based prevention: Logic and theory. *Psychology in the Schools, 47*(1), 71–88. https://doi.org/10.1002/pits.20452

Ezeonwu, M., & Berkowitz, B. (2014). A collaborative communitywide health fair: The process and impacts on the community. *Journal of Community Health Nursing, 31*(2), 118–129. https://doi.org/10.1080/07370016.2014.901092

Finnegan, L., & Ervin, N. E. (1989). An epidemiological approach to community assessment. *Public Health Nursing, 6*(3), 147–151.

Green, L., & Kreuter, M. (1999). *Health promotion planning: An educational and environmental approach* (3rd ed.). Mayfield Publishing. http://www.courseweb.uottawa.ca/pop8910/Outline/Models/Model-Green.PDF.

Green, L. W., & Kreuter, M. W. (2005). *Health promotion planning: An educational and ecological approach* (3rd ed.). McGraw-Hill.

Issel, L. M. (2008). *Health program planning and evaluation: A practical systematic approach for community health* (2nd ed.). Jones & Bartlett.

McKenzie, J. F., Neiger, B. L., & Thackeray, R. (2016). *Planning, implementing, and evaluating health promotion programs: A primer* (7th ed.). Pearson.

Public Health Agency of Canada. (2008). *Program evaluation tool kit.* http://www.phac-aspc.gc.ca.

Ranjbaran, S., Dehdari, T., Sadeghniiat-Haghighi, K., et al. (2015). Poor sleep quality in patients after coronary artery bypass graft surgery: An intervention study using the PRECEDE-PROCEED model. *The Journal of Tehran University Heart Center, 10*(1), 1–8.

Rossi, P., Lipsey, M., & Henry, G. T. (2018). *Evaluation: A systematic approach* (8th ed.). Sage.

Veney, A., & Kaluzny, J. (2005). *Evaluation and decision making for health services* (4th ed.). Health Administration Press.

Vollman, A. R., Anderson, E. T., & McFarlane, J. (2017). *Canadian community as partner: Theory and multidisciplinary practice in nursing* (4th ed.). Lippincott Williams & Wilkins.

Stakeholders and Populations of Community Health Practice

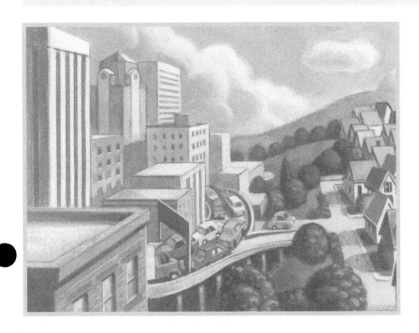

11

Working With the Individual as Client: Health and Wellness Across the Lifespan

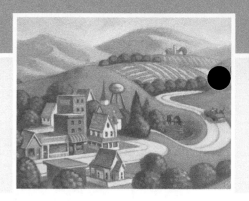

OUTLINE

Healthy Living Approach, 246
Early Child Development as a Determinant of Health, 247
Child and Adolescent Health, 248
  Overweight and Obesity, 251
  Physical Activity, 252
  Nutrition, 252
  The Comprehensive School Health Approach, 254
  Unintentional Injuries and Accidents, 256
  Tobacco Use, 257

Immunization, 258
Adult Health, 259
  Women's Health, 259
  Men's Health, 264
Older Persons' Health, 266
  The Role of the Community Health Nurse in Caring for Older Persons, 268
  Resources for Community Health Nurses, 270

OBJECTIVES

After reading this chapter, you should be able to:

11.1 Examine the impact of a healthy living approach throughout the lifespan.

11.2 Understand some of the influences on healthy child development.

11.3 Discuss the major health issues of children and adolescents and describe the role of the community health nurse (CHN) in promoting their health in the community.

11.4 Compare and contrast the major health issues of men and women.

11.5 Explain the chronic health problems that are often experienced by older persons and describe the role of the CHN in caring for them.

KEY TERMS*

ageism, 266
aging, 266
gerontological nursing, 266
gerontology, 266
healthy living, 246
menopause, 260

neglect, 269
primordial prevention, 255
testicular self-examination (TSE), 265
three Ds, 269
women's health, 259
vaccine hesitancy, 258

*See the Glossary on page 468 for definitions.

This chapter examines the health status of populations and of individuals across the lifespan. The emphasis is on population health and health promotion, but consideration is also given to health status, health risks, and the effects of lifestyle on health.

HEALTHY LIVING APPROACH

The healthy living approach to health promotion and disease prevention can help to reduce the occurrence and outcomes of certain chronic illnesses and therefore contribute to the quality of life for Canadians. However, it is necessary to keep in mind that healthy living is affected by factors such as the determinants of health and societal foci, and that public policies can also influence the development and impact of chronic illnesses in the population. A healthy living approach should encompass not only behavioural change, but also a strong policy framework that creates a supportive environment for change and empowers populations to gain more control over lifestyle decisions (Laverack, 2017). **Healthy living** at the population health level refers to the practice of health enhancing behaviours that support, improve, maintain, and enhance population health.

In Canada, greater focus on a socioenvironmental approach with a population focus, health disparities, and the need for policy changes has led to greater "big picture" thinking on healthy living. In 2005, federal, provincial, and territorial ministers of health approved a collaborative healthy living strategy called the Integrated Pan-Canadian Healthy Living Strategy (HLS), which provides a conceptual framework for sustained action to promote healthy living. In Canada, the Public Health Agency of Canada (PHAC) Healthy Living Unit works with the Centre for Health Promotion to help coordinate and deliver the HLS, including an Integrated Strategy on Healthy Living and Chronic Disease. The strategy for chronic diseases consists of three pillars: promoting health by addressing the conditions that lead to unhealthy eating, physical inactivity, and unhealthy weights; preventing chronic disease through focused and integrated action on major chronic diseases and their risk factors; and supporting the early detection and management of chronic diseases.

The healthy living approach was further supported in 2010, when Canada's ministers of health and of health promotion/healthy living produced the Declaration on Prevention and Promotion. The declaration outlined five principles to guide healthy living: (1) prevention is a priority; (2) prevention is the hallmark of a quality health system; (3) prevention is the first step in management; (4) many approaches can be used in health promotion; and (5) health promotion is everyone's business. The promotion of health and the prevention of disease, disability, and injury are priorities and necessary to sustain the health system (PHAC, 2015a).

Preventing major chronic illnesses in adults, such as cancer, diabetes, and respiratory and cardiovascular diseases, is a priority health concern globally. The leading causes of death worldwide in 2012 were cardiovascular disease (46.2%), cancer (21.7%), respiratory disease (10.7%), and diabetes (4%) (World Health Organization [WHO], 2014). Cancer is the leading cause of death in Canada (Government of Canada, 2017). In an effort to address this concern, the WHO (2014) developed nine voluntary global targets to be attained by 2025, including (1) a reduction in overall mortality from cardiovascular disease, cancer, diabetes, or chronic respiratory diseases; (2) a reduction in the harmful use of alcohol; (3) a reduction in the prevalence of insufficient physical activity; (4) a reduction in the intake of salt; (5) a reduction in the prevalence of tobacco use in people 15 years and older; (6) a reduction in the prevalence of high blood pressure; (7) an end to the rise in obesity and diabetes; (8) improved coverage of treatment for prevention of heart attacks and strokes; and (9) greater availability of affordable basic technologies and medicines. Many of these targets are based in prevention and health promotion strategies that are consistent with a healthy living approach to address chronic illness.

The economic burden of chronic illness in Canada is enormous. For example, increased visits to the emergency room and hospitalization rates for patients experiencing chronic heart failure has contributed to a $2.8 billion per year increase in the health care costs Heart & Stroke Foundation (2016). In North America, a healthy living approach is being taken to improve health outcomes by reducing preventable risk factors for diseases, such as regular physical activity, healthy eating, and nonsmoking. Current thinking holds that healthy living is learned in childhood; therefore, prevention is key during the formative years to work toward reducing the number of chronic illnesses that occur in adulthood. More recently, in the *Chief Public*

Health Officer's Report on the State of Public Health in Canada in 2017, the priorities for healthy living focused on "designing" healthy living environments because of the tremendous potential that changing the built environment can have on helping Canadians live healthier lives (PHAC, 2017).

As mentioned earlier, Canada developed a conceptual framework for sustained action based on healthy living. The current priorities of the HLS are in areas such as physical activity and healthy eating and their relation to weight; tobacco reduction; and prevention of diabetes and other chronic illnesses (PHAC, 2007). The vision is to create a healthy Canadian population based on healthy living. The two primary goals are to reduce health disparities and improve overall health outcomes in each of the areas of emphasis. The objectives of the HLS (priority 1) are to increase by 20% the number of Canadians who eat healthily, participate in regular physical activity, and have healthy body weights. The HLS has provided support for the development of health living initiatives, and reports have been generated that demonstrate that the goals of the HLS continue to be supported (e.g., in the areas of improved cooking and preparation skills in Canada and abroad) (Health Canada, 2010). Since the emphasis in the HLS is a population health approach, consideration has been given to the interrelationship between a person's behaviour and socioeconomic factors such as environment, poverty, education, and employment. Actions on these social determinants of health will contribute to improved population health instead of only focusing on changing individual behaviours. The strategies to reach the objectives include intersectoral collaboration for policy and community development, research development and transfer, and providing public information. Healthy living priorities for mental health and injury prevention are part of the long-term planning and priorities for the PHAC. Four strategic directions have been identified in the HLS: leadership and policy development, knowledge development and transfer, community development and infrastructure, and public information (PHAC, 2007). Fig. 11.1 presents a diagram depicting the Integrated Pan-Canadian Healthy Living Strategy framework.

Throughout this chapter, the areas of emphasis identified in the HLS conceptual framework are addressed within the following lifespan groups: children and youth, adults, women, men, and older persons. Consideration is given to populations and individuals within a socioecological context with attention to the strategic directions as outlined in the framework. Within each age group, certain health issues, conditions, and concerns are discussed in more detail because of their higher risk at certain time frames in the lifespan. For further information on the integration of the healthy living strategies in Canada, see the PHAC "Healthy Living Fund" link on the Evolve website.

EARLY CHILD DEVELOPMENT AS A DETERMINANT OF HEALTH

Early child development means creating the conditions for children (from gestation to 8 years of age) to thrive in their

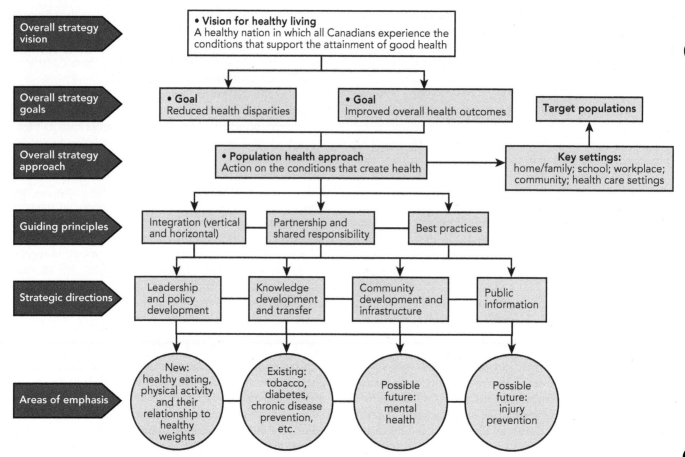

Fig. 11.1 Integrated Pan-Canadian Healthy Living Strategy Framework Diagram. (From Public Health Agency of Canada. [2005]. *The Integrated Pan-Canadian Healthy Living Strategy.* Adapted and reproduced with permission from the Minister of Health, 2016.)

physical, socioemotional, and language/cognitive development. There are three elements of healthy child development, which include: (1) stable, responsive, and nurturing caring; (2) safe, supportive environments; and (3) appropriate nutrition (WHO, 2019). According to the National Collaborating Centre for Determinants of Health (2009), early child development is one of the most important determinants of health.

For further support of this position, see the WHO's *Total Environment Assessment Model for Early Child Development* link on the Evolve website. This model, which is geared to health care providers, researchers, and policymakers, describes how the socioenvironmental determinant is fundamental to early child development.

Some influences on healthy child development are found in Box 11.1. Key factors that contribute to health inequities are discussed in more depth in the document titled *Report on the State of Public Health in Canada 2009: Growing Up Well—Priorities for a Healthy Future* (PHAC, 2009b). This report (see the PHAC link on the Evolve website) highlights six areas of concern that have the greatest impact on the health of Canadian children: (1) socioeconomic status and developmental opportunities; (2) abuse and neglect; (3) prenatal risks; (4) mental health and disorders; (5) obesity; and (6) unintentional injuries (PHAC, 2009b).

CHILD AND ADOLESCENT HEALTH

Children's health includes the health of children from infancy to adolescence. The future of Canada depends on how our children are cared for. Focusing on the health needs of children increases the chances of future adults who value and practise healthy lifestyles and who are healthier (PHAC, 2009b). See the PHAC *Report on the State of Public Health in Canada 2009: Growing Up Well—Priorities for a Healthy Future* (the link is on the Evolve website). Specifically, see Chapter 3, which describes some key considerations about Canadian children's health; Chapter 4, which discusses, family and environmental factors influencing health; and Chapter 5, which provides information on various community and government programs available in Canada and internationally that have been implemented to facilitate a healthy life for children and their families.

CHNs have the following two major roles to fulfill in the area of child and adolescent health:
1. Provision of direct services to children and their families: assessment, management of care, education, and counselling.
2. Assessment of the community and the establishment of programs to ensure a healthy environment for its children.

Many opportunities arise for CHNs to teach healthy lifestyles to children and caregivers and to provide family-centred

BOX 11.1   Influences on Healthy Child Development

- Although playtime is essential for healthy child development, many children do not get enough time to play due to increased academic demands, fewer and/or shorter recesses at school, hurried lifestyles, and changes in family structure.* Play positively influences children's physical (e.g., provides exercise), cognitive (e.g., enhances problem-solving skills), social (e.g., establishes interpersonal relationships), mental (e.g., helps build self-esteem), and psychometric (e.g., develops and improves muscle strength) development.[†]
- There is limited government support for social integration of persons with disabilities into Canadian society.[§] In fact, in this area Canada ranks twenty-seventh among the 29 Organisation for Economic Co-operation and Development nations on public spending, and these authors identify the need for federal government policies to "meet the costs."[§]
- The demand for quality child care has grown steadily in Canada over the past three decades, with a notable increase in one-parent and stepfamilies. In 2011, almost half (46%) of parents reported using some type of child care, with 33% using day care centres, 31% home daycares, and 21% private arrangements.[°]

- Regulated child care is accessible to only 17% of Canadians. Since regulated child care is important for early child development, government policies need to ensure Canadian families have access to affordable and quality child care, regardless of socioeconomic status.[§]
- Abused children are more likely to experience poor health in adulthood.[‖]
- In Canada, 12% of children under the age of 12 live in poverty.[#]
- Low birth weights, disability and death, behavioural problems, and mental health disorders are more likely to occur in children born into low socioeconomic environments, and these conditions can contribute to poor health for the rest of their lives.[**]
- The material, social, structural, or community environments that influence the socioeconomic status of children lead to poor health as adults.[††]
- "All Canadians would benefit from improved early childhood development in terms of improved community quality of life, reduced social problems, and improved Canadian economic performance"[§] (p. 24).

Sources: *Ginsburg, K. R. (2007). The importance of play in promoting healthy child development and maintaining strong parent-child bonds. *Pediatrics, 119*(1), 182–191.
[†]Beckmann Murray, R., Proctor Zentner, J., Pangman, V., et al. (2009). *Health promotion strategies through the lifespan* (2nd Cdn. ed.). Pearson Prentice Hall.
[°]Sinha, M. (2014). *Child care in Canada* (Catalogue No. 89-652-X - No. 005; ISBN 978-1-100-24896-7). Statistics Canada: Social and Aboriginal Statistics Division. https://www150.statcan.gc.ca/n1/pub/89-652-x/89-652-x2014005-eng.htm
[§]Mikkonen, J., & Raphael, D. (2010). *Social determinants of health: The Canadian facts*. York University School of Health Policy and Management. www.thecanadianfacts.org/
[‖]Cromer, K. R., & Sachs-Ericsson, N. (2006). The association between childhood abuse, PTSD, and the occurrence of adult health problems: Moderation via current life stress. *Journal of Traumatic Stress, 19*(6), 967–971.
[#]Public Health Agency of Canada (PHAC). (2009b). The chief public health officer's report on the state of public health in Canada 2009: Growing up well—Priorities for a healthy future. http://www.phac-aspc.gc.ca/cphorsphc-respcacsp/2009/fr-rc/index-eng.php
[**]Canadian Institute for Health Information. (2008). *Reducing gaps in health: A focus on socio-economic status in urban Canada.* https://secure.cihi.ca/free_products/Reducing_Gaps_in_Health_Report_EN_081009.pdf
[††]Conroy, K., Sandel, M., & Zuckerman, B. (2010). Poverty grown up: How childhood socioeconomic status impacts adult health. *Journal of Developmental & Behavioral Pediatrics, 31*(2), 154–160.

care in the community. Specific issues that may arise during adolescence such as teenage pregnancy and sexually transmitted infections were discussed later in Chapter 15 and will be discussed again in Chapter 16 of this text.

Ongoing growth and development make this age group unique. Table 11.1 provides a brief review of some common health concerns from infancy to adolescence. Physical, cognitive, and emotional changes occur more rapidly during childhood and adolescence than at any other time in the lifespan. Health visits should be scheduled at key ages to monitor these changes. A community health nursing assessment for child health (Box 11.2) includes assessing growth and health status, development, quality of the parent–child relationship, and family support systems.

CHNs such as nurse practitioners in a community clinic or a public health nurse visiting with families (newborns and other age groups) may need to conduct an assessment of any of the following age groups: infant, toddler, schoolchild, and adolescent (some individual assessment tools

are provided in Appendix E.5 "Infant, Child, and Youth Screening Tools" on the Evolve website). CHNs need to actively involve the parent(s) throughout the assessment process, and the developmental stages need to be part of the assessment. This parental involvement will facilitate data collection, empower the parent(s), and encourage parental identification of health concerns. The CHN and parent(s) partner to identify appropriate interventions to address all health concerns and to plan follow-up and evaluation strategies. The CHN, in collaboration with the parent(s), may determine the need for a referral to a specific community agency. The CHN would follow the referral process as outlined in Chapter 3.

The CHN considers the developmental stages previously mentioned to be part of child and family assessment (Table 11.2). Also, the developmental stages are considered by the CHN to provide anticipatory guidance to parents so that developmental stage progression is maximized. For example, during a home visit to a family with a newborn, a CHN

TABLE 11.1   Common Health Concerns—Infancy Through Adolescence

Age Group	Common Health Concerns	Age Group	Common Health Concerns
Newborn (1 to 4 weeks)	• Seborrheic dermatitis ("cradle cap") • Oral candidiasis ("thrush") • Constipation • Iron-deficiency anemia • Roseola infantum • Colic	School child (6 to 12 years)	• Accommodative esophoria • Otitis externa • Serous otitis media • Allergic rhinitis • Asthma • Herpes type 1 • Contact dermatitis
Infant (1 to 12 months)	• Atopic dermatitis • Diaper dermatitis		• Tinea corporis (ringworm of the nonhairy skin)
Toddler (12 months to 3 years)	• Umbilical cord granuloma • Myopia • Astigmatism • Strabismus • Hearing impairment • Otitis media • Dental caries • Malabsorption syndrome • Impetigo • Pharyngitis • Acute nonspecific gastroenteritis (simple diarrhea) • Varicella (chickenpox) • Rubella (3-day measles) • Pinworms (Enterobius vermicularis) • Miliaria rubra ("heat rash" or "prickly heat") • Viral croup (laryngotracheobronchitis)	Adolescents (13 to 21 years)	• Tinea capitis (ringworm of the head) • Warts • Pediculus humanus capitis (head lice) • Mumps • Diabetes type 1 • Fifth disease (erythema infectiosum) • Hand-foot-and-mouth disease • Pityriasis rosea • Hordeolum (stye) • Epistaxis (nosebleed) • Acne vulgaris • Dental caries and gingivitis • Aphthous stomatitis • Tinea cruris • Tinea pedis (athlete's foot) • Infectious mononucleosis • Hepatitis A, B, and C virus • Rocky Mountain spotted fever • Lyme disease • Sexually transmitted infections
Preschooler (3 to 5 years)	• Measles • Diarrhea • Postural problems • Juvenile hypertension • Hypochromic anemia		

Source: Adapted from Beckmann Murray, R., Proctor Zentner, J., Pangman, V., et al. (2006). Health promotion strategies through the lifespan (Cdn. ed.). Pearson Canada.

BOX 11.2   Community Health Nursing Assessment for Child Health

• Physical assessment
• Psychosocial assessment
• Nutritional needs
• Elimination patterns
• Sleep behaviours
• Development and behaviour
• Safety issues
• Parenting concerns

would most likely assess for indicators of the development of trust between the parent(s) and the newborn. The CHN could counsel the parent(s) on ways to promote the development of trust during parent–newborn interactions. The CHN would also discuss issues surrounding development of trust during infancy. Provision of resources to the parent(s) may be indicated to assist in acquiring parental skills to promote the development of trust. One resource that could be provided is the PHAC First Connections … Make All the Difference resource kit (the link is in the Tool Box on the Evolve website). This kit includes resources for health care providers and information for parents and primary caregivers on promoting infant attachment.

Transitions are life events that occur from infancy and continue as a person ages. These transitions, often referred to as turning points in life (with the potential to create crisis), can present as challenges that sometimes require support to move forward. The Health Canada resource Growing Healthy Canadians: A Guide for Positive Child Development (the link is in the Tool Box on the Evolve website) is an excellent source of information on transition from infancy to adulthood. Information is provided on the role of communities, research on the determinants of health, and factors that influence development.

TABLE 11.2 Developmental Stages—Infancy Through Adolescence				
Age Group	Freud (Psychosexual)	Erickson (Psychosocial)	Piaget (Logical, Cognitive, and Moral)	Kohlberg (Moral)
Newborn (1 to 4 weeks)			Beginning development of motor and cognitive skills	
Infant (1 to 12 months)	Oral stage	Trust versus mistrust	Period I (sensorimotor)	
Toddler (12 months to 3 years)	Anal stage	Autonomy versus shame and doubt	Period I (sensorimotor) (beginning of preoperational): child is egocentric; beginning of parallel play	Level 1 (preconventional) Stage 1: punishment and obedience orientation
Preschooler (3 to 5 years)	Phallic stage (Oedipus complex; Electra complex)	Initiative versus guilt	Period II (preoperational): rapid language development	
Schoolchild (6 to 12 years)	Latent stage	Industry versus inferiority	Period III (concrete operations) Ability to perform mental operations	Level 1 (preconventional) Stage 2: instrumental relativist orientation
Adolescents (13 to 21 years)	Genital stage	Identity versus identity diffusion	Period IV (formal operations): stages -abstract thinking develops -increased ability to reason about consequences	Level 2 (conventional) Stage 3: good boy, nice girl orientation Stage 4: society maintaining orientation Level 3 (postconventional) Stage 5: social contact orientation Stage 6: universal ethical principle orientation

Source: Adapted from Astle, B. J., Duggleby, W., Potter, P. A., et al. (2019). *Canadian fundamentals of nursing* (6th ed., pp. 347–351). Elsevier Canada.

Overweight and Obesity

"Overweight and obesity are conditions that occur at different points of weight gain, can have very different outcomes, and possibly different determinants and risk factors" (Clinton, 2009, p. 7). Over one in four Canadians adults are obese (24.3 to 25.4%) and of children and youth aged 6 to 17 years, 8.6% are obese (PHAC and Canadian Institute for Health Information, 2011). The majority of Canadians are at increased health risks due to excess weight. "Obesity is sometimes defined as the condition of an individual who is 20% or more above ideal weight" (Beckmann Murray et al., 2009, p. 362). However, obesity is more than an individual health issue. Many factors contribute to obesity. Societal changes led to the proliferation of fast-food availability to meet the demands of working families, easier access to vending machines containing fast foods, and increased plate sizes, which has led to increased portions or "supersizing" with extra calories. Vending machines with fast-food choices are common in schools. Soft drinks and sugary fruit punch add empty calories. Snacking on high-sugar and high-fat foods is a problem. Advertising directed at children also promotes poor food choices.

Additionally, because of increased awareness for child safety pertaining to walking to school and out-of-school activities, parents have increasingly taken to driving their children to school and to after-school activities. Also, transportation for taking children to school through busing rather than walking has resulted in decreased physical activity levels of children and adolescents. In Canada, over 50% of school children and adolescents (5 to 17 years of age) are driven to school either by car or by bus (Mahon, 2006). Furthermore, there has been an increase in sedentary lifestyle of children and youth due to technological changes that have precipitated increased time spent in nonphysical activities such as watching television and playing video or online games (PHAC and Canadian Institute for Health Information, 2011). More than half of Canadian children are not active enough for optimal health and development (Heart and Stroke Foundation, 2021). In an effort to address this problem, most schools have maintained or reintroduced physical activity education programs, as well as increased healthy food choices in schools. Governments have introduced new health promotion policies such as bans on trans fats and the introduction of the Children's Fitness Tax Credit. Communities are planning for and providing physical activity opportunities, such as connecting neighbourhoods with walking trails. There is also more control over advertising targeting children and adolescents. For further information on the influence of the built environment on promoting healthier outcomes for Canadians, see the

PHAC link on the Evolve website: "Bringing Health to the Planning Table—A Profile of Promising Practices in Canada and Abroad." For information on alternatives for physical activity and modes of travel to school, see the School Travel Planning News link on the Evolve website.

The medical consequences of obesity vary, with obese children and teens having an increased prevalence of:

- Hypertension
- Respiratory problems
- Hyperlipidemia
- Bone and joint difficulties
- Hyperinsulinemia
- Menstrual problems

The psychosocial disadvantages of being overweight in the young may include the following:

- Teasing
- Scholastic discrimination
- Low self-esteem
- Negative body image

There is a downward spiral of overweight, poor self-image, increasing isolation, and decreasing activity, which together lead to obesity. Long-term risks include heart disease, diabetes, and cancer. For further information on the issue of overweight and obesity in Canada and the ecological approach to addressing obesity and its determinants, see the link for the Canadian Population Health Initiative report on the Evolve website. The Government of Canada document *Healthy Weights for Healthy Kids: Report of the Standing Committee on Health* contains information on what determines healthy weights, what works for healthy weight control, and issues pertaining to Indigenous populations (see the link on the Evolve website).

Physical Activity

As previously indicated, television and screen time contribute to a sedentary lifestyle and increase the tendency of children and youth to be overweight and obese (PHAC and Canadian Institute for Health Information, 2005, 2011). As the time spent on these passive activities increases in relation to time spent playing actively with others, obesity in Canadian children and youth also increase (PHAC and Canadian Institute for Health Information, 2011). Interventions need to be based on goals of lifestyle changes for the entire family. The goal is to modify the way the family eats, exercises, and plans daily activities. Guidelines for managing childhood obesity are discussed in Box 11.3. The goal of managing weight in children and adolescents is to normalize weight. This may involve:

- Slowing the rate of weight gain
- Allowing children to "grow into" their weight
- Improving dietary habits
- Increasing physical activity
- Improving self-esteem
- Improving parent relationships

Physical activity and adequate rest for all ages are important factors in preventing disease and promoting health. The Canadian Society for Exercise Physiology, in cooperation

---

BOX 11.3   Guidelines for Managing Childhood Obesity

- Set goals related to healthier lifestyle, not dieting.
- Keep objectives realistic and obtainable.
- Modify family eating habits to include low-fat food choices. Serve calorie-dense foods that incorporate *Canada's Dietary Guidelines*: whole grains, fruits, vegetables, lean-protein foods, and low-fat dairy products.
- Encourage family members to stop eating when they are satisfied. Encourage recognizing hunger and satiation cues.
- Schedule regular times for meals and snacks. Include breakfast and do not skip meals.
- Have low-calorie, nutritious snacks ready and available. Avoid having empty-calorie junk foods in the home.
- Encourage the keeping of food intake and activity diaries.
- Promote physical activity. Make daily exercise a priority. Encourage family participation. Find ways to make the activity fun. Include peers.
- Limit television viewing. Do not allow snacking while watching television.
- Scale back screen time. Replace sedentary time with hobbies, activities, and chores.
- Recognize healthier food choices when eating out. Order broiled, roasted, grilled, or baked items. Split orders or take home "doggy bags."
- Praise and reward children for the progress they make in reaching nutrition and activity goals. Emphasize the unique positive qualities of each child.
- Understand the genetic features of the child's or adolescent's body type. Acceptance of the child who has a higher range of abdominal girth measurement may be a part of reaching health goals.

---

with the Healthy Active Living and Obesity Research Group at the University of Alberta and the PHAC, have developed the world's first *24-hour Movement Guidelines* to integrate physical activity, sedentary behaviour, and sleep guidelines for each age group (Table 11.3). The *Guidelines* consider the important interrelationship between all three behaviours and include guidelines for pregnancy and multiple sclerosis.

For more information on the recommended activity and sleep levels for all Canadians, see the link for the Canadian Society for Exercise Physiology; https://csepguidelines.ca on the Evolve website. Along with the guides are resources and videos that CHNs can use to plan health promotion programs to promote healthy lifestyles across the lifespan.

Nutrition

Promoting good nutrition and dietary habits is one of the most important aspects of maintaining child health. The first six years in a child's life are the most important for developing sound lifetime eating habits. The quality of nutrition has been widely accepted as an important influence on growth and development. It is now recognized as an important factor in disease prevention.

Atherosclerosis begins during childhood. Other diseases such as obesity, diabetes, osteoporosis, and cancer may have early beginnings also. Low-income and minority families are

TABLE 11.3 The Canadian 24-Hour Movement Guidelines

Age	Physical Activity	Sleep	Sedentary Behaviour (sitting, screen time)
Toddlers 1–2 years	Several times per day (e.g., interactive floor-based play, 30 minutes of tummy time)	0–3 months (14–17 hrs) 12–16 months (12–16 hrs) Including naps	Not being restrained more than 1 hour at a time (e.g., in stroller, highchair)
Preschoolers 3–4 years	180 minutes of activity, of which 60 minutes is energetic play	10–13 hours Including naps	
Children and Youth 5–17 years	60 minutes per day of moderate to vigorous activity Include muscle and bone strengthening 3 times /wk Plus several hours of light activity	5–13 years (9–11 hrs) 14–17 years (8–10 hrs)	No more than 2 hours per day of screen time
Adults 18–64 years	150 minutes of moderate to vigorous activity per week Muscle and bone strengthening twice a week		

Source: Summarized from Canadian 24-Hour Movement Guidelines (https://csepguidelines.ca/)

at increased risk for poor nutrition, but all groups show poor dietary habits.

The child and family both provide a range of variables that influence nutritional habits. Ethnic, racial, cultural, and socioeconomic factors influence what the parents eat and how they feed their children. The child brings individual issues to the nutritional arena, such as:

- Slow eating
- Picky patterns
- Food preferences
- Allergies
- Acute or chronic health problems
- Changes with acceleration and deceleration of growth

Parents often have unrealistic expectations of what children should eat. *Canada's Dietary Guidelines* (see the link on the Evolve website) offers guidelines for daily food requirements for all ages. The latest version addresses, for the first time, gender difference in nutritional requirements and suggests portion sizes and food choices based on quality. Physical growth serves as an excellent measure of adequacy of the diet. Height, weight, and head circumference of children younger than 3 years are plotted on appropriate growth curves at regular intervals to allow assessment of growth patterns. Good nutritional intake supports physical growth at a steady rate.

A 24-hour diet recall by the parent is a helpful screening tool to assess the amount and variety of food intake of children. If the recall is fairly typical for the child, the CHN can compare the intake with basic recommendations for the child's age. CHNs will want to ask about the family's and the child's concerns regarding diet and look at the family's meal patterns. In some situations, the CHN could direct the family to the interactive website for *Canada's Dietary Guidelines*, where the family can plan meals based on food choices and healthy eating habits. The site also provides tips for healthy eating at home and school.

Growth charts are one tool available to assess whether a child is growing within the "normal" range for age. They also provide the opportunity to monitor a child's growth over time. These charts are used during well-child assessments.

The results can be used to reassure parents regarding their child's growth and also to provide an opportunity to teach about the normal range that contributes to individual child differences. Further information about the health of children, including calculating growth using growth charts and height calculators, see the *WHO Child Growth Standards* (the link is in the Tool Box on the Evolve website).

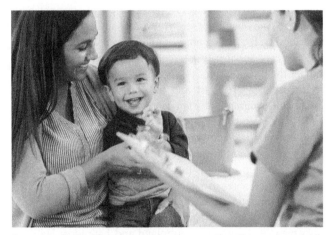

A community health nurse explains the growth patterns on a growth chart to a child and her mother. (iStockphoto/SDI Productions)

The increased occurrence of type 2 diabetes in childhood, especially in children who are obese, supports the need for school and other community programs to promote healthy lifestyles and therefore diabetes prevention in this population. One study in Nova Scotia explored the risk factors for childhood weight problems based on school and family factors (Veugelers & Fitzgerald, 2005). A notable finding was that students who skipped breakfast were more likely to have weight issues and to eat unhealthy foods at lunch at school. One recommendation by the study authors that relates to one of the determinants of health and families was that "preventive public health actions should be targeted first toward low-income neighbourhoods" (p. 612). Poverty puts populations at increased risk for poorer health.

Community and government interventions are needed to address the health disparities in which poor Canadians live and work if their health is to be improved. Food is one of the prerequisites for health identified in the Ottawa Charter for Health Promotion. CHNs can advocate for healthy public policies to reduce inequities in income. This might be accomplished by partnering with other community groups to influence the various government levels and through involvement with nursing professional organizations to advocate for change. Of particular note for CHNs is the Joint Report from the PHAC and the Canadian Institute for Health Information (PHAC & Canadian Institute for Health Information [CIHI], 2011) which outlines opportunities for obesity prevention and management, including community-based interventions and the development of healthy public policies. Public policy strategies discussed include subsidy programs (e.g., the Food Mail program for northern Canada) and the regulation of marketing food to children.

Any discussions on food inequalities should include recognition of the determinants of health, such as food insecurity; inequitable access to physical activity; and environmental determinants of health. For example, rural and Indigenous children tend to be overweight and obese because of living on lower incomes and residing in areas where nutritious foods are either unavailable or very expensive and unaffordable (PHAC, 2009b). The PHAC's (2009c) document *Obesity: An Overview of Current Landscape and Prevention-Related Activities in Ontario* presents statistics on overweight and obesity in Canadian children, youth, and adults, as well as the contributing factors to obesity and related health concerns and presents an obesity-prevention approach. CHNs could initiate the development of community-based interventions such as school breakfast and healthy snack programs and food bank programs at higher-education institutions. They could also offer health educational programs on nutritious foods and physical activity requirements in the community.

One of the national research initiatives of significance for Canadian communities is the Early Learning and Child Care (ELCC) experiences in selected cities across the nation. The study was funded by Social Development Canada and the cities of Toronto and Vancouver (Mahon, 2006). Participating cities were St. John's, Newfoundland and Labrador; Halifax, Nova Scotia; Montreal, Quebec; Sherbrooke, Quebec; Toronto, Ontario; Sudbury, Ontario; Winnipeg, Manitoba; Saskatoon, Saskatchewan; Calgary, Alberta; Vancouver, British Columbia; and Whitehorse, Yukon. It was found that (1) most successful programs target all children under 12 years and not just the high-risk groups; (2) even with community partnerships, ELCC requires more support than is offered by cities to be able to expand services to all children and families; (3) inconsistency exists across the cities in relation to the sufficiency of the provision of child programs; (4) cities with more resources are better able to access funding; (5) high-quality programs are needed for out-of-school children, such as programs before and after the school day; and (6) cities are responsible for recreational facilities for this latter group. The study findings showed that these city programs require government funding at all levels so that parents are supported and early learning and childcare needs are met. As well, the study findings indicate the need for cities to form partnerships that focus on health promotion and population health if communities are to address lifestyle changes through supportive environments.

The Comprehensive School Health Approach

Healthy child development can be promoted through the Comprehensive School Health Framework (CSHF). This approach to child health moves beyond the behavioural and healthy living approach, to, as its name implies, a comprehensive framework for health promotion. Central to the philosophy of Comprehensive School Health (CSH) is the belief that "healthy learners are better learners" (Murray, Low, Hollis, et al., 2007). The link between CSH and academic success is evidenced by research (Dukowski, 2009; Murray et al., 2007). CSH focuses on school children as a population; the use of the CSHF is relevant as children spend approximately one-third of each weekday in school. Thus, opportunities to access the population and build capacity are plentiful (Canadian Association for School Health, 2006). The concept of CSH has been endorsed by WHO and is recognized internationally. The term *comprehensive school health* is most commonly used in Canada. Similar frameworks exist in other countries and are known as "health promoting schools" or "coordinated school health" (Canadian Association for School Health, 2006).

CSH has its roots in population health, particularly the 1986 WHO's seminal Ottawa Charter for Health Promotion. The Ottawa Charter helped change the focus of health promotion by deemphasizing individual responsibility and lifestyle change and emphasizing the importance of understanding the broader influences on health. In line with the Ottawa Charter, the CSH approach promotes health in and out of the classroom. CSH drew particularly on the Ottawa Charter's focus on development of personal skills (Stewart-Brown, 2006). This and the other four tenets of the Ottawa Charter remain one part of the population health promotion model (Hamilton & Bhatti, 1996) discussed in Chapter 4. CHNs practising within CSHF recognize that programs that focus on helping individual children in the classroom, without acknowledging the importance of the environments within which the children live, as well as the sociopolitical context of those environments, will not be as effective in long-term promotion of health (Health Nexus, 2008; Labonte, 2003). For example, a CHN working within the CSHF might want to provide students with some health information about nutrition. Therefore, a classroom presentation about nutrition might be supplemented by a school breakfast program and a district-wide nutrition policy that supports provision of healthy foods to the children in the schools. In addition, the CHN might work with parent or guardian support groups at the school to encourage fundraisers that do not involve foods with a low nutritional rating (e.g., selling gift baskets instead of chocolate bars). The CHN might educate teachers and staff about alternatives to food rewards (e.g., stickers or other low-cost items). The CHN might also participate as a member of a multidisciplinary group that advocates for legislation of a nationwide breakfast program for children.

Children's health is recognized as being influenced by the relationships of children with family, school, and community. CHNs who work within the CSHF must be supportive of these relationships, as well as be cognizant of the following four CSH cornerstones:

- Social and physical environment (e.g., programs support physical activity, environments are inclusive and welcoming, schools are built in environmentally safe areas).
- Teaching and learning (programs are typically universal and upstream in their approach; programs build developmental assets, nurture development of protective factors and resiliency, and target students' knowledge, attitudes, skills, and behaviours).
- Healthy school policy (e.g., nutrition policies, tobacco-free policies).
- Partnerships and services (e.g., programs involve intersectoral and interprofessional partnerships between the school and community; and the accessibility of health services in the school, particularly primary and secondary preventions, are considered) (Avison, 2009; Joint Consortium for School Health, 2010; PHAC, 2008).

Stewart-Brown (2006), commissioned by WHO, conducted an extensive literature review that focused on the evidence-informed practice of CSH. The report concluded that, to be most effective, CHNs who work within the CSHF should promote injury prevention, nutrition, physical activity, and mental health. Programs should involve families, the community, and the school when possible. In addition, CHNs should support programs that are delivered by students to students (peer-delivered) because they can be as effective as those facilitated by an adult.

Comprehensive school health CHNs spend significant amounts of time engaging in both primordial and primary prevention. Although the concept of primary prevention is commonly found in health promotion literature, the concept of *primordial prevention*, or preventing risk factors for health issues from ever occurring, is seen less often. A similar pattern exists in discussions about the CSHF. Ironically, the concept is not new and was first suggested by Strasser (1978). **Primordial prevention** includes broader activities that focus on preventing the emergence of risk factors that are known to create the conditions for disease. It includes creating supportive environments and helping populations develop personal life skills, such as healthy eating and smoking cessation (Centers for Disease Control and Prevention [CDC], 2008). This level of prevention was used in a significant study titled "The Children and Adolescent Trial of Health (CATCH)." Randomized control trials were conducted on elementary school children between 1987 and 2000. Researchers engaged schoolchildren in activities designed to promote cardiovascular health. Programs focused on physical activity, nutrition, and smoking (Mahon, 2006). Research about the importance of primordial prevention continues to demonstrate its importance for policy development and population health

promotion. Findings from the Labarthe, Dai, Day, et al. (2009) longitudinal study on children aged 8 to 18 years supported the effectiveness of obesity-prevention programs beginning in the elementary school population.

Comprehensive School Health Project in New Brunswick

Since the early 2000s, New Brunswick has been using a comprehensive healthy school approach to support a number of initiatives in the province to address child health. One such initiative is the partnering of nursing students at the University of New Brunswick with local CHNs to create and implement health promotion presentations grounded in primordial and primary prevention. Content for each presentation is based on epidemiology and surveillance literature (Canadian Council on Social Development, 2007; Leitch, 2007; PHAC, 2008) and supported by evidence from the New Brunswick Grades 6–12 Student Wellness Survey and the Elementary Student Wellness Survey (New Brunswick Health Council, 2017). Outcomes for each presentation are matched to the provincial education curriculum outcomes for each grade. Some topics include handwashing, healthy active learning, nutrition, injury prevention, healthy friendships, smoking prevention, and hygiene. Nursing students visit the same classrooms each week and build relationships with schoolchildren and school staff. Presentations follow a predictable pattern, beginning with deep breathing and stretching activities. Nursing students also build capacity by becoming involved with the home and school, drawing on experts within the community (e.g., a mother whose daughter has severe allergies discusses her experiences and demonstrates the use of an anaphylaxis kit), and contributing to the school newsletter. Nursing students include both teachers and the children in the evaluation of the presentations. Preparation for the clinical experience encourages nursing students to transfer knowledge from previous and current coursework and to build on their own strengths and interests. For example, they draw on theory from the previous years about healthy child development, common pediatric chronic and acute health challenges, and mental health challenges. Knowledge transfer from concurrent theory courses includes epidemiology, immunizations, communicable diseases, leadership, effective communication and presentation skills, community development, and more.

As the nursing students learn in the classroom about community assessment through asset mapping (Ryan & Bourke, 2008), they learn in the clinical site about the Developmental Asset Framework that is supported by school districts across the province (Ryan & Bourke, 2008). The focus for presentations is strengths based and positive in approach. Students learn in the theory courses about population health and the importance of evidence-informed practice, and they use epidemiology and research when creating or modifying their clinical classroom presentations. As well, they learn about the importance of building capacity, relationship building, and working with the community. In the clinical settings, they have the opportunity to build relationships by visiting the same classrooms each week, including the voices of the children and teachers in evaluating the presentations, and extending the relationship outside the classroom to the broader school community. As students learn in the theory courses about primary health care, social justice, and citizenship, they learn in clinical settings about healthy public policy within the school district and across Canada. They also discuss poverty, inclusion, citizenship initiatives, and capacity-building initiatives at the school (e.g., "Leader in Me Program"). Nursing students are also encouraged to bring their strengths and interests to the program. One example is of a student who loved to sing and had a degree in music, and who was able to record herself singing safety and hand-washing songs for future presentations. Another student who enjoyed sewing was able to make beanbags for a game that was developed by the group.

Nursing students have commented positively about the experience, and other schools have requested partnerships. The direction for the ongoing planning of the partnership is based on recent, local research (Morrison, Kirby, Losier, et al., 2009). For example, in 2006 and 2007, wellness behaviours of students from grades 5 to 12 were surveyed provincially by the New Brunswick Department of Wellness, Culture and Sport in collaboration with the New Brunswick Department of Education, the University of New Brunswick, and the Université de Moncton. Students' mental fitness needs were assessed. The researchers concluded that there is substantial evidence that students who meet their needs for relatedness, competence, and autonomy are more likely to participate in healthy lifestyle choices. More work in the field of mental fitness is developing in schools and through the Department of Wellness, Culture and Sport. Comprehensive school health CHNs continue to be inspired by the belief that "children are critically important. We must keep them healthy and help them when they are not" (Leitch, 2007, p. 17).

Unintentional Injuries and Accidents

Injuries and accidents are the most common causes of preventable disease, disability, and death in people under 60 years of age worldwide. Most accidents occur in the home; therefore, measures to promote home safety are important. In Canada between 2001 and 2007, a total of 51 178 deaths occurred due to unintentional injury, which accounted for 4.2% of all deaths. Unintentional injuries are also the leading cause of death among Canadian children and youth from 1 to 19 years of age (PHAC, 2009a). Most injuries and accidents are preventable. A 2006 Safe Kids Canada survey found that most parents were unaware of the serious risks of injury to children under 14 years of age (Safe Kids Canada, 2007). The key to changing behaviours is teaching age-appropriate safety. Often, CHNs take the lead role in providing education on the prevention of accidents and injuries and work with partners such as teachers, police safety officers, and social workers. The CHN identifies risk factors by assessing the characteristics of the child, family, and environment. Interventions include anticipatory guidance, environmental modification, and safety education. Education should focus on age-appropriate interventions based on knowledge of the leading causes of death and risk factors. Injury prevention topics are listed

---

BOX 11.4   Injury Prevention Topics

- All-terrain vehicle and snowmobile safety
- Bicycle safety
- Bunk beds involving the top bunk
- Car restraints, seat belts, airbag safety
- Crime prevention
- Dangling blind or curtain cords—strangulation hazard
- Decreasing gang activities
- Drowning and near drowning associated with bath seats
- Gun control
- Magnet-related injuries including the ingestion of a magnet from a toy
- Pedestrian safety
- Playground safety
- Preventing drowning; water safety
- Preventing falls—including falls from trampolines
- Preventing fires, burns, frostbite
- Preventing poisoning
- Rail safety
- Safe driving practices
- School bus safety
- Sports safety
- Substance-abuse prevention

---

in Box 11.4. For further information on preventing unintentional injuries, see the website for Parachute, a national organization dedicated to preventing injuries and saving lives (the link is on the Evolve website). This website provides information and resources on a variety of injury topics that would be useful to CHNs, other health care providers working in the area of safety, and parents.

Canadian Nurses Association (CNA) provides a summary of the issues in relation to the built environment and injury prevention. Injury is a significant issue in Canadian public health because of the morbidity and mortality implications, including premature mortality. The various age groups are discussed in reference to economic implications based on the types of injuries that most commonly occur in Canada. See the CNA backgrounder *The Built Environment, Injury Prevention and Nursing: A Summary of the Issues* (the link is on the Evolve website), which provides information on the role of the nurse in primary, secondary, and tertiary unintentional injury prevention.

Another injury prevention topic that can have an impact on the role of CHNs is crime prevention. CHNs support the creation of safe communities and the reduction of the risk for injury by supporting strategies that reduce crime in their communities. From a safe community perspective, the National Crime Prevention Strategy has been established by the Government of Canada to provide national leadership on effective ways to prevent and reduce crime (Government of Canada, 2016). In 2015, a report was released on 10 crime prevention programs supported by that strategy for 12- to 17-year-olds. That report showed that there were positive results from those programs, including improved academic performance and parenting (Public Safety Canada, 2015). CHNs need to be aware of their role in supporting strategies to prevent crime and promote safe communities and building on those strategies to develop safe communities (see the Public Safety Canada link on the Evolve website).

Injury in children and youth is an important community issue and requires continued injury prevention strategies to reduce and prevent its occurrence. More government programs are required, as well as policies instituted to reduce income disparities. At a community level, strategies need to be directed toward environmental improvements such as safe playgrounds; mass educational programs on home, vehicle, and community safety measures; and safer highways. One issue raised is whether these government programs should be directed to aggregate groups such as "high-risk" groups or provided to the total population in this age group. See the PHAC "Child Health" link on the Evolve website, which provides several links to information on child and youth health as well as child and youth community programs. For resources on safety topics in relation to childcare (e.g., water safety, toy safety, playground safety) for families and practitioners, see the Canadian Child Care Federation link on the Evolve website. The federation is a bilingual provincial and territorial association that promotes the use of the best health care practices.

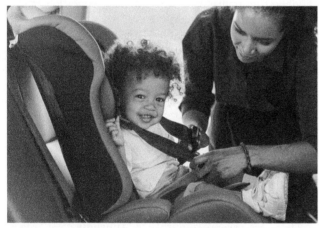

Children should always be restrained while riding in a vehicle. (iStockphoto/Youngoldman)

Tobacco Use

Smoking is a risk factor for cardiovascular disease (CVD), cancer, and lung disease. Smoking has been identified as one of the major preventable causes of morbidity and mortality in Canada.

In 2017, 16.2% of Canadians aged 12 and older (approximately 5 million) smoked either daily or occasionally and the prevalence of cigarette smoking in youth aged 15–19 years was 8%, unchanged from 2015 (Statistics Canada, 2017). Electronic cigarettes are emerging as a new trend in youth smoking behaviours, with 6% or 127 000 of youth aged 15–19 years reporting past-30-day use of e-cigarettes (Statistics Canada, 2017).

Second-hand smoke—smoke exhaled or given off by a burning cigarette—is toxic. Second-hand smoke is also referred to as "environmental tobacco smoke" or "passive smoking". In Canada, the proportion of nonsmokers aged 12 and older exposed to second-hand smoke in the home has decreased from 5.5% in 2011 to 4.7% in 2012 (Statistics Canada, 2017). However, children exposed to second-hand smoke experience increased episodes of ear and upper-respiratory-tract infections and are more likely to take up smoking. Tobacco use is the single most preventable cause of lung cancer (Lung Association of Saskatchewan, 2009). Primary prevention is of utmost importance. Smoking-cessation strategies such as national ad campaigns aimed at altering the perception of smoking as "cool," education, and self-help groups have led to decreased tobacco use. Therefore, these efforts need to be continued. Lung cancer is the leading cause of cancer death for both men and women, but the incidence of lung cancer remains higher in males than in females (PHAC, 2019). and the total cases of lung cancer in men and women combined are greater than those for breast cancer and prostate cancer (Canadian Cancer Society, 2019).

Advertisements in the media and on billboards of tobacco products have been eliminated, and public display of tobacco products has been banned or restricted. Efforts to manage the media exposure of youth and adults to tobacco advertising is one strategy in the campaign to prevent individuals from starting to smoke and to encourage them and support them in their efforts to quit. CHNs spend a great deal of time working with clients to assist them to deal with the effects of smoking or of second-hand smoke. The CHN is in a strategic position to support and act as a positive role model when working to reduce smoking behaviours.

Interventions to discourage smoking focus on the parent, the child or adolescent, and public policy. CHNs need to offer the following:

- Educational programs dealing with the negative health effects of second-hand smoking on children
- Interventions to stop smoking
- Ways to create a smoke-free environment
- Behaviour-modification techniques

Antismoking programs directed at children and teenagers are more successful if the focus is on short-term rather than long-term effects. Developmentally, children and teenagers cannot visualize the future to imagine the consequences of smoking. Also, teenagers often perceive themselves to be invincible and believe "it will not happen to me." The immediate health risks and the cosmetic effects need to be emphasized. Music, sports, and other activities, including stress-reducing techniques, need to be encouraged. Teaching social skills to resist peer pressure is critical. Recently, a concern has emerged regarding smoking electronic cigarettes (e-cigarettes) versus tobacco cigarettes, especially in children and teenagers. E-cigarettes replace the act and taste of smoking, but there are pros and cons to using e-cigarettes. Legislation that regulates e-cigarettes is just beginning to be developed. Regardless of whether they smoke cigarettes or e-cigarettes, children and teenagers need to be aware of the short- and long-term health risks of smoking and be encouraged to quit. For information on the Quit4Life smoking cessation program for youth, see the Health Canada "Quit4Life" link on the Evolve website. This site provides information on and links to several smoking prevention and cessation programs targeted at youth.

CHNs can become politically active by advocating for:
- Enforcement of restrictions on the sale of tobacco to minors
- An increase in funds for antismoking education
- A ban on the sale of e-cigarettes to youth under the minimum age for tobacco consumption

For further information on tobacco and health, see the Physicians for a Smoke-Free Canada link on the Evolve website, which contains information on who smokes in Canada and provides statistics on the leading causes of preventable deaths and the health impacts of smoking.

Immunization

Immunization is an important preventive measure that needs to be initiated in infancy and continued throughout the lifespan as recommended for specific ages. Routine immunization of children has been very successful in preventing selected diseases, such as measles, mumps, and rubella; however, 2019 reports from the U.S. Centers for Disease Control and Prevention (CDC) have reported measles outbreaks (three or more cases) in eight American jurisdictions, including the states of New York and California. The PHAC has also reported measles in Canada in week 18 of 2019, with 48 cases of measles in five provinces and one territory (PHAC, 2019). These outbreaks have been linked to travellers who brought measles back from Ukraine, Israel, and the Philippines, where large outbreaks were occurring in 2019. Fortunately, Canada continues to have a low rate of reported cases of vaccine preventable diseases (Fig. 11.2).

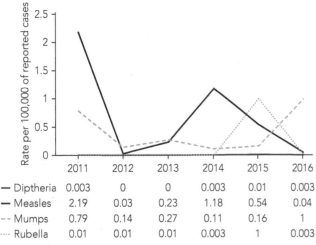

	2011	2012	2013	2014	2015	2016
— Diptheria	0.003	0	0	0.003	0.01	0.003
— Measles	2.19	0.03	0.23	1.18	0.54	0.04
-- Mumps	0.79	0.14	0.27	0.11	0.16	1
.... Rubella	0.01	0.01	0.01	0.003	1	0.003

Fig. 11.2 Reported Cases of Vaccine Preventable Disease in Canada: 2011–2016. (From Canadian Notifiable Diseases Surveillance System [CNDSS], Public Health Agency of Canada [PHAC]. [2018]. *Reported cases from 1924–2016 in Canada—Notifiable diseases on-line.* https://diseases.canada.ca/notifiable/charts?c=pl)

One of the factors that can have a negative impact on the uptake rates of early childhood immunizations is **vaccine hesitancy,** which is a delay in obtaining vaccines or refusal to get vaccinated despite the availability of vaccination services (Strategic Advisory Group of Experts on Immunizations [SAGE], 2014). Vaccine hesitancy is often specific to the vaccine, and varies by time and place, and from production to the arm. CHNs use communication and intervention strategies to address parental and client concerns about safety, risks, fear of needles or other issues. The Canadian Paediatric Society provides up-to-date and accurate information for CHNs, parents, and clients on the risks and responsibilities of vaccinations (https://caringforkids.cps.ca).

In 2015, the Canadian Childhood National Immunization Survey showed that by the age of two years 89% of Canadian children had received the measles vaccine and 77% had received the diphtheria, pertussis, and tetanus vaccines (Statistics Canada, 2017). Although Canada has a publicly funded vaccination program, the national uptake rate of childhood immunizations is only 84% as compared to Finland at 95% (MacDonald, 2016). Vaccine hesitancy is an important issue that needs to be addressed by CHNs to avoid outbreaks of vaccine-preventable diseases. One way for CHNs to address vaccine hesitancy is by promoting routine childhood immunizations and providing education on the risks and benefits of vaccines.

The routine immunization schedules for Canadians are presented in Appendix E-4 "Canadian Required Immunization Schedule" on the Evolve website. These schedules provide Canadian immunization guidelines; however, variations occur within provinces and territories. For further information on the administration of vaccines and the latest immunization schedules, see the PHAC "National Advisory Committee on Immunization" link on the Evolve website. This source provides information on timely medical, scientific, and public health advice pertaining to vaccines and their use in Canada, as well as a link to the latest *Canadian Immunization Guide.*

There are several resources in Appendix E-5 "Infant, Child, and Youth Screening Tools" on the Evolve website that the CHN can use to assess and screen children and youth: "Accident Prevention in Children," "Screening for Common Orthopedic Problems," "Vision and Hearing Screening Procedures," "Development Characteristics: Summary for Children," "Development Behaviours: Summary for School-Age Children," and "Tanner Stages of Puberty."

For information on priority areas for action regarding children and youth, see the PHAC link *The Chief Public Health Officer's Report on the State of Public Health in* Canada 2009: *Growing Up Well—Priorities for a Healthy Future* on the Evolve website. Specifically, Chapter 6 of the report provides information on the following four priority areas for action: "better data and information; improved and ongoing education and awareness; healthy and supportive environments; and coordinated, multi-pronged and sustained strategies" (PHAC, 2009b, p. 70).

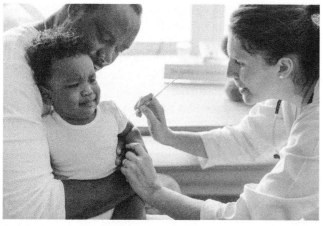

An infant receives a regularly scheduled immunization. (iStockphoto/ Rawpixel)

ADULT HEALTH

Increases in adult overweight and obesity are major public health concerns in Canada and other developed countries. Lifestyle practices such as a sedentary lifestyle, smoking, and alcohol use place these adults at increased risk for type 2 diabetes, hypertension, certain cancers, and cardiovascular diseases due to dyslipidemia. Preventive community health nursing strategies directed at aggregates, populations, communities, and individuals are needed to address the increase in unhealthy lifestyle practices.

Women's Health

To understand women's health issues, one must first understand the term *women's health*. **Women's health** addresses health promotion, health protection, disease prevention, and health maintenance in women. This term recognizes that the health of women is holistic and is related to the biological, psychosocial, spiritual, and cultural dimensions of women's lives. Moreover, women's normal life events or rites of passage, such as menstruation, childbirth, and menopause, are considered part of normal female development rather than syndromes or diseases requiring medical treatment only. This broad emphasis on women's health is in contrast to the view of women solely in relation to their reproductive health or their role in parenting children.

Unfortunately, millions of people, particularly women, do not have access to basic health-related resources. In most countries, women live longer than men, but women are generally less healthy. This gender difference in health is often related to poverty, and helping poor women helps poor children. When children are poor, it is usually because their mother is poor. The number of lone-parent families is on the rise in Canada, and 80% of all lone parent families are headed by women (Canadian Women's Association, 2015). Worldwide, the education of women is the single most important factor in the improvement of the health of women and their families. When women are educated, their socioeconomic status improves and mortality rates decline. Because women's financial stability is closely linked to health outcomes, it is essential to promote policies that support the advancement of women. Because CHNs are visible and involved in the community with individual and groups of women, there are many opportunities to provide women with the knowledge and skills to take charge of their own health. For example, CHNs can influence women through their assessments, educate women about primary prevention strategies, and advocate for policy change through their professional associations and other avenues.

Breast Self-Examination

In 2011, the Canadian Task Force on Preventive Health Care recommended new breast cancer screening guidelines that include no routine mammography screening for women aged 40 to 49 years and screening every 2 to 3 years for women aged 50 to 74. The guidelines also recommended against routine clinical breast self-exam (BSE) and breast self-examination in asymptomatic women (Canadian Medical Association Journal [CMAJ], 2011). Systematic reviews and meta-analysis in the literature support the task-force decision that there is no evidence to support performing routine BSE and there is good evidence that exists to show that harm could occur. The harm referred to for some women is the result of having a false-positive test, the breast biopsy procedure, or the emotional response when a lump is found and there is a need for additional testing (CMAJ, 2011).

Despite this debate on self-exams, the National Breast Cancer Foundation recommends that women have an annual clinical breast exam by a family physician or gynecologist, as well as conduct a monthly BSE. Refer to the Canadian Cancer Society website listed in the Tool Box on the Evolve website for information on the recommended screening guidelines and the technique for BSE. CHNs can help women learn the correct technique for BSE and help them understand what to look for when conducting a BSE. Clients should know how, when, and why to do BSE and what are the expected normal findings and early signs of cancer. They must also understand the importance of reporting any changes or concerns immediately. Often, the CHN has the skills to do this teaching; however, referrals can be made to family physicians or breast screening programs in communities.

Reproductive Issues

Women often use health care services for reproductive issues or problems, and CHNs are often the health care providers they encounter. CHNs are in a unique position to advocate for policies that increase women's access to services for reproductive health. In addition, many CHNs discuss contraception with women of child-bearing age. Contraceptive counselling requires accurate knowledge of current contraceptive choices and a nonjudgemental approach. The goal of contraceptive counselling is to ensure that women have appropriate instruction to make informed choices about reproduction. The choice of method depends on many factors, including the woman's health, frequency of sexual activity, number of partners, and plans to have children.

CHNs must not assume that all women are fully informed about contraception and that a method is used correctly and consistently. Unintended pregnancies can occur among adolescents as well as women. The CHN needs to consider many factors when planning for contraceptive assessment and education. Some of these factors are culture, health status, socioeconomic status, and client literacy. Preconception counselling addresses risks before conception and includes education, assessment, diagnosis, and interventions. The purpose is to reduce or eliminate health risks for women and infants.

Another concern critical to preconception awareness is exposure to health-endangering substances, including alcohol. A major preventable cause of birth defects, intellectual disability, and neurodevelopmental health disorders is fetal exposure to alcohol during pregnancy. Community health nursing interventions need to address substance use. They also need to address other factors that can affect well-being, such as nutrition, physical activity, environmental exposures, and intimate-partner violence.

Related to women's reproductive health is access to prenatal care. For many women, barriers to prenatal care include:
- Lack of transportation
- Difficulty accessing the health care system
- Lack of child care

CHNs can serve as advocates not only to encourage their clients to use prenatal care services but also to work toward the establishment of services that are available, accessible, and affordable to all pregnant women. CHNs also need to be able to respond to clients who may be experiencing fertility issues. Smaller communities often do not have fertility experts, and women may need to travel for specialized care. The CHN needs to consider how to support women experiencing fertility issues through individual counselling sessions or the establishment of community self-help support groups.

Menopause

Another developmental phase for women is **menopause,** also referred to as *the change* or *change of life,* the time when the levels of the hormones estrogen and progesterone change in a woman's body. Women's attitudes toward menopause vary greatly and are influenced by culture, age, support, and the recounted experiences of other women. Menopause has been viewed on a continuum from a normal progression of aging, to a disease state, a time of imbalance, or ill health.

Hormone replacement therapy (HRT) was approved by Health Canada for the relief of some of the menopausal symptoms experienced by women (Health Canada, 2006a). Many women started taking these medications, and the benefits were remarkable for the majority. Most women continued HRT for several years, some up to 20 years. Some early research studies suggested that HRT had the added value of heart protection and the prevention of osteoporosis. However, a longitudinal study (1991 to 2004) by the Women's Health Initiative in the United States concluded that HRT provides no benefit of heart protection (Health Canada, 2006a). The study results led to changes in the use of HRT; for example, in

Canada, HRT with combined estrogen and progestin is now recommended only in specific individual client situations. The decision to use HRT in postmenopausal women is based on consideration of benefits versus harm, and HRT is aimed at improving quality of life using the lowest possible effective dosage in the short term (Health Canada, 2006a). Some study findings have suggested a possible increase in mild cognitive impairment and dementia in some women over 65 years of age taking the combined HRT of estrogen and progestin (Health Canada, 2006a). This possible outcome continues to be monitored.

With the change in hormones during menopause, women are at risk for bone mass and tissue deterioration, which can lead to osteoporosis. Approximately 11.9% of Canadians 40 years and older were living with diagnosed osterporosis in 2015-2016 (PHAC, 2021). Measures that can significantly reduce osteoporosis in the future are for children, youth, and young adults to eat foods high in calcium, to take vitamin D, to be physically active with weight-bearing exercises and involvement in sports, and to avoid smoking and excessive intake of caffeine and alcohol (Osteoporosis Canada, 2010).

Primary osteoporosis-prevention activities aimed at women need to include:
- Diets rich in calcium and vitamin D
- Exposure to sunlight for 20 minutes a day, recommended as an alternative source of vitamin D
- Daily intake of vitamin D based on age
- Exercise, especially weight-bearing activities such as walking, running, stair climbing, and weightlifting, to improve bone density.

Osteoporosis Canada developed "Osteoporosis Canada's 10-Year Fracture Risk Assessment Tool," an app for Apple devices that helps health care providers calculate a client's 10-year risk of fracture and includes treatment and management recommendations for osteoporosis (see the link in the Tool Box on the Evolve website).

Heart Disease

Once considered a disease of men, heart disease is now the second leading cause of death for women (and men) aged 45–65 years in Canada, and is in the top five causes of death for women aged 20–44 years, although mortality rates for women are consistently lower than for men (Bushnik, 2016). In 2013/2014, an estimated 230 000 women aged 20–64 reported that they had been diagnosed with heart disease by a health care professional. Factors that may be contributing to this include:
- women aged 20–39 had a six-fold increase in their obesity rate from 1981 to 2013 (4% to 24%), while women aged 40–59 had a twofold increase (13% to 29%),
- fitness levels of younger and middle-aged women have continued to decline during the past three decades,
- despite improvements in hypertension awareness and control over the past 20 years, older women are significantly less likely than older men to have their blood pressure controlled with antihypertensive medication (Bushnik, 2016).

Women not only wait longer than men to go to an emergency department but may also have a different clinical presentation for myocardial infarction. Both genders may present with chest pain (Health Canada, 2006b; Heart & Stroke Foundation, 2007); however, women may be more vague in describing their pain, and women more often present with nonspecific chest pain and atypical symptoms than men (Heart & Stroke Foundation, 2007). Also, compared with men, women may experience symptoms such as nausea, back pain, and indigestion (Health Canada, 2006b). Other symptoms specific to women are fatigue, sleep disturbance, and weakness (McSweeney, Cody, O'Sullivan, et al., 2003; University of Michigan, 2008).

Many factors predispose women to CVD. Factors that are thought to contribute to the development of CVD in women include (Edwards, 2012):

- Smoking
- Elevated triglyceride levels (>200 mg/dL)
- Low levels of high-density lipoprotein (HDL) cholesterol (<50 mg/dL)
- Hormonal alterations—low estrogen levels, elevated testosterone levels
- Inflammation as manifested by elevated high-sensitivity C-reactive protein (hs-CRP)
- Type 2 diabetes
- Abdominal obesity waist circumference >35 inches "apple shape"
- Hypertension
- Diets high in fat and low in fibre
- Physical inactivity
- Family history

Sociocultural factors have a significant influence on women and heart disease. A lower socioeconomic status correlates with low levels of knowledge and understanding about health, limited health maintenance and preventive care, and decreased access to care.

The key to addressing the alarming epidemic of heart disease is education aimed at certain populations and focusing on risk-factor modification, such as diet, smoking, physical activity, and stress management. CHNs can partner with communities to promote heart health initiatives. Community heart health initiatives need to address all income levels with a focus on the determinants of health, such as unemployment and education. As well, communities need to provide supportive environments such as walking paths. Public policies dealing with health should be initiated. CHNs need to be aware that heart disease is a health concern not just for men. Dissemination of information about the various factors that influence the development of CVD can be accomplished through prevention and outreach activities. Intervention efforts should reflect the diversity of age, environment, and ethnicity in the community. CHNs can also do a careful family history assessment, which can highlight situations that might place an individual at a higher level of risk. CHNs can initiate the development of heart health programs for groups. Group education programs for high-risk individuals save money, reach greater numbers with time savings, and have the benefit of sharing experiences among group members that might allay fears and provide support.

Diabetes Mellitus

In 2017 approximately 2.3 million Canadian adults, or 7.3% of the population reported being diagnosed with diabetes mellitus, but those proportions were higher than the national average in New Brunswick (9.5%) and Ontario (8.0%). Canadian females (6.3%) were less likely than males (8.4%) to report they had diabetes (PHAC, 2018). Ninety percent of all adults with diabetes have type 2, while among children and youth the majority have type 1. Obesity and physical inactivity increase the risk of onset of type 2 diabetes mellitus and also affect the progression of this disease. Preventing or managing obesity and increasing physical activity can prevent or delay the onset of type 2 diabetes. Although type 1 diabetes is not preventable, it can be controlled (PHAC, 2018).

Social, environmental, and behavioural factors have resulted in inequalities in the prevalence of diabetes mellitus between Indigenous and non-Indigenous adults in Canada. The prevalence of diabetes in Indigenous adults living off reserve is 1.9 times higher than among non-Indigenous adults (PHAC, 2018). The inequalities experienced by igenous people in Canada is linked to factors such as the loss of Indigenous culture and language, as well as the unaddressed intergenerational trauma resulting from colonial policies and practices. Inequalities in diabetes could be at least partially addressed by improving those factors that perpetuate the inequalities, including low income, lack of employment, poor working conditions, and preventive services (PHAC, 2018).

Based on a higher prevalence of diabetes in the Indigenous population, the impact of diabetes on the health of current and future generations of Indigenous people is of concern. In response to the high rates of diabetes and its risk factors in Indigenous populations, the Canadian government launched the Aboriginal Diabetes Initiative (ADI) in 1999, as part of the Canadian Diabetes Strategy. ADI is a community-based initiative designed for children, youth, parents, and families that includes plans to improve access to healthy foods, including traditional foods, and enhanced training for home and community care nurses on clinical practice guidelines. Unfortunately, the third phase of ADI ended in 2015, but the website resources remain available (see https://www.fnha.ca/Documents/ADI_Resources.pdf) and can be used by CHNs to design diabetes education programs with Indigenous populations (see the Health Canada "First Nations, Inuit and Aboriginal Health: Diabetes" link on the Evolve website).

In the general population, risk factors for diabetes mellitus are more prevalent in women than in men (PHAC and Canadian Institute for Health Information, 2011). Risk factors include low socioeconomic status, less formal education, smoking, decreased physical activity, pregnancy, and being overweight (Diabetes Canada, 2018). Diabetes is a potentially debilitating disease and, if not properly controlled, can lead to life-long health concerns. One example of a program designed to help pregnant women control gestational diabetes is the Canadian Diabetes Association's Ontario Monitoring for Health Program, which provides funding for the supplies needed for the treatment of diabetes including needles, lancets, and blood glucose meters (the link is on the Evolve website). Such programs can help to address the health needs of women living with diabetes and promote their health and well-being.

Gestational diabetes mellitus (GDM) is a condition characterized by a carbohydrate intolerance that is first identified or first develops during pregnancy. Recent data shows that a higher proportion of women are diagnosed with gestational diabetes in First Nations (4.8%), Inuit (4.0%), and Métis (2.2%) populations as compared with the non-Indigenous population (0.5%) (PHAC and Canadian Institute for Health Information, 2011). When a mother has diabetes, the birth weight of her newborn is very likely to be high (Reading, 2009). For those children, obesity can lead to diabetes in later life. As well, maternal obesity may be a factor in determining a child's obesity (Boney, Verma, Tucker, et al., 2005).

Community and government interventions are needed to address the health disparities that exist for women who are at risk for developing diabetes, if their health is to be improved. CHNs can become advocates for change as they initiate the development of community programs that promote women's health in general and, more specifically, programs to prevent complications from gestational diabetes. Nutrition education programs that target Indigenous women should consider the impact of traditional diets on diabetes and incorporate appropriate content. CHNs are in a position to have a positive effect on the lives of women who are living with diabetes and thus reduce the burden of this disease.

CHNs can take preventive measures when caring for women at risk for developing diabetes, such as assessing for a history of GDM in women, especially Indigenous women. Focusing on family history as well as personal health history provides an opportunity for the CHN to identify those at high risk. Primary prevention activities include interventions aimed at educating women about diabetes, nutrition, and the risks of obesity, smoking, and physical inactivity. Community interventions that address healthy eating, exercise, and weight reduction benefit women who are at risk for diabetes. Screening for diabetes is an example of secondary prevention. Screening activities include a finger-stick blood glucose test or a full glucose-tolerance test. Screening is also accomplished through a thorough history-taking and physical examination. CHNs need to be well versed in understanding the health disparities among women to target those at greater risk. Tertiary prevention includes activities that are aimed at reducing the complications of the disease process. Examples of tertiary prevention for women with diabetes include intense monitoring of blood glucose levels, modification of diet and medications as indicated, and efforts to prevent long-term complications. As noted, Indigenous women are at a high risk for developing diabetes, and CHNs must be aware of the need for cross-cultural communication when caring for Indigenous populations (see the "Evidence-Informed Practice" box).

EVIDENCE-INFORMED PRACTICE

Diabetes is more common among Indigenous people than it is among the general population. A qualitative research study by Bird, Wiles, Okalik, et al. (2008) focused on the experiences and perceptions of Inuit participants who live with diabetes. A case-study approach was undertaken, with four in-depth interviews, field observations, and informal interviews. Data were transcribed and analyzed using a holistic thematic analysis and open coding. Participants described accessibility issues related to the inability to obtain healthy foods and health services. Language interpretation was also an issue. The importance of cross-cultural communication was predominant in the findings, as were issues related to trust and rapport when diabetes care was discussed. Findings suggested a paucity of health education and services in Inuit communities. The importance of including the voices of Inuit people when providing and directing diabetes education and health services delivery was stressed.

Application for CHNs

Partnering with clients is extremely important as a CHN, and this article reinforces how essential this undertaking is when working with clients with diabetes. For clients residing in rural and remote areas, a lack of healthy and affordable foods is a barrier to healthy eating as a diabetic. Cross-cultural communication, cultural differences, and a lack of health services can present challenges for CHNs in their nursing practice.

Questions for Reflection and Discussion

1. What questions might you ask a person who lives in a rural and remote community about their experience living with diabetes?
2. How does this research study relate to what you have read about rural and remote community health nursing practice?
3. What key terms would you use to find the latest evidence on cross-cultural competence in Inuit communities?

Source: Bird, S., Wiles, J., Okalik, L., et al. (2008). Living with diabetes on Baffin Island: Inuit storytellers share their experiences. *Canadian Journal of Public Health, 99*(1), 17–21.

For further information on diabetes, see the Diabetes Canada's *2018 Clinical Practice Guidelines for the Prevention and Management of Diabetes in Canada* (see the link on the Evolve website). It provides professional guidelines for all aspects of management of diabetes. A second document worth exploring is the PHAC's *Diabetes in Canada: Facts and Figures from a Public Health* Perspective 2011 (see the link on the Evolve website). It provides extensive data on age-standardized statistical findings from Canada's national diabetes surveillance system; these data include prevalence and incidence rates, hospitalizations, and mortality related to diabetes.

Mental Illness

CHNs who view health holistically recognize that mental health is as important as physical health in the daily functioning of all individual clients. Individual clients who have physical illnesses often develop mental health problems as they endeavour to cope with their physical health challenges, and those who have mental health problems may also experience physical health challenges. Mental illness occurs when a person has changes in thinking, mood, or behaviour that result in impaired functioning or difficulty coping over a period of time. Although both men and women suffer from mental illness, women experience certain conditions more often than men.

🌐 CULTURAL CONSIDERATIONS

Caregiving Patterns and Toxic Stress in Children

Maternal care giving patterns, such as acquiring the behaviours and values of an ethnic group, can help to protect young children from the negative consequences of toxic stress. Condon, Holland, Slade, and colleagues (2017) conducted a cross-sectional study to examine the relationships among maternal caregiving patterns and children's toxic stress response in a multiethnic, urban sample of maternal-child dyads (n=54). Toxic stress is the result of persistent exposure to stress, causing significant physiological disruptions including a prolonged activation of the body's stress response. Participants self-identified as Black (46.3%), Hispanic (46.3%), and mixed (7.4%). Data were collected from participants on caregiving patterns, including racial socialization (acquiring the behaviours, perceptions, values, and attitudes of an ethic group), parental behaviours, and indicators of toxic stress in the children (e.g., systolic blood pressure, salivary interleukin-6, and seasonal allergies). Findings show that higher (more positive) maternal racial socialization was associated with lower child systolic blood pressure and lower odds of childhood seasonal allergies. These findings suggest that positive maternal racial socialization behaviours could be protective against the negative consequences of toxic stress in young children. Future research should explore the causal relationship between caregiver patterns and indicators of toxic stress in young children. These findings could help CHNs plan interventions to help families promote health and address the negative consequences of toxic stress in young children.

Questions to Consider
1. What are "ethnic behaviours"?
2. How can CHNs promote positive maternal caregiving patterns?

Source: Condon, E., Holland, M., Slade, A., et al. (2017). The influence of maternal caregiving practices on indicators of toxic stress in children. *Journal of Pediatric Health, 32*(4), 330. doi:10.1016/j.pedhc.2018.04.012

Depression is a particularly serious health concern for women. A number of factors contribute to depression in women; possible contributors being researched are biological factors, including genetics and gonadal (sex) hormones, and psychosocial factors such as life stress, trauma, and interpersonal relationships. Risk factors for depression include being female, having a family history of depression, being unemployed, and having a chronic illness. CHNs can encourage health care providers in their communities to screen and treat depression among women and to work for the development of other services that decrease stress and generally improve the mental well-being of women.

The PHAC's *Report from the Canadian Chronic Disease Surveillance System: Mental Illness in* Canada, 2015 is the first national report of its kind to present administrative data and data on adolescents under the age of 15 years (PHAC, 2015b). It provides statistics and information on various forms of mental illness and additional information, such as hospitalization rates. The report shows that Canadian women are more likely than men to use mental health services, especially those who are 25 to 39 years old (see the link on the Evolve website). WHO's *Mental Health: New Understandings, New Hope* discusses socioeconomic factors, demographic factors, family environment, the presence of major physical diseases, and serious threats as factors affecting mental health (see the link on the Evolve website).

Cancer

A diagnosis of cancer is a life-changing event and is considered a life transition. Upon diagnosis, a woman is confronted with many decisions that often leave her feeling overwhelmed and out of control (in crisis). Cancer is the leading cause of death in Canada, and breast cancer is the most common cause of death from cancer in women. The incidence rate for all cancers combined is on the increase in Canadian women, and this increase is partly explained by the rise in incidence rates for melanoma, thyroid, uterine, and liver cancer (Canadian Cancer Society's Advisory Committee on Cancer Statistics, 2014). Although women suffer from other cancers, such as lung, pancreatic, and ovarian cancer, and non-Hodgkin's lymphoma, this section will address the three leading causes of death from cancer: lung, breast, and colorectal cancer. Cervical cancer and the role of the CHN in screening will also be discussed.

Lung cancer is the leading cause of death for both sexes in Canada, but from 2001 to 2010, the overall age-standardized incidence rates for women rose by 0.5%. Tobacco consumption in women began to drop in the mid-1980s and since 2006, lung cancer incidence rates for women are no longer increasing (Canadian Cancer Society's Advisory Committee on Cancer Statistics, 2014). Health public policies that ban smoking in public places and primary prevention measures, including smoking cessation and prevention programs, are key initiatives that have helped to reduce tobacco consumption in both men and women.

Breast cancer is the second leading cause of cancer deaths among Canadian women (Canadian Cancer Society, 2019a), and this type of cancer has had screening programs devoted to its detection. Screening activities (the secondary level of prevention) include mammography and breast examination by a health care provider. Early detection may mean cure, whereas late detection often means a limited prognosis.

Colorectal cancer is the third leading cause of cancer deaths among Canadian women (Brenner, D. et al. 2020). Primary prevention and early detection are the keys to surviving colorectal cancer. CHNs can inform women of their risks, the signs and symptoms to be aware of, and screening opportunities in their communities.

Cervical cancer is another common cancer diagnosis for Canadian women. However, mortality and incidence rates for cervical cancer decreased between 2001 and 2010, largely due to Pap test screening (Canadian Cancer Society, 2019b). Common risk factors for cervical cancer are inadequate screening, multiple sexual partners, smoking, the sexual behaviour of a male partner(s), a young age at first intercourse, infection with human papillomavirus (HPV), a weakened immune system, multiple births, and long-term use of birth control pills (Canadian Cancer Society, 2019b). For further information on the prevention of cervical cancer, see the PHAC "Cervical Cancer" link on the Evolve website, which provides information on the incidence, risk factors, and management of cervical cancer in Canada.

Obesity

The prevalence of obesity in both women and men generally increases up to age 65 years, after which the prevalence starts to decline. Based on self-reported heights and weights, obesity was more prevalent in Canadian men than women in 2007/2008, and even more prevalent in Indigenous women than non-Indigenous women (PHAC & CIHI, 2011). Obesity is a major health concern because it is linked to the development of diabetes mellitus, hypertension, CVD, and other medical problems. The CHN can provide education about the risks to health from overweight and obesity. The educational offerings can be fashioned after a community health model, using the levels of prevention to establish effective interventions for women at risk for weight-control issues.

Because obesity in women is such a stigma in Western culture, women are at high risk for suffering adverse social and psychological consequences of obesity. Even as children, women begin to fear obesity. The consequences of obesity can also include social and financial discrimination. More women enter weight-loss programs for their perceived loss of attractiveness than for health concerns. In today's North American culture, being thin is often identified with competence, success, control, power, and sexual attractiveness. The culture's focus on and preoccupation with a woman's thinness and physical shape can be seen in the media and the entertainment industry, where beauty is equated with very thin women. These idealistic and often unrealistic images can perpetuate women's dissatisfaction and preoccupation with their bodies.

CHNs are in a key position to include assessment for eating disorders and referral for treatment into their routine clinical practices. Included in this assessment would be an abdominal girth measurement (waist circumference) and waist-to-hip ratio measurement. It is important to note that calculation of body mass index is often replaced with measuring waist circumference to calculate body fat. The goal of the CHN is to identify not only women who have eating disorders but also those women at risk for developing eating disorders. Through a comprehensive physical and psychosocial assessment, as well as a history of dietary practices, the

CHN may be able to identify women with an eating disorder and provide appropriate referrals. CHNs can promote healthy eating habits and regular physical activity as a weight-control strategy. At a population level, CHNs can discourage advertising that promotes exceptionally thin bodies for women. They can also promote exercise and healthy eating programs in their communities.

Men's Health

Men have a lower life expectancy than women and a higher mortality rate (Mikkonen & Raphael, 2010). When compared with women, men show the following differences:

- Men have fewer episodes of chronic illnesses
- Men are more prone to accidents
- Men experience more extreme forms of social exclusion, such as homelessness and substance abuse
- Men have a suicide rate that is four times greater
- Men are more often perpetrators of robbery and physical assault
- Men are more prone to engage in antisocial behaviour and criminal offences (particularly disadvantaged young males) (Mikkonen & Raphael, 2010)

Moreover, men's health is sometimes negatively affected by unhealthy ideas of masculinity that favours aggressiveness, dominance, and excessive self-reliance (Mikkonen & Raphael, 2010).

Although men and women have similar ideas about health, there are some distinct differences. Most people view health as being closely associated with well-being. Both men and women define *health* comprehensively and refer to it as a state or condition of well-being, and they often relate this condition to capacity, performance, and function. In some cultures, men's health values can influence individual health behaviours ("Cultural Considerations" box). See the Canadian Institutes of Health Research (CIHR) document *Gender and Sex-Based Analysis in Health Research: A Guide for CIHR Researchers and Reviewers* (see the link on the Evolve website) for some of the research based on sex and gender, specifically men's health.

CULTURAL CONSIDERATIONS

South Asian Men's View of Physical Activity
An ethnographic, qualitative study determined that traditional South Asian cultural values influenced older immigrant men's preference for walking to socially connect with other men as compared with participating in strenuous exercise together. Participants associated strenuous exercise with paid labour.

Question to Consider
How would the CHN use this cultural consideration to plan a population health intervention to target physical activity in older South Asian immigrant men?

Source: Oliffe, J., Grewal, S., Bottorff, J., et al. (2009). Connecting masculinities and physical activity among senior South Asian Canadian immigrant men. *Critical Public Health, 19*(3/4), 383–397. doi:10.1080/09581590902951605.

Men often engage in compensatory, aggressive, and risk-taking behaviour predisposing them to illness, injury, and even death. Men tend to avoid medical help as long as possible, leading to serious health problems. A preventive focus is wise because men have been identified as a high-risk group.

Men need to openly express their health concerns. Health care providers can help men explore their concerns by encouraging them to discuss nonhealth problems as well as health problems and by promoting preventive health care. Although some men are apprehensive about discussing health concerns with professionals, strategies can be used to reduce men's anxiety. CHNs can remove physical barriers separating themselves from the client, use handouts and other written information to support verbal instructions, and show a genuine interest in men's needs.

There have been significant gains in global life expectancy at birth in recent years, with an increase of 3 years between 2010 and 2015, from 67 to 70 years (United Nations, Department of Economic and Social Affairs, Population Division, 2015). Table 11.4 lists life expectancies for men and women in selected countries. Accidents, homicides and other violence, cancers, circulatory system diseases, and infectious and parasitic diseases account for most deaths in developed countries. See Table 11.5 for facts on cancer in Canada.

Testicular cancer is a commonly found solid tumour malignancy that most often occurs in men 15 to 35 years of age. The etiology of this cancer, the testicular germ cell, is unknown. Many possible explanations exist:

- Age
- Family history
- Endocrine problems
- Genetic disorders
- Human immunodeficiency virus
- Cryptorchidism
- Occupational factors

The most common presenting symptom is a painless, firm scrotal mass or swelling that is accidentally discovered. Low back pain may result, with retroperitoneal lymph node involvement. The CHN needs to teach men who are at risk for testicular cancer a preventive strategy as part of a comprehensive testicular educational program. Instructions on how to perform a monthly **testicular self-examination (TSE)** (a self-examination of the testicles to assess for any unusual lumps or bumps) are provided in Fig. 11.3 and in Box 11.5. A program may consist of audiovisual aids and pamphlets followed by step-by-step procedures and return demonstrations. These approaches lead to increased frequency of TSE and enhanced comfort levels of the men performing the procedure. If tumours are found, the most common form of

TABLE 11.4 Life Expectancies at Birth by Sex for Men and Women in Selected Countries, 2018

Country	Men (Years)	Women (Years)	Total
Canada	79.9	84.0	82.0
United Kingdom	79.5	83.1	81.3
United States	76.1	81.1	78.6
Japan	81.1	87.3	84.2
France	79.6	85.6	82.6
Norway	81.0	84.3	82.7
Sweden	80.8	84.1	82.5

Source: Organisation for Economic Cooperation and Development (OEDC). (2018). *Life Expectancy at Birth.* https://data.oecd.org/healthstat/life-expectancy-at-birth.htm

TABLE 11-5 Projected Estimates of New Cases and Age-Standardized Incidence Rates, Canada, 2020

Type of Cancer	No. of New Cases (2020 estimates)	ASIR*
Breast (Most common cancer among Canadian women)		
Females	27,700	66.9
Prostate (Most common cancer among Canadian men)		
Males	23,300	NA
Lung and bronchus		
Females	14,800	59.3
Males	15,000	64.8
Colorectal		
Females	12,000	50.8
Males	14,900	71.5

*ASIR, age-standardized incidence rates

Brenner, D. et al. (2020). Projected estimates of cancer in Canada in 2020. *CMAJ*, 2020;192(9):E199–E205; DOI: https://doi.org/10.1503/cmaj.191292.

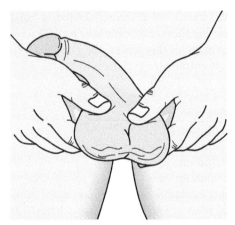

Fig. 11.3 Performing a Testicular Self-Examination.

BOX 11.5   Performing a Step-by-Step Monthly Testicular Self-Examination

1. Perform the testicular self-examination during a warm bath or shower. Be sure your hands are warm.
2. Roll each testicle between your thumb and fingers. Testicles should be egg-shaped, 4 cm, oblong, and similar in size and have a rubbery texture; the left dangles lower than the right.
3. Check the epididymis for softness and slight tenderness.
4. Check the spermatic cord for firm, smooth, tubular structure.

---

management is retroperitoneal lymph node dissection and chemotherapy for metastases larger than 3 cm.

See the Canadian Cancer Society's "Prostate Cancer" link in the Tool Box on the Evolve website for statistics, signs, and symptoms, as well as management of prostate cancer. The Health Canada "Just for You—Men" link on the Evolve website has information pertaining to several health issues for men, such as heart health, mental health, work-life balance, and diseases and conditions.

OLDER PERSONS' HEALTH

The growth of the population aged 65 years and older in Canada has steadily increased since the turn of the century. The Canadian population is aging, with the median age in Canada in 1971 being 26.2 years and in 2011 being 39.9 years. Older persons make up the fastest-growing age group, and by 2051 it is expected that one in every four Canadians will be over the age of 65 years (Statistics Canada, 2010). Currently, many older persons live into their 80s and 90s (Touhy, Jett, Boscart et al., 2019), and an increased number of older persons are reaching 100 years of age. This latter group is referred to as *centenarians*. Since most health care for older persons is now delivered outside of an acute-care setting, CHNs in particular provide nursing care to an increased proportion of the aging population, which involves specialized knowledge, skills, and abilities in gerontology. Furthermore, the increasing proportion of those over 65 years of age will continue, a change that has implications for health promotion

strategies such as creating healthy environments, reorienting health services, and increasing prevention. Also, increasing health care resources, such as skilled home care personnel (Boal & Loengard, 2007) to meet the needs of this aggregate group may prove challenging with the current limited fiscal resources.

Aging, if defined purely from a physiological perspective, has been described as a process of deterioration of body systems. This definition is obviously inadequate to describe the multidimensional aging process in older persons. **Aging** can be more appropriately defined as the total of all changes that occur in a person with the passing of time. Aging starts from the time of birth, not when a person reaches age 65 years. Influences on how one ages come from several domains, including physiological, psychological, sociological, and spiritual processes. The physiological declines associated with aging have been easier to understand than aging as a process of growth and development.

Myths associated with aging have evolved over time. Some common myths are that all older persons are infirm and senile and cannot adapt to change and learn new behaviours or skills. These myths are easily debunked by older persons who run marathons, learn to use the Internet, and are vibrant members of society. **Ageism,** a term coined by Robert Butler in the 1960s, denotes discrimination toward older people because of their age (Millar, 2014; Touhy et al., 2019). Ageism may be obvious or subtle, and it fosters a stereotype that does not allow older persons to be viewed realistically and denies the diversity of aging. It classifies all older persons as being the same (a homogeneous group) and therefore denies the individuality of older persons (a heterogeneous group).

Gerontology is the specialized study of the processes of aging (Beckmann Murray et al., 2006; Meiner & Lueckenotte, 2006), with a focus on what is "normal" and "successful" aging (Millar, 2014). *Geriatrics* is the study of disease in old age. **Gerontological nursing** is the specialty of nursing concerned with assessment of the health and functional statuses of older persons, planning and implementing health care and services to meet the identified needs, and evaluating the effectiveness of such care (Meiner & Lueckenotte, 2006).

A client experiences aging physiologically, psychologically, sociologically, and spiritually. Physiological changes occur in all body systems with the passing of time. How and when these processes occur varies widely among individuals. Moreover, the degree of aging within various body systems in the same individual varies as well. Table 11.6 highlights common physiological changes with the aging of body systems and the nursing implications of these changes. The effect of these physiological changes overall may result in a diminished physiological reserve, a decrease in homeostatic mechanisms, and a decline in immunological response. These changes require adaptation by older persons, but it is also important to recognize that aging is not a disease (Meiner & Lueckenotte, 2006; Touhy et al., 2019). Intellectual capacity does not usually decline with age.

No known intrinsic psychological change occurs with aging. The influences of the environment and culture on

TABLE 11.6 Physiological Age-Related Changes in Body Systems

System	Age-Related Changes	Implications for Nursing
Skin	Thinning of the skin	Skin breakdown and injury
	Atrophy of sweat glands	Increased risk of heat stroke
	Decrease in vascularity	Frequent pruritus, dry skin
Respiratory	Decreased elasticity of lung tissue	Reduced efficiency of ventilation
	Decreased respiratory muscle strength	Atelectasis and infection
Cardiovascular	Decrease in baroreceptor sensitivity	Orthostatic hypotension and falls
	Decrease in number of pacemaker cells	Increased prevalence of dysrhythmias
Gastrointestinal	Dental enamel thins; loss of teeth and presence of caries	Periodontal disease
		Swallowing dysfunction
	Gums recede	Constipation
	Delay in esophageal emptying	
	Decreased muscle tone	
	Altered peristalsis	
Genitourinary	Decreased number of functioning nephrons	Modifications in drug dosing may be required
	Reduced bladder tone and capacity	Incontinence more common
	Prostate enlargement	Possible compromise of urinary function
Neuromuscular	Decrease in muscle mass	Decrease in muscle strength
	Decrease in bone mass	Osteoporosis, increased risk of fracture
Sensory	Loss of neurons and nerve fibres	Altered sensitivity to pain that may pose safety issues
	Decreased visual acuity, depth perception, adaptation to light changes	Hearing loss that may cause limitation in activities
	Loss of auditory neurons	Possible change in food preferences and intake
	Altered taste sensation	
Immune	Decrease in T-cell function	Increased incidence of infection
	Appearance of autoantibodies	Increased prevalence of autoimmune disorders

personal development and maturation are substantial and further limit the ability of the CHN to predict how an individual ages psychologically. Some known and some disputed changes in brain function over time may influence cognition and behaviour. Reaction speed and psychomotor response are somewhat slower, both of which can be related to the neurological changes with aging. This is demonstrated particularly during timed tests of performance in which speed is an influencing variable. It has also been demonstrated in simulated tests of driving skills, where speed of response, perception, and attention slow with age. Typically, older individuals can learn and perform as well as younger individuals, although they may be slower, and it may take them longer to accomplish a specific task. It is therefore important for CHNs to consider these changes when providing education programs to older persons.

Intellectual capacity does not normally decline with age as was previously thought. An age-associated memory impairment, benign senescent forgetfulness, involves very minor memory loss. This is not progressive and does not cause dysfunction in daily living. Reassurance by formal caregivers such as CHNs is important for the older person and families since anxiety often exacerbates the problem of mild memory impairment. Memory aids (e.g., mnemonics, signs, and notes) may help the older person compensate for this type of impairment.

The later years for many older persons mark a period of changing social dynamics. Social networks provide the structure for social support. Most older people continue to respond to life situations as they did earlier in their lives. Aging does not bring about radical changes in beliefs and values. How individuals stay involved in activities and with people who bring their lives meaning and support is a major factor that can contribute to ongoing health and vitality.

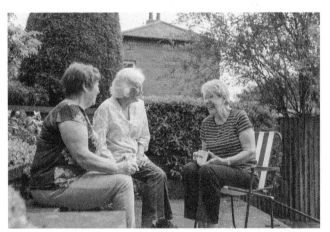

Older adults may be at an increased risk for depression and should be encouraged to participate in social experiences. (iStockphoto/SolStock)

As older persons adapt and cope with the challenge of aging, especially the successive losses and changes that occur for many, an increased spiritual awareness and consciousness can occur (Touhy et al., 2019). *Spirituality* refers to the need to transcend physical, psychological, and social identities to experience love, hope, and meaning in life, and it is more than religion. Having a purpose in life, religious affiliations, and religious rituals are aspects of spirituality that can include other activities and relationships. Caring for pets and plants or experiencing nature through a walk outdoors can also foster spiritual growth. Physical and functional impairments and fear of death may challenge one's spiritual integrity. Having a strong sense of spirituality enables individuals who are physically and functionally dependent on others to avoid despair by appreciating that they are still capable of giving and deserving of receiving love, respect, and dignity.

The Role of the Community Health Nurse in Caring for Older Persons

CHNs are pivotal to older persons having access to health care services. It is important to build relationships in a caring manner. Once that relationship is developed, the CHN can work with the individual and family to promote the health of the older person, to initiate actions to prevent disease, to facilitate access to community resources, and in many cases to provide palliation ("Ethical Considerations" box). The Canadian Community Health Nursing Standard of Practice 4, "Professional Relationships," notes the principle of connecting with others to promote maximum participation and self-determination and provides the CHN with communication strategies for building relationships such as face-to-face, telephone, group, print, or electronic methods (Appendix 1).

ETHICAL CONSIDERATIONS

An older person who has been diagnosed with final-stage lung cancer asks the CHN whether she should go to the palliative-care unit "when my time is near" or die at home. She appears to wish to die at home, even if it might require her to spend her own money to do it. Her family members have said that they would prefer that she go to the palliative-care unit.

Ethical principles that apply to this scenario are:

- *Promoting and respecting informed decision-making (CNA Code of Ethics).* According to this primary value, CHNs recognize and promote a person's right to be informed and involved in decision making about his or her health. Therefore, CHNs value the giving of health information to clients in their care in an open, accurate, and transparent manner.
- *Preserving dignity (CNA Code of Ethics).* This primary value requires that CHNs relate to all persons with respect and, during decision making, take into account their unique values, beliefs, and social and economic circumstances.
- *Distributive justice.* If the decision is for the client to die at home, are the necessary resources accessible in her community to support her and her family?

Questions to Consider

1. What information can the CHN provide to the client and her family that might help them reach a decision together?
2. The client asks the CHN to explain the differences between the three acronyms CPR, DNAR, as well as AND so that she can make an informed decision. What are the ethical principles to consider in these three end-of-life decisions?

Health care in general is oriented toward acute illness. Chronic illness requires a shift in perspective compared with the rapid onset and focus on curing an acute problem. In chronic illness, cure is not expected, so community health nursing activities need to be more holistic, addressing function, wellness, and psychosocial issues. With chronic illness, the focus is on *healing* (a unique process resulting in a shift in the body, mind, and spirit system) rather than *curing* (elimination of the signs and symptoms of disease).

Chronic illnesses occur over a long period with occasional acute exacerbations and remissions. They can affect several systems and be discouraging because of symptoms such as persistent pain and also because of losses in functioning, and often, social interactions. The prevalence of chronic illness rises with the lengthening of the lifespan and highly technical medical care. Not only do chronic illnesses cause disability and activity restriction, they also often require frequent hospitalizations for exacerbations.

Many older persons adjust to the changes associated with aging and actually experience health and wellness with aging. Often, their definitions of health change with aging. Touhy et al. (2019) maintain that even though many older persons experience chronic illnesses, they can experience wellness. It is also noteworthy that not all older persons have a chronic illness. It has become evident that to be effective in the prevention of chronic illnesses and the promotion of health, the focus on education at individual and population levels also requires supportive environments (Touhy et al., 2019). Supportive physical environments are needed to allow older persons to stay physically active and to eat nutritious meals. Supportive social environments—for example, family members, the availability of older person centres, and government pensions based on financial need—are needed to assist older persons in communities.

Touhy et al. (2019) indicate the importance of mobility for older persons and the role the CHN can play in partnership with older persons to restore and maintain wellness. Communities with a commitment to health promotion for older persons provide safe sidewalks for walking, shopping malls for winter walking, and parks with walking trails. Also, communities need to ensure that home services such as Meals on Wheels and outdoor home-maintenance services are available. The CHN might partner with the community for planning these services if they are lacking in the community. CHNs provide education programs to individual and aggregate older persons about the benefits of nutritious eating and physical activity. Health Canada's *Physical Activity Guide to Healthy Active Living for Older Adults* (see the link on the Evolve website) provides information about choices concerning physical activity to promote health and to prevent disease in older persons.

Immobility can be caused by a variety of chronic illnesses, such as degenerative joint disease, osteoporosis, cerebrovascular accidents, Parkinson's disease, and neuromotor disorders (Touhy et al., 2019). Chronic illnesses can result in pain, stiffness, loss of balance, psychological problems, a fear of falling, and falls, all of which may contribute to immobility. Many factors contribute to older persons falling, and several of them can be prevented. For information on falls, see the Registered Nurses' Association of Ontario (RNAO) guideline *Prevention of Falls and Fall Injuries in the Older Adult* (the link is on the Evolve website). The PHAC's *Safe Living Guide* (the link is in the Tool Box on the Evolve website) can be used by CHNs in the home setting to assess the home environment for safety, including risk of falls. CHNs are in a prime position to educate the public, older persons and their caregivers, and aggregates of older persons in the community about fall prevention.

Management of some of the chronic illnesses can be aided by the provision of opportunities for physical activity through community recreational programs such as swimming, water aquatics for older persons, and mall walking. For many older persons, these activities can prevent or at least slow down disabilities from chronic illness. In addition, physical activity can contribute to an improved sense of well-being (Touhy et al., 2019). Also, involvement in these activities encourages independence.

In the management of chronic illness, the focus is on the development of self-management skills. The CHN is in partnership with the client, paying attention to the client's self-concept and self-esteem as well as to the resources that are needed to manage the disease outside the medical system. Goals for care are structured to help clients adjust their day-to-day choices to maintain the highest level of functional ability possible within the limits of their conditions (Millar, 2014; Touhy et al., 2019). The motivation to make the lifestyle changes that are necessary to cope with chronic illness may stem from a fear of death, disability, pain, negative effects on activities of daily living, and family.

Chronic illness can have an impact on an individual's ability to function at the highest possible level of health. For example, urinary incontinence in a client experiencing dementia can complicate nursing care and result in social isolation. The CHN can play a role in partnership with older persons to help restore and maintain wellness by implementing interventions to address urinary incontinence in this population to prevent institutionalization.

Another area of concern for older persons is minor memory loss, or "forgetfulness," that can be due to "normal" aging changes. However, more than a minor loss is possible due to disease processes, and this can interfere with the ability to carry out activities of daily living. New cognitive theories of aging are developing, and the current debate is whether intellectual skills—for example, memory games and other forms of memory training—can enhance cognitive functioning and perhaps even prevent cognitive deterioration (Millar, 2014). A significant memory loss in older persons is likely because of one or more of the **three D**s of intellectual impairment (Touhy et al., 2019):

- *Dementia* (progressive intellectual impairment)
- *Depression* (mood disorder)
- *Delirium* (acute confusion)

Delirium and dementia are often referred to as cognitive impairment. See the RNAO best practice guidelines "Screening for Delirium, Dementia and Depression in the Older Adult" and "Caregiving Strategies for Older Adults with Delirium, Dementia and Depression" (the links are on the Evolve website). These guidelines were developed for nurses who work with older persons experiencing cognitive impairment and their caregivers. These two guidelines differentiate between the three *D*s, provide screening tools for use with older persons, and discuss nursing considerations in caring for these older persons and in working with their caregivers.

For older persons experiencing any of the three *D*s, CHNs need to be aware of the existing community services such as outpatient clinics, daycare services, and self-help groups. If services are lacking and needed in the community, CHNs (based on input from clients) can initiate partnerships in the communities so that these services become available. As well, CHNs can initiate education programs at the aggregate and community levels.

Medication use in older persons is an important consideration for CHNs. The changes that come with aging can alter the pharmacokinetics and pharmacodynamics of medications in older persons and can result in health and safety issues. In addition, many older persons take several prescription and over-the-counter medications for the treatment of their chronic illnesses and are thus at an increased risk for iatrogenic drug reactions (Millar, 2014; Touhy et al., 2019). Nonadherence to prescribed medications is often identified in the literature as a concern with older persons.

CHNs need to assess medication use with older persons and educate this aggregate group as necessary. One strategy is to ask to see the medications that older persons are taking and to discuss with the older persons their understanding of these medications and their pattern of use. If not visiting the older person in their homes, many CHNs use the "brown bag approach"—older persons are asked to bring all their medications (prescription and nonprescription) to the CHN. Together, the CHN and the older person review the medications to determine client knowledge and skill in taking medications, which provides an opportunity for safety issues to be addressed.

One often-overlooked concern of older persons is that of abuse. *Elder abuse* encompasses physical, psychological, financial or material, spiritual, and sexual abuse as well as neglect (Health Canada, 2008). *Abuse* consists of the willful infliction of physical pain or injury, debilitating mental anguish and fear, theft or mismanagement of money or resources, or unreasonable confinement or the deprivation of services. **Neglect** refers to intentionally or unintentionally not providing care or to a lack of services that are necessary for the physical, spiritual, social, and mental health of an older person who is dependent on a caregiver. Older persons can make independent choices with which others may disagree. Their right to self-determination can be taken from them if they are declared incompetent. *Exploitation* is the illegal or improper use of a person or their resources for another's profit or advantage. During the assessment process, CHNs need to be aware of incongruence between injuries and the explanation of their causes, dependency issues between the client and caregiver, and substance abuse by the caregiver. See the Department of Justice Canada's "Elder Abuse Is Wrong" link on the Evolve website.

The majority of older persons live in homes alone, with spouses, or with other family or friends. Female spouses represent the largest group of family caregivers of the older person family caregivers. *Stress, strain,* and *burnout* are words that are used to reflect the negative effects of the family caregiver burden. Issues involve the work itself, past and present relationships, the effect on others, and the caregiver's lifestyle and well-being. For many families, the caregiving experience is a positive, rewarding, and fulfilling one. Community health nursing intervention can facilitate good health for older persons and their caregivers and contribute to meaningful family relationships during this period. Caregiving situations can vary from grandparents caring for grandchildren or other relatives to older person spouses taking care of their partners or their own older parents (Touhy et al., 2019). Older persons are living longer, with many older persons delaying institutionalization, and some family members and friends are assuming the caregiver role at home.

Caregiving roles can be formal (professional or personal care providers) or informal (family and friends). Women are often caregivers, with women who are employed outside the home acting as informal caregivers as often as women who work in the home (Beckmann Murray et al., 2006). Caring for someone in the home, such as someone with Alzheimer's disease, on a continual basis can be very stressful and challenging. Family and friend caregivers are often not health care providers, and the stress they experience may not be recognized. CHNs need to be alert for signs of caregiver stress and assist caregivers to reduce their stress or refer caregivers to community resources for support and assistance in dealing with their stress and their caregiving responsibilities, such as adult daycare services, Meals on Wheels, and respite care in the home and in many institutions. Some signs of caregiver stress are denial, anger, withdrawing socially, anxiety, depression, exhaustion, sleeplessness, emotional reactions, lack of concentration, and health concerns (Alzheimer Society of Canada, 2015). Further information on these signs and ways to reduce caregiver stress is available on the Alzheimer Society of Canada website (the link is on the Evolve website). The information is directed to those who care for people with Alzheimer's disease; however, the signs of stress and the ways to reduce stress are applicable to all caregiver situations. The CHN needs to be familiar with the respite care available in the community and refer caregivers as needed.

There is an abundance of health information and related resources for older persons and health care providers on numerous topics such as health promotion and injury prevention. See the Government of Canada's "Seniors" and the PHAC's "Aging and Seniors" links on the Evolve website.

Resources for Community Health Nurses

CHNs have many resources available to assist them in their many roles and to facilitate and support clients in striving to achieve healthy living throughout the life stages. The RNAO website (see the link on the Evolve website) provides best practice guidelines that direct nurses in their practice with clients. These guidelines include breastfeeding best practice guidelines for nurses, enhancing adolescent development, nursing management of hypertension, prevention of falls and fall injuries in the older person, and supporting and strengthening families through expected and unexpected life events. Many other Web-based resources provide information pertaining to various age groups that is useful to CHNs. Working with individuals and families experiencing life's developmental stages is challenging for any CHN; however, it is also a very rewarding experience as the CHN has the opportunity to influence and facilitate healthy life choices at the micro and macro levels.

When working with all clients, CHNs need to continue to put an emphasis on illness prevention and on promotion of healthy living. Doing so requires maintaining an "upstream" comprehensive approach that considers the influence of the determinants of health and provision of socioenvironmental multilevel strategies that are evidence informed. Healthy living patterns are learned, acquired behaviours; therefore, if the trend of decreasing health is to be reversed, efforts must be directed toward the Canadian population, especially families and children.

👤 STUDENT EXPERIENCE

Early childhood development can be influenced by many factors, including genetics, family structure and relationships, nutrition, education, and the environment. The quality of early environments can affect development and behaviour of children and can have both short- and long-term implications on health. The "Total Environment Assessment Model for Early Child Development" (TEAM-ECD) is one model that illustrates the importance of considering the association between a child's early development and their environments. A WHO report entitled *Total Environment Assessment Model for Early Child Development* presents a research brief on the TEAM-ECD model and explains why it is important to consider environmental effects on early childhood development (see the link on the Evolve website).

Read through the WHO research brief and familiarize yourself with the guiding principles of the model, model components, and model application. Answer the following questions:

1. List and explain how each of the environmental levels identified in the model can support or undermine early child development. Give examples.
2. What is a "nurturant" environment and how can it impact a child's early development?
3. How can the TEAM-ECD model be used to guide outcome measures for health promotion and prevention programs?

CHAPTER SUMMARY

11.1 A healthy lifestyle across the lifespan can reduce the occurrence and outcomes of certain chronic illnesses and therefore contributes to quality of life. A healthy lifestyle is affected by factors such as the determinants of health and societal foci, as well as public policies. A life course approach considers *latent effects,* which relate to biological and developmental events that take place during the fetal or infancy stage that affect health later in life; *pathway effects,* which relate to early life events and environments, especially the social environment, that place an individual on a particular life path that affects health later in life; and *cumulative effects,* which relate to multiple environmental risks experienced at different ages that together increase the risk of disease in adulthood.

11.2 Some of the influences on healthy child development include lack of good nutrition, lack of social support, unintentional injuries and accidents, overweight and obesity, lack of physical activity, and tobacco use.

11.3 The major health issues of children and adolescents include overweight and obesity, insufficient physical activity, poor nutrition, unintentional injuries and accidents, tobacco use, and the need for completed immunizations. CHNs can promote child and adolescent health in the community by providing direct services to children and their families; assessing the needs of children in the community; establishing programs to ensure a healthy environment for children; managing child and adolescent care, health education, and promotion programs; counselling; and advocating for a comprehensive school health approach.

11.4 Gender affects health. Men engage in more risk-taking behaviours than women, such as physical challenges, and they tend to avoid the diagnosis and treatment of illnesses, as compared with women. Men's health issues can include testicular cancer, and they are more prone to injuries. Women's health issues can include breast cancer, and reproductive health issues (e.g., contraception, fertility issues, menopause). Both men and women experience chronic illnesses such as heart disease, cancer, and diabetes.

11.5 The chronic health problems that are often experienced by older adults include heart disease, diabetes, cancer, mobility issues, and urinary incontinence, depression, and dementia. The role of CHNs caring for older persons includes striving to maximize functional status and minimize costs through direct care and appropriate referrals to community resources.

CHN IN PRACTICE: A CASE STUDY

Older Persons' Issues

Sonya, a 79-year-old widow, lives alone in an older persons' high-rise apartment building. Sonya's neighbours and the administrator of the apartment building reported to the CHN who visits residents in the apartment building that no one had been observed coming or going from Sonya's apartment recently. The neighbours reported that when they did see Sonya, she appeared unkempt and did not appear to recognize them.

When the CHN made a visit to the apartment, Sonya answered the door and was very pleasant. The CHN validated the unkempt appearance of both Sonya and the apartment and detected an odour of urine. Sonya was mobile without the use of aids. Sonya was hesitant and unsure in her answers. Her history revealed medical problems. Sonya said that she has a son and daughter-in-law living in the next town who usually phone her at least once a week. Their phone number was taped on a table beside the phone.

Information found in the family assessment was that Sonya's son is an alcoholic, her daughter-in-law has the beginning symptoms of heart disease, and her great-grandchild has asthma and is cared for by Sonya's son and daughter-in-law. Several pill bottles were observed on the kitchen counter, with the names of a local physician and pharmacist.

The CHN noted that both Sonya and her clothes were dirty and that she moved without aids and appeared steady on her feet. The kitchen was littered with unwashed dishes and empty fast-food boxes. Sonya could not recall buying or having the dinners delivered. A billfold with several bills was lying open on the kitchen counter, as well as an uncashed Canada pension cheque.

Think About It

1. What should the CHN do about this situation?
2. What factors make this a difficult situation?

☞ TOOL BOX

The Tool Box contains useful resources that can be applied in community health nursing practice. These related resources are found either in the appendices at the back of this text or on the Evolve website at http://evolve.elsevier.com/Canada/Stanhope/community/.

Appendices

- Appendix 1: Canadian Community Health Nursing Professional Practice Model and Standards of Practice
- Appendix E-4: Canadian Required Immunization Schedule
- Appendix E-5: Infant, Child, and Youth Screening Tools

Tools

Canadian Cancer Society. Prostate Cancer.

This site provides information on prostate cancer, with statistics, advice for managing with prostate cancer, and the risk factors.

Dietitians of Canada, Canadian Paediatric Society, The College of Family Physicians of Canada, Community Health Nurses of Canada. *Promoting Optimal Monitoring of Child Growth in Canada: Using the New WHO Growth Charts.* (www.dietitians.ca/growthcharts)

This site provides access to WHO growth charts for Canada, which can be used to monitor and assess the growth of Canadian infants and children in primary care and public health.

Health Canada. Canadian Guidelines for Bodyweight Classification in Adults: Quick Reference Tool for Professionals. (http://www.hc-sc.gc.ca/fn-an/nutrition/weights-poids/guide-ld-adult/index-eng.php)

This site provides a tool that gives the calculations for the body mass index and the waist circumference measure.

Health Canada. Growing Healthy Canadians: A Guide for Positive Child Development. (https://www.healthyfam-iliesbc.ca/home/blog/growing-healthy-kids)

This guide is a collection of information to promote the well-being of children.

Health Canada. Healthy Living. Reaching for the Top: A Report by the Advisor on Healthy Children and Youth. (http://www.hc-sc.gc.ca/hl-vs/pubs/child-enfant/advisor-conseillere/index-eng.php)

This Health Canada report presents five key recommendations and 95 sub-recommendations that will have an impact on health care programs to improve the health of children and youth.

National Breast Cancer Foundation. Breast Self-Exam. (https://www.nationalbreastcancer.org/breast-self-exam)

This site contains information and a video that can be used to teach women about breast self-exams and how to perform them.

Osteoporosis Canada. (http://www.osteoporosis.ca/)

Choose the link "Calcium Requirements" to access a calcium calculator. This is an excellent tool to share with clients because they can enter their daily food and fluid intake and then calculate the amount of calcium taken. Also, clients will likely find the list of foods and their calcium content helpful.

Public Health Agency of Canada. Family Front and Centre: A Support Resource Promoting Healthy Child Development. (https://www.canada.ca/content/dam/phac-aspc/migration/phac-aspc/hp-ps/dca-dea/publications/ffc-ief/assets/pdf/ffc_attachment.pdf)

This resource provides a checklist of information for health care providers to assess infant attachment.

Public Health Agency of Canada. The Safe Living Guide—A Guide to Home Safety for Seniors. (http://www.phac-aspc.gc.ca/seniors-aines/publications/public/injury-blessure/safelive-securite/index-eng.php)

This tool can be used by CHNs to assess a home environment for safety, including falls.

REFERENCES

Alzheimer Society of Canada. (2015). *Caregiver stress checklist.* http://www.alzheimer.ca/en/Living-with-dementia/Caring-for-someone/Self-care-for-the-caregiver/Caregiver-stress.

Astle, B. J., Duggleby, W., Potter, P. A., et al. (2019). *Canadian fundamentals of nursing* (6th ed.). Elsevier Canada.

Avison, C. (2009). Comprehensive school health in Canada. *The Canadian Association of Principals Journal, 17*(2), 6–7.

Beckmann Murray, R., Proctor Zentner, J., Pangman, V., et al. (2006). *Health promotion strategies through the lifespan* (Cdn ed.). Pearson Canada.

Beckmann Murray, R., Proctor Zentner, J., Pangman, V., et al. (2009). *Health promotion strategies through the lifespan* (2nd Cdn ed.). Pearson Prentice Hall.

Bird, S., Wiles, J., Okalik, L., et al. (2008). Living with diabetes on Baffin Island: Inuit storytellers share their experiences. *Canadian Journal of Public Health, 99*(1), 17–21.

Boal, J., & Loengard, A. (2007). Home care. In R. J. Ham, P. D. Sloane, G. A. Warshaw, et al. (Eds.), *Primary care geriatrics: A case-based approach* (5th ed.) (pp. 172–178). Mosby.

Boney, C. M., Verma, A., Tucker, R., et al. (2005). Metabolic syndrome in childhood: Association with birth weight, maternal obesity, and gestational diabetes mellitus. *Pediatrics, 115*(3), e290–e296.

Brenner, D., et al. (2020). Projected estimates of cancer in Canada in 2020 Canadian. *Canadian Medical Association Journal, 192(9),E199–E205;* https://doi.org/10.1503/cmaj.191292. March 02, 2020.

Bushnik, S. (2016). *The health of girls and women (Catalogue no. 89-503-X).* Statistics Canada. https://www150.statcan.gc.ca/n1/en/pub/89-503-x/2015001/article/14324-eng.pdf?st=OVZ_NMyM.

Canadian Cancer Society. (2019a). *Breast cancer statistics 2009.* https://www.cancer.ca/en/cancer-information/cancer-type/breast/statistics/?region=on.

Canadian Cancer Society. (2019b). *Cervical cancer.* http://www.cancer.ca.

Canadian Cancer Society's Advisory Committee on Cancer Statistics. (2014). *Canadian cancer statistics 2014.* http://www.cancer.ca/~/media/cancer.ca/CW/cancer%20information/cancer%20101/Canadian%20cancer%20statistics/Canadian-Cancer-Statistics-2014–EN.pdf.

Canadian Council on Social Development. (2007). *Growing up In North America: Child health and safety in Canada, the United States and Mexico.* https://folio.iupui.edu/bitstream/handle/10244/124/DA3622H5035.pdf?sequence=1.

Canadian Institute for Health Information. (2008). *Reducing gaps in health: A focus on socio-economic status in urban Canada.* https://secure.cihi.ca/free_products/Reducing_Gaps_in_Health_Report_EN_081009.pdf.

Canadian Task Force on Preventive Health Care. (2011). Recommendations on screening for breast cancer in average-risk women aged 40–74 year. *Canadian Medical Association Journal, 183(17).* https://doi.org/10.1503/cmaj.110334. November 22.

Canadian Notifiable Diseases Surveillance System (CNDSS), Public Health Agency of Canada (PHAC). (2018). *Reported cases from 1924–2016 in Canada—Notifiable diseases on-line.* https://diseases.canada.ca/notifiable/charts?c=pl.

Canadian Women's Association. (2015). *Fact Sheet: Women and poverty in Canada.* https://canadianwomen.org/wp-content/uploads/2018/09/Fact-Sheet-WOMEN-POVERTY-September-2018.pdf.

Centers for Disease Control and Prevention. (2008). *A public health plan to prevent heart disease and stroke.* http://www.cdc.gov/dhdsp/action_plan/.

Clinton, K. (2009). Preventing youth overweight and obesity: A population health perspective. *Transdisciplinary Studies in Population Health Series, 1*(1), 7–21.

Condon, E., Holland, M., Slade, A., et al. (2017). The influence of maternal caregiving practices on indicators of toxic stress in children. *Journal of Pediatric Health*, *32*(4), 330. https://doi.org/10.1016/j.pedhc.2018.04.012

Conroy, K., Sandel, M., & Zuckerman, B. (2010). Poverty grown up: How childhood socioeconomic status impacts adult health. *Journal of Developmental and Behavioral Pediatrics*, *31*(2), 154–160.

Cromer, K. R., & Sachs-Ericsson, N. (2006). The association between childhood abuse, PTSD, and the occurrence of adult health problems: Moderation via current life stress. *Journal of Traumatic Stress*, *19*(6), 967–971.

Diabetes Canada. (2018). *Are you at risk?* https://www.diabetes.ca/DiabetesCanadaWebsite/media/Managing-My-Diabetes/Tools%20and%20Resources/are-you-at-risk.pdf?ext=.pdf.

Dukowski, L. (2009). Comprehensive school health—why should we care? *Canadian Association of Principals Journal*, *17*(2), 4–5.

Edwards, M. L. (2012). The enigma of heart disease in women: New insights may precipitate diagnosis and improve patient outcomes. *Journal of the American Academy of Nurse Practitioners*, *24*(10), 574–578. https://doi.org/10.1111/j.1745-7599.2012.00773.x.

Ginsburg, K. R. (2007). The importance of play in promoting healthy child development and maintaining strong parent-child bonds. *Pediatrics*, *119*(1), 182–191.

Government of Canada & Canadian Cancer Society. (2019c). *Canadian cancer statistics 2019*. Toronto: Canadian Cancer Society. http://www.cancer.ca/~/media/cancer.ca/CW/cancer%20information/cancer%20101/Canadian%20cancer%20statistics/Canadian-Cancer-Statistics-2019-EN.pdf?la=en.

Government of Canada. (2016). *National crime prevention strategy*. http://www.publicsafety.gc.ca/cnt/cntrng-crm/crm-prvntn/strtg-en.aspx.

Government of Canada. (2017). *Canadian cancer statistics*. Retrieved from https://www.canada.ca/en/public-health/services/chronic-diseases/cancer/canadian-cancer-statistics.html.

Hamilton, N., & Bhatti, T. (1996). *Population health promotion: An integrated model of population health and health promotion*. Health Canada: Health Promotion Development Division.

Health Canada. (2006a). *Benefits and risks of hormone replacement therapy (estrogen with or without progestin)*. https://www.canada.ca/en/health-canada/services/healthy-living/your-health/medical-information/benefits-risks-hormone-replacement-therapy-estrogen-without-progestin.html.

Health Canada. (2006b). *Women and heart health*. https://www.canada.ca/content/dam/hc-sc/migration/hc-sc/hl-vs/alt_formats/hpb-dgps/pdf/facts_heart.pdf.

Health Canada. (2008). *Just for you—Seniors*. http://www.hc-sc.gc.ca/hl-vs/jfy-spv/seniors-aines-eng.php.

Health Canada. (2010). *Improving cooking and food preparation skills: A profile of promising practices in Canada and abroad*. http://www.hc-sc.gc.ca/fn-an/nutrition/child-enfant/cfps-acc-profil-apercu-eng.php.

Health Nexus, & Ontario Chronic Disease Prevention Alliance. (2008). *Primer to action: Social determinants of health*.

Heart & Stroke Foundation. (2007). *Heart attack warning signs*. https://www.heartandstroke.ca/heart-disease/emergency-signs.

Heart and Stroke FOundation Canada. (2021). *Heart health activity*. Retrieved from https://www.heartandstroke.ca/healthy-living/healthy-kids/heart-healthy-activity.

Heart & Stroke Foundation. (2016). *The burden of heart failure*. https://www.heartandstroke.ca/-/media/pdf-files/canada/2017-heart-month/heartandstroke-reportonhealth-2016.ashx?la=en&hash=91708486C1BC014E24AB4E719B47AEEB8C5EB93E.

Joint Consortium for School Health. (2010). *What is a comprehensive school health approach?* http://www.jcsh-cces.ca/index.php/about/comprehensive-school-health/what-is-csh.

Labarthe, D. R., Dai, S., Day, S., et al. (2009). Findings from project heartbeat! Their importance for CVD prevention. *American Journal of Preventive Medicine*, *37*(1S), S105–S115.

Labonte, R. (2003). *How our programs affect population health determinants: A workbook for better planning and accountability*. Population Health and Evaluation Research Unit for Health Canada.

Laverack, G. (2017). The challenge of behaviour change and health promotion. *Challenges*, *8*(25). https://doi.org/10.3390/challe8020025.

Leitch, K. (2007). *Reaching for the top: A report by the advisor on healthy children and youth*. Health Canada. http://www.hc-sc.gc.ca/hl-vs/pubs/child-enfant/advisor-conseillere/index-eng.php.

Lung Association of Saskatchewan. (2009). *Lung cancer*. http://www.sk.lung.ca.

MacDonald, N. (2016). The long and winding road to improving immunization rates: Sharing best practices in Canada. *Canada Communicable Disease Report*, *42*(12), 243–245.

Mahon, R. (2006). Of scalar hierarchies and welfare redesign: Child care in three Canadian cities. *Transactions of the Institute of British Geographers (1965)*, *31*(4), 452–466.

McSweeney, J. C., Cody, M., O'Sullivan, P., et al. (2003). Women's early warning symptoms of acute myocardial infarction. *Circulation*, *108*(21), 2619–2623. http://circ.ahajournals.org/content/108/21/2619.full.

Meiner, S. E., & Lueckenotte, A. G. (2006). *Gerontological nursing* (3rd ed.). Mosby.

Mikkonen, J., & Raphael, D. (2010). *Social determinants of health: The Canadian facts*. York University School of Health Policy and Management. www.thecanadianfacts.org/.

Millar, C. A. (2014). *Nursing for wellness in older adults: Theory and practice* (7th ed.). Lippincott Williams & Wilkins.

Morrison, W., Kirby, P., Losier, G., et al. (2009). Conceptualizing psychological wellness: Addressing mental fitness needs. *Canadian Association of Principals Journal*, *17*(2), 19–21.

Murray, N., Low, B., Hollis, C., et al. (2007). Coordinated school health programs and academic achievement: A systematic review of the literature. *Journal of School Health*, *77*(9), 589–599.

National Collaborating Centre for Determinants of Health. (2009). *Early child development as a determinant of health*. [PowerPoint] https://nccdh.ca/resources/entry/antoinettes-story.

New Brunswick Health Council. (2017). New Brunswick student wellness survey. https://nbhc.ca/new-brunswick-student-wellness-survey.

Oliffe, J., Grewal, S., Bottorff, J., et al. (2009). Connecting masculinities and physical activity among senior South Asian Canadian immigrant men. *Critical Public Health*, *19*(3/4), 383–397. https://doi.org/10.1080/09581590902951605

Osteoporosis Canada. (2010). *Osteoporosis facts and statistics*. https://osteoporosis.ca/about-the-disease/fast-facts/.

Perry, C., Sellers, D., Johnson, C., et al. (1998). The Child and Adolescent Trial for Cardiovascular Health (CATCH): Intervention, Implementation, and Feasibility for Elementary

Schools in the United States. *Health Education & Behavior*, 24(6), 716–735. https://doi.org/10.1177/109019819702400607.

PHAC. (2021). *Osteoporisis and related fractures in Canada.* Retrieved from https://www.canada.ca/content/dam/phac-aspc/documents/services/publications/diseases-conditions/osteoporosis-related-fractures-2020/osteoporosis-related-fractures-2020.pdf.

Public Health Agency of Canada (PHAC) & Canadian Institute for Health Information (CIHI). (2011). *Obesity in Canada.* http://www.phac-aspc.gc.ca/hp-ps/hl-mvs/oic-oac/assets/pdf/oic-oac-eng.pdf.

Public Health Agency of Canada (PHAC). (2005). *Integrated strategy on healthy living and chronic disease.* http://www.phac-aspc.gc.ca/about_apropos/reports/2008-09/hlcd-vsmc/surveillance/index-eng.php.

Public Health Agency of Canada (PHAC). (2007). *The 2007 report on the integrated pan-Canadian healthy living strategy.* http://publications.gc.ca/collections/collection_2011/aspc-phac/HP10-1-2007-eng.pdf.

Public Health Agency of Canada (PHAC). (2009a). *Child and youth injury in review, 2009.* http://www.phac-aspc.gc.ca/publicat/cyi-bej/2009/index-eng.php.

Public Health Agency of Canada (PHAC). (2009b). *The chief public health officer's report on the state of public health in Canada 2009: Growing up well—priorities for a healthy future.* http://www.phac-aspc.gc.ca/cphorsphc-respcacsp/2009/fr-rc/index-eng.php.

Public Health Agency of Canada (PHAC). (2009c). *Obesity: An overview of current landscape and prevention-related activities in Ontario.* https://www.ocdpa.ca/publications/obesity-overview-current-landscape-and-prevention-related-activities-ontario.

Public Health Agency of Canada (PHAC). (2015a). *Creating a healthier Canada: Making prevention a priority.* http://www.phac-aspc.gc.ca/hp-ps/hl-mvs/declaration/index-eng.php.

Public Health Agency of Canada (PHAC). (2015b). *Report from the Canadian chronic disease surveillance system: Mental illness in Canada, 2015.* http://healthycanadians.gc.ca/publications/diseases-conditions-maladies-affections/mental-illness-2015-maladies-mentales/alt/mental-illness-2015-maladies-mentales-eng.pdf.

Public Health Agency of Canada (PHAC). (2017). *The public health officer's report on the state of public health in Canada 2017.* https://www.canada.ca/content/dam/phac-aspc/documents/services/publications/chief-public-health-officer-reports-state-public-health-canada/2017-designing-healthy-living/PHAC_CPHO-2017_Report_E.pdf.

Public Health Agency of Canada (PHAC). (2018). *Key health inequalities in Canada: A national portrait.* https://www.canada.ca/en/public-health/services/publications/science-research-data/inequalities-diabetes-infographic.html.

Public Health Agency of Canada (PHAC). (2019). *Lung cancer.* Retrieved from https://www.canada.ca/en/public-health-services/chronic-diseases/cancer/lung-cancer.html.

Public Health Agency of Canada (PHAC). (2019). *Measles and rubella weekly monitoring report: Week 18:April 28 to May 4, 2019.* https://www.canada.ca/en/public-health/services/publications/diseases-conditions/measles-rubella-surveillance/2019/week-18.html.

PHAC. (2021). *Osteoporisis and related fractures in Canada.* Retrieved from https://www.canada.ca/content/dam/phac-aspc/documents/services/publications/diseases-conditions/osteoporosis-related-fractures-2020/osteoporosis-related-fractures-2020.pdf.

Public Safety Canada. (2015). *Results of crime prevention programs for 12–17-year-olds.* http://www.publicsafety.gc.ca/cnt/rsrcs/pblctns/rslts-crm-prvntn-12-17/smmry-eng.pdf.

Reading, J. (2009). *A life course approach to the social determinants of health for Aboriginal Peoples for the Senate Sub-Committee on Population Health.* http://www.parl.gc.ca/40/2/parlbus/commbus/senate/com-e/popu-e/rep-e/appendixAjun09-e.pdf.

Ryan, G., & Bourke, C. (2008). *Community connection asset mapping process.* The Connecticut Assets Network.

Safe Kids Canada. (2007). *Child & youth unintentional injury, 1994 to 2003: 10 years in review.* http://www.ccsd.ca/resources/ProgressChildrenYouth/pdf/skc_injuries.pdf.

Sinha, M. (2014). *Child care in Canada (Catalogue No. 89-652-X - No. 005; ISBN 978-1-100-24896-7). Statistics Canada: Social and Aboriginal statistics Division.* https://www150.statcan.gc.ca/n1/pub/89-652-x/89-652-x2014005-eng.htm.

Statistics Canada. (2010). *Estimates of population, by age group and sex for July 1, Canada, provinces and territories, annual (CANSIM Table 051-0001).* http://www5.statcan.gc.ca/cansim/a26?lang=eng&id=510001.

Statistics Canada. (2017). *Canadian tobacco, alcohol and drugs survey summary results.* https://www.canada.ca/en/health-canada/services/canadian-tobacco-alcohol-drugs-survey/2017-summary.html.

Stewart-Brown, S. (2006). *What is the evidence on school health promotion in improving health or preventing disease and specifically, what is the effectiveness of the health-promoting schools approach?* WHO Regional Office for Europe (Health Evidence Network report). http://www.euro.who.int/document/e88185.pdf.

Strasser, T. (1978). Reflections on cardiovascular diseases. *Interdisciplinary Science Review, 3,* 225–230.

Strategic Advisory group of experts on immunization (SAGE). (2014). *Report of the SAGE Working Group on Vaccine Hesitancy* [Internet]. World Health Organization. https://www.who.int/immunization/sage/meetings/2014/october/1_Report_WORKING_GROUP_vaccine_hesitancy_final.pdf.

Touhy, T., Jett, K., Boscart, V., et al. (2019). *Ebersole and Hess' gerontological nursing & healthy aging* (2nd Cdn ed.). Elsevier Canada.

United Nations, Department of Economic and Social Affairs, Population Division. (2015). *World population prospects: The 2015 revision, volume I: Comprehensive tables* (ST/ESA/SER.A/379).

Veugelers, P. J., & Fitzgerald, A. L. (2005). Prevalence of and risk factors for childhood overweight and obesity. *Canadian Medical Association Journal, 173*(6), 607–613.

World Health Organization (WHO). (2014). *Global status report on noncommunicable diseases.* http://www.who.int/nmh/publications/ncd-status-report-2014/en/.

World Health Organization (WHO). (2019). *Ten facts about early child development as a social determinant of health.* https://www.who.int/maternal_child_adolescent/topics/child/development/10facts/en/.

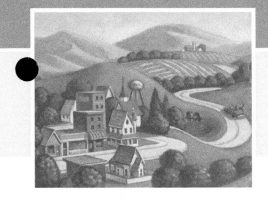

12

Working With Families

OUTLINE

Family Nursing in the Community, 276
The Canadian Family, 277
    Definition of Family, 277
    Family Demography, 277
    Family Structure, 278
    Determinants of Health, 278
Family Health, 280
    Family Health and Functionality, 280
Four Approaches to Family Nursing, 281
Theoretical Frameworks for Family Nursing, 281
Family Assessment Models and Approaches, 287
    Friedman Family Assessment Model (Short Form), 287
    Calgary Family Assessment Model, 287
    McGill Model of Nursing, 287
    McMaster Model of Family Functioning, 288
    Relational Practice, 288
Family Home Visits, 290
    Planning for Home Visits, 290

Engagement, 291
Family Assessment, 293
Interventions, 294
Termination and Evaluation, 294
Postvisit Documentation, 295
Appraisal of Family Health Risks and Capacity, 295
    Biological Risk Assessment, 295
    Environmental Risk Assessment, 297
    Behavioural Risk Assessment, 299
Family Interventions, 299
    Calgary Family Intervention Model, 300
    Family Health Risk Reduction, 301
    Family Empowerment, 302
    Family Resiliency, 302
    Care Planning With Families, 303
    Advantages and Challenges of Mutual Goal Setting, 303
    Clinical Judgement, 304
    Community Resources, 305

OBJECTIVES

After reading this chapter, you should be able to:

12.1 Explain the importance of family nursing in the community setting.

12.2 Define *family* and *family structure* and explain the role of the determinants of health in family health.

12.3 Analyze how family health and functioning are established.

12.4 Compare and contrast four approaches to family nursing.

12.5 Compare and contrast social science theoretical frameworks for family nursing.

12.6 Explain the primary family assessment models and approaches.

12.7 Outline the various phases of family home visits.

12.8 Outline the major risks to family health.

12.9 Explain how to apply the Calgary Intervention Model, reduce family health risks, and plan care with families.

KEY TERMS*

behavioural risk, 299
biological risk, 295
circular communication, 301
commendations, 301
ecomap, 298
economic risk, 297
engagement, 291
family, 277
family assessment, 293
family crisis, 302
family demography, 277
family functions, 297

family health, 280
family nursing, 276
family nursing theory, 281
family resiliency, 302
family strengths, 300
family structure, 278
family systems nursing model, 287
functional families, 280
genogram, 295
health risk appraisal, 301
health risk reduction, 302
health risks, 301

home visit, 291
relational practice, 288
risk, 301

social risks, 301
termination phase, 294
transition, 287

*See the Glossary on page 468 for definitions.

The family as a patient unit is fundamental to the practice of community health nursing, and community health nurses (CHNs) are responsible for promoting healthy families in society. Family nursing is practised in all settings. The trend in the delivery of health care has been to move health care to community settings; thus, family nursing is incorporated in community health nursing practice. CHNs work with families as an essential social unit, recognizing that individuals are connected to their communities and community health through a number of often-complex relationships and competing demands. CHNs support family health across the lifespan, including prenatal health care, infants or children with complex health challenges, adolescent mental health, and older persons with mobility needs.

Family nursing is a specialty area that has a strong theory base and is more than just "common sense" or viewing the family as the context for individual health care. Family nursing consists of CHNs and families working together to ensure the success of the family and its members in adapting to health and illness.

Working as partners with families, CHNs focus on capacity building; that is, CHNs recognize family strengths and use these strengths to deal with health concerns. The family as a patient unit is fundamental to the practice of community health nursing, and CHNs are responsible for promoting healthy families in society. Societal support contributes to healthier families. CHNs need to be involved in community assessment, planning, development, and evaluation activities that emphasize family issues and the family's ability to sustain itself.

The family is both an important environment affecting the health of individuals and a social unit whose health is basic to that of the community and the larger population. It is within the family that behaviour—including health values, habits, and risk perceptions—is developed, organized, and performed. Individuals' health behaviours are both affected by and experienced within the family environment, the larger community, and society. For example, if a child is raised in a home where the parents demonstrate healthy eating with daily physical activity and are nonsmokers, the child is more likely to adopt these healthy behaviours and to maintain them into adulthood. The risks to individual and family health are affected by the family social norms—in this example, the norm is practising healthy living. In the same manner, it is in the context of community systems, norms, and values that family health habits are developed. For example, communities with walking trails, bicycle paths, affordable housing and day care, and community gardens are supportive environments for family health and in turn impact community well-being.

To intervene effectively and appropriately with families to reduce their health risk and promote their health, it is necessary to view the family as the unit of care and to understand family structure and functioning, family theory, nursing theory, and models of health risk. It is usually necessary to go beyond the individual and family to also understand the complex environment in which the family exists. Increasing evidence of the effects of social, biological, economic, and life events on health suggests a broader approach be taken in addressing health risks for families.

The purpose of this chapter is to present a current overview of families and family nursing, theoretical frameworks, and strategies for assessing and intervening with families in the community; to note the influences, both individual and in society, that place families at risk for poor health outcomes; and to discuss how positive outcomes for families can be accomplished based on family strengths. Options are explored for structuring community health nursing interventions with families to decrease health risks and to promote health and well-being. The Calgary Family Assessment Model (CFAM) is introduced as an assessment and an organizing framework for working with families and The Calgary Family Intervention Model (CFIM) is discussed in regard to promoting healthy family functioning (Shajani & Snell, 2019). Both models are summarized in Appendix 7.

FAMILY NURSING IN THE COMMUNITY

Health care decisions are made within the family, the basic social unit of society. Families are responsible for providing or managing the care of family members. In the current health care system, families are significant members of health care teams since they are the ever-present factor. Currently, families are expected to take more responsibility for assisting in the health care of ill family members.

CHNs partnering with families are responsible for:
- Helping families promote their health and healing
- Assisting with the identification of family strengths and health concerns
- Assisting and supporting families to cope with health concerns within the context of the existing family structure, family strengths, and community resources
- Identifying, enhancing, and promoting family resiliency
- Collaborating with families to develop useful interventions
- Referring to community resources as agreed upon by the family
- Facilitating family evaluation of strengths and progress made in reference to health concerns

CHNs need to be knowledgeable about family structures, family developmental stages, functions, processes, and roles. As a partner, it is important that the CHN acknowledge that the family is the expert in relation to their health concern and in the selection of interventions that are most likely to work. Although the family is also the expert in relation to what is most important to it and the health of its members, the CHN uses evidence-informed practice when working with the family in decision making about health intervention choices. In addition, CHNs need to be aware of and understand their own personal values and attitudes pertaining to their own families, as well as being open to different family structures and cultures. Reflexivity is central to the CHN's work with families and in all home visiting encounters. Exploring one's biases, assumptions, and expectations with diverse families (see Chapter 7) and understanding how these influence care are essential standards of CHN practice (Community Health Nurses of Canada [CHNC], 2019). This essential starting place of the CHN's practice with families means that the nurse can bring a practice of reflection and responsiveness to families and can model relational practice with families who may also strive to be more relational and responsive within the family unit.

THE CANADIAN FAMILY

In Canadian community health nursing, the family as patient encompasses a varied unit of people who comprise their own mini community. They have a culture and practices and ways of being that must be understood by the CHN to provide effective family nursing and to support individual and family health.

Definition of Family

The definition of *family* is critical to the practice of community health nursing. Family has traditionally been defined using the legal concepts of relationships such as genetic ties, adoption, guardianship, or marriage. Since the 1980s, a broader definition of family has been used that moves beyond the traditional blood, marriage, and legal constrictions. "**Family** refers to two or more individuals who depend on one another for emotional, physical, and/or financial support. The members of the family are self-defined" (Kaakinen & Harmon Hanson, 2018, p. 5). Shajani and Snell (2019) state, "The family is who they say they are" (p. 55), which moves beyond the traditional definitions. Based on these definitions, it is important to recognize that a family is a group and is therefore two or more people, with membership being defined by the family. Therefore, it is critical that CHNs working with families ask the family members who they consider to be their family and then include those members in health care planning. The family may range from traditional nuclear and extended families to a variety of family structures as lone-parent families, stepfamilies, same-sex couples with or without children, foster families, friends, or neighbours, including street family for people who experience homelessness and may be estranged from other family members. Pets or animals may also be important members of the family, providing a source of support or activity for people (International Federation on Ageing, 2020).

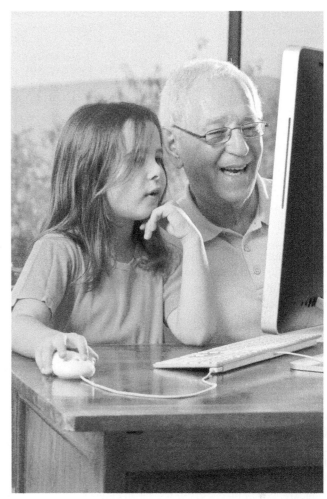

People view families and their experiences based on their own family of origin. However, the varied configurations of family are limitless and of all shapes, sizes, and colours. (CanStock Photo Inc./pisu)

Family Demography

Family demography is the study of the structure of families and households and the family-related events, such as marriage and divorce, that alter structure through their number, timing, and sequencing. An important use of family demography by CHNs is to forecast stresses and developmental changes experienced by families and to identify possible solutions to family health concerns. It is important to note that the structure of families has changed over time from traditionally defined families (e.g., nuclear and extended families) to include blended families, cohabitating heterosexual or homosexual/same-sex partners, sibling-led households, foster families, and, more recently, couples living apart or commuter families as well as "skipped-generation" families (grandparents caring for grandchildren).

Table 12.1 provides examples of the various family forms most common in Canada. In Canada, same-sex marriages

TABLE 12.1 Examples of Different Family Forms in Canada

Type of Family	Description
Nuclear	• Parents and children living together
Lone parent (single parent or one parent)	• Unmarried, separated, or divorced mother or father living alone with their children
Extended	• Nuclear family and relatives of the nuclear family
Blended (stepfamily)	• A widowed or divorced spouse with some or all of their children lives with a new spouse from another union with some or all of their children
Commuter	• Couple with or without children who live in separate residences in two different geographical locations most of the time because of work commitments. They are in a committed relationship as a couple.
Living apart together (LAT)	• A couple who are in a caring relationship, and for a variety of reasons, keep their own residences
Same sex	• Partners of the same sex living together who may or may not have children
Grandparent-led (skipped generation)	• A grandparent who is caring for grandchild/children within a three-generation family
Cohabiting (common-law)	• Unmarried couples living together

Source: Vanier Institute of the Family. (2018). *A snapshot of family diversity in Canada*. https://vanierinstitute.ca/a-snapshot-of-family-diversity-in-canada-february-2018/

were legalized nationally in July 2005 (Government of Canada, 2018). Most persons view families and their experiences through the lens of their own family of origin. It is important to be aware of and attempt to understand other family variations. The rapid changes in family form that have occurred in recent decades are increasingly being studied and understood for the implications to family and community health. For instance, many studies have demonstrated that children's development, education, and well-being within families of same-sex parents is much the same, or better than, those in traditional family arrangements (Mazrekaj, De Witte, & Cabus, 2020). The Vanier Institute of the Family (2018) reported major changes in the Canadian family in the following aspects: structural, functional, and affective. Some of the changes, based on Canadian census data, are:

- 66% of families in Canada include a married couple (down from 83% in 1981)
- 18% are living common-law (this number has tripled since 1981)
- 16% are lone-parent families—diverse family structures that continuously evolve (up from 11% in 1981, though relatively unchanged since 2001)
- In 2016, there were nearly 73 000 same-sex-couple families in Canada, 12% of whom are raising children (up from 8.6% in 2001).
- In 2016, there were nearly 404 000 multi-generational households in Canada—the *fastest-growing household type* since 2001 (+38%).
- In 2016, nearly 33 000 children in Canada aged 0 to 14 lived in skip-generation households (i.e., living with grandparent(s) with no middle [i.e., parent] generation present).
- In 2011, 22% of Inuk (Inuit) grandparents, 14% of First Nations grandparents, and 5% of Métis grandparents lived with their grandchildren, compared with 3.9% of non-Indigenous grandparents.

For more detailed description and discussion of the changing patterns in the Canadian family, refer to the Vanier Institute's *Snapshot of Family Diversity in Canada* (the link is on the Evolve website: https://vanierinstitute.ca/a-snapshot-of-family-diversity-in-canada-february-2018/).

Family Structure

Family structure refers to the characteristics and demographics (gender, age, number) of individual members who make up a family unit. More specifically, the family structure defines who the family members are (who is in this family), what the relationships are between these members, and family context. Shajani and Snell (2019) further divide family structure into internal, external, and contextual categories, with additional subcategories. Fig. 12.1 is a branching diagram from the CFAM that outlines the structural, developmental, and functional categories of family assessment, as well as associated subcategories.

Determinants of Health

Social determinants of health raise questions of social justice for nurses who are engaged with families (Deatrick, 2017). The determinants of health need to be considered when working within everyday, embodied practice with families in the community. Determinants such as housing are part of the physical (built) environment, which is one of the determinants of health, and a is a deeply personal and embodied experience to be at home and in patients' homes as a CHN. Income is another determinant of health. Adequate income is related to the ability to purchase affordable housing and to meet food security and other needs. The determinants of health "personal health practices and coping skills" incorporate lifestyle choices that affect the family. Gender and social environments are determinants of health that also have an impact on the family. The "Determinants of Health" box provides examples of information on the determinants of health for CHNs to consider when working with families.

Family-Level Determinants of Health

- *Socioeconomic status is a consistent and reliable predictor of a vast array of outcomes across the life span, including physical and psychological health. Children and youth under 18 are particularly vulnerable to conditions of poverty.* In Canada, 1.3 million children (1 in 5) live in conditions of poverty. In comparison, 40% of Indigenous children in Canada live in poverty, and 60% of Indigenous children on reserves live in poverty.
- *One aspect of poverty is not having enough food or having limited access to nutritious and healthy food.* In 2017–2018, 1 in 8 households in Canada was food insecure, amounting to 4.4 million people, including more than 1.2 million children living in food-insecure households.
- Residents in Nunavut spend twice as much on food as the rest of the country on average ($14,800 vs. $7,300 annually) and in Nunavut, 7 of 10 Inuit preschoolers live in food-insecure households.
- Food insecure households were 80% more likely to report having diabetes, 60% more likely to report high blood pressure, and 70% more likely to report food allergies.
- *Canada does not yet have a strategy on affordable housing, and vulnerable populations are most affected by this lack of policy.* An estimated 235 000 people in Canada experienced homelessness in 2016, with roughly 35 000 people being homeless on any given night.
- Nearly 1 in 5 households experience serious housing affordability issues (spending over 50% of their low income on rent), which puts them at risk of homelessness.
- *Inadequate housing and income are linked with domestic violence. Women with lower incomes experience physical abuse more frequently than women with higher incomes.*
- Police-reported family violence against children and youth increased in nearly all provinces and territories between 2017–2018, with family violence increasing the risk for psychological and behavioural problems. *As such, more community strategies are needed to prevent, reduce, and eliminate these and all social threats (such as poverty, lack of food security, housing instability, and violence) to family health.*

Sources: Canadian Observatory on Homelessness. (2019). *What is homelessness?* https://www.homelesshub.ca/about-homelessness/homelessness-101/what-homelessness; Statistics Canada. (2018). *Family violence in Canada: A statistical profile*. https://www150.statcan.gc.ca/n1/pub/85-002-x/2019001/article/00018-eng.htm; Statistics Canada. (2020). *Dimensions of poverty hub*. https://www.statcan.gc.ca/eng/topics-start/poverty; Tarasuk, V., & Mitchell, A. (2020). *Household food insecurity in Canada, 2017–2018*. Research to Identify Policy Options to Reduce Food Insecurity (PROOF). https://proof.utoronto.ca/wp-content/uploads/2020/03/Household-Food-Insecurity-in-Canada-2017-2018-Full-Reportpdf.pdf

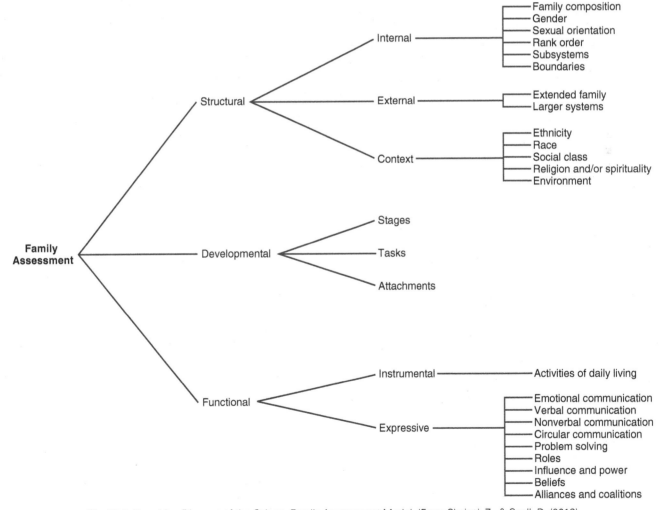

Fig. 12.1 Branching Diagram of the Calgary Family Assessment Model. (From Shajani, Z., & Snell, D. (2019). *Wright & Leahey's nurses and families: A guide to family assessment and intervention* (7th ed.). F.A. Davis Company, Philadelphia, with permission.)

FAMILY HEALTH

Despite the focus on family health within nursing, the meaning of family health lacks consensus and is not precise. The term *family health* is often used interchangeably with the concepts of family functioning, healthy families, or familial health. **Family health** refers to the health of a family system that is ever changing and encompasses a holistic focus that includes biological, psychological, sociological, cultural, and spiritual factors (Kaakinen & Harmon Hanson, 2018).

This holistic approach refers to individual members as well as the family unit as a whole. An individual's health (wellness–illness continuum) affects the entire family's functioning, and, in turn, the family's functioning affects the health of the individuals. Thus, assessment of family health involves simultaneous assessment of individual family members and the family system as a whole. For CHNs, it is important in clinical practice to distinguish between caring for "the individual as patient," with the family as the context for care, and the "family as patient" and, therefore, as the unit of care. For example, in the former instance, the individual family member is the unit of care, with family members in the background; in the latter instance, the family is the unit of care and the individual is in the background (Kaakinen, Coehlo, Steele, et al., 2018; Shajani & Snell, 2019).

Family Health and Functionality

Family functioning is described in various ways in the literature. Table 12.2 presents features of family functioning, from lower to higher functioning. Health care providers have tended to classify families dependent on their coping skills as a unit into two groups: "good families," or functional families, and "bad families," or dysfunctional families. In reality, aspects of family functioning are not static and occur along a continuum. **Functional families** demonstrate effective coping within the family unit, provide autonomy, and are responsive to the particular interests and needs of individual family members. Dysfunctional families demonstrate ineffective coping within the family unit that inhibits clear communication and does not provide psychological support for individual members. Unhealthy families have been referred to as *dysfunctional families*; they have also been referred to

TABLE 12.2 Features of Lower and Higher Functioning Families	
Lower Functioning	**Higher Functioning**
• The family is unstable with ineffective family coping to meet family needs.	• The family is stable and copes with its physical, psychosocial, and spiritual needs, and growth and development needs.
• Family members do not support one another and may act as if other family members do not matter.	• The family works together, members are sensitive, encourage and support each other, especially during problem solving and decision making, thereby strengthening family relationships and unity.
• Member individuality is often lost because of extremely close or distant relationships among some members in the family.	
• There is lack of problem solving and decision making by the family.	
• Families with children are too permissive or restrictive with child-rearing practices. One example of unhealthy practices would be child abuse.	• Families with children practise healthy child-rearing and discipline.
• The family lacks positive parental role modelling. Children assume parental roles because parents are unable to do so.	• Parents are positive role models for children in the family.
• The boundary is too rigid so that there is very limited family and individual member contacts with external systems, or boundary is too flexible and family system is overwhelmed with information from outside sources.	• The boundary is flexible so family and its external systems are able to exchange information.
• Unclear lines of authority with roles and rules that are unclear and/or not relevant often result in derogatory comments among family members.	• Power structure, roles, and rules are clear and relevant.
• Family members are domineering with one another and do not respect individuals' rights and abilities.	• Power is appropriately shared with family members.
• Communication among family members is lacking; family arguments occur that negate family members.	• Communication among family members is open and direct; members actively listen to one another and are respectful of member individuality.
• The family home is insecure with high anxiety levels; scapegoating and blaming of others for individual and/or family problems is common.	• The family is sufficiently open, flexible, adaptable, and resilient so it can manage a variety of demands on the unit.
• The family has limited or no involvement with the community.	• The family's demonstration of growth produces community relationships.
• The family often denies problems or tries to solve all of its own problems and is unwilling to accept outside help.	• The family is open to accepting outside help when appropriate and recognizes limitations.

Source: Adapted from McEwen, M., & Pullis, B. (2009). *Community-based nursing: An introduction* (3rd ed.). Saunders.

as *noncompliant, resistant,* or *unmotivated families.* These terms denote families that are not functioning well within the family unit or in society. The use of the term *dysfunctional family* has been challenged by some family writers (Bell, 1995; Cooley, 2013). CHNs would be well advised to avoid thinking in these terms because it suggests pathology with deficits versus family capacity building based on strengths. Therefore, this terminology tends to encourage helplessness in the family. It also encourages CHNs to assign blame and to use "why" questions, which are linear and suggest causation, instead of "how" questions to explore possible interventions. CHNs might consider referring to these families as families with health challenges. Although the two terms *functional* and *dysfunctional* are far from ideal when referring to family functioning, they are often used in the family and nursing literature.

FOUR APPROACHES TO FAMILY NURSING

Central to the practice of family nursing is conceptualizing and approaching the family from four perspectives (Kaakinen et al., 2018). All have legitimate implications for nursing assessment and intervention (Figs. 12.2 and 12.3). Which approach CHNs use is determined by many factors, including the health care setting, family circumstances, and CHN values, beliefs, and resources:

1. *Family as context, or structure.* This approach has a traditional focus that places the individual first and the family second. The family as context serves as either a resource or a stressor to individual health and illness. A CHN using this focus might ask an individual patient, "How has your diagnosis of insulin-dependent diabetes affected your family?" or "Will your need for medication at night be a problem for your family?"

2. *Family as patient.* The family is first, and individuals are second. The family is seen as the sum of individual family members. The focus is on each individual as he or she affects the family as a whole. From this perspective, a CHN might say to a family member who has just become ill, "Tell me about what has been going on with your own health and how you perceive each family member responding to your mother's recent diagnosis of liver cancer."

3. *Family as system.* The focus is on the family as patient, and the family is viewed as an interacting system in which the whole is more than the sum of its parts. This approach simultaneously focuses on individual members and the family as a whole. The interactions between family members become the target for nursing interventions (e.g., the direct interactions between the parents, or the indirect interaction between the parents and the child). The systems approach to family always implies that when something happens to one family member, the other members of the family system are affected. Questions CHNs ask when approaching a family as system are "What has changed between you and your spouse since your child's head injury?" or "How do you feel about the fact that your son's long-term rehabilitation will affect the ways in which the members of your family are functioning and getting along with one another?"

4. *Family as component of society.* The family is seen as one of many institutions in society, along with health, education, religious, and financial institutions. The family is a basic or primary unit of society, as are all the other units, and they are all a part of the larger system of society. The family as a whole interacts with other institutions to receive, exchange, or give services and communicate. CHNs have drawn many of their tenets from this perspective as they focus on the interface between families and community agencies.

THEORETICAL FRAMEWORKS FOR FAMILY NURSING

The theoretical frameworks used in family nursing are based in family theory. Within the family social science tradition, four conceptual approaches have dominated the field of marriage and family: structure–function theory, systems theory, developmental theory, and interactional theory (Nies & McEwen, 2019). These theories are constantly evolving and being tested, which helps make this knowledge base stronger and more user-friendly when working with families. Table 12.3 summarizes the four major family social theories and what they have contributed to **family nursing theory,** whose function is to characterize, explain, and predict phenomena (events) evident within family nursing. Table 12.4 provides information on assessment and interventions in relation to each theory as well as the advantages and limitations of each theory.

Structure–function theory is a framework that is useful for assessing families and health. Illness of a family member results in the alteration of the family structure and function. If a single mother is ill, she cannot carry out her various roles, so grandparents or siblings may have to assume childcare responsibilities. Family power structures and communication

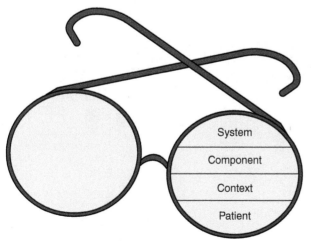

Fig. 12.2 Four Views of the Family. (From Coehlo, D., Hanson, S., Kaakinen, J., Steele, R., & Tabacco, A. (2018). *Family Health Care Nursing: Theory, Practice, and Research* (6th ed.). F.A. Davis Company, Philadelphia, PA with permission.)

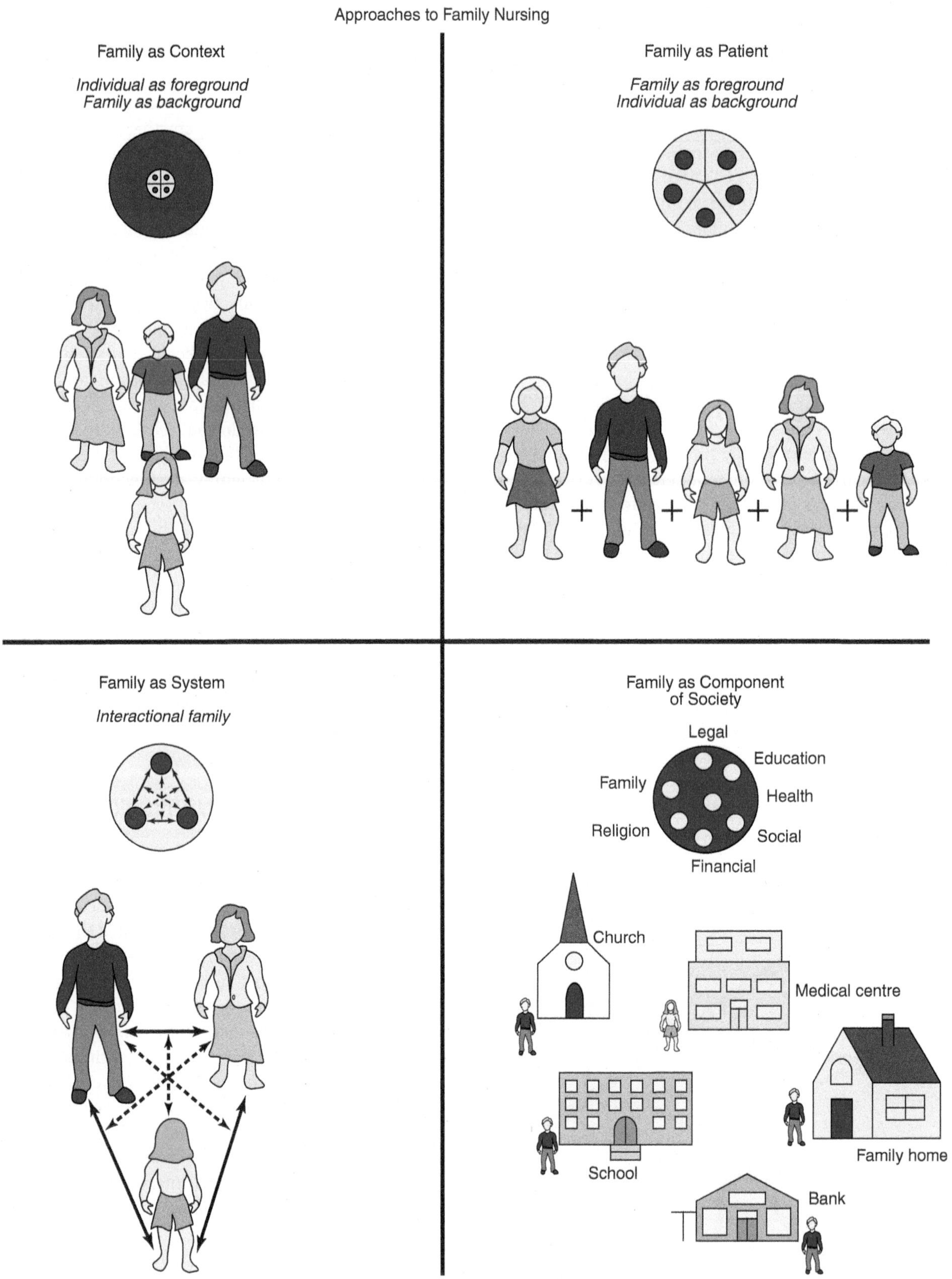

Approaches to Family Nursing

Family as Context

Individual as foreground
Family as background

Family as Patient

Family as foreground
Individual as background

Family as System

Interactional family

Family as Component
of Society

Legal

Education

Family

Health

Religion

Social

Financial

Church

Medical centre

School

Family home

Bank

Fig. 12.3 Approaches to Family Nursing. (From Coehlo, D., Hanson, S., Kaakinen, J., Steele, R., & Tabacco, A. (2018). *Family Health Care Nursing: Theory, Practice, and Research* (6th ed.). F.A. Davis Company, Philadelphia, PA with permission.)

TABLE 12.3 Key Points and Assumptions of Selected Theoretical Frameworks for Family Nursing

Theory	Key Points	Assumptions

Structure–Function Theory	• It defines family as a social system.
	• Family is viewed as open to the outside system, but boundaries are maintained.
	• Family is viewed as passive in adapting to outside system and therefore is not viewed as a change agent.
	• It examines families in terms of
	  1. Relationships with, for example, government, health care, and religious institutions
	  2. Family patterns in relation to society
	  3. How well the family structure performs its functions
		• A family is a social system with functional requirements.
		• A family is a small group that has basic features common to all small groups.
		• Social systems, such as families, accomplish functions that serve the individuals in addition to those that serve society.
		• Individuals act within a set of internal norms and values that are learned primarily in the family through socialization.

Systems Theory	• It is influenced by theory from physics and biology. • A system is composed of a set of interacting elements. • Each system can be identified and is distinct from the environment in which it exists. • An open system exchanges energy and matter with the environment (negentropy). • A closed system is isolated from its environment (entropy). • Systems depend on both positive and negative feedback to maintain a steady state (homeostasis). • Seeking therapy when the marital relationship is strained is an example of using negative feedback to maintain a steady state.	• Family systems are greater than and different from the sum of their parts. • There are many hierarchies within family systems and logical relationships between subsystems (e.g., mother–child, family–community). • There are boundaries in the family system that can be open, closed, or random. • Family systems increase in complexity over time, evolving to allow greater adaptability, tolerance to change, and growth by differentiation. • Family systems change constantly in response to stresses and strains from within and from outside environments. There are structural similarities in different family systems (isomorphism). • Change in one part of family systems affects the total system. • Causality is modified by feedback; therefore, causality never exists in the real world. • Family systems patterns are circular rather than linear; change must be directed toward the cycle. • Family systems are an organized whole; therefore, individuals within the family are interdependent. • Family systems have homeostasis features to maintain stable patterns that can be adaptive or maladaptive.
Developmental Theory	• Principles of individual development are applied to the family unit. • The stage of the family unit is determined by age of the oldest child. • Identified family tasks need to be accomplished during each stage of family development. • Developmental concepts include moving to a different level of functioning, implying progress in a single direction. • Family disequilibrium and conflicts are described as occurring during transition periods from one stage to another. The family has a predictable natural history designated by stages, beginning with the simple husband–wife pair. • The group becomes more complex with the addition of each new child. • The group again becomes simple and less complex as the younger generation leaves home. • The group comes full circle to the original husband–wife pair. • At each family life-cycle stage, there are developmental needs of the family and tasks that must be performed. • Achievement of family developmental tasks helps individual members accomplish their tasks.	• In every family, there are both individual and family developmental tasks that need to be accomplished for every stage of the individual and family life cycle that are unique to that particular group. • Families change and develop in different ways because of internal and environmental stimulations. • Developmental tasks are goals to work toward rather than specific jobs to be completed at once. • Each family is unique in its composition and complexity of age–role expectations and positions. • Individuals and families are a function of their history, as well as the current social structure. • Families have commonalities despite the way they develop over the family lifespan. • Families may arrive at similar developmental levels through different processes.

Continued

TABLE 12.3   Key Points and Assumptions of Selected Theoretical Frameworks for Family Nursing—cont'd

Theory	Key Points	Assumptions
Interactional Theory	• Family is viewed as interacting personalities. • Family is examined by the symbolic communications by which family members relate to one another. • Within the family, each member occupies a position to which a number of roles are assigned. • Members define their role expectations in each situation through their perceptions of the role demands. • Members judge their own behaviour by assessing and interpreting the actions of others toward them. • Central to the interaction approach is the process of role taking. • The ability to predict other family members' expectations for one's role enables each member to have some knowledge of how to react in the role and indicates how other members will react to performing the role.	• Complex sets of symbols having common meanings are acquired through living in a symbolic environment. • Individuals distinguish, evaluate, and assign meaning to symbols. • Behaviour is influenced by meanings of symbols or ideas rather than by instincts, needs, or drives; therefore, the meaning an individual assigns to symbols is important to understanding behaviour. • The self continues to change and evolve over time through introspection caused by experience and activity. • The evolving self has several dimensions: the physical body and characteristics and a complex social self. The "me" is a conventional, habitual self that consists of learned, repetitious responses. The "I" is spontaneous to the individual. • Individuals are actors as well as reactors; they select and interpret the environment to which they respond. • Individuals are born into a dynamic society. • Individuals learn from the culture and become the society. • Individuals' behaviour is a product of their history, which is continually being modified by new information.

TABLE 12.4 Information on Assessment and Interventions, Advantages and Limitations of Selected Theoretical Frameworks for Family Nursing

Theory	Assessment and Interventions	Advantages	Limitations
Structure–Function	• Determine whether changes resulting from the illness influence the family's ability to carry out its functions. • Sample assessment questions are "How did the death alter the family structure?" and "What family roles were changed with the onset of the chronic illness?" • Interventions become necessary when a change in the family structure alters the family's ability to function. • Examples of interventions using this theory include helping families use existing support structures and helping families modify the way they are organized so that role responsibilities can be distributed.	• Comprehensive approach that views families in the broader community in which they live	• Static picture of the family, which does not allow for dynamic change over time
Systems	• Assessment is made of: • Individual members • Subsystems • Boundaries • Openness • Inputs and outputs • Family interactions • Family processing • Adaptation or change abilities • Assessment questions include "Who is in the family system?" and "How has one member's critical illness affected the entire family system?" • Interventions need to assist individual, subsystem, and whole family functioning. • Examples include establishing a mechanism for providing families with information about their family members on a regular basis and discussing ways to provide for a "normal" family life for family members after someone has become ill.	• Views families from both a subsystem and a suprasystem approach • Views the interactions within and among family subsystems as well as the interactions among families and the larger suprasystems, such as community, world, and universe • Focus is on the interaction of the family with other systems rather than on the individual, which is sometimes more important.	

Continued

TABLE 12.4   Information on Assessment and Interventions, Advantages and Limitations of Selected Theoretical Frameworks for Family Nursing—cont'd

Theory	Assessment and Interventions	Advantages	Limitations
Developmental	• Several questions can be asked, for example, "Where does this family place on the continuum of the family life cycle?" and "What are the developmental tasks that are not being accomplished?" • Typical kinds of community health nursing intervention strategies using this perspective help the family understand individual and family growth and development stages and deal with the normal transitions between developmental periods (e.g., tasks of the school-age family member versus tasks of the adolescent family member).	• Provides a basis for forecasting what a family will be experiencing at any period in the family life cycle (e.g., role transitions and family structure changes)	• Model was developed at a time when the traditional nuclear family was emphasized
Interactional	• Emphasis is placed on interaction between and among family members and family communication patterns about health and illness behaviours appropriate for different roles. • Nursing strategies focus on:* • Effectiveness of communication among members • Ability to establish communication between community health nurses and families • Clear and concise messages between members • Similarities between verbal and nonverbal communication patterns • Directions of the interaction • Observe how family members interact with one another to help explain family communication, roles, decision making, and problem solving†.	• Focus on internal processes within families, such as roles, conflict, status, communication, responses to stress, decision making, and socialization • Processes, rather than end products, of social interactions are major focus; thus, this framework used by many nurse scholars	• Broadness and lack of agreement about concepts and assumptions of the theory, which has made it difficult to refine • Families considered as closed units with little relation to the outside society

Sources: *Barnes, Hanson, Novilla, et al., 2020.
†Friedman, Bowden, & Jones, 2003.

patterns are affected when a parent is ill. However, *systems theory* encourages CHNs to view patients as participating members of a family. CHNs using this perspective determine the effects of illness or injury on the entire family system—that is, the family as the unit of care. Emphasis is on the whole rather than on individuals. In comparison, *developmental theory* assists CHNs in anticipating clinical health concerns in families; identifying family strengths; assessing the family's developmental stage; assessing the extent to which the family is fulfilling the tasks associated with its respective stage; assessing the family's developmental history; and assessing the availability of resources essential for performing developmental tasks. Finally, CHNs using *interactional theory* would explore individual family members' perceptions and their interactions and communication processes with other members. Believing that "illness is a family affair," CHNs would analyze family roles, expectations, conflicts, problem solving, and decision making (Wright, 2019, p. 610).

FAMILY ASSESSMENT MODELS AND APPROACHES

Each family assessment model and approach is unique and can be used to create a database upon which to plan interventions. Many family assessment models and approaches are available, and five of these are discussed next.

Friedman Family Assessment Model (Short Form)

The Friedman Family Assessment Model (Short Form) integrates the structure–function framework and developmental and systems theories. The Friedman Family Assessment Model (Short Form) is presented in Appendix E.3 on the Evolve website. The model takes a broad approach to family assessment and views the family as a subsystem of society. The family is viewed as an open social system. The family's structure (organization) and functions (activities and purposes) and the family's relationship to other social systems are the focus of this approach. The assumptions of systems theory underlying this model are presented in Table 12.3.

This assessment approach is important for CHNs because it enables them to evaluate the family system as a whole, as part of the whole of society, and as an interactive system. The guidelines for the Friedman Family Assessment Model (Short Form) consist of the following six broad categories of interview questions:

1. Identifying data
2. Developmental family stage and history
3. Environmental data
4. Family structure, including communication, power structures, role structures, and family values
5. Family functions, including affective functions, socialization, and health care
6. Family coping (Friedman et al., 2003, p. 319)

Each category has several subcategories. The Friedman model was developed to provide guidelines for family nurses who are interviewing a family to gain an overall view of what is going on in the family. The questions are extensive, and it may not be possible to collect all the data at one visit. All the categories may not be pertinent for every family.

Calgary Family Assessment Model

The Calgary Family Assessment Model (CFAM) is a **family systems nursing model** that takes a holistic approach to assessment of family health (see Appendix 7) (Shajani & Snell, 2019). As a family systems nursing model, the focus is on the family unit as patient. This family systems nursing approach consists of a structural, developmental, and functional assessment of the family. The structural assessment includes the categories of the internal and external structures and context of the family. See Fig. 12.1 for the branching diagram of CFAM, which outlines the subcategories in the structural assessment. The genogram and ecomap are two commonly used structural assessment tools used in this model; they are presented later in this chapter.

The developmental assessment contains the family life-cycle stages, tasks usually achieved in relation to life-cycle stages, and attachments for the family. The family life-cycle stages are as follows: leaving home as a single young adult, family joining as a new couple, families with children, families with adolescents, children leaving home and moving forward, and families in later life. The hypothesis is that the family is always at a new stage and facing new transitions as it deals with new issues of development (Shajani & Snell, 2019). **Transition** is the movement from one developmental or health stage or condition to another that may be a time of potential risk for families. For example, a family with an adolescent and a young child is developmentally at the stage of "families with adolescents." *Attachments* refers to particular emotional bonds formed between specific members and does not refer to right or wrong attachments (Shajani & Snell, 2019). CHNs seek to understand these attachments in relation to family development.

Functional assessment includes the categories of instrumental and expressive functioning. *Instrumental family functioning* refers to the activities of everyday living. *Expressive family functioning* refers to the emotional functioning, communication types, and other areas as outlined in the CFAM branching diagram.

McGill Model of Nursing

The McGill Model of Nursing was initially developed by Dr. Moyra Allen and others and then was further developed by Dr. Marilyn Ford-Gilboe and colleagues (Ford-Gilboe, 2002). This developmental model of health in nursing explores contextual factors of health work, health potential, style of nursing, competence in health behaviour, and health status. It is described by Barnes et al. (2020) as having the potential to become a health promotion model as it focuses on increasing the unity of the family unit and also its quality of life. Kaakinen et al. (2018) describe this interactional model as a family health promotion model that empowers patients toward improvements in their health. Rather than focus on the deficits or dysfunctional aspects of a family, the CHN uses this assessment model to identify family strengths in relation to individual family members, the family as the unit of care, and external resources.

McMaster Model of Family Functioning

Another assessment model, the McMaster Model of Family Functioning (MMFF), holds the basic premise that the family's role is to provide support for one another so individuals can develop and maintain functioning in three areas: social, psychological, and biological (Harrawood, 2017). While helping to care for one another, families have three task areas to address: the basic task area, the developmental task area, and the hazardous task area. The basic task area addresses instrumental issues that are family members' fundamental needs, such as food, money, and shelter. The developmental task area encompasses issues that pertain to life stages such as marriage, pregnancy, and launching children. Finally, the hazardous task area involves managing crises like illness and job loss. Optimal family functioning is the ability to adequately address all three tasks.

According to the MMFF, the three task areas are addressed through six overlapping dimensions: problem-solving, communication, roles, affective responsiveness, affective involvement, and behaviour control. Problem-solving has to do with the way that families solve two types of problems: instrumental and affective. *Instrumental problems* are problems related to the instrumental task described above, while *affective issues* relate to problems surrounding emotions and feelings. Families must effectively handle instrumental problems before they can effectively deal with those that are affective in nature. Within the MMFF there is a seven-step model of effective problem-solving: identifying the problem, appropriately communicating the problem, developing a set of solutions, deciding on one solution, carrying out the action, monitoring, and evaluating the effectiveness of the choice. All families, whether they are functioning effectively or not, have problems; however, effective families have the ability to resolve their problems.

The next dimension in the MMFF is that of communication. Here, patterns of communication encompass only that which is exchanged verbally and is assessed in relation to the instrumental and affective areas that are addressed in the problem-solving domain. Communication is assessed on two continuums: clear to masked and direct to indirect. Clear communication is communication that is distinct, while masked communication is disguised and vague. Direct communication is communicating toward the appropriate person, while indirect communication is routed to other people. Communication patterns can fall into four discrete patterns: clear and direct, clear and indirect, masked and direct, masked and indirect.

Family roles are patterns of behaviors that guide how family members fulfill family functions and are also part of assessing family functions. The MMFF examines the following five roles: (1) provision of resources, (2) nurturance and support, (3) adult sexual gratification, (4) personal development, and (5) maintenance and management of the family system. Patterns of behaviour control are said to occur in three types of situations: those that are physically dangerous, those that address meeting and expressing psychobiological needs and drives, and those involving interpersonal socializing behaviour. When addressing these areas, four types of behaviour control emerge: rigid, flexible, laissez-faire, and chaotic. Rigid patterns of behaviour are marked by narrow responses with little variation. Flexible patterns manifest as reasonable behaviours with room for negotiation and are seen as the most effective. Laissez-faire patterns possess no set of standards for responding and are extreme and erratic. Chaotic behaviour control is described as random shifting between rigid, flexible, and laissez-faire styles; family members have no way of knowing which standards apply, causing confusion.

Relational Practice

Finally, **relational practice** (Hartrick Doane & Varcoe, 2005, 2020) is an approach to inquiry for family nursing that is guided by conscious participation with patients using a number of relational skills including listening, questioning, empathy, mutuality, reciprocity, self-observation, reflection, and a sensitivity to emotional contexts. Relational practice encompasses therapeutic nurse–patient relationships and relationships among health care providers. Approaching family nursing as relational inquiry aims to build on family strengths, recognize differences among family members without taking sides, or reinforcing power relationships. Hartrick Doane and Varcoe (2005, 2007, 2020) describe this approach as acknowledging that power and differences are important features of relationships that must not be made visible. This sort of practice begins by entering into relation, inquiring into the family health and healing experience, following the lead of families, and learning to let be (Box 12.1). Inquiring and listening for what is meaningful and important to the family is central relational family nursing practice and requires considerable awareness of both self and others. Drawing on this model in your own practice, consider how you can look beyond the surface of the patients and families and enter your practice with an approach of inquiry.

◢ EVIDENCE-INFORMED PRACTICE

Rural living may compound marginalization and create additional challenges for young mothers who are experiencing structural vulnerabilities. Nurse-Family Partnership (NFP) is an intervention program that starts early in pregnancy with intensive and purposeful home visits that continue until the child's second birthday. It was thought that having public health nurses (PHNs) deliver the NFP to mothers living in rural communities might help to improve outcomes for these families. This interpretive descriptive study sought to explore the influence of rural contexts on the delivery of NFP in British Columbia, Canada. A total of 10 PHNs and 11 supervisors who were providing the NFP program in rural communities were interviewed for the study.

In the study, PHNs noted the importance the intensive nursing home visiting partnership, and the relationship in the lives of their rural patients, especially in the face of extreme financial and social inequities for some families. Remaining flexible in their approach and protecting time for the partnership work and intensive home visiting supported nurses practising in rural environments. Rural PHNs were often the sole NFP nurse in their offices, however, and with the intensive scope of the work, they struggled to remain connected to their supervisors and other colleagues. Challenges

EVIDENCE-INFORMED PRACTICE—CONT'D

concentrated on negotiating boundaries of the relationship that are routine aspects of rural practice, and included poor weather, reduced accessibility, and long travel distances, all features that are also common in rural community health practice.

It was concluded that PHNs are well-positioned to identify the modifications that are required to support the delivery of this intensive partnership program for rural families, particularly for people who experience structural vulnerabilities such as those explored in *Chapter 15*.

Application for CHNs

The study findings indicate that establishing an intensive committed partnership program with families who are in early pregnancy though to early parenting year establishes a unique support for people isolated and lacking other resources in rural communities.

An intensive and intentionally longer relationship can provide opportunities for CHNs, and negotiating boundaries with both the families and office and supervisors will support success.

Questions for Reflection and Discussion

1. How might you apply these lessons learned to different areas of community health nursing practice, where more intensive and longer-term home visiting could be beneficial?
2. What has been your experience in working with the family as unit of care?
3. Find additional research on approaches to longer term with families. What findings and approaches could be applied to your CHN practice negotiating longer term relationships and intensive home visits and outreach in rural communities?

Source: Campbell, K., MacKinnon, K., Dobbins, M., Van Borek, N., & Jack, S. (2019). Weathering the rural reality: delivery of the Nurse-Family Partnership home visitation program in rural British Columbia, Canada. *BMC Nursing, 18*(1), 1–14. https://doaj.org/article/8ca698486fcf49389135a3bb6b2e0a0d

BOX 12.1 Relational Nursing Practice: Assessing and Intervening Processes.

1. Entering Into Relation: Getting "in Sync" With a Family
   - Conscious and intentional participation
   - Stopping to look, listen, and hear
   - Unconditional positive regard
   - Being in sync
   - Walking alongside family
2. Being in Collaborative Relation: Staying "in Sync"
   - Family collaborating with nurse
   - Family and nurse working together to assess and intervene
3. Inquiring Into the Family Health and Healing Experience
   - Inquiry into what is meaningful and significant to the family
   - Keeping family at the centre of view
4. Following the Lead of Families
   - Taking cues from families
   - Taking a stance of unknowing and uncertainty
   - Using theoretical knowledge to enhance sensitivity to family experience
   - Scrutinizing theoretical and expert knowledge against family experience
5. Listening To and For
   - Listening through phenomenological, critical, and spiritual lenses
   - Listening through a socioenvironmental health-promotion lens
6. Self-observation
   - Participating consciously and intentionally
   - Self-knowing
7. Letting Be and Change
   - Letting be to know who this family is and what is happening for them
   - Creating the opportunity for family to come to know more about their own experience, patterns, capacities, challenges, and contextual constraints
8. Collaborative Knowledge Development
   - Drawing on family knowledge (experiential, historical, sociocultural)
   - Drawing on nursing knowledge (scientific, theoretical, biomedical, political, practical)
9. Pattern Recognition
   - Identifying underlying patterns of experience
   - Identifying the family's responses
   - Identifying patterns of capacity
   - Identifying capacity-adversity patterns
10. Naming and Supporting Capacity
    - Seeing and recognizing capacity
    - Looking beyond the surface
    - Honouring the family's version of the story
    - Working with the family to enhance capacity and address adversity
11. Emancipatory Action
    - Recognizing and naming inequities
    - Recognizing and naming structural conditions
    - Drawing on and sharing contextual knowledge
    - Introducing alternative discourses
    - Devoting energy to remedying structural inequities
    - Creating coalitions

Source: Hartrick Doane, G., & Varcoe, C. (2005). *Family nursing as relational inquiry: Developing health promoting practice* (Box 7.1, p. 288). Lippincott, Williams & Wilkins.

Many other family assessment models exist, but the focus in this text is on the CFAM, one of the most frequently used in Canada (Bell, 2015). Using a family assessment model is one of the first steps CHNs take in identifying family strengths, health risks, and health concerns when working with the family to implement health promotion interventions. The overall family nursing approach a CHN takes with CFAM is one of continued relationship building, following the phases of the helping relationship (see "Care Planning With Families" later in this chapter). The intervention work of mutual goal setting and planning within the relationship may include including intensive and longer-term CHN care, as well as negotiating the relationship boundaries of living in the same rural communities (Campbell, MacKinnon, Dobbins, et al., 2019), and unlimited other scenarios.

While the people and contexts a CHN works with are unlimited, there are also principles and standards, as well as the nursing process, to hold on to as an anchor. For instance, before the first meeting with a family, the CHN creates a plan for the assessment process (see the "How to" box).

✴ HOW TO …

Plan for the Assessment Process
Planning includes answering the following key questions:
1. What is the reason for the visit?
2. Who will be present during the interview?
3. Where will the visit take place, and how will the space be arranged?
4. What is going to be assessed?
5. How are the data going to be collected?
6. What will be done with the data collected?

FAMILY HOME VISITS

CHNs work with families in a variety of settings, including clinics, schools, support groups, and offices. However, an important aspect of the CHN's role in reducing health risks and promoting the health of populations has been the tradition of providing services to families in their homes.

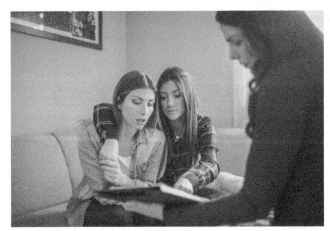

An advantage of the community health nurse meeting the family in the home is that it allows family members to feel comfortable and be themselves. Home visits also allow the nurse to witness the everyday realities, relationships, and habits of family members, especially if these are over the course of several visits over time. (iStockphoto/ NoSystem Images)

Planning for Home Visits

Before making arrangements with the family for the initial appointment, the CHN decides the best place to meet with the family, which might be in the home, clinic, or office. Often this decision is dictated by the type of agency with which the CHN works (e.g., home health is conducted in the home, or a mental health agency may choose to have the family meet in the neighbourhood clinic office). The CHN needs to review the agency policy about home

visiting before the decision is made to contact the family to make arrangements regarding where and when to meet.

Meeting in the family home has a number of advantages, including:
- It allows for viewing the everyday family environment.
- Family members are likely to feel more relaxed and therefore demonstrate typical family interactions.
- It emphasizes that the health concern is the responsibility of the whole family and not one family member.
- It may increase the probability of having more family members present during a family interview.

At the same time, meeting in the family home has two possible disadvantages:
- The family may perceive the visit as an invasion of privacy. The home may be the only sanctuary or safe place for the family or individual family members to be away from the scrutiny of others.
- Meeting with a family on its home ground means that it may take greater effort for the CHN to establish the helping relationship. The CHN must be highly self-reflective and skilled in communication while guiding the interaction. The CHN must also remain goal oriented and realistic about the CHN's and the family's roles and capacities.

Conducting the family appointment in the office or clinic allows easier access to other health care providers for consultation. An advantage of using the clinic may be that the family situation is so intense that a more formal, less personal setting may be necessary for the family to begin discussion of emotionally charged issues. A disadvantage of not seeing the everyday family environment is that it may reinforce a possible power differential or culture gap between the family and the CHN.

After the decision is made regarding where to meet the family, the CHN contacts the family. It is important to remember that the family gathers information about the CHN from this initial phone call to arrange a meeting, so the CHN should be confident and organized. After the introduction, the CHN concisely states the reason for requesting the family visit and encourages all family members to attend the meeting. Several possible times for the appointment can be offered, including late afternoon or evening, allowing the family to select the most convenient time for all members to be present (see the "How to" box).

✴ HOW TO …

Set an Appointment With the Family
The assessment process starts immediately upon referral. The following are suggestions that will make the process of arranging a meeting with the family easier:
1. Remember that the assessment is reciprocal and the family will be making judgements about you when you call to make the appointment.
2. Introduce yourself and state the purpose for the contact.
3. Do not apologize for contacting the family. Be clear, direct, and specific about the need for an appointment.
4. Arrange a time that is convenient for the greatest possible number of family members.
5. Confirm the place, time, date, and directions to the selected meeting place.

Usually, a home visit is initiated as the result of a referral from a health or social agency. A **home visit** is the provision of community health nursing care where the patient resides. However, a family may request services, or the CHN may initiate the home visit as a result of case-finding activities. The CHN would need to clarify with the referral agency and family the reason for the visit request. The first contact between the CHN and the family provides the foundation for an effective therapeutic relationship. The CHN needs to be aware that families may feel that they are being "checked up on," that they are seen as being inadequate or dysfunctional, or that their privacy is being impinged on. These potential areas of concern underlie the need for sensitivity on the part of the CHN, the need to clarify information regarding the reason for visits, and the need to establish collaborative, trusting relationships with family members. Subsequent home visits should be based on need and mutual agreement between the CHN and the family. Often, CHNs are not sure of the reason for the visit. This carries with it the potential for the visit to be compromised and to come aimlessly or abruptly to a premature halt. Regardless of the reason for the home visit, it is necessary that the CHN be clear about the purpose for the visit and that this purpose or understanding be shared with the family.

Preparing for the visit has several components. For the most part, these are best accomplished in order, as presented in the "How to" box.

HOW TO ...

Prepare for the Home Visit
- First, if at all possible, the CHN needs to contact the family by telephone before the home visit to introduce themself, to identify the reason for the contact, and to schedule the home visit. A first telephone contact should be a maximum of 15 minutes. The CHN needs to give their name and professional identity—for example, "This is Karen Smith. I'm a community health nurse from the [health unit or health authority]."
- The family needs to be informed of how they came to the attention of the CHN—for example, as the result of a referral or a contact from observations or records in the school setting. If a referral has been received, it is important and useful to ascertain whether the family is aware of the referral.
- A brief summary of the CHN's knowledge about the family's situation will allow family members to clarify their health concerns. For example, the CHN might say, "I understand that your baby was discharged from the hospital yesterday and that you requested some assistance with learning more about how to care for your baby at home."
- A visit needs to be scheduled as soon as possible. Letting the family know agency hours available for visits, the approximate length of the visit, and the purpose of the visit is helpful to the family in determining when to set the visit. Although the lengths of home visits may vary, depending on circumstances, approximately 30 minutes to 1 hour is usual.
- If possible, the visit needs to be arranged for a time when as many family members as possible will be available for the entire visit.
- The telephone call can terminate with a review by the CHN of the time, place, and purpose for the visit, directions to the meeting place, and a means for the family to contact the CHN in case they need to verify or change the time for the visit, or to ask questions. If the family does not have a telephone, another method for setting up the visit can be used. A note can be dropped off at the family home or sent by mail informing the family of when and why the home visit will occur and providing a way for the family to contact the CHN if necessary.

The possibility exists that the family may refuse a home visit. Less experienced CHNs or students may mistakenly interpret this as a personal rejection. Families make decisions about when and which outsiders are allowed entry into their homes. The CHN needs to explore the reasons for the refusal, considering the following:
- The family may not feel comfortable with the way in which the CHN presented themself for any number of reasons (i.e., overfamiliarity or poor attention to the orientation stage of the relationship; perceived sense of CHN control or paternalism; lack of clarity regarding expectation or information about services; or lack of cultural awareness).
- There may be a misunderstanding about the reason for the visit.

As the CHN plans for the first family visit, they begin by seeking to understand what the possible family health concern(s) might be from the family's unique perspective. The objective of seeking to understand starts in the planning stage and continues throughout the home visits. See Box 12.2 for questions the CHN could ask when seeking to understand the family and its health concern(s). Based on the information gathered, the CHN will be able to validate or invalidate hunches and explore possible interventions with the family.

The stages of a home visit using CFAM and CFIM are summarized in Table 12.5. Building a trusting relationship with the family as patient is the cornerstone of successful home visits. The following five skills are fundamental to effective home visits:
1. Observing
2. Listening
3. Questioning
4. Probing
5. Prompting

The need for these skills is evident in all stages of the home visit process.

Engagement

Engagement is the beginning of the interview process with a family, where the focus is on the establishment of the nurse–patient relationship. The first visit to the home affords the CHN the opportunity to assess the family's neighbourhood and community resources, as well as the home and

BOX 12.2   Questions That Seek to Understand the Family (System) and Its Health Concern (Problem)

Who
- Who is in the system? Who are the key players?
- Who first noticed the health concern?
- Who is concerned about the health concern?
- Who is affected by the health concern? (most, least)
- Who referred the family?

What
- What is the health concern at this time?
- What is the meaning that the health concern has for the family and for different members of the family?
- What solutions have been attempted?
- What question(s) do I feel obliged to ask?
- What beliefs perpetuate the health concern?
- What beliefs might be identified as core beliefs?
- What beliefs are perpetuated by the health concern?
- What concerns and solutions perpetuate the beliefs?

Why
- Why is the family presenting at this time?

Where
- Where has the information about this health concern come from?
- Where does the family see the health concern originating?
- Where does the family see the health concern and the family going if there is no change or if there is change?

When
- When did the health concern begin?
- When does the health concern begin in relation to another phenomenon of the family?
- When does the health concern not occur?

How
- How might a change in the health concern affect other parts of the family (key members, relationships, beliefs)?
- How does a change in one part of the family affect another part of the family or the health concern?
- How will I know when my work with this family is over?
- How might my work with this family constrain the system from finding its solution?

Source: From Shajani, Z., & Snell, D. (2019). *Wright & Leahey's nurses and families: A guide to family assessment and intervention* (7th ed.). F.A. Davis Company, Philadelphia, PA with permission.

TABLE 12.5   Stages and Activities of a Home Visit

Stage	Activity
1. Engagement	• Introduce yourself and your professional identity • Clarify the source of referral for the visit • Clarify the purpose for the home visit • Share information on the reason and purpose of the home visit with the family • Establish a shared perception of purpose with the family • Establish the nurse–patient relationship
2. Family assessment	• Apply the CFAM to identify family health concerns • Work with the family to identify mutually agreeable goals • Work with the family to identify solutions
3. Family intervention	• Implement nursing interventions using the CFIM • Continue to work on the nurse–patient relationship
4. Termination and evaluation	• Review the visit with the family • Evaluate the extent to which the goals have been met • Provide referrals to other community resources as needed • Plan for future visits (if the need is identified during evaluation)
5. Postvisit documentation	• Document the visit

CFAM, Calgary Family Assessment Model; *CFIM*, Calgary Family Intervention Model.

family interactions. The actual home visit includes several components:
- The CHN provides professional identification and tells the patient the location of the agency.
- A brief social conversation helps establish rapport.
- The CHN describes their role, responsibilities, and limitations.
- The CHN determines the patient's expectations (an important step).

The major portion of the home visit involves establishing the relationship and implementing the community health nursing process. Too much disclosure of personal family information during early contacts between the family and CHN may threaten the family. The CHN needs to slow the process down and take time to build trust. Assessment, planning, intervention, and evaluation are ongoing. Assessment is interactive. As the CHN evaluates families, the families evaluate the CHN. The reason for the visit determines what then occurs in the home visit.

It is important that the CHN be realistic about what can be accomplished in a home visit. In some situations, one visit may be all that is possible or appropriate. In this instance, health concerns and the resources available to meet them are explored with the family, and it is determined whether further services are desired or indicated. If further services are indicated and the CHN's agency is not appropriate, the CHN can assist the family in identifying other services available in the community and can help in initiating referrals. Although it is not unusual to have only one home visit with a family, often multiple visits are made. The frequency and intensity of home visits vary, depending on not only the health concerns of the family but also the eligibility of the family for services as defined by agency policies and priorities. It is realistic for CHNs to expect that a first visit would include an initial family assessment and at least the beginning of building a relationship with the family.

Families may or may not be able to control interruptions during the visit. Telephones ring, pets join in the visit, people come and go, and televisions are left on. The CHN can ask that, for a limited time, televisions be turned off or that other disruptive activities be limited. Families may be so accustomed to the background noises and routine activities that they do not recognize them as being potentially disruptive.

Personal safety is an issue that may arise either in approaching the family home or once the family has opened the door to the CHN:

- CHNs need to examine personal fears and objective threats to determine whether safety is indeed an issue.
- Precautions (e.g., carry a cellphone, visit with an escort or in CHN pairs or teams, or—in rare circumstances—accompanied by a police or security officer) can be taken in known high-risk situations such as when violence has occurred or is suspected in the home.
- Readily identifiable uniforms may be required.
- A sign-out process indicating the timing and location of home visits may be used routinely.
- CHNs' driving routes can be registered with the agency.

CHNs are most often perceived as helpful, caring health professionals with specialized skills working with patients in the community in a supportive capacity. As guests in patient homes, CHNs are usually perceived as nonthreatening (Smith, 2013). While home visits are generally safe, as with all worksites, the possibility of violence exists and CHNs need to use caution. If a reasonable question exists about the safety of making a visit, a CHN should not make the visit alone. Box 12.3 outlines some safety concerns and precautions that can help CHNs avoid dangerous situations.

Family Assessment

Family assessment is the cornerstone for family nursing interventions. By using a systematic process, family health concerns are identified, and family strengths and capacities are emphasized as the building blocks for interventions. Building the interventions with family-identified health concerns and strengths allows for equal family and provider commitment to the solutions and ensures more successful interventions.

CHNs need to use a systematic format for family assessment. At times, the CHN may need to make modifications to a framework so that a complete individualized family assessment can be conducted. Keep in mind that cultural assessments are conducted with the patient as individual, family, and community. History and culture contribute in a number of ways to individual and family health. For example, refer to the "Cultural Considerations" box.

CULTURAL CONSIDERATIONS

Culture, Food, and Family Health
Cultural meanings of food and health can have a major impact on family functioning and ultimately on family and individual food practices. Eating patterns and how families make decisions about food practices are influenced by distinctive cultural values, especially if those food practices are linked to maintaining a cultural identity.* Changing negative family food practices that are embedded in culture could be perceived as changing one's cultural identity. For example a traditional Newfoundland "Jiggs' Dinner" boils salt beef and vegetables in the same pot, which results in a meal that is high in salt and fat content. The cultural meaning of food and health can also influence how individuals develop opinions on the norms and standards set by society, such as what is a "normal" body weight and body shape.† The cultural eating pattern and health should be assessed and understood by CHNs when designing health promotion interventions that focus on changing harmful family food practices in multicultural populations. The plate of food presented in Canada's Food Guide 2019 mainly includes westernized foods with little recognition of traditional or ethnic foods, which patients may interpret as classifying their traditional foods as unhealthy.‡

Question to Consider
How could a CHN design an effective intervention that takes into consideration the cultural influences on food practices?

Sources: * Beagan & Chapman, 2012.
† Ristovski-Slijepcevic, Bell, Chapman, et al., 2010.
‡ Lapum, St-Amant, Garcia., et al., 2019.

Therefore, when conducting a family assessment, CHNs need to consider culture and should include relevant areas based on a cultural nursing assessment (see Chapter 7). For example, a more in-depth cultural or spiritual assessment might be indicated, and, therefore, might be integrated into the family assessment model. During the family visit, it is critical that the CHN be sufficiently familiar with the chosen family assessment model so that complete data are collected during the development of the nurse–patient relationship.

Many family assessment frameworks exist, but the focus of this chapter is on the CFAM. The CFAM process may be quite simple and fit naturally in conversation; and a brief family assessment interview of 15 minutes or less can be entirely appropriate and effective (Bell, 2015, 2016). Many people do not have the time or tolerance for long in-depth interviews—and a developmental approach to getting to know a family may better support the relationship over several brief interviews. Following the collection of data, a CHN analyzes the data collected and develops a prioritized list of family health concerns and strengths; nursing interventions are planned and implemented in partnership with the family (whenever possible). All interviews and family visits, whether

BOX 12.3   Safety Concerns and Precautions for Family Home Visits

1. Possible unsafe situations
   - Patients or family members have a pattern of violent behaviour such as domestic violence (physical, verbal, emotional).
   - Patients or family members who are known to use substances.
   - Persons with communicable diseases are in the home.
   - Settings in which there are environmental risks, such as an unsafe physical environment (e.g., extreme hoarding, water damage or mold contamination, threatening animals, and second-hand smoke).
2. Actions taken to promote safety
   - Arrange the visit by telephone or virtual meeting system with the family so family members have given permission to visit.
   - Have another CHN accompany you on the visit, if necessary.
   - If the neighbourhood is considered unsafe (e.g., it has a high rate of random violence or is an isolated wilderness setting), arrange to meet the family in a neutral, safe area such as a clinic if the family health conditions allow.
   - Leave a schedule of your home visits with the supervisor at your agency (and communicate any schedule changes).
   - Certain areas may be safer during certain times of the day (e.g., during morning or early afternoon hours), so consider timing when planning home visits.
   - Know the directions to the family home.
   - Dress in a professional manner.
   - In the home, use indoor footwear and remove your outdoor boots or shoes; do not put bags on the floor—being careful to avoid cross-contamination when visiting multiple homes.
   - Have a cellphone that is readily accessible and functional.
   - Drive on main highways or roads and drive or walk in heavily travelled areas.
   - When walking, avoid areas where people are loitering.

   - Keep supplies, equipment, and other necessary items easily accessible in the vehicle rather than in the trunk to avoid taking time to locate them.
   - Keep a purse or other valuables locked and out of sight in the vehicle's trunk or a locked compartment.
   - Keep keys accessible in your pocket to enable entrance to your vehicle quickly.
   - Do not wear expensive jewellery.
   - Check the front and back seats before getting into your vehicle.
   - Keep a nearly full tank of gasoline.
   - Keep your vehicle well-maintained, in working order, with a spare tire and a well-equipped roadside safety bag with a blanket, water, flashlight, and so on.
   - Park your vehicle in such a way that a quick exit may be possible.
   - Look for suspicious behaviour such as individuals following you and contact the police.
   - Avoid offering rides to home visit family members or strangers.
   - Keep the vehicle locked with the windows up at all times.
   - If vehicle problems occur, remain in your vehicle and phone for help.
3. Precautions to use in the home
   - When ascending stairs, follow the patient.
   - If you have concerns about patient behaviour, always visit when other family members are present.
   - Listen to your intuition and if you are feeling unsafe, leave the family situation.
   - If the family or visitors behave in a threatening or inappropriate manner, terminate the home visit immediately.
   - Ask that pets be moved to another room if they are threatening or bothersome; have the family pets join in the visit if they are important or calming companions for the family members.

Sources: Adapted from McEwen, M., & Pullis, B. (2009). *Community-based nursing: An introduction* (3rd ed.). Saunders; Smith, C. M. (2013). Home visiting: Opening the doors for family health. In F. A. Maurer & C. M. Smith (Eds.), *Community/public health nursing practice: Health for families and populations* (5th ed., pp. 302–325). Saunders/Elsevier.

brief or more in-depth, are goal oriented (e.g., establishing the engagement/orientation phase of the helping relationship, engaging in assessment processes, establishing goals and interventions, evaluating interventions). A variety of assessment strategies are explored in "Appraisal of Family Health Risks and Capacity," later in this chapter.

Interventions

The Canadian Community Health Nursing Professional Practice Model and Standards of Practice provides guidance on the CHN's responsibilities under the various standards when intervening with the family as patient (CHNC, 2019). The standards also provide direction on the strategies to use when working with families, such as forming partnerships, promoting capacity building, empowering families, and advocating for families. See "Family Interventions," later in this chapter, for a detailed discussion of this topic.

Termination and Evaluation

When the purpose of the visit has been accomplished, the CHN reviews with the family what has occurred and what has been accomplished. This is the major focus of the **termination phase,** and it provides a basis for evaluating whether further home visits are needed or referrals to community resources are required:

- Ideally, termination of the visit and, ultimately, termination of service begin at the first contact with the establishment of a goal or purpose.
- If communication has been clear to this point, the family and CHN can now plan for future visits, specifically the next visit.

CHNs need to engage in evaluation that involves critical, creative, and concurrent reflection about the patient situation. Evaluation has two components: process (formative) and outcome (summative). The termination home visit phase involves outcome evaluation (summative).

Postvisit Documentation

Even though the CHN has now concluded the home visit and left the patient's home, the responsibility for the visit is not complete until the interaction has been recorded. Visit recording is a basic element needed for legal and clinical purposes. It is important that the recording be current, dated, and signed. The format may consist of:

- Narratives
- Flow sheets
- Problem-oriented medical records
- Subjective, objective, assessment plans
- A combination of formats

Postvisit documentation should be based on a family-centred community health nursing process with the family as the unit of care. Therefore, the health concern needs to be documented as a family health concern and not an individual health concern. Examples are the following: a family that needs to accomplish the stage-appropriate task of providing a safe environment for a preschooler; a couple with communication difficulties that has a desire for improved communication with an adolescent daughter; a couple interested in improving their parenting skills with their toddler; or adult children seeking ways to support their mother, an older person who is recovering from a fall. At times, it may be necessary to address individual health concerns, for example the mother's broken wrist from her fall, or fall prevention within the home, too. However, as mentioned, the emphasis must be on the individual as a member of and within the structure of the family as a unit, such as the family conversations about roles and capacities to support aging in place despite fall risks.

APPRAISAL OF FAMILY HEALTH RISKS AND CAPACITY

Risks to a family's health arise in three major areas:
1. Biological and age-related risks
2. Environmental risks
3. Behavioural risks

In most instances, a risk in one of these areas may not be enough to threaten family health, but a combination of risks from two or more categories could lead to a family crisis. For example, if a family presents with a family history of cardiovascular disease, this health risk is often increased by an unhealthy lifestyle and the presence of determinants of health such as coping skills and social environment. An understanding of the three major areas of risk provides the basis for a comprehensive approach to family health risk assessment and intervention.

In addition, it is crucial for CHNs to have a broad contextual understanding of "risk" and the complexities and capacities of families' everyday lives (Browne, Hartrick Doane, Reimer, et al., 2010). Based on a broad contextual understanding, risk and disadvantage are not simply situated with individuals and the family; instead, they are viewed as part of structural inequities (e.g., poverty, unemployment, and geographical isolation) that influence the health of individuals and families (Hartrick Doane & Varcoe 2005, 2007, 2020).

Family nursing practice must then assess both risk and capacity and base interventions on these assessments. CHNs can support this balanced approach by being self-aware, transparent, collaborative, and flexible in their work with families (Browne et al., 2010).

Biological Risk Assessment

The family plays an important role in both the development and management of a disease or condition. Some illnesses can be related to either genetics or lifestyle patterns. These factors contribute to the biological risk for certain conditions. Patterns of cardiovascular disease, for example, can often be traced through several generations of a family; such families are said to be at risk for cardiovascular disease. How or whether cardiovascular disease is found in a family is often influenced by the lifestyle of the family. CHNs, as family nurses, need to recognize that family history data can provide the genetic information required by families to make relevant decisions.

One of the most widely used techniques for assessing the patterns of health and illness in families is the genogram (Harrawood, 2017). Briefly, a genogram is a drawing that shows the family unit of immediate interest to the CHN and includes at least three generations of family members with gender and age, their relationships, health status, and mortality, using a series of circles, squares, and connecting lines. Basic information about the family, relationships in the family, and patterns of health and illness can be obtained by completing the genogram with the family (McGoldrick, Gerson & Petry, 2020). The following is shown in Fig. 12.4:

- A square indicates a male.
- A circle indicates a female.
- An X through either a square or a circle indicates a death.
- Marriage is indicated by a solid horizontal line.
- Offspring or children are noted by a solid vertical line.
- A broken horizontal line indicates a divorce or separation.
- Dates of birth, marriage, death, and other important events can be indicated where appropriate.
- Major illness or conditions can be listed for each individual family member.

It is important to include a legend on the genogram that conveys the meaning of the various symbols used—this is because there are variations in acceptable symbols and by providing a legend, communication is enhanced. Patterns can be quickly assessed by reviewing the genogram information and providing a guide for the health interviewer about health areas that need further exploring.

The genogram in Fig. 12.4 was completed for a fictional family, the Grahams. Some of the interesting health patterns that can be seen from the genogram are the repetition of the following:

- Hypertension
- Adult-onset diabetes
- Cancer
- Hypercholesterolemia

Completing a genogram requires interviews with as many family members as possible. If possible, it is important to

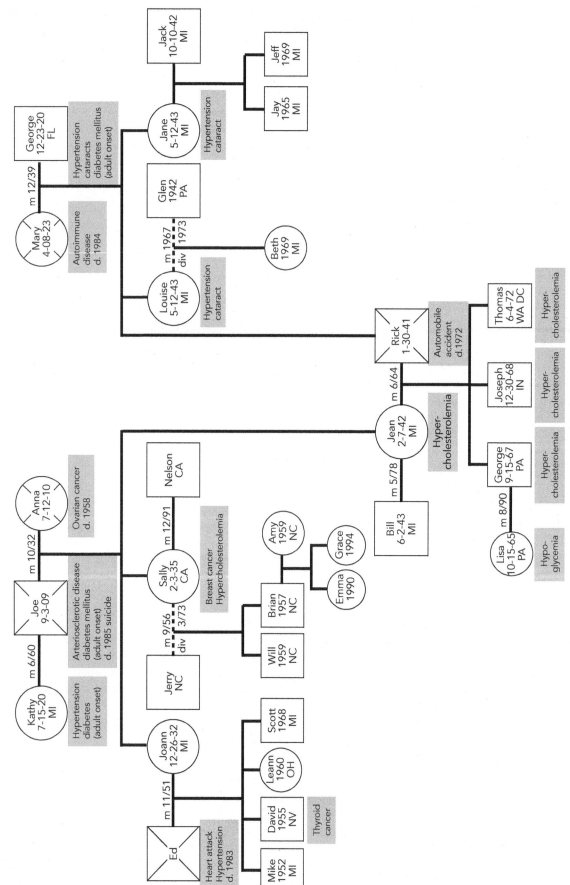

Fig. 12.4 Genogram of the Graham Family. (The two letter abbreviations under each person indicate their state of birth.) (Developed by Carol Loveland-Cherry in Stanhope, M., & Lancaster, J. [2019]. *Public health nursing: Population-centered health care in the community* [10th ed.]. Mosby.)

collect family history data dating back three generations to develop a complete picture of the family and their health patterns. Often, as families complete the genogram with the CHN, they experience an awareness of strengths in their family health status. This can have an empowering effect.

A more intensive and quantitative assessment of a family's biological risk can be achieved through the use of a standard family risk assessment. Because such assessments involve other areas in addition to biological risk, one will be described later, after the description of other types of risk assessment.

Both normative and non-normative life events pose potential risks to the health of families. Even events that are generally viewed as being positive require changes and can place stress on a family. The normative event of the birth of a child, for example, requires considerable changes in family structures and roles (see the "CHN in Practice: A Case Study, Adolescent Prenatal Community Nursing: A Family Assessment" box). Furthermore, family functions are expanded from previous levels, requiring families to add new skills and establish additional resources. **Family functions** are behaviours or activities performed to maintain the integrity of the family unit and to meet the family's needs, individual members' needs, and society's expectations. These changes can in turn result in strain and—if adequate resources are not available—stress. Therefore, to adequately assess life risks, both normative and non-normative events occurring in the family need to be considered. Community-level support groups have been successful in assisting families in dealing with a variety of stressful situations and crises (e.g., Families Anonymous; Bereaved Parents; Parents, Families and Friends of Lesbians and Gays; and One Parent Families Association of Canada) that arise from both life events and age-related events. CHNs have been instrumental in developing and moderating such groups.

CHN IN PRACTICE: A CASE STUDY

Adolescent Prenatal Community Nursing: A Family Assessment

The Valley View Health Clinic was notified that Tori, age 16, had been referred by the school counsellor at the local high school for prenatal community health nursing. Tori, who is just completing Grade 10, is 4 months pregnant, in apparently good health, and living at home with her mother, stepfather, and younger sister. The family lives in a rural area outside of a small farming community. The father of the baby, Dustin, also lives with his parents and farms in the same rural community. Dustin continues to see Tori on a regular basis. The referral information provides the CHN with a beginning, but limited, assessment of the family situation.

Think About It

1. Describe how a family assessment is different from an individual patient assessment for this CHN in practice.
2. What kind of difficulties could you anticipate when arranging for a family assessment interview?
3. Discuss factors to be considered when determining the place to conduct a family assessment interview. Include pros and cons.
4. Consider a broader contextual assessment of risk and search an article in the literature for an assessment and intervention relevant to this case study. Summarize the findings of the article and include your reflections on the new learning gained from this article.

Environmental Risk Assessment

The importance of social risks to family health is gaining increased recognition. A family's health risk increases if they are living in:

- Neighbourhoods that experience high crime rates
- Communities without adequate recreation or health resources
- Communities that have major noise pollution or chemical pollution
- Other high-stress environments

Information on environmental health is discussed in *Chapter 17*. Family preparedness in disaster management is discussed in *Chapter 18*.

Significant social stress is experienced through oppression and discrimination, whether racism, cultural or religious discrimination, ageism, ableism, misogyny, homophobia, transphobia, or other types. The psychological burden resulting from discrimination is itself a stressor, and it adds to the effects of other stress experiences. The implication of these examples of risky social situations is that they contribute to the stressors experienced by families. If adequate resources and coping processes are not available, distress and disruption in health can and do occur from oppression and discrimination.

Persons with a low income are at a greater risk for health problems. **Economic risk,** which is related to social risk, is determined by the relationship between family financial resources and the demands on those resources. Having adequate financial resources means that a family is able to purchase the necessary services and goods related to health, such as:

- Adequate housing
- Clothing
- Food
- Education
- Health or illness care

The amount of money that a family has available is related to situational, cultural, social, and other structural factors. A family may have an income well above the poverty level, but because of the illness of a family member, they may not be able to meet financial demands. Likewise, families from ethnic groups or families with same-sex parents may experience discrimination in finding housing. Even if they find housing, they may not be welcome and may be harassed, resulting in increased stress.

The assessment of environmental health risk is less defined and developed. An ecomap can be used to assess information on relationships that the family has with others such as relatives and neighbours; family connections with other social units such as a religious community, school, work, clubs, and organizations; and the flow of energy, positive or negative, in the family. It is also important to assess the environmental social risks that a family may be influenced by, such as neighbourhoods with high rates of crime, communities without adequate recreation and health resources, or communities that have major noise pollution or chemical pollution.

An **ecomap** represents the family's interactions with other groups and organizations, accomplished by using a series of circles and lines. In Fig. 12.5, a legend box is included in the bottom left corner. Consider the family of interest (the Graham family [see Fig. 12.5]):

- It is represented by a circle in the middle of the page.
- Other groups and organizations are then indicated by other circles.

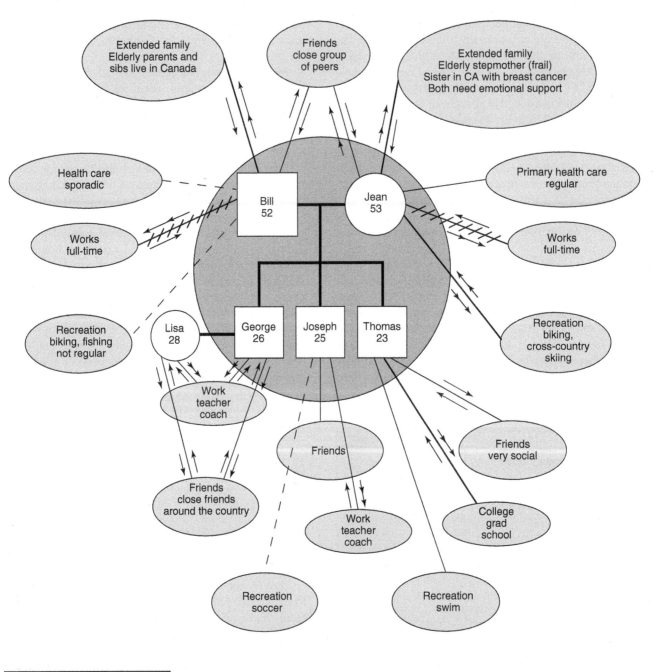

Fig. 12.5 Ecomap of the Graham Family. (Developed by Carol Loveland-Cherry in Stanhope, M., & Lancaster, J. [2019]. *Public health nursing: Population-centered health care in the community* [10th ed.]. Mosby.)

- Lines, representing the flow of energy, are drawn between the family circle and the circles representing other groups and organizations.
- An arrowhead at the end of each line indicates the direction of the flow of energy (into or out of the family).
- The weight of the line indicates the intensity of the energy.

The Graham family ecomap indicates that much of the family energy goes into work (also a source of stress for the parents). Major sources of energy for the Grahams are their immediate and extended families and friends.

In addition to the support network shown by the ecomap, other aspects of social risk include characteristics of the neighbourhood and community where the family lives. A CHN who has worked in the general geographical area may already have conducted a community health assessment and have a working knowledge of the neighbourhood and community. It is important, however, for the CHN to obtain information from the family to understand their perceptions of the community; information about the origins of the family, which is useful to understand other social resources and stressors; information about how long the family has lived in their current location; and the immigration patterns of the family and their ancestors, which provide insight into pressures they may experience.

Economic risk is one of the foremost predictors of health. Families often consider financial information private, and both the CHN and the family may be uncomfortable when discussing finances. It is not necessary to know actual family income, except in instances when it is needed to determine whether families are eligible for programs or benefits. It is useful to know whether the family's resources are adequate to meet their needs. And it is important to understand that the family may be quite comfortable with their finances and standard of living, which may be different from those of the health care provider. CHNs should not impose their financial values onto the family.

With regard to health risk, it is important to understand the resources that families have to obtain health and illness care; adequate shelter, clothing, and food; and access to recreation. Families with limited resources may qualify for social programs. Unfortunately, in a growing number of families, the main wage earner is employed but receives no additional health care insurance benefits, and the salary is not sufficient for supportive health promotion or illness-related care. This is a policy issue, and CHNs can contribute to the drafting of legislation and provide testimony related to the stories of families in their caseloads.

Behavioural Risk Assessment

Personal health habits also contribute to the major causes of morbidity and mortality in Canada. The pattern of personal health habits, known as **behavioural risk,** defines individual and family health status. Families maintain major responsibility for:

- Determining what food is purchased and prepared

- Setting sleep patterns
- Planning family activities
- Setting and monitoring norms about health and health risk behaviours
- Determining when a family member is ill
- Determining when health care should be obtained
- Carrying out treatment regimens

Individuals can, in some instances, structure priorities and make choices, and families can structure time and activities for other family members. However, there are multiple levels of intervention beyond individuals and families that establish the conditions for health and wellbeing. For example, a community in which a family lives can promote family recreation and activity by having accessible parks and walking or biking paths. It is these conditions that help families select activities that provide moderate, regular physical exercise rather than sedentary activities in the home setting.

When we look at factors that promote or inhibit positive lifestyles, families and patterns within families do play a role in health promotion. They regulate time and energy and the boundaries of the system. A number of tools exist for assessing individuals' lifestyle risks, but few are available for assessing family lifestyle patterns. Although assessment of individual lifestyle contributes to determining the lifestyle risk of a family, it is important to look at risks for the family as a unit. One approach is to identify family patterns for lifestyle components. In the areas of health promotion, health protection, and preventive services, lifestyle can be assessed in several dimensions. From the literature on health behaviour research, the critical dimensions include

- The value that a family places on the behaviour
- The family's knowledge of the behaviour and its consequences
- The effect of the behaviour on the family
- The effect of the behaviour on the individual
- Barriers to performing the behaviour
- Benefits of the behaviour

It is important to assess the frequency, intensity, and regularity of specific behaviours, as well as to evaluate the resources available to the family for implementing behaviours. Thus, items for assessment of physical activity include:

- The value that a family places on physical activity
- The hours that a family spends exercising
- The kinds of exercise the family does
- Resources available for exercise

FAMILY INTERVENTIONS

Family interventions take place at primary, secondary, and tertiary levels (see the "Levels of Prevention" box). Building on strengths at all these levels, the CHN considers how to facilitate disease prevention and health promotion.

LEVELS OF PREVENTION

Related to Families Experiencing Violence or Abuse

Primary Prevention

A CHN uses a family genogram in an assessment to identify family strengths and health risks and plan with the family strategies to prevent disease.

A CHN provides programs in child development for families at risk for child or elder abuse, such as poverty, history of violence, or solo parenting or family caregiving.

Secondary Prevention

During a home visit, a CHN screens for warning signs of abuse in the family.

A CHN provides programs in child development and behaviour management for families who have not abused their children but whose children are brought to the attention of social work authorities for aggressive behaviour problems.

Tertiary Prevention

A CHN develops programs with the family to change nutritional patterns to reduce complications from obesity.

A CHN refers families experiencing relationship violence or abuse to family therapy.

BOX 12.4 Family Intervention Tips

- Interventions (held in partnership and conversation) are the core of clinical work with families.
- They are offered in the context of collaborative, therapeutic conversations as the CHN supports the family to, together, devise solutions to their health challenge, addressing what might lead or contribute to that challenge. In this way there can be potential for solutions that fit the family context and circumstances.
- They must be approached within the training, skill, and capacity of the CHN.
- They must be devised with respect for the family's values and cultural background in a way to support cultural safety.
- They are not *done to* families and can only be *offered for* families. The CHN cannot direct change but can create a context for family deliberation, decisions, and actions where change can occur.
- The CHN should inquire with the family with an open mind, avoid advice giving, while respectfully providing information and correcting any misinformation.
- The CHN should receive feedback without becoming defensive, and offer feedback with respect and asking permission, avoiding any blaming of self or the family.

SOURCES: Broekema, S., Paans, W., Roodbol, P.F., Luttik, M.L.A. (2019). Nurses' application of the components of family nursing conversations in home health care: a qualitative content analysis. *Scandinavian Journal of Caring Sciences, 34*(2), 322–331. https://doi.org/10.1111/scs.12731; Greenwood, S., Wright, T., & Nielsen, H. (2006). Conversations in context: Cultural safety and reflexivity in child and family health nursing. *Journal of Family Nursing, 12*(2), 201–224. https://doi.org/10.1177/1074840706287405; Levac, A.M.C., Wright, L.M., & Leahey, M. (2002). Children and families: Models for assessment and intervention. In J.A. Fox (Ed.), *Primary health care of infants, children, and adolescents* (2nd ed., pp. 10–19). Mosby.

Risk assessment tends to focus on the needs or problems of the family. By contrast, family interventions concentrate more on family assets and strengths rather than family risks and deficits. In particular, the CFAM, CFIM, and the McGill Model of Nursing encompass this asset-based approach. The right column of Table 12.2 identifies features of higher functioning in families that CHNs need to consider when engaging in family interventions. Understanding whether these features (family strengths) are present or were present in the family in the past would be helpful when planning interventions to promote, protect, or maintain family health. **Family strengths** are "positive behaviours or qualities that help maintain family health" (Smith, 2013, p. 355). Family strengths, capacities, and resources can be used to help families deal with health concerns and to promote their health. Health promotion is most likely to occur when a family is able to define health holistically and with a wellness or well-being focus rather than health as the absence of disease. For example, a family with a parent who has been newly diagnosed with celiac disease agrees to maintain a gluten-free household as a family to promote family health and wellness. Another example is a family concerned about well-being who prioritizes spending limited resources on a family membership at the local community recreation centre. The family commits to participating in the public swimming programming for families.

Boxes 12.4 and 12.5 provide the CHN with considerations in relation to family interventions. A CHN's family interventions may include roles such as direct clinical care, health promotion, health education, counselling, and advocacy. These interventions and additional roles for CHNs when partnering with families is presented by the International Council of Nurses (see the link in the Tool Box on the Evolve website).

BOX 12.5 Factors to Consider When Planning Interventions

- What is the agreed-on health concern to change?
- At what domain of family functioning is the intervention aimed?
- How does the intervention match the family's style of relating?
- How is the intervention linked to the family's strengths and previously useful solution strategies?
- How is the intervention consistent with the family's ethnic and religious beliefs?
- How is the intervention new or different for the family?

Source: From Shajani, Z., & Snell, D. (2019). *Wright & Leahey's nurses and families: A guide to family assessment and intervention* (7th ed.). F.A. Davis Company, Philadelphia, PA with permission.

Calgary Family Intervention Model

When the family assessment is completed and intervention is warranted to facilitate positive family change, the CHN may want to use the Calgary Family Intervention Model (CFIM). This model helps CHNs identify solutions in partnership with the family to promote, improve, or sustain family functioning

TABLE 12.6   Circular Questions to Invite Change in the Domains of Family Functioning

Type of Question	Cognitive	Affective	Behavioural
Difference Question Explores differences between people, relationships, time, ideas, or beliefs	What is the best advice given to you about supporting your son with morbid obesity? What is the worst advice that you received?	Who in the family is most worried about the medical treatments for obesity and your upcoming bariatric surgery?	Which family member is best at discussing the concerns around obesity and supporting reflection or motivation with the family?
Behavioural Effect Question Explores communications between how one family member's behaviour affects other members	What do you know about the effect of life-threatening illness on children?	How does your son show that he is afraid of dying?	What could you do to show your son that you understand his fears?
Hypothetical/Future-Oriented Question Explores family options and alternative actions or meanings in the future	What do you think will happen if these skin grafts continue to be painful for your son?	If your son's skin grafts are not successful, what do you think his mood will be? Angry? Resigned?	When will your son engage in treatment for his contractures?
Triadic Question Explores the relationship between two people through a third person	If your father were not drinking daily, what would your mother think about his receiving treatment for alcoholism?	What does your father do that makes your mother less anxious about his condition?	If your father were willing to talk with your mother about solutions to his addiction, what could he say?

Source: From Shajani, Z., & Snell, D. (2019). *Wright & Leahey's nurses and families: A guide to family assessment and intervention* (7th ed.). F.A. Davis Company, Philadelphia, PA with permission.

in the cognitive, affective, and behavioural domains (Shajani & Snell, 2019). A change in one domain can lead to changes in the others. A CHN can focus on developing interventions that focus on one or more domains.

In the CFIM, family strengths are identified through the use of **commendations,** a practice where the CHN praises the family for patterns in behaviour that are family strengths within the family unit. Using commendations as an intervention helps change family functioning in the cognitive domain. Commendations often help family members begin viewing the family unit in a different, more positive light. In fact, Moules and Johnstone (2010) indicate that when nurses use a family-strengths approach with commendations and conversation at the centre, the family focuses on its visions and hopes for the future. These practices enable a shift from focusing on factors related to family health concerns, and these concerns can become integrated so that life and family relationships beyond illness can take hold once again.

Circular communication is reciprocal communication between people, whereby each person influences the behaviour of the other. Difference, behavioural effect, hypothetical and future-oriented, and triadic questions are the four types of circular questions used to invite change in the three domains of family functioning (Shajani & Snell, 2019). Examples for each type of question are presented in Table 12.6. Shajani and Snell (2019) provide a detailed discussion of CFAM and CFIM.

Family Health Risk Reduction

Several factors contribute to the development of healthy or unhealthy outcomes. Clearly, not everyone exposed to the same event will have the same outcome. The factors that determine or influence whether disease or other unhealthy results occur are called **health risks. Risk** is the probability of some event or outcome occurring within a specified period of time. Controlling health risks is done through disease prevention and health promotion efforts.

Although single risk factors can influence outcomes, the combined effect of several risks has greater influence. For example, a family history of cardiovascular disease is a single biological risk factor that is affected by smoking (a behavioural risk that is more likely to occur if other family members also smoke) and by diet and exercise. Diet and exercise are influenced by family and society's norms. The determinants of health such as culture, biology, and income can also influence diet and exercise. The combined effect of a family history, determinants of health, family behavioural risks, and society's influences is greater than each of the three individual risk factors (smoking, diet, exercise). **Social risks** refer to risky social situations that can contribute to the stressors experienced by families. If adequate resources and coping processes are not available, breakdowns in health can occur.

Health risk appraisal refers to the process of assessing and analyzing for the presence of specific factors in each of the categories that have been identified as being associated with an increased likelihood of an illness developing such as cancer, or *an unhealthy event,* such as an automobile accident.

Health risk reduction is based on the assumption that decreasing the number of risks or the magnitude of risk will result in a lower probability of an undesired event. For example, to decrease the likelihood of adolescent substance abuse, family behaviours such as parents not drinking, alcohol not being available in the home, and family contracts related to alcohol and drug use may be useful. Health risks can be reduced through a variety of approaches. It is important to note the specific risk and the family's tolerance of it. Risk reduction is a complex process that requires knowledge of the specific risk and the family's perceptions of the nature of the risk.

A **family crisis** occurs when the family is not able to cope with an event and becomes disorganized; the demands of the situation exceed the resources of the family. When families experience a crisis or a crisis-producing event, they attempt to gather their resources to deal with the demands created by the situation. Examples of family resources are money and extended family who are available to them. Families cope by using known processes and behaviours to help them manage or adapt to the problem. Thus, if a family's main wage earner were to experience an unexpected illness, family resources might include financial assistance or emotional support from relatives. Family coping strategies, in contrast, would include whether the family were able to ask a relative to loan them emergency funds or were able to talk with relatives about the worries they were experiencing. (See the Registered Nurses' Association of Ontario [RNAO] Best Practice Guidelines *Crisis Intervention* and *Supporting and Strengthening Families Through Expected and Unexpected Life Events* links on the Evolve website.)

Family Empowerment

Empowerment is a process that CHNs use to promote and protect the health of families, encourage autonomy, and provide families with information to actively involve them so that they can make informed choices about their health (Murdaugh, Parsons & Pender, 2018). Help-giving interventions do not always have positive outcomes for patients. If families do not perceive a situation as a health concern, offers of help may cause resentment. Help-giving also may have negative consequences if there is no match between what is expected and what is offered. A CHN's failure to recognize a family's capacities (strengths) and to not define an active role for them can contribute to the family's dependency and lack of growth. This can be frustrating for both the CHN and the family. For families to become active participants, they need to feel a sense of personal competence and a desire for and willingness to take action. Definitions of *empowerment* reflect the following three characteristics of the empowered family seeking help:
- Access and control over needed resources
- Decision-making and problem-solving abilities
- Abilities to communicate and obtain needed resources

Empowerment requires a viewpoint that may conflict with the views of many helping professions, including nursing. Empowerment's underlying assumption is one of a partnership between the professional and the patient as opposed to one in which the professional is dominant. Families are assumed to be either competent or capable of becoming competent. This implies that the professional is not an unchallenged authority who is in control. Empowerment promotes an environment that creates opportunities for competencies to be used. Finally, families need to identify that their actions result in behaviour change. A community health nursing intervention that incorporates the principles of empowerment meets the following requirements:
- It is directed toward the building of nurse–family partnerships.
- It emphasizes health risk reduction and health promotion.

The CHN's approach to the family needs to be positive and focused on capacity building, competencies, and strengths rather than on health concerns, deficits, or pathology. The interventions need to be consistent with family cultural norms and the family's perception of the health concern. Rather than making decisions for the family, the CHN supports the family in primary decision making and bolsters their self-esteem by recognizing and using family strengths and support networks. Interventions that promote desired family behaviours increase family competency, decrease the need for outside help, and result in families seeing themselves as being actively responsible for bringing about desired changes. The goal of such an empowering approach is to create a partnership between the CHN and the family characterized by cooperation and shared responsibility. Family Systems Nursing occurs in a relationship between an individual/family and a nonjudgemental nurse who focuses on how family members can be supportive to each other, how to identify strengths and resources of the family, and how to share and reflect on the experiences of everyday life together while living with health challenges.

Family Resiliency

Family resilience helps families adapt to a crisis. **Family resiliency** is defined as "the ability to cope with expected and unexpected stressors" (West & Jakubec, 2019, p. 300). In 1993, McCubbin and McCubbin developed the Family Resiliency Model to assess family stress and family adjustment and adaptation. This model was a further development of the previously available family stress theories such as the Family Adjustment and Adaptation Response Model. The McCubbin and McCubbin model explores family adaptation as it adjusts to stressors on the family system in an attempt to regain equilibrium. This model considers family strengths as the family copes with their changed situation and attempts to maintain family functioning (Hadfield & Ungar, 2018).

Black and Lobo (2008) describe family resiliency as "the successful coping of family members under adversity that enables them to flourish with warmth, support, and cohesion" (p. 33). These authors reviewed the family literature and found that the prominent factors of resilient families include:
- *Positive outlook.* They overcome challenges with an optimistic lens; a sense of humour is present.
- *Spirituality.* They use a sense of purpose to deal with stressors.
- *Family member accord.* Family members work together in a supportive manner.
- *Flexibility.* Family members show an ability to adapt to interchangeable roles and functions when needed, such as during times of change.

- *Family communication.* They use collaboration to problem solve; they also use direct, open channels of communication and openly express emotion.
- *Financial management.* They are able to manage family finances; when confronted with financial challenges, family caring is maintained.
- *Family time.* Family members work together to complete daily family tasks and functions.
- *Shared recreation.* Leisure activities are enjoyed as a family.
- *Routines and rituals.* Routines and rituals are maintained even during times of stress.
- *Support networks.* They use and contribute to the maintenance of support networks (Black & Lobo, 2008).

Care Planning With Families

Increasingly, health care providers work with patients in an interactive, collaborative style. This approach is consistent with a more knowledgeable public and the recent self-care movement. However, it may not be consistent with cultures that look to health care providers for more direct guidance; therefore, it is important to determine the family's value system before assuming whether a care plan will work.

Mutual goal setting for the care plan involves a shift in responsibility and control toward a shared effort by the patient and CHN as opposed to an effort by the CHN alone. The premise of goal setting and care planning is family control. It is assumed that when the family has legitimate control, its ability to make healthful choices is increased. Mutual goal setting is a strategy aimed at formally involving the family in the care plan and community health nursing process. Through mutual goal setting, the CHN and the family jointly define the roles of both the family members and the CHN.

The care plan, then, is a working agreement that is continuously renegotiable and may or may not be written.

For family health risk reduction, it is essential that the care plan be made with all responsible and appropriate members of the family. Involving only one individual is not sufficient if the goal is family health risk reduction, which requires a total family system effort and change. Scheduling a visit with all family members present may require extra effort; if meeting with the entire family is not possible, each family member can collaborate in motivational interviewing and support the CHN in mutual goal setting and care planning.

Mutual goal setting is a learned skill on the part of both the CHN and the family. All persons involved need to know the purpose and process of goal setting and care planning within the helping relationship. The three general phases of the helping relationship are *beginning, working,* and *termination.* These three phases can be further divided into a total of eight sets of activities, as summarized in Table 12.7.

In the beginning phase, mutual goal setting starts with the collection and analysis of data, and it involves both the family and the CHN. An important aspect of this step is obtaining the family's view of the situation and its health concerns. The CHN can:

- Present his or her observations
- Validate the observations with the family
- Obtain the family's view

TABLE 12.7 Phases of Relationship and Activities in Mutual Goal Setting and Care Planning

Phase	Activity
1. Beginning phase	• Mutual data collection and exploration of needs and problems • Mutual establishment of goals • Mutual development of a plan
2. Working phase	• Mutual division of responsibilities • Mutual setting of time limits • Mutual implementation of plan • Mutual evaluation and renegotiation
3. Termination	• Mutual closure of the helping relationship

In the working phase, it is important that goals be mutually set and realistic. A pitfall for CHNs and patients who are new to collaborative care planning is to set overly ambitious goals that can lead to a sense of failure or disappointment with both the family and CHN. The CHN needs to recognize that there may be discrepancies between professional priorities and those of the patient and determine whether negotiating is required. Because mutual goal setting is a process characterized by renegotiating, the goals are not static.

Throughout the process, the CHN and family continually learn and recognize what each can contribute to meeting health concerns. The exploring of resources allows both parties to become aware of their own and one another's strengths and requires a review of the CHN's skills and knowledge, the family support systems, and community resources.

Developing a plan to meet the goals involves:
- Specifying activities
- Prioritizing goals
- Selecting a starting point
- Deciding who will be responsible for which activities (the decision is made by the CHN and the family)
- Setting time limits that involve deciding on a deadline for accomplishing (or evaluating progress toward accomplishing) a goal and the frequency of contacts

At the agreed-on time, the CHN and family together evaluate the progress in both process and outcome. The care plan can be modified, renegotiated, or terminated on the basis of the evaluation.

In the termination phase, acknowledgement of achievement or planning for next steps can be useful. This phase may entail writing a therapeutic letter or some written form of acknowledgement (of both suffering and success) that highlights the mutual work of the family and the CHN.

Advantages and Challenges of Mutual Goal Setting

Mutual goal setting takes time and effort and may require the family and CHN to reorient their roles. Increased control on the part of the family also means increased family responsibility for implementation and outcomes. Some CHNs may have difficulty relinquishing the role of the controlling expert professional. Care plans are not always successful, and mutual goal setting is neither appropriate nor possible in some cases. Some patients do not want to have this kind of involvement; they prefer to defer to the "authority" of the professional. The following are included in this group:

- Individuals with minimal cognitive skills
- Those who are involved in an emergency situation
- Those who are unwilling to be more active in their care
- Those who do not see control of or authority for health concerns as being within their domain

Some of these patients may gain motivation to set goals with the CHN for their family's health, while others never will. Motivational goal setting depends on:

- The value of input from both the CHN and the family
- The competency of the family
- The family's ability to be responsible
- The dynamic nature of the process

Mutual goal setting not only allows for but also requires continual renegotiating. Although it may not be appropriate in all situations or with all families, collaborative care planning can give direction and structure to health risk reduction and health promotion in families.

The initial contact between a community health nursing service and a family may provide limited information, and the situation that develops may be much more complex than anticipated. The "CHN in Practice: Case Study, Mutual Goal Setting and Problem Solving During Prenatal Community Health Nursing" box illustrates the issues and approaches to ongoing assessment, mutual goal setting, and collaborative care planning outlined in this chapter.

📋 CHN IN PRACTICE: A CASE STUDY

Mutual Goal Setting and Problem Solving During Prenatal Community Health Nursing

Amy, a student who has just started grade 11, had been referred by her school counsellor at the local high school for prenatal community health nursing at the Valley View Health Clinic. You have been supporting Amy and the family as the CHN in collaboration with the general practitioner and obstetrician. Amy is now 8 months pregnant and, due to vaginal bleeding, will need to be monitored in hospital while on bedrest. She is being transferred to the hospital in a city over 100 km from the rural farming community where her mother, stepfather, and younger sister reside, as well as her boyfriend and the baby's father, Taylor, and his family.

Think About It

1. What would you do next as the CHN assigned to this family who is facing this new situation related to Amy's pregnancy?
2. How would you help this family empower themselves to manage the current situation?
3. After the initial contact, how would you extend the assessment to the entire family system?
4. How would you establish mutual goals and care planning with this family? On what terms?
5. What developmental stage is this family in? Use the Calgary Family Assessment Model (CFAM) to guide your decision.

Clinical Judgement

Critical thinking and clinical judgements are required throughout the application of the community health nursing process when working with families. In making clinical judgements or evaluating outcomes, CHNs engage in critical thinking with awareness of ethical and equity-oriented concerns. When an outcome is not achieved, the CHN and the family work together to examine the challenges and barriers to success. Barriers can be systemic as well as coming directly from within the family unit. If there are material or resource needs, these must be addressed; however, this can occur as part of—and not separate from—the family interventions. The CHN's clinical judgement must come into the interventions to determine therapeutic questions and to support family strengths through any challenges and barriers. Building these assets and capacities together as a family builds resilience (Walsh, 2016). Family apathy and indecision are also known to be key barriers in family nursing interventions and can break down some of the functioning and resilience within a family unit (Kaakinen et al., 2018). Other identified barriers include the family's sense of hopelessness; fear of failure; fear and mistrust of the health care system; minimal access to monetary resources; and minimal access to other resources and support (Kaakinen et al., 2018). Friedman et al. (2003) also identified the following nurse-related barriers to achieving the outcome:

- CHN imposes ideas
- CHN uses negative labels
- CHN does not identify family strengths
- CHN neglects cultural or gender implications

Family apathy may occur because of value differences between the CHN and the family (e.g., in relation to religious, cultural, or social values), because the family is overcome with a sense of hopelessness, because the family views the health concerns as too overwhelming, or because family members have a fear of failure (Kaakinen et al., 2018). By giving commendations, the CHN can help the family identify its strengths, which can make the family feel empowered and hopeful. In addition, a family may be indecisive because:

- Members cannot determine which course of action is better.
- They have an unexpressed fear or concern.
- They have a pattern of making decisions only when faced with a crisis.

An important part of clinical judgement when working with families is deciding when to terminate the relationship between the CHN and the family. *Termination* is phasing out the CHN from family involvement. When termination is built into the interventions, the family benefits from a smooth transition process. The family is given credit for the outcomes of the interventions that they helped design. Strategies often used in the termination component are:

- Decreasing contact with the CHN
- Extending invitations to the family for follow-up
- Making referrals when appropriate

The termination should include a summative evaluation meeting in which the CHN and family put a formal closure to their relationship. When termination with a family occurs suddenly, it is important for the CHN to determine the forces bringing about the closure. The family may be initiating the termination prematurely, which requires a renegotiating process. Regardless of how termination comes about, it is an important aspect in working with families.

Community Resources

Families have varied and complex health concerns. Sometimes peoples' needs are best met directly in communities and the CHN role can be to assist the family in identifying the social, community needs and resources that may prevent and resolve health challenges. For instance, while working with the family who is concerned about their mother's risk and fall at home, it may be discovered that a neighbourhood association has a supportive walking group for older persons who want to get out of the house, but no longer want to walk alone, after falls or for other reasons. The CHN is often involved in mobilizing several referral resources to effectively and appropriately meet family health promotion issues. Identifying resources in a community requires time and effort. One valuable source is the Internet. Often community service organizations, such as the local Chamber of Commerce and municipality, or the community health unit or regional health authority, publish community resource listings that are available in print, on webpages, or in health apps. Regardless of how a resource is identified, the CHN needs to be familiar with the types of services offered and any requirements or costs involved. If this information is not available, the CHN can contact the resource.

Locating and using these systems often requires skills in identifying key words, appraising quality and potential ethical issues with organizations that may take advantage of vulnerable people, and the time and patience to review volumes of information that many families lack. CHNs work with families to identify community resources, and as patient advocates they help families learn to use the resources. This may involve:

- Sharing information on resources with families
- Rehearsing with families what questions to ask of a resource
- Preparing required materials
- Making the initial contact
- Arranging transportation to the resource

The appropriateness and effectiveness of resources need to be evaluated with families afterward. It is important to remember that navigating the maze of resources is often difficult for the CHN as well. If a family is in crisis or does not have a phone or a home base from which to call or receive return calls, this process is even more difficult, and the family's sense of helplessness may be increased. Sometimes the family is comprised of "street family" members. Therefore, the CHN's assistance, while promoting the family's sense of empowerment, is both necessary and complex.

Each family is an unexplored mystery, unique in the ways in which it meets the needs of its members and of society. We are social beings and operate in our family units. Healthy and vital families are essential to the world's future because family members are affected by what their families have invested in them or failed to provide for their growth and well-being. Families will continue to survive challenges and changes in norms, expectations, forms, structure, and function, and will continue to serve as the foundational social unit of society.

STUDENT EXPERIENCE

1. Define your family or a family you visited in the community in terms of its family structure.
2. a. Develop a genogram for your family. The following website may prove useful: http://www.strongbonds.jss.org.au/workers/families/genograms.html. Be sure to include a legend in the genogram.
   b. What have you found out about your family's health and illness patterns?

3. a. Develop an ecomap for your family. The previous site also includes an ecomap, located at http://www.strongbonds.jss.org.au/workers/cultures/ecomaps.html. Be sure to include a legend in the ecomap.
   b. What have you found out about your family's connections outside their family boundary with the community?

CHAPTER SUMMARY

12.1 Families are the context within which health care decisions are made. The importance of the family as a major patient system for CHNs in reducing health risks and promoting the health of individuals and populations is well documented. Family nursing is practised in all settings. CHNs are responsible for assisting families in meeting health care needs.

12.2 Traditionally, *family* has been defined as a nuclear family: mother, father, and young children. A wider variety of family forms exist now more than the nuclear tradition. These forms include lone parent, extended, blended, commuter, living apart together, same sex, grandparent-led, as well as cohabitating friends and couples. CHNs need to ask patients whom they consider to be their family and then include those members in the family interviews. *Family structure* refers to the characteristics and demographics (gender, age, number) of individual members who make up a family unit.

12.3 Families have varied and complex health concerns. Several social determinants contribute to the experience of healthy or unhealthy outcomes. Not everyone exposed to the same event will have the same outcome. Rather than refer to families with ineffective coping skills as "dysfunctional," CHNs might consider thinking about referring to these families as families with health challenges related to family functioning.

12.4 Four approaches to conceptualizing families are (1) family as context, (2) family as patient, (3) family as a system, and (4) family as component of society.

12.5 Family nursing is a specialty area that has a strong theoretical base and is more than just common sense. *Structure–function theory* views the family as a social system with members who have specific roles and functions. *Systems theory* describes families as a unit of the whole, composed of members whose interactional patterns are the focus of attention. *Developmental theory* emphasizes how families change over time and focuses on interactions and relationships among family members. *Interactional theory* focuses on the family as a unit of interacting personalities and examines the communication processes by which family members relate to one another.

12.6 The Friedman Family Assessment Model integrates the structure–function framework and developmental and systems theories. The Calgary Family Assessment Model (CFAM) takes a holistic approach to assessment of family health. Using the McGill Model of Nursing, the CHN identifies family strengths in relation to individual family members, the family as the unit of care, and external resources. Relational practice is an approach to inquiry for family nursing that is guided by collaboration with patients using a number of relational skills including listening, questioning, empathy, mutuality, reciprocity, self-observation, reflection, and sensitivity to emotional and social contexts and power relations.

12.7 Home visits afford the opportunity to gain a more accurate assessment of the family structure and behaviour in the natural environment. Home visits also provide opportunities to observe the home environment and to identify both barriers and supports to reducing health risks and reaching family health goals.

12.8 Risks to a family's health arise in three major areas: biological and age-related risks, environmental risks, and behavioural risks. These factors contribute to the biological risk for certain conditions.

12.9 Increasingly, health care providers are working with patients in a more interactive, collaborative style. The Calgary Family Intervention Model (CFIM) proposes family interventions focused on strengths and individual and family assets. An asset-based approach focuses on family competencies and family strengths rather than risks and deficits. Mutual goal setting and collaborative care planning involve a shift in responsibility and control from the professional alone to a shared effort by patient and professional. Relational practice emphasizes the awareness and attention to power within relationship and context. Relational inquiry invites exploration of health concerns with power and context being in the foreground. Family strengths and resources can be used to help families deal with their health concerns and to promote health. It is important for the CHN to recognize that the family has the right to make its own health decisions.

🗎 CHN IN PRACTICE: A CASE STUDY

Supporting a Family—and the Wider Community—Through Difficult News

The Mamudu family consists of David (father, 47 years old) and Becca (mother, 43 years old) and their children Ann (18 years old), Michelle (15 years old), David Jr. (13 years old), and Michael (7 years old). David is the pastor of Faith Baptist Church in the suburb of a large Canadian city, where he has served the past 15 years. Becca is a homemaker and the primary caretaker for the children.

For the past year, Becca has felt tired and "run down." At her annual physical, she describes her symptoms to her physician. After several tests, Becca is diagnosed with stomach cancer. She starts to cry and says, "How will I tell my family?"

Becca's primary physician refers the family to Trisha, a CHN. Trisha calls the household and speaks with Becca to arrange a home visit. Becca confides to Trisha that it has been 2 weeks since she received the cancer diagnosis, but she has yet to tell her husband and children. Becca asks Trisha if she can help her tell her family and explain what it all means. Trisha makes an appointment for a home visit with the family.

Think About It

1. If you were the CHN, how would you plan for this home visit?
2. What life-cycle stage is this family in? Use the CFAM (see Appendix 7) to guide your decision.
3. Using the CFAM, what data would you plan to collect in your family assessment under structural, developmental, and functional areas?
4. What specific community health nursing interventions would you use? Provide a rationale.

🛜 TOOL BOX

The Tool Box contains useful resources that can be applied in community health nursing practice. These related resources are found either in the appendices at the back of this text or on the text's Evolve website at http://evolve.elsevier.com/Canada/Stanhope/community/.

Appendices

- Appendix E.3: Friedman Family Assessment Model (Short Form)
- Appendix 7: The Calgary Family Assessment Model and the Calgary Family Intervention Model

Tools

Ecomap Construction. (http://www.strongbonds.jss.org.au/workers/cultures/ecomaps.html)

This site contains an example of an ecomap, which is used to delineate the external structure of the family.

Introduction to the Genogram. (http://www.genopro.com/genogram/)

This site contains information on the background for use of genograms.

How to Draw Genograms (video posted by Wilma Schroeder, MMFT, BN, RN). (https://youtu.be/wH-uP1UiJWY)

This video contains instructions on constructing genograms.

Understanding Families: Simple Guide to Genograms. (http://www.strongbonds.jss.org.au/workers/families/genograms.html)

This site contains instructions for constructing genograms.

REFERENCES

Barnes, M. D., Hanson, C. L., Novilla, L. B., et al. (2020). Family-centered health promotion: Perspectives for engaging families and achieving better health outcomes. *Inquiry: The Journal of Health Care Organization, Provision, and Financing, 57,* 46958020923537. https://doi.org/10.1177/0046958020923537.

Beagan, B. L., & Chapman, G. E. (2012). Meanings of food, eating and health among african nova scotians: "Certain things aren't meant for black folk. *Ethnicity and Health, 17*(5), 513–529. https://doi.org/10.1080/13557858.2012.661844.

Bell, J. M. (1995). The dysfunction of "dysfunctional. *Journal of Family Nursing, 1*(3), 235–237.

Bell, J. M. (2015). Growing the science of family systems nursing: Family health intervention research focused on illness suffering and family healing [L'avancement de la recherché sur l'intervention infirmiere systémique en santé familiale: Bilan]. In F. Duhamel (Ed.), *La santé et la famille: Une approche systémique en soins infirmiers [families and health: A systemic approach in nursing care]* (3rd ed.) (pp. 102–125) Chenelière Éducation. [In French] English language translation available from U of C Institutional Repository, PRISM. http://hdl.handle.net/1880/51114.

Bell, J. (2016). The central importance of therapeutic conversations in family nursing: Can talking be healing? *Journal of Family Nursing, 22*(4), 439–449.

Black, K., & Lobo, M. (2008). A conceptual review of family resilience factors. *Journal of Family Nursing, 14*(1), 33–55.

Broekema, S., Paans, W., Roodbol, P. F., et al. (2019). Nurses' application of the components of family nursing conversations in home health care: A qualitative content analysis. *Scandinavian Journal of Caring Sciences, 34*(2), 322–331. https://doi.org/10.1111/scs.12731.

Browne, A. J., Hartrick Doane, G., Reimer, J., et al. (2010). Public health nursing practice with "high priority" families: The significance of contextualizing "risk. *Nursing Inquiry, 17,* 27–38.

Campbell, K., MacKinnon, K., Dobbins, M., et al. (2019). Weathering the rural reality: Delivery of the nurse-family partnership home visitation program in rural British Columbia, Canada. *BMC Nursing, 18*(1), 1–14. https://doaj.org/article/8ca698486fcf49389135a3bb6b2e0a0d.

Canadian Observatory on Homelessness. (2019). *What is homelessness?* https://www.homelesshub.ca/about-homelessness/homelessness-101/what-homelessness.

Coehlo, D., Hanson, S., Kaakinen, J., et al. (2018). *Family health care nursing: Theory, practice, and research* (6th ed.). Philadelphia, PA: F.A. Davis Company.

Community Health Nurses of Canada. (2019). *Canadian community health nursing professional practice model and standards of practice.* https://www.chnc.ca/standards-of-practice.

Cooley, M. L. (2013). A family perspective in community/public health nursing. In F. A. Maurer, & C. M. Smith (Eds.), *Community/public health nursing practice: Health for families and populations* (5th ed.) (pp. 327–344). Saunders/Elsevier.

Deatrick, J. (2017). Where is "family" in the social determinants of health? Implications for family nursing practice, research, education, and policy. *Journal of Family Nursing, 23*(4), 423–433.

Ford-Gilboe, M. (2002). Developing knowledge about family health promotion by testing the developmental model of health and nursing. *Journal of Family Nursing, 8*(2), 140–156.

Friedman, M. M., Bowden, V. R., & Jones, E. G. (2003). *Family nursing: Research, theory and practice* (5th ed.). Prentice Hall.

Government of Canada. (2018). *Rights of LGBTI persons.* https://www.canada.ca/en/canadian-heritage/services/rights-lgbti-persons.html.

Greenwood, S., Wright, T., & Nielsen, H. (2006). Conversations in context: Cultural safety and reflexivity in child and family health nursing. *Journal of Family Nursing, 12*(2), 201–224. https://doi.org/10.1177/1074840706287405.

Hadfield, K., & Ungar, M. (2018). Family resilience: Emerging trends in theory and practice. *Journal of Family Social Work, 21*(2), 81–84.

Harrawood, L. (2017). Models of family assessment. In J. Carlson, & S. Dermer (Eds.), *The Sage encyclopedia of marriage, family, and couples counseling* (Vol. 2) (pp. 603–610). Sage Publications.

Hartrick Doane, G., & Varcoe, C. (2005). *Family nursing as relational inquiry: Developing health promoting practice.* Lippincott, Williams & Wilkins.

Hartrick Doane, G., & Varcoe, C. (2007). Relational practice and nursing obligations. *Advances in Nursing Science, 30,* 192–205.

Hartrick Doane, G., & Varcoe, C. (2020). *How to nurse: Relational inquiry in action* (2nd ed.). Wolters Kluwer.

International Federation on Ageing. (2020). *Companion animals and the health of older persons.* https://ifa.ngo/publication/health/companion-animals-and-the-health-of-older-persons/.

Kaakinen, J. R., Coehlo, D. P., Steele, R., et al. (2018). *Family health care nursing: Theory, practice, and research* (6th ed.). Davis: F. A.

Kaakinen, J. R., & Harmon Hanson, S. M. (2018). Family health care nursing: An introduction. In J. R. Kaakinen, D. P. Coehlo, R. Steele, et al. (Eds.), *Family health care nursing: Theory, practice, and research* (6th ed.) (pp. 3–32). Davis: F. A.

Lapum, J. L., St-Amant, O., Garcia, W., et al. (2019). *Interpreting Canada's 2019 food guide and food labelling for health professionals.* https://ecampusontario.pressbooks.pub/foodguide/.

Levac, A. M. C., Wright, L. M., & Leahey, M. (2002). Children and families: Models for assessment and intervention. In J. A. Fox (Ed.), *Primary health care of infants, children, and adolescents* (2nd ed.) (pp. 10–19). Mosby.

Mazrekaj, D., De Witte, K., & Cabus, S. (2020). School outcomes of children raised by same-sex parents: Evidence from administrative panel data. *American Sociological Review*, *85*(5), 830–856. https://doi.org/10.1177/0003122420957249.

McEwen, M., & Pullis, B. (2009). *Community-based nursing: An introduction* (3rd ed.). Saunders.

McGoldrick, M., Gerson, R., & Petry, S. (2020). *Genograms: Assessment and intervention* (4th ed.). W. W. Norton.

Moules, J., & Johnstone, H. (2010). Commendations, conversations, and life-changing realizations: Teaching and practicing family nursing. *Journal of Family Nursing*, *16*(2), 146–160. https://doi.org/10.1177/1074840710365148.

Murdaugh, C. L., Parsons, M. A., & Pender, N. J. (2018). *Health promotion in nursing practice* (8th ed.). Pearson.

Nies, M. A., & McEwen, M. (2019). *Community/public health nursing: Promoting the health of populations* (6th ed.). Elsevier.

Ristovski-Slijepcevic, S., Bell, K., Chapman, G., et al. (2010). Being "thick" indicates you are eating, you are healthy and you have an attractive body shape: Perspectives on fatness and food choice amongst Black and White men and women in Canada. *Health Sociology Review*, *19*(3), 317–329. https://doi.org/10.5172/hesr.2010.19.3.317.

Shajani, Z., & Snell, D. (2019). *Wright & Leahey's nurses and families: A guide to family assessment and intervention* (7th ed.). F.A. Davis Company.

Smith, C. M. (2013). Home visiting: Opening the doors for family health. In F. A. Maurer, & C. M. Smith (Eds.), *Community/public health nursing practice: Health for families and populations* (5th ed.) (pp. 302–325). Saunders/Elsevier.

Statistics Canada. (2018). *Family violence in Canada: A statistical profile*. https://www150.statcan.gc.ca/n1/pub/85-002-x/2019001/article/00018-eng.htm.

Statistics Canada. (2020). *Dimensions of poverty hub*. https://www.statcan.gc.ca/eng/topics-start/poverty.

Tarasuk, V., & Mitchell, A. (2020). *Household food insecurity in Canada, 2017–18. Research to identify policy Options to reduce food insecurity (PROOF)*. https://proof.utoronto.ca/resources/proof-annual-reports/household-food-insecurity-in-canada-2017-2018/.

Vanier Institute of the Family. (2018). *A snapshot of family diversity in Canada*. https://vanierinstitute.ca/a-snapshot-of-family-diversity-in-canada-february-2018/.

Walsh, F. (2016). Family resilience: A developmental systems framework. *European Journal of Developmental Psychology*, *13*(3), 313–324.

West, C., & Jakubec, S. L. (2019). Family nursing. In B. J. Astle, & W. Duggleby (Eds.), *Canadian fundamentals of nursing* (6th ed.) (pp. 307–323). Elsevier.

Wright, L. (2019). Older adults and their families: An interactional intervention that brings forth love and softens suffering. *Journal of Family Nursing*, *25*(4), 610–626.

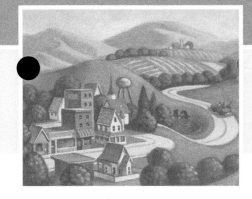

13

Working With Groups, Teams, and Partners

OUTLINE

Groups, Teams, and Partners, 309
   Principles of a Group Process, 311
   A Model for Group Development, 312
   Task and Maintenance Roles, 313
   Group Rules and Standards, 313
   Leadership Behaviours, 314
   Conflict Transformation, 315

Group Evaluation, 317
Working with Health Care Teams and Partners, 317
   Team Building in the Community, 317
   Forming Community Partnerships, 319
   Interprofessional Partnerships, 319
   Interprofessional Education, 320

OBJECTIVES

After reading this chapter, you should be able to:

13.1 Examine the professional roles and partnerships created by CHNs.
13.2 Identify the five dimensions that influence group process.
13.2 Describe the five stages of group development.
13.3 Understand the roles assumed by group members.
13.4 Understand the importance of the rules and standards for groups.
13.5 Describe various leadership styles and behaviours.

13.6 Describe different types of conflict in groups and give examples of group conflict resolution strategies.
13.7 Evaluate the composition and performance of a group.
13.8 Discuss key concepts of effective team building.
13.9 Identify some principles that can create effective and sustainable partnerships.
13.10 Discuss the benefits of working with groups, teams, and partners in the community.

KEY TERMS*

collaborative patient-centred practice, 320
group, 310
group process, 311
interprofessional health care teams, 310

leadership, 314
partnership, 319
team, 310

*See the Glossary on page 468 for definitions.

The Community Health Nurses of Canada Practice Model (Community Health Nurses of Canada [CHNC, 2019) defines the patient as individuals, families, groups, communities, populations, and systems. Therefore, community health nurse (CHN) practice involves working with diverse groups, teams, and partners to address the health needs of patients. CHNs need to understand groups, group dynamics, and team building. The Canadian Community Health Nursing Standards of Practice (CCHN Standards) (CHNC, 2019) identify the practice expectations for CHNs when working with groups, teams, and partners (see Appendix 1). Some of the information required to work with groups is provided in this chapter; however, readers are encouraged to consult other resources that provide detailed information on group structure and function.

GROUPS, TEAMS, AND PARTNERS

CHNs work with a variety of small patient groups from families to self-help groups, community groups, health care teams, professional associations, and committees. CHNs practice in health care teams, using a case management approach and family-centred care. Therefore, working with small groups is an important part of everyday CNH practice (CHNC, 2019). Regardless of the type of group, the structure and functioning of the group is of utmost importance. Groups can be instrumental in bringing about changes to improve the health and well-being of individuals, populations, and communities. Table 13.1 presents selected examples of how CHNs can work with a variety of groups, teams, and partners.

TABLE 13.1   Working With Groups, Teams, and Partners

Group, Team, or Partner	Purpose	Application to Practice
Family	• To promote family and individual health behaviours to manage health challenges and promote health	• Assist family to adapt to the birth of a high-risk neonate • Monitor immunization status • Tuberculosis monitoring and follow up • Follow up on outbreak of measles • Provide health education for expectant parents
Self-Help Community Groups	• To engage in disease prevention • To engage in health promotion • To support and empower patients • To provide health teaching	• Nutrition education • Coordinate occupational therapy for patients who are experiencing immobility • Empower members of a mental health support group with knowledge of available services
Workplace groups	• To promote a healthy lifestyle • To engage in advocating for health policy to support a healthy workplace	• Advocate for ergonomic assessments at the worksite
Primary health care teams	• To coordinate and deliver the most effective patient interventions by an interprofessional team	• Hold regular team meetings • Collaborate with professional and nonprofessional team members to address issues related to heart health in the community
Palliative care team	• To coordinate and deliver the most effective patient interventions	• Medication reviews • Pain management • Discussion of MAID protocol
Professional associations, e.g., CNA	• To advocate for healthy public policy	• Provide position statement on crib safety • Develop policy on breastfeeding-friendly spaces

CNA, Canadian Nurses Association; *MAID,* Medical assistance in dying.

Working effectively with groups, teams, and partners requires that CHNs understand and apply group concepts. When working with groups, it is important to consider the purpose of the group, group membership, group dynamics, group process, group leadership, group size, and group task and maintenance functions.

Throughout this text, *patient* is defined as the individuals, families, groups, communities, populations, and systems. The term *aggregate* refers to a group within a population, such as a group of schoolchildren or older persons. The CHN may also work with a subgroup of aggregates, often referred to as a small group. Usually, a small group comprises fewer than 20 members; 12 group members is considered ideal. However, every group is unique, and the level of involvement of all members and the purpose of the group often influences the size of the group (e.g., a prenatal group versus a family experiencing measles).

A group should contain the least number of members needed to accomplish the task, to build and maintain the group, and to accomplish the group purpose (Dimock & Kass, 2008). A **group** is a collection of two or more individuals in face-to-face interactions with a common purpose and who are in an interdependent relationship (Maurer & Smith, 2013). Each group member influences and is, in turn, influenced by every other member. Also, since relationships exist and affect a group, the group needs to work at relationship building if it is to be an effective group. Key elements in this definition of *group* are member interaction, group purpose, and interdependence. Therefore, a random collection of individuals, such as people standing at a bus stop or sharing an elevator, is not usually considered a group, unless there is interaction or a group purpose present.

CHNs work with many patient groups and practice a "care process approach" with **interpersonal health care teams** of nurses, intraprofessional teams of professionals, primary health care teams, and case management teams (CHNC, 2019). Interprofessional collaborative models for health service delivery are critical to improving care in the community. Collaboration among teams of health care professionals can ensure that the patient receives care at the right time and in the right place. Many factors can facilitate joint efforts among professions and professionals in the community, including patient-centred care, evidence-informed practice, access to the right service at the right time and place, and using epidemiology to identify services (CNA, 2019) (see the "Evidence-Informed Practice" box).

EVIDENCE-INFORMED PRACTICE

In a grounded theory study, McCallin and Bamford (2007) describe some of the factors that can facilitate interprofessional collaboration, including the emotional intelligence of the team and professional competence. To be effective, a team requires "both emotional intelligence and expertise, including technical, clinical, social and interactional skills" (p. 386). In this study, the purposes were to identify the main concerns of health care providers from different professions working on interprofessional teams in two main acute care teaching hospital settings and to explain how these team members handled workplace practice concerns. The sample consisted of 44 health team members from seven disciplines. Data were collected by interview and participant observation.

EVIDENCE-INFORMED PRACTICE—CONT'D

It was found that in interprofessional teams, professional competence was especially valued; personalities often contributed to having to deal with problems and dysfunctional team members; team members focused less on social factors affecting team process and outcome; team members focused more on tasks that affected team effectiveness; many team members focused on individuality and individual expertise; avoidance of conflict was used; support for interprofessional colleagues was seldom provided; psychosocial safety within the teams was threatened as new discipline alignments were formed; professional boundaries were blurred; and technical expertise, cognitive intelligence, and emotional intelligence were identified as required to work effectively with all other team members.

Application for CHNs

CHNs use an "interdisciplinary approach and cooperate with other organizations as needed, based on how complex the circumstances are" (Canadian Public Health Association [CPHA], 2010, p. 21). Therefore, it is important for CHNs to consider the factors that facilitate collaboration among professions and strengthen those factors as needed.

Questions for Reflection and Discussion

1. Analyze the findings from this study in relation to the CNA (2019) principles that facilitate interprofessional collaboration. Which factors are facilitating or hindering the interprofessional collaboration?
2. Explore recommendations that could support and sustain interprofessional collaboration with this health care team, e.g., recruitment and workplace interprofessional education to support human resources.
3. How would you approach group conflict as an interprofessional team member?
4. What keywords would you use to search the evidence-informed practice literature about the effectiveness of interprofessional teams? Explain your choices.

Sources: McCallin, A., & Bamford, A. (2007). Interdisciplinary teamwork: Is the influence of emotional intelligence fully appreciated? *Journal of Nursing Management, 15*(4), 386–391; Canadian Public Health Association (CPHA). (2010). *Public health—community health nursing practice in Canada: Roles and activities* (4th ed.). https://www.cpha.ca/sites/default/files/assets/pubs/3-1bk04214.pdf

Principles of a Group Process

Group process refers to how the group as a unit is working and how group members interact with one another (Dimock & Kass, 2007). CHNs can apply the principles of group process at every group interaction with patients and the health care team. When interacting with groups, it is important for CHNs to be aware of the interrelated dimensions in a group that can significantly influence group process, including group physical and emotional climate, involvement, interaction, cohesion, and productivity (Dimock & Kass, 2007).

Group physical and emotional climate refers to the physical milieu the group meets in and the emotional atmosphere of the group. For group meetings, CHNs need to consider physical milieu factors such as adequate lighting, appropriate temperature and ventilation, comfortable chairs, and limiting distractions. Another factor is the physical arrangement of the seating for group members; it should encourage and support decision making, verbal and nonverbal communication, and expression of feelings. The CHN, in selecting the type of seating arrangement, needs to consider the group and its purpose. For example, if it is a committee meeting where note taking and decision making are required, a table and chairs are suggested; however, if it is a self-help group meeting, an open circle of chairs is suggested so that all members can see and hear one another. This latter approach is more likely to encourage expression of feelings (Dimock & Kass, 2007). It is important to meet the safety and security needs of group members through the group's emotional atmosphere. The CHN contributes to this emotional atmosphere by being welcoming and open to contributions from all members and being respectful and supportive, thereby increasing trust and decreasing member anxiety. This kind of emotional atmosphere encourages group members to participate, take risks, and share resources.

Group involvement refers to the degree of attraction and commitment by group members to the achievement of group goals. The extent of group member involvement is demonstrated by respecting group meeting times, group participation, and commitment to group work. Effective groups are groups in which members are highly involved and have therefore developed group cohesiveness and solidarity. The CHN as group facilitator can encourage involvement by acknowledging the unique contributions to the group by members. The leadership style of the CHN can also contribute to group involvement; for example, the CHN can encourage members to take part in setting group goals and processes.

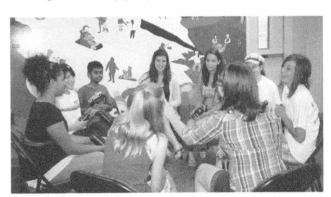

Group members interact and influence one another, whether formally or informally, such as in this youth group meeting at a community centre. (Courtesy Gloria Viverais-Dresler & Heather Jessup-Falcioni)

Group interaction refers to how the group members connect and relate to one another. The physical and emotional climate has an impact on group interaction. Therefore, the CHN needs to influence the physical and emotional climate. The more frequent the interactions, the more likely it is that the groups will be productive. The CHN needs to assess the patterns of communication and the roles of group members to gain a sense of the level of group interaction and intervene as needed.

Group cohesion is the attraction between individual members and the group, a sense of togetherness often described as a sense of "we-ness" (Boyd & Ewashen, 2008). Similarity in members' goals and values tends to increase group cohesion. For example, members of a coalition advocating for school policies to eliminate junk food in the school cafeteria may come from diverse backgrounds, such as teachers, social workers, and parents, but they have the common goal of preventing childhood obesity and work together as a cohesive group to accomplish that goal. Groups that are supportive of their members, set and work toward the same goals, see themselves as a work group, work through challenges, and celebrate successes are often seen as a highly unified group. Often, group work is attractive to members when there are clearly stated group goals, and the group is cohesive. Dimock and Kass (2007) identify cohesion as a product of the first three group dimensions that significantly influence group process. CHNs support group cohesion by assisting the group to identify its purpose. They can also assess the extent that the group perceives itself and its sense of "we-ness."

Group productivity refers to the activities that a group uses to reach its task and process goals and, therefore, to accomplish maximum effectiveness. Productivity is a motivator for retaining group membership and maintaining positive group interaction. Leadership style and the sharing of group member roles influence productivity. The CHN needs to consider the leadership style in the group and also evaluate the group member roles and their influence on group productivity so that appropriate interventions can be implemented if required.

A Model for Group Development

A classic model of group development is the Tuckman's stages of group development model (Tuckman, 1965; Tuckman & Jensen, 1977; Whittingham, 2018). This model can help CHNs understand the group process, especially during the formation of new groups, and includes new therapeutic groups (Whittingham, 2018). It has long been applied to small-group development and has been established as a valid model to guide practice. This model is outlined in Box 13.1.

BOX 13.1 Five Stages of Group Development

Stage 1: Forming. Group members, as strangers, focus on getting to know one another.
Stage 2: Storming. Group members begin to express their feelings as real issues are focused on.
Stage 3: Norming. Group members start to feel part of the group and recognize the benefits of the group reaching its goal.
Stage 4: Performing. Group members focus on the group work and share ideas in a supportive group environment.
Stage 5: Adjourning. Group members recognize the need for termination of the group and therefore work toward completion of the tasks and disengage from other group members.

Sources: Based on Tuckman, B. W., & Jensen, M. A. C. (1977). Stages of small group development revisited. *Group and Organizational Studies, 2*(4), 419–427.

Stage 1, *forming,* starts when the group has its first meeting. Usually, group members are polite to one another and cautious about expressing their own opinions and feelings, so conflict is avoided. The group tends to take a task focus—for example, setting meeting times, clarifying its purpose, and setting the agenda for the next meeting. This is a good time for the CHN to encourage group members to develop a common purpose for the group (e.g., develop a position statement on breastfeeding, conduct heart health education).

Stage 2, *storming,* occurs as the group works on the task and related issues and some comfort is established; feelings and thoughts are expressed by some group members, with some of this expression possibly causing conflict over goals and procedures. Sometimes, this is referred to as "testing others." Some group members will be very silent during this expression of conflict. Some members are passive, and others respond to the threat by expressing anger (Smith, Meyer, & Wylie, 2006). The perception of power and threat in the group may influence the kind of group member behaviour (Kamans, Otten, & Gordijn, 2011). CHNs can work to ensure that all members of the group have input into the tasks and issues by encouraging all members to voice their opinions and by managing any conflict that arises in the group.

Stage 3, *norming,* occurs when group members recognize the benefits of group work, and group members begin to accept differing members' viewpoints, skills, and experiences. A sense of "we-ness" exists. In an effective group, conflict is dealt with (Marquis & Huston, 2017).

Stage 4, *performing,* is the stage in which the group works together, demonstrates trust among members, gets the work done, and shows flexibility (Marquis & Huston, 2017). Interdependence within the group is evident as task and maintenance roles are shared by group members. The group is described as effective and well-functioning. Although this stage is the aim of all groups, it is important to note that not all groups reach this stage. CHNs can support the performing stage by ensuring the work of the group is documented in meeting minutes or within any documents being produced. CHNs also "perform" or implement appropriate nursing interventions during this phase (e.g., education sessions, policy formation, care planning).

Stage 5, *adjourning,* occurs when, based on group evaluation, it is determined that the group's purpose has been met and therefore the group will be terminated (Tuckman & Jensen, 1977). Although group members are usually satisfied with the group and its accomplishments, some members may feel sad about the loss of their group, experience the grieving process, and begin to withdraw from the task and emotional aspects of group interactions. CHNs can use this phase to evaluate the effectiveness of the group and whether or not it achieved its purpose (e.g., position statements were created, health education sessions were conducted, policies were developed).

The five-stage model continues to be used today in many settings to analyze group processes, and according to Seck and Helton (2014) the principles of the model can be applied to the task of small groups and can effectively analyze and help to enhance the small group process. CHNs can apply this model to the creation of any new group in an effort to enhance group productivity and accomplish maximum effectiveness of the group's work.

Task and Maintenance Roles

Group members usually assume task, maintenance, or nonfunctional roles within the group. As Table 13.2 indicates, task and maintenance roles are facilitators to group functioning, while nonfunctional roles are barriers (Dimock & Kass, 2007). Examining group roles, a part of group process, provides the CHN with an understanding of how well the group is functioning and achieving the purpose. Task roles help the group accomplish tasks and therefore meet its purpose. For example, a group member who assumes the task role of problem definer ensures that the group begins with a clear purpose; and a group member who assumes the task role of information seeker helps clarify any unclear areas so that the group can keep working effectively on the task. In task roles, the focus is on problem solving and decision

making (Dimock & Kass, 2008). Maintenance roles help create a positive working climate and facilitate group interaction. For example, a group member who assumes the maintenance role of encourager provides praise to group members for their contributions; and a group member who assumes the role of compromiser helps decrease group conflict. Nonfunctional roles are individual-oriented roles that hinder group cohesiveness and productivity. For example, the aggressor who verbally attacks other group members or makes jokes about the group task is likely to hinder the group process; and the dominator may take over the task and present his or her point of view as the best and only worthwhile way to proceed.

Group Rules and Standards

Group rules and standards govern how the group makes decisions, how work is assigned, and what is acceptable member behaviour. In an effective group:

- Members show respect and trust by actively listening to others' points of view.
- Members are transparent and avoid hidden agendas.

TABLE 13.2 Selected Examples of Roles Assumed in Groups

Type	Example	Explanation
Task roles	Problem definer	Clarifies and defines the purpose of the group Explores best evidence for practice
	Information seeker	Asks for factual information about group work, procedures, or suggestions made
	Information giver	Offers information about group work, procedures, or suggestions Presents the best evidence for practice
	Opinion seeker	Asks for group members' opinions about group work
	Opinion giver	Offers own opinions related to group work
	Elaborator	Provides examples related to suggestions on how these might work
	Recorder	Tracks in writing the activities and accomplishments of the group
	Evaluator	Raises questions about group activities and accomplishments and compares group activities to an expected standard of group work
	Feasibility tester	Checks for reality and how practical suggested solutions are
Group-building and maintenance roles	Coordinator	Clarifies and relates statements to previous comments made
	Harmonizer	Mediates differences and attempts to reconcile these, often by pointing out similarities in views
	Encourager	Demonstrates warmth and responsiveness to viewpoints and conveys praise for contributions made
	Orienter	Monitors the group so it stays focused; identifies departures from goals, procedures, etc. May make suggestions for improvements in group functioning
	Follower	Listens and accepts suggestions of group members and expresses agreement
	Compromiser	Decides to go along with the group in a group conflict situation
	Gatekeeper	Encourages participation and open communication by all group members
	Commentator	Tracks in writing group process and conveys findings to the group
Individual-oriented roles (nonfunctional roles)	Blocker	Hinders group functioning by arguing, disagreeing, or not accepting ideas beyond reason or focusing on dead issues
	Aggressor	Conveys disapproval of group members' beliefs or feelings
	Digressor	Moves the group away from group work by digressing from the topic under discussion
	Recognition seeker	Focuses attention on self
	Dominator	Focuses on controlling and manipulating the group
	Confessor	Expresses personal situation in the group
	Help seeker	Focuses on self-weaknesses to gain group sympathy
	Withdrawer	Uses behaviours to withdraw from group such as daydreaming, whispering to another group member, or leaving the group temporarily

Sources: Adapted from Dimock, H. G., & Kass, R. (2007). *How to observe your group* (4th ed.). Captus Press; Marquis, B. L., & Huston, C. J. (2017). *Leadership roles and management functions in nursing: Theory and application* (9th ed.). Lippincott Williams & Wilkins.

- Meetings start on time and end on time.
- Members are open and share positive and negative feelings about what is happening in the group.
- Members focus on the task so that the group's purpose and goals are reached.
- Members demonstrate accountability and responsibility to the group.

Group standards and rules often follow a standard form of decision making. One standard process for governing formal meetings can be found in the parliamentary procedures known as *Robert's Rules of Order*. Those rules address policies and procedures on how to conduct a formal group meeting and topics such as the order of business for the meeting, approval of minutes, and agenda setting.

All groups need to determine the decision-making process, and whether it will be as consensus decision making, majority decisions, or leader-only or single-member-only decisions. Consensus decision making is the most difficult and most time-consuming method; however, all the resources in the group are used, each member has supported the decision, and therefore each member is committed to the decision, which encourages group solidarity. Decision making by majority vote is less time consuming, and those group members (the majority) who supported the decision will commit to it; however, those who did not support the motion or abstained may or may not be committed to the decision. If a decision is made by the leader only or a single member only, group support and commitment to follow through on the decision will vary depending on how much the group supports the leader or individual member's decision. CHNs need to be cognizant of group rules and standards and how to conduct meetings. They also need to know how to determine when consensus decision-making in groups is feasible, such as when approving a new policy or procedure.

Leadership Behaviours

Leadership refers to the act of influencing and directing others; it includes assisting the group to meet its goal(s) (Dimock & Kass, 2007) and maintaining group cohesiveness. Group leaders play an active role in helping the group fulfill its purpose and goals (Boyd & Ewashen, 2008). Leaders are constantly attentive to the group process and facilitate it; they also monitor when interventions should be directed at an individual or the group as a whole (Boyd & Ewashen, 2008). Strong leadership is essential for groups to function effectively. It may come from one person or may be shared by a number of people, depending on the situation. Some of the advantages of shared leadership are increased productivity, enhanced group cohesion, and satisfaction with group membership. When working with groups, CHN can engage in various leadership behaviours, as Box 13.2 indicates.

There are four generally accepted leadership styles, including autocratic, laissez-faire, democratic, and shared. However, there is growing interest in transformational and transactional leadership styles in nursing management and leadership theories (Marquis & Huston, 2017). Transformational and transactional leadership styles complement each other, as the transactional leader deals with the day-to-day tasks

---

> **BOX 13.2   Examples of CHN Leadership Behaviours**
>
> - *Advising:* Providing direction based on knowledgeable opinion (e.g., vaccine schedules)
> - *Analyzing:* Reviewing what has occurred as encouragement to examine behaviour and its meaning (e.g., dietary recall, evaluation of programs and policies)
> - *Clarifying:* Checking the meanings of interaction and communication through questions and restatement (e.g., medication review)
> - *Confronting:* Presenting behaviour and its effects to the individual and the group to challenge existing perceptions (e.g., advocating for up-to-date vaccinations in school-aged children)
> - *Evaluating:* Analyzing the effect or outcome of action or the value of an idea based on some standard (e.g., impact of a health education program on dietary behaviours)
> - *Initiating:* Introducing topics, beginning work, or changing the focus of a group (e.g., assessing patients' home care needs postsurgery)
> - *Questioning:* Encouraging analysis of a view or views through questions that support examination (e.g., evidence-based practice in wound care)
> - *Reflecting behaviour:* Reflecting on how a certain behaviour can impact care (e.g., using best practice standards to guide care)
> - *Reflecting feelings:* Naming the feelings that may be behind what is said or done (e.g., the stages of grieving, coping strategies)
> - *Suggesting:* Proposing or bringing an idea to a group (e.g., modifying or creating new policies)
> - *Summarizing:* Restating discussion or group action in brief form, highlighting important points (e.g., updating the patient care plan post health care team meeting)
> - *Supporting:* Giving emotionally comforting feedback that helps a person or group continue actions (e.g., encouraging comments)

Sources: Lassiter, P. G. (2006). Working with groups in the community. In M. Stanhope & J. Lancaster (Eds.), *Foundations of nursing in the community: Community oriented practice* (pp. 301–317). Mosby/Elsevier.

---

and the transformational leader focuses on motivating and inspiring followers (Table 13.3). The benefits of CHNs using a transformational leadership style could include creating healthy workplaces and addressing problems experienced in practice. Green, Miller, and Aarons (2013) examined the relationship between transformational leaders and the emotional exhaustion and turnover intention among community mental health providers. They found that managers who used a transformational leadership style including individual consideration and intellectual stimulation helped to buffer the effect of exhaustion and turnover. They recommended that organizations should invest in developing leaders who use transformational leadership styles to address the problems being experienced by community mental health providers.

The four leadership styles of autocratic, laissez-faire, democratic, and shared leadership can be used effectively by CHNs and are briefly discussed next. The first is the *autocratic leadership style,* also referred to as *authoritarian*

TABLE 13.3 Comparison of Transformational and Transactional Leadership

Transformational Leadership	Transactional Leadership
• Considers individual needs and wants • Promotes intellectual stimulation of followers • Empowers others through change, innovation, and growth • Raises others to higher levels of motivation and morality by identifying shared values • Uses personal charisma to motivate followers	• Focuses on day-to-day tasks • Focuses on organizational goals and not the individual • Examines cause-and-effect relationships to promote change and growth • Does not identify shared values • Uses rewards to engage others

or *paternalistic leadership style.* In this style of leadership, the leader maintains control in the group; communication is from the leader to the members; coercion of the group members is the motivator; work demands and not work requests are made; decision making does not involve others; the leader makes the decisions; the leader is the "I" and the group members are the "you"; and punitive criticism is often used (Marquis & Huston, 2017). This leadership style is best used in situations where decisions need to be made quickly or when high productivity is needed. For example, this style of leadership is best used in emergency or crisis situations, such as when CHNs are involved in disaster management (such as the SARS outbreak), or CHNs are working on projects with short project deadlines (such as planning a vaccination program for H1N1 immunizations). Autocratic leadership may help reduce group member frustration, but it can also stifle member's creativity, self-motivation, and autonomy (Marquis & Huston, 2017). It does not foster the development of group cohesion, and members do not learn independence or value the benefits of group work.

The second is the *laissez-faire leadership style,* which is a nondirected delegative leadership style. In this style of leadership, the leader assumes little or no group control; permissiveness prevails; minimal or no direction is provided by the leader; two-way communication occurs among group members; decision making is shared by the group; the emphasis is on the "you" for the group; and criticism is usually withheld (Marquis & Huston, 2017). This leadership style is best used by CHNs in situations when problem solving requires generating alternative solutions and when group members are self-directed and committed to the goal without strict time constraints. For example, this style of leadership could be used by a group of CHNs brainstorming how to address a measles outbreak in the community. This leadership style can encourage creativity and increase productivity when group members are self-directed and committed; however, it can result in group frustration, apathy, and loss of interest if not implemented properly (Marquis & Huston, 2017).

The third is the *democratic* or *participative leadership style.* In this style of leadership, the leader maintains some group control; communication is two-way; suggestions and guidance direct group members; group members are involved in decision-making; the emphasis is on the "we" for the group; and constructive criticism is used. This leadership style is best used in groups who meet for a long period of time, whose members have a variety of experiences, when coordination and cooperation is needed, and when thorough problem solving

is required and promotes group member growth (Marquis & Huston, 2017). This leadership style is time consuming, may be frustrating for group members looking for quick solutions, or can be ineffective if all group members are inexperienced, such as a CHN working with a school's student council to develop sexual-health curriculum content delivery strategies.

The fourth is *shared leadership.* In this style of leadership, there is a balance of power between leaders and members; the group has a common purpose or goal; leadership roles are shared so that work is done; the emphasis is on working together with a "we" approach; members share information, follow a collaborative decision-making process, and engage in cooperative interactions and constructive criticism (Pearce, Conger, & Locke, 2007). This leadership style works well in groups that have worked together for an extended period of time, are knowledgeable, and are highly committed to the group's goal. Shared leadership can empower members of the group, which can lead to increased productivity, a positive group climate, and group cohesiveness. However, a shared leadership style can be time consuming and may create conflict among group members who want a designated leader. This leadership style could be used by a CHN when organizing an interprofessional primary health care team meeting, because it encourages each member to participate in organizing, assessing, and planning patient care.

One example of a CHN who aspired to a national leadership role is Katie Dilworth, the 2018–2019 president of Community Health Nurses of Canada (CHNC). Katie started her leadership path as a community health nurse in the home health sector and then moved into public health as a frontline nurse and nurse administrator. As president of CHNC, Katie is the chair of the board of directors and represents CHNC at CNA and PHAC. The new standards for practice were passed in 2019 under her leadership. Other CHN leaders on the CHNC Board include Julia Lukewich, assistant professor of nursing from the Faculty of Nursing, Memorial University of Newfoundland, whose research interests are in the area of the integration and optimization of the nurse's role within primary health care. Angela Luciani from Nunavut is also a CHNC board member who participates on the national research and health policy committee. Each of these CHNs has demonstrated leadership behaviour by participating as a board member on a national nursing association.

Conflict Transformation

Conflict is an inevitable part of most group interactions, and most group members do not welcome conflict (Chinn, 2008;

Dimock & Kass, 2007). Chinn (2008) maintains that conflict can be transformed so that the group addresses the issue constructively and learns from it. Conflict transformation draws on three types of power:

- *The power of diversity,* which refers to supporting flexibility, creativity, and diverse viewpoints;
- *The power of solidarity,* which refers to incorporating variety within the group through sharing of leadership and promoting communication skill development; and
- *The power of shared responsibility,* which refers to group member accountability for their own actions, encouraging reflection and evaluation of self and group based on concern for the group and individual members (Chinn, 2008).

Group conflict can be intrapersonal, interpersonal, or intergroup. *Intrapersonal conflict* refers to conflict that occurs within an individual (Barr & Dowding, 2008; Pangman & Pangman, 2010). For example, a CHN working with a group of teenagers regarding sexual health and pregnancy may not personally support abortion and therefore experiences internal conflict about providing information about this option and the available community clinics that provide abortion ("Ethical Considerations" box). *Interpersonal conflict* refers to conflict between two or more people who have different values and beliefs (Barr & Dowding, 2008; Pangman & Pangman, 2010). For example, a home health nurse supports a palliative care patient's decision to die at home; however, the family physician and the social worker both believe that the patient should be hospitalized. *Intergroup conflict* refers to conflict between two or more groups (Barr & Dowding, 2008; Pangman & Pangman, 2010). For example, a municipal council has decided to close a community swimming pool, and a Healthy Communities citizens' group is opposing this decision.

Questions to Consider

1. The CHN finds in the course of working with teenagers that they do not share her beliefs about abortion. In relation to each of the ethical considerations noted, how should the CHN respond?
2. When working with this aggregate, what are some strategies CHNs can use to demonstrate integrity in their practice?

Additionally, conflict in groups can arise because of relationship, task, and process difficulties. Relationship conflicts arise when interpersonal friction develops among group members with differing personalities. For example, some competitive group members disagree with each other on many topics, which can affect group dynamics. Task conflicts arise when group members disagree about the work to be done. For example, some group members may be reflective and want to defer decision making on an issue so that more time is spent on a review, whereas others may want a quick decision without further discussion. Process conflicts arise when group members disagree about how to manage and complete the work. For example, all group members refuse to assume the role of recorder due to their time commitments, so it has been suggested that a secretary be hired for this role. Conflict occurs because some group members support the financing of the secretary, whereas others do not.

When conflict occurs within a group, the group must respond to it if it is to be resolved (Chinn, 2008). Some common group-conflict strategies are avoidance, competing, compromising, accommodating, and collaborating (Barr & Dowding, 2008). See Table 13.4 for examples of group conflict resolution strategies. As Figure 13.1 shows, the order of the strategies progresses from a concern for self to a concern for the group.

ETHICAL CONSIDERATIONS

A CHN working with a group of teenagers regarding sexual health and pregnancy does not personally support abortion. Ethical principles that apply to this interpersonal conflict are:

- *Social justice.* This principle recognizes that all citizens have an equal opportunity in the benefits and burdens in society. When providing care, CHNs do not discriminate based on a person's race, ethnicity, culture, political and spiritual beliefs, social or marital status, gender, sexual orientation, age, health status, place of origin, lifestyle, mental or physical ability, or socioeconomic status or any other attribute.
- *Veracity.* The principle of veracity identifies the need to be truthful, which promotes trust in the CHN–patient relationship. CHNs are honest and practise with integrity in all their professional interactions.
- *Autonomy.* CHNs, to the extent possible, provide persons in their care with the information they need to make informed decisions related to their health and well-being. They also work to ensure that health information is given to individuals, families, groups, populations, and communities in their care in an open, accurate, and transparent manner.
- *Autonomy.* CHNs in their professional capacity relate to all persons with respect. The CHN permits the individuals to choose those actions and goals that fulfill their life plans.

HOW TO …

Handle Group Conflict

- Remain calm and positive.
- Use direct and objective communication.
- Use positive body language and tone of voice.
- Focus on the problem not the group member(s).
- Recognize that outcomes of conflict can result in member and group growth.
- Group members need to express their feelings about the conflict without blaming. Start statements with "I feel …"
- Group members need to clarify in a factual manner what happened in the conflict situation without blaming. Start statements with "When (such and such happened) …"
- Each group member shares (preferably seated in a circle) how they wish the group to proceed so the conflict situation is resolved. Start statements with "I want …"
- Group members verbalize the mutually shared beliefs and agreements that are evident in the conflict situation and how the conflict situation will influence or positively change the group's principles of solidarity. Start statements with "Because …"

Sources: Barr, J., & Dowding, L. (2008). *Leadership in health care.* Sage Publications; Chinn, P. L. (2008). *Peace and power: Creative leadership for building community* (7th ed.). Jones & Bartlett.

TABLE 13.4 Examples of Group Conflict Resolution Strategies

Type	Description	Example
Avoidance	Group members are aware of the conflict but do not address it	Conflict has occurred and further discussion of this topic does not occur, with the group moving in another direction
Competing	Some group members use power to have their own needs met rather than the needs of the group	A newly established group trying to determine meeting times and frequency has members in conflict over availability. The leader in the organization uses power and states that they are available only on Tuesday mornings, so that is when the meetings must be held
Compromising	Group members explore solutions to a conflict and negotiate a solution where members have equal gain	Group A and Group B need to meet. The travel distance between the two groups is 200 km, and neither group wants to spend the resources or time to travel. After considerable negotiation, both groups decide to meet halfway
Accommodating	Group members who are in conflict resolve the difference by one member cooperating and giving in to the other members for the benefit of the group	Conflict has occurred between group members about group goals. The group members in the conflict situation agree to the suggested goals so that the team can move the task forward
Collaborating	Group members examine the differences that exist and work together to establish an acceptable solution that is beneficial to all group members	A group of community members at their first meeting are planning location of meetings, and a member suggests that travelling to the proposed meeting site is not equitable for all group members for time spent and resources spent to travel. Rotation of meeting sites among member agencies is suggested. The group discusses this idea and agrees to rotate the sites so that all members share in the travel expenses and time spent to get to meetings

Sources: Based on Barr, J., & Dowding, L. (2008). *Leadership in health care.* Sage Publications.

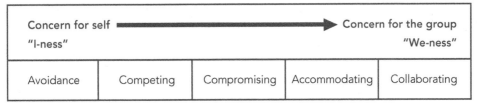

Fig. 13.1 Examples of Group Conflict Resolution Strategies. (Based on Barr, J., & Dowding, L. (2008). *Leadership in health care.* Sage Publications.)

Group Evaluation

When working with groups, the CHN needs to observe and examine how the group is functioning to determine group effectiveness. The CHN could also have each group member complete the group evaluation form in Fig. 13.2 so that group strengths and weaknesses are identified, and interventions initiated to improve group effectiveness. The group evaluation form can be used for the formative and summative evaluation of a group.

WORKING WITH HEALTH CARE TEAMS AND PARTNERS

Team Building in the Community

Team building is discussed in this chapter with reference to CHNs working with interprofessional health care teams and families, self-help groups, community groups, professional associations, and committees. Interprofessional health care teams consist of health care providers with a variety of knowledge, skills, and areas of expertise who work together with the patient. Moreover,

an interprofessional team has a group structure and group process and can experience group conflict. Since it is a group, it has a clearly stated team purpose and goals and performs at a more advanced level of unity than what is usually required of a group (Barr & Dowding, 2008). The CHN can apply these principles of team building to the interprofessional team and to families, self-help groups, community groups, professional associations, and committees. According to Kreitner, Kinicki, and Cole (2007), as cited in Pangman & Pangman, 2010, the goal of team building is to develop high-performing teams with the following characteristics:

- *Participative leadership.* The team leader consults with team members when making decisions, empowers team members, and promotes their interdependence.
- *Shared responsibility.* All team members take responsibility for team performance.
- *Aligned on purpose.* The team shares a common goal.
- *Strong communication.* The team has an atmosphere of openness, and respect, trust, and honest communication exists among all team members.

GROUP EVALUATION FORM

Group: _____   Date: _____

Time: _____   Observer: _____

For each area, place an "X" in the box that most nearly describes the group.

1. **UNITY** (degree of unity, cohesion, or "we-ness")

   ❐ Group is just a collection of individuals or subgroups; little group feeling.

   ❐ Group is very close, and there is little room or felt need for other contacts and experience.

   ❐ Some group feeling. Unity stems more from external factors than from friendship.

   ❐ Strong common purpose and spirit based on real friendships. Group usually sticks together.

2. **SELF-DIRECTION** (group's own motive power)

   ❐ Little drive from anywhere, either from members or designated leader.

   ❐ Domination from a strong single member, a clique, or the designated leader.

   ❐ Group has some self-propulsion but needs considerable push from designated leader.

   ❐ Initiation, planning, executing, and evaluating comes from total group.

3. **GROUP CLIMATE** (extent to which members feel free to be themselves)

   ❐ Climate inhibits good fun, behaviour, and expression of desire, fears, and opinions.

   ❐ Members freely express needs and desires: joke, tease, and argue to detriment of the group.

   ❐ Members express themselves but without observing interests of total group.

   ❐ Members feel free to express themselves but limit expression to total group welfare.

4. **DISTRIBUTION OF LEADERSHIP** (extent to which leadership roles are distributed among members)

   ❐ A few members always take leadership roles. The rest are passive.

   ❐ Many members take leadership, but one or two are continually followers.

   ❐ Some of the members take leadership roles, but many remain passive followers.

   ❐ Leadership is shared by all members of the group.

5. **DISTRIBUTION OF RESPONSIBILITY** (extent to which responsibility is shared among members)

   ❐ Everyone tries to get out of jobs.

   ❐ Many members accept responsibilities but do not carry them out.

   ❐ Responsibility is carried by a few members.

   ❐ Responsibilities are distributed among and carried out by nearly all members.

6. **PROBLEM SOLVING** (group's ability to think straight, make use of everyone's ideas, and decide creatively about its problems)

   ❐ Not much thinking as a group. Decisions made hastily, or group lets leader or worker do most of the thinking.

   ❐ Some thinking as a group but not yet an orderly process.

   ❐ Some cooperative thinking, but group gets tangled up in pet ideas of a few. Confused movement toward solutions.

   ❐ Good pooling of ideas and orderly thought. Everyone's ideas are used to reach final plan.

7. **METHOD OF RESOLVING DISAGREEMENTS WITH GROUP** (how group works out disagreements)

   ❐ Group waits for the designated leader to resolve disagreements.

   ❐ Compromises are affected by each subgroup giving up something.

   ❐ Strongest subgroup dominates through a vote and majority rule.

   ❐ Group as a whole arrives at a solution that satisfies all members and that is better than any single suggestion.

8. **MEETS BASIC NEEDS** (extent to which group gives a sense of security, achievement, approval, recognition, and belonging)

   ❐ Group experience adds little to the meeting of most members' needs.

   ❐ Group experience contributes substantially to basic needs of most members.

   ❐ Group experience contributes to some degree to basic needs of most members.

   ❐ Group contributes substantially to basic needs of all members.

9. **VARIETY OF ACTIVITIES**

   ❐ Little variety in activities—stick to same things.

   ❐ Considerable variety in activities. Try out new activities.

   ❐ Some variety in activities.

   ❐ Great variety in activities. Continually trying out new ones.

Fig. 13.2 Group Evaluation Form. (Reprinted with permission from Dimock, H. & Kass, R. (2007). *How to observe your group* (4th ed.). Captus Press Inc. (http://www.captus.com.)

10. DEPTH OF ACTIVITIES (extent to which activities are gone into in such a way that members can use full potentials, skills, and creativity)

❏ Little depth in activities—just scratching the surface.

❏ Some depth but members are not increasing their skills.

❏ Considerable depth in activities. Members able to utilize some of their abilities.

❏ Great depth in activities. Members find each a challenge to develop their abilities.

11. LEADER–MEMBER RAPPORT (relations between the group and the designated leader)

❏ Antagonistic or resentful.

❏ Indifferent toward leader. Friendship neither sought nor rejected. Noncommunicative.

❏ Friendly and interested. Attentive to leader's suggestions.

❏ Intimate relations: openness and sharing. Strong rapport.

12. ROLE OF THE LEADER (extent to which the group is centred around the designated leader)

❏ Activities, discussion, and decisions revolve around interests, desires, and needs of leader.

❏ Group looks to leader for suggestions and ideas. Leader decides when member gets in a jam.

❏ Leader acts as stimulator—suggests ideas or other ways of doing things. Helps group find ways of making own decisions.

❏ Leader stays out of discussion and makes few suggestions of things to do. Lets members carry the ball themselves.

13. STABILITY

❏ High absenteeism and turnover; influences group a great deal.

❏ High absenteeism and turnover; little influence on group growth.

❏ Some absenteeism and turnover with minor influence on group.

❏ Low absenteeism rate and turnover. Group very stable.

Fig. 13.2—cont'd

- *Future focused.* Change is seen as an opportunity for professional and personal growth.
- *Focused on task.* The team is results oriented and stays on task.
- *Creative talents.* Each member's creativity and talents are encouraged and applied.
- *Rapid response.* Possibilities are identified and acted upon promptly.

CHNs often fulfill the role of team facilitator, meaning they organize, coordinate, and evaluate the work of the teams. Based on the role of facilitator as described by Kelly and Crawford (2013), the CHN needs to reflect on the following questions:

- How has the atmosphere or environment contributed to successful team building?
- How have team members demonstrated mutual respect, trust, and honesty with one another?
- How have team members actively participated in the problem-solving and decision-making work of the team?
- Is each team member familiar with the purpose, goal, and objectives of the team?
- How do all team members encourage and support creativity and new ideas?
- How productive is the team?
- How is the team progressing toward goal attainment?
- Do team meetings begin and end on time?
- How does the team leader motivate the team?
- How is the team vision promoted by the leader?

For information on health teams, see the Health Council of Canada report, *Teams in Action* and the Canadian Health Services Research Foundation report, *Teamwork in Healthcare* (the links are in the Tool Box on the Evolve website).

Forming Community Partnerships

CHNs form partnerships in the community for a variety of reasons, but some of the most common are to build capacity in the system in the most appropriate ways, to reduce and contain costs, to avoid duplication of services, to coordinate services, and to most effectively address patient health care concerns. A **partnership** is a relationship between individuals, groups, or organizations, in which the partners actively work together in all stages of planning, implementation, and evaluation. For example, CHNs may form a partnership with local high-school teachers to design, implement, and evaluate a smoking cessation program for youths.

A number of general principles contribute to creating effective and sustainable partnerships (Box 13.3). CHNs need to be aware of these principles when working with partners.

Interprofessional Partnerships

Interprofessional partnerships are important for community health nursing practice. Some of the attributes found to contribute to effective interprofessional partnerships are:

- Each partner recognizes the purpose and the need for the partnership.

BOX 13.3   Principles for Creating Effective and Sustainable Partnerships

- Partnership members discuss and agree on the mission, values, goals, outcomes, and activities (e.g., the outcome of a smoking cessation program is increased knowledge).
- Partners agree that partnerships take time to develop.
- Communication between partners is clear, frequent, open, and evaluative (e.g., a schedule of meetings is developed, and minutes are recorded and circulated).
- All communication and activities will take into consideration the principles of social justice and equity (e.g., equal access to naloxone kits).
- Partner relationships are built on mutual respect, trust, caring, acceptance, and commitment.

- Partnerships work with strengths and assets and address weaknesses.
- Recognition of the diverse and vital contributions of partner members is acknowledged.
- Partners share resources and agree on power distribution and use within the partnership (power may not be equally distributed).
- All members agree to be partners, share the recognition for the successes, and accept responsibility for any associated risks.
- All partners review and determine partner roles and responsibilities.
- Flexibility in the partnership structure will allow for changing needs.

Sources: Centre for Addiction and Mental Health. (2008). *Recommendations of the building equitable partnerships (BEP) symposium 2008.* http://www.camh.net; Vollman, A. R., Anderson, E. T., & McFarlane, J. (2017). *Canadian community as partner: Theory & multidisciplinary practice* (4th ed.). Lippincott, Williams & Wilkins.

- A collegial relationship is valued, and partner members convey reciprocity, mutual respect, trust, genuineness, open communication, and equality, and are committed to conflict management.
- Interdependence exists among partner members and includes sharing, cooperation, "presence of synergy," and flexible boundaries.
- Power and leadership are shared by the partners and are based on the knowledge and expertise of partners, and decision making is by consensus and is egalitarian (Butt, Markle-Reid, & Browne, 2008).

Interprofessional partners engage in collaborative work (Butt et al., 2008; Vollman et al., 2017). *Collaboration* is defined as the commitment of two or more partners—such as agency and patient—who are in a power-sharing partnership. Collaboration is distinct from coordination and cooperation; coordination and cooperation are often part of the collaborative process (Vollman et al., 2017). However, all three concepts are interdependent and essential to building relationships in interprofessional partnerships. Vollman et al. (2017) include partnerships as a link to strengthening community action, one of the Ottawa Charter strategies to reach Canada's population health goals. **Collaborative patient-centred practice** is the active involvement of health care providers from various professions working together collaboratively to improve patient health outcomes with the patient as a partner (e.g., CHNs, family physicians, social workers, and dieticians work collaboratively with teachers and students to advocate for healthy school nutrition policies). This model of health care practice facilitates improvement of population health; patient health; access to health care; communication among health care providers; patient and health care provider satisfaction; and better utilization of human health care resources (Health Canada, 2004). For further information on interprofessional collaboration in

primary health care, refer to the Canadian Health Services Research Foundation's *CHSRF Synthesis: Interprofessional Collaboration and Quality Primary Healthcare* (see the link on the Evolve website).

Interprofessional Education

Butt et al. (2008) identified interprofessional education as one of the systematic moderating factors in interprofessional health and social service partnerships. *Interprofessional education* (IPE) has been defined as "occasions when two or more professions learn with, from, and about each other to improve collaboration and the quality of care" (Barr, Freeth, Hammick, et al., 2006, p. 1).

Since 2003, an interprofessional health care education movement has been active in Canada (Health Canada, 2004). This movement focuses on IPE, providing the opportunity for learning with and about a variety of disciplines through students sharing their discipline perspectives in learning environments (Buring, Bhushan, Broeseker, et al., 2009). Cusack and O'Donoghue (2012) examined health science students' perceptions of an IPE module with 92 students from nursing, physiotherapy, medicine, and diagnostic imaging. They found that the module was well received, and 91% reported high satisfaction with the learning approach. The students also reported that they were able to collaborate with and learn from the other disciplines. IPE promotes collaboration, communication, and teamwork in the practice setting.

This chapter has provided information on the knowledge and skills that CHNs need to work effectively in partnership with health care providers and patients. Health care reform in Canada has placed a greater emphasis on teams and partnerships as a future direction for community health care nursing practice. Therefore, it is vital that CHNs develop team-building skills and initiate partnership development that is effective and sustainable.

STUDENT EXPERIENCE

Form a group of at least four students. You are part of a newly formed team of interagency health care partners from social and health agencies who have identified the issue of low literacy levels in their community. Community health assessment data that led to identification of this issue were higher population of newcomers, higher incidence of high school dropouts, lower educational levels in the community, higher unemployment rates, and poorer levels of health based on census data.

1. Identify who the key interagency partners are in this team. Each student member will assume a role for one of the identified agencies.

2. The overall team goal is to increase literacy in the community.

3. As a group of students, each wearing an interagency hat, collaborate to assess and plan how your team will work together to meet this goal. Included in this planning should be consideration of the required group processes and team building, other partners that may need to be invited to join the team, and additional required assessment data, etc.

4. Evaluate how your team functioned, using the group evaluation form in Figure 13.2.

5. Discuss the team task and maintenance roles assumed by group members and the effect on team functioning.

CHAPTER SUMMARY

13.1 Five dimensions that significantly influence group process are group physical and emotional climate, group involvement, group interaction, group cohesion, and group productivity.

13.2 The five stages of group development are (1) forming—group members focus on getting to know one another, (2) storming—group members begin to express their feelings as real issues are focused on, (3) norming—group members start to feel part of the group, (4) performing—group members focus on the group work and share ideas, and (5) adjourning—group members recognize the need for termination of the group and therefore work toward completion of the tasks.

13.3 The kinds of roles group members assume as the group develops are task roles (problem definer, information seeker, information giver, opinion seeker, opinion giver, elaborator, recorder, evaluator, feasibility tester); group-building and maintenance roles (coordinator, harmonizer, encourager, orienter, follower, compromiser, gatekeeper, commentator), and individual-oriented roles (blocker, aggressor, digressor, recognition seeker, dominator, confessor, help seeker, withdrawer).

13.4 Group rules and standards govern how the group makes decisions, how work is assigned, and what is acceptable member behaviour. It is important for CHNs to understand group rules and standards because they can influence the role of the CHN when conducting meetings and making decisions.

13.5 Examples of leadership styles are autocratic, laissez-faire, democratic, shared, transformational, and transactional.

Leadership behaviours include advising, analyzing, clarifying, confronting, evaluating, initiating, questioning, reflecting behaviour and feelings, suggesting, summarizing, and supporting.

13.6 There are three types of group conflict: intrapersonal, interpersonal, and intergroup. Examples of group conflict resolution strategies include avoidance, competing, compromising, accommodating, and collaborating.

13.7 The composition and performance of a group can be evaluated through observation of strengths and weaknesses and group activities such as degree of unity, self-direction, climate, distribution of leadership and responsibility, problem solving, and method of resolving disagreements.

13.8 The goal of team building is to develop high-performing teams with the following characteristics: participative leadership, shared responsibility, aligned on purpose, strong communication, future focused, focused on task, creative talents, and rapid response.

13.9 The principles that can create effective and sustainable partnerships include clear, frequent, and open communication; mutual respect, trust, caring, acceptance, and commitment among partners; sharing resources and agreeing on power distribution and use within the partnership; and agreement among all to be partners, share the recognition for the successes, and accept responsibility for any associated risks. Interprofessional education is one of the systematic moderating factors in interprofessional education (IPE) and social service partnerships. More opportunities for IPE would be beneficial because it can lead to more effective teams in the clinical setting.

CHN IN PRACTICE: A CASE STUDY

Group Work With the Parents of Teenagers Who Have Discipline Problems

Mark, a community health nurse (CHN), and Mary, a social worker, conduct parenting classes for parents of teenagers with discipline problems. The 2-hour class meets every Wednesday for 5 weeks. At the first class, Mark and Mary outline to the parents

that the classes will cover areas such as enhancing teen self-esteem; developing good decision-making skills; developing cooperation and successful attitudes; using effective disciplining; and dealing with teens' angry and disruptive behaviours.

At the beginning of each class, Mark and Mary ask the group if they have any questions or concerns they would like to

Continued

CHN IN PRACTICE: A CASE STUDY—CONT'D

discuss with the class. Generally, the first hour includes Mark and Mary lecturing with the aid of a PowerPoint presentation of key points and often includes video vignettes of parent–teen interactions. The second hour of the class is a group discussion of an assigned parenting challenge with some role playing on how to intervene with the challenge.

During week 4, Andrea, a 33-year-old lone parent of a 15-year-old daughter, starts to cry when the class is assigned the topic of handling angry, disruptive teens. Andrea shares with the group that her daughter left home that evening in an angry state and will not be back. It is not the first time this has happened, but Andrea is worried because the first time her daughter left, the weather was warmer. This time, the weather is cold, and she is worried about how her daughter was dressed and where she was going, as most of her friends do not live with their parents. Susan, a fellow group member, leans over and hugs Andrea and says, "I had that experience with my daughter 2 months ago and that is why I am here—to try and figure out how to cope with this type of situation. You're not alone. If you ever want to talk, we can meet at Tim Hortons for coffee anytime."

The discussion that follows focuses on how to find support when it is needed and how to cope with a teen who leaves

home when she is angry. Mark and Mary identify agencies in the area that provide ongoing services for parents, such as discipline classes and educational support resources, as well as 1–800 numbers for telecounselling services that are available 24 hours a day.

The class ends on a positive note, with the members agreeing to talk more about their worries and feelings about parenting at the start of the next class.

Think About It

1. Identify the task and maintenance behaviours evident in this group meeting.
2. What are Mark and Mary's roles when working with (a) parents and (b) in group situations, such as the parenting classes?
3. Find an evidence-informed article about the role of the CHN in working with parents of teenagers as a group. What do the findings indicate about the role of the CHN?
4. Do you think that Susan's response to Andrea would be reassuring? Provide a rationale for your answer.
5. If you were the CHN, how would you have handled Andrea's sharing of her personal story so that the group continues to move forward? Provide specific examples with rationales.

 TOOL BOX

The Tool Box contains useful resources that can be applied in community health nursing practice. These related resources are found either in the appendices at the back of this text or on the Evolve website at http://evolve.elsevier.com/Canada/Stanhope/community/.

Appendix
- Appendix 1: Canadian Community Health Nursing Professional Practice Model and Standards of Practice

Tools

The Community Toolbox. Building Teams: Broadening the Base for Leadership. (http://ctb.ku.edu/en/table-of-contents/leadership/leadership-ideas/team-building/checklist)

This Tool Box site contains further links to sites with information, such as group facilitation, team building, and what makes a good team.

ELL Tool Box. (http://www.elltoolbox.com/)

This Tool Box provides examples of activities that group members can practice to enhance their group skills, such as listening, providing clear directions, and information analysis.

Manitoba Health, Healthy Living and Seniors. *Primary Care Interprofessional Team Toolkit.* (http://www.gov.mb.ca/health/primarycare/providers/pin/docs/pinit.pdf)

This tool kit provides instructions and resources on building an interprofessional team to meet the practice goals and profiles of Manitoba health care providers. It also outlines the scope of practice for various professionals, such as registered nurses, speech pathologists, counsellors, and dieticians and presents a three-step process to help integrate health care providers into a primary health care team.

REFERENCES

Barr, J., & Dowding, L. (2008). *Leadership in health care.* Sage Publications.

Barr, H., Freeth, D., Hammick, M., et al. (2006). The evidence base and recommendations for interprofessional education in health and social care. *Journal of Interprofessional Care, 20*(1), 75–78.

Boyd, M. A., & Ewashen, C. (2008). Interventions with groups. In W. Austin, & M. A. Boyd (Eds.), *Psychiatric nursing for Canadian practice* (pp. 255–269). Lippincott, Williams & Wilkins.

Buring, S. M., Bhushan, A., Broeseker, A., et al. (2009). Interprofessional education: Definitions, student competencies, and guidelines for implementation. *American Journal of Pharmaceutical Education, 73*(4), 59–64.

Butt, G., Markle-Reid, M., & Browne, G. (2008). Interprofessional partnerships in chronic illness care: A conceptual model for measuring partnership effectiveness. *International Journal of Integrated Care, 8*(14). http://www.ncbi.nlm.nih.gov/pmc/articles/PMC2387190/.

Canadian Public Health Association (CPHA). (2010). *Public health—community health nursing practice in Canada: Roles and activities* (4th ed.). Canadian Public Health Association. https://www.cpha.ca/sites/default/files/assets/pubs/3-1bk04214.pdf.

Canadian Nurses Association (CNA). (2019). *Position Statement: Interprofessional collaboration.* https://www.cna-aiic.ca/-/media/cna/page-content/pdf-en/cna-position-statement_interprofessional-collaboration.pdf

Centre for Addiction and Mental Health. (2008). *Recommendations of the building equitable partnerships (BEP) symposium 2008.* http://www.camh.net.

Chinn, P. L. (2008). *Peace and power: Creative leadership for building community* (7th ed.). Jones & Bartlett.

Community Health Nurses of Canada (CHNC). (2019). *Canadian community health nursing: Professional practice model and standards of practice.* https://www.chnc.ca/standards-of-practice.

Cusack, T., & O'Donoghue, G. (2012). The introduction of an interprofessional education module: Students' perceptions. *Quality in Primary Care, 20*(3), 231–238.

Dimock, H. G., & Kass, R. (2007). *How to observe your group* (4th ed.). Captus Press.

Dimock, H. G., & Kass, R. (2008). *Leading and managing dynamic groups* (4th ed.). Captus Press.

Green, A., Miller, E., & Aarons, G. (2013). Transformational leadership moderates the relationship between emotional exhaustion and turnover intention among community mental health providers. *Community Mental Health Journal, 49*(4), 373–379. https://doi.org/10.1007/s10597-011-9463-0.

Health Canada. (2004). *Interprofessional education for collaborative patient-centred practice: Research synthesis paper*. https://www.med.mun.ca/getdoc/58a756d2-1442-42ed-915b-9295b6d315c6/Curran--Resarch-Synthesis-Paper.aspx.

Kamans, E., Otten, S., & Gordijn, E. H. (2011). Power and threat in intergroup conflict: How emotional and behavioural responses depend on amount and content of threat. *Group Processes & Intergroup Relations, 14*(3), 293–310.

Kelly, P., & Crawford, H. (2013). *Nursing leadership and management* (2nd Cdn ed.). Canada: Nelson education.

Lassiter, P. G. (2006). Working with groups in the community. In M. Stanhope, & J. Lancaster (Eds.), *Foundations of nursing in the community: Community oriented practice* (pp. 301–317). Mosby/Elsevier.

Marquis, B. L., & Huston, C. J. (2017). *Leadership roles and management functions in nursing: Theory and application* (9th ed.). Lippincott Williams & Wilkins.

Maurer, F. A., & Smith, C. M. (2013). *Community/public health practice: Health for families and populations* (5th ed.). Elsevier.

McCallin, A., & Bamford, A. (2007). Interdisciplinary teamwork: Is the influence of emotional intelligence fully appreciated? *Journal of Nursing Management, 15*(4), 386–391.

Pangman, V. C., & Pangman, C. (2010). *Nursing leadership from a Canadian perspective*. Lippincott, Williams & Wilkins.

Pearce, C. L., Conger, J. A., & Locke, E. A. (2007). Theoretical and practitioner letters: Shared leadership theory. *The Leadership Quarterly, 18*, 281–288.

Seck, M., & Helton, L. (2014). Faculty development of a joint MSW program utilizing Tuckman's model of stages of group development. *Social Work with Groups, 37*(2), 158–168.

Smith, D., Meyer, S., & Wylie, D. (2006). In J. M. Hibberd, & D. L. Smith (Eds.), *Nursing leadership and management in Canada* (3rd ed.) (pp. 519–547). Elsevier Canada.

Tuckman, B. W. (1965). Developmental sequence in small groups. *Psychological Bulletin, 63*, 384–399.

Tuckman, B. W., & Jensen, M. A. C. (1977). Stages of small group development revisited. *Group & Organization Studies, 2*(4), 419–427.

Vollman, A. R., Anderson, E. T., & McFarlane, J. (2017). *Canadian community as partner: Theory & multidisciplinary practice* (4th ed.). Lippincott, Williams & Wilkins.

Whittingham, M. (2018). Interpersonal theory and group therapy: Validating the social microcosm. *International Journal of Group Psychotherapy, 68*, 93–98.

14

Indigenous Health: Working With First Nations People, Inuit, and Métis

R. L. Bourque Bearskin and S.L. Jakubec

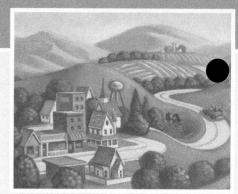

OUTLINE

Indigenous Peoples in Canada: Definitions, 325
Population Snapshot of Indigenous Peoples, 325
The Health Status of Indigenous People, 326
The Historical and Legislative Context of Indigenous Health Issues, 327
  Precolonization and Colonization, 327
  Key Events and Legislation, 328
  First Nations Peoples Treaties, 328
  The *Indian Act*, 330
The Consequences of Colonization and Historical Trauma, 330
  Residential School Legacy, 330
  The Sixties Scoop, 332
  Indigenous Health Advocacy Actions, 332

Indigenous Nursing in Canada, 332
  The Truth and Reconciliation Commission of Canada, 333
  Decolonization, 333
Indigenous Determinants of Health, 334
  Proximal Determinants of Health, 334
  Intermediate Determinants of Health, 335
  Distal Determinants of Health, 335
CHN in Practice: a Comprehensive Case Study, 336
  Developing an Exercise and Wellness Program for Indigenous Women in Northern Creek, 336
  Background, 336
  Community Health Assessment, 336
  Planning for a Community Health Nursing Intervention, 337

OBJECTIVES

After reading this chapter, you should be able to:
14.1 Understand the terminology used to identify Indigenous peoples.
14.2 Provide a snapshot of the Indigenous population.
14.3 Discuss the health status of Indigenous peoples.
14.4 Describe the historical experiences faced by First Nations people, Inuit, and Métis in Canada.

14.5 Explain the consequences of colonization and historical trauma for Indigenous peoples.
14.6 List the determinants of health specific to First Nations people, Inuit, and Métis.
14.7 Describe the application of the community health nursing process to promote wellness in an Indigenous community using a rights-based, trauma-informed, strengths-based, and capacity-building approach.

KEY TERMS*

Aboriginal, 325
colonialism, 327
decolonization, 333
distal determinants of health, 334
First Peoples, 325
Indian, 325
Indigenous, 325
Indigenous peoples, 325
Indigenous ways of knowing, 326

intergenerational trauma, 336
intermediate determinants of health, 334
native, 325
proximal determinants of health, 334
residential schools, 330
self-determination, 336
Sixties Scoop, 332
trauma-informed care, 334
treaty, 328

*See the Glossary on page 468 for definitions.

This chapter provides an overview of Indigenous people's experiences in relation to community health. It covers key concepts of Indigenous ways of knowing and being, and the continued effects of colonialism. A comprehensive case study illustrating a community health nursing intervention with a First Nation community is explored in the second half of this chapter.

It is important to begin this chapter and all engagement with communities and their health with point of entry, an invitation to learn about community and health, and with a land acknowledgement. This is part of actions for reconciliation to honour the traditional lands, Indigenous knowledge, and relationships cultivated by Indigenous Peoples for thousands of years. In this way, we acknowledge the traditional territories where this textbook is published in Milton, Ontario, Canada, the traditional home of many Nations including the Mississaugas of the Credit First Nation, the Anishinaabe, the Attawandaron, the Haudenosaunee, and the Métis. You are reading from a place and connected to land that you will acknowledge, especially in your community nursing work as well.

In respect for tradition of one's self in place and community, we also introduce ourselves, so the reader knows our positionalities and locations (Bourque Bearskin, Kennedy, Bourque, et al., 2020). We are two nursing scholars who are passionate about community health. Bourque Bearskin is a nêhiyaw-iskwêw (Cree Woman) from Beaver Lake Cree Nation, rooted in Métis identity. As Canadian Institutes of Health Research (CIHR) Indigenous Health Research Chair in Nursing in British Columbia, her work stems from her lived experience and relationship with First Nations, Inuit, and Métis Peoples. Jakubec is of European Settler ancestry; now a visitor in Treaty 7 traditional lands, she is originally from the unceded territory of the Syilx/Okanagan Nation where learning and respect for the land was baked in with the Okanagan sun. She has also lived and learned as a nurse in Treaty 6, in unceded Witsuwit'en territory and alongside Indigenous people in Aotearoa/New Zealand, West Africa, and South India. We come together to promote Indigenous health equity.

In acknowledging the original Peoples known as the traditional right holders and custodians upon which we live, work, and play, we want to honour and respect all those whose historical relationships with the land continue to this day. We hold up our hands in respect to the Elders, both past, present, and future, for they hold the memories, the traditions, the culture, and the hopes of Indigenous Peoples. To our ancestors, teachers, mentors, and mentees who have contributed to this growing nursing approach for culturally and trauma-informed and safe practice: we thank you.

INDIGENOUS PEOPLES IN CANADA: DEFINITIONS

The term **Indigenous** refers to the First Nations, Inuit, and Métis Peoples in Canada, replacing the term Aboriginal. However, the term Aboriginal is used to acknowledge the rights of Indigenous Peoples in the *Constitution Act*, which assigned the term **Indian** as the legal identification of those who were not Inuit or Métis (Indigenous and Northern Affairs Canada, 2012). **First Peoples** is another collective term used to refer to the original inhabitants of Canada (Younging, 2018). The term *Indian* is rarely used outside of reference to the *Indian Act* in Canada, and its use—aside from a legal context—could be considered offensive. The term **native** was considered appropriate in earlier years; it refers to people who originate from a specific place or local

territory and is now used only in that context. Over the years the use of these terms changed to refer to Indigenous people as **Aboriginal**, meaning the original inhabitants of a country (including First Nations, Inuit, and Métis people). This was confirmed in 1985 in the Canadian Constitution. The term *Aboriginal* remains in common use; however, it does not fully recognize the diversity of **Indigenous Peoples**. The Canadian government's official agreement to the United Nations' Declaration of the Rights of Indigenous Peoples in 2016, which is now being implemented into British Columbia's legislation to align provincial, municipal, and federal laws to provide a framework for decision making (Government of British Columbia, n.d.).

Whenever possible, it is best to understand, describe, and relate to people through their specific and preferred ways of being identified, for example: "Louise is a First Nation elder and a member of the Haida community of Atewaas (Old Masset)." "Paul is a Moose Cree and Métis from Moose Factory Island," or "Dan is Musuau Innu from one of the two Innu communities of Labrador." Note that Innu and Inuit do not describe the same group. Innu are part of a First Nation of eastern Quebec and southern Labrador, whereas Inuit are not First Nation, but rather a distinct Indigenous cultural group originating from the North West Territories and Nunavut.

POPULATION SNAPSHOT OF INDIGENOUS PEOPLES

According to the Office of the United Nations High Commissioner for Human Rights (OHCHR, 2020), the population of Indigenous peoples worldwide is over 370 million. Indigenous peoples live in 70 countries and are acknowledged as the inheritors, practitioners, and holders of unique cultural ways of relating to other people and their environment. Indigenous peoples have retained social, cultural, economic, and political characteristics that are distinct from those of the dominant societies in which they live and represent a rich diversity of religions, traditions, languages, and histories (Hovey, Delormier, & McComber, 2014).

In 2016, the Indigenous Peoples were the fastest-growing population in Canada. First Nations, Inuit, and Métis Peoples represent 1,673,785 million people, accounting for 4.9% of Canada's population. A total of 58.4% self-identify as First Nations people, 35.1% as Métis, and 3.9% as Inuit. Since 2006, the Indigenous population has grown 42.5%; this is four times higher than the growth rate of the non-Indigenous population. The largest proportion of Indigenous people live in Ontario (24.2%), and 56.8% live in one of the western provinces. Moreover, 29.2% of the total Indigenous population is 14 years of age or younger (Statistics Canada, 2017). These statistics are an indicator of the resurgence and strength of Indigenous ways of knowing and Indigenous peoples in Canada.

The "Cultural Considerations" box looks at Indigenous ways of knowing in relation to community health nursing practice.

CULTURAL CONSIDERATIONS

Indigenous Ways of Knowing and Being

Indigenous peoples and their ways of knowing have survived extensive oppression throughout North America.* The Truth and Reconciliation Commission of Canada† and the Office of the United Nations High Commissioner for Human Rights‡ refer to the Indigenous experience as cultural genocide. However, Indigenous ways of knowing and being have survived, and they are linked through language and constructed from everyday events, relationships, environmental and spiritual dimensions of thought, and storytelling practices.§ **Indigenous ways of knowing** are approaches to understanding life that underscore the histories, experiences, and teachings of the people who originate from a land.‖ For community health nurses (CHNs), understanding Indigenous ways of knowing and being is essential for culturally safe, relational nursing practice.

Questions to Consider

1. How can Indigenous ways of knowing and scientific ways of knowing work together for the advancement of community health?
2. What are some of the barriers to integrating Indigenous and scientific ways of knowing for community health care?
3. What actions can a CHN take to facilitate the integration of Indigenous and scientific ways of knowing for community health care?

* *Sources*: Battiste, 2013; Bourque Bearskin, Cameron, King, et al., 2016; Jakubec & Bourque Bearskin, 2020.
† Truth and Reconciliation Commission of Canada, 2015.
‡ Office of the United Nations High Commissioner for Human Rights, 2020.
§ Sinclair, Doerfler, & Stark, 2013.
‖ Absolon, 2008.

THE HEALTH STATUS OF INDIGENOUS PEOPLE

It is widely acknowledged that the health status of First Nations, Inuit, and Métis populations in Canada falls below that of the general Canadian population (Health Canada, 2018). The projected life expectancy of the general population in 2017 is 79 for men and 83 for women. By contrast, the projected life expectancy in 2017 of First Nations and Métis men was 73 to 74; and the projected life expectancy in 2017 of First Nations and Métis women was 78 to 80. Lower still was the projected life expectancy in 2017 of Inuit men (64 years) and Inuit women (73 years) (Health Canada, 2018).

Food insecurity, sexual health, addictions (smoking, alcohol, and prescription drug use), mental health conditions, and spiritual health problems continue to influence the overall wellness of First Nations people and Inuit, with devastating impacts (National Collaborating Centre for Aboriginal Health, 2014). Suicides among First Nations peoples, Métis peoples, and Inuit peoples are three, two, and nine times the national average, respectively (Statistics Canada, 2019). The overall rate of death from injury is much higher in the Indigenous population than it is in the non-Indigenous population and a primary cause of death in youth (Lachance,

Hossack, Wijayasinghe, et al., 2009). Indigenous infants are 1.7 times more likely to be born with congenital anomalies, 2.6 times more likely to experience infection, and First Nations and Inuit infants are 7 times more likely to experience sudden infant death syndrome (Sheppard, Shapiro, Bushnik et al., 2017).

Current research shows that some Indigenous groups around the world are rapidly acquiring lifestyle diseases such as obesity, type 2 diabetes, and heart disease, as well as physical and mental health illnesses related to alcohol and drug use (WHO, 2020). Moreover, the low standards of health experienced by Indigenous people are related to poverty, malnutrition, overcrowding, environmental contamination, and inadequate clinical care (Greenwood, de Leeuw & Lindsay, 2018).

Historically, the federal government has provided a limited range of health services to First Nations people living on-reserve. In recent years, health policy has shifted to increased First Nations control of health services with a view to building local capacity and more culturally appropriate health planning and delivery (Smith & Lavoie, 2008). As introduced in Chapter 2, British Columbia's First Nations Health Authority (FNHA, n.d.a) was established in 2013 to reform the delivery of health care to BC First Nations to improve their health. The FNHA is now responsible for the planning, management, service delivery, and funding of health programs in British Columbia that were previously provided by the federal government. The federal government is responsible for covering a number of health-related goods and services to First Nations people and Inuit in other provinces under the Non-Insured Health Benefit program. This program does not provide health-related goods and services to Métis, First Nations people living off-reserve, or First Nations people who are not registered under the *Indian Act*, despite the fact that these groups are affected by the same determinants of health (Allan & Smylie, 2015). Most primary care and all secondary and tertiary care services, however, are provided through provincially operated services, which are less available in rural and isolated parts of the country (Lavoie, Wong, Katz, et al., 2016). For Indigenous peoples, structural racism is rooted in colonial systems and policies that create unequal access to power and resources and devalue Indigenous perspectives. Studies on the experiences of Indigenous Peoples' access to services have shown that delaying or avoiding access to health care is related to anticipated racism and the reporting of past negative experiences that involved health care providers' discrimination, stigmatization, and stereotyping (Horrill, McMillan, Schultz, et al., 2018; Turpel-Lanfond, 2020).

CHNs face many compounding factors that affect their ability to work effectively in the current approach to nursing service delivery in First Nations, Inuit, and Métis communities (Canadian Nurses Association, 2014). CHNs working with First Nations, Inuit, and Métis populations must understand the historical considerations that have led to growing health disparities and ineffective health care policies (Cameron, Camargo Plazas, Santo Salas, et al., 2014).

For further information on the health of Indigenous peoples in Canada, visit the National Collaborating Centre for Aboriginal Health (NCCAH) website (the link is on the Evolve website.)

THE HISTORICAL AND LEGISLATIVE CONTEXT OF INDIGENOUS HEALTH ISSUES

What factors have contributed to the health disparities and conditions of Indigenous populations in Canada? Colonization, key events, and legislation have significantly influenced the current conditions of Indigenous health. An understanding of these factors should inform community health nursing practice with First Nation, Inuit, and Métis peoples.

Precolonization and Colonization
Precolonization

Prior to the arrival of European settlers, indigenous people lived and flourished in the lands now called Canada. Indigenous communities were found to have had innovative ideas on education, hunting, fishing, and gathering foods alongside sophisticated and complex social and cultural governance strategies to manage and preserve food, shelter, medicine, and democracy of their nation-to-nation states (Dickason & McNab, 2009).

Over 500 years ago in the area of what has become Canada, it is estimated that the Indigenous population was between 200 000 and 2 million (with the most widely accepted estimate being 500 000) (Royal Commission on Aboriginal Peoples, 1996). These population figures suggest that effective systems of hygiene, nutrition, medicine, and healing practices existed that ensured survival, health, and wellness. The diet of the original people included staples such as corn, beans, squash, nuts, and meat. Moreover, in almost every region, indigenous people possessed knowledge of the various vitamins and minerals needed for good health. Indigenous people were strong, healthy, and well-organized people, and no historical records or data exist that suggest they suffered from rampant diseases or epidemics. Infectious diseases were absent prior to European contact, and dental caries accounted for less than 1% of all teeth according to paleopathological evidence. The first recorded outbreaks of infectious disease in original communities occurred between 1734 and 1741 (Obomsawin, 2007).

Colonization

The first known contact between Indigenous people and Europeans in what is now Canada took place in the tenth century when the Vikings reached the Atlantic Coast. Contact grew by the late sixteenth century, when Scandinavians, Bretons, Basques, and Normans became regular visitors to North Atlantic fishing grounds. The French (who founded the city of Quebec in 1608) and British were the primary colonizers of what is now Canada and competed for control of lands in North America ("European Colonization and the Native peoples," n.d.; Indigenous and Northern Affairs Canada, 2010). Starting in 1701, the British Crown entered into treaties to foster peaceful relations between Indigenous people and Europeans (Indigenous and Northern Affairs Canada, 2010). Despite the spirit and intent of treaties, much of indigenous land fell under the control of European settlers (Lawrence, 2002). By the 1760s, the British became the dominant colonial power in North America (Indigenous and Northern Affairs Canada, 2010). **Colonialism** is a policy of acquiring or maintaining colonies; it involves a wealthier power controlling and exploiting another society. In the case of Indigenous peoples in Canada, colonialism resulted in the erosion of social bonds and trust and the dispossession of original people from the land (Alfred, 2009). *Colonization* refers to the settlement of colonies and the imposition of one power's culture on another. According to the Royal Commission on Aboriginal Peoples (1996), four stages of colonization in Canada are characterized as having taken place in three waves:

1. *Legal wave.* Control of the Indigenous population was undertaken with legislation that suppressed legal rights.
2. *Administrative wave.* A reserve system was created to isolate Indigenous people and claim traditional lands.
3. *Ideological wave.* The residential school system and foster-parent system were intended to assimilate and isolate Indigenous people.

Table 14.1 indicates the stages and negative effects of colonization on Indigenous people identified by Thira (2014). The Royal Commission evolved to address the waves as the foundation for four phases of colonization, first moving from separate worlds, then to contact and cooperation, to displacement and assimilation, and finally, to negotiation and renewal (Carruth, 2013).

Around the world, colonization has led to the devaluing of Indigenous knowledge systems relative to dominant cultural knowledge, including health knowledge. Indigenous

TABLE 14.1 The Stages and Negative Impact of Colonization

Relocation/Reserves	Theft of Rights and Criminalization of Culture	Residential School System
• Theft of home/belonging	• Theft of cultural traditions	• Theft of family
• Theft of economy/food source	• Theft of ceremonial artefacts	• Theft of culture and language
• Theft of localized spiritual places/culture/identity	• Theft of history	• Theft of identity/social role
• Theft of lifestyle and freedom	• Theft of sociocultural identity	• Theft of parenting and life skills
	• Theft of livelihood	• Theft of self-esteem/spirit
		• Theft of value (internalized racism)

Source: Thira, D. (2014). *Beyond the four waves of colonization.* https://thira.ca/files/2014/08/Colonization-Article-CNPR-Revised1.pdf

people are often seen as deficient, dysfunctional, diseased, or damaged. These beliefs do very little to recognize the ongoing oppression of Indigenous people in the health care system. Much of the advocacy in Indigenous health (which is discussed further in the examination of antioppressive practices in Chapter 15) has been about understanding Indigenous people *by and with* Indigenous people within a colonial context to prevent further marginalization (Funnel, Tanuseputro, Letendre et al., 2019; Sockbeson, 2011).

Key Events and Legislation

CHNs need to be acutely aware of the historical context of Indigenous people in Canada. This awareness provides the contextual understanding of many of the factors that contribute to the growing health disparities seen in the Indigenous population. Table 14.2 introduces key events and legislation that have influenced the health of Indigenous people today.

First Nations Peoples Treaties

The historical context is punctuated by treaty making. The treaties were nation-to-nation agreements intended to remind people to live in peace and friendship and share the resources

of the land equally (The Canadian Encyclopedia, 2020). The Dish With One Spoon Wampum represents the first Treaty made in North America. This treaty symbolizes unity and was used to establish peace among Indigenous nations prior to the arrival of the Europeans.

During the years of war between the French and the British in North America (1754–1763), the Canadian government (on behalf of the British Crown) forced the signing of Treaties with various First Nations groups, after the implementation of strategies that led to the starvation and ravages of disease of First Nations Peoples (Starblanket, 2020). Treaties were then misinterpreted as a means by which the government could obtain large tracts of land and resources. Treaties between First Nations peoples and the Crown have been contentious because a number of treaty obligations, including those that impact community health, were not fulfilled by the government. In the context of Aboriginal–European history in Canada, a **Treaty** came to be an agreement between First Nations Peoples and the Crown in which First Nations Peoples agreed to coexist and share the land and resources. It was an understanding that Treaties were a negotiation on sharing of the land and protecting their culture:

TABLE 14.2	Key Events and Legislation That Have Influenced Indigenous Health
Year	**Events and Legislation**
1500	Early contact between original peoples and Europeans developed out of mutual curiosity; an exchange of goods; military and trade alliances; and friendship and intermarriage. This was a time of cooperation and independence, with each group able to negotiate its own trade and military alliances.
1763	The *Royal Proclamation of 1763* summarized the rules regarding land ownership. It stated that Aboriginal people were not to be *molested or disturbed* on their lands and that any transactions had to be properly negotiated between the Crown and Aboriginal representatives. Lands were only to be acquired by treaty or purchase by the Crown. The *Royal Proclamation of 1763* was the first time the Crown acknowledged the title and rights of Indigenous peoples.
1800s	The First Nations and European relationship shifted from one of partnership to one of domination of the former by the latter. The number of European settlers increased, shifting the economy from the fur trade to timber, minerals, and agricultural production; colonial governments no longer needed First Nations as military allies; an ideology of European superiority took hold.
1849	The first residential school was established in Alderville, Ontario. First Nations children were removed from their homes at age 5 and placed in church-run schools as a means to civilize them.
1850	The purpose of the Robinson-Huron and Robinson-Superior treaties were for the Anishinaabe Nations ("Ojibwe Indians") to give up their rights to land title to the Crown, and in return they would receive reserves, annuities, and sustained rights to fish and hunt on unoccupied Crown lands. These two treaties became the prototype for the "Numbered Treaties" which took place after Confederation.
1857	The Province of Canada passed "An Act to Encourage the Gradual Civilization of the Indian Tribes in This Province, and to Amend the Laws Respecting Indians." First Nations people *of good character* were declared non-Indians and invited into Canadian society.
1867	Confederation was declared with a new partnership between English and French colonists to manage lands in Canada. First Nations were not mentioned in Confederation documents. The *British North America Act* made "Indians and Lands Reserved for Indians" subject to government regulation. Parliament passed laws to replace traditional First Nations governments with elected band councils with limited powers, taking control of valuable resources on reserve lands and applying non-First Nations concepts of marriage and parenting. Traditional potlach and sun dance ceremonies were banned, and a pass system was instituted where, in some cases, First Nations people could not leave reserves without permission from a federal agent. Starvation, violence, abuse, infectious diseases, cultural suppression, relocation, and family and community disruption were all experienced during this time. By 1871, the First Nations population had been reduced to 102000.
1876	According to the *Indian Act*, Status Indians are wards of the federal government. The Act defines who is entitled to be registered as an Indian under the Act. It also regulates aspects of First Nations and Inuit peoples' lives without their input.

Continued

TABLE 14.2   Key Events and Legislation That Have Influenced Indigenous Health—cont'd

Year	Events and Legislation
1920	The federal government made residential school attendance compulsory for all First Nations, Inuit, and some Métis children between the ages of 7 and 15. Over 100 residential schools were built and operated until 1996. Children were removed from their homes and communities to attend school 10 months a year. Many children died of disease; suffered abuse; were separated from their siblings; were punished for speaking their languages; and were forbidden to use traditional practices.
1950s and 1960s	A 1951 amendment to the *Indian Act* meant that provinces were guaranteed federal funding for each First Nations, Inuit, and Metis child apprehended by child protection agencies. The result was a ballooning in the number of First Nations, Inuit and some Métis children taken into care by the mid-1960s—a phenomenon known as the "Sixties Scoop." The number of First Nations, Inuit, and Métis children in care rose from 1% in 1959 to 30 to 40% in the 1960s.
1969	The federal government released its White Paper on Indian Policy, which proposed the dismantling of the *Indian Act* and the elimination of Indian status to enable First Nations and Inuit peoples to have the same rights, opportunities, and responsibilities as other Canadians. First Nations, Inuit, and Métis groups resoundingly rejected this proposal, seeing it as the end of their existence as distinct peoples, spawning a new era focused on the recognition of Indigenous survival despite assimilation efforts.
1982	After years of political struggle by First Nations, Inuit, and Métis peoples, the *Constitution Act, 1982* recognized existing Aboriginal and treaty rights.
1990	The Oka Crisis took place over land claims agreements. A conflict in the Kanesatake reserve was sparked by plans to expand a golf course in the neighbouring community of Oka on land the Mohawk claimed as a traditional burial ground.
1996	The last federally run residential school, White Calf Collegiate, in Saskatchewan, closed.
1999	The new territory of Nunavut, which is self-governed, was created on April 1.
2007	The first settlement agreements were made to residential school survivors. Jordan's Principle was passed in the House of Commons; this principle is meant to help settle disputes between provincial and federal governments over payment of health care services delivered to First Nations children.
2008	Prime Minister Stephen Harper offered a full apology on behalf of Canadians for the Indian residential school system. Bill C-21 *(An Act to Amend the Canadian Human Rights Act)* corrects the fundamental injustice of denying people governed by the *Indian Act* recourse against human rights violations; it was given royal assent. The Canadian Human Rights Commission's National Aboriginal Initiative was established to strengthen the human rights protection of First Nation and Inuit peoples. First Nations and Inuit peoples are able to take action against First Nations governments as well as the federal government if they experience discrimination in decisions affecting their daily lives.
2012	The grassroots movement Idle No More was launched by four Indigenous women. In 2012, Indigenous and non-Indigenous people mobilized in response to growing frustration over sweeping federal legislative changes regarding control over land and environmental regulations that threatened the rights of Indigenous people in Canada.
2015	The Truth and Reconciliation Commission of Canada released 94 calls to action, encouraging federal, provincial, territorial, and First Nation, Inuit, and Métis peoples to work together toward changing policies and programs to repair the harm caused by residential schools.
2016	Canadian Human Rights case in inequitable provision of child welfare was upheld.
2019	Reclaiming Power and Place: The Final Report of the National Inquiry into Missing and Murdered Indigenous Women and Girls; Defining and naming genocide; *Their Voices Will Guide Us* Education Guide was released.
2020	The Canadian Human Rights Tribunal (CHRT) ruled that all First Nations children living on and off reserve are eligible for funding under the Jordan Principle: legislation that recognizes the inequities that Indigenous children face and calls on the government to pay for a child's services and seek reimbursement later, so the child does not get caught in the middle of a similar dispute.
2020	The Government of Canada introduced legislation to adopt the United Nations Rights of Indigenous Peoples as an overarching framework to work on nation-to-nation agreements in support of self-determination and sovereignty.

Sources: Blackstock, C. (2016). The Complainant: The Canadian Human Rights Tribunal on First Nations Child Welfare. *McGill Law Journal*, *62*(2), 285–328; Bourque Bearskin, R. L. (2011). A critical lens on culture in nursing practice. *Nursing Ethics, 18*(4), 548–559. https://doi.org/10.1177/0969733011408048; Coats, K. (2015). *Idle No More and the remaking of Canada*. University of Regina Press; First Nations Studies Program at University of British Columbia. (n.d.). *Sixties scoop.* http://indigenousfoundations.arts.ubc.ca/sixties_scoop/; First Nations Studies Program at University of British Columbia. (n.d.b.). *The White Paper 1969.* https://indigenousfoundations.arts.ubc.ca/the_white_paper_1969/; Government of Canada. (2020a). *Highlights from the Report of the Royal Commission on Aboriginal Peoples.* https://www.rcaanc-cirnac.gc.ca/eng/1100100014597/1572547985018; Government of Canada. (2020b). *Guide to the Canadian Charter of Rights and Freedoms.* https://www.canada.ca/en/canadian-heritage/services/how-rights-protected/guide-canadian-charter-rights-freedoms.html; Government of Canada. (2020c). *Implementing the United Nations Declaration on the Rights of Indigenous Peoples in Canada.* https://www.justice.gc.ca/eng/declaration/index.html; Higginbottom, G. M. A., Caine, V., Salway, S., et al. (2011). *Providing culturally safe and competent health care—A self-directed workbook and digital resource.* Faculty of Nursing, University of Alberta; Indigenous and Northern Affairs Canada. (2010). *A history of treaty-making in Canada.*https://www.rcaanc-cirnac.gc.ca/DAM/DAM-CIRNAC-RCAANC/DAM-TAG/STAGING/texte-text/ap_htmc_treatliv_1314921040169_eng.pdf; Mas, S. (2015). Truth and reconciliation offers 94 "calls to action." *CBC News*, December 14. http://www.cbc.ca/news/politics/truth-and-reconciliation-94-calls-to-action-1.3362258; National Inquiry into Missing and Murdered Indigenous Women and Girls. (2019). R*eclaiming power and place: The final report of the national inquiry into missing and murdered indigenous women and girls.* https://www.mmiwg-ffada.ca/wp-content/uploads/2019/06/Final_Report_Vol_1a-1.pdf.

laws, language, education, and health systems of governance. Fig. 14.1 shows a map of the evolving treaties and land agreements in Canada. The 11 numbered treaties (or post-Confederation treaties) were signed by First Nations and the Crown between 1871 and 1921. Treaty 6 (which encompassed much of Alberta and Saskatchewan) specifically promised access to health care through the "medicine chest" clause, a right that chiefs have sought with mixed results over the years since (Taylor, 1999).

Dislocation and disease from the beginning of the early fur-trading days through the expansion of the West took a heavy toll on First Nations peoples. They suffered despair, persecution, and deaths in the hundreds. As a result, they were forced into a situation where their survival relied on signing treaties that, paradoxically, only further damaged the health of their communities yesterday, today, and will continue into the future, unless fundamental truths are recognized and acted upon (Daschuk, 2013; Truth and Reconciliation Commission of Canada, 2015).

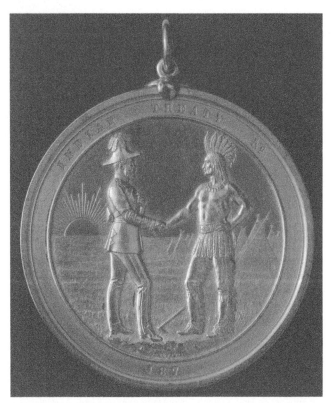

An Indian Chiefs Medal, which was presented to commemorate Treaties 3, 4, 5, 6, 7. Medals were important in treaty ceremonies and served as reminders to all participants of the commitments made. (Library and Archives Canada, Acc. No. 1964-1-1M)

The *Indian Act*

The misinterpretation of the Treaties and demonization of the colonial state resulted in the creation of the *Indian Act* in 1876. Beginning with the amalgamation of two key pieces of British citizenship legislation: the *Gradual Civilization Act* of 1857 and the *Gradual Enfranchisement Act* of 1869. The *Indian Act* was a policy that forced assimilation of First Nation peoples who lost their independent self-governing

approaches. The *Indian Act* exists today and is still used to set out certain federal government obligations and to continue to exert power and control over all aspects of Indian life, such as reserve lands, Indian money, and resources, and who has Indian status and who does not (Helin, 2006; McDonald & Steenbeek, 2015).

In 1985, Bill C-31 was introduced into legislation and the *Indian Act* was amended to remove any form of discrimination against Indian women who married non-Indian men. Previously, an Indian woman who married a non-Indian man would lose her Indian status. However, an Indian man who married a non-Indian woman did not lose his Indian status; in fact, a non-Indian wife gained the benefits of Indian status. The *Indian Act* was amended to allow women who had lost Indian status (along with their children) to regain it. However, this amendment to the Act created a new form of discrimination in that the grandchildren of the women who had originally lost their status would continue to lose their status if they married a person without official Indian status. The *Indian Act* not only dissociated Indian women from their communities but also created opportunities to develop policies that would allow the dissociation of Indian women from their first families. Indigenous identity and health care remain closely linked to the *Indian Act* (Government of Canada, 2020a; Lavoie, Forget, & Browne, 2010).

Introduced briefly in Chapter 1, five federal agencies are responsible for delivering health care services to First Nations peoples. Over the years, the federal government Department of Indian Affairs continued to employ nurses and doctors to provide health care services, and in 1944, the National Health and Welfare Department was formed and then assumed responsibility for all health services (Boyer, 2014). First Nations and Inuit Health (FNIH) currently provides funding to all First Nations communities. Non-Insured Health Benefits are provided to all First Nations people who are registered as "Status Indians" both on- and off-reserve. Indigenous and Northern Affairs Canada provide health care services in First Nations and Inuit communities. FNIH has worked with communities to begin to transfer responsibility for service provision of on-reserve health care to communities and band councils, and since 2013 the First Nations Health Authority in BC became the first to assume governance and responsibility for the programs and services formerly delivered by Health Canada (Lavoie, Forget, & O'Neil, 2007; FNHA, n.d.a.).

THE CONSEQUENCES OF COLONIZATION AND HISTORICAL TRAUMA

Residential School Legacy

Attempts to assimilate and colonize First Nations people resulted in the destruction and suppression of language, ceremonies, and culture. The residential school system, in particular, led to these outcomes and the disconnection of families (Legacy of Hope Foundation, 2009; Milloy, 1999). **Residential schools** were religious schools established and funded by the federal government to assimilate Aboriginal children (Truth and Reconciliation Commission of Canada,

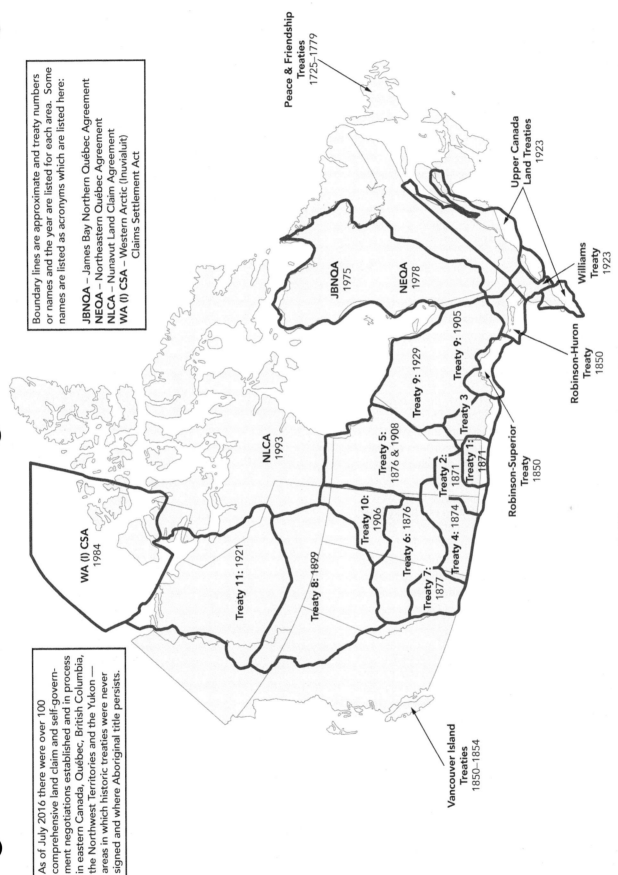

As of July 2016 there were over 100 comprehensive land claim and self-government negotiations established and in process in eastern Canada, Québec, British Columbia, the Northwest Territories and the Yukon — areas in which historic treaties were never signed and where Aboriginal title persists.

Boundary lines are approximate and treaty numbers or names and the year are listed for each area. Some names are listed as acronyms which are listed here:

JBNQA – James Bay Northern Québec Agreement
NEQA – Northeastern Québec Agreement
NLCA – Nunavut Land Claim Agreement
WA (I) CSA – Western Arctic (Inuvialuit) Claims Settlement Act

Peace & Friendship Treaties 1725–1779

Upper Canada Land Treaties 1923

Williams Treaty 1923

Robinson-Huron Treaty 1850

Robinson-Superior Treaty 1850

JBNQA 1975

NEQA 1978

Treaty 9: 1905

Treaty 9: 1929

Treaty 3

Treaty 5: 1876 & 1908

Treaty 2: 1871

Treaty 1: 1871

NLCA 1993

WA (I) CSA 1984

Treaty 11: 1921

Treaty 8: 1899

Treaty 10: 1906

Treaty 6: 1876

Treaty 7: 1877

Treaty 4: 1874

Vancouver Island Treaties 1850–1854

Fig. 14.1 Evolving Treaties and Land Agreements in Canada. (*Map credit:* © Can Stock Photo Inc./Lirch. *Data sources:* Canadian Northern Economic Development Agency. [2016]. *Modern Treaties of the North.* http://www.cannor.gc.ca/eng/1458573988380/1458574067957; Indigenous and Northern Affairs Canada. [2015]. *Comprehensive Claims.* https://www.aadnc-aandc.gc.ca/eng/1100100030577/1100100030578; Southern Chief's Organization. [2016]. *Treaty Maps.* http://scoinc.mb.ca/treaties/)

2015; Miller, 2015). Residential schools became compulsory in 1920. Children were often seized by force from their homes and sent away to live in impersonal and oppressive institutions run by churches. The schools had a multigenerational effect because children did not grow up learning about their traditional roles as children or parents. Rather, children were raised in an abusive and unsafe environment where adults frequently exerted power and control in positions of authority (Bourassa, McKay-McNabb, Hampton, 2004; Dion Stout & Kipling, 2003). First Nations and Inuit children in residential schools learned that their culture and language were of no value within a European-dominated society (Dutcher, 2008). Many First Nations and Inuit people who attended these schools carry the psychological damage from all forms of abuse, which they pass on to subsequent generations (National Inquiry into Missing and Murdered Indigenous Women and Girls, 2019).

The Sixties Scoop

The **Sixties Scoop** was a practice of removing or "scooping" large numbers of Indigenous children from their families and either sending them to foster homes or adopting them out, usually into non-Indigenous families in Canada and the United States. The program was active from the 1960s to the mid-1980s (First Nations Studies Program at University of British Columbia, n.d.a). Much like the practice of residential schools, this practice was largely hidden. To this day, survivors and their children continue to suffer from the institutionalized separation of their families. A disproportionate number of Indigenous children are in the care of welfare systems, which further isolates family members from one another. A 2007 hearing of the Canadian Human Rights Tribunal on First Nations child welfare reported that an estimated 27 000 First Nations children account for 30 to 40% of all children in the child welfare system (Blackstock, 2011). In 2017, the Government of Canada recognized the loss of cultural identity of survivors of the Sixties Scoop and established financial compensation; as well, a healing foundation was formed to assist in survivors' healing and education of Canadians.

Indigenous Health Advocacy Actions

In the early 1970s, a resurgence of political advocacy began, and Indigenous people were standing up for their treaty rights. Indigenous leaders began by seeking control of their children's education. In 1972, the National Indian Brotherhood wrote a policy document advocating for Indian control of Indian education and for parental control over their own children. Today, control over education and health remains for the most part a federal responsibility. Beginning in the early 1980s, constitutional amendments have affirmed existing Indigenous and treaty rights and as mentioned earlier, reinstated the status of First Nations women who were originally disenfranchised from their communities.

Concerted advocacy has been directed at the issue of missing and murdered First Nations, Inuit, and Métis women and girls. According to a report by the Royal Canadian Mounted Police (2014), the number of Indigenous female homicides and unresolved cases of missing Indigenous females between 1980 and 2012 is 1 181. This issue has raised awareness about violence and injustice that Indigenous people, particularly females, continue to face. Advocacy has taken a variety of forms to raise public awareness and demand government action on the matter. In 2015, the Minister of Justice and Attorney General of Canada, Minister of Status of Women, and Minister of Indigenous and Northern Affairs announced a national inquiry into missing and murdered Indigenous women and girls.

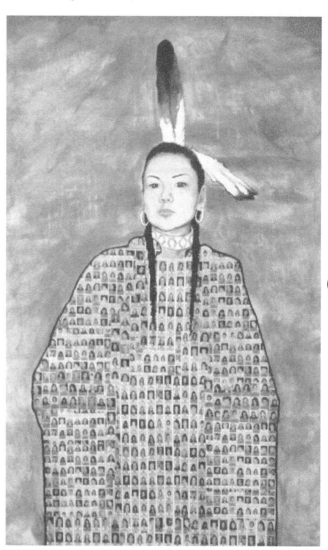

Jonathan Labillois' artwork Still Dancing depicts images of many missing and murdered First Nations, Inuit, and Métis women and girls. (Jonathan Labillois)

Indigenous Nursing in Canada

In the late 1800s, the relationship between missionaries and the Indigenous healers was not clearly understood, and the rapid influx of settlers changed the social and political economies for both the Indigenous peoples and nursing (Burnett, 2010; Cashman, 1966; Lux, 2016). Indigenous people taught their traditional medicine and healing practices to missionaries who befriended them. Missionaries drew on Indigenous knowledge for their own medical and nursing work. The growth of

European settlements and Western advances in medicine fundamentally transformed the relationship between Indigenous people and early nursing pioneers (Jesuit missionaries), who are credited with the genesis of health care in Canada.

Registered nursing education remained closed to First Nations, Inuit, and Métis women until the late 1930s. By the early 1960s, increasing numbers of First Nations women were pressuring Indian and Northern Affairs to support their education (McCallum, 2014). At this time, when the nursing profession opened its doors to men and married women, the number of licensed practical nurse and nursing aid or assistance programs grew, as did the role of community health representatives. Many First Nations, Inuit, and Métis people undertook this training or took up positions as community health representatives, which furthered higher education in health and community development and inspired leaders in Indigenous health. During the 1960s, Indigenous nurses worked mainly in hospital settings.

Determined Indigenous nursing students had to attain special permission from the Government of Canada to attend college or university, which was not the case for the average Canadian. Moreover, a degree was required for outpost and northern nursing with the federal government. Indigenous nurses continue to face barriers in terms of isolation and racism in the context of professional practice. They also face structural barriers in nursing education due to masked forms of ethnocentrism in nursing curricula (Vukic, Jesty, Mathews, et al., 2012).

The Aboriginal Nurses Association of Canada (ANAC, 2005) had its first official gathering of nurses in 1975, during which 41 Indigenous nurses started to map out their own destiny. They expressed their concerns on matters related to Indigenous health, supported one another, and began to build a bridge within and outside the nation. Jean Goodwill and Jocelyn Bruyere, both Cree nurses, were founding members of the ANAC. They were instrumental in focusing attention on the gaps in Indigenous health and nursing education and advocated for ways to deliver nursing interventions to First Nations, Inuit, and Métis populations. Over the past 40-plus years, Indigenous nurses in Canada have been combining their Western education with a firm grounding in their own languages, cultures, and healing traditions. While advances have been made, representation and equitable access to education and professional life remain concerns, as Indigenous nurses make up only 3% of the nursing workforce in Canada, yet the Indigenous population makes up 4.9% of the Canadian population (University of Saskatchewan, 2016). Indigenous nurses are in a unique position to facilitate change and ways of thinking about community health for Indigenous people (Bourque Bearskin et al., 2016; Hart Wasekeesikaw, Bourque Bearskin, & McDonald, 2020).

The Truth and Reconciliation Commission of Canada

The Truth and Reconciliation Commission of Canada emerged from the Residential Schools Settlement Agreement, which settled the legal actions against the Canadian government and various religious groups that operated residential schools. It was

BOX 14.1 Steps to Decolonizing Thinking

1. Acknowledge that colonization has occurred and continues to occur.
2. Examine how your own perceptions may be framed by colonial thinking—explore what evidence supports your perceptions.
3. Examine different perspectives and sources of evidence and knowledge.
4. Explore the implications and outcomes (Hostility? Respect? Separation? Allegiance?) of different perceptions and ways of thinking.
5. Commit to actions and outcomes that promote solidarity and build allegiances.
6. Continually reflect and recommit to solidarity.

Source: Based on Walia, 2012.

not until 1996 that the last government-run residential school closed. The abuse and unhealthy conditions in residential schools were virtually unknown to the public and health care providers until the commission's reports were presented in 2015.

Over six years, the commission travelled across Canada to hear from former residential school students who had been taken from their families as children, and residential school staff. The unique and shared stories provided powerful teaching tools so that the consequences of colonialism will be forever remembered by Canadian society, and so that Indigenous people can begin to shed the historical shame and dissociation from their culture, reviving pride in their traditions (Truth and Reconciliation Commission of Canada, 2015). A foundation for the resistance and resiliency necessary for decolonization has arisen from the intense experiences shared by residential school survivors in the commission's work.

Decolonization

The process of undoing the impact of a colonial state is referred to as **decolonization**. Decolonization entails engaging in critical reflexive thought processes that address social issues in the wider framework of Indigenous self-determination, sovereignty, and social justice within the context of Indigenous histories, struggles, and ideals (Tuhiwai Smith, 2012). The process of decolonization reveals how our assumptions and perceptions inform our practice in the context of the social determinants of health and knowledge transfer in nursing (Racine & Petrucka, 2011). Decolonization is an active process whereby we connect thinking to practice in an effort to better understand the truths of others as they are, rather than as they would be viewed through Western perspectives of community health. It involves deconstructing original narratives about Indigenous Peoples and the domination of neoliberal policies (McFarlane & Schabus, 2017). The steps in Box 14.1 provide insight into how to move oneself beyond colonizing perceptions of Indigenous people.

Decolonizing approaches are not just conceptual; they can be applied by CHNs in nursing practice. Alongside Indigenous people and communities, CHNs might engage in shared storytelling, critical questioning of policies governing health care delivery, responding to verbal and nonverbal

---

| BOX 14.2 | **Approaches to Trauma-Informed Care** |

Residential school and historical experiences have impeded Indigenous people's abilities to adopt positive coping responses and may create negative relationships with community health care providers. CHNs must possess a high level of cultural understanding of the residual effects that span generations of Indigenous people. Without this understanding, CHNs run the risk of retraumatizing Indigenous patients without even knowing that they are doing so.* Trauma-informed care is not focused on the treatment of psychological symptoms of trauma. Rather this care seeks to enable the broader commitment with training and support for health and social care practitioners, to provide services in a manner that is welcoming and responsive to the special needs of those affected by trauma.[†]

Sources: * Alberta Health Services, 2020;
[†] Levine, Varcoe & Browne, 2020.

---

expressions of resistance, and building collaborative relationships that recognize Indigenous people as inherent right holders rather than needy victims.

Trauma-informed care (Box 14.2) is another decolonizing practice CHNs can draw upon for culturally safe work with Indigenous people. **Trauma-informed care** refers to care that attends to a patient's past experiences of violence or trauma and the role it currently plays in their lives.

INDIGENOUS DETERMINANTS OF HEALTH

While Canadians are among the healthiest in the world, the health status of Indigenous peoples in Canada is lower, largely due to their dramatically different circumstances. The determinants of health influence people's lives in complex and dynamic ways. While the Public Health Agency of Canada (PHAC) recognizes a number of determinants of health that affect all Canadians, Indigenous people's organizations and researchers have identified additional determinants of health that affect Indigenous people specifically.

Across the globe, Indigenous peoples express similar health struggles and, according to the World Health Organization (WHO, 2016), their health issues are also influenced by social determinants of health. The social determinants of health are categorized as proximal, intermediate, and distal (Hackett, Feeny, & Tompa, 2016; Loppie Reading & Wien, 2009; National Collaborating Centre for Aboriginal Health, 2013; Riva, Plusquellec, Juster, et al., 2014). **Proximal determinants of health** are conditions that directly affect the health of individuals, such as health behaviours, physical environments, employment and income, social status, education, and food insecurity. **Intermediate determinants of health** are the conditions that give rise to the proximal determinants, such as health care systems; educational systems; community infrastructure, resources, and capacities; environmental stewardship; and cultural continuity. **Distal determinants of health** arise from political, economic, and social realities and include colonialism, racism and social exclusion, and repression of self-determination.

Proximal Determinants of Health
Health Behaviours

Health behaviours are individual behaviours that directly affect people's health and may affect the health of those around them (Short & Mollborn, 2015). Examples include dietary choices, physical activity, smoking, drug use, alcohol use, and sexual behaviours. The overall daily smoking rate for First Nations adults is higher than the Canadian rate (43.2 versus 19.0%). These behaviours are complex, and it is acknowledged that health behaviours are profoundly influenced by social, economic, and environmental factors such as personal life skills, stress, culture, social relationships and belonging, sense of control, education, and income (Bourque Bearskin, 2011; Health Canada, 2014; Stewart, Castleden, King, et al., 2015).

Physical Environments

Physical environments include housing, air and water quality, and sanitation services. Poor sanitation and contaminants in the air, water, or soil can cause a variety of health ailments of the respiratory and gastrointestinal system, as well as cancers and birth defects (Health Canada, 2014, 2018). Housing shortages in First Nations have led to overcrowding. Moreover, many on-reserve homes lack access to clean water, proper sanitation services, and adequate ventilation. Over half of the people living in First Nations communities reported the presence of mould and mildew in their homes. Over 33% of on-reserve dwellings required major repairs compared with 7.5% of non-Aboriginal dwellings (Sanderson, Mirza, Polacca, et al., 2020; Loppie Reading & Wien, 2009).

Employment, Income, and Social Status

Income and social status are considered to be the most important determinants of health (Public Health Agency of Canada [PHAC], 2011). Inadequate income leads to poverty, which inhibits the ability of people to obtain the material goods needed to survive, such as housing, nutrient-rich foods, and clean water. A lack of employment (and the purpose and meaning associated with it) and inadequate income are detrimental to individual and community physical health as well as individual psychosocial and mental wellness (Loppie Reading & Wien, 2009; Bingham, Moniruzzaman, Patterson et al, 2019).

Education

In 2016, the proportion of Indigenous people aged 25 to 64 with a high school diploma or equivalent as their highest level of educational attainment was 25%. The corresponding proportion for non-Indigenous people was 24%. Whereas in the Inuit and Metis population 18 and 27% respectively achieved a high school diploma. The main difference between the Indigenous and non-Indigenous populations in terms of postsecondary qualifications was the proportion of university graduates: 11% of Indigenous adults had a university-level education, whereas 29% of non-Indigenous adults had a university-level education, the same is true for certificate, diploma, or degree attainment. The largest gap in educational attainment is for Inuit students (Statistics Canada, 2017).

Access to Adequate Food

Economic disparity is a significant contributing factor to both psychological distress and the ability to access adequate food (Hajizadeh, Bombay, & Asada, 2019; Hossain & Lamb, 2019). Considering the median annual income for Indigenous people living in First Nations communities is lower than that of the general Canadian population ($20 000 versus $27 600 after tax), obtaining nutrient-rich foods is often impossible (Statistics Canada, 2011). Structural food procurement, environmental concerns for food growth and delivery, as well as social and cultural aspects of food preparation, and eating habits are all important access issues of Indigenous communities whether rural, remote, or urban (Goettke & Reynolds 2019). Between 24–60% of First Nations experience food insecurity, which is three to five times higher than food insecurity experienced in the general Canadian population. Food insecurity and malnutrition have a significant impact on the overall health of First Nations citizens. The lack of nutrient-rich foods can lead to increased rates of obesity, distress, depression, and multiple physical conditions such as vitamin and mineral deficiencies and diabetes (Chan, Batal, Sadik, et al., 2019).

Intermediate Determinants of Health
Health Care Systems

Individuals must have physical, political, and social access to health care services to realize their benefits. In rural communities specifically, physical access to health care services is limited, and public health programs are fragmented. In terms of priorities and funding, changes have been slow to shift focus because Indigenous morbidity and mortality are increasingly resulting from chronic illness and not from communicable disease. Social access to health care is limited for Indigenous people because the health care system is often unable to accommodate the cultural or language needs of Indigenous patients. Limited social access has meant that some Indigenous people are unwilling to use the services of the health care system. The most commonly reported barriers to access to health care are timeliness (e.g., long wait lists) and the effectiveness of health care services (Loppie Reading & Wien, 2009; Stewart et al., 2015; Stewart, King, Blood, et al., 2012).

Educational Systems

Education has an important and profound impact on the potential employment, income, and social status of all individuals. Often, mainstream education does not address the social determinants that may act as obstacles for Indigenous children and youth, and curriculum addressing Indigenous content and learning styles are often underdeveloped and underfunded. In 2006, 35% of First Nations adults living on-reserve had successfully completed a postsecondary education program, a 5% increase from 1996 (Health Canada, 2014; Rowan, Rukholm, Bourque Bearskin, et al., 2013).

Community Infrastructure, Resources, and Capacities

Limited opportunities for infrastructure and resource development contribute to economic insecurity and marginalization and, subsequently, deprivation among community members. Limited social resources (e.g., qualified individuals who can plan and implement programs) reduce the access a community has to program funding. When a community has limited resources, underfunded programs, and greater community responsibilities without an increase in self-determination, the result can be community-level stress and community stagnation (Loppie Reading & Wien, 2009).

Environmental Stewardship

Indigenous people continue to face significant struggles to exert authority over their traditional environments. Within Indigenous tradition and culture, the natural environment is a resource for good health. Colonization created a huge disconnect between Indigenous people and the land. Indigenous people are no longer stewards of their traditional lands and do not share in the profits from resource extraction from those lands. Moreover, the contamination of air, land, water, and wildlife have combined to reduce the supply of traditional foods and medicines that once sustained communities (Astle, Bourque Bearskin, Dordunno et al., 2020; Loppie Reading & Wien, 2009). Morrison (2020) discusses the rapidly expanding Indigenous food system networks and the correlation between Indigenous wellness and transformational learning. Indigenous approaches to health and well-being are strengthened in networks where increased activities related to giving, sharing, and trading of food, knowledge, and services are present within a complex system of Indigenous biodiversity and cultural heritage.

Cultural Continuity

Cultural continuity is the extent of social and cultural cohesion within a community. It involves traditional and intergenerational connectedness maintained through intact families and the engagement of elders, enabling the passing of knowledge to subsequent generations (Loppie Reading & Wien, 2009). The preservation and presence of culture can be difficult to measure due to its multifaceted and varied dimensions. However, the most common indicator of First Nation cultural continuity is the use of Indigenous language: 44.9% of all First Nations people living in First Nations communities had an Indigenous language as their mother tongue, compared to 13.4 % living off reserve (Statistics Canada, 2017). Cultural continuity as a protective factor was found to moderate suicide risk among Indigenous people in Canada (Bingham et al, 2019; Chandler & Lalonde, 1998).

Distal Determinants of Health
Colonialism

Colonialism has impacted and continues to impact the health of Indigenous peoples by creating social, political, and economic inequities that influence the creation of unfavourable intermediate and proximal determinants of health. Assimilation policies damaged families and the tie between culture, language, and social networks. The compounded effects of colonialism are directly related to trauma. Trauma experienced in one generation that is unresolved or ignored, or receives little to no support, results in intergenerational trauma (Legacy of Hope Foundation, 2009). **Intergenerational trauma** is "the transmission of a collective emotional and psychological injury over the lifespan and across generations among Aboriginal people and continues to affect the health and well-being of young Aboriginal men and women" (Mehrabadi, Paterson, Pearce, et al., 2008) All types of abuse were experienced in residential schools, including (and arguably most often) sexual abuse. Survivors of sexual abuse may demonstrate a wide range of effects: low self-esteem, self-blame, guilt, depression, substance use, social withdrawal, and family and relationship problems. These problems can be passed on from one generation to the next. Frequent substance use was reported by those who had experienced sexual abuse, and living on-reserve was the strongest factor associated with Indigenous young people and sexual behaviour (O'Neill, Fraser, Kitchenham et al., 2018; Devries, Free, Morison, et al., 2009).

Racism and Social Exclusion

Colonialism is maintained through power and privilege over Indigenous Peoples; *anticolonial knowledge* helps health care providers address the *oppression* of imposed and unjust colonial rule by challenging assumptions that normalize and privilege (Van Herk, Smith & Andrew, 2011). With colonialism came social stratification based on ethnic grounds. The resulting societal hierarchy created an imbalance in the way resources, power, freedom, and control were distributed, which affected Indigenous people in many ways, including their access to education, health services, and physical environments. It also led to the social exclusion of Indigenous people. Increased alcohol and drug use in adolescence and decreased self-esteem have been observed as negative health outcomes from the stress of living with social exclusion and racial discrimination. Indigenous people are more likely to abstain from alcohol consumption than non-Indigenous people; however, a higher proportion of those who consume alcohol, consume it heavily (Lachance et al., 2009). Urban Indigenous people, especially women, are more likely to die from alcohol-related diseases (Tjepkema, Wilkins, Senécal, et al., 2010). Indigenous youth in British Columbia identified substance use as the strongest factor associated with sexual behaviour and reported higher incidents of practising unsafe sex compared with those living off-reserve (Devries et al., 2009). Krieger's (2016) examination of the multiple crossroads of structural racism's impacts on health issues such as substance use highlights the lived experience, emphasizing that ultimately "there is nothing 'distal' about structural discrimination because it is intimately encountered and embodied, day in and day out" (p. 833).

Self-Determination

Self-determination is the ability of a group to decide how its needs will be met without the interference of outside governance. Self-determination greatly impacts health determinants such as housing, education, and health care, and allows communities and groups to participate equally in political and economic decision making. Colonialism impacted self-determination by creating a situation in which Indigenous peoples have unequal access to and control over their own governance, properties, economic assets, health services, education, and so on (Bourque Bearskin et al., 2016; Loppie Reading & Wien, 2009).

CHN IN PRACTICE: A COMPREHENSIVE CASE STUDY

Developing an Exercise and Wellness Program for Indigenous Women in Northern Creek

This section of the chapter is a case study that examines the processes CHNs follow to develop a wellness program with Indigenous women in the fictitious town of "Northern Creek." This case study describes the application of a collaborative, community-based program planning process that incorporates strategies to build capacity and improve the health and wellness outcomes of Indigenous women living in an urban community and in nearby reserves. The CHNs in this case study are Marina, an advanced practice master's-prepared nurse who works at the Northern Creek Wellness Project (NCWP), and Jaida, who is a support worker at the Northern Creek Community Health Centre (NCCHC) of the largest First Nations community in the area.

Background

Marina and Jaida are meeting Sarah, a fourth-year nursing student who is completing her community health clinical assignment. Marina is the preceptor, but Sarah will spend some time with Jaida at the NCCHC and accompany Jaida on monthly visits to the smaller and more remote reserves in the area. Sarah is from the Mohawk Nation, whereas the First Nations in this region are Ojibwe and members of the Anishinabek Nation. Sarah grew up in an urban setting, but she has a mentor from the ANAC mentorship project who lives in one of the First Nation communities. The purpose of this initial meeting is to confirm working arrangements and to introduce Sarah to the NCWP, which launched last year. The meeting begins with Marina providing an overview of the initial community health assessment and planning process, which is ongoing. She explains that there are cycles within cycles of the community health nursing process.

Community Health Assessment

Northern Creek is a small industrial town in northern Ontario with a population of 100 000. The town is a major transportation hub for the region, which is rich in natural resources. In recent years, the forestry, manufacturing, and mining industries have been depressed and are making a very slow recovery. The population is stagnant, and many families have members who have lost their jobs. The town has a rich multicultural European heritage and is home to approximately 8 000 Indigenous peoples—mainly First Nations people. One large and two small First Nations communities lie within a 200-km radius of the town. The many lakes and forests in the area make it an ideal place for outdoor pursuits in the summer, but it is not as easy to maintain an active lifestyle through the long, cold winters and in the context of physical distancing requirements owing to pandemic virus spread.

Over the past year, the regional public health unit and the NCWP have formed a network of groups interested in community health who want to see low-wage earners in the region have better access to health promotion and disease prevention activities. The community health network, whose members have a common interest in physical activity programming, include community health and resource centres, recreational facilities, neighbourhood organizations, churches, schools, the local university, and local industry. To date, the community health network has identified several pre-existing initiatives relevant to physical activity:

- Advocacy for people on social assistance or receiving low wages who may not have access to organized exercise or healthy eating programs
- A Healthy Babies Healthy Children program
- Walking programs in the town's local parks, mall, and older persons' centres with training of lay fitness instructors by the town's recreation department
- Community gardening programs through the town's community association alongside a horticulture program with a nearby community college
- A public library lending program for pedometers, exercise DVDs, and other fitness technology and equipment
- Healthy workplace initiatives: Personalized health information on healthy eating, physical activity, smoking cessation, and stress management offered by several employers, including a large mining company

The community health network aims to promote physical activity to low-wage earners as a means of increasing their wellness and preventing the onset of chronic illnesses like diabetes. This strategy is informed by Canadian Community Health Survey data that confirm that people with higher incomes and education report better levels of health overall, are more likely to be physically active, are less likely to have diabetes and other chronic conditions, and live longer (Public Health Agency of Canada, 2018).

Network members want to expand the reach of their community health programs to priority populations. In this area, the priority populations have been identified as First Nations individuals, youth living independently, parents of young children, homeless and underhoused community members, and older persons living in isolated situations. Recently, the community health network received special project funding. Funds were specifically dedicated toward strategies to increase physical activity in the First Nations population; in particular, focusing on exercise during winter and on the urgent health and well-being concerns of the pandemic (First Nations Health Authority, n.d.b.; National Collaborating Centre for Indigenous Health, 2020; Power, Wilson, Best et al., 2020).

The public health unit compiled a community profile that compared urban and rural First Nations populations with the total urban population. It drew information from several sources: the 2016 census community profile, the First Nations population profile for the Census Metropolitan Area (CMA),

the public health unit (Statistics Canada, 2017), and profiles of First Nations living on-reserve in the region (Health Canada, 2018). To make comparison easier, the results were summarized in a table. Table 14.3 illustrates the type of information that might be gathered from the sources mentioned for the community of Northern Creek. (For a tool kit providing "steps" and "tools" to facilitate the health assessment process in Canadian communities where mining is a major industry, see the MiningWatch Canada link in the Tool Box on the Evolve website. For information on assessing the community health needs of First Nations and Inuit, see the Health Canada link on the Evolve website.)

The public health manager explained that it was difficult to find comparative health information on small communities. While several Indigenous communities across the country have participated in regional health surveys, access to survey data is often restricted to the participating community, part of a global concern for Indigenous data sovereignty (Taylor & Kukutai, 2016). The restricted access to data conforms to principles of ownership, control, access, and possession (OCAP) governing the collection and use of Indigenous health information (First Nations Health Authority, 2019).

Planning for a Community Health Nursing Intervention

The community health network is guided by a vision of improving the health of the population by reducing inequities and increasing access and control over the factors that determine health—social determinants such as economic resources, education, social support, and a clean physical environment. The network is focused on individuals who are either essentially healthy or at risk for disease. By increasing resources for all concerned populations, including subpopulations living under high-risk conditions, the group aims to increase the health and well-being of the local Indigenous population as a whole.

Network members subscribe to the view that health is embodied, a reserve of biopsychosocial resources that people can access in order to participate in society (Williamson & Carr, 2009). They are committed to using strategies that build capacity for this embodied participation, either as their main goal or as a means to an end. This entails working with strengths and maximizing the assets and resources of individuals, groups, and collectives to deal with life challenges and changes. Integral to strategies like community development and empowerment, community capacity building is about increasing the capabilities of people to articulate and address community health issues and to overcome barriers to achieve improved outcomes in their quality of life. Community participation is an essential component of capacity building and is explored as part of health promotion strategies in Chapter 4. A community's capacity to participate must be supported at individual, community, and societal levels (Bell, 2012). The community network intends to build capacity at both community and individual levels for this project. The network will bring together organizations in the community to share skills and resources, identify opportunities for collaboration, and

TABLE 14.3   Northern Creek Area: Population Estimates, 2016

	URBAN COMMUNITY			URBAN FIRST NATIONS PROFILE			RURAL FIRST NATIONS PROFILE		
	Total	Male	Female	Total	Male	Female	Total	Male	Female
Population Data (Age in Years)									
Total population	122 910	59 885	63 025	10 055	4 655	5 400	2 015	1 062	953
15	20 235	10 350	9 885	2 995	1 475	1 520	602	271	331
15–64	82 980	41 015	41 960	6 670	2 985	3 680	1 335	647	688
64	19 680	8 515	11 165	385	200	190	77	44	33
Median age	42	41	41	26	23	28	24	21	26
% aged 15 and over	84	83	84	70	68	72	72	69	73
Health Indicators									
Well-being									
Perceived health, very good or excellent	66 740 (54.3%)	(56.6%)	(53.9%)	5 571 (55.4%)	*	*	806 (40.0%)	*	*
Health Conditions									
Overweight or obese	72 640 (59.1%)	(70.9%)	(53.8%)	6 355 (63.2%)	*	*	1 470 (73.0%)	*	*
Health Behaviours									
Leisure-time physical activity, moderately active or active	73 992 (60.2%)	(62.6%)	(58.4%)	6 103 (60.7%)	*	*	429 (21.3%)	*	*
Personal Resources									
Sense of community belonging	90 585 (73.7%)	(80.5%)	(78.4%)	7 993 (79.5%)	*	*	1 621 (80.5%)	*	*

*Data not available.

make plans to work together to strengthen the community. Complementing the community-level activities, the network will support capacity-building approaches at the individual level by involving the people using the services in the planning and evaluation of those services.

Primary Prevention: Health Promotion and Risk Reduction

Whenever possible, population-based practice focuses on primary prevention. This level of prevention includes promoting health and reducing risk. The community health network members have conducted a literature review to identify factors to consider when developing the physical activity program to increase wellness and decrease the prevalence of type 2 diabetes. They understand that regular exercise can help a person feel stronger and fitter, have more energy, feel more relaxed, and sleep better. As well, inactivity is a known risk factor for chronic health problems (National Collaborating Centre for Indigenous Health, 2020). So, increasing physical activity has the potential to both promote health and reduce the risk of disease. A risk-reduction approach hinges on knowing which factors increase the likelihood of specific chronic diseases. Some risk factors, such as age, sex, and genetic inheritance, are nonmodifiable. Others, such as body type (weight distribution) and activity levels, are potentially modifiable. A risk-reduction approach entails identifying the at-risk population and tailoring interventions to inform susceptible people about the risks and preventive measures. For example, type 2 diabetes, the most common form of diabetes, is increasing at higher-than-expected rates; however, it can be effectively delayed and prevented through lifestyle changes,

in particular regular exercise (WHO, 2020). The Diabetes Prevention Program found that people at risk for developing this condition were able to cut their risk by 58% with moderate physical activity (30 minutes a day) and weight loss (5 to 7% of body weight). For people over age 60, the risk was cut by almost 71% (Diabetes Prevention Program Research Group, 2002). However, despite knowledge of health and related social inequities for Indigenous peoples, equitable access to preventative and structural care is, sadly, not the norm (Browne, Varcoe, Lavoie et al., 2016; Polanco & Arbour, 2018). This notion speaks to the importance of using equity-informed strategies within capacity-building approaches that foster broad community participation.

CHN Considerations Regarding Planning

The CHNs shared the following observations at the community health network planning session:

- The network already has links with the First Nations of Northern Creek. One First Nations organization is represented in the network, and the professor of kinesiology representing the local college is Indigenous.
- The NCWP has many connections to the urban and rural Indigenous community, and several staff members are Indigenous. Over the past 3 years, the NCCHC has built an effective working relationship with most of the local chiefs and the band council. At least one member of the band council attends the quarterly NCCHC health committee meeting.
- The potential users of an exercise program are not represented on the network; however, three women attending a

well women's clinic on the largest reserve have approached Jaida about setting up an exercise class.

- The NCCHC offers group classes on healthy nutrition, which it would like to expand to include an exercise component, particularly if it could train volunteer leaders, as is the case in the local mall's walking programs.
- The mall walking program attracts women only. The community outreach workers at the NCWP say their patients have not joined the program because it is on the outskirts of town and because the people going there "are all dressed in fancy sports outfits."
- The special project funding will be sufficient to conduct a pilot project, the results of which can be used to seek additional resources.

After the CHNs shared their observations with the community health network, and after much deliberation by the network, the network decided to develop a 6-week exercise and wellness program focused specifically on Indigenous women on two sites: the largest reserve, which is closest to the town, and the NCWP in town, which provides services to First Nations people living on- and off-reserve, and Métis. The network acknowledges the importance of more fully involving Indigenous people, especially women, within the region in the planning process.

Preparing to Implement the Exercise and Wellness Program for Indigenous Women

Marina will lead the pilot project from the AWC. She is assisted by Jaida. The student nurse, Sarah, who will be with Marina and Jaida for 3 months, and two community health representatives (CHRs) from the NCWP are assigned to the project. In addition, Jaida has invited the three women (Patsy, Darlene, and Shania) who had approached her community about setting up an exercise class to join the planning team. At the first planning meeting, Jaida (taking on the leadership role of facilitator and resource) welcomed everyone and made introductions. The steering group sat around a table so they could see one another and feel encouraged to talk and ask questions.

The steering group began the meeting with a question that would encourage discussion: What would attract women to an exercise class? Patsy, Darlene, and Shania offered several reasons for their interest: to stay healthy; to get balance in their lives and set an example for their children; to lose weight; and to have something to do. They said that people like to be outdoors in the summer and walk a lot but that there is little to do in the winter. Because of television and the Internet, people are more sedentary than in the past, particularly so during pandemic restrictions when activities and formal exercise programs have stalled. They noted that women would benefit from the regular social interaction, which was also strained during the pandemic. The group had a brainstorming session about what makes it easy and what makes it hard to keep fit.

Jaida handed out copies of the *Canadian 24-Hour Movement Guidelines for Adults*, which was developed by the PHAC in association with the Canadian Society for Exercise

Physiology, along with the FNHA's practical exercise samples and tools from their *Being Active Making Exercise More Convenient* resource. These tools and resources were a starting place for the group to look for ideas on what types of exercise they could include in the pilot project. (These toolkits can be accessed through links at the Evolve website.) Apologetically, she explained that efforts to tailor the guide for First Nations people, Inuit, and Métis have experienced starts and stops over many years (Kesäniemi, Riddoch, Reeder et al., 2010; Tremblay, Katzmarzyk, Colley et al., 2017; Young & Katzmarzyk, 2007). Sarah commented that she was pleased to see that her exercise group at the university had all the elements of a good fitness program—strength training, cardiovascular fitness, and balance. Everyone agreed that the handbook had some good ideas and that their steering group could determine which activities would be suitable for Indigenous women.

From there, the discussion turned to questions about how formal the exercise and wellness program should be, where it would be held, and when it could be held (the best time of day and day of week). The group identified two possible settings: the church hall, which was more central, and the health centre meeting room, which could provide childcare on some days of the week. The question of whether to charge a small admission fee was also discussed. Jaida explained that they had funding to run the exercise class and that she could help with the organization but did not have the skills or the time to run the class herself. One CHR, a trained fitness instructor, said she could lead the class if volunteers could help set up. The CHR explained that traditional practices were respected with groups at the NCWP; usually gatherings started with a snack and an opening prayer and, on some occasions, there would be a smudging ceremony. The steering group decided that it would be best to ask the elders on-reserve for advice on these matters.

Jaida summarized the steering group's discussion and proposed that the group gather further information from the community on the proposed exercise and wellness program. This additional information would provide specifics on what women wanted and did not want in the program, which could be used to guide planning. At the same time, informing community members about the exercise and wellness program would raise awareness about it and create interest. Each group member agreed to approach three Indigenous women from Northern Creek with the following questions:

1. Which of the following activities (e.g., walking, bicycle riding, gardening, fitness class, dancing, weightlifting) have you participated in during the last 12 months?
2. What sort of exercises would you like to see included in an exercise class?
3. Where would be the most convenient place to hold an exercise and wellness class—in the church hall or in the health centre?

To keep it simple, the steering group decided that it would record the answers in point form and give the notes to Sarah to summarize for the next meeting, which was in 2 weeks' time.

At the second steering group meeting, Jaida welcomed everyone and explained that the task for this meeting was to plan the exercise class in more detail. The group had three main sources of information:

1. The summary of key themes from the interviews with local Indigenous women.
2. An overview of recommended activity levels in adults (Canadian Society for Exercise Physiology, 2020).
3. A review of patterns of physical activity, their determinants and consequences, and the results of various interventions designed to increase the physical activity of Indigenous people in Canada and the United States (Foulds, Warburton, & Bredin, 2013).

Sarah presented a summary of the 24 completed interviews. (Note: The themes are based on findings from the Women Warriors program [Pelletier, Smith-Forrester, & Klassen-Ross, 2019], as well as intervention studies by Klomp, Dyck & Sheppard, [2003], Gellert, Aubert, & Mikami [2010], and health and wellness planning tools [First Nations Health Authority, 2019]).

The key themes from the interviews are:

- The program should be for Indigenous women only.
- People like it when gatherings include food as well as growing and preparing food; it brings people together.
- Recognition and support for childcare and other caregiving and home responsibilities.
- It is good to have time to talk to the exercise leader about the exercises, to find out if you are doing them properly; other suggestions were to include information on what to eat and possibly traditional healing practices to support fitness, health, and well-being.
- There should be time to socialize afterward and encouragement to meet more often outside of the group for recreation and socialization.
- Everyday activities such as walking and at-home fitness should also be encouraged in simple ways that can be visible to encourage others in the community.
- It is easier to exercise with people and everyday environments—and also with music that has a good rhythm, music that gets you moving.
- Participants should be taught how to do the exercises so they get the most out of them and so they do not hurt themselves.
- The exercises and activities should not be too strenuous at the beginning of the program, so participants can keep up.

Jaida explained that the review of best practices in other communities provided useful information on how to put together a program for their town and the largest reserve nearby. She presented Table 14.4 to the steering group, which lists an inventory of existing urban community programs that support a healthy lifestyle.

In relation to the review of patterns of physical activity, Jaida explained that there was limited research on physical activity interventions and outcomes among Indigenous peoples in Canada, and none have been specifically developed with Indigenous women (Pelletier et al, 2017; Wicklum, Sampsom, Henderson et al., 2019). Moreover, the group did

TABLE 14.4 Inventory of Urban Community Programs That Support a Healthy Lifestyle

Program Type	Program Organizer
Walking programs	Municipal recreation department (programs take place at local parks, recreation fields, malls, and older persons' centres)
Fitness classes/ swimming	YMCA-YWCA and local fitness centres
Sports programs	Universities and schools
Pedometers for lease	Main library
Camping, canoeing	Youth organizations (e.g., Boy Scouts, Girl Guides)
Skating	Municipal rinks, local rinks
Sponsored walks	Charities

not yet have sufficient information on program participants to assess the applicability of the studies to this community (Bell, 2012). Relatively little is known about the patterns and levels of physical activity in Indigenous populations or about the determinants and barriers to physical activity in different environmental and cultural contexts (Foulds et al., 2013; Giles & Darroch, 2014; Ironside, Ferguson, Katapally et al., 2020).

The steering group decided that it would be best to use the identified themes as a guide for planning. As well, it would consider using programs and strategies that had some claim of being effective, despite the incomplete information. The group felt that it had made some progress. Group members reasoned that if they built on strengths and worked with the resources they had and in partnership with community members, they would be more likely to develop an exercise and wellness program that the community needs and wants. Evidence indicates that capacity-building approaches have been successful with Indigenous and other communities (Savard & Todd, 2020). A large systematic review found that interventions that use community-based participatory approaches and strong community engagement activities throughout the process were more successful in building capacity and creating and sustaining positive health outcomes than those that involve people to a lesser degree as consultants (Funnel et al., 2019).

Jaida then introduced the steering group to the Community Capacity Building Tool (CCBT) (PHAC & Alberta/NWT Region, 2008). The CCBT was designed to assist community-based health projects integrate community capacity building into their work. The tool uses a definition of *community capacity* developed in Australia (Hawe, King, Noort, et al., 2000):

An approach to the development of sustainable skills, organizational structures, resources, and commitment to health improvement in health and other sectors, to prolong and multiply health gains many times over (New South Wales Health Department, 2001, p. i).

Drawing on this definition, the CCBT identifies nine features of community capacity building:

1. Participation
2. Leadership
3. Community structures
4. Role of external support
5. Asking why
6. Obtaining resources
7. Skills, knowledge, and learning
8. Linking with others
9. Sense of community

Jaida proposed that the steering group use the tool to determine the capacity-building actions it needs to take and to check its progress toward capacity building.

The steering group focused on the first feature: participation.

Participation is the active involvement of people in improving their own and their community's health and well-being. Participating in a project means the target population, community members, and other stakeholders are involved in project activities, such as making decisions and evaluation. (PHAC & Alberta/NWT Region, 2008, p. 1)

Sarah recorded group members' answers to the participation questions that follow. She also mapped the group's location in its health-project journey by noting "just started," "on the road," "nearly there," or "we're there" to document the phases and growth of the project.

- Have we actively involved community organizations? *On the road:* The project team is a subcommittee of a community-wide network of health, social services, education groups, and various organizations with an interest in physical activity programming. Our first step in linking to the First Nations community organizations will be to talk to the chief and council and get their support.

- Have we actively involved the priority community? *On the road:* Three members of our planning group live on the largest First Nation community in the area. One woman (Shania) is a member of the health committee and a member of the board of the urban NCWP, so she has a voice in decision making about health matters. We need to recruit Indigenous women from the town and from the smaller reserves in the area. Also, we do not have representation from Indigenous women in their middle years.

- Have we identified and overcome barriers to the priority group participating in project meetings? *On the road:* The project meetings are being held in the community to make it easy for First Nations women to attend. Virtual meeting options will be available for physical distancing requirements and for ongoing remote meeting convenience as we cannot provide childcare regularly, and transportation may be a barrier to participation for Indigenous women from the town and from the smaller reserves.

- Are we using different methods to keep everyone informed about the project? *Just started:* The project team will communicate by email and by word of mouth. They have not thought about how they will keep others informed.

Addressing all of the features in the CCBT, the steering group engaged in one particularly valuable discussion of the "Asking Why" feature, which is a community process that uncovers the root causes of community health issues. During this process, the steering group explored what had changed over time and the social contexts and situations that contributed to less exercise, increased obesity, and related concerns in health and well-being. Shania commented: "There is a lot to do in our community. We want people to want to live here, young and old. We don't really get together much. When I was a girl, my family was active all year round—there was always something going on. We didn't exercise but we walked, went out on the land, danced, and had fun." Jaida responded that it is only through dialogue and sharing what we know about exercise and well-being together, and in participation with the community that we will find the right approach to an exercise program for the community. The group acknowledged the importance of community dialogue but felt they were not ready to go to the community with a plan just yet. Jaida suggested that they leave it for now and come back to it next time to avoid being overwhelmed. The group decided to start the next meeting with a discussion on the topic of engaging the community in dialogue as part of their program planning.

To support the community dialogue, the CHR suggested inviting various stakeholders from the community and using a Talking Circle, where everyone has an opportunity to express themselves if they want to. The aim of Talking Circles is to create an inclusive atmosphere so that everyone can have a voice; the purpose is not debate but to hear different opinions (Brown & Di Lallo, 2020).

For the remainder of the meeting, group members planned the exercise and wellness program based on identified best practices for physical activity programming (Law, Williams, Langley et al, 2020; Moore, Warburton, O'Halloran et al. 2016; NCCIH, 2020). The program would include exercise classes and proven health promotion strategies (e.g., an emphasis on regular exercise, behaviour modification such as movement, food intake, sleep, and emotions journaling). Group members agreed to the following:

- As pandemic physical distancing measures allow, run group exercise classes for 6 weeks, with 2 in-person classes per week, modelled on exercise programs offered in town, and to offer virtual options.

- As part of each exercise class, include a warm-up, cardio, and a cool-down, with a mix of exercises to increase strength and flexibility.

- Invite the CHR from the NCWP, who is a trained fitness instructor, to run the exercise classes with help from Sarah and volunteers.

- Recruit volunteers to help set up equipment, set up recording/streaming, and organize social activities after each class in person or for virtual group visiting.

- Address equity and trauma-informed principles in the program development and implementation (see *Trauma and Violence-Informed Physical Activity Toolkit (TVIPA)* in the Toolkit resources at the end of this chapter).

- Include 15 minutes of health information on topics selected by participants during each class or in response to pandemic or other current public health measures or disaster responses. Incorporate tools and techniques on taking charge of health based on self-management concepts (Registered Nurses' Association of Ontario, 2010; 2018).

- Make it fun! Use Indigenous dance traditions and music from traditional and contemporary Indigenous musicians (National Collaborating Centre for Indigenous Health, 2020). For information on Indigenous dance traditions across Canada, see the Carleton University *Native Dance* link: https://carleton.ca/circle/2016/native-dance/

Implementation and Evaluation

Jaida provided a progress report at the next community health network meeting in Northern Creek. Shania, Susan, and the CHR attended the meeting for information and to get to know the network partners. Jaida had put together their ideas in a logic model (Table 14.5). The logic model identifies three components of the program: partnership building, skills development, and exercise classes. It also links the main activities under each component with the intended results. This model is intended to help everyone concerned understand how the program is supposed to work. It will also guide actions and allow different people to be involved in the delivery of the program without losing direction (Watson, Broemeling & Wong, 2009).

Evaluation Report

The exercise and wellness program—named *Northern Creek Naturally Fit and Active*—was delivered over 6 weeks in the early fall, almost as planned but with one or two adjustments to accommodate delays, pandemic physical distancing restrictions that were mandated part way through, and unexpected findings from the initial focus group. An interim program evaluation was conducted after the final session. The findings from this evaluation provided feedback on the program and a baseline measurement on physical activity levels for the second session (Table 14.6).

The evaluation plan was derived from the program logic model but took into consideration that the program was being implemented in stages and that some components might take longer to implement than others, particularly owing to the priority pandemic response in the community.

The planning group identified indicators of success for each question and located or developed tools to gather the required information. In keeping with the capacity-building intent of the program, the Indigenous women in the steering group were involved in designing the evaluation. In addition, they helped gather and interpret the data and played a key role in presenting the findings to the intervention group and

TABLE 14.5 **Program Logic Model for an Exercise and Wellness Program for Indigenous Women in Northern Creek**

Components	Partnership Building	Program Development Activities	Program (Exercise Class) Activities
Priority group	Urban and rural community groups and organizations	Target First Nations women living inside and outside of the community and other Indigenous women	Develop exercise classes for First Nations women, living inside and outside of the community and other Indigenous women. Age group: 25–70.
Activities	Build partnerships with urban and rural groups and organizations to encourage physical activity	Recruit women to the project planning group and build skills: • Build organizational skills of steering committee • Develop exercise leadership skills and training	Recruit 10–15 participants: • Advertise in community stores, on social media and on community radio • Use word of mouth
	Engage community groups: a. Inside the community: • Make a presentation to the chief and band council about the program • Hold community information sessions b. Outside the community: • Meet with partners from community health and recreation services about the program and linkages	Engage women in project steering group activities: • Arrange meetings at a convenient time and place • Encourage participation by being friendly and informal • Seek feedback on what works and what does not	Eliminate or reduce barriers to participation: • Offer exercise classes in an easily accessible location, at minimal cost to participants • Provide an opportunity for socialization • Conduct a focus group with participants to identify needs, interests, and the perceived barriers to participation • Customize the program for women on-reserve to meet their needs
	Develop a communication strategy to keep community partners informed	Train women as exercise leaders	Engage women in a 6-week, 2-hour/week exercise and wellness program that builds fitness and skills, provides health information (e.g., nutrition, proper footwear, traditional practices), and is fun

TABLE 14.5   Program Logic Model for an Exercise and Wellness Program for Indigenous Women in Northern Creek—cont'd

Components	Partnership Building	Program Development Activities	Program (Exercise Class) Activities
Process indicators	Community participation: • A number of community meetings • Involvement of a number of organizations and sectors	Planning team: • A number of Indigenous women in the steering group • Meetings every 2–4 weeks, documented in the minutes	Fitness program in progress: • A number of group exercise sessions established • A number of people participating per group exercise session
Short-term outcomes		Identify perceived benefits for participants belonging to the steering group and training as exercise leaders and gather suggestions for improvement (focus group)	Support participants in the following: • Increased engagement in a regimen of physical activity • Increased awareness of risk factors for poor health and chronic disease such as diabetes (low level of physical activity and poor nutrition) Identify and address barriers to physical activity. Tailor the program to participant needs (e.g., transportation). Customize strategies (e.g., for pregnant women and older persons).
Intermediate outcomes		Develop community leaders: • Women have the necessary skills to sustain physical activity initiatives in their respective communities	Enhance participant health: • Increased participation in physical activity • Reduced social isolation
Long-term outcomes	Increase fitness and well-being of community members. Decrease risk factors for chronic disease. Increase community capacity to organize and to address local concerns for health and well-being. Increase environmental support of members being physically active—normalize outdoor, indoor, and home activities and exercise.		

TABLE 14.6   Northern Creek Naturally Fit and Active Program Evaluation Plan

Question	Project Activity/Indicator of Success	Interventions and Evaluation Strategies	Who Has the Information?
Was the First Nations community engaged in decision making about the program?	• Three First Nations women were recruited to the steering group and participated in the development and evaluation of the program • The women represented two First Nations community organizations (health committee and school board) • The women said they found the steering group meetings long at times but felt they had been able to contribute more with each meeting and were satisfied with the decision-making process • Women from the reserve were consulted on the design of the activity program • Community leaders were kept informed about the project	• Steering group minutes • Steering group meeting evaluation	Steering group chair • The minutes record meeting attendance, key discussion points, outcomes, and action items • At the end of each meeting, the chair sought feedback on the meeting, going around the table. Everyone preferred this approach to completing an evaluation form*.
Was the exercise and wellness program implemented as planned (with pandemic contingency backup)?	• The exercise classes were advertised in local stores, on social media, and on local radio, but most people heard about them from their friends and family (word of mouth)	• Poster (hard copy and digitized for social media) • Radio announcement • Registration feedback	• Steering group chair • Recruitment successes and challenges are tracked and recorded in the meeting minutes

Continued

TABLE 14.6   Northern Creek Naturally Fit and Active Program Evaluation Plan—cont'd

Question	Project Activity/Indicator of Success	Interventions and Evaluation Strategies	Who Has the Information?
	• The community health representative (CHR) led the classes with assistance from the nursing student and two First Nations women recruited and paid as helpers • In total, 12 women registered for the classes; 9 of the women completed the session; 3 women had dropped out by week 3, one because her child was ill, the other 2 because they found the exercises too strenuous • The exercise portion of the class was followed as planned. Different types of indoor and outdoor exercises were added for variety, e.g., dance routines, nature walks. • The social gatherings after class were well attended in person and/or virtually	• Physical activity/ exercise class record	• CHR/project coordinator • The CHR tracks the number of women attending each session and make notes of any changes to the program
Were the barriers to access identified and addressed?	• The results of the focus group at the end of week 1 were used to tailor the program • The main barriers to participation identified were the lack of childcare along with access to the technology and space at home for virtual activities. Women were encouraged to bring their children to the class, but doing so meant they might have to temporarily leave the group to attend to them. Once or twice a sitter was available on site for in-person classes.	• Focus group summary of barriers • Steering group minutes • Program adaptation	• Project coordinator • Steering group chair
Did the program achieve its goal?	• At the end of the 6-week session, a focus group of 9 participants said they felt they had benefited from the group and were more active • They found the health information sessions interesting, appreciated the attempts to bring in traditional practices, and valued access to the class virtually/online when travel to the class or pandemic restrictions required. Participants enjoyed the topics and focus areas of discussion and socializing, suggested additional topics for discussions, and shared resources and other books, virtual fitness classes, and other opportunities. • All women said the social and outdoor activities were especially enjoyable and kept them coming back	Focus group summary	Project coordinator

*Diem, E., & Moyer, A. (2015). *Community and public health nursing: Learning to make a Difference through teamwork* (2nd ed.). Canadian Scholars' Press.

at a community health network meeting. The results of the evaluation are summarized in Table 14.6.

Lessons learned and recommendations for future programs were also shared with the steering group and at a community health network meeting. One unanticipated result from the exercise program generated much discussion. Two or three participants had arranged to walk together on the weekends. They used the pedometers from the main library to keep track of their mileage, and the gadgets had generated a lot of interest from families. Everybody wanted one! Before

long, there was talk about a "community walk" around the lake. The old path around the lake had become overgrown, so the community planned to get together one weekend to clear it. The intervention (exercise program) was a small beginning, but it was starting to bring the community together and build a sustainable capacity for healthy living and a healthier natural environment too.

The authors acknowledge the contributions of Alwyn Moyer and Elizabeth Diem for the original case study section of the chapter.

STUDENT EXPERIENCE

Form a small group and complete one of the following experiences:

1. Consider how you might prepare to take part in an Indigenous cultural experience such as a smudging ceremony? Develop a 10-minute health information session for use in a physical activity program incorporating smudging in a culturally safe and appropriate manner.
2. Reflect on how to work with an elder who has offered to help designing a physical activity program based on the medicine wheel. Consider how to organize the program around the medicine wheel philosophy and practices.

Log on to the Four Directions Teaching website at http://www.fourdirectionsteachings.com. After listening to the introduction, click on "Ojibwe" to hear the teachings on the medicine wheel. (For an example of using the medicine wheel in program planning, see the Ontario Aboriginal Diabetes Strategy link on the Evolve website.)

CHAPTER SUMMARY

14.1 The term *indigenous* means "native to the area"; it is often used by the United Nations to refer to peoples of long settlement and connection to specific lands. *Indian* is the legal identity of Indigenous people in Canada who are not Inuit or Métis; aside from a legal context, using this term could be considered offensive.

14.2 In 2016, the population of First Nations people, Inuit, and Métis in Canada was 1 673 785. Indigenous people represent almost 4.9% of Canada's population and are the fastest-growing population in the country.

14.3 The health status of First Nations people, Inuit, and Métis in Canada is disproportionately poor, a situation impacted by a number of social, political, and historical factors.

14.4 The colonial history of Indigenous peoples in Canada is a context of trauma and oppression that has impacted the contemporary community health of Indigenous populations.

14.5 Historical patterns of trauma and oppression have left many Indigenous people in Canada mistrustful of authorities and community health care providers. Trauma-informed care addresses the role previous trauma plays in current conditions and problems. Culturally safe relational practice is particularly relevant for Indigenous community health care.

14.6 The determinants of health for Indigenous populations include proximal (i.e., health behaviours, physical environments, employment and income, social status, education, and food insecurity), intermediate (i.e., health care systems; educational systems; community infrastructure, resources, and capacities; environmental stewardship; and cultural continuity), and distal (i.e., colonialism, racism and social exclusion, and repression of self-determination).

14.7 Analyzing health concerns and community health nursing interventions for First Nations, Inuit, and Métis populations in Canada requires a trauma-informed, relational, capacity-building approach. The determinants of health, population-based practice, health promotion, risk reduction, chronic disease prevention/management, capacity building, teamwork, program planning, and evaluation and sustainability of health programming are all elements of planning for Indigenous health. Capacity-building processes engage Indigenous community members as community partners in all aspects of decision making and intervention. CHNs draw on rights-based, strengths-based, and capacity-building approaches to promote wellness in an Indigenous community.

CHN IN PRACTICE: A CASE STUDY

Sarah's Developing Indigenous Community Health Practice

Marina has noticed that Sarah is able to explain her work when they meet one-on-one but seems reluctant to present the same ideas at the steering group meetings. Marina wants Sarah to practise her leadership skills at these meetings. She wonders whether Sarah's hesitation to speak is a personal characteristic or whether there are cross-cultural influences at play. Having read the ANAC (2009) framework for First Nations, Inuit, and Métis nursing, Marina is intrigued by the emphasis on providing a culturally safe environment for learning. Traditionally, nurses have been encouraged to be sensitive to cultural influences on health behaviour and respect different ways of knowing. However, some argue that culture is socially constructed, arising within a historical context, and maintained by complex power relationships, which are not readily visible and can serve to marginalize people (Browne et al., 2016; Bourque Bearskin et al., 2020). They argue that it is not sufficient to merely accommodate differences because it can perpetuate inequities. CHNs are advised to question how cultural differences have arisen, what purpose they serve, and how they are perpetuated in order to take action and provide a health care environment where different cultures can feel safe and begin to shape a system responsive to their needs.

Think About It

1. How might Marina convey her observations to Sarah and provide a culturally safe environment to explore this situation?
2. A grocery store in town wants to donate day-old doughnuts to the Northern Creek exercise program. Discuss the pros and cons of accepting this offer.

📶 TOOL BOX

The Tool Box contains useful resources that can be applied in community health nursing practice. These related resources are found either in the appendices at the back of this text or on the Evolve website at http://evolve.elsevier.com/stanhope/community/.

Appendix

- Appendix 2: CNA Backgrounder: "Social Determinants of Health and Nursing: A Summary of the Issues"

Tools

Health Canada. Assessment and Planning Tool Kit for Suicide Prevention in First Nations Communities. (http://www.naho.ca/documents/fnc/english/FNC_SuicidePreventionToolkit.pdf)

This tool kit has been prepared to assist First Nations peoples address suicide in their communities. The tool kit provides information and research on suicide prevention such as community assessment, community risk factors, and how to develop a healing plan.

Canadian Society for Exercise Physiology with the Public Health Agency of Canada: Canadian 24 Hour Movement Guidelines for Adults (https://csepguidelines.ca/adults-18-64)

These are Canada's first guidelines of this kind, offering clear direction about what a healthy 24 hours looks like for Canadian adults aged 18–64 years. Moving more, reducing sedentary time, and sleeping well are the centrepieces of the guidelines.

First Nation Health Authority: *Being Active—Making Exercise More Convenient* (https://www.fnha.ca/wellness/wellness-and-the-first-nations-health-authority/wellness-streams/being-active/)

This weblink hosts a collection of resources, including tips for individuals, community group activities, simple exercise program cards, a prevention graphic novel, and an important diabetes information resource and research papers.

Trauma- and Violence-Informed Physical Activity Toolkit (TVIPA) (https://equiphealthcare.ca/resources/trauma-and-violence-informed-physical-activity-toolkit/)

This collection of tools is part of the Equipping Health and Social Services for Equity (EQUIP) program, and includes project reports, documentary film, listings of resources and programs as well as tips and strategies for people both planning and seeking responsive physical activity programs.

REFERENCES

Aboriginal Nurses Association of Canada. (2005). *30 years of community*. Author.

Aboriginal Nurses Association of Canada. (2009). *Cultural competence and cultural safety in nursing education: A framework for first nations, Inuit, and Métis nursing.* Author https://www.cna-aiic.ca/en/nursing-practice/evidence-based-practice/indigenous-knowing/indigenous-knowing-resources/cultural-components-overview.

Absolon, K. E. (2008). *Kaandosswin: How we come to know.* Fernwood Publishing.

Alberta Health Services. (2020). *Trauma informed care (TIC): For individuals who help those impacted by trauma provide patient centred care.* https://www.albertahealthservices.ca/info/Page15526.aspx.

Alfred, T. (2009). Colonialism and state dependency. *Journal of Aboriginal Health*, 5(2), 42–60.

Allan, B., & Smylie, J. (2015). *First Peoples, second class treatment.* The Well Living House Action Research Centre for Indigenous Infant, Child, and Family Health and Wellbeing, St. Michael's Hospital, Toronto.

Astle, B., Bourque Bearskin, R. L., Dordunno, D., et al. (2020). *Nurses for planetary health: A call to action. Nurses and nurse practitioners of British Columbia.* https://www.nnpbc.com/nurses-for-planetary-health-a-call-to-action/.

Battiste, M. (2013). *Decolonizing education: Nourishing the learing spirit.* Purich Publishing.

Bell, G. R. (2012). *A framework for community engagement in primary health. Primary health and chronic disease management Saskatoon health region.* https://www.saskatoonhealthregion.ca/locations_services/Services/Primary-Health/Documents/SHR%20framework%20for%20community%20engagement.pdf.

Bingham, B., Moniruzzaman, A., Patterson, M., et al. (2019). Indigenous and non-indigenous people experiencing homelessness and mental illness in two Canadian cities: A retrospective analysis and implications for culturally informed action. *BMJ Open*, 9(4), e024748–e024748. https://doi.org/10.1136/bmjopen-2018-024748.

Blackstock, C. (2011). *The Canadian Human rights Tribunal on first nations child welfare: Why if Canada wins, equality and justice lose. Children and youth services review*, 33(1), 187–194. https://cwrp.ca/publications/canadian-human-rights-tribunal-first-nations-child-welfare-why-if-canada-wins-equality.

Blackstock, C. (2016). The complainant: The Canadian human rights tribunal on first nations child welfare. *McGill Law Journal*, 62(2), 285–328.

Bourassa, C., McKay-McNabb, K., & Hampton, M. (2004). Racism, sexism and colonialism: The impact on the health of Aboriginal women in Canada. *Canadian Woman Studies*, 24(1), 23–30.

Bourque Bearskin, R. L. (2011). A critical lens on culture in nursing practice. *Nursing Ethics*, 18(4), 548–559. https://doi.org/10.1177/0969733011408048.

Bourque Bearskin, R. L., Cameron, B. L., King, M., et al. (2016). Mamawoh kamatowin "coming together to help each other in wellness": Honouring indigenous nursing knowledge. *International Journal of Indigenous Health*, 11(1), 5–19.

Bourque Bearskin, R. L., Kennedy, A., Bourque, D. H., & Bourque, D. E. (2020). Nursing leadership in Indigenous health. In J. I. Waddell, & N. A. Walton (Eds.), *Yoder-Wise's leading and managing in Canadian nursing* (2nd ed.)(pp. 54–89). Elsevier Inc.

Boyer, Y. (2014). *Moving Aboriginal health forward: Discarding Canada's legal barriers.* UBC Press.

Brown, D., & Di Lallo, S. (2020). Talking circles: A culturally responsive evaluation practice. *American Journal of Evaluation*, 41(3), 367–383. https://doi.org/10.1177/1098214019899164.

Browne, V., Varcoe, C., Lavoie, J., et al. (2016). Enhancing health care equity with indigenous populations: Evidence-based strategies from an ethnographic study. *BMC Health Services Research*, 16(1), 544–544. https://doi.org/10.1186/s12913-016-1707-9.

Burnett, K. (2010). *Taking medicine: Women's healing work and colonial contact in southern Alberta, 1830–1930.* UBC Press.

Cameron, B. L., Camargo Plazas, M. P., Santo Salas, A., et al. (2014). Understanding inequalities in access to health care services for Aboriginal people: A call for nursing action. *Advances in Nursing Science, 37,* 3.

Canadian Nurses Association. (2014). *Aboriginal health nursing and Aboriginal health: Charting policy direction for nursing in Canada.* https://www.cna-aiic.ca/~/media/cna/page-content/pdf-en/aboriginal-health-nursing-and-aboriginal-health_charting-policy-direction-for-nursing-in-canada.pdf?la=en.

Canadian Society for Exercise Physiology. (2020). *Canadian 24-Hour movement guidelines for adults ages 18–64 years: An integration of physical activity, sedentary behaviour, and sleep.* https://csepguidelines.ca/wp-content/uploads/2020/10/24HMovementGuidelines-Adults18-64-2020-ENG.pdf.

Carruth, A. M. (2013). *NDG4m online classroom notes: Report of the Royal Commission on Aboriginal peoples stage 1 and 2. Trillium Lakelands District school board, Lindsay, Ontario.* http://ndg4m.weebly.com/uploads/1/7/0/1/17010548/report_of_the_royal_commission_on_aboriginal_peoples_stage_1_and_2.pdf.

Cashman, T. (1966). *Heritage of service the history of nursing in Alberta.* Alberta Association of Registered Nurses. [Seminal Reference].

Chan, L., Batal, M., Sadik, L., et al. (2019). *FNFNES final report for Eight Assembly of first nations regions: Draft comprehensive Technical report. Assembly of first nations.* University of Ottawa, Université de Montréal. http://www.fnfnes.ca/docs/FNFNES_draft_technical_report_Nov_2__2019.pdf.

Chandler, J. J., & Lalonde, C. (1998). Cultural continuity as a hedge against suicide in Canada's First Nations. *Transcultural Psychiatry, 35*(2), 191–219.

Coats, K. (2015). *Idle No more and the remaking of Canada.* University of Regina Press.

Daschuk, J. (2013). *Clearing the plains: Disease, politics of starvation, and the loss of Aboriginal life.* University of Regina Press.

Devries, K. M., Free, C. J., Morison, L., et al. (2009). Factors associated with the sexual behavior of Canadian Aboriginal young people and their implications for health promotion. *American Journal of Public Health, 99*(5), 855–964.

Diabetes Prevention Program Research Group. (2002). Reduction in the incidence of type 2 diabetes with lifestyle intervention or metformin. *New England Journal of Medicine, 346*(6), 393–403.

Dickason, O., & McNab, D. (2009). *Canada's first nations: A history of founding peoples from earliest times.* Oxford University Press.

Diem, E., & Moyer, A. (2015). *Community and public health nursing: Learning to make a difference through teamwork* (2nd ed.). Canadian Scholars' Press.

Dion Stout, M., & Kipling, G. (2003). *Aboriginal people, resilience and the residential school legacy.* The Aboriginal Healing Foundation.

Dutcher, L. (2008). *Colonization and the health impacts on Aboriginal people in Canada.* Unpublished course paper for History 3374. University of New Brunswick.

European colonization and the Native peoples. (n.d.). https://slmc.uottawa.ca/?q=european_colonization.

First Nations Child and Family Caring Society. (2015). *Jordan's Principle.* https://fncaringsociety.com/jordans-principle.

First Nations Child and Family Caring Society of Canada. (2020). *Tribunal rules on four categories of Jordan's Principle eligibility to ensure substantive equality.* https://fncaringsociety.com/sites/default/files/2020_chrt_36_information_sheet_jr_update.pdf.

First Nations Health Authority. (2019). *Health and wellness planning: A tool kit for BC first nations* (1st ed.). https://www.fnha.ca/WellnessSite/WellnessDocuments/FNHA-Health-and-Wellness-Planning-A-Toolkit-for-BC-First-Nations.pdf.

First Nations Health Authority. (n.d. b). *Being active—making exercise more convenient.* https://www.fnha.ca/wellness/wellness-and-the-first-nations-health-authority/wellness-streams/being-active.

First Nations Health Authority. (n.d.a). *About the FNHA.* http://www.fnha.ca/about.

First Nations Studies program at university of British Columbia. (n.d.a). *Sixties scoop.* http://indigenousfoundations.arts.ubc.ca/sixties_scoop/.

First Nations Studies program at university of British Columbia. (n.d.b). *The White Paper 1969.* https://indigenousfoundations.arts.ubc.ca/the_white_paper_1969/.

First Nations Studies Program at University of British Columbia. (2009). *Terminology.* http://indigenousfoundations.arts.ubc.ca/home/identity/terminology.html#indigenous.

Foulds et al., 2013 Foulds, W., Warburton, D. E. R., & Bredin, S. S. D. (2013). A systematic review of physical activity levels in Native American populations in Canada and the United States in the last 50 years. *Obesity Reviews, 14*(7), 593–603. https://doi.org/10.1111/obr.12032.

Funnel, S., Tanuseputro, P., Letendre, A., Bourque Bearskin, R. L., & Walker, J., (2019). "Nothing about us without us." How community-based participatory research methods were adapted in an Indigenous end-of-life study using previously collected data. *Canadian Journal on Aging, 39*(2), 145–155. https://doi.org/10.1017/s0714980819000291.

Gellert, K. S., Aubert, R. E., & Mikami, R. E. (2010). Ke "Ano Ola: Moloka"i's community-based healthy lifestyle modification program. *American Journal of Public Health (1971), 100*(5), 779–783. https://doi.org/10.2105/AJPH.2009.176222.

Giles, D., & Darroch, F. E. (2014). The need for culturally safe physical activity promotion and programs. *Canadian Journal of Public Health, 105*(4), e317–e319. https://doi.org/10.17269/cjph.105.4439.

Goettke, E., & Reynolds, J. (2019). "It's all interconnected… like a spider web": A qualitative study of the meanings of food and healthy eating in an indigenous community. *International Journal of Circumpolar Health, 78*(1), 1648969–1648969. https://doi.org/10.1080/22423982.2019.1648969.

Government of British Columbia. (n.d.). *BC declaration on the rights of indigenous peoples act.* https://www2.gov.bc.ca/gov/content/governments/indigenous-people/new-relationship/united-nations-declaration-on-the-rights-of-indigenous-peoples.

Government of Canada. (2020a). *Highlights from the report of the Royal commission on Aboriginal peoples.* https://www.rcaanc-cirnac.gc.ca/eng/1100100014597/1572547985018.

Government of Canada. (2020b). *Guide to the Canadian Charter of rights and freedoms.* https://www.canada.ca/en/canadian-heritage/services/how-rights-protected/guide-canadian-charter-rights-freedoms.html.

Government of Canada. (2020c). *Implementing the united nations declaration on the rights of indigenous peoples in Canada.* https://www.justice.gc.ca/eng/declaration/index.html.

Greenwood, M., de Leeuw, S., & Lindsay, N. M. (2018). *Determinants of indigenous peoples' health in Canada: Beyond the social.* Canadian Scholars' Press.

Hackett, C., Feeny, D., & Tompa, E. (2016). Canada's residential school system: Measuring the intergenerational impact of familial attendance on health and mental health outcomes. *Journal of Epidemiology & Community Health (1979)*, *70*(11), 1096–1105. https://doi.org/10.1136/jech-2016-207380.

Hajizadeh, M., Bombay, A., & Asada, Y. (2019). Socioeconomic inequalities in psychological distress and suicidal behaviours among Indigenous peoples living off-reserve in Canada. *Canadian Medical Association Journal*, *191*(12), E325–E336. https://doi.org/10.1503/cmaj.181374.

Hart Wasekeesikaw, F., Bourque Bearskin, R.L., & McDonald, C. (2020). The legacy of colonization for the health and well-being of indigenous people: Towards reconciliation. In C. McDonald & M. McIntyre (eds.), *Realities of Canadian nursing: Professional, practice, and power issues* (5th ed.) (pp. 64–82). Wolters Kluwer.

Hawe, P., King, L., Noort, M., et al. (2000). *Indicators to help with capacity building in health promotion* (No. SHPN: 990099). Australian Centre for Health Promotion. Better Health Good Health Care.

Health Canada. (2014). *A statistical profile on the health of first nations in Canada: Determinants of health, 2006 to 2010. her Majesty the queen in right of Canada*. http://publications.gc.ca/collections/collection_2014/sc-hc/H34-193-1-2014-eng.pdf.

Health Canada. (2018). *First Nations and Inuit health and wellness indicators*. https://health-infobase.canada.ca/fnih/.

Helin, C. (2006). *Dances with dependency: Indigenous success through self-reliance*. Orca Spirit Publishing and Communications.

Higginbottom, G. M. A., Caine, V., Salway, S., et al. (2011). *Providing culturally safe and competent health care—a self-directed workbook and digital resource*. Faculty of Nursing, University of Alberta.

Horrill, T., McMillan, D. E., Schultz, A., & Thompson, G. (2018). Understanding access to healthcare among indigenous peoples: A comparative analysis of biomedical and postcolonial perspectives. *Nursing Inquiry*, *25*(3), e12237. https://doi.org/10.1111/nin.12237.

Hossain, B., & Lamb, L. (2019). Economic insecurity and psychological distress among Indigenous Canadians. *The Journal of Developing Areas*, *53*(1), 109–125. https://doi.org/10.1353/jda.2019.0007.

Hovey, R. B., Delormier, T., & McComber, A. (2014). Social-relational understandings of health and well-being from an Indigenous perspective. *International Journal of Indigenous Health*, *10*(1), 35–54.

Indigenous, & Northern Affairs Canada. (2015). *Comprehensive claims*. https://www.aadnc-aandc.gc.ca/eng/1100100030577/1100100030578.

Indigenous and Northern Affairs Canada. (2010). *A history of treaty-making in Canada*. https://www.rcaanc-cirnac.gc.ca/DAM/DAM-CIRNAC-RCAANC/DAM-TAG/STAGING/texte-text/ap_htmc_treatliv_1314921040169_eng.pdf.

Indigenous and Northern Affairs Canada. (2012). *Terminology*. https://www.aadnc-aandc.gc.ca/eng/1358879361384/1358879407462.

Ironside, F., Ferguson, L.J., Katapally, T.R., & Foulds, H.J.A. (2020). Cultural connectedness as a determinant of physical activity among Indigenous adults in Saskatchewan. *Applied Physiology Nutrition and Metabolism*, *45*(9), 937–947. https://doi.org/10.1139/apnm-2019-0793.

Jakubec, S., & Bearskin, B. (2020). Decolonizing and anti-oppressive nursing practice: Awareness, allyship, and action.

In L. McCleary, & T. McParland (Eds.), *Ross-kerr and Wood's Canadian nursing: Issues and perspectives* (6th ed.) (pp. 243–268). Elsevier Inc.

Kesäniemi, A., Riddoch, C. J., Reeder, B., Blair, S. N., & Sørensen, T. I. A. (2010). Advancing the future of physical activity guidelines in Canada: An independent expert panel interpretation of the evidence. *International Journal of Behavioral Nutrition and Physical Activity*, *7*(1), 41–41. https://doi.org/10.1186/1479-5868-7-41.

Klomp, H., Dyck, R. F., & Sheppard, S. (2003). Description and evaluation of a prenatal exercise program for urban Aboriginal women. *Canadian Journal of Diabetes*, *27*(3), 231–238.

Krieger, N. (2016). Living and dying at the crossroads: Racism, embodiment, and why theory is essential for a public health of consequence. *American Journal of Public Health (1971)*, *106*(5), 832–833. https://doi.org/10.2105/AJPH.2016.303100.

Lachance, N., Hossack, N., Wijayasinghe, C., et al. (2009). *Health determinants for first nations in Alberta 2010*. Health Canada.

Lavoie, J. G., Forget, E. L., & Browne, A. J. (2010). Caught at the crossroad: First Nations, health care, and the legacy of the Indian Act. *Pimatisiwin: A Journal of Aboriginal and Indigenous Community Health*, *8*(1), 83–100.

Lavoie, J. G., Forget, E. L., & O'Neil, J. D. (2007). Why equity in financing first nation on-reserve health services matters: Findings from the 2005 national evaluation of the health transfer policy. *Healthcare Policy*, *2*(4), 79–96.

Lavoie, J. G., Wong, S., Katz, A., & Sinclair, S. (2016). Opportunities and barriers to rural, remote and first nation health services research in Canada: Comparing access to administrative claims data in manitoba and British Columbia. Appuis et obstacles à la recherche sur les services de santé en milieu rural, éloigné et autochtone au Canada: Comparaison de l'accès aux données administratives sur les demandes de remboursement au manitoba et en colombie-britannique. *Healthcare Policy = Politiques de sante*, *12*(1), 52–58.

Lawrence, B. (2002). Re-writing histories of the land: Colonization and indigenous resistance in eastern Canada. In S. Razack (Ed.), *Race, space, and the law: Unmapping a white settler society* (pp. 21–47). Between the Lines Books.

Law, R., Williams, L., Langley, J., et al. (2020). 'Function first—Be active, stay Independent'—promoting physical activity and physical function in people with long-term conditions by primary care: A protocol for a realist synthesis with embedded co-production and co-design. *BMJ Open*, *10*, e035686. https://doi.org/10.1136/bmjopen-2019-035686.

Legacy of Hope Foundation. (2009). *Where are the children? Exhibit: Intergenerational impacts*. https://legacyofhope.ca/wherearethechildren/.

Levine, S., Varcoe, C., & Browne, A. J. (2020). "We went as a team closer to the truth": Impacts of interprofessional education on trauma- and violence- informed care for staff in primary care settings. *Journal of Interprofessional Care*, 1–9. https://doi.org/10.1080/13561820.2019.1708871.

Loppie Reading, C., & Wien, F. (2009). *Health inequalities and the social determinants of Aboriginal peoples' health*. National Collaborating Centre for Aboriginal Health.

Lux, M. K. (2016). *Separate beds: A history of Indian hospitals in Canada, 1920s–1980s*. University of Toronto Press.

Mas, S. (2015). *Truth and reconciliation offers 94 "calls to action."* *CBC News*. December 14. http://www.cbc.ca/news/politics/truth-and-reconciliation-94-calls-to-action-1.3362258.

McCallum, L. M. (2014). *Indigenous women, work, and history.* University of Manitoba Press.

McDonald, C., & Steenbeek, A. (2015). The impact of colonization and Western assimilation on health and wellbeing of Canadian Aboriginal people. *International Journal of Regional and Local History, 10*(1), 32–46. https://doi.org/10.1179/205145301 5Z.00000000023.

McFarlane, P., & Schabus, N. (Eds.). (2017). *Whose land is it anyway? A manual for decolonization.* Federation of Post-Secondary Educators of BC.

Mehrabadi, A., Paterson, K., Pearce, M., et al. (2008). Gender differences in HIV and Hepatitis C related vulnerabilities among Aboriginal young people who use street drugs in two Canadian cities. *Women & Health, 48*(3), 235–260. https://doi. org/10.1080/03630240802463186.

Miller, J. R. (2015). *Residential schools.* http://www. thecanadianencyclopedia.ca/en/article/residential-schools/.

Milloy, S. J. (1999). *A national crime: The Canadian government and the residential school system 1879–1986.* University of Manitoba Press.

Moore, M., Warburton, J., O'Halloran, P. D., Shields, N., & Kingsley, M. (2016). Effective community-based physical activity interventions for older adults living in rural and regional areas: A systematic review. *Journal of Aging and Physical Activity, 24*(1), 158–167. https://doi.org/10.1123/japa.2014-0218.

Morrison, D. (2020). *Back to the roots: Restoring Indigenous food landscapes.* Cultural Survival Quarterly Magazine. September https://www.culturalsurvival.org/publications/cultural-survival-quarterly/back-roots-restoring-indigenous-food-landscapes.

National Collaborating Centre for Aboriginal Health. (2013). *Physical activity.* http://www.nccah-ccnsa.ca/Publications/Lists/Publications/ Attachments/72/1791_NCCAH_fs_physactivity_EN.pdf.

National Collaborating Centre for Aboriginal Health. (2014). *Landscapes of First Nations, Inuit, and Métis health: An environmental scan of organizations, literature, and research* (3rd ed.). literature, and research. http://www.nccah-ccnsa.ca/ Publications/Lists/Publications/Attachments/134/2014_12_09_ RPTScan_LandscapesofHealth_EN_Web.pdf.

National Collaborating Centre for Indigenous Health (NCCIH). (2020). *Physical activity during winter and COVID-19.* https:// www.nccih.ca/docs/diseases/2020-10-30-How%20to%20stay%20 active%20in%20winter%20during%20COVID-19-EN.pdf.

National Inquiry into Missing and Murdered Indigenous Women and Girls. (2019). *Reclaiming power and place: The final report of the national inquiry into missing and murdered Indigenous women and girls.* https://www.mmiwg-ffada.ca/wp-content/ uploads/2019/06/Final_Report_Vol_1a-1.pdf.

New South Wales Health Department. (2001). *A framework for building capacity to improve health (No. SHPN: 990226).* New South Wales Health Department. https://yeah.org.au/wp-content/uploads/2014/07/A-Framework-for-Building-Capacity-to-Improve-Health.pdf.

Obomsawin, R. (2007). *Historical and scientific perspectives on the health of Canada's First Peoples.* https://soilandhealth.org/wp-content/uploads/02/0203CAT/020335.obomsawin.pdf.

Office of the United Nations High Commissioner for Human Rights. (2020). *Special rapporteur on the rights of Indigenous peoples.* http://www.ohchr.org/en/issues/ipeoples/ srindigenouspeoples/pages/sripeoplesindex.aspx.

O'Neill, L., Fraser, T., Kitchenham, A., & McDonald, V. (2016). Hidden burdens: A review of intergenerational, historical and complex trauma, implications for indigenous families. *Journal of Child & Adolescent Trauma, 11*(2), 173–186. https://doi. org/10.1007/s40653-016-0117-9.

Pelletier, C. A., Smith-Forrester, J., & Klassen-Ross, T. (2017). A systematic review of physical activity interventions to improve physical fitness and health outcomes among Indigenous adults living in Canada. *Preventive Medicine Reports, 8*, 242–249. https://doi.org/10.1016/j.pmedr.2017.11.002.

Polanco, F., & Arbour, L. (2018). Type 2 diabetes in Indigenous populations: Why a focus on genetic susceptibility is not enough. In M. Greenwood, S. de Leeuw, & N. M. Lindsay (Eds.), *Determinants of indigenous peoples' health in Canada: Beyond the social* (pp. 296–311). Canadian Scholars' Press.

Power, T., Wilson, D., Best, O., et al. (2020). COVID–19 and Indigenous Peoples: An imperative for action. *Journal of Clinical Nursing, 29*, 15–16. https://doi.org/10.1111/jocn.15320.

Public Health Agency of Canada. (2011). *What determines health?* http://www.phac-aspc.gc.ca/ph-sp/determinants/index-eng.php.

Public Health Agency of Canada. (2018). *Key health inequalities in Canada: A national portrait—executive summary.* https:// www.canada.ca/en/public-health/services/publications/science-research-data/key-health-inequalities-canada-national-portrait-executive-summary.html.

Public Health Agency of Canada, & Alberta/NWT Region. (2008). *Community capacity building tool.* https://www.canada.ca/ en/public-health/corporate/mandate/about-agency/regional-operations/community-capacity-building-tool.html.

Racine, L., & Petrucka, P. (2011). Enhancing decolonization and knowledge transfer in nursing research with non-western populations: Examining the congruence between primary healthcare and postcolonial feminist approaches. *Nursing Inquiry, 18*(1), 12–20. https://doi.org/10.1111/j.1440-1800.2010.00504.x.

Registered Nurses' Association of Ontario. (2010). *Strategies to support self-management in chronic conditions: Collaboration with patients.* Author.

Registered Nurses' Association of Ontario. (2018). *RNAO best practices evidence Booster: Strategies to support self-management in chronic conditions: Collaboration with patients.* https://rnao. ca/sites/rnao-ca/files/Strategies_to_Support_Self-Management_ in_Chronic_Conditions_-_Collaboration_with_Patients.pdf.

Riva, M., Plusquellec, P., Juster, R. P., et al. (2014). Household crowding is associated with higher allostatic load among Inuit. *Journal of Epidemiology & Community Health, 68*, 363–369.

Rowan, M. S., Rukholm, E., Bourque-Bearskin, R. L., et al. (2013). Cultural competence and cultural safety in Canadian schools of nursing: A mixed methods study. *International Journal of Nursing Education Scholarship, 10*(1), 1–10. https://doi. org/10.1515/ijnes-2012-0043

Royal Canadian Mounted Police. (2014). *Missing and murdered Aboriginal women: A national operational overview. Her Majesty the queen in right of Canada.* https://www.rcmp-grc. gc.ca/en/missing-and-murdered-aboriginal-women-national-operational-overview.

Royal Commission on Aboriginal Peoples. (1996). *Highlights from the report of Royal commission on Aboriginal peoples: People to people and nation to nation.* https://www.rcaanc-cirnac.gc.ca/en g/1100100014597/1572547985018.

Sanderson, D., Mirza, N., Polacca, M., Kennedy, A., & Bourque Bearskin, R. L. (2020). Nursing, Indigenous health, water, and climate change. *Witness: The Canadian Journal of Critical Nursing Discourse, 2*(1), 66–83. https://witness.journals.yorku.ca/index. php/default/article/view/55/28.

Savard, S., & Todd, S. (2020). *Canadian perspectives on community development*. University of Ottawa Press.

Sheppard, A., Shapiro, G., Bushnik, T., et al. (2017). *Birth outcomes among first nations, Inuit and Métis populations (Catalogue no. 82-003-X)*. *Health reports*. Statistics Canada. Canadian Centre for Health Information. https://www150.statcan.gc.ca/n1/en/pub/82-003-x/2017011/article/54886-eng.pdf?st=6cWIomZ-.

Short, S. E., & Mollborn, S. (2015). Social determinants and health behaviors: Conceptual frames and empirical advances. *Current Opinion in Psychology, 5*, 78–84. https://doi.org/10.1016/j.copsyc.2015.05.002.

Sinclair, N. J., Doerfler, J., & Stark, H. K. (2013). *Centering Anishinaabeg studies: Understanding the world through stories*. Michigan State University Press.

Smith, R., & Lavoie, J. (2008). First nations health networks: A collaborative system approach to health transfer. *Healthcare Policy, 4*(2), 101–112.

Sockbeson, R. C. (2011). *Cipenuk red hope: Weaving policy toward decolonization & beyond*. University of Alberta. Unpublished PhD dissertation.

Southern Chief's Organization. (2016). *Treaty maps*. http://scoinc.mb.ca/treaties/.

Starblanket, T. (2020). *Suffer the little children: Genocide, Indigenous nations and the Canadian state*. Clarity Press Inc.

Statistics Canada. (2011). *National household survey 2011*. https://www12.statcan.gc.ca/nhs-enm/2011/dp-pd/prof/index.cfm?Lang=E.

Statistics Canada. (2017). *Aboriginal peoples in Canada: Key results from the 2016 census*. https://www150.statcan.gc.ca/n1/en/daily-quotidien/171025/dq171025a-eng.pdf?st=zfhgdrAt.

Statistics Canada. (2019). *Suicide among First Nations people, Métis and Inuit (2011–2016): Findings from the 2011 Canadian census health and environment cohort (CanCHEC)*. https://www150.statcan.gc.ca/n1/en/pub/99-011-x/99-011-x2019001-eng.pdf?st=DQezdteG.

Stewart, M. J., Castleden, H., King, M., et al. (2015). Supporting parents of Aboriginal children with asthma: Preferences and pilot interventions. *International Journal of Indigenous Health, 10*(2), 131–149.

Stewart, M., King, M., Blood, R., et al. (2012). Health inequities experienced by Aboriginal children with respiratory problems and their parents. *Canadian Journal of Nursing Research, 45*, 6–27.

Taylor, J. L. (1999). Two views on the meaning of the treaties six and seven. In R. T. Price (Ed.), *The spirit of the Alberta Indian treaties* (pp. 9–45). University of Alberta Press.

Taylor, J., & Kukutai, T. (2016). Indigenous data sovereignty: Toward an agenda. *Indigenous data sovereignty: Toward an agenda* (Vol. 38). ANU Press. https://doi.org/10.22459/CAEPR38.11.2016.

The Canadian Encyclopedia. (2020). *Treaties in Canada education guide and worksheets*. https://www.thecanadianencyclopedia.ca/en/studyguide/treaties-in-canada-learning-guide-and-worksheets.

Thira, D. (2014). *Beyond the four waves of colonization*. https://thira.ca/files/2014/08/Colonization-Article-CNPR-Revised1.pdf.

Tjepkema, M., Wilkins, R., Senécal, S., et al. (2010). Mortality of urban Aboriginal adults in Canada, 1991–2001. *Chronic Diseases in Canada, 31*(1), 4–21.

Tremblay, M. S., Katzmarzyk, P. T., Colley, R. C., & Janssen, I. (2017). *A 50th anniversary celebration of CSEP member contributions to the understanding of exercise physiology: A focus on physical activity and fitness epidemiology*. Canadian Society for Exercise Physiology. https://csep.ca//news.asp?a=view&id=178.

Truth, & Reconciliation Commission of Canada. (2015). *TRC findings*. http://www.trc.ca/websites/trcinstitution/index.php?p=893.

Tuhiwai Smith, L. (2012). *Decolonizing methodologies: Research and indigenous peoples* (2nd ed.). University of Otago Press.

Turpel-Lafond (Aki-Kwe), M. E. (2020). *In Plain sight: addressing Indigenous–specific racism and discrimination in B.C. Health Care*. British Columbia Health Ministry. https://engage.gov.bc.ca/app/uploads/sites/613/2020/11/In-Plain-Sight-Full-Report.pdf.

University of Saskatchewan. (2016). *Aboriginal nursing in Canada ("Professional Occupations in nursing" NOC 2016-301)*. https://nursing.usask.ca/documents/aboriginal/AboriginalRNWorkforceFactsheet.pdf.

Van Herk, K. A., Smith, D., & Andrew, C. (2011). Examining our privileges and oppressions: Incorporating an intersectionality paradigm into nursing. *Nursing Inquiry, 18*(1), 29–39. https://doi.org/10.1111/j.1440-1800.2011.00539.x

Vukic, A., Jesty, C., Mathews, S. V., et al. (2012). Understanding race and racism in nursing: Insights from Aboriginal nurses. *International Scholarly Research Nursing, 2012,* Article ID 196437.

Walia, H. (2012). *Decolonizing together. Moving beyond a politics of solidarity toward a practice of decolonizationBriarpatch Magazine*. http://briarpatchmagazine.com/articles/view/decolonizing-together.

Watson, B. E., Broemeling, A. M., & Wong, S. T. (2009). A results-based logic model for primary healthcare: A conceptual foundation for population-based information systems. *Healthcare Policy/Politiques de Santé, 5*(SP), 33–46. https://doi.org/10.12927/hcpol.2009.21184.

Wicklum, S., Sampson, M., Henderson, R., et al. (2019). Results of a culturally relevant, physical activity-based wellness program for urban Indigenous women in Alberta, Canada. *International Journal of Indigenous Health, 14*(2), 169–204. https://doi.org/10.32799/ijih.v14i2.31890.

Williamson, C., & Carr, J. (2009). Health as a resource for everyday life: Advancing the conceptualization. *Critical Public Health, 19*(1), 107–122. https://doi.org/10.1080/09581590802376234.

World Health Organization. (2016). *Fact sheet: Health of indigenous peoples*. https://www.who.int/gender-equity-rights/knowledge/factsheet-indigenous-healthn-nov2007-eng.pdf.

World Health Organization. (2020). *Fact sheet: Diabetes*. https://www.who.int/news-room/fact-sheets/detail/diabetes.

Younging, G. (2018). *Elements of indigenous style: A guide for writing by and about indigenous peoples*. Brush Education.

Young, T. K., & Katzmarzyk, P. T. (2007). Physical activity of Aboriginal people in Canada. *Canadian Journal of Public Health, 98*, 148–160.

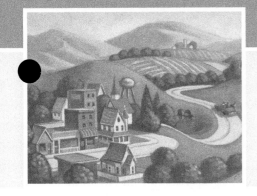

Working With People Who Experience Structural Vulnerabilities

OUTLINE

Vulnerability: Definition and Influencing Factors, 352
Determinants of Health, 355
Factors Predisposing People to Vulnerability (Health Inequities), 355
Poverty, 356
Poverty and Health, 356
Homelessness and Housing Instability, 358
Understanding the Concept of Homelessness, 358
Effects of Housing Instability on Health, 359
Homelessness and At-Risk Populations, 359
Violence, 360
Homicides, 360
Social and Community Factors That Influence Violence, 360
Violence as a Form of Abuse, 361
Assault, 364

Community Mental Health, 366
At-Risk Populations for Mental Illness, 367
Determinants of Mental Health, 369
The Community Health Nurse's Collaborative Role in Community Mental Health Care, 369
Substance use and Community Health, 372
Promotion of Healthy Lifestyles and Resiliency Factors, 373
Harm Reduction in Prevention Strategies, 373
Vulnerability of Children and Youth, 375
Adolescent Sexual Behaviour and Pregnancy, 375
Community Health Nurses Caring for People Experiencing Structural Vulnerabilities: Roles and Levels of Prevention, 377
The Roles of the Community Health Nurse, 380
Levels of Prevention and the Community Health Nurse, 383

OBJECTIVES

After reading this chapter, you should be able to:

15.1 Define the experience of *structural vulnerabilities* with a focus on oppression, inequity, social justice, and the complex determinants of health that impact populations.

15.2 Discuss the effects of poverty on the health and well-being of individuals, families, and communities.

15.3 Discuss how experiencing homelessness is influenced by and extends vulnerability and affects the health and well-being of individuals, families, and communities.

15.4 Discuss how structural vulnerabilities influence violence in Canadian communities.

15.5 Explain how structural vulnerabilities influence mental illness and substance use.

15.6 Explain the effects of mental illness and substance use on individuals, families, and the community as a whole.

15.7 Understand the risk and resiliency factors related to adolescent pregnancy and the role of community health nurses in health promotion for pregnant adolescents.

15.8 Explain the roles and practices of community health nurses working with populations who experience structural vulnerabilities and for social justice, harm reduction, and trauma-informed care.

KEY TERMS*

absolute homelessness, 358
absolute poverty, 356
concurrent disorder, 372
comprehensive services, 381
domestic violence, 362
harm reduction, 372
health disparities, 352
health inequities, 353
hidden homelessness, 358
"honour" killing, 364
inequalities, 352

inequity, 356
intimate partner violence, 363
nonsuicidal self-injury, 370
poverty, 356
probability, 353
racism, 352
risk factors, 353
relative poverty, 356
resiliency, 353
secondary victimization, 362
sex workers, 360

sexual assault, 364
sheltered homelessness, 358
subjective poverty, 356

structural violence, 353
structural vulnerability, 352
violence, 360

*See the Glossary on page 468 for definitions.

In Canada and around the world you often hear about community health care for "vulnerable groups" or working with "vulnerable populations" (National Collaborating Centre for Determinants of Health [NCCDH], 2014; 2020). The COVID-19 pandemic highlighted the language and terminology related to vulnerability, as well as risks and resiliency factors for populations. Throughout the pandemic, people who were considered vulnerable to becoming seriously ill from the virus, for instance older persons and people with certain chronic medical conditions, were identified for public health planning and interventions. You will see the term "vulnerable populations" in many organizational vision statements or targets, on websites, in academic papers, newsletters, and textbooks much like this one. You may also hear about indicators of vulnerability (such as health status) and inequities (for example, unjust policies placing one group's health status at greater risk than another's). What you do not so often hear is precisely what people are vulnerable to, the origins of that vulnerability, how it is produced, and by whom. What you also do not often hear is that no population or group of people is inherently vulnerable.

To consider vulnerability as caused by, or intrinsic to, individuals or a result of personal deficits causes harm and results in interventions that will, at best, only partially address the needs of people. A harm-reduction and equity-informed approach seeks to understand and respond to vulnerability from how and where it originates, how it is sustained and organized, and attempts to address who and what is responsible (Katz, Hardy, Firestone, et al., 2019). Consider the children who are structurally vulnerable to climate change and environmental policy, for example (see Chapter 17). The production of a vulnerability that originates from environmental policy requires multiple levels of community health interventions. From this perspective of vulnerability, you can then proceed to understand and address the causes and effects of vulnerability experienced by populations in your community health nurse (CHN) practice.

This chapter provides a discussion of the wider scope of inequities and the effects of **structural vulnerability** (risks for negative health outcomes because of the interface of socioeconomic, political, and societal hierarchies of dominance and oppression) (Bourgois, Holmes, Sue, et al., 2017). How these systems of oppression contribute to vulnerabilities that span a number of populations and aggregates is also highlighted (though not exhaustively) in this chapter. Structural vulnerabilities impact people of all ages who face systematic oppression and discrimination, for example: Indigenous people (see Chapter 14); recent immigrants to Canada and refugees; people with disabilities; people who are gender and sexually diverse (see Chapter 7); people who are experiencing homelessness or housing instability; people who live with

mental illness; people with low literacy skills; and people living in poor, rural, or remote communities (Canadian Index of Wellbeing Network, 2016; Public Health Agency of Canada [PHAC], 2020a). Definitions, experiences, vulnerability indicators, and CHN interventions to address vulnerabilities at multiple levels are discussed in light of a growing body of research and examples.

VULNERABILITY: DEFINITION AND INFLUENCING FACTORS

Vulnerable populations are groups and communities who are at a higher risk for poor health as a result of the barriers they experience to social, economic, political, and environmental resources, as well as limitations due to illness or disability (NCCDH, 2020).

The terms *equity seeking, marginalized,* and *high priority* are also used to discuss the positions of people and groups who suffer from injustice and inequitable access to health care. Because health injustice, disparities, and inequities persist in society, affected populations can be considered a *high priority* for community health care and for social or policy change (Raphael, Bryant, Mikkonen, & Raphael, 2020). These terms are also contentious in that they do not fully address the oppression and power relationships that place people at the margins instead of at the centre of decision making for community health. For example, the term *equity seeking* implies a responsibility on the part of people who are already disadvantaged by health disparities (Katz et al., 2019). At times, equity discourses fail to address the **racism** and white supremacy that are implied within well-intentioned individualistic community health practices and language, and therefore antiracist, antidiscrimination practices must be explicitly applied (Blanchet Garneau, Browne, & Varcoe, 2019).

Health disparities are wide variations in health services and health status among certain populations defined by specific characteristics (National Collaborating Centres for Public Health, 2020). Health disparities exist throughout Canada and relate to key factors such as socioeconomic status, education, literacy, employment and working conditions, food security, and genetics. The Public Health Agency of Canada's 2020 annual report (PHAC, 2020a) details these key factors and other contributing factors that lead to health disparities.

The health status of populations also underscores inequalities, with indicators such as morbidity, mortality, self-rated health, psychiatric hospitalizations, and suicides. **Inequalities** are simply the uneven distribution of health outcomes or health resources; however, these distributions shine the light on structural and social determinants of health (SDOH), as well as inequities (Pickett & Wilkinson, 2017). Indicators of health inequalities are found in socioeconomic measures of income, education levels, employment and occupational status, and so on (PHAC, 2018). When disparities in health status within or between groups are shown to be systematic and avoidable, they are unjust. These systematic and avoidable differences in health status are called health inequities. The determinants of health are mostly responsible for **health inequities**—the unfair and avoidable differences in health status seen within and between people and between countries (Blas, Roebbel, Rajan, et al., 2016). For example, certain population subgroups are at higher risk of experiencing mental health issues because of greater exposure and vulnerability to unfavourable social, economic, and environmental circumstances, interrelated with gender (World Health Organization, 2014). The COVID-19 pandemic pointed to this vulnerability in the area of women and violence (VAW Learning Network, 2020) and mental health (Pfefferbaum & North, 2020; Public Health Agency of Canada, 2020a). These inequities spark moral outrage as also witnessed during the COVID-19 pandemic, when systematic, unfair, avoidable differences resulted in death and disease arising from ageism, racism, and other forms of discrimination.

Experiences of unequal power, restricted access to resources, and oppression from a system-level approach resulting in the denial of basic needs are referred to as **structural violence**. Experiences of violence in this way shape individual experiences and violations of human rights. Most importantly, structural violence normalizes harms done to people and communities, laying down patterns of systematic oppression (Farmer, Nizeye, Stulac & Keshaviee, 2006; Gerlach, Browne, Sinha et al, 2017). Practices such as harm reduction and trauma-informed care and policy are some of the vehicles used to mitigate structural harms to both individuals and communities. Indeed, communities as a whole can experience the impacts of structural violence. **Trauma-informed care** is an approach that recognizes the impacts of previous violent and traumatic events on current health and mental health situations. This approach concentrates on relationship building; engagement and choice; awareness; and skills building across individual, interpersonal, and system levels of health service. As was discussed in Chapter 14, a key aspect of trauma-informed practice is understanding how trauma can be experienced differently by different populations, such as Indigenous peoples, immigrants and refugees, people with developmental disabilities, women, men, children and youth, and other populations (Kimberg & Wheeler, 2019). CHNs use these approaches to care with numerous individuals and groups, across many settings, including the home. Because CHNs are in key positions to detect and intervene in violence that is experienced at multiple levels, they need to understand how community-level influences can affect all types of violence. Preventing trauma and violence and mitigating their adverse effects promotes health equity at community and individual levels of intervention.

Practices that support mitigation and prevention rely on addressing risk and resiliency factors. Again, most often, these factors are systemic. People who experience poverty are often exposed to multiple risk factors that accumulate and can contribute to violence and lead to poor health. CHNs are concerned with these risk factors and ways to mitigate them and improve individual and community health. **Risk factors** are those conditions that have a direct effect on the likelihood of an adverse outcome; that is, they increase the probability of a poor health outcome. **Probability** is an aspect of risk (and the risk continuum, discussed in Chapter 4). It is an estimation of the likelihood an event will occur. Take one straightforward example: wearing a seatbelt reduces the probability of fatal injury in a motor vehicle accident; therefore, wearing a seatbelt decreases the risk of fatal injury in a motor vehicle. However, causal patterns of probability are more complex in relation to the effect of diet on coronary disease, where diet interacts with numerous other risk factors. Age, or rather changes that occur with age, is an example of a risk factor. Risk factors are not isolated; they often interact and have causes, referred to as *determinants;* for example, low income leads to difficulty finding affordable housing, which forces people to live in poorer neighbourhoods that typically have increased crime rates (social risk); inadequate housing may contribute to lead poisoning from exposure to peeling lead-based paint (environmental risk); and food insecurity leads to poor nutritional status (behavioural risk) and stress that can lead to family violence (behavioural risk) (Sebastian, 2014). Food insecurity is an example of how vulnerability results from many interacting factors over which individuals have little control.

CHNs often work with patients who experience structural vulnerabilities and the impact of health disparities, including structural violence. Because not all individuals and communities have the same vulnerabilities (as witnessed around the world during the COVID-19 pandemic), addressing structural factors requires a comprehensive understanding of risk and resiliency in these populations. Both risk and resiliency factors are often structural and, as such, individually targeted interventions may be insufficient. **Resiliency** refers to the capacity of people, communities, and organizations to cope effectively when faced with considerable adversity or risk. Resiliency applies to any vulnerable populations as part of communities and is not simply a matter of resources or funding—more money or additional staff resources do not necessarily build resilience when inequities are system-wide. In the case of food insecurity, the vulnerable population could be individuals, households, and communities in remote locations who have access only to costly and preserved/packaged foods; an approach based on resiliency would focus on addressing procurement and other issues of community access to nutritious food, as well as individual knowledge of how to source and prepare locally available foods. Individual resiliency factors are just one aspect of interventions that must be considered in addition to broader social justice, environmental, economic, and political aspects of food security. The interplay of different levels of intervention cannot be overemphasized. When the CHN places emphasis on patient, community, and systemic strengths and assets, rather than on deficits and susceptibility, resiliency is more likely to increase.

The "Evidence-Informed Practice" box describes a pan-Canadian research project that explored the effects of COVID-19 on people's perceived mental health and well-being.

EVIDENCE-INFORMED PRACTICE

Risk and resilience factors at multiple levels influence mental health and well-being in people's everyday lives during disaster or outbreak situations, including the COVID-19 pandemic, which is a novel, community, and globally experienced crisis. This Canadian study sought to discover if and how potential risk factors (i.e., reduction in income, job insecurity, feelings of vulnerability to contracting the virus, lack of confidence in avoiding COVID-19, adherence to preventative policies) and resilience factors (i.e., trait resilience, family functioning, social support, social participation, and trust in health care institutions) are associated with mental health and well-being outcomes, and whether these resilience factors buffer (i.e., moderate) the associations between risk factors and said outcomes.

Following the first two weeks of government-recommended preventative measures, 1,122 Canadian workers completed an online questionnaire that included multiple well-being outcome scales, in addition to measures of potential risk and resilience factors. Structural equation modelling analysis revealed that, overall, the risk factors were associated with poorer well-being outcomes, except social distancing, which was associated with lower levels of stress. In general, resilience factors did not buffer the risk factors. In summary, this study found that the COVID-19 crisis encompassed several stressors related to the virus as well as to its impact on one's social, occupational, and financial situation, which put people at risk for lower well-being as early as 1 to 2 weeks after the crisis began. While several resilience factors emerged as being positively related to well-being, such factors may not be enough, or be sufficiently activated at that time, to buffer the effects of the numerous life changes required by COVID-19.

Application for CHNs While CHNs and public health decision-makers should offer and design services that are directly focused on mental health and well-being, it is important they go beyond promoting and celebrating individuals' inner potential for resilience. CHNs can support individuals in activating sustained, supportive environmental resources during a pandemic. Crisis experiences, when well-managed, can reorganize environmental and structural resources for sustained health-promoting practices and programs beyond the crisis.

Questions for Reflection and Discussion
1. In what ways are the mental health risks from a pandemic particularly significant for people with structural vulnerabilities (e.g., poverty, housing instability, racialized discrimination, disability, and other inequities)?
2. Mental health resiliency during a pandemic depends on much more than individual strengths; for example, an individual who is living in poverty may need to access a safe house or an apartment after eviction, adding additional risk factors for coping. What CHN supports can be instrumental to addressing resiliency factors (such as the example of safe housing for individuals on a limited income, or others, such as children and youth, older persons, or veterans)?

Source: Coulombe, S., Pacheco, T., Cox, E., Khalil, C., Doucerain, M.M., et al. (2020). Risk and resilience factors during the COVID-19 pandemic: A snapshot of the experiences of Canadian workers early on in the crisis. *Frontiers in Psychology, 11*, 580702. https://doi.org/10.3389/fpsyg.2020.580702

Traditionally, CHNs have focused on identifying the health concerns of and the risk and resiliency factors for the populations with whom they work. Social justice and political actions have also become aspects of community development in the effort to create meaningful solutions to social inequities (see Chapter 9). Focusing on patient strengths, assets, and capabilities, and working with patients to find resolutions to individual and community health needs remains an area of focus of CHN practice (see the "CHN in Practice: A Case Study, "Buns in the Oven": A Prenatal Nutrition Program" box). This assets-based approach is discussed in more detail in Chapters 4 and 9.

CHN IN PRACTICE: A CASE STUDY

"Buns in the Oven": A Prenatal Nutrition Program
"Buns in the Oven" is a weekly program that offers prenatal nutrition support for pregnant women through all of Ottawa's community health centres. The program is sponsored by Ottawa Public Health, the Canadian Prenatal Nutrition Program, and numerous partner agencies. All Buns in the Oven programs have the same goals and objectives. However, each program adapts to the unique needs of the patients and setting it serves; for example, one program offers access to satellite food banks and baby supplies, and another runs late into the afternoon/early evening and has made services more accessible for women who work several jobs or take local transit to reach the program site. The overall program is focused on food security and nutritional factors related to preventing low birth weight of newborns and preterm deliveries as well as promoting healthy infant feeding practices. Some programs are scheduled so that participants have the opportunity to meet with CHNs and other clinicians and to join in other programs (e.g., social support and recreational activities, and parenting education sessions that cover topics such as early childhood development).

Think About It
1. How could a targeted food security program such as Buns in the Oven promote individual resiliency for patients? How could it promote assets and strengths? Explain.
2. What is the connection of resiliency to the sociocultural and economic concerns of people who access a nutrition program such as Buns in the Oven?
3. How do determinants of health influence the resiliency of participants in a program such as Buns in the Oven?

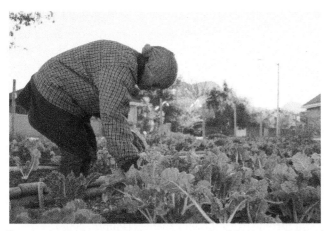

Community garden programs are an example of the integrated food security projects that community nurses may support. (iStockphoto/nattrass)

Determinants of Health

Many factors affect the health of populations: individual factors such as gender, biology, and behavioural factors, as well as social and environmental factors such as housing and food security. Various SDOH have an even greater influence on health than biomedical and behavioural risk factors (Raphael et al., 2020). Many decades of research on the determinants of health demonstrate that the vast majority of avoidable deaths are attributable to factors that are tied to the distribution of resources in society and to daily living conditions (WHO, 2017). These determinants of health have been discussed throughout this text. See the "Determinants of Health" box for highlights on income, gender, and biological determinants of health to consider in relation to structurally vulnerable populations.

DETERMINANTS OF HEALTH

Income, Age, Gender, Racism, and Biology

- In 2019, the average hourly minimum wage in Canada was $11.45.* Over the past 40 years, change has been marginal—and most wages have not increased in step with inflated costs of living.[†]
- Food banks and charities have stepped in to fill gaps created by inadequate social and income programs; however, the food security needs of one in eight Canadians who are considered to be food insecure are not being sufficiently met.[†]
- Early childhood development and learning, especially in the first 3 years of life, are negatively affected by food insecurity.[‖] Children under 18 now represent 34.1% of those served by food banks, a stunning overrepresentation compared to the general population, where they sit at 19.4% of the population. Single-person households have increased and now account for close to half (48%) of all recipients of food bank services.[#]
- Being employed does not ensure a means to overcome poverty.** In all, 7.6% of adult Canadians are considered "working poor" or struggle to make ends meet. They have less stable jobs, unpredictable working hours, fewer benefits, and increased health problems.[††]

- Canadians with low incomes usually belong to one of three groups that have significantly reduced well-being (Indigenous peoples, racialized groups, and people with disabilities):
  23.6% of Indigenous peoples experienced poverty in 2016 compared to 13.8% for non-Indigenous people.
  Racialized people experienced poverty rates of 20.8% in 2016, compared to 12.2% of white people.
  In 2014, 23.2% of people with a disability lived in poverty, compared to 8.6% of those without a disability.[††]
  Canadians earning less than $20 000 annually are three times more likely to experience a decline in self-rated health when compared to Canadians in the highest income bracket.[‡‡] Low-income Canadians have the highest mortality rates, hospitalization rates, and emergency visit rates as well as the lowest life expectancy rates.[‡‡]
  In 2016, 81.3 % of all lone-parent families were headed by women. These households had half the median income of male lone-parent families.[††]
- The rate of child poverty declined less than half a percentage point between 2017–2018, from 18.6 to 18.2%, leaving nearly 1 in 5 children experiencing the harsh long-term consequences that poverty and discrimination have on social, mental, and physical health and well-being.**

Sources: * Government of Canada, 2019. [†] Tarasuk, & McIntyre, 2020. [#] Food Banks Canada, 2019. ** Campaign 2000, 2020. [††] Citizens for Public Justice, 2020. [‡‡] Canadian Index of Wellbeing Network, 2016.

Population health disparities continue in Canada, despite some broad improvements in individual health (Raphael et al., 2020). Determinants of health such as income and social status, social support networks, social environments, and employment/working conditions influence the health of Canadians (see Chapter 1 for a discussion about the determinants of health).

Factors Predisposing People to Vulnerability (Health Inequities)

Considering the key determinant of income and social status, it is clear that disparities contribute to health inequities. Some people do not have the financial resources to pay for costs related to medical care, such as medical supplies, transportation to health centres, and associated costs such as meals and accommodation. Others who are self-employed or work in small businesses may not have health benefits. A lack of financial resources or health benefits may cause some to avoid preventive health services. Doing so leaves them at an increased risk of experiencing the effects of preventable illnesses. Certain preventive health tests are not covered by many government health insurance plans, such as the prostate-specific antigen test for prostate cancer detection.

Dental health may also be compromised for some because it is not covered by government health insurance plans. People living with low income are the group that is most marginalized by the current dental care system, which relies on employment benefits, health insurance, or personal funds for payment. While oral health greatly impacts a person's overall physical and mental health, and contributes to time lost from work or school, over 32% of Canadians have no dental insurance (Canadian Dental Association, 2017). Groups subjected to structural vulnerabilities, including people given low incomes, are found to be systematically disadvantaged from accessing dental care that is organized around private purchase and provision of services. Other populations who experience inequities and harms include young children living in low-income families; young adults and others working without dental insurance; elderly people living in institutions or with low incomes; Indigenous peoples; refugees and immigrants; people with disabilities; and people living in rural and remote regions (Canadian Academy of Health Sciences, 2014). In a large sample of people experiencing social and health inequities, the prevalence of self-rated poor oral health was found to be high and dramatically worse than what is found in the general population. Significant relationships were observed between poor oral health and vulnerabilities related to mental health, trauma, and housing instability (Wallace, Browne, Varcoe, et al., 2015).

Low income and poverty increase health disparities and inequities across a number of health issues. Income inequality greatly impacts overall living standards and well-being (Canadian Index of Wellbeing Network, 2016), so structurally vulnerable populations are disadvantaged, and widespread health disparities exist for these populations. The severity of these determinants of health on people who are structurally vulnerable varies depending on factors such as geography, support systems, and policies. Understanding poverty and its relationship to health is crucial for effective CHN practice.

Age is another factor that contributes to increased vulnerability. For example, the very young and the very old have fewer coping resources (physiological, sociological, psychological), resulting in enhanced health risks such as opportunistic infections and chronic diseases. The features of **inequity** are experienced across other key determinants of health, but for the purposes of this text, poverty and age will be highlighted.

POVERTY

Around the world, people living in poverty tend to have the worst health. Evidence shows that health and social status are intimately linked. Studying these inequalities reveals that people with higher social status tend to have better health, while those with lower social status tend to have worse health outcomes (PHAC, 2018; Raphael et al., 2020). In general, **poverty** refers to having insufficient financial resources to meet basic living expenses: food, shelter, clothing, transportation, and medical expenses. Other items such as personal-care products, school supplies, and cellphones or Internet that are very much a part of social functioning, are not usually factored in. The Ottawa Charter for Health Promotion (WHO, 1986) indicates that one of the basic prerequisites for health

is income. For years, income level has been used as the criterion that determines whether someone is considered to be poor. People who experience poverty are more likely to live in unsafe environments, work at high-risk jobs, eat less nutritious foods, and have multiple stressors.

The term *poverty* can be more specifically defined as *absolute poverty, relative poverty,* and *subjective poverty.* **Absolute poverty** refers to "a deprivation of resources that is life-threatening" while **relative poverty** "refers to a deprivation of some individuals in relation to those who have more" and in this way is a measure of inequity (Beckmann Murray, Proctor Zentner, Pangman, et al., 2009, p. 15). **Subjective poverty** refers to the accounts of individuals and families of insufficient income to meet their expenses (Phipps, 2003).

Canada, in contrast to the United States, does not have an official poverty line. Instead, Canadian researchers use Statistics Canada's before-tax low-income cut-offs, or LICOs, to determine poverty status. LICOs are "income thresholds below which a family will likely devote a larger share of its income on the necessities of food, shelter and clothing than the average family" (Statistics Canada, 2020).

In 2018, 8.7% of the Canadian population lived on a low income, a rate that has been trending downward since 2015 when just over 12% of the population was officially recorded as living in poverty (Statistics Canada, 2020). Hourly wages have increased over time, along with trends upwards in economic resiliency. Poverty is tracked through Canadian statistics and advocacy agencies. The national poverty rate in Canada dropped to 8.7% in 2018 compared with 9.5% a year earlier, with poverty among older persons at 6.7%. However, the child poverty rate changed very little at 8.2%, with 566 000 children living in poverty compared to one million at a peak in 2012 (Statistics Canada, 2020). Related measures of housing needs and food insecurity, however, are increasing, along with overall income disparity. As such, vulnerabilities related to poverty and income warrant careful attention, assessment, and advocacy from CHNs.

Most people experiencing poverty in Canada endure the effects of constant deprivation: a persistent feeling of being trapped and that life is about surviving each day. In this way of life, there is no choice, there is no flexibility, and, if something unexpected happens—a sickness, accident, family death, fire, theft, or rent increase—there is no buffer to deal with the emergency. It is essential for CHNs to show respect for patients and attempt to understand how patients' life situations, such as the determinants of health, influence their health and well-being. Poverty is one health determinant that must be measured against the presence of other determinants that may increase or decrease the negative effects of poverty. The causes of poverty are complex and interrelated, as are the outcomes.

Poverty and Health

Canadians who live with low income experience greater health inequities compared with Canadians who have higher income. A variety of tools bring together information about the links between social determinants and health, including income and social status, that inform community health interventions and social planning. They include mapping strategies (Canadian Council on Social Determinants of Health, 2014) and social science approaches to program implementation and evaluation (Gruß Bunce, Davis, et al., 2021).

Understanding the impact and resulting vulnerabilities from poverty is an important starting place for CHNs to provide care to people in the community. Although it is difficult to change a family's economic circumstances as one individual CHN, nurses can play a critical role to address SDOH through screening and effective coordination of care, and they can and do influence morbidity and mortality. Across the lifespan, poverty plays an important role in health, adding to the disparities and health inequities. Those who are living in poverty have higher rates of infant morbidity and mortality, a shorter life expectancy, and more complex health problems (Raphael et al., 2020). The role of the CHN is to minimize the effects of SDOH, including poverty, on health and well-being through practice, research, and professional education. The "CHN Support and Care for a Family Living with Poverty" box discusses how a CHN can support a family living with poverty that seeks to improve its health.

CHN IN PRACTICE: A CASE STUDY

CHN Support and Care for a Family Living with Poverty

Jayda lives with her children—a daughter, 12; a son, 5; and infant twin girls—and her common-law husband, Jack, in subsidized housing. The CHN, Vanessa, has been impressed with Jayda's friendliness and confidence despite the many challenges she faces, including uncontrolled diabetes, chronic fatigue syndrome, and now, a prolapsed uterus. Jayda's 12-year-old daughter has recently been diagnosed with attention deficit hyperactivity disorder, depression, and a hearing deficit. At age 5, Jayda's son has struggled with learning basic letters and numbers. Neither adult is currently employed and finances are very tight, with social assistance benefits being their sole income. They cannot afford a cellphone, and often rely on the local food bank. Jayda's family lives close by and provides some help when they can.

Vanessa began working with this family because one twin was diagnosed with failure to thrive at her 6-month checkup. A priority was to determine whether there was enough food in the home and why one twin was so much smaller than the other. The CHN communicated her compassion for the family by listening carefully when taking histories on each family member. She demonstrated concern and care by monitoring the smaller twin's growth and development each week. In addition, it was a priority to improve Jayda's health so that she could take care of her children and herself in the future.

Vanessa's interventions included assessing Jayda's blood sugar level and the family's food intake and access to food at each visit. Vanessa discussed meal planning with the whole family based on food bank and other temporary supports. Vanessa also located local tutoring programs to help the older children with their learning needs and arranged for hearing aids for the older daughter, as well as visits to a community mental health nurse to treat Jayda's depression. Vanessa found an infant development program with family

support workers who do home visits and are able to show Jayda how to stimulate the twins' development. When summer approached, Vanessa also found community children's programs that would provide the two older children with learning opportunities, recreation, and supervision while Jayda recuperated from a scheduled hysterectomy to repair her prolapsed uterus. Vanessa showed Jayda and Jack materials to assist them with pursuing employment that could fit with their family responsibilities and qualifications. Over time, one step at a time, through a strong CHN-patient relationship, listening, and providing the right referrals at the right time, support is possible even when there are numerous cumulative vulnerabilities for a family to address.

Think About It

1. Identify the strengths in this family. Consider how to work with these strengths, even when there are overwhelming cumulative vulnerabilities.
2. Based on this patient situation, which actions by the CHN relate to the Canadian Community Health Nursing Professional Practice Model and Standards of Practice (see Appendix 1)?

Poor health outcomes often result from barriers that impede access to health care, such as geographical location, language barriers, access to a health care provider, transportation difficulties, inconvenient clinic hours, lack of health information, stigma, and the negative attitudes of health care providers toward patients living with poverty (Bhatt & Bathija, 2018). Poverty adds to barriers to people's access to health care and can be especially difficult for those considered to be working poor for whom many employers, especially those paying low or minimum wage, do not provide extended health benefits to their employees. Poverty, while presenting a significant obstacle to health across the lifespan, has an especially negative effect on women. Women, due to their gender, are highly vulnerable to poverty as they are more likely to be working in jobs that pay the minimum wage. In addition, they often have lone-parenting responsibilities. These factors may result in women being more dependent than men on social services (Raphael et al., 2020). Women are disproportionately impacted by poverty, as are children. According to Campaign 2000 (2020), which is a public education movement working to reduce child poverty, in 2018, 8.2% of children in Canada lived in poverty, a rate that has gone down steadily over the past 6 years. Unfortunately, 1.2 million children were food insecure in 2017–2018, representing the highest number recorded since food insecurity monitoring began in Canada (Campaign 2000, 2020).

Poverty affects child growth, development, and well-being in ways such as increased chronic illness and accidental injury, as well as low birth weight, and decreased language acquisition and reading development. Poverty also leads to longer-term problems with diet and mental health (Desapriya & Khoshpouri, 2018). Income-based inequalities in accessing mental health services are notable in Canada, where many psychosocial services are provided on a fee-for-service basis. Employment benefit programs provide only limited support for these mental health supports, and many people are unable to access these evidence-based therapies at all (Bartram, 2019). Poverty intersects and impacts access to health services and many other determinants, for example, homelessness and housing stability.

HOMELESSNESS AND HOUSING INSTABILITY

Related to poverty, access to housing is marked with inequalities in Canada and throughout the world. Homelessness is increasing globally, and, not surprisingly, homelessness in Canada is following the same trend. The number of homeless people in Canada is difficult to determine for many reasons, with one of the main difficulties being that census data are collected through enumeration of people with an address. With limitations of the record keeping and surveys in mind, it is estimated that in Canada between 150 000 and 300 000 individuals are homeless (Employment and Social Development Canada, 2017). Identification of people experiencing homelessness often relies on shelters and other homeless-serving organizations, where several groups are not represented, however (for example, homeless women, who represent 27.3% of people experiencing homelessness in Canada). Studies show that homeless women are at higher risk of violence and assault, sexual exploitation, and abuse. Many women experience what is referred to as hidden homelessness because they prefer to avoid the shelter system and the streets, even if it means staying in dangerous situations, including ones where there is domestic violence. While the risk of violence is present for women experiencing homelessness, domestic violence is also a major *cause* of homelessness for women, alongside other factors of gender inequality, such as poverty related to income inequality, sole parenting, and family responsibilities, which also contribute to food insecurity and other health problems. The complex and interconnected nature of vulnerabilities is vital to understanding the concept of homelessness.

Understanding the Concept of Homelessness

Many contributing factors can lead to homelessness. Box 15.1 presents a few of these factors. For example, if there is limited housing, accommodation prices usually increase and, therefore, housing becomes unaffordable for the population that is living on a limited income. Homelessness and poverty are interrelated, and both are affected by other inequities, such as employment. When companies close or relocate, former employees may go long periods without a steady income. Often these displaced workers seek out full-time work but may be able to find part-time work only; these individuals are considered to be underemployed. An increase in part-time jobs may mean that a higher number of people are underemployed. Sometimes workers take any job they can find because they are facing economic hardship. Some workers may be overqualified for the job they do. This kind of employment scenario frequently occurs with newcomers who, for a variety of reasons (e.g., a language barrier and qualifications from their homeland that are not recognized in Canada), may be unable to work in their field of expertise. Factors such as unemployment,

> **BOX 15.1 Contributing Factors to Homelessness**
>
> - Lack of affordable housing
> - Low income or poverty
> - Mental health issues
> - Substance use
> - Unemployment or underemployment
> - Immigration
> - Violence and criminal history
> - Family conflict

underemployment, overwork (such as having numerous jobs or working more than 40 hours a week), and stress at work are associated with poor health that may impact housing stability (Canadian Observatory on Homelessness, 2021).

Many segments of the population experience homelessness. Homelessness can be considered as absolute homelessness, sheltered homelessness, and hidden homelessness (Gaetz, Barr, Friesen, et al., 2012). **Absolute homelessness** describes the condition of people who are perpetually homeless; they are sometimes referred to as the *chronic homeless*. Absolutely homeless people are often observed sleeping on park benches or sidewalks and begging on the streets. They experience chronic and persistent poverty along with other risk factors (i.e., mental or physical disabilities, substance use problems, severe mental illness, other chronic health problems, and chronic family difficulties, poverty, limited social support).

Sheltered homelessness describes the condition of people who need to use emergency shelters either occasionally or regularly for sleeping purposes. **Hidden homelessness** describes the condition of people who may be sleeping in their vehicles and/or using the couch or other temporary sleeping cot at a friend's home. As noted earlier, the visible homeless population is between 150 000 to 300 000, but the hidden homeless population is considered to be at least three times higher, between 450 000 and 900 000 (Gaetz, Dej, Richter, et al., 2016). People who experience hidden homelessness may be affected by crisis poverty (temporary transient poverty):

- Lives are generally marked by hardship and struggle
- Homelessness is often transient or episodic
- The homeless person may resort to brief stays in shelters or other temporary accommodations
- Homelessness may result from lack of employment opportunities, lack of education, obsolete job skills, or domestic violence. These issues lead to persistent poverty and need to be addressed, along with efforts to find stable housing.

CHNs may have the opportunity to work with homeless patients in emergency shelters, while home visiting a family who has a homeless person temporarily living with them, or when other community agencies refer homeless patients to CHNs. Although people who have never been homeless usually cannot truly understand what it means to be homeless, CHNs can increase their sensitivity toward the homeless population by examining their own personal beliefs, values, and knowledge of homelessness. The "How to" box presents questions CHNs can reflect on.

HOW TO ...

Evaluate the Concept of Homelessness
- What is it like to live on the streets?
- What issues might confront a young mother and her children inside a homeless shelter?
- How is it that people are so poor that they have no place to go?
- What really causes homelessness?
- How do you respond to a person on the street asking for money to buy a sandwich or catch a bus?
- How is your response different (or not) when a young mother with children asks you for money?
- How do you react to the smell of urine in a stairwell or elevator?

The "CHN in Practice: A Case Study, Street Outreach to King Street Supported Housing Units" box identifies some of the concerns related to a street outreach setting.

CHN IN PRACTICE: A CASE STUDY

Street Outreach to King Street Supported Housing Units
Lisa is a CHN working with an outreach community health service in a mid-sized Canadian city. One of the settings Lisa visits is a collection of supported housing units in the urban core. One of these units is for adolescent women leaving sex work. Shawna is an 18-year-old woman who has been at the housing unit for less than a month and is currently being treated for sexually transmitted infections (STIs). Lisa is providing Shawna information about the medication regime and follow-up care for STIs, as well as other supportive counselling. While Shawna is also receiving social services and vocational supports in pursuit of work and longer-term housing, she is overwhelmed by the transition and loneliness of semi-independent living after two years of living with a pimp and a group of sex workers.

Think About It
1. What community health nursing interventions could Lisa employ that might have a positive impact on the determinants of health currently affecting Shawna and other populations who are structurally vulnerable populations, such as people leaving sex work?
2. How can Lisa help Shawna become more empowered, considering the complex individual and social determinants of health Shawna is experiencing?

For further information on homelessness and poverty, see the Homeless Hub, a large web-based resource centre for knowledge, mobilization, and networking in the field of homelessness research in Canada, and also the Government of Canada's Homelessness Strategy Directives (the links are on the Evolve website).

Effects of Housing Instability on Health

Homelessness has important health implications. People experiencing homelessness have an increased risk for a wide range of health concerns, such as problematic substance use, mental illness, human immunodeficiency virus (HIV) and acquired immunodeficiency syndrome (AIDS), tuberculosis (TB), STIs, unplanned pregnancies, seizures, chronic obstructive pulmonary disease, musculoskeletal disorders, and skin and foot problems (Guirguis-Younger, McNeil, & Hwang, 2014). Access to health care services is a problem for many homeless people. For example, a man with type 1 diabetes who lives on the street may sleep in a shelter. Getting adequate rest and exercise, taking insulin on a schedule, eating regular meals, attending to foot and skin care, and following a prescribed diet are virtually impossible. How does one purchase an antibiotic without money? How is a child treated for scabies and pediculosis when there are no bathing facilities? How does an older person with peripheral vascular disease elevate his legs when he must be out of the shelter at 7 a.m. and on the streets all day? These health concerns are often related to gross inequities and limited access to basic health and social care. People experiencing homelessness devote a large portion of their time to just trying to survive. Health promotion activities in these circumstances are far from the everyday reality for many people.

People living on the streets spend many hours on their feet and often sleep in positions that compromise their peripheral circulation. Hypertension is exacerbated by high rates of alcohol use and high sodium content foods served in fast-food restaurants, shelters, and other meal sites. Crowded living conditions put homeless people at risk for exposure to viruses and bacteria that cause pneumonia and TB. Hepatitis and HIV are also growing concerns among the homeless population. In addition to its effects on physical health, homelessness also affects psychological, social, and spiritual well-being. Becoming homeless means more than losing a home or a regular place to sleep and eat; it also means losing friends, personal possessions, and familiar surroundings. People without stable homes often live in constant change, chaos, confusion, and fear. Many describe experiencing a loss of dignity, low self-esteem, a lack of social support, and generalized despair. Furthermore, homelessness contributes to early death; it is estimated to erase as much as 25 years off a person's life, and inequitable access to palliative and end-of-life care leaves many people to die in the streets, in shelters, and in encampments without basic rights to comfort and compassion (Reimer-Kirkham, Stajduhar, Pauly, et al., 2016; Stajduhar & Mollison, 2018).

Homelessness and At-Risk Populations

Being homeless affects health across the lifespan, from pregnancy to childhood, adolescence, and older adulthood, at end of life, and during grief and bereavement. Each group has different needs, and CHNs need to be aware of the unique needs of homeless patients at every age. CHNs need to identify the precursors to homelessness; anticipate the effects of homelessness on physical, emotional, and spiritual well-being; become knowledgeable about resources to assist those without housing stability; assist those without homes to gain access to needed health care services; work with communities to build capacity to work with this population and to address health inequities; participate in activities that will facilitate the building of healthy public policies to address homelessness; and work toward reorienting the health system so that it focuses on a socioenvironmental street approach for the homeless population. The work of street nurse Cathy Crowe, discussed in Chapter 3, provides CHNs with a strong example of the importance of the advocacy role of CHNs for people experiencing structural vulnerabilities and of working with them to empower, support, and encourage change in the sociopolitical community environment.

VIOLENCE

The intersecting social determinants of poverty (socioeconomic status), urban crowding (housing), unemployment, gender inequality, ageism, and racism are identified as factors that influence violence. **Violence** is generally defined as nonaccidental acts, interpersonal or intrapersonal, that result in physical or psychological injury to one or more persons. Violence can be physical, psychological, sexual, financial, or spiritual abuse. In this section, homicides, social and community factors that influence violence, and violence as a form of abuse are discussed.

Violence is a major cause of premature mortality and lifelong disability, and violence-related morbidity is a significant factor in health care costs. CHNs often care for the victims, the perpetrators, and those who witness physical and psychological violence. CHNs also can take an active role in the development of community responses to violence by contributing to the development of public policy and needed resources.

Homicides

In 2018, Canadian police services reported 651 homicides—15 fewer victims than the previous year. Although the homicide rate fell 4% in 2018 (to 1.76 per 100 000 population), it remains higher than the national average for the previous decade. While homicide continues to be a relatively rare occurrence, representing less than 0.2% of all violent crimes in Canada in 2018, homicide rates are considered benchmarks for levels of violent activity both in Canada and internationally. Disparities do exist between provinces and territories with regard to homicide rates; while all other provinces saw a decline in the rate of homicides, in 2018 there was a record number for Ontario, with an increase of 49 homicides that occurred in the census metropolitan area (CMA) of Toronto.

The national rate of firearm-related homicides declined 8% in 2018. This marks the first decrease of homicides committed with a firearm since 2013, with Prince Edward Island, Yukon, the Northwest Territories, and Nunavut reporting no firearm-related homicides in 2018.

Disparities also exist for structurally vulnerable groups, and there were 140 Indigenous victims of homicide reported in 2018, representing 22% of all homicide victims throughout Canada (Statistics Canada, 2019a).

Although much of the focus is often on homicides linked to criminal activity, the majority of homicides in Canada

are committed by an acquaintance (34%), a family member (33%), a stranger (19%), or by someone with whom the victim had a current or former intimate relationship—nonspousal (6%). In 2018, only 8% of victims were killed by someone with whom they had a criminal relationship. (Statistics Canada, 2019a).

Social and Community Factors That Influence Violence

Many factors in a community can support or minimize violence and contribute to resiliency, whether it relates to the examples given of homicide, or related to bullying, domestic violence, or other forms of abuse. Changing social conditions, multiple demands on people, economic conditions, and social institutions influence the level of violence and human abuse. Population characteristics, community resources, and community design and facilities can all influence the potential for violence, and mediate effects of violence in communities.

Population Characteristics

A community's structure can influence the potential for violence. For example, when people live in crowded conditions and in poverty, the potential is greater for community tensions and violence. Communities with a high population density can positively or negatively influence violence. Those with a sense of cohesiveness may have a lower crime rate than areas of similar size that lack social and cultural groups to support unity among members. For example, residents of public housing often form neighbourhood associations to deal with situations common to many or all residents. Tension can often be released in a productive way through projects carried out by the neighbourhood association.

Fear and apathy may cause community residents to withdraw from social contact. Withdrawal can foster crime because many residents assume someone else will report suspicious behaviour, or they fear reprisals for such reports. This tends to happen in larger communities in which the neighbourhood does not lend itself to social interaction and sharing because of highly mobile population patterns or where there is an environment that does not promote opportunities for neighbours to interact.

High population density areas may be characterized by a sense of confusion, resulting in disintegration and disorganization. These areas often have transient populations that have limited physical or emotional investment in the community. Lack of community concern allows crime and violence to go unchecked and may become a norm for the area. For instance, apathy and stereotyping about **sex workers** (or people who work for street or brothel prostitution, cybersex, pornography, massage parlours, and other areas of the sex industry) places these workers at even higher risk for violence. Also, as crime increases, residents who are able to move leave the area, contributing to higher concentrations of violence and community disintegration, as residents who leave are often the most capable of taking action within the population.

Community Resources and Facilities

Communities differ in the resources and facilities they provide to residents. Some communities are more desirable places to live, work, and raise families and have facilities that can reduce the potential for crime and violence. Recreational resources such as playgrounds, parks, swimming pools, movie theatres, tennis courts, basketball courts, walking trails, and bicycle paths provide socially acceptable outlets for a variety of feelings. These resources are adjuncts that residents can use for pleasure, personal enrichment, and group development. Spectator sports, such as football or hockey, also allow community members to express feelings of anger and frustration. However, viewing and playing physically aggressive sports can also encourage a sense of violence and contribute to higher rates of violence and substance use (Kingsland, Wiggers, Vashum, al., 2016). Familiarity with factors contributing to a community's violence or potential for violence enables CHNs to recognize those factors and intervene accordingly. It is the CHN's responsibility to work with the citizens and agencies of the community to correct or improve deficits. Factors to be included when assessing a community for violence are shown in Box 15.2.

Violence as a Form of Abuse

The potential for violence against individuals or groups (e.g., homicide, robbery, bullying, assault, and sexual assault) or oneself (e.g., suicide) is directly related to the level of violence in the community. Persons living in areas with high rates of crime and violence are more likely to become victims than those in more peaceful areas. The forms of violence that are most common are homicide and suicide. Homicide was discussed earlier in this chapter; suicide is discussed later in this chapter's discussion of community mental health. Next is a discussion of bullying, domestic violence, female genital mutilation, "honour"-based violence, assault, and sexual assault.

Bullying

Bullying is common across the lifespan: as many as 75% of people report that they have been affected by bullying, and one in five adolescents report being victimized through cyberbullying (PREVNet, 2019). Bullying can take many forms, such as physical, verbal, and social bullying, as well as cyberbullying, and it causes many ill effects including headaches, depression, anxiety, and risk of suicide. The incidence of school violence, such as bullying and violent fighting, by school-aged children and adolescents has increased and the overall solutions to this problem in Canada lag behind those of other countries (PREVNet, 2019; Public Safety Canada, 2018). Alongside schools, workplaces and older persons' lodges and assisted living environments are sites of commonplace and troubling bullying behaviours. Close to 20% of people describe workplace bullying or harassment experiences, with women reporting higher levels of harassment than men (Hango & Moyser, 2018), and 25% of older persons reporting having experienced bullying in a study of peer bullying in subsidized apartments in Canada (Goodridge , Heal-Salahub, PausJenssen, et al., 2017).

BOX 15.2 Indicators of Violence in Individual, Family, and Community Contexts

Individual Factors
- Signs of physical abuse (abrasions, contusions, burns)
- Physical symptoms related to emotional distress
- Developmental and behavioural difficulties
- Presence of physical disability
- Social isolation
- Decreased role performance within the family and in job- or school-related activities
- Mental health concerns such as depression, low self-esteem, and anxiety
- Fear of intimacy with others
- Substance abuse

Familial Factors
- Economic stressors
- Presence of some form of family violence
- Poor communication
- Problems with child rearing
- Lack of family cohesion
- Recurrent familial conflict
- Lack of social support networks
- Poor social integration into the community
- Multiple changes of residence
- Access to guns
- Homelessness
- Family needs require members to work, even though the work may be demoralizing or otherwise damaging

Community Characteristics
- High crime rate
- High levels of unemployment
- Lack of neighbourhood resources and support systems
- Lack of community cohesiveness
- Media glamorization or sensationalization of violence

Schools provide many programs to help students learn to deal with violence—for example, classes on bullying and its management—and have policies of zero tolerance for violence. Informed parents can assist and support their children to apply what they have learned about handling violence. Research shows that fighting back on bullying behaviours tends to worsen bullying, and children should be encouraged to be assertive and clear that the bullying behaviour is not okay. Reporting with the explicit goal of stopping the bullying is recommended, with effective use of role-play in practising both reporting and responding back to bullying behaviour. Practice with children and adolescents in this way can provide some skills and language that can then be available to them during a more emotionally-laden experience. Overall promotion and support of healthy relationships serves to prevent bullying and supports children and adolescents with communication and social skills, understanding and respecting social responsibility, and empathy for others. Reporting the violent behaviours, and demonstrating and practising respect for self and others, is the best prevention (PREVNet, 2019).

Domestic Violence

Violence or abuse that occurs between people who are related to each other or who have a relationship with each other is referred to as **domestic violence**. Domestic violence includes relationship or dating violence, spousal abuse, family violence, intimate partner violence, and gender-based violence. It can be perpetrated by one person over another in a single act or a series of acts that form a pattern of abuse that causes fear or physical and/or psychological harm. The violence or harm can take many forms (e.g., physical, verbal, sexual, emotional and psychological, and financial) and people may experience more than one kind of violence or harm. Five categories of maltreatment or abuse are:

- *Physical abuse.* It involves applying force to any part of another person's body. It includes grabbing, pushing, hitting, shaking, choking, biting, kicking, burning, poisoning, or other dangerous use of force.
- *Sexual abuse.* It involves using a child or other person for sexual purposes and exploitation. It might include fondling, intercourse, incest, sodomy, exhibitionism, prostitution, or pornographic exposure.
- *Emotional and psychological abuse.* It involves using emotional behaviours to decrease a person's or child's self-esteem and self-image. It might include verbal threats, social isolation, intimidation, exploitation, terrorizing, manipulation, or consistently making unreasonable demands.
- *Financial abuse.* It involves the misuse of a person's funds and assets. It includes theft of funds from a bank account or obtaining property or other purchases without full knowledge and consent. In the case of a victim who is not competent, abuse may also involve using the person's funds or making financial choices that are not in the best interests of that person.
- *Neglect.* It involves, intentionally or not, failing to provide care for those who are dependent. It might include not attending to their physical, emotional, educational, and medical needs, and abandonment (Department of Justice, 2017a).

Victims of domestic violence can be children, women, men, same-sex partners, and older persons. The majority of victims of family violence are females. Approximately 57% of child and youth victims are females and 43% are males. For the 18 965 children and youth victimized by a family member, a parent was the most common perpetrator (59% of the time) (Statistics Canada, 2019b). Consider the following 2018 statistics on family violence:

- Rates of police-reported family violence and domestic homicide are generally declining.
- Rural rates of police-reported family violence against children and youth are nearly twice as high as urban rates.
- Spousal violence was the most common form of family violence, with nearly half of family violence occurring at the hands of a current or former spouse (married or common-law), and women remain four times more likely to be victims of spousal homicide than men.
- Police-reported family-related sexual offences are nearly five times higher for female children and youth than their male counterparts.

BOX 15.3 Risk and Resiliency Factors for Mental Health Problems After Intimate Partner Violence

Key Risk Factors

- A history of childhood sexual abuse
- The use of avoidance coping
- Having maladaptive negative beliefs, such as self-blame
- Receiving negative reactions or support, including negative religious coping
- Having experienced psychological violence or sexual violence, especially if combined with physical violence

Key Factors in Resiliency

- The availability of positive support systems (i.e., informal and formal)
- Positive religious support
- Higher education
- Marriage versus cohabitation
- Having some control over the legal process

Source: Adapted from Carter-Snell, C., & Jakubec, S. (2013). Exploring influences on mental health after interpersonal violence against women. *International Journal of Child, Youth and Family Studies, 1,* 72–99.

- Rates of family violence are highest among females aged 30 to 34 and males aged 15 to 19.
- Older persons represented a relatively small proportion (3%) of all family violence victims. Older persons who experienced family violence most often experienced family violence by their adult children. (Statistics Canada, 2019b).

Violence that can cause significant injury and death takes the following three forms: sexual abuse, emotional abuse, and physical abuse. Generally, violence within families is perpetrated by the most powerful members against the least powerful ones. Intimate partner violence is directed primarily toward the partner who may be perceived as being the nondominant partner in the relationship (although this partner may fight back physically). Partners can be heterosexual or homosexual and may or may not be married. Intimate partner violence, including both spousal and dating violence, accounts for one in every four violent crimes reported to police.

Understanding domestic violence, mental health consequences, and contributing factors is helpful in preventing **secondary victimization,** which is when survivors experience further stress or trauma at the hands of social and health care workers who engage in discrimination, victim blaming, insensitive communication techniques, disbelief, shaming, stigmatization, or minimization of the experience (Fleckinger, 2020). Because of the high rate of the patterns of secondary victimization and discrimination, CHNs' understanding of sexual assault and its effects, trauma- and violence-informed care, prevention, and treatment are important mental health and public health concerns. Risk and resiliency factors for mental health problems after intimate partner violence are presented in Box 15.3.

CHNs need to be alert for signs and symptoms of potential abuse. A variety of risk-assessment tools exist for **intimate partner violence,** which is physical or sexual harassment or psychological aggression by a current or former intimate partner (including a spouse, dating partner, or domestic living partner). The reason for the assessment should determine which tool to select (Northcott, 2012). For example, is it to determine a risk assessment of a spousal assault offender, to determine lethality, or to determine spousal assault recidivism? (*Recidivism* refers to a person's relapse into crime.) The Ontario Domestic Assault Risk Assessment (ODARA) is the first validated domestic-violence risk-assessment tool available to assess the likelihood of wife assault. This 13-question (yes-or-no answer) tool calculates the likelihood of assault based on assaults that are known to police; it can then be used to predict the risk of repeated domestic assault of females by males. The tool compares the male under study with other males who have assaulted their wives. A Likert scale of 0 to 7 ranks the likelihood for repeat domestic assault by the male, with a higher number indicating a greater likelihood of assault. There are two ODARA tools: the ODARA-LE (Ontario Domestic Assault Risk Assessment—Law Enforcement) for police use and the ODARA-C (Ontario Domestic Assault Risk Assessment—Clinical) for use by health care providers (Department of Justice, 2015; Northcott, 2012).

For further information on domestic violence (all forms of abuse), refer to the Government of Canada's "About Family Violence" link on the Evolve website. This website covers topics related to identifying family violence (with information on different age groups), and legal and governmental resources. A tab to quickly exit the site is available for those who may be searching the site seeking safety and concerned about being identified.

All individuals in Canada who suspect child abuse are required to report it to the proper child protection agencies as mandated by law (Department of Justice, 2017b). Indigenous peoples have their own child protection agencies (Department of Justice, 2015). The Department of Justice (2017b) has an information site called *Child Abuse is Wrong: What Can I Do?* that defines and discusses the various types of child abuse, prevalence of child abuse, law, as well as prevention and management. Identifying abusive parents and recognizing child abuse are topics covered in the "How to" boxes that follow.

✳ HOW TO …

Identify Warning Signs for Needed Support and Early Intervention to Prevent Child Abuse

The following characteristics constitute warning signs of actual or potential child abuse:
- Denial of the reality of the pregnancy—that is, refusal to talk about the impending birth or to think of a name for the child
- An obvious concern or fear that the baby will not meet desired expectations: sex, hair colour, temperament, or resemblance to family members
- Failure to follow through on the desire for an abortion
- An initial decision to place the child for adoption and a change of mind
- Rejection of the mother by the father of the baby
- Family experiencing stress and numerous crises, and the birth of a child may be the "last straw"
- Initial and unresolved negative feelings about having a child
- Lack of support for the new parents
- Isolation from friends, neighbours, or family
- Parental evidence of poor impulse control or fear of losing control
- Contradictory history
- Appearance of detachment
- Appearance of misusing medications or alcohol
- Shopping for hospitals or health care providers
- Unrealistic expectations of the child
- Verbal, physical, or sexual abuse of mother by father, especially during pregnancy
- Child not biological offspring of stepfather or mother's current partner
- Excessive talk of needing to "discipline" children and plans to use harsh physical punishment to enforce discipline

---

✳ HOW TO …

Recognize Actual or Potential Child Abuse

Be alert to the following:
- An unexplained injury
- Injuries to the skin: burns, old or recent scars, ecchymosis, soft tissue swelling, human bites
- Fractures: recent or older ones that have healed
- Subdural hematomas
- Trauma to genitalia
- Whiplash (caused by shaking small children)
- Dehydration or malnourishment without obvious cause
- Provision of inappropriate food or medications (alcohol, tobacco, medication prescribed for someone else, foods not appropriate for the age)
- Evidence of poor general care: poor hygiene and grooming or dirty clothes
- Unusual fear of CHN and others
- Evidence that child is considered to be a "bad" child
- Inappropriate dress for the season or weather conditions
- Reports or evidence shown by child of sexual abuse
- Injuries not mentioned in history
- Apparent need to take care of the parent and speak for the parent
- Maternal depression
- Maladjustment of older siblings

Female Genital Mutilation

Female genital mutilation (FGM) is "any procedure that injures or removes all or part of the external female genital organs for non-medical reasons." In Canada, FGM of a child is a crime and is considered to be a form of child abuse (Department of Justice, 2017b). FGM is a practice that is centuries old and is common in many African countries and certain Asian and Middle Eastern countries. Justification for FGM is related to tradition, power inequities, and the desire for women to adhere to community norms or law (WHO, 2016).

Harmful—and at times life-threatening—this act of violence is practised against women in violation of human rights, FGM can take several forms. The extent of mutilation can vary, ranging from the excision of the clitoris with partial or total removal of the labia minora, to the severe form, in which the labia majora are fused following the removal of the clitoris and labia minora. These procedures are associated with morbidity related to substantial complications such as severe pain, hemorrhage, infection, tetanus, and septicemia. Long-term effects of FGM include impaired urinary and menstrual functioning, chronic genital pain, cysts, and risk of childbirth complication and newborn deaths (WHO, 2016). Increasingly, women who were mutilated are immigrating to Canada, mostly residing in urban centres. Performing this procedure has been illegal in Canada since 1997, when the Criminal Code was amended to include the practice. CHNs need to be familiar with the practices of newcomers to Canada and also for Canadian practices of male circumcision, which is no longer a recommended medical practice (Dave, Afshar, Braga et al., 2018). Cultural practices can impact health in ways that may be supportive or harmful. For further information, see the WHO and UNICEF links on female genital mutilation, found on the Evolve website.

"Honour"-Based Violence: Honour Killings

"Honour"-based violence (HBV) is considered a distinct form of family violence. Most often, the victim is female. Occurring within the family and community sphere, it is an act that is deliberately intended to restore "honour" to the family and is rooted in men's efforts to control women's sexual and social lives (Department of Justice, 2016; Gill, 2014). HBV occurs across a wide range of communities, ethnic groups, and religions. In an **"honour" killing**, a family member or a self-appointed community leader kills another person perceived as having brought dishonour to the family or community by breaking from traditional social conduct (e.g., by dating or having a relationship with someone not approved by the family, being sexually assaulted, identifying too much with Western culture and ideas, defying family guidance or refusing an arranged marriage, pursuing a higher education or career, or leaving an abusive spouse). "Honour" killings are homicides, but because the motives behind this form of violence are in honour of tradition, religion, or culture, the term *honour* is used. Nonetheless, no honour exists in "honour" killing.

Assault

In large urban centres, CHNs in home health care may encounter patients who have been assaulted and have long-term health problems such as head injuries, spinal cord injuries, or stomas from traumas such as motor vehicle crashes or abdominal gunshot wounds. In addition to physical care, CHNs also address the emotional trauma resulting from violence. They can support victims as they make sense of their traumatic experiences, identify strengths and community supports, and refer them for further counselling if anxiety, sleeping problems, substance use or depression become persistent and interfere with functioning.

Sexual Assault

Sexual assault is sexual contact with another person without that person's consent. Often, physically abused women are also forced into sex. Sexual assault has implications for the prevention of unintended and adolescent pregnancies, HIV, AIDS, and STIs as well as for women's healthy sexuality and self-esteem. The term *rape* is no longer used in Canada. Instead, based on the terminology used in the Criminal Code of Canada, the term *sexual assault* is used. Sexual assault offences include sexual assault, sexual assault with a weapon, and aggravated sexual assault.

Sexual assault is one of the most underreported forms of human violence. The majority of violence against women is intimate partner violence. Sexual assault also happens to men, especially boys and young men, but the statistics on the incidence of male sexual assault vary. In the majority of cases, sexual offenders are known to their victims. Prevention of sexual assault, like that of other forms of human abuse, requires a broad-based community focus for educating both the community as a whole and key groups such as police, health care providers, educators, and social workers.

A first step in intervening in the incidence and treatment of sexual assault survivors is to change and clarify misconceptions about sexual assault and its survivors. Sexual assault is a crime of violence, not a crime of passion. The underlying issues are hostility, power, and control rather than sexual desire. The defining issue is lack of consent of the victim. When a woman or man refuses any sexual activity, that refusal means "no." People have the right to change their mind, even when they seemed initially agreeable. Pressure from physical contact, threats, or deliberate inducement of drug or alcohol intoxication is a violation of the law. The myths continue that women say no to sex when they really mean yes, and that the victims of sexual assault are culpable because of the way they dress or act. On campuses and workplaces throughout the country and elsewhere, negative attitudes toward acquaintance or "date rape" have been slow to change, as highlighted in several high-profile cases and media explorations of the issue.

During the act of sexual assault, the person assaulted is often hit, kicked, stabbed, and severely beaten. This violence further traumatizes victims because in addition to the violation of the sense of self, they fear for their life and are inundated with feelings of helplessness, lack of control, and vulnerability. People react to sexual assault differently, depending on their personality, past experiences, background, and the support received after the trauma. Some cry, shout, or discuss the experience. Others withdraw or may be confused and may be ashamed or otherwise fearful about discussing the attack. During the immediate as well as follow-up stages, victims tend to blame themselves for what happened. Effective prevention of secondary adverse mental health consequences depends on the identification of resiliency factors. The CHN can draw on the victim's strengths to promote patient agency and shape interventions. For example, the CHN could help the individual reframe events to reduce self-blame and identify individuals or agencies that may provide supportive reactions, therapy, and legal advice and resources.

It is important while working with sexual assault victims to help them identify the issues behind self-blame. Although fault should not be placed on survivors, they should be encouraged to take control, learn assertiveness, and therefore believe that they can take certain actions to prevent future sexual assaults. Survivors need to talk about what happened and to express their feelings and fears in a nonjudgemental

atmosphere. Nonjudgemental listening is important. In any psychological trauma, the right to privacy and confidentiality is crucial. Sexual assault victims should be given privacy, respect, and assurance of confidentiality; told about health care procedures conducted immediately after the sexual assault; and offered a complete physical examination, possibly by a sexual assault nurse examiner (SANE), a role discussed in Chapter 3.

People in rural communities do not regularly receive comprehensive health care following sexual assaults, which can result in higher rates of mental illness, substance abuse, revictimization, and chronic health problems. Rural victims are also at risk for secondary victimization, the stigmatization and revictimization that results from the responses of others to the assault. The potential for secondary victimization increases when rural victims must be transported out of their community for treatment, face delays in services, and encounter health care providers who react negatively toward them or provide incomplete services (Carter-Snell, Jakubec & Hagen, 2020) (see Evidence-Informed Practice box, below).

EVIDENCE-INFORMED PRACTICE

After a recent sexual assault, patients in many rural and remote communities do not typically receive comprehensive services. Delays in service with staff shortages, lack of familiarity with procedures, negative responses such as disbelief regarding the assault, and even turning patients away and requiring them to travel elsewhere—away from their support systems—are all too frequently experienced by people who live in rural and remote communities. These experiences increase their risks for mental health disorders and chronic diseases, placing a significant burden both on the patient's health and on the community.

Supporting the capacity of rural crisis and health care providers to provide comprehensive sexual assault services is a priority for reducing the risks of secondary victimization and other mental health impacts for sexual assault victims. A research study by Carter-Snell, Jakubec, and Hagen (2020) sought to find ways of addressing these risks, understanding, and implementing the educational resources needed for crisis care workers in rural and Indigenous communities in Alberta. A participatory action research approach was used in five Canadian communities to find collaborative solutions to their unique community challenges. Mixed methods were used to collect data about the impact of community-identified interventions on knowledge, service quality, and comfort level in providing services. Interventions included support for multidisciplinary advisory teams, resource development, and education sessions for service providers. The specific and unique education selected by these communities provided trauma-informed knowledge of collaborative and comprehensive services in their community. Both focus group and survey data demonstrated increased collaboration and shared knowledge, enhanced communication, and

improved services such as provision of increased privacy for patients. Knowledge increased in all key areas of services and service quality. The data suggested that changes were sustained for at least 6 months post-training. Findings support the effectiveness of establishing a multidisciplinary community development program. Increased knowledge, comfort, and teamwork can improve the services that patients receive, influencing the health of both the individuals and the community.

Application for CHNs Recognize that comprehensive sexual assault response in any community is part of any usual holistic practice. Collaboration with the medical, policing, victim support, and community resources teams will support a comprehensive response. CHNs play an important role in understanding the collaborative team, making connections, referrals, and providing information for patients to enhance access to services and for services to respond with compassion and regard for promoting both health and justice. Regardless of whether a victim chooses to seek criminal charges in the short or longer term, CHNs can prevent secondary victimization with immediate, private, comprehensive, trauma- and violence-informed care.

Questions for Reflection and Discussion
1. What are some of the roles CHNs could be involved in as part of a comprehensive sexual assault service to people in rural communities?
2. How can CHNs prevent revictimization of rural patients who have experienced sexual assault?
3. How might CHNs collaborate with other members of the community health, social care, policing, and justice systems to support people in rural communities following sexual assault?

Source: Carter-Snell, C., Jakubec, S. L., & Hagen, B. (2020). Collaboration with rural and remote communities to improve sexual assault services. *Journal of Community Health, 45*(2), 377–387.

CHNs often provide continuous care once a sexual assault victim enters the health care system. Disclosure may occur to a CHN through a mental health nursing role, an STI program role, or other community health service. Because many victims deny the sexual assault once the initial crisis is past, a single-session debriefing should be completed during the initial examination. The health assessment and debriefing should be carried out by specially trained providers who have obtained the consent of the victim prior to using the sexual assault evidence kit (SAEK). In some provinces and territories, SANEs perform the health assessment in the emergency department to gather evidence, usually using a SAEK for criminal prosecution of sexual assault. This is an important community health nursing intervention, and it often takes time, which allows the SANE the opportunity to begin communication with the victim. The evidence collected by the SANE is credible and effective in resultant court proceedings. Certain tests should be offered to all sexual assault victims, such as a pregnancy test and tests for STIs. Sexual assault is a situational crisis for which advance preparation by the victim is rarely possible. Therefore, CHNs need to help victims cope with the stress and disruption of their lives caused by the attack. Counselling focuses on the crisis and the fears, feelings, and issues involved. CHNs help survivors learn how to regain their personal strength and reduce the immediate anxiety and confusion. If post-traumatic stress disorder (PTSD) has developed, professional psychological or psychiatric treatment is indicated.

Many sexual assault victims need follow-up mental health services to help them cope with the short-term and long-term effects of the crisis. The time after a sexual assault is one of disequilibrium, psychological breakdown, and reorganization of attitudes about the safety of the world. Common, everyday tasks often tax a person's resources and many individuals forget or fail to keep appointments. CHNs need to make appropriate referrals and obtain permission from the sexual assault victim to remain in contact through telephone conversations, which allows for ongoing assessment of the victim's needs and opportunities to intervene when needed.

COMMUNITY MENTAL HEALTH

Mental health is defined as more than the absence of illness; it is "a state of well-being in which the individual realizes his or her own potential, can cope with the normal stresses of life, can work productively and fruitfully, and is able to make a contribution to his or her own community" (WHO, 2018). Good mental health is an asset because it helps individuals manage stresses in daily living and, therefore, helps to protect them from mental health issues.

One in five Canadians will experience *mental illness* in their lifetime (Canadian Mental Health Association, 2021). All people will be affected by the mental illness of a friend, family member, coworker, or neighbour. Mental illness affects all individuals of all ages and does not discriminate between race, culture, sex, socioeconomic status, or educational level. Over half of Canadians (53%) consider anxiety and depression to be "epidemic" in Canada, with that perception spiking amongst younger people, according to a new survey commissioned by the Canadian Mental Health Association (CMHA): 59% of 18- to 34-year-olds consider anxiety and depression to be "epidemic" in Canada, followed closely by addiction (56%), and ahead of physical illnesses such as cancer, heart disease and stroke, as well as diabetes (Canadian Mental Health Association, 2018). Legislation is required to address unmet mental health needs and bring mental health care into balance with physical health care.

A variety of mental health terms are used by family, patients, police, community members. They include *mental health patient* and *mental health consumer* (meaning service user or consumer). Those who resist psychiatric labels and who may have endured maltreatment and discrimination may self-identify as a "mental health survivor" or "survivor of psychiatry." It is best for the CHN to take guidance from the patient as to how they self-identify and avoid marginalizing and stigmatizing labels. In this text, the term "person(s) with a mental illness" (PMI) is used because it is familiar to those who have lived with mental illness and is the "people-first" terminology that CHNs commonly use to refer to a patient who is affected by mental illness. People who are living with mental health problems and illnesses have been the key drivers for, and are themselves at the heart of, the current momentum for change in mental health (Mental Health Commission of Canada, 2016).

In Canada, the response to persons with mental illness has evolved and continues to respond to critiques as well as growing needs. Historically, persons with mental illness were institutionalized and subjected to treatments that are no longer considered ethical or effective. In the 1960s, changes in mental health policy initiated the movement of care from large, isolating, specialized psychiatric institutions into the community. The catalysts for this change included social reform, the goal of reducing the cost of institutional care, the positive effects of new medications on symptom control, and advocacy for patient autonomy and social inclusion (Goldner, Jenkins & Bilsker, 2016). Although these changes were intended to be positive, community support resources have not always been sufficient or accessible for individuals who are living with mental illness in the community. More often than not, PMI experienced gaps in service, along with poverty-level disability incomes and workplace or employment discrimination that has diminished their quality of life. Taken together, these circumstances have heightened discrimination and the marginalized social status of many PMI. This inequity is also correlated with a higher risk for negative health outcomes (Bartram, 2019). Potential consequences of inequitable access to mental health care encompass biological, psychological, and social domains (see Box 15.4).

Recognition of the importance of the SDOH and equitable access to treatment and preventative care has led to significant shifts in mental health policy, practice, and research. Strides have been made in recent decades in terms of evidence-informed treatments that improve outcomes for mental illness and health promotion for those who are able to access

BOX 15.4 Potential Consequences of Having Inequitable Access to Mental Health Care

- Greater disability rates over a lifetime than those with physical illnesses
- Underemployment and unemployment rates that are high, which contribute to many living in poverty
- More risk for poverty; this may lead to inappropriate dress and unkempt appearance, which can contribute to stigmatization
- Higher suicide rates, substance abuse and accidental overdoses, and early death from treatable medical conditions, contributing to a higher mortality rate
- Greater risk for homelessness
- Greater risk for personal injury, medical comorbidities, including HIV/AIDS, hepatitis B and C, hypothyroidism, heart or chronic lung disease, diabetes, and skin conditions
- Increased interactions with law enforcement
- Increased hospital and associated costs
- Increased caregiver burden

Source: Adapted from Goldner, E., Jenkins, E., & Bilsker, D. (2016). *A Concise Introduction to Mental Health in Canada* (2nd ed.). Canadian Scholars' Press.

this care. However, access to this care is not equitably distributed, and treating the social determinants of mental health involves focusing more on systemic change than on medical treatments. It entails creating public policies that improve these issues and changing social norms to place greater value on giving everyone an equal chance at living a fulfilling and healthy life (Shim & Compton, 2018).

In the Canadian public policy context, the past two decades have been punctuated by important changes in this regard. Firstly, in 2006, three major reports related to mental health in Canada were published. The Canadian Alliance on Mental Illness and Mental Health (2006) published its report *Framework for Action on Mental Health and Mental Illness*. The major recommendation to health and social policy leaders of Canada was to develop a national action plan on mental illness and mental health. At that time, Canada was the only G8 country without a national mental health strategy. The Kirby report, *Out of the Shadows at Last* (Kirby, 2006), is considered one of the premier documents with regard to mental health and mental illness development in the country (see the link on the Evolve website). Finally, *The Human Face of Mental Health and Mental Illness in Canada* (PHAC, 2006) had as its purpose to raise awareness and increase knowledge and understanding about mental health and mental illness in Canada.

In 2007, the federal government formed the Mental Health Commission of Canada (MHCC). The commission, which is a nonprofit agency, is dedicated to improving the mental health system and changing attitudes and behaviours on mental health issues, with a view to implementing a national strategy for mental health. The MHCC began its work with four key initiatives. The first initiative was to create the framework of the first national mental health strategy for Canada;

it released its strategy *Changing Directions, Changing Lives* in 2012 (MHCC, 2012). The second initiative was the 10-year antistigma and antidiscrimination initiative called "Opening Minds"; it deals with the dual notions of hope and recovery. The goal is to eliminate the stigma and fear related to mental illness within four target groups: youth, health care providers, the workforce, and the media. The third initiative was an extensive research demonstration project on mental health and homelessness, which studied the housing-first initiative for homeless individuals across the country. The fourth initiative was the establishment of a knowledge exchange centre to provide the general public, researchers, educators, and scientists with a web-based resource for education and exchange of information (MHCC, 2012). In the following decade, in-depth work took place to develop and implement workplace standards, attention to school and university mental health, the housing-first initiative, the recovery model, as well as targeted programs for Indigenous peoples, veterans, caregivers, seniors, and emerging or young adults (MHCC, 2017). These initiatives have been transformative for the mental health and well-being of all Canadians, recognizing that the continuum of mental health and illness all requires commitment and strategy across sectors and populations (MHCC, 2021).

At-Risk Populations for Mental Illness
Children and Youth

Childhood is a time of establishing the foundation for mental health and resiliency, however 70% of PMI also see their symptoms begin to develop during adolescence. It is also estimated that 20% of children will experience a mental health disorder that will have a significant negative impact on their functioning (CIHI, 2020a). Types of mental health problems typically diagnosed during childhood are depression, anxiety, and attention deficit disorders. Hospitalizations for mental health problems and illnesses increased by over 60% for people between ages 5–24 years during the decade between 2008–2018 (CIHI, 2020a). Currently, it is estimated that less than 20% of children and youth who need it are able to access mental health treatment; further, there is a shortage of programs designed to prevent mental health problems in children. The *National Standard of Canada for Mental Health and Well-Being for Post-Secondary Students* was launched in 2020 and is the first framework of its kind in the world. It is designed to enhance and expand strategies already put in place by Canada's universities, colleges, institutes, CEGEPs, and polytechnics as they work to foster positive mental health for students (MHCC, 2021).

Older Persons

In Canada, the population of adults older than 65 years has been steadily increasing. As the life expectancy of individuals continues to grow, the number of people experiencing mental illness in later life will increase. This trend will be expensive and will challenge communities to deliver the needed mental health services for older persons. Many older persons maintain highly functional lives. However, some have mental health deficits associated with normal age-related sensory losses, failing physical health, and social deprivation or isolation that can make it difficult to perform the activities of daily living. Life changes related to work roles and retirement often result in reduced social contact and support. Other losses are associated with the death of a spouse, other family members, or friends. Reduced social networks and contact brought about by these life events can influence mood and contribute to serious states of depression. However, depression is not a normal part of aging (Touhy, McCleary & Boscart, 2019).

It is important for CHNs to recognize that older persons who are depressed usually have a clinically different presentation from depressed patients in other age groups. Older persons who are depressed tend to present with many bodily complaints, such as persistent pain, nausea and vomiting, and insomnia, and usually do not express feelings of sadness, guilt, or worthlessness (Touhy et al., 2019).

Activities to improve the mental health status of and support for older persons include public education programs, prevention approaches, and the provision of mental health services in primary care. Specific approaches to reduce stress include the use of community support groups, education about lifestyle management, and workplace programs for family members. Nevertheless, most programs currently available for older persons with mental health problems as well as their families and caregivers are primarily concerned with monitoring or restoring mental health, rather than with preventing distress or illness.

People With Serious and Persistent Mental Illness

Community mental health nurses (CMHNs) may work in Assertive Community Treatment teams developed to care for individuals with serious and persistent mental illness when deinstitutionalized from long-term psychiatric facilities. Research has found that this type of intensive community support alongside recovery (a model that advances patient autonomy and choice with a view that people with mental illness can and do get better [MHCC, 2015]) resulted in a decrease of psychiatric symptoms and hospital stays and an improvement in quality of life, social inclusion, and housing stability (Morse, Monroe-Devita, York, et al., 2020). CMHNs are also employed at community health centres and with community agencies to provide intensive case management and coordination of care for patients experiencing mental illness and their families. Again, the balance of intensive support with PMI and their autonomy and choice at the centre of community care is the focus for the CHN when working with patients who have persistent illness, and the relationship with the patient is key.

Alongside the evolution of the National Strategy for Mental Health, the Canadian Nurses Association (CNA, 2005) issued a backgrounder on mental health in "Mental Health and Nursing: A Summary of the Issues" and a "Position Statement on Mental Health Services" (CNA, 2012). (See the links to these documents on the Evolve website.) In these documents, the CNA does the following:

- Distinguishes between mental illness and mental health.
- Describes the changes in mental health care over the past 40 years in Canada (e.g., the evolution of treatment regimens; the movement of care from institutions to the community, where programs address mental illness and promote mental health; the advocacy by consumers and families for appropriate therapeutic regimens; and the recognition that stigma underlies the discrimination associated with mental illness).
- Describes the coordination of mental health services through projects such as the Canadian Collaborative Mental Health Initiative.

The Psychiatric/Mental Health Nursing group is a specialty within the Canadian Federation of Mental Health Nurses, and there are nursing competencies for this group within the CNA certification program. CMHNs work in communities across Canada, and their focus and scope of practice are evolving.

All CHNs have the community nursing responsibility of directing efforts at prevention of mental illness (e.g., educate the public about mental health and promote positive attitudes); supporting recovery; treatment and management (e.g., include the SDOH in planning care and be informed about the latest interventions); and advocacy (e.g., fight for continuity of care and more community resources).

Tertiary prevention targeted at persons with serious mental illness has sought to reduce the proportion of homeless adults who have serious mental illness, to increase their employment, and to decrease the number of adults with mental health disorders who are incarcerated. Brief hospital stays and inadequate community resources have resulted in an increased number of persons with serious mental illness living on the streets or in jail. According to a CIHI (2019) report, people from poorer neighbourhoods were more likely to be hospitalized for mental health and addictions reasons. More men were admitted to hospital, but older women had longer hospitalizations for mental health and addictions. Currently, many people with severe mental health disorders live in poverty and enter the criminal justice system because they lack the ability to earn or maintain a suitable standard of living. Living alone or with limited community support may increase risk of vulnerabilities. Even people who live with family caregivers or in supervised housing are at risk for inadequate services because the long-term care they require often depletes human and fiscal resources.

The Canadian Mental Health Association (CMHA) and the Schizophrenia Society of Canada are national organizations that have chapters across Canada. They are resources CHNs might access and refer patients to as needed. These organizations influence policy on mental health concerns, provide support to patients and their families, provide public education, and support mental health research (CMHA, 2021; Schizophrenia Society of Canada, 2021). CHNs should be aware of the community mental health resources available in their community so that they can make appropriate referrals to patients and their families. For a comprehensive discussion of specific mental illnesses, refer to a Canadian psychiatric nursing textbook.

Determinants of Mental Health

The 12 determinants of health (Government of Canada, 2020) are important factors to consider in relation to persons with severe and persistent mental health disorders. Goldner, Jenkins and Bilsker (2016) indicate that poverty and social isolation are viewed as both a cause and effect of psychiatric symptoms. They also associate the PHAC's determinants of health with persons with mental health disorders. Goldner et al. (2016) point out that although biology and genetic endowment are determinants of health and genetics and biological factors play a role in some mental health problems, many of the other determinants also affect people with mental health disorders and represent areas where CHNs can help patients. When it comes to mental health, three social determinants are particularly significant: racism, biological impacts of chronic stress, and socioeconomic status. See the "Determinants of Health" box.

DETERMINANTS OF HEALTH

Mental Health

Freedom From Discrimination and Violence

With regard to freedom from violence, this determinant also relates to the determinant of healthy child development. A range of adult mental health problems are the result of childhood trauma.

Social Inclusion

Social support is associated with better health outcomes. The PHAC notes that there is a buffering effect against health problems from the caring and respect of social relationships, and the resulting sense of satisfaction and well-being.* Unfortunately, a large number of people diagnosed with mental health disorders face isolation and exclusion, stigma being a major contributing factor. Others face unsafe social environments: psychiatric patients who live in poor, inner-city neighbourhoods are more likely to be physically and sexually assaulted.

Access to Economic Resources

Socioeconomic and educational status are strongly associated with better health. Persons with serious mental health disorders face high rates of unemployment and poverty-level incomes. With the onset of a disorder such as schizophrenia occurring in early adulthood, university education and early career trajectories are cut short in many instances.[†] This determinant also relates to the determinant of physical environments. Decent, affordable housing may pose an urgent need for mental health patients who face chronic homelessness, which itself is associated with a host of negative health outcomes.

Sources: * PHAC, 2018. [†] Goldner, Jenkins & Bilsker, 2016.

Different communities or populations have different experiences with the social determinants of mental health. The impact of these differences can be health inequities: entire communities that experience poorer health or mental health than the general population. A large review of the evidence found the main individual factors that were demonstrated to have a statistically significant independent association with worse mental health were low income, not living with a partner, lack of social support, female gender, low level of education, low income, low socioeconomic status, unemployment, financial strain, and racism or discrimination. Community-level factors included neighbourhood socioeconomic conditions, social capital, geographical distribution and built environment, neighbourhood problems, and ethnic composition (Silva, Loureiro, & Cardoso, 2016).

The Community Health Nurse's Collaborative Role in Community Mental Health Care

CHNs and CMHNs can assist in targeted assessment and interventions of at-risk populations. In some communities, CHNs and CMHNs collaborate. In communities where there are no CMHNs, CHNs have the option of seeking the support of CMHNs from outside communities in order to plan interventions. It is important that CHNs and CMHNs be involved in the establishment of educational programs and mental health first aid for the recognition of symptoms, with follow-up assessment for depression and/or psychosis (Mental Health First Aid Canada, 2021). CHNs and CMHNs also require knowledge of available community services such as teen health clinics, crisis help lines, and emergency department mental health services so that referrals can be made as needed.

Collaboration With Law Enforcement

Law-enforcement agencies have taken steps to educate their staff in dealing sensitively with individuals who have a mental illness, and high-profile cases of excessive force and discrimination have provided a catalyst for greater integration of community health and policing services and skills. The traditional approach was to arrest persons with a mental illness and put them in jail so that they could have access to mental health assessment and treatment. Opportunities exist for CHNs to collaborate with the police and for law enforcement agencies to integrate mental health awareness and trauma-informed approaches in their services (CAMH, 2018). For example, a CHN may be supporting a person who is the victim or perpetrator of a crime; addressing a patient's emotional distress or substance use; working on an accident investigation; or working with the police on other community health concerns (Coleman & Cotton, 2014). CMHNs have the ability to collaborate with the police in determining the best plan for community follow-up and thus provide more appropriate care and treatment, potentially avoiding incarceration.

Collaboration in Crisis Intervention and Prevention

CHNs play an important role in identifying stressful events, assessing stress responses, educating communities, and intervening to prevent or alleviate disability and disease resulting from stress or acute crises. Although everyone is vulnerable to stressful life events and may develop mental illness, persons with chronic and persistent mental illness have numerous problems. They may not have access to adequate health services or suitable housing. Many accessible and coordinated services are needed to enable people with chronic mental illness to stay in the community, yet these are not always available. Interventions for community survival for those with chronic and persistent mental illness can require a broad range of well-coordinated services, including mental and physical health services, housing assistance, substance abuse treatment (for some), and social and vocational rehabilitation. Many mental health service systems exist. The CHN, by partnering with other community health care providers and service providers, can facilitate the coordination of these services in the community. The CHN can be an advocate for persons with chronic and persistent mental illness. The CHN may also assess the need for or engage in crisis intervention; for example, when people experience suicidal ideation or distress that is so disabling as to limit functioning or safety in the community.

CHNs working in community settings, child health or school clinics, antenatal and prenatal care, and home health are well positioned to conduct early mental health assessments of children and adolescents that can positively affect their mental health. Because many children and adolescents lack specialized services or access to them, community mental health assessment activities are essential as part of routine CHN practice and can support early identification of needs and assist in service advocacy. Assessment activities include identifying types of programs available or lacking in places where children and adolescents spend time. Assessments should be performed in schools and in the homes of patients served, as well as in daycare centres, churches, and organizations that plan and guide age-specific play and entertainment programs. Assessment data are essential for planning and developing programs that address mental health concerns prevalent from the prenatal period through adolescence. Addressing concerns during these developmental periods can reduce mental health problems in adulthood.

How can CHNs intervene? The general medical sector—including primary care clinics, hospitals, and nursing homes—has long been identified as the initial point of contact for many adults with mental illness; for some, these providers may be the only source of mental health services. Early detection of and intervention for mental health problems can be increased if persons presenting in primary care are assessed for mental health problems. CHNs who work in the general medical sector and in other community settings are in an ideal position to assess and detect mental health problems. CHNs conduct comprehensive biopsychosocial assessments and are often the professionals most trusted with sensitive information by patients in these settings. Screening tools for depression, anxiety, substance use, and cognitive impairment can assist the CHN in early detection of and intervention for mental illness. Health Canada provides information on tools that are used for substance abuse screening and mental health screening. This information is found on the Health Canada websites listed on the Evolve website.

Suicide

Like mental illness, suicide in present-day society is stigmatizing. This chapter uses definitions that represent more current thinking in reference to suicide and suicidal behaviours. The words *suicide* or *death by suicide* are used to describe the act of taking one's own life. Terms such as *committed suicide, failed suicide,* and *successful suicide* that use the terms *commit* and *attempt* intimate criminality and, as such, are stigmatizing to those people who are impacted. Changing the language that we use to describe suicide and suicidal behaviour is a first step in addressing the ways in which nurses can sensitively and empathically begin working with individuals who are suicidal (Beaton, Forster & Maple, 2012).

The term *suicidal behaviour* is used to describe the potentially self-harming behaviours of a suicidal individual. **Nonsuicidal self-injury** (NSSI) is a term used to describe self-directed, deliberate harm or alteration of bodily tissue without the presence of suicidal intent and includes behaviours such as self-cutting, head banging, burning, self-hitting, and scratching or picking skin or hair to the point of bleeding, often as a compulsion to relieve anxiety or other experiences of distress (Doyle, Sheridan, & Treacy, 2017; Taylor, Jomar, Dhingra, et al., 2018). Estimates based on community and clinical inpatient samples indicate that as many as 30 to 40% of adolescents (and 4 to 6% of adults) engage in NSSI (Hamza, Steward, & Willoughby, 2012).

In Canada, 5 000 people were admitted to hospital or died because of self-harm in 2018–2019, and close to 4 000 people (11 people every day) died by suicide. Hospitalization rates were highest among girls and women aged 10–24, who were three times more likely to be in hospital due to self-harm than males in that same age category. Death rates from suicide were highest among men 45 years and older (CIHI, 2020b).

Suicide rates in Canada show great disparities between genders and age, although suicide occurs in all age groups, cultures, and social classes. On a per-capita basis, suicide rates in Canada are on a downward trend; however, suicide rates among Indigenous peoples were significantly higher than the rate among non-Indigenous peoples.

The suicide rate among First Nations peoples (24.3 deaths per 100 000 person-years at risk) was three times higher than the rate among non-Indigenous peoples (8.0 deaths per 100 000 person-years at risk). Among First Nations people living on reserve, the rate was about twice as high as among those living off reserve. However, suicide rates varied by First Nations band, with just over 60% of bands having a zero-suicide rate. The rate among Métis people was approximately twice as high as the rate among non-Indigenous people. Among Inuit peoples, the rate was approximately nine times higher than the non-Indigenous rate (72.3 versus 8.0 deaths per 100 000 person-years at risk). Suicide rates and disparities were highest among youth and young adults (aged 15–24 years) for First Nations males and Inuit males and females (Kumar & Tjepkema, 2019). The social determinants and enduring trauma and discrimination that contribute to these alarming statistics are discussed further in Chapter 14.

BOX 15.5   Suicide Risk and Protective Factors

Risk Factors

- Suicidal ideation with intent
- Lethal suicide plan
- History of previous suicide attempt
- Co-occurring psychiatric illness
- Co-occurring medical illness
- History of childhood abuse
- Family history of suicide
- Lack of social support
- Unemployment
- Recent stressful life event (e.g., death, other loss)
- Hopelessness
- Helplessness
- Panic attacks
- Feeling of shame or humiliation
- Impulsivity
- Aggressiveness
- Loss of cognitive function (e.g., loss of impulse control)
- Access to firearms and other lethal means
- Substance abuse (without formal disorder)
- Impending incarceration
- Low frustration tolerance
- Sexual orientation issues
- Social isolation

Key demographic risk (widowed, divorced, single, white, elderly, adolescent, young adult, Indigenous, LGBTQ2).

Protective Factors

- Sense of responsibility to family (e.g., spouse, children) or to others
- Pregnancy
- Personal, social, cultural, and religious beliefs that discourage suicide and support self-preservation
- Satisfaction with life
- Positive social support
- Access to health care
- Supportive living arrangements
- Effective coping skills
- Effective problem-solving skills
- Intact reality testing
- Connection with others
- Sense of purpose and meaning in life

Source: Adapted from Jakubec, S.L. (2019). Chapter 22: Suicide and nonsuicidal self-injury. In C.L. Pollard, S.L. Jakubec, and M.J. Halter (Editors), *Varcarolis's Canadian Psychiatric Mental Health Nursing: A Clinical Approach* (2nd ed., p. 499). Elsevier Canada.

Every suicide is tragic because it can often be prevented, and such a loss causes complicated, enduring grief for family members, friends, and entire communities. Mental illness and life crises such as unemployment and relationship break-ups are two factors that precipitate risk for suicide in men and women (Halter, Pollard & Jakubec, 2018). Other risk factors associated with the distress that can trigger suicidal behaviour include pathological gambling, incarceration, discrimination, and victimization by bullying. Box 15.5 shows selected suicide risk and protective factors.

Many deaths by suicide can be prevented by early recognition and interventions. Recent MHCC professional and public education in the areas of mental health first aid (Mental Health First Aid Canada, 2021) and suicide prevention (MHCC, 2021) are examples of national efforts to address the crisis. Often there are warning signs prior to suicide, and CHNs need to be aware of these warning signs and educate those at risk (Halter et al., 2018). CHNs can establish patients at risk, provide early patient intervention, and advocate for suicide-prevention programs (CAMH, 2020). Some common warning signs for people at risk for suicide are found in the Registered Nurses' Association of Ontario best practices guideline "Assessment and Care of Adults at Risk for Suicidal Ideation and Behaviour" (see the link on the Evolve website). This guideline presents information on risk factors for and warning signs of suicide, suicide assessment considerations, and interventions to consider. For example, some of the warning signs for suicide are making statements about death, describing methods of harming self, developing a suicide plan, giving possessions away, mood changes, and withdrawal and social isolation (Registered Nurses' Association of Ontario [RNAO], 2009). These signs may apply to any person who is at risk for suicide, who has problems with daily interactions such as family relationships, or who is experiencing personal problems. Many available tools are also included and discussed on the RNAO website. Warning signs for adolescent suicide ideation could include a loss of interest in usual activities, acting-out behaviours, and unnecessary risk taking. For more information on suicide and adolescents, see The Centre for Suicide Prevention's *Teen Suicide Resource Toolkit* (see the link on the Evolve website).

Despite the widespread use of telephone crisis lines, school-based intervention programs, and antidepressants, high rates of suicide, particularly among adolescents, middle-aged men, older persons, and Indigenous peoples continue (to be in agreement with high rates of suicide) (Mental Health Commission of Canada, 2021). All suicide attempts should be taken seriously. The CHN's goals are to:

- Detect risk factors
- Promote safety (establish agreements for seeking help if the person is impulsive, provide supportive environments, and decrease access to lethal means)
- Prevent self-harm (identify and discuss risk factors and risk-reduction strategies)
- Make appropriate referrals (support groups, mental health services)
- Help people return to health (empower patients to promote hopefulness).

At a community level, CHNs need to be involved in a coordinated response to the prevention of suicide and the care of those who have attempted suicide. In their roles in community health nursing, CHNs need to be involved in the development of policies and protocols for suicide prevention across the lifespan. Community health nursing care may focus on family members and friends of suicide victims. Survivors often feel anger toward the dead person, yet often turn the anger inward. Likewise, survivors often question their own liability for the death. The impact of suicide can affect family, friends, coworkers, and the community. Beyond the anger some survivors feel, they and others may have difficulty dealing with their feelings toward the dead person. They may have difficulty concentrating and may limit their social activities because it is difficult for both survivors and their friends to talk about the suicide. CHNs help survivors cope with the trauma of the loss and make referrals to a counsellor or support group. Suicide affects the community. For information on community assessment, planning, and implementation considerations in Indigenous communities, see the Health Canada tool kit listed in the Tool Box on the Evolve website. This tool kit was prepared to assist Indigenous peoples address suicide in their communities.

At a primary prevention and societal level, see WHO's *Preventing Suicide: A Global Imperative* (the link is on the Evolve website). Important discussions and strategies are being explored internationally because suicide is indeed a global crisis. For other primary prevention risk assessment tools, see the Mental Health Commission of Canada's *Suicide Risk Assessment Toolkit* resource (on the Evolve site); for secondary and tertiary prevention, the Mental Health Commission of Canada has developed the *Toolkit for People Who Have Been Impacted by a Suicide Attempt* (see link on the Evolve website).

SUBSTANCE USE AND COMMUNITY HEALTH

CHNs seek to identify groups for whom substance use may be problematic in order to design programs that meet specific needs, mobilize community resources, and reduce harms. Managing risk and reducing harm—whether it involves substance use or other common but risky human behaviours—requires understanding the unique people you work with as a CHN. Substance use is different for everyone, and often there is a combination of biological, psychological, and social factors that can contribute to why a person may be struggling with addiction or substance use. For example, some of the risk factors for addiction include: a person's genes, the way a person's brain functions, previous experiences of trauma, cultural influences, social issues such as poverty and other barriers to accessing the SDOH. While the SDOH may contribute to addiction or substance use, there is no single set of factors that cause substance use and addiction (Canadian Mental Health Association of Ontario, n.d.; PHAC, 2020b).

One important factor to consider is how mental health and addictions are linked and impact one another. A mental health issue, in conjunction with addiction or substance use, is known as a **concurrent disorder**. While it is difficult to obtain an accurate statistic of people living with concurrent disorders, research shows that more than 50% of those who are seeking help for an addiction also have a mental illness (Centre for Addiction and Mental Health [CAMH], 2021).

Since substance use often begins during youth, researchers have focused on this age group as a way to understand which factors put people at risk and which factors protect them from substance use problems. Box 15.6 shows selected youth substance use risk and protective factors.

> **BOX 15.6   Selected Risk Factors and Protective Factors for Substance Use in Youths**
>
> *Risk factors for substance use problems in youth include:*
> - Alcohol or other drug problems among family members
> - Poor school performance
> - Poverty, family conflicts, chaos, or stress
> - Having friends who drink or use drugs
> - Not fitting in socially or being excluded because of factors such as race, ethnicity, gender, or sexual orientation
> - Emotional, physical, or sexual abuse
> - Experiencing discrimination or oppression
>
> *The protective factors for substance use problems include:*
> - Having a positive adult role model
> - Good parental or other caregiver supervision
> - Having a strong attachment to family, school, and community
> - Having goals and dreams
> - Being involved in meaningful, well-supervised activities (e.g., sports, volunteer work)
>
> *Source*: Centre for Addiction and Mental Health. (2021). *Addiction.* https://www.camh.ca/en/health-info/mental-illness-and-addiction-index/addiction

Although people may find themselves at greater or lesser risk of substance use, all patients are *people* before the problem (Canadian Centre on Substance Use & Addiction, 2019). Studies show that hazardous alcohol and drug use disorders are among the most stigmatized conditions, and that stigma impedes effective prevention and treatment (Collins, Bluthenthal, Boyd et al., 2018). Stigmatizing language and disrespectful behaviour affect how people see themselves and how they are treated by society as a whole. It is important to remember that a substance use disorder should be treated as a medical condition. Shifting language to more accurately reflect the nature of the health condition and the primary concern for the person and their community context can lead to wider support of life-saving interventions. Through a "person first" point of view—rather than addressing the patient through labels (e.g., "addict" or "alcoholic"), CHNs can begin to meet their patients where they are, to understand their needs and their contexts, and to reduce harms resulting from both stigma and substance use (PHAC, 2020b).

Harm reduction is a strategy used widely in health policy and practice to reduce harm to an individual or society by modifying hazardous behaviours that are difficult, and in some cases impossible, to prevent. Examples include requiring drivers to wear seatbelts or snowboarders and bicyclists to use helmets; promoting safer sexual practices; and providing needle-exchange programs to reduce the risk of blood-borne infections among people who use intravenous drugs. Although prominent since the 1970s and 1980s in response to infectious diseases such as hepatitis B and HIV, the history of this approach extends as far back as the early 1900s with narcotic maintenance clinics. In Canada, the history of federal endorsement and provincial implementation of harm reduction for substance use has a more recent history, starting from the late 1980s. Until now, however, provincial uptake has varied and central principles of this approach (including a focus on preventing harm rather than on substance use per se, tailoring approaches to specific needs of populations, addressing underlying causes of drug-related harm, involving people using substances in decision-making for the evidence-based, rights-orientated models) have not been universally implemented (Hyshka, Anderson-Baron, Pugh et al., 2019).

The harm reduction approach disentangles the notion that drug use equals harm and instead identifies the *negative consequences* of drug use as the target for intervention, rather than drug use itself. Harm reduction as an approach stands in opposition to the traditional medical model of addiction, which labels any illicit substance use as abuse, as well as to the moral model, which labels drug use as wrong and therefore illegal. While it is most often applied in treatment for substance use, harm reduction is increasingly being employed in different settings and with a variety of populations, and in instances where there is motivation to reduce the negative effects of substances or behaviours. Examples of harm reduction programs can be found in tobacco smoking reduction and e-cigarette substitution programs, managed alcohol, and even in some eating disorder and other health programs (Hawk, Coulter, Egan, et al., 2017)

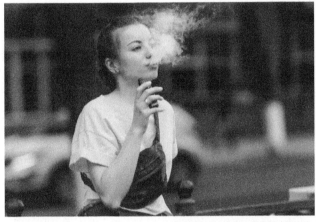

Electronic cigarettes, while considered part of harm reduction strategy by some, are considered a new community health concern by others. (iStockphoto/licsiren)

Promotion of Healthy Lifestyles and Resiliency Factors

Assisting patients to achieve optimal health includes identifying interventions other than or in addition to the use of medications as being possible. Supporting assertiveness and decision-making skills and awareness of various options helps patients increase their capacities for managing their health. Nagging health concerns, such as difficulty sleeping, muscle tension, and lack of energy, are common responses to chronic stress.

CHNs need to help patients understand when developing skills and personal practices can ameliorate symptoms, and when higher levels of intervention may be necessary. At times that intervention may be a referral to social care and

support—legal, financial, or medical. CHNs also provide useful information to community groups that can build health promotion and resiliency within existing community services (for instance, urban and smaller community libraries that offer direct and indirect social care and social support for people of all ages). Assisting the development of community recreational resources or directly facilitating or referring patients to health-promoting activities such as stress-reduction, relaxation, or exercise groups are all primary health-promoting activities to which CHNs may contribute.

Lack of educational opportunities, job training, or both can contribute to socioeconomic stress and poor self-esteem, which can lead to substance use to escape the situation or temporarily manage distress. CHNs help patients identify community resources and solve problems to meet basic needs rather than avoid them. In addition to decreasing risk factors associated with alcohol, tobacco, and other substance problems, it is important to increase protective or resiliency factors.

Substance Use Education

Substance use education for community health should be more about developing health literacy (the knowledge and skills needed to manage substance use) than about lifestyle marketing and teaching about "good" and "bad" behaviours. Prevention programs should focus on minimizing harm and promoting resiliency to prevent harmful patterns of use rather than "teaching" on drug use per se. In most cases of smoking cessation, for example, the patient will know very well about the harmful effects—and will have potentially made many efforts to change the behaviour. The CHN will not be the bearer of all the latest news on the subject but a resource to support health literacy and honest individual and group self-appraisal. CHNs may also be educators or advisors to school systems or community groups to ensure that all relevant aspects of individual, group, and community education can be designed and implemented. Health promotion and education should be designed to focus on motivation and self-awareness so individuals can address their own readiness to change and build resiliency as they select their own goals and the services that will meet their individual needs and develop their personal skills.

Across all services at the individual, group, program, or community level, the focus should be on developing individual and community capacities, giving adequate attention to both healthy public policy and community action rather than on preventing or "fixing" individual problems that will have very complex influences and causes.

Harm Reduction in Prevention Strategies

As introduced earlier, a harm reduction approach includes policies and programs that aim to help people who use substances to be safer and healthier without requiring abstinence or reduction in use. Health promotion that employs harm reduction strategies includes (1) the promotion of resiliency factors and (2) education about drugs and guidelines for use. CHNs are in an ideal position to use health promotion strategies such as promoting and facilitating healthy alternatives to dangerous drug-use practices and providing education about drugs to decrease harm from irresponsible or unsafe drug-use practices.

To identify substance abuse problems and plan appropriate interventions, CHNs can assess each patient individually. Think of the "4 *Hs*" to remember what to ask when assessing substance use patterns: *how* taken (route), *how* much, *how* often, and *how* long. When substance use problems are identified, the CHN can assist patients in understanding the connection between their substance-use patterns and the negative consequences on their health, their family, and the community. Motivational interviewing approaches are useful in understanding the readiness for change and motivations of the patient (Miller & Rollnick, 2012). The CHN may consider patient participation in a self-help group. Referrals to any number of programs that meet the patient where they are in terms of their readiness for change may be necessary for some patients. Community programs and services that CHNs might refer patients to include managed alcohol programs and other medical management such as methadone clinics, supervised injection programs, peer support programs, detoxification centres, smoking-cessation programs, behavioural addiction programs, or substance use awareness programs offered by local mental health or addiction centres.

When assessing substance use or behavioural patterns, CHNs need to determine the factors influencing and maintaining the behaviours and substance use. Some underlying health problems (e.g., pain, stress, insomnia) may be relieved by nonpharmaceutical interventions. Ask about the amount, frequency, and duration of use and the route of administration of each drug. To establish the presence of a substance use disorder, determine whether the substance use or behaviour is causing any negative health consequences or problems with relationships, employment, finances, or the legal system. The "How to" box lists examples of questions to ask to determine any socioeconomic concerns that are often secondary to substance abuse. If a pattern of chronic, regular, and frequent use of a drug exists, CHNs need to assess the patient for a history of withdrawal symptoms to determine whether there is physical dependence on the drug. A progression in substance use patterns and related problems warns about the possibility of compulsive or out-of-control behaviour. Denial is common during the change process and, in the case of substance use disorders, it is largely due to the shame and stigma surrounding substance use. Signs of denial include:

- Lying about use
- Minimizing use patterns
- Blaming or rationalizing
- Intellectualizing
- Changing the subject
- Using anger or humour
- "Going with the flow" (agreeing that a problem exists and stating that the behaviour will change but not demonstrating any behaviour changes)

Nonstigmatizing language, the guidance of motivational interviewing, and a trauma-informed approach are important for CHNs to use in order to build trust, especially when there may be signs of denial.

❊ HOW TO ...

Assess Socioeconomic Concerns Resulting From Substance Use Disorders

If a patient admits to using alcohol, tobacco, or other substances, ask the following questions:
- Do your family or friends worry or complain about your drinking or using drugs?
- Has a family member gone for help about your drinking or using drugs?
- Have you neglected family obligations as a result of drinking or using drugs?
- Have you missed work because of your drinking or using drugs?
- Does your boss complain about your drinking or using drugs?
- Do you drink or use drugs before or during work?
- Have you ever been fired or quit because of drinking or using drugs?
- Have you ever been charged with driving under the influence or being drunk in public?
- Have you ever had any other legal problems related to drinking and using drugs, such as assault and battery, breaking and entering, or theft?
- Have you had any accidents while intoxicated, such as falls, burns, or motor vehicle accidents?
- Have you spent your money on alcohol or other drugs instead of paying your bills (e.g., telephone, electricity, rent)?

Suspect a problem if the patient becomes defensive or exhibits other behaviours indicating denial when asked about alcohol or other substance use. Refer to the screening tools found at the Canadian Centre on Substance Abuse's *Collaboration for Addiction and Mental Health Care: Best Advice* link on the Evolve website.

The CHN is in a key position to support people who are experiencing substance use problems and their families. The CHN's knowledge of community and medical resources and how to navigate them can significantly influence the quality of care patients receive. The CHN's knowledge can be used to refer the patient to the appropriate community resource(s).

Substance use intervention strategies used with patients can vary, depending on their readiness for change. Understanding the stages of change (see Chapter 4) and assessing the stage of change that a patient is at facilitate successful outcomes as discussed in relation to the defence mechanism of denial. After the patient has received treatment, the CHN needs to coordinate aftercare referrals and follow up with the patient for any next steps and maintenance support. The CHN needs to provide additional support in the home as the patient and family adjust to changing roles and manage the stress involved with such changes. The CHN supports people with substance use disorders who have relapsed by reminding them that relapses may well occur but that they and their families can continue to work toward recovery and an improved quality of life. The CHN assesses and encourages patients, based on readiness, to return for treatment or seek other supports.

Problematic substance use is often a family and community concern. People in a close relationship with a person experiencing substance use problems often develop unhealthy coping mechanisms in order to continue the relationship, and many conflicting emotions such as anger and fear may need some integration. The CHN helps families integrate the complex experiences, recognize the problematic substance use, and understand and communicate with the person in a caring manner. Whether the person with the substance use disorder is agreeable to treatment or not, family members need to be given some guidance about services that are available to support resiliency. CHNs help identify treatment options, counselling assistance, pharmacy support, financial assistance, support services, and (if necessary) legal services for the family members (see the "CHN in Practice: A Case Study, Home Care for a High-Priority Family" box).

CHN IN PRACTICE: A CASE STUDY

Home Care for a High-Priority Family

Yasmin, a CHN, is a home health case manager in a large, low-income housing area in her community. She designs care plans and coordinates health care services for patients who need health care at home. She makes the initial visits to determine the level and frequency of care needed and then acts as supervisor of the volunteers and health care workers who perform most of the day-to-day care. Lone-parent families are the norm, and drug trafficking and sex trade are commonplace in this housing area.

Yasmin makes a home visit to Anne, a 26-year-old mother of three. Anne takes care of her 68-year-old maternal grandfather, Gino, who is recovering from cardiac bypass surgery. A widower for 5 years, Gino now lives with his granddaughter and her children. Gino has a smoking history of two packs per day for almost 50 years. Since his surgery, he has decreased to one pack per day, but he refuses to quit. He had a history of heavy alcohol use, reportedly consuming up to "a 40 ouncer" (1.1 L) of liquor a day, with a pattern of withdrawal seizures. Four years ago, Gino went through alcohol detoxification, but he refused to stay at the facility for continued treatment, stating he could stay sober on his own. Since that time, he has had several binge episodes, but Anne says he has not been drinking since the surgery.

Anne is a widow and has two sons, ages 3 and 9, and a daughter, age 5. The oldest son's father has substance use problems and is currently incarcerated for manslaughter (while driving under the influence of alcohol), and the father of her two youngest children was killed by a stray bullet in a drug raid 3 years ago. She and her husband had smoked crack cocaine for several months, but both stopped when she became pregnant with their youngest child, and she has continued to abstain from cocaine use. Anne has been angry at the community and frightened of police officers ever since the drug raid in which her husband was killed. Other residents were also hurt, and less than $500 worth of cocaine was found three apartments away from hers.

Anne does not consume alcohol, but she vapes nicotine intermittently throughout the day. She quit smoking cigarettes after her first pregnancy but resumed vaping soon after the births of her children.

Think About It

1. What type of interventions can Yasmin provide for Gino regarding his smoking?
2. How can Yasmin help Anne cope with the potential risk of Gino's substance use when he progresses to more independence?
3. How can Yasmin help Anne with her substance use (vaping nicotine)?
4. Aware of the genetic link to alcoholism and of the high rate of substance use in the housing area, how can Yasmin help prevent Anne and her children from developing substance use problems?
5. What can Yasmin do to support resiliency for the children and family as a whole?

VULNERABILITY OF CHILDREN AND YOUTH

Children and youth are considered structurally vulnerable populations. Regardless of socioeconomic status, gender, age, race, ethnicity, cultural identity, spirituality, personality, gender identity, sexual orientation, or physical or mental abilities, children are vulnerable to maltreatment (Department of Justice, 2015; 2017a, 2017b). The factors that influence children's and adolescent's well-being are discussed in Chapter 11.

Adolescent pregnancy rates have steadily declined, yet approximately 13 000 infants are born to adolescent parents (young people under age 20) each year. Adolescent parents and their children receive care from CHNs as two pediatric patients, each with unique health care needs. Young parents and their children may be at risk for negative health outcomes, not directly as a consequence of parental age but because of poverty and other inequities in the SDOH that they may experience. This section focuses on adolescent pregnancy because it is a primary public health concern that has a significant effect on both the individual and the community over the long term.

Adolescent Sexual Behaviour and Pregnancy

While some serious health risks are involved in pregnancy in young people under 15, the majority of negative outcomes of young pregnancy and parenting can be ameliorated by quality service provision focused on youth-specific needs. A large Canadian cohort study confirmed that, when compared with adults, adolescents have improved outcomes such as lower rates of gestational hypertension, gestational diabetes, antepartum hemorrhage, and operative deliveries. However, adolescents also have significantly higher sociodemographic risk factors and seek prenatal care later than adults do. These risk factors, in combination with young age, lead to other important maternal, obstetrical, and neonatal adverse outcomes.

CHNs who provide school, community, outpatient clinic, and home care have a role in addressing high-risk needs to ensure healthy pregnancies, and to reduce adverse perinatal outcomes (Fleming, Ng & Osborne, 2013). Early parenthood is associated with challenging life trajectories including decreased educational, occupational, and economic attainment. Young parents are more likely to live in poverty, have poorer mental health, and have higher rates of substance use. Peer influences are important to the potential for and outcomes of adolescent pregnancy. Other factors influencing young pregnancy are a history of sexual victimization, family structure, and parental influences (Wong, Twynstra, Gilliland, et al., 2020). Improving outcomes for pregnant and parenting adolescents also improves the prospects that their children will live healthy and happy lives. Understanding risks and resiliency factors with adolescent pregnancy is a starting place for the CHN.

Early Identification of the Pregnant Adolescent

Adolescents may delay seeking pregnancy services because they do not recognize early signs of pregnancy or they may falsely hope that the pregnancy will just go away. An adolescent may also delay seeking care to keep the pregnancy a secret from family members, who may pressure the adolescent to either maintain or terminate the pregnancy, or because the adolescent does not want to have a gynecological examination.

Attention needs to be paid to subtle cues that a young person may offer about sexuality and pregnancy concerns, such as questions about one's fertile period or requests for confirmation that one need not miss a period to be pregnant. Once the CHN identifies the specific concern, information can be provided about how and when to obtain pregnancy testing. The CHN needs to determine how an adolescent would react to the possible pregnancy before completing the test. If the test is negative, the CHN needs to take the opportunity to assess whether the young person would consider birth control counselling to prevent pregnancy. A follow-up visit is important after a negative test to determine whether retesting is necessary or whether another concern exists.

If the pregnancy test is positive, the CHN needs to refer the pregnant adolescent to the family physician or nurse practitioner for a health assessment and pregnancy counselling. Pregnancy counselling usually includes:

- Information on adoption, pregnancy termination, and early parenting
- Assessment of support systems for the pregnant young person
- Identification of the immediate concerns the pregnant adolescent might have

Often it is difficult to focus on counselling in any depth at the time of the initial pregnancy testing results. A follow-up visit is usually more productive and should be arranged as soon as possible. A pregnant adolescent may be referred to a CHN for follow-up counselling, which could be provided at a public health clinic or school setting. This pregnancy counselling requires that the CHN and pregnant young person explore strengths and weaknesses for personal care and pregnancy options such as pregnancy termination or parenting

the child. If parenting is the choice, the responsibilities of early parenting are discussed during pregnancy and postpartum. Young people vary in their interest in including the partner or their parents in this discussion. Issues to discuss include education and career plans, family finances and qualifications for outside assistance, and personal values about pregnancy and parenting at this time in life. The CHN needs to ask about violence at each visit because pregnant adolescents are more vulnerable to violence. Violence that begins in pregnancy may continue for several years after, with increasing severity. The CHN needs to observe for physical signs of abuse, as well as for controlling behaviour of partners. As decisions are made about the course of the pregnancy, the CHN is instrumental in referral to appropriate programs. The CHN can also begin prenatal education and counselling on nutrition, substance use, exercise, and any special medical concerns.

Special Issues in Caring for Pregnant Adolescents and Their Children

Community health nursing interventions through education and early identification of concerns may dramatically alter the course of the pregnancy and the birth outcome for pregnant adolescents.

The nutritional needs of a pregnant adolescent are especially important. The CHN needs to assess the pregnant youth's current eating pattern and provide creative guidance to address the issue of the demands of pregnancy on a normally changing adolescent's body and their nutritional habits, which may include fast foods. For example, protein can be increased at fast-food establishments by ordering milkshakes instead of soft drinks and broiled chicken sandwiches instead of hamburgers. Healthy snack foods such as granola bars and dried fruits and nuts are suggested. The CHN needs to be familiar with Canada's Food Guide (see the Health Canada "Food and Nutrition" link on the Evolve website) and the links to various resources, and needs to discuss nutritional food choices with the pregnant young person.

Government-funded programs have been developed across Canada to address the nutritional needs of structurally vulnerable people. Some of the programs developed across Canada are Healthy Moms, Healthy Babies in Whitehorse, Yukon; *Centre Cap enfants* (a family resource centre) in Wellington, Prince Edward Island; and BOND: Babies Open New Doors in Powell River, British Columbia. These programs are similar and include education on a variety of topics related to pregnancy and postpartum issues and childcare offered in individual and group sessions. The programs are usually offered to pregnant people under 20 years of age who are considered to be structurally vulnerable based on the determinants of health. These programs are presented under the PHAC project titled "Canada Prenatal Nutrition Program (CPNP)" (see the link on the Evolve website).

The CHN can help prepare the pregnant young people for the transition to parenthood while still pregnant—for example, at childbirth education classes. The trend toward early discharge from the hospital has made prenatal preparation even more important. The CHN can enlist the support of the young person's parents in education about infant care and stimulation. Both young parents-to-be would benefit from this education. Adolescents may not know how to establish early parenting practices, care, and routines or how to communicate with an infant. The CHN can assist in this health education to promote parent–child attachment. Young parents may lack information on newborn and infant growth and development or may have preconceived ideas and unrealistic expectations about their child's development (O'Brien, Greyson, Chabot, et al., 2018). See the "CHN in Practice: A Case Study, A Program for Young Parents" box for a description of a high school–based program. These skills can be taught and may prevent the child from later developing academic or behavioural problems.

CHN IN PRACTICE: A CASE STUDY

A Program for Young Parents

A local agency for youth requested the assistance of Kristen, a CHN, in the implementation of a new high school–based program for young people who are parents. The primary goal of the program is to keep these adolescents in school through graduation. The secondary goal is to provide knowledge and skills about healthy pregnancy, labour and delivery, and parenting. After delivery, students enrolled in this program were paid for school attendance; this money could be used to defray the costs of childcare.

A CHN was the ideal choice to conduct the educational sessions. The group met weekly during the lunch hour. The curriculum that was developed had topics from early pregnancy through the toddler years. Occasionally, Kristen brought in outside speakers such as a labour and delivery nurse or an early intervention specialist.

Kristen also met individually with each enrolled student to provide case management services. Ideally, she would ensure that each student had a health care provider for prenatal care, that each student was visited at home by a CHN, and that both the pregnant adolescent and their partner knew about other parenting and support groups.

One educational session that was particularly interesting was the discussion about the postpartum course—provided 6 weeks after delivery. There were many lively discussions about labour experiences, as well as some emotional discussions about the reality of coming home with a baby and changes in the relationship with their partner. Many young people benefited from understanding the normalcy of postpartum blues, but one youth recognized that they had a more serious and persistent depression with severe anxiety and privately approached Kristen for assistance.

At the end of the first school year, the dropout rate for pregnant and parenting adolescents had been reduced by half, and preterm labour rates had also declined. The local school board and a local agency serving youth joined together to provide financial support to continue this program for an additional 2 years. Kristen was asked to expand the educational programs and interventions she had developed.

Think About It

• What are some directions in which Kristen might expand the program? List four.

After the birth of the baby, the CHN needs to observe how the young parent responds to infant and toddler cues for basic needs and distress. See Healthy Child Manitoba's *Making Connections: Your First Two Years With Baby* (the link is on the Evolve website) for specific techniques that the new mother can be instructed to use in early child care. This website provides information on how to promote infant attachment and how to evaluate normal infant or child milestones. The CHN could also direct caregivers to this site for information on what infant attachment is and how to promote infant attachment.

The stresses associated with a new role and additional responsibilities of childcare can interfere with young parents' ability to concentrate on their school work. There are many community and educational resources that a CHN needs to be familiar with when working in partnership with the school so that young parents are provided with the appropriate supports to achieve school success.

COMMUNITY HEALTH NURSES CARING FOR PEOPLE EXPERIENCING STRUCTURAL VULNERABILITIES: ROLES AND LEVELS OF PREVENTION

CHNs who work with people experiencing vulnerabilities need well-developed assessment skills, current knowledge of available resources, and the ability to plan care based on patient concerns and receptivity to help. They also need to be able to show respect for the patient as being more than the vulnerabilities they experience, and use a trauma-informed approach to care. CHNs need to assess the *living environment* and *neighbourhood surroundings* of families and groups who are structurally vulnerable for environmental hazards such as lead-based paint, asbestos, water and air quality, industrial wastes, and the incidence of crime. Working with community leaders, CHNs are able to assess community strengths and assets, identify structural vulnerabilities with a health plan, and identify what will be required to address patient concerns.

Because people experiencing structural vulnerabilities often experience multiple stressors, assessment must balance the need to be comprehensive with a focus on only the information that a CHN needs and that the patient is willing to provide. The CHN needs to include questions about the patient's perceptions of his or her *socioeconomic resources,* including identifying people who can provide support and financial resources. Support from other people may include caregiving, emotional support, and help with instrumental activities of daily living, such as transportation, shopping, and babysitting. Financial resources may include the extent to which the patient can pay for any additional health services and medications, as well as questions about eligibility for third-party payment. The CHN needs to ask the patient about the perceived adequacy of both formal and informal support networks, including identifying areas of discrimination.

Structurally vulnerable populations need to be assessed for *congenital* and *genetic predisposition* to illness and either receive education and counselling as appropriate or be referred to other health care providers as necessary. For example, pregnant adolescents who use substances need to be referred to programs to support harm reduction during their pregnancy and, ideally, after delivery of their infant as well.

When necessary, assessment may include evaluation of a patient's *preventive health needs,* including age-appropriate screening tests, such as immunization status, blood pressure, weight, serum cholesterol, Papanicolaou smears, breast examinations, mammograms, prostate examinations, glaucoma screening, and dental evaluations. It may be necessary to make referrals to have some of these tests done for patients.

The CHN needs to also assess the amount of *stress* the person or family is experiencing. Does the family have healthy coping skills and family interaction? Are some family members able and willing to care for others? What is the level of mental health in each member? Also, are diet, exercise, and rest and sleep patterns conducive to good health? Exploring these questions and linkages are essential to effective CHN practice. Beyond physical health assessment, assessing structural vulnerabilities may require more nuanced probing, as is illustrated in the "How To…Assess Structural Vulnerability" box. This assessment tool consists of initial screening questions followed by qualitative assessment probes to help CHNs quickly understand and begin to intervene and address a patient's structural vulnerability.

❄ HOW TO …

Assess Structural Vulnerability
Financial Security
Do you have enough money to live comfortably—pay rent, get food, pay utilities/telephone?
- How do you make money? Do you have a hard time doing this work?
- Do you run out of money at the end of the month/week?
- Do you receive any forms of government assistance?
- Are there other ways you make money?
- Do you depend on anyone else for income?
- Have you ever been unable to pay for medical care or for medicines at the pharmacy?

Residence:
- Do you have a safe, stable place to sleep and store your possessions?
- How long have you lived/stayed there?
- Is the place where you live/stay clean/private/quiet/protected by a lease?

Risk Environments
Do the places where you spend your time each day feel safe and healthy?
- Are you worried about being injured while working/trying to earn money?
- Are you exposed to any toxins or chemicals in your day-to-day environment?
- Are you exposed to violence? Are you exposed regularly to drug use and criminal activity?
- Are you scared to walk around your neighborhood at night/day?
- Have you been attacked/mugged/beaten/chased?

Food access:
- Do you have adequate nutrition and access to healthy food?
- What do you eat on most days?
- What did you eat yesterday?
- What are your favorite foods?
- Do you have cooking facilities?

Social Network
Do you have friends, family, or other people who help you when you need it?
- Who are the members of your social network, family, and friends? Do you feel this network is helpful or unhelpful to you?

- In what ways?
- Is anyone trying to hurt you?
- Do you have a primary care provider/other health professionals?

Legal Status
Do you have any legal problems?
- Are you scared of getting in trouble because of your legal status?
- Are you scared the police might find you?
- Are you eligible for public services? Do you need help accessing these services?
- Have you ever been arrested and/or incarcerated?

Education
Can you read?
- In what language(s)? What level of education have you reached?
- Do you understand the documents and papers you must read and submit to obtain the services and resources you need?

Discrimination
[Ask the patient directly] Have you experienced discrimination?
- Have you experienced discrimination based on your skin colour, your accent, or where you are from?
- Have you experienced discrimination based on your gender or sexual orientation?
- Have you experienced discrimination for any other reason?

[Ask yourself silently] May some service providers (including me) find it difficult to work with this patient?
- Could the interactional style of this patient alienate some service providers, eliciting potential stigma, stereotypical biases, or negative moral judgments?
- Could aspects of this patient's appearance, ethnicity, accent, etiquette, addiction status, personality, or behaviors cause some service providers to think this patient does not deserve/want or care about receiving top quality care?
- Is this patient likely to elicit distrust because of his/her behavior or appearance?
- May some service providers assume this patient deserves his/her plight in life because of his/her lifestyle or aspects of appearance?

SOURCE: Bourgois, P., Holmes, S., Sue, K., & Quesada, J. (2017). Structural vulnerability: Operationalizing the concept to address health disparities in clinical care. *Academic Medicine, 92*(3), 299–307.

In some situations, the CHN works with individual patients; in others, the CHN develops programs and policies for structurally vulnerable populations. In both cases, planning and implementing care for members of vulnerable populations involve a partnership between the CHN and the patient. CHNs who direct and control the patient's care cannot establish a trusting relationship and may inadvertently foster a cycle of dependency and lack of personal health control. In fact, the most important initial step is for CHNs to establish that they are trustworthy and dependable. For example, CHNs working in a community clinic for substance abusers must overcome any suspicion that patients may have of them and eliminate any fears patients may have of being manipulated.

The relationship with the patient depends on the nature of the contact. Some are seen in clinics, others in homes, in schools, or at work. Regardless of the setting, the following key community health nursing actions need to be used:

- *Create a trusting environment.* Trust is essential since many of these individuals have previously been disappointed in their interactions with health care and social systems. It is important to follow through and do what you say you are going to do. If you do not know the answer to a question, the best reply is "I do not know, but I will try to find out."
- *Show respect, compassion, and concern.* Structurally vulnerable persons have been defeated again and again by life's circumstances. They may have reached a point where they question if they even deserve to get care. Listen carefully, since listening is a form of respect as well as a way to gather information to plan care.
- *Do not make assumptions.* Assess each person and family. No two people or groups are alike.
- *Coordinate services and providers.* Getting health and social services is not always easy. Often patients feel like they are travelling through a maze. In most communities, a large number of useful services exist. Patients who need them may simply not know how to find them. For example, patients may need help finding a food bank, a health centre, or a social services agency. They may also need help obtaining low-cost or free clothing through churches or in second-hand stores. Patients often need help determining whether they meet the eligibility requirements. If gaps in service are found, CHNs can work with others to try to get the needed services established.
- *Advocate for accessible health care services.* Structurally vulnerable patients have trouble getting access to services. Neighbourhood clinics, mobile vans, and home visits can be valuable for them. Also, coordinating services at a central location is helpful. These multiservice centres can provide health care, social services, daycare, drug and alcohol recovery programs, and case management. When working with structurally vulnerable populations, it is a good idea to arrange to have as many services as possible available in a single location and at convenient times. This "one-stop shopping" approach to care delivery is helpful for populations experiencing multiple social, economic, and health-related stresses.

- *Focus on prevention.* Use every opportunity to teach about preventive health care. Primary prevention may include child and adult immunization and education about nutrition, foot care, safer sex, contraception, and the prevention of injuries or chronic illness. It may also include providing prophylactic anti-TB drug therapy for HIV-positive patients who live in homeless shelters or giving the influenza vaccine to people who are immunocompromised or adults older than 65. Secondary prevention would include screening for health problems such as TB, diabetes, hypertension, foot problems, anemia, drug use, or abuse.
- *Know when to "walk beside" the patient and when to encourage the patient to "walk ahead."* At times it is hard to know when to do something for patients and when to teach or encourage them to do it for themselves. Community health nursing actions range from providing encouragement and support to providing information and active intervention. It is important to assess for the presence of strength and the ability to problem solve, cope, and access services. For example, CHNs may provide information and encouragement to patients about immunization and influenza clinics and schedule the clinics at varying times and places in the community that are easy to access. It is then up to the patient to access these clinics to acquire the intervention.
- *Know what resources are available.* It is important to be familiar with community agencies that offer health and social services to structurally vulnerable populations. Also, follow up after you make a referral to ensure the patient was able to obtain the needed help. Examples of agencies found in most communities are health units or authorities; community mental health centres; voluntary organizations such as the Canadian Red Cross, missions, shelters, soup kitchens, and food banks; nurse-managed or free clinics; social service agencies such as the Salvation Army; and church-sponsored health and social services.
- *Develop your own support network.* Working with structurally vulnerable populations can be challenging, rewarding, and at times exhausting. CHNs need to find their sources of support and strength. This can come from friends, colleagues, hobbies, exercise, poetry, music, and other sources.

In addition to the community health nursing actions described in the preceding list, the "How to" box summarizes goals, interventions, and evaluating outcomes with structurally vulnerable populations.

✳ HOW TO ...

Intervene With Structurally Vulnerable Patients
Goals
- Set reasonable goals that are based on the baseline assessment of health needs. Focus on reducing disparities in health status among structurally vulnerable populations.
- Work toward setting manageable goals with the patient. Goals that seem unattainable may be discouraging.
- Set goals collaboratively with the patient as a first step toward patient empowerment
- Set family-centred, culturally sensitive goals

Continued

✳ HOW TO ...—cont'd

Interventions

- Set up outreach and case-finding programs to help increase access to health services for structurally vulnerable populations
- Do everything you can to minimize the "hassle factor" connected with the interventions planned. Structurally vulnerable populations may not have the extra energy, money, or time to cope with unnecessary waits, complicated treatment plans, or confusion. CHNs, as advocates for patients, need to identify what hassles may occur and develop ways to avoid them. For example, CHNs might provide comprehensive services during a single encounter rather than ask the patient to return for multiple visits. Multiple visits for more specialized aspects of the health concerns of a patient, whether individual or family group, reinforce a perception that health care is fragmented and organized for the professional's convenience, rather than the patient's.
- Work with patients to ensure that interventions are culturally sensitive and competent
- Focus on teaching patients skills in health promotion and disease prevention. Also, teach them how to be effective health care consumers. For example, role-play with a patient on how to ask questions when in a physician's office or with other health care providers.
- Help patients learn what to do if they cannot keep an appointment with a health care or social service professional

Outcomes

Know that it is often difficult for structurally vulnerable patients to return for follow-up care. Help patients develop self-care strategies for evaluating outcomes. For example, teach homeless patients the signs and symptoms of infection and intervention strategies they can use or when to seek additional assistance.

- Remember to evaluate outcomes in terms of the goals you have mutually agreed on with the patient. For example, one outcome for a homeless person receiving isoniazid therapy for TB might be that the person return to the clinic daily for direct observation of adherence with the drug therapy.

In general, the need exists for more agencies that provide comprehensive services with nonrestrictive eligibility requirements. Communities often have many agencies that restrict eligibility to make it difficult for more people to receive services. For example, shelters may prohibit people who have been drinking alcohol from staying overnight and sometimes limit the number of sequential nights a person can stay. Food banks usually limit the number of times a person can receive free food. Agencies are often specialized as well. The result is that individuals and families who are structurally vulnerable must go to several agencies to obtain services for which they qualify and that meet their health concerns. Having to do so is tiring and discouraging, and people may forgo help because of these difficulties, which also include the added expense of travel.

The Roles of the Community Health Nurse

In a society that values self-reliance, individual responsibility, and personal accountability, members of structurally vulnerable populations may not get the respect they deserve. It is important for CHNs to understand their own beliefs about people experiencing structural vulnerability. As well, CHNs must understand the issues surrounding the illness and personal situation of a patient experiencing structural vulnerability. To be able to interact effectively with structurally vulnerable populations, CHNs need to identify health care needs, barriers to care, and essential health care services for these individuals, their families, and communities.

As discussed in Chapter 3, CHNs fulfill a variety of roles. CHNs need to know about community agencies that offer various health and social services. They also need to follow up with the patient after a referral to ensure that the desired outcomes were achieved. Sometimes, excellent community resources may be available but impractical because of transportation or other access issues. CHNs need to identify these potential concerns by following through with referrals, and they can also work with other team members to make referrals as convenient and realistic as possible. Although patients with social problems such as financial needs should be referred to social workers, it is useful for CHNs to understand the close connections between health and social problems and to know how to work effectively with other professionals. A list of community resources can often be found online or in a telephone book. The following agency resources are available in most communities:

- Health units or health authorities
- Community mental health centres and outpatient programs
- Detox and drug/alcohol treatment centres
- Canadian Red Cross and other voluntary organizations
- Food and clothing banks
- Missions and shelters
- Nurse-managed neighbourhood clinics
- Social service agencies such as vocational retraining programs
- Church-sponsored assistance such as the Salvation Army and others
- Cultural group, immigrant, refugee, or veteran agency sponsored assistance (e.g., Indigenous Friendship Centres)

Specific populations are often resourceful in managing multiple stressors. CHNs work with patients to help them identify and draw on their own strengths when managing their health concerns. Also, patients may be able to depend on informal support networks. Even though social isolation is a health concern for many vulnerable patients, CHNs should not assume that patients have no one who can or will help them.

CHNs link patients with health services by making appropriate referrals and by following up with patients to ensure that the desired outcomes from the referral were achieved. See the "How to" box on coordinating health and social services for patients from structurally vulnerable populations. CHNs are effective case managers in community nursing clinics, health departments, hospitals, and various other health care agencies. They emphasize health promotion and illness prevention with patients who are structurally vulnerable and focus on helping them avoid unnecessary hospitalization. Most importantly, they support patients while navigating complex care, offering guidance, and advocating where barriers may exist, and challenging discrimination if necessary.

❋ HOW TO …

Care Navigation for People Experiencing Structural Vulnerabilities

CHNs who work with people experiencing vulnerabilities often need to coordinate services across several agencies for members of these groups. It is helpful to have a strong professional network of people who work in other agencies and to support the navigation of care. Strong professional networks make it easier to coordinate care smoothly and in ways that do not add to patient stress. CHNs can develop strong professional networks by participating in community coalitions and attending professional meetings.

When one is making referrals to other agencies, a phone call can be a helpful way to obtain information that patients will need for the visit. When possible, having an interprofessional, interagency team plan of care for patients at high risk for health problems can be effective. It is crucial to obtain patients' written and informed consent before engaging in this kind of planning because of confidentiality issues. The following list of tips can be helpful:

- Be sure to involve patients in making decisions about the kinds of services they will find beneficial and can use
- Work with community coalitions to develop plans for service coordination for targeted structurally vulnerable populations
- Collaborate with legal counsel from the agencies involved in the coalitions to ensure that legal and ethical issues related to care coordination have been properly addressed. Examples of issues to address include privacy and security of clinical data.
- Develop policies and protocols for making referrals, following up on referrals, and ensuring that patients receiving care from several agencies experience the process as smooth and seamless

---

Many CHN actions in relation to structurally vulnerable populations are in the realm of case management and care navigation; that is, the CHN assesses and evaluates needs, makes referrals, and links patients with other community services, continuing to coordinate, monitor, and evaluate the outcomes of care. In the case manager role, the CHN is often an advocate for the patient or family. The CHN serves as an advocate when referring patients to other agencies, when working with others to develop health programs, and when trying to influence legislation and health policies that affect structurally vulnerable groups or populations. Referring patients to community agencies involves much more than simply making a phone call or completing a form. CHNs need to ensure that the agency to which a patient is referred is the right one that will meet the patient's concerns. CHNs can do more harm than good by referring stressed, discouraged patients to an agency from which they are not actually

eligible to receive services. The CHN helps patients navigate and access often numerous social and health care agencies. See the "How to" box on support care navigation in working with people experiencing vulnerabilities.

It is helpful to provide comprehensive services in locations where people live and work, including schools, churches, neighbourhoods, and workplaces. **Comprehensive services** are health services that focus on more than one health concern. For example, some CHNs use mobile outreach clinics to provide a wide array of health promotion, illness prevention, and illness management services to geographically remote areas. A single patient visit may focus on an acute health concern such as influenza, but it may also include health education about diet and exercise, counselling for smoking cessation, and a follow-up appointment for immunizations once the influenza is over. The shift away from hospital-based care includes a renewed commitment to the health services that structurally vulnerable populations need to prevent illness and promote health, such as the reduction of environmental hazards and violence and assurance of safe food and water. Navigation of multiple social and health care agencies requires strong communication and collaboration practices.

❋ HOW TO …

Support Care Navigation in Working With People Experiencing Structural Vulnerabilities
- Know available services and resources
- Find out what is missing; look for creative solutions
- Use your clinical skills
- Develop long-term relationships with the families you are caring for
- Assess and build upon the family's resilience and resourcefulness
- Be the road map that guides the family to services and helps it get the services it needs
- Communicate openly with the family and the agencies that can help the family
- Advocate to change the environment and the policies that create the conditions of vulnerability for your patients

---

Beginning with harm reduction and trauma- and violence-informed approaches, CHNs can provide care to patients, families, and groups in a number of ways. The following are examples: (1) a CHN in a mobile clinic might administer a tetanus booster to a patient who has been injured by a piece of farm machinery and may also check the patient's blood pressure during the same visit; (2) a home health nurse seeing a family referred by the courts for child abuse might weigh the child, conduct a nutritional assessment, and help the family learn how to manage behavioural problems or other challenges; (3) a public health nurse working in a school might lead a support group for pregnant adolescents and conduct a birthing class; and (4) a public health nurse working with patients in the community being treated for TB might monitor drug treatment to ensure that patients are best able to complete their full course of therapy.

CHNs also focus on advocacy and social justice concerns. CHNs may function as advocates for structurally vulnerable populations by working for the passage and implementation of policies that lead to improved public health services for these populations. For example, one CHN may serve on a local coalition for homeless people who do not have provincial or territorial health insurance plans. Another may work to develop a plan for sharing the provision of free or low-cost dental health care by local health care organizations and providers. CHNs who function in an advocacy role and facilitate change in public policy are intervening to promote social justice. CHNs need to bring forward evidence and accounts from the everyday realities of practice to advocate for policy changes to improve social, economic, and environmental factors that predispose populations to poor health.

CHNs have a critical role in the delivery of health care to those who experience poverty, homelessness, mental health, or substance use problems, and impacts of vulnerability. To be effective, CHNs need strong physical and psychosocial assessment skills, current knowledge of available resources, and an ability to convey respect, dignity, and value to each person. CHNs need to be able to work with their patients to prevent illness and promote, maintain, and restore health. CHNs need to be prepared to look at the whole picture (upstream thinking): the person, the family, and the community interacting with the environment (refer to the *Canadian Community Health Nursing: Professional Practice Model and Standards of Practice* [Community Health Nurses of Canada, 2019]).

An assessment may take place in the home or in a community site. Visiting in the home provides a great deal of useful information about the family, its resources, its support systems, and its knowledge of common housekeeping and health issues (see the roles and activities of public health nurses and CHNs in *Public Health–Community Health Nursing Practice in Canada: Roles and Activities* [the link is on the Evolve website]). For example, the CHN needs to assess for the adequacy of heating and cooling, water supply, cleanliness, cooking facilities, food storage, sleeping arrangements, and safety issues such as loose rugs, fire extinguishers, and fire alarms.

CHNs who work with people experiencing structural vulnerabilities may fill numerous roles, as Box 15.7 indicates.

The nature of a CHN's role depends on whether the patient is an individual, a family, a group, a community, or a population. For example, a CHN might teach a patient with HIV about the need for prevention of opportunistic infections, may help a family with an HIV-positive member understand myths about the transmission of HIV, may work with a community group concerned about HIV transmission among students in the schools, and may work with the community to identify priorities for action to prevent and reduce transmission of HIV. In each case, the CHN teaches how to prevent infectious and communicable disease and considers that the size of the group and the teaching methods will differ for each group.

Health education is often employed when working with people experiencing vulnerabilities. The CHN can support

---

BOX 15.7 Community Health Nurse Roles When Working With People Experiencing Vulnerabilities

- *Case finder.* Identify individuals, families, and groups at risk for disease or other community health concerns through outreach and encourage them to obtain health services
- *Health educator.* Teach patients who experience structural vulnerabilities strategies to prevent illness and promote health
- *Counsellor.* Counsel patients who experience structural vulnerabilities about ways to increase their sense of personal power and help them identify strengths and resources
- *Direct-care provider.* Provide direct care in a variety of settings, including storefront clinics, mobile clinics, shelters, homes, neighbourhoods, worksites, churches, and schools to patients who experience structural vulnerabilities
- *Community assessor and developer.* Collaborate with other community members to assess community health needs and develop approaches to meeting these needs
- *Monitor and evaluator of care.* Review and analyze results about community health interventions to determine outcomes, whether needs are met, and whether changes may be required in care or programs
- *Case manager and care navigator.* Function as a case manager for vulnerable patients, making referrals and linking them with available and accessible community services—navigating sometimes complex health and social care agency policies and practices
- *Advocate.* Serve as an advocate for patients who experience structural vulnerability with other agencies when making a referral to ensure that they get the services they need
- *Health program planner.* Develop community programs that respond to health concerns of patients who experience structural vulnerability; work with patients and other health care providers to develop and advocate for these programs
- *Participant in developing health policies.* Work with local, provincial or territorial, or federal groups to develop and implement healthy public policy. Influence legislation that affects structurally vulnerable populations

---

members of a population with limited health literacy or basic literacy through needs assessment along with direct teaching and provision or development of educational materials that fit the patient needs. It may be necessary to collaborate with a health educator, an interpreter or translator, or an expert in health communications to design messages that structurally vulnerable populations can best relate to, understand and use.

CHNs must consider the determinants of health in all program planning and health care interventions, using knowledge of the health disparities of people experiencing vulnerabilities. This level of health promotion requires more than health teaching. It is not enough to teach people how to be healthy if the social or economic conditions in which they live undermine their ability or motivation to engage in health actions. Instead, it requires attention to supporting health opportunity, health equity, and broader social justice.

It means advocating for policies and practices that acknowledge the complex circumstances that affect people's actions and abilities. It means advocating for policies and programs such as affordable housing, community outreach services, preventive health services, and other assistance programs for patients, in communities and society. It means advocating for health-supporting environments free from childhood trauma and other factors that increase the likelihood of substance use problems in youth and adulthood; and health-supporting living and working environments free from hazards and poor conditions that place people at risk for illness and injury. It means promoting social connectedness that increases meaningful opportunities and reduces isolation and antisocial behaviour.

Levels of Prevention and the Community Health Nurse

Primary prevention services include affordable housing, housing subsidies, effective job-training programs, employer incentives, preventive health care services, multisystem case management, birth control services, safer-sex education, needle-exchange programs, safe drug consumption sites, parent education, and counselling programs. As a primary prevention for mental health problems, CHNs could provide education about stress-reduction techniques to older persons attending a health fair. In this primary prevention work, CHNs form networks with other health care providers to educate policymakers and the public about the value of these preventive services. These services could provide health education and other forms of care to build individual and community resilience and consequently prevent many devastating problems. It is important to know about the social and political environments in which these problems occur. While health disparities can be addressed at multiple levels, including the individual level, CHNs also intervene in policy, health care system, and environmental improvement strategies designed to improve the places where people live, learn, work, and play. Examples of these intervention approaches may include the following: a voluntary school wellness policy that ensures food and beverage offerings meet certain standards; the integration of depression screening and referral

supports in a workplace; and a change to street infrastructure that enhances connectivity and promotes physical activity (Centers for Disease Control and Prevention, 2013). CHNs may work to influence politicians and other policymakers at the federal, provincial and territorial, and local levels about the plight of vulnerable populations in their community.

Secondary prevention activities are aimed at reducing the prevalence or pathological nature of a condition. They involve early diagnosis, prompt treatment, and the limitation of disability. For example, these services might target those exposed to higher risks because of the threat of homelessness, as well as those who are newly homeless. Examples include supportive and emergency housing, targeted case management, housing subsidies, soup kitchens and meal sites, and comprehensive physical and mental health services. CHNs can work with people experiencing homelessness and housing instability to provide education about existing services and develop strategies toward influencing public policy that will provide more comprehensive services for people experiencing homelessness and housing instability.

Tertiary prevention activities attempt to restore and enhance functioning and reduce disabilities. At a community level, these activities might include supporting affordable housing, promoting psychosocial rehabilitation programs, and participation in advocacy groups for persons with a mental illness or the homeless population. Tertiary prevention of homelessness includes comprehensive case management, physical and mental health services, emergency-shelter housing, needle-exchange programs, drug and alcohol detoxification, and treatment for substance use disorders.

Health initiatives need to focus on the elimination of health disparities by expanding access to health care for vulnerable or high-priority populations. The determinants of health need to be addressed before the health of vulnerable populations in Canada can be improved. CHNs can play an important role in multiple levels of intervention and prevention.

It is important for CHNs to understand the three levels of prevention and health promotion related to vulnerable populations (see the "Levels of Prevention" box related to vulnerable populations, below).

LEVELS OF PREVENTION

Related to Structurally Vulnerable Populations
Primary Prevention
A CHN provides influenza and pneumococcal vaccinations to structurally vulnerable populations such as older person patients and people recovering from cancer who are immunocompromised (unless contraindicated) or structurally vulnerable populations prone to communicable diseases.

Secondary Prevention
A CHN conducts screening clinics for structurally vulnerable populations. For example, the CHN who works in homeless

shelters, prisons, and substance abuse treatment facilities needs to know that these groups are at high risk for acquiring communicable diseases. For example, both patients and staff need routine screening for TB.

Tertiary Prevention
- A CHN refers severely mentally ill adults to a therapy group
- A CHN works with women who have left violent or abusive relationships to support growth and enhance self-esteem
- A CHN advocates for rehabilitation and recovery services for structurally vulnerable populations

STUDENT EXPERIENCE

1. Using web-based resources, examine health statistics and demographic data for your geographical area to determine which structurally vulnerable populations are predominant. Look through a local telephone book for examples of agencies that you think provide services to these structurally vulnerable populations. Prepare a table with your findings. Do a literature search to identify recommended state-of-the-art interventions for people who experience poverty or homelessness. Compare the recommended programs and interventions with those available in your target area. How does your area measure up? Give some specific recommendations about how you would fill the gaps.

2. For 1 week, keep a list of incidents related to mental health problems that you learn about in the local media. Categorize the incidents according to age, sex, and socioeconomic, ethnic, or minority status.

3. Explore the resources in your community that are available for patients and families requiring mental health services. Prepare a chart of these services with the contact information and eligibility criteria to share with your classmates.

4. Select one of the structurally vulnerable populations discussed in this chapter. Search the literature for two evidence-informed articles that identify one aspect of community health nursing care for that population. Prepare a summary of your articles, outlining the health care components for CHN use.

5. Search the literature for information pertaining to the vulnerabilities experienced by Indigenous women and children. Identify and list your findings and bring them to class.

CHAPTER SUMMARY

15.1 People experiencing structural vulnerabilities are more sensitive to risk factors than those who are more resilient since they are often exposed to cumulative risk factors. Socioeconomic problems, including poverty and social isolation, physiological and developmental aspects of age, poor health status, and highly stressful life experiences, predispose people to vulnerability. Vulnerability can become a cycle, where the predisposing factors and inequities lead to poor health outcomes, chronic stress, and hopelessness. These outcomes increase vulnerability. Addressing health inequities requires that the focus be on developing individual and community capacities, giving adequate attention to both healthy public policy and community action rather than on preventing or "fixing" problems that will have complex influences and causes.

15.2 Poverty has a direct effect on health and well-being across the lifespan. People who experience poverty have higher rates of chronic illness and infant morbidity and mortality, a shorter life expectancy, and more complex health problems.

15.3 Factors that contribute to homelessness include an increase in the number of persons living in poverty, diminishing availability of low-cost housing, increased unemployment, lack of treatment facilities for mental health and substance use problems, domestic violence, and relationship violence. The complex health concerns of homeless persons include the inability to get adequate rest, exercise, and nutrition; environmental exposure; infectious diseases; acute and chronic illnesses; trauma; and mental health concerns.

15.4 Significant mortality and morbidity result from violence. CHNs provide care for victims, perpetrators, and those who witness physical and psychological violence, and also take an active role in the development of community responses to violence, such as the development of public policy and needed resources.

15.5 Incidence rates and prevalence rates for mental health problems are very high, and people are at risk for threats to mental health at all ages across the lifespan. Low-income and minority groups are often at an increased risk for mental health problems because they often lack access to services. Mental health care has increasingly moved into the community.

15.6 Social conditions such as a fast-paced life, excessive stress, and the availability of drugs influence the incidence of problematic substance use. Problematic substance use is a major community health concern, linked to numerous forms of morbidity and mortality. Harm reduction is an approach to problems with alcohol, tobacco, and other substances; it deals with problematic substance use primarily as a health concern rather than as a criminal problem.

15.7 Children and youth are considered to be structurally vulnerable populations. Adolescents, especially those who become pregnant, have special nutritional needs. Youth who are pregnant will need support during and after the pregnancy from family and friends, from the other parent of the baby, and from health care providers including CHNs.

15.8 CHNs assess structurally vulnerable individuals, families, groups, aggregates, populations, and communities to determine which socioeconomic, physical, biological, psychological, and environmental factors are problematic for patients. They work as partners with patients who experience structural vulnerabilities to identify patient strengths, assets, and health concerns and to develop intervention strategies designed to break the cycle of vulnerability.

CHN IN PRACTICE: A CASE STUDY

High-Priority Pregnancy Care in the Community

Tanis, a 46-year-old farm worker pregnant with her fifth child, has come to the clinic requesting treatment for swollen ankles. During your assessment, you learned that she had seen the primary health care nurse practitioner (PHC-NP) at the local health unit 2 months ago. The PHC-NP gave her some sample vitamins, but Tanis lost them. She has not received regular prenatal care and has no plans to do so. Her previous pregnancies were essentially normal, although she said she was "toxic" with her last child. She also said that her middle child was "not quite right." He is in grade 7 at 15 years old. Tanis is 157 cm (5 ft. 2 in.) tall, weighs 81.6 kg (180 lb.), and has a blood pressure of 160/90. She has pitting edema of the ankles and a mild headache.

Tanis says that she usually takes the antipsychotic medication risperidone (Risperdal), but has run out of it and cannot afford to have her prescription refilled. She says that she has been a patient in several psychiatric inpatient units in the past and that she has become more agitated and now has problems managing her daily activities. As her agitation grows, she says that she usually hears voices, and this really makes her aggressive.

None of Tanis's children live with her, and she has no plans for taking care of the infant. She thinks she will ask the child's father, a truck driver, to help her since she often travels around the country with him.

Think About It
1. What additional information do you need to help you adequately assess Tanis's health status and current needs?
2. What community health nursing activities would you suggest, given her history, physical examination, and psychological descriptions?

📶 TOOL BOX

The Tool Box contains useful resources that can be applied in community health nursing practice. These related resources are found either in the appendices at the back of this text or on the Evolve website at http://evolve.elsevier.com/stanhope/community/.

Appendix
- Appendix 1: Canadian Community Health Nursing: Professional Practice Model and Standards of Practice

Tools

Gender and Health Collaborative Curriculum. Gender and Health Modules

This website provides interactive learning modules about gender and health in reference to poverty and diseases such as cardiovascular disease and depression. It also includes modules on "gender, sex, and sexuality" and "gender and trauma."

SexualityandU.ca.

This website contains links to tools useful for health care providers and educators when teaching about sexual health.

REFERENCES

Bartram, M. (2019). Income-based inequities in access to mental health services in Canada. *Canadian Journal of Public Health*, *110*(4), 395–403. https://doi.org/10.17269/s41997-019-00204-5.

Beaton, S., Forster, P., & Maple, M. (2012). The language of suicide. *The Psychologist, 25*, 731. https://www.psychology.org.au/publications/inpsych/2013/february/beaton.

Beckmann Murray, R., Proctor Zentner, J., Pangman, V., et al. (2009). *Health promotion strategies through the lifespan* (2nd ed.). Pearson Prentice Hall.

Bhatt, J., & Bathija, P. (2018). Ensuring access to quality health care in vulnerable communities. *Academic Medicine, 93*(9), 1271–1275. https://doi.org/10.1097/acm.0000000000002254.

Blanchet Garneau, A., Browne, A., & Varcoe, C. (2019). Understanding competing discourses as a basis for promoting equity in primary health care. *BMC Health Services Research, 19*(1), 764–764. https://doi.org/10.1186/s12913-019-4602-3.

Blas, E., Roebbel, N., Rajan, D., et al. (2016). Intersectoral planning for health and health equity. In G. Schmets, D. Rajan, &

S. Kadandale (Ed.), *Strategizing national health in the 21st century: A handbook*. World Health Organization. https://www.researchgate.net/publication/319464919_Chapter_12_Intersectoral_planning_for_health_and_health_equity.

Bourgois, P., Holmes, S., Sue, K., et al. (2017). Structural vulnerability: operationalizing the concept to address health disparities in clinical care. *Academic Medicine, 92*(3), 299–307. https://doi.org/10.1097/acm.0000000000001294.

Campaign 2000. (2020). *Setting the stage for a poverty-free Canada*. https://campaign2000.ca/campaign-2000s-new-national-report-card-on-child-and-family-poverty-sets-the-stage-for-a-poverty-free-canada/.

Canadian Academy of Health Sciences. (2014). *Improving access to oral health care for vulnerable people living in Canada*. https://cahs-acss.ca/wp-content/uploads/2015/07/Access_to_Oral_Care_FINAL_REPORT_EN.pdf.

Canadian Alliance on Mental Illness and Mental Health. (2006). *Framework for action on mental health and mental illness*. http://www.cmha.ca/public_policy/framework-for-action-on-mental-illness-and-mental-health/.

Canadian Centre on Substance Use and Addiction. (2019). *Overcoming stigma through language: A primer*. https://www.ccsa.ca/sites/default/files/2019-09/CCSA-Language-and-Stigma-in-Substance-Use-Addiction-Guide-2019-en.pdf.

Canadian Council on Social Determinants of Health. (2014). *Maps to inform intersectoral planning and action: A technical report*. http://ccsdh.ca/images/uploads/Maps_to_Inform_Intersectoral_Planning_and_Action_Technical_Report.pdf.

Canadian Dental Association. (2017). *A snapshot of oral health in Canada*. https://www.cda-adc.ca/stateoforalhealth/snap/.

Canadian Index of Wellbeing Network. (2016). *How are Canadians really doing? The CIW 2016 national report*. https://uwaterloo.ca/canadian-index-wellbeing/reports.

Canadian Institute for Health Information (CIHI). (2019). *Common challenges, Shared priorities measuring access to home and community care and to mental health and addictions services in Canada*. https://www.cihi.ca/sites/default/files/document/shp-companion-report-en.pdf.

Canadian Institute for Health Information (CIHI). (2020a). *Child and youth mental health in Canada [infographic]*. https://www.cihi.ca/en/child-and-youth-mental-health-in-canada-infographic.

Canadian Institute for Health Information (CIHI). (2020b). *Thousands of Canadians a year are hospitalized or die after intentionally harming themselves*. https://www.cihi.ca/en/new-data-available-on-mental-health-and-addictions-services-and-home-and-community-care.

Canadian Mental Health Association. (2018). *Over half of Canadians consider anxiety and depression "epidemic", September 17*. https://cmha.ca/documents/over-half-of-canadians-consider-anxiety-and-depression-epidemic.

Canadian Mental Health Association. (2021). *About CMHA*. http://www.cmha.ca/about-cmha/.

Canadian Mental Health Association of Ontario (n.d.). Factors that impact addiction and problematic substance use. https://ontario.cmha.ca/factors-that-impact-addiction-and-substance-misuse/.

Canadian Nurses Association (CNA). (2005). *CNA backgrounder: Mental health and nursing: A summary of the issues*. https://www.cna-aiic.ca/~/media/cna/page-content/pdf-en/bg6_mental_health_e.pdf?la=en.

Canadian Nurses Association (CNA). (2012). *Position statement on mental health services*. https://www.cna-aiic.ca/~/media/cna/page-content/pdf-en/ps85_mental_health_e.pdf?la=en.

Canadian Observatory on Homelessness. (2021). *About homelessness: Employment*. https://www.homelesshub.ca/about-homelessness/education-training-employment/employment.

Carter-Snell, C., & Jakubec, S. (2013). Exploring influences on mental health after interpersonal violence against women. *International Journal of Child, Youth and Family Studies, 1*, 72–99.

Carter-Snell, C., Jakubec, S. L., & Hagen, B. (2020). Collaboration with rural and remote communities to improve sexual assault services. *Journal of Community Health, 45*(2), 377–387. https://doi.org/10.1007/s10900-019-00744-4.

Centers for Disease Control and Prevention. (2013). *A practitioner's guide for advancing health equity: Community strategies for preventing chronic disease*. https://www.cdc.gov/nccdphp/dch/pdf/healthequityguide.pdf.

Centre for Addiction and Mental Health (CAMH). (2018). *Police mental health: A discussion paper*. https://www.camh.ca/-/media/files/pdfs---public-policy-submissions/police-mental-health-discussion-paper-oct2018-pdf.

Centre for Addiction and Mental Health (CAMH). (2020). *Suicide prevention: A review and policy recommendations*. https://www.camh.ca/-/media/files/pdfs---public-policy-submissions/suicide-prevention-review-and-policy-recommendations-pdf.

Centre for Addiction and Mental Health (CAMH). (2021). *Addiction*. https://www.camh.ca/en/health-info/mental-illness-and-addiction-index/addiction.

Citizens for Public Justice. (2020). *Poverty trends Canada 2020*. https://cpj.ca/wp-content/uploads/2020/09/Poverty-Trends-2020.pdf.

Coleman, T., & Cotton, D. (2014). Tempo: police interactions—a report towards improving interactions between police and people living with mental health problems. *Mental Health Commission of Canada*. https://www.mentalhealthcommission.ca/sites/default/files/TEMPO%252520Police%252520Interactions%252520082014_0.pdf.

Collins, A. B., Bluthenthal, R. N., Boyd, J., et al. (2018). Harnessing the language of overdose prevention to advance evidence-based responses to the opioid crisis. *International journal of drug policy, 55*, 77–79. https://doi.org/10.1016/j.drugpo.2018.02.013.

Community Health Nurses of Canada. (2019). *Canadian community health nursing: Professional practice model and standards of practice*. https://www.chnc.ca/en/standards-of-practice.

Coulombe, S., Pacheco, T., Cox, E., et al. (2020). Risk and resilience factors during the COVID-19 pandemic: a snapshot of the experiences of Canadian workers early on in the crisis. *Frontiers in Psychology, 11*, 580–702. https://doi.org/10.3389/fpsyg.2020.580702.

Dave, S., Afshar, K., Braga, L. H., et al. (2018). Canadian Urological Association guideline on the care of the normal foreskin and neonatal circumcision in Canadian infants (full version). *Canadian urological association journal/journal de l'association des urologues du Canada, 12*(2), E76–E99. https://doi.org/10.5489/cuaj.5033.

Department of Justice. (2015). *Inventory of spousal violence risk assessment tools used in Canada*. https://www.justice.gc.ca/eng/rp-pr/cj-jp/fv-vf/rr09_7/p4.html.

Department of Justice. (2016). *Preliminary examination of so-called "honour killings" in Canada*. https://www.justice.gc.ca/eng/rp-pr/cj-jp/fv-vf/hk-ch/p5.html.

Department of Justice. (2017a). *About family violence*. https://www.justice.gc.ca/eng/cj-jp/fv-vf/about-apropos.html.

Department of Justice. (2017b). *Child abuse is wrong: What can I do?*. https://www.justice.gc.ca/eng/rp-pr/cj-jp/fv-vf/caw-mei/toc-tdm.html.

Desapriya, E., & Khoshpour, P. (2018). Letters: investing appropriately to alleviate child poverty in Canada. *Canadian Medical Association Journal, 190*(26), E805–E806. https://www.cmaj.ca/content/cmaj/190/26/E805.full.pdf.

Doyle, L., Sheridan, A., & Treacy, M. P. (2017). Motivations for adolescent self-harm and the implications for mental health nurses. *Journal of psychiatric and mental health nursing, 24*(2–3), 134–142. https://doi.org/10.1111/jpm.12360.

Employment and Social Development Canada. (2017). *Homeless shelters*. https://www23.statcan.gc.ca/imdb/p2SV.pl?Function=getSurvey&SDDS=7538.

Farmer, P. E., Nizeye, B., Stulac, S., et al. (2006). Structural violence and clinical medicine. *PLoS Medicine, 3*(10), e449 https://dx.doi.org/10.1371%2Fjournal.pmed.0030449.

Fleckinger, A. (2020). The dynamics of secondary victimization: When social workers blame mothers. *Research on social work practice, 30*(5), 515–523. https://doi.org/10.1177%2F1049731519898525.

Fleming, N., Ng, N., Osborne, C., et al. (2013). Adolescent pregnancy outcomes in the province of Ontario: a cohort study. *Journal of obstetrics and gynaecology canada, 35*(3), 234–245. https://doi.org/10.1016/s1701-2163(15)30995-6.

Food Banks Canada. (2019). *Hunger count 2019*. https://www.foodbankscanada.ca/Research-Advocacy/HungerCount.aspx.

Gaetz, S., Barr, C., Friesen, A., et al. (2012). *Canadian definition of homelessness*. Canadian Observatory on Homelessness Press. https://www.homelesshub.ca/sites/default/files/COHhomelessdefinition.pdf.

Gaetz, S., Dej, E., Richter, T., et al. (2016). *The state of homelessness in Canada 2016*. Canadian Observatory on Homelessness Press. https://www.homelesshub.ca/sites/default/files/attachments/SOHC16_final_20Oct2016.pdf.

Gerlach, A. G., Browne, A. J., Sinha, V., et al. (2017). Navigating structural violence with Indigenous families: the contested terrain of early childhood intervention and the child welfare system in Canada. *International Indigenous Policy Journal, 8*(3). https://doi.org/10.18584/iipj.2017.8.3.6. Article 6.

Gill, A. (2014). "Honour," "honour"-based violence and so-called "honour" killings. In A. Gill, K. Roberts, & C. Strange (Ed.), *"Honour" killing and violence: Theory, policy and practice*. Palgrave Macmillan.

Goldner, E., Jenkins, E., & Bilsker, D. (2016). *A concise introduction to mental health in Canada* (2nd ed.). Canadian Scholars' Press.

Goodridge, D., Heal–Salahub, J., PausJenssen, E., et al. (2017). Peer bullying in seniors' subsidized apartment communities in Saskatoon, Canada: participatory research. *Health and Social Care in the Community, 25*(4), 1439–1447. https://doi.org/10.1111/hsc.12444.

Government of Canada. (2019). *Federal minimum wage: Issue paper.* https://www.canada.ca/en/employment-social-development/services/labour-standards/reports/federal-minimum-wage.html.

Government of Canada. (2020). *Social determinants of health and health inequalities.* https://www.canada.ca/en/public-health/services/health-promotion/population-health/what-determines-health.html.

Gruß, I., Bunce, A., Davis, J., et al. (2021). Initiating and implementing social determinants of health data collection in community health centers. *Population Health Management, 24*(1), 52–58. https://doi.org/10.1089/pop.2019.0205.

Guirguis-Younger, M., McNeil, R., & Hwang, S. W. (2014). *Homelessness & health in Canada.* University of Ottawa Press.

Halter, M., Pollard, C., & Jakubec, S. L. (Eds.). (2018). *Varcarolis's Canadian psychiatric mental health nursing* (2nd ed.) Elsevier Canada.

Hamza, C. A., Stewart, S. L., & Willoughby, T. (2012). Examining the link between nonsuicidal self-injury and suicidal behavior: a review of the literature and an integrated model. *Clinical psychology review, 32*(6), 482–495. https://doi.org/10.1016/j.cpr.2012.05.003.

Hango, D., & Moyser, M. (2018). *Insights on Canadian society: Harassment in Canadian workplaces.* https://www150.statcan.gc.ca/n1/pub/75-006-x/2018001/article/54982-eng.htm.

Hawk, M., Coulter, R. W. S., Egan, J. E., et al. (2017). Harm reduction principles for healthcare settings. *Harm Reduction Journal, 14*(7). https://doi.org/10.1186/s12954-017-0196-4.

Hyshka, E., Anderson-Baron, J., Pugh, A., et al. (2019). Principles, practice, and policy vacuums: Policy actor views on provincial/territorial harm reduction policy in Canada. *International Journal of Drug Policy, 71,* 142–149. https://doi.org/10.1016/j.drugpo.2018.12.014.

Jakubec, S. L. (2019). Suicide and nonsuicidal self-injury. In C. L. Pollard, S. L. Jakubec, & M. J. Halter (Ed.), *Varcarolis's Canadian psychiatric mental health nursing: A clinical approach* (2nd ed.) (p. 499). Elsevier Canada.

Katz, A., Hardy, B., Firestone, M., et al. (2019). Vagueness, power and public health: Use of "vulnerable" in public health literature. *Critical Public Health, 30*(5), 601–611. https://doi.org/10.1080/09581596.2019.1656800.

Kimberg, L., & Wheeler, M. (2019). Trauma and trauma-informed care. In M. R. Gerber (Ed.), *Trauma-informed healthcare approaches: A guide for primary care.* Springer International Publishing. https://doi.org/10.1007/978-3-030-04342-1.

Kingsland, M., Wiggers, J., Vashum, K., et al. (2016). Interventions in sports settings to reduce risky alcohol consumption and alcohol-related harm: a systematic review. *Systematic reviews, 5*(1), 12. https://doi.org/10.1186/s13643-016-0183-y.

Kirby, M. J. L. (2006). *Out of the shadows at last: Highlights and recommendations Final report of the standing senate committee on social Affairs and Technology.* http://www.parl.gc.ca/39/1/parlbus/commbus/senate/com-e/soci-e/rep-e/pdf/rep02may06part1-e.pdf.

Kumar, M. B., & Tjepkema, M. (2019). *Suicide among first Nations people, Métis and Inuit (2011–2016): Findings from the 2011*

Canadian Census Health and Environment Cohort (CanCHEC). https://www150.statcan.gc.ca/n1/en/pub/99-011-x/99-011-x2019001-eng.pdf?st=zuDcCbuh.

Learning Network, V. A. W. (2020). *COVID-19 and gender-based violence in Canada.* http://vawlearningnetwork.ca/docs/COVID-gbv-canada-recommendations.pdf.

Mental Health Commission of Canada. (2012). *Changing directions, changing lives.* https://www.mentalhealthcommission.ca/sites/default/files/MHStrategy_Strategy_ENG_0_1.pdf.

Mental Health Commission of Canada. (2015). *Recovery guidelines.* https://www.mentalhealthcommission.ca/sites/default/files/2016-07/MHCC_Recovery_Guidelines_2016_ENG.PDF.

Mental Health Commission of Canada. (2016). *Advancing the mental health strategy for Canada: A framework for action (2017–2022).* https://www.mentalhealthcommission.ca/sites/default/files/2016-08/advancing_the_mental_health_strategy_for_canada_a_framework_for_action.pdf.

Mental Health Commission of Canada. (2017). *Strengthening the case for investing in Canada's mental health system: Economic considerations.* https://www.mentalhealthcommission.ca/sites/default/files/2017-03/case_for_investment_eng.pdf.

Mental Health Commission of Canada. (2021). *Suicide risk assessment toolkit: A resource for healthcare workers and organizations.* https://www.mentalhealthcommission.ca/sites/default/files/2021-01/mhcc_cpsi_suicide_risk_assessment_toolkit_eng.pdf.

Mental Health First Aid Canada. (2021). *Mental health first aid: Big picture.* https://www.mhfa.ca/en/big-picture.

Miller, W. R., & Rollnick, S. (Eds.). (2012). *Motivational interviewing: Preparing people for change* (3rd ed.) Guilford Press.

Morse, G., Monroe-DeVita, M., York, M. M., et al. (2020). Implementing illness management and recovery within assertive community treatment teams: a qualitative study. *Psychiatric Rehabilitation Journal, 43*(2), 121–131. https://doi.org/10.1037/prj0000387.

National Collaborating Centre for Determinants of Health. (2014). *Let's talk: Populations and the power of language.* https://nccdh.ca/resources/entry/lets-talk-populations.

National Collaborating Centre for Determinants of Health. (2020). *Glossary: Vulnerable populations.* https://nccdh.ca/glossary/entry/vulnerable-populations.

National Collaborating Centres for Public Health. (2020). *What are the social determinants of health?.* https://nccdh.ca/images/uploads/comments/NCCPHSDOHFactsheet_EN_May2012.pdf.

Northcott, M. (2012). *Intimate partner violence risk assessment tools: A review.* Department of Justice Canada. https://www.justice.gc.ca/eng/rp-pr/cj-jp/fv-vf/rr12_8/rr12_8.pdf.

O'Brien, H. L., Greyson, D. L., Chabot, C., et al. (2018). Young parents' personal and social information contexts for child feeding practices: an ethnographic study in British Columbia, Canada. *Journal of Documentation, 74*(3), 608–623. https://open.library.ubc.ca/cIRcle/collections/facultyresearchandpublications/52383/items/1.0363925.

Pfefferbaum, B., & North, C. S. (2020). Mental health and the COVID-19 pandemic. *New England Journal of Medicine, 383*(6), 510–512. https://doi.org/10.1056/nejmp2008017.

Phipps, S. (2003). *The impact of poverty on health: A scan of research literature.* https://secure.cihi.ca/free_products/CPHIImpactonPoverty_e.pdf.

Pickett, K. E., & Wilkenson, R. G. (2017). Editorial: immorality of inaction on inequality. *BMJ, 356,* j556. https://doi.org/10.1136/bmj.j556.

PREVNet. (2019). *Bullying: What we know and what we can do.* https://www.prevnet.ca/.

Public Health Agency of Canada. (2020b). *Communicating about substance use in compassionate, safe and non-stigmatizing ways: A resource for Canadian health professional organizations and their membership.* https://www.canada.ca/en/public-health/services/publications/healthy-living/communicating-about-substance-use-compassionate-safe-non-stigmatizing-ways-2019.html.

Public Health Agency of Canada (PHAC). (2006). *The human face of mental health and mental illness in Canada, 2006.* http://phac-aspc.gc.ca/publicat/human-humain06/index-eng.php.

Public Health Agency of Canada (PHAC). (2018). *Key health inequalities in Canada: A national portrait.* https://www.canada.ca/content/dam/phac-aspc/documents/services/publications/science-research/key-health-inequalities-canada-national-portrait-executive-summary/key_health_inequalities_full_report-eng.pdf.

Public Health Agency of Canada (PHAC). (2020a). *Chief Public Health Officer of Canada's report on the state of public health in Canada 2020: From risk to resilience: An equity approach to COVID-19.* https://www.canada.ca/en/public-health/corporate/publications/chief-public-health-officer-reports-state-public-health-canada/from-risk-resilience-equity-approach-COVID-19.html.

Public Safety Canada. (2018). *Bullying prevention: Nature and extent of bullying in Canada.* https://www.publicsafety.gc.ca/cnt/rsrcs/pblctns/bllng-prvntn/index-en.aspx#a05.

Raphael, D., Bryant, T., Mikkonen, J., et al. (2020). *Social determinants of health: The Canadian facts.* Ontario Tech University Faculty of Health Sciences and York University School of Health Policy and Management.

Registered Nurses' Association of Ontario (RNAO). (2009). *Assessment and care of adults at risk for suicide ideation and behaviour.* http://rnao.ca/bpg/guidelines/assessment-and-care-adults-risk-suicidal-ideation-and-behaviour.

Reimer-Kirkham, S., Stajduhar, K., Pauly, B., et al. (2016). Death is a social justice issue: perspectives on equity-informed palliative care. *Advances in Nursing Science, 39*(4), 293–307. https://doi.org/10.1097/ans.0000000000000146.

Schizophrenia Society of Canada. (2021). About. https://schizophrenia.ca/about/.

Sebastian, J. G. (2014). Vulnerability and vulnerable populations: An overview. In M. Stanhope, & J. Lancaster (Ed.), *Foundations for population health in community/Public health nursing* (pp. 374–388). Mosby/Elsevier.

Shim, R., & Compton, M. (2018). Addressing the social determinants of mental health: if not now, when? If not us, who? *Psychiatric Services, 69*(8), 844–846. https://doi.org/10.1176/appi.ps.201800060.

Silva, M., Loureiro, A., & Cardoso, G. (2016). Social determinants of mental health: a review of the evidence. *European Journal of Psychiatry, 30*(4), 259–292.

Stajduhar, K. I., & Mollison, A. (2018). *Too little, too late: How we fail vulnerable Canadians as they die and what to do about it.* University of Victoria Institute on Aging and Lifelong Health. https://www.uvic.ca/research/groups/peol/assets/docs/too-little-too-late.pdf.

Statistics Canada. (2019a). *Homicide in Canada, 2018.* https://www150.statcan.gc.ca/n1/en/daily-quotidien/191127/dq191127a-eng.pdf?st=0UpE0Bik.

Statistics Canada. (2019b). *Family violence in Canada: A statistical profile, 2018.* https://www150.statcan.gc.ca/n1/en/pub/85-002-x/2019001/article/00018-eng.pdf?st=2GsOps0D.

Statistics Canada. (2020). *Canada's official poverty dashboard, February 2020.* https://www150.statcan.gc.ca/n1/pub/11-627-m/11-627-m2020018-eng.htm.

Tarasuk, V., & McIntyre, L. (2020). *Food insecurity in Canada. The Canadian Encyclopedia.* https://www.thecanadianencyclopedia.ca/en/article/food-insecurity-in-canada.

Taylor, P., Jomar, K., Dhingra, K., et al. (2018). A meta-analysis of the prevalence of different functions of non-suicidal self-injury. *Journal of Affective Disorders, 227,* 759–769. https://doi.org/10.1016/j.jad.2017.11.073.

Touhy, T. A., McLeary, L., & Boscart, V. (2019). Mental health and wellness in later life. In T. A. Touhy, K. F. Jett, V. Boscart, et al. (Ed.), *Ebersole and Hess' gerontological nursing & healthy aging* (2nd ed.) (pp. 409–438). Elsevier Canada.

Wallace, B., Browne, A. J., Varcoe, C., et al. (2015). Self-reported oral health among a community sample of people experiencing social and health inequities: implications for the primary health care sector. *BMJ Open, 5*(12), 1–10. https://doi.org/10.1136/bmjopen-2015-009519.

Wong, S. P. W., Twynstra, J., Gilliland, J. A., et al. (2020). Risk factors and birth outcomes associated with teenage pregnancy: a Canadian sample. *Journal of Pediatric and Adolescent Gynecology, 33*(2), 153–159. https://doi.org/10.1016/j.jpag.2019.10.006.

World Health Organization (WHO). (1986). The Ottawa charter for health promotion. http://www.who.int/healthpromotion/conferences/previous/ottawa/en/.

World Health Organization (WHO). (2014). *Social determinants of health.* https://apps.who.int/iris/bitstream/handle/10665/112828/9789241506809_eng.pdf?sequence=1.

World Health Organization (WHO). (2016). *Media centre fact sheet: Female genital mutilation.* http://www.who.int/mediacentre/factsheets/fs241/en/.

World Health Organization (WHO). (2017). *Q & A detail: Determinants of health.* https://www.who.int/news-room/q-a-detail/determinants-of-health.

World Health Organization (WHO). (2018). *Mental health: Strengthening our response.* https://www.who.int/news-room/fact-sheets/detail/mental-health-strengthening-our-response.

Specific Domains of Community Health Practice

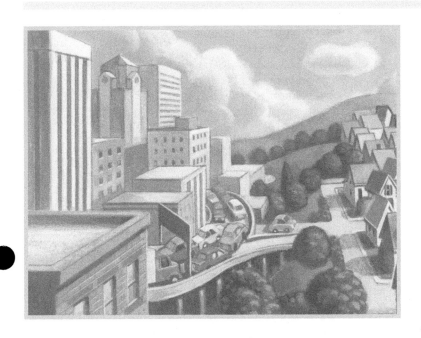

Communicable and Infectious Disease Prevention and Control

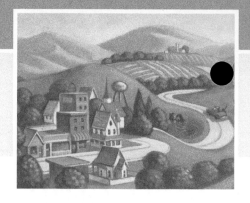

OUTLINE

Historical Perspectives, 391
Determinants of Health, 392
Communicable Diseases, 394
  Agent, Host, and Environment, 394
  Modes of Transmission, 395
  Disease Development, 395
  Disease Spectrum, 395
Surveillance of Communicable Diseases, 396
  List of Notifiable Diseases, 396
  Primary, Secondary, and Tertiary Prevention, 397
  The Role of Community Health Nurses in Disease
    Prevention and Control, 398
  Vaccine-Preventable Diseases, 398
  Non–Vaccine-Preventable Diseases, 404

Sexually Transmitted Infections, 405
Infectious Diseases, 410
  Viral Hepatitis, 410
  Ebola Virus Disease, 411
  Waterborne and Foodborne Diseases, 412
  Vectorborne Diseases, 414
  Diseases of Travellers, 415
  Zoonoses, 416
Parasitic Diseases, 416
The Community Health Nurse's Role in Providing
  Preventive Care, 416
  Primary Prevention, 416
  Secondary Prevention, 418
  Tertiary Prevention, 419

OBJECTIVES

After reading this chapter, you should be able to:

16.1 Discuss the past and current effects and threats of communicable and infectious diseases on society.

16.2 Identify the determinants of health that affect communicable diseases, infectious diseases, and sexually transmitted infections.

16.3 Explain how the factors that make up the epidemiological triangle can interact to cause the transmission and development of communicable diseases.

16.4 Define *surveillance* and discuss the role of the community health nurse (CHN) in communicable disease prevention and control.

16.5 Identify and describe common infectious diseases.

16.6 Discuss the risk and diagnosis of parasitic diseases in Canada.

16.7 Explain the CHN's role in primary, secondary, and tertiary preventive care of patients with communicable and infectious diseases.

KEY TERMS*

acquired immunity, 394
acquired immunodeficiency syndrome (AIDS), 405
active immunization, 394
anthrax, 391
chlamydia, 405
common vehicle, 395
communicable disease, 394
communicable period, 395
contact tracing, 419
directly observed therapy (DOT), 419
disease, 395
Ebola virus disease, 411
elimination, 394
emerging infectious diseases, 391
environment, 394

eradication, 394
gonorrhea, 405
hantavirus pulmonary syndrome (HPS), 391
hepatitis A virus (HAV), 410
hepatitis B virus (HBV), 411
hepatitis C virus (HCV), 411
herd immunity, 394
HIV antibody test, 419
horizontal transmission, 395
incubation period, 395
infection, 395
infectious disease, 410
infectiousness, 394
natural immunity, 394
partner notification, 419

passive immunization, 394

resistance, 394

severe acute respiratory syndrome (SARS), 392

surveillance, 396

vaccine, 394

vector, 395

vertical transmission, 395

*See the Glossary on page 468 for definitions.

Concern about the widespread effects of communicable and infectious diseases requires that community health nurses (CHNs) stay current about communicable and infectious disease guidelines and implement those guidelines in practice. This chapter presents an overview of the communicable and infectious diseases CHNs deal with most often. It also presents information on nursing management of communicable and infectious diseases, including primary, secondary, and tertiary prevention.

Communicable and infectious diseases are often acquired through behaviours that can be avoided or changed. For this reason, community health nursing interventions tend to focus on disease prevention. Prevention can take the form of vaccine administration (e.g., for hepatitis A and B), early detection (e.g., for tuberculosis), or teaching patients about abstinence or safer sex (for the prevention of sexually transmitted infections [STIs]).

HISTORICAL PERSPECTIVES

In the 1900s, communicable and infectious diseases were the leading causes of death in Canada. Improved nutrition, vaccines, and antibiotics have put an end to the epidemics that once ravaged entire populations. For example, in 1926, tuberculosis (TB) caused 7% of all deaths in Canada; by 1990, less than 1% of deaths occurred due to TB (Lung Association, 2006). In the early 1900s in Canada, patients with TB were being treated on an in-patient basis, and the minimum length of treatment was at least 1 year. Antimicrobial medications were discovered for the effective treatment of TB in 1948, and by the 1980s, the downward trend in TB had levelled off. For more information on the history of TB in Canada, see the Canadian Public Health Association's "History of Tuberculosis" web page and the Canadian Lung Association's "Who We Are" web page (the links are on the Evolve website).

However, chronic diseases—such as heart disease, cancer, and stroke—have replaced communicable and infectious diseases as the leading causes of death. In fact, each year in Canada, the majority of deaths occur from noncommunicable diseases such as cardiovascular disease, cancer, and diabetes (WHO, 2011).

The Public Health Agency of Canada (PHAC) works to prevent and control communicable diseases through the Centre for Communicable Diseases and Infection Control (CCDIC), which has four divisions: Surveillance and Epidemiology Division; Professional Guidelines and Public Health Practice Division; Programs and Partnerships Division; and Strategic Issues and Integrated Management Division. The CCDIC is involved in creating and sharing knowledge and facilitating action on communicable diseases such as human immunodeficiency virus/acquired immunodeficiency syndrome (HIV/AIDS), TB, STIs, hepatitis B and C, and health care infections (Public Health Agency of Canada [PHAC], 2013).

Despite better surveillance, control, and treatment, communicable and infectious diseases are a global concern. **Emerging infectious diseases** are those in which the incidence has actually increased in the past two decades or has the potential to increase in the near future. Emerging infectious diseases may include new or known infectious diseases. Consider the following examples: (1) Ebola virus is a virus with a frightening mortality rate that is highly contagious; (2) HIV and AIDS are associated with a rising number of previously rare opportunistic infections such as cryptosporidiosis, toxoplasmosis, and *Pneumocystis* pneumonia; (3) West Nile virus (WNV) and Zika are viruses that are new to Canada and transmitted mainly by infected mosquitoes; (4) **anthrax** is an acute disease caused by the spore-forming bacterium *Bacillus anthracis* that is highly resistant to disinfection and environmental destruction and may remain in contaminated soil for many years; (5) avian influenza virus is a contagious viral infection that most often affects birds but can infect mammals; (6) the H1N1 flu virus is a strain of influenza virus that is transmissible to humans (who have developed little or no immunity to it) and could result in an influenza pandemic; (7) Middle East respiratory syndrome (MERS) is a viral respiratory illness that is new to humans—it was first reported in Saudi Arabia in 2012; and (8) cryptococcal disease is a rare but treatable fungal infection that has emerged on Vancouver Island, British Columbia (British Columbia Centre for Disease Control, 2014).

As the following examples indicate, new killers are emerging, and old, familiar diseases are taking on different and more virulent characteristics.

Hantavirus pulmonary syndrome (HPS), also referred to as *hantavirus disease,* is an infectious disease caused by the hantavirus. Until recently, only four to six cases of HPS occurred in Canada per year, but from 2013 to 2015, cases of HPS in Canada increased substantially (Drebot, Jones, Grolla, et al., 2015). HPS begins with flu-like symptoms that can become life-threatening when the virus affects the lungs and causes respiratory problems (PHAC, 2014b). In Canada, deer mice (*Peromyscus maniculatus*) are the principal carriers of HPS. Infected mice shed the virus in fresh urine, droppings, and saliva. Humans become infected from the inhalation of the virus if exposed to heavily contaminated materials in which mice have nested. Also, but less often, ingestion of contaminated food or water by humans can lead to HPS. Seldom are people infected as a result of having been bitten by a mouse. Since 1989, there have been 109 confirmed cases and 27 deaths of HPS in Canada (PHAC, 2014b).

Necrotizing fasciitis, most commonly referred to as *flesh-eating disease,* is a severe condition that has a high fatality rate. A skin injury usually precedes the development of the disease. Most often, the bacteria causing the disease are group A streptococci. This condition is common in temperate zones and semitropics, although rare cases have occurred in Canada. It is estimated that between 90 and 200 cases occur in Canada per year (Thunder Bay District Health Unit, 2021). Since January 2005, this disease has been under surveillance by Health Canada.

Escherichia coli (E. coli) O157:H7 is a highly toxic strain of the *E. coli* bacterium and is most frequently transmitted by consumption of contaminated food (e.g., contaminated ground beef, contaminated unpasteurized milk, contaminated fresh produce). One of the most common medical problems associated with *E. coli* is severe diarrhea, but it can also cause kidney damage. This disease arises often as a result of lower standards of water quality, sanitation, and food preparation. Outbreaks have occurred in the United States, Canada, and Europe (via contaminated sprout seeds from Egypt) (Marler Clark, n.d.).

Bovine spongiform encephalopathy (BSE), also known as *mad cow disease,* can be transmitted to humans through the consumption of contaminated beef. The origin of BSE remains unconfirmed, but it is believed to be related to feeding cattle meat and bone meal that has been contaminated with BSE. BSE was identified in Canada in 1993 in a beef cow that had been brought into Canada from Britain in 1987. The disease also appeared in the United States in 2003, when a BSE-infected animal was imported from Canada. BSE has been reported in many other countries, including several European countries, Japan, and Israel. BSE is a federally notifiable disease in Canada, which means that all suspected cases must be reported to the Canadian Food Inspection Agency. New cases of BSE were found in Canadian beef as recently as 2015 (Canadian Food Inspection Agency, 2015). Numerous measures have been taken to prevent further cases and the spread of BSE, such as surveillance programs, feeding product controls, and cattle identification programs.

Creutzfeldt-Jakob disease (CJD) is a rare disease that affects the central nervous system and can be fatal in humans. There are two forms of CJD: classic and variant (vCJD). Classic CJD occurs in the general population at a rate of about one case per million people worldwide. Most cases have no known cause or triggering event. By contrast, vCJD is a new disease in humans linked to eating beef products from cattle known to be infected with the same organism that causes BSE. CJD and vCJD are federally notifiable diseases in Canada. Figure 16.1 identifies the definite and probable cases of CJD cases in Canada by province and territory. In Canada, the number of suspected cases of CJD from 1998 to 2019 were 2 008, and there were 194 deaths of CJD from 2015 to 2017 (PHAC,

2019a, g). The data on CJD is updated frequently. For the latest updates, see the PHAC's "Creutzfeldt-Jakob Disease (CJD)/Variant Creutzfeldt-Jakob Disease (vCJD)" link on the Evolve website.

West Nile virus (WNV) is a mosquito-transmitted illness that can affect livestock, birds, and humans, and was first identified in New York City in 1999. The first confirmed human cases of WNV in Canada were reported in Ontario and Quebec in 2002. In 2018, there were 367 clinical cases of WNV reported in 4 provinces: Alberta (45), Ontario (126), Manitoba (33), Quebec (163), with 26 deaths reported (PHAC, 2019c).

Severe acute respiratory syndrome (SARS) is a disease of undetermined etiology with no definitive treatment. In early 2003, SARS was first reported in China and Hong Kong. Then in March 2003, the first Canadian cases were reported in patients who were identified as Canadians returning from Hong Kong. WHO and the PHAC worked collaboratively to monitor and control the SARS outbreak in Canada. Further information about SARS is provided in Chapter 18.

MERS-CoV, which is caused by a coronavirus, was reported in Saudi Arabia in 2012. Since then, all cases have been linked to patients living in or travelling to the Middle East. Symptoms are severe and include fever, cough, and shortness of breath, with complications including kidney failure and death. Since 2012, WHO has been notified of 2 374 laboratory-confirmed cases of MERS-CoV globally, with the majority of those cases coming from Saudi Arabia. To date there have been no reported cases in Canada (WHO, 2019).

SARS-CoV-2 (coronavirus disease 2019 or COVID-19) which is caused by a novel coronavirus, was first reported as an epidemic in mainland China in February 2020 and declared a pandemic by the WHO on March 11, 2020. (Dos Santos, 2020). The origin and source remain unknown, although initial cases were associated with snakes, birds, and bats. Human to human transmission has been supported and the disease has spread rapidly around the world. As of July 2021, world-wide there were 191 148 056 confirmed cases (WHO, 2021a) and in Canada there were 1 424 715 cases with 1 393 117 of those cases resolved (Government of Canada, 2021).

DETERMINANTS OF HEALTH

Several determinants of health affect well-being, illness, health promotion, and disease prevention. For example, poverty and low literacy may lead individuals with communicable diseases to become socially excluded because they have limited access to health services and programs for treatment. Gender is a factor in the incidence and prevalence of several STIs. The CHN role is to create a supportive environment—for example, by providing information sessions and accessible health services such as clinics. The "Determinants of Health" box presents the influence of health services, poverty, education and literacy, and gender on communicable and infectious diseases.

DETERMINANTS OF HEALTH

The Influence of the Determinants of Health on Communicable and Infectious Diseases

- In Canada, 220 697 to 245 987 people live with chronic hepatitis C virus (HCV), and 44% of those infected do not know.* It has been found that one in five people in Canada who experienced HCV is an immigrant who has difficulties with access to health care. As a chronic disease, HCV places a substantial economic burden on Canadians.[†]
- In Canada, about 3 million people obtain their drinking water from private wells, and these wells can become contaminated from poor construction, improper location, or if surface water is contaminated.[‡]

- In Canada, approximately 4 million (1 in 8) people are affected annually by a food-borne illness and, of these, there are about 11 600 hospitalizations and 238 deaths.[§]
- Globally, approximately 55 000 people die of rabies annually, and approximately 95% of these deaths are in Asia and Africa.[‖]
- Reported cases of STIs are steadily increasing in Canada, with a 49% increase in chlamydia, an 81% increase in gonorrhea, and a 92% increase in syphilis between 2007 and 2016. Multiresistant gonorrhea is also an emerging issue, especially for the 15- to 29-year-old age group.[#]

Sources: *Canadian AIDS Treatment Information Exchange. (2019). *Fact sheets: The epidemiology of hepatitis C in Canada.* https://www.catie.ca/en/fact-sheets/epidemiology/epidemiology-hepatitis-c-canada

[†] Sherman, M., Shafran, S., Burak, K., et al. (2007). Management of chronic hepatitis C: Consensus guidelines. *Canadian Journal of Gastroenterology, 21*(Suppl. C), 25C–34C.

[‡] Government of Canada. (2019). Be well aware -information for private well owners. https://www.canada.ca/en/health-canada/services/publications/healthy-living/water-talk-information-private-well-owners.html.

[§] Government of Canada. (2016). Yearly food-borne illness estimates for Canada. https://www.canada.ca/en/public-health/services/food-borne-illness-canada/yearly-food-borne-illness-estimates-canada.html.

[‖] World Health Organization (WHO). (2009b). *Rabies.* http://www.who.int/topics/rabies/en/.

[#] Public Health Agency of Canada (PHAC). (2009b). *Polio (Poliomyelitis).* http://travel.gc.ca/travelling/health-safety/diseases/polio

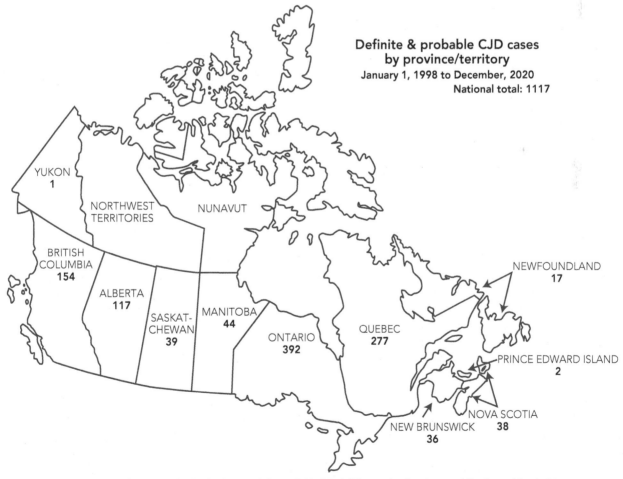

Definite & probable CJD cases by province/territory
January 1, 1998 to December, 2020
National total: 1117

YUKON 1
NORTHWEST TERRITORIES
NUNAVUT
BRITISH COLUMBIA 154
ALBERTA 117
SASKATCHEWAN 39
MANITOBA 44
ONTARIO 392
QUEBEC 277
NEWFOUNDLAND 17
PRINCE EDWARD ISLAND 2
NOVA SCOTIA 38
NEW BRUNSWICK 36

Fig. 16.1 Definite and Probable Cases of Creutzfeldt-Jakob Disease by Province and Territory, March 31, 2019. *CJD,* Creutzfeldt-Jakob disease. (Public Health Agency of Canada. [2019a]. Creutzfeldt-Jakob Disease. CJD-Surveillance System: Statistics—Referrals of Suspected CJD Reported by CJDSS, 1998–2019 as of March 31, 2019. https://www.canada.ca/en/public-health/services/surveillance/blood-safety-contribution-program/creutzfeldt-jakob-disease/cjd-surveillance-system.html#pycases)

COMMUNICABLE DISEASES

A **communicable disease** is a contagious disease of human or animal origin caused by an infectious agent. Its transmission depends on the successful interaction of the infectious agent, the host, and the environment, the factors that make up the epidemiological triangle (see Chapter 3). Communicable diseases can be prevented and controlled. The goal of prevention and control programs is to reduce the prevalence of a disease to a level at which it no longer poses a major public health problem. In some cases, diseases may even be eliminated or eradicated. The goal of **elimination** is to remove a disease from a large geographical area such as a country or region of the world. **Eradication** is the permanent elimination of a disease worldwide. WHO officially declared the global eradication of smallpox on May 8, 1980 (WHO, 1999). After the successful eradication of smallpox, the eradication of other communicable diseases became a realistic goal.

Agent, Host, and Environment

Changes in the characteristics of any of the factors may result in disease transmission. Consider the following examples. Antibiotic therapy may not only eliminate a specific pathological agent but also alter the balance of normally occurring organisms in the body. As a result, one of these agents overruns another, and disease, such as a yeast infection, occurs. Individuals living in the temperate climate of Canada do not contract malaria at home, but they may become infected if they travel to a climate where malaria-carrying mosquitoes thrive. As these examples illustrate, the balance among agent, host, and environment is often precarious and may be unintentionally disrupted. In the twenty-first century, the potential results of such disruption require attention as advances in science and technology, destruction of natural habitats, explosive population growth, political instability, and a worldwide transportation network combine to alter the balance among the environment, people, and the agents that produce disease.

Agent Factor

Four main categories of infectious agents can cause infection or disease: bacteria, fungi, parasites, and viruses. The individual agent may be described by its ability to cause disease and by the nature and the severity of the disease. *Infectivity, pathogenicity, virulence, toxicity, invasiveness,* and *antigenicity* are terms commonly used to characterize infectious agents and their unique impact on the epidemiological triangle (i.e., rate of transmission, severity of illness and so on). These terms are defined in Box 16.1.

Host Factor

A human or animal host can harbour an infectious agent. The characteristics of the host that may influence the spread of disease are host resistance, immunity, herd immunity, and infectiousness. **Resistance** is the ability of the host to withstand infection, and it may involve natural or acquired immunity. **Natural immunity** refers to species-determined, innate resistance to an infectious agent. For example, coyotes in Saskatchewan rarely contract rabies, because that species has developed a natural immunity to rabies. **Acquired immunity**

> ### BOX 16.1   Six Characteristics and Impacts of an Infectious Agent
>
> 1. *Infectivity:* The ability to enter and multiply in the host
> 2. *Pathogenicity:* The ability to produce a specific clinical reaction after infection occurs
> 3. *Virulence:* The ability to produce a severe pathological reaction
> 4. *Toxicity:* The ability to produce a poisonous reaction
> 5. *Invasiveness:* The ability to penetrate and spread throughout a body tissue
> 6. *Antigenicity:* The ability to stimulate an immunological response

is the resistance acquired by a host as a result of previous natural exposure to an infectious agent. Having measles once protects against future infection. Acquired immunity may be induced by active or passive immunization. **Active immunization** refers to the immunization of an individual by the administration of an antigen (infectious agent or **vaccine** [a preparation of killed microorganisms, living attenuated organisms, or living fully virulent organisms]) to stimulate an active response by the host's immunological system, which is usually characterized by the presence of antibodies produced by the individual host, therefore providing complete protection against the specific disease. Vaccinating children against childhood diseases is an example of inducing active immunity. **Passive immunization** refers to immunization through the transfer of a specific antibody from an immunized individual to a nonimmunized individual, such as the transfer of antibodies from mother to infant or the administration of an antibody-containing preparation (immune globulin or antiserum). Passive immunity from immune globulin is almost immediate but short-lived. It is often induced as a stopgap measure until active immunity has time to develop after vaccination. Examples of commonly used immune globulins include those for hepatitis A, rabies, and tetanus.

Herd immunity refers to the immunity of a group or community. It is the resistance of a group of people to the invasion and spread of an infectious agent. Herd immunity is based on the resistance of a high proportion of individual members of a group to infection. It is the basis for increasing immunization coverage for vaccine-preventable diseases. Higher immunization coverage will lead to greater herd immunity, which in turn will block the further spread of the disease. For example, the national immunization campaign for the administration of the H1N1 vaccine was an effort to achieve herd immunity.

Infectiousness is a measure of the potential ability of an infected host to transmit the infection to other hosts. It reflects the relative ease with which the infectious agent is transmitted to others. Individuals with measles are extremely infectious; the virus spreads readily via airborne droplets. A person with Lyme disease cannot spread the disease to other people (although the infected tick can).

Environmental Factor

In the context of communicable diseases, the **environment** refers to all that is external to the human host, including social and physical factors. These environmental factors facilitate the transmission of an infectious agent from an infected host to other susceptible hosts. Reduction in communicable disease risk can be achieved by altering these environmental factors. Using mosquito nets and insect repellents to avoid insect bites, installing sewage systems to prevent fecal contamination of water supplies, and washing utensils after contact with raw meat to reduce bacterial contamination are all examples of altering the environment to prevent disease.

Modes of Transmission

Communicable diseases can be transmitted vertically or horizontally. **Vertical transmission** is the passing of an infection from parent to offspring via sperm, placenta, milk, or contact in the vaginal canal at birth. Examples of vertical transmission are transplacental transmission of HIV and syphilis. **Horizontal transmission** is the person-to-person spread of infection through one or more of the following four routes: direct or indirect contact, common vehicle, airborne, or vectorborne. Most STIs are spread by direct sexual contact. Enterobiasis, or pinworm infection, can be acquired through direct contact or indirect contact with contaminated objects such as toys, clothing, and bedding. **Common vehicle** refers to the transportation of the infectious agent from an infected host to a susceptible host via food, water, milk, blood, serum, saliva, or plasma. Hepatitis A can be transmitted through contaminated food and water; hepatitis B can be transmitted through contaminated blood. Legionellosis and TB are both spread via contaminated droplets in the air. A **vector** is a non-human organism, often an insect, that either mechanically or biologically plays a role in the transmission of an infectious agent from source to host. For example, a vector can be an arthropod, such as a tick or mosquito, or other invertebrate, such as a snail, that can transmit the infectious agent by biting or depositing the infective material near the host.

Disease Development

Exposure to an infectious agent does not always lead to an infection. Similarly, infection does not always lead to disease. Infection depends on the infective dose, the infectivity of the infectious agent, and the immunocompetence of the host. It is important to differentiate infection from disease, as clearly illustrated by the HIV/AIDS epidemic. **Infection** refers to the state produced by the invasion of a host by an infectious agent. Infection involves the entry, development, and multiplication of the infectious agent in the susceptible host. Such infection may or may not produce clinical signs. **Disease** refers to the presence of abnormal alterations in the structure or functioning of the human body that fits within the medical model. It is one of the possible outcomes of infection, and it may indicate a physiological dysfunction or pathological reaction. For example, individuals who test positive for HIV are infected, but if they do not exhibit clinical signs, they are not considered at that time to have the disease. If individuals test positive for HIV and also exhibit clinical signs of AIDS, they are infected and have the disease.

Incubation period and *communicable period* are not synonymous. **Incubation period** is the time interval between the invasion by an infectious agent and the first appearance of signs and symptoms of the disease. The incubation periods of infectious diseases vary from between 2 and 4 hours for staphylococcal food poisoning to between 10 and 15 years for AIDS. **Communicable period** is the interval during which an infectious agent may be transferred directly or indirectly from an infected person to another person. The period of communicability for influenza is 3 to 5 days after the clinical onset of symptoms. Hepatitis B–infected people are infectious many weeks before the onset of the first symptoms and remain infective during the acute phase and chronic carrier state, which may persist for life.

Disease Spectrum

People with communicable diseases may exhibit a broad spectrum of disease that ranges from subclinical infection to severe and fatal disease. Those with subclinical or nonapparent infections are important from the public health point of view because they are a source of infection but may not be receiving the care that those with a clinical disease receive. They should be targeted for early diagnosis and treatment. Those with a clinical disease may exhibit localized or systemic symptoms and mild to severe illness. The final outcome of a disease may be recovery, death, or something in between, including a carrier state; complications requiring an extended hospital stay; or disability requiring rehabilitation.

At the community level, the disease may occur in endemic, epidemic, or pandemic proportion. *Endemic* refers to the constant presence of a disease in a particular population or geographical area. For example, pertussis is endemic in the United States. *Epidemic* refers to the occurrence of a greater number of cases of a disease, an injury, or other condition than expected in a particular area or group. Although people tend to associate large numbers with epidemics, even one case can be termed *epidemic* if the disease was considered previously eliminated from that area. For example, one case of polio, a disease considered eliminated from Canada, would be considered epidemic. *Pandemic* refers to an epidemic occurring in a geographically widespread area or in a large population. HIV/AIDS is both epidemic and pandemic because the number of cases is growing rapidly across various regions of the world. SARS emerged as a communicable disease and is an example of a pandemic. In February 2003, the world learned of a mysterious respiratory disease primarily infecting travellers and health care workers in Southeast Asia (Katz & Hirsch, 2003). Thought at first to be a form of influenza, this illness was soon recognized as an atypical and sometimes deadly pneumonia, transmitted easily through close contact and seemingly unresponsive to treatment with antibiotics and antiviral medications. Initially confined to mainland China, this disease of unknown etiology and no respect for national borders spread to Hong Kong and then quickly to Hanoi, Singapore, and Toronto, prompting WHO in 2003 to release a rare emergency travel advisory that heightened the surveillance of patients with atypical pneumonia around the globe. Intense international investigation revealed that SARS was associated with a new strain of coronavirus. Common symptoms included cough, dyspnea, malaise, and fever. By the end of July 2003, more than 8 000 cases with more than 800 deaths had been reported to WHO from approximately 30 countries.

In March of 2020, WHO declared the novel coronavirus SARS-CoV-2 (coronavirus disease 2019 or COVID-19) a pandemic due to the speed and scale of transmission. COVID-19 is transmitted human to human by respiratory droplets, close contact with diseased patients, and aerosol contact, with the dominant route being airborne. The majority of individuals are asymptomatic or present with mild symptoms, but those who are symptomatic present with cough, sore throat, headache, fever, myalgia, dyspnea, loss of taste or smell, nausea, vomiting, and diarrhea. Disease severity is related to immune status and underlying conditions such as age, hypertension, diabetes, and cancer (Dos Santos, 2020). As of July 2021, world-wide there were 191 148 056 confirmed cases and 4 109 303 deaths, and in Canada there were 1 423 889 confirmed cases and 26 504 deaths (WHO, 2021a).

In an effort to reduce mortality and morbidity from COVID-19, public health and social measures were implemented around the world, including personal protective measures (e.g., physical distancing, avoiding crowded settings, hand hygiene, respiratory etiquette, mask-wearing); environmental measures (e.g., cleaning, disinfection, ventilation); surveillance and response measures (e.g., testing, genetic sequencing, contact tracing, isolation, and quarantine); physical distancing measures (e.g., regulating the number and flow of people attending gatherings, maintaining distance in public or workplaces, domestic movement restrictions); and international travel-related measures (WHO, 2021b). In an unprecedented timeline, three two-dose vaccines were developed, tested, and administered worldwide. As of July 2021, 43% of the total population of Canada was fully vaccinated and 68% were partially vaccinated (Government of Canada, 2021).

The "Ethical Considerations" box discusses safety precautions during a communicable disease outbreak.

ETHICAL CONSIDERATIONS

The Canadian Nurses Association's *Code of Ethics* states the following: "During a natural or human-made disaster, including a communicable disease outbreak, nurses provide care using appropriate safety precautions in accordance with legislation, regulations, and guidelines..."* This duty raises ethical concerns for CHNs who might be worried about the adequacy of safety precautions when caring for a patient who has a communicable disease.

Ethical principles that apply to this duty include:
- *Distributive justice.* This ethical principle has to do with fairness. During an outbreak, CHNs should ensure that patients receive their fair share of services and resources based on their need and that those services and resources are not withheld or limited because of the risk of contracting the disease.
- *Beneficence.* CHNs have a general duty to perform actions that maintain or enhance the dignity of patients whenever those actions do not place undue burden on CHNs.

Question to Consider
- What are the CHN's responsibilities in preventing the spread of measles to populations at risk, such as people infected with HIV?

Source: *Canadian Nurses Association (CNA). (2017). *Code of ethics for registered nurses, 2017 edition* (p. 37). http://www.cna-aiic.ca/

SURVEILLANCE OF COMMUNICABLE DISEASES

Depending on the type of organism involved, the conditions of spread and the target population, outbreaks can be acute and fast-moving (e.g., gastroenteritis in a nursery school or long-term care facility) or evolve more slowly (e.g., the AIDS pandemic). While public health authorities are ultimately responsible for ensuring the detection and control of outbreaks, CHNs are important in surveillance. They are often a first point of contact with the affected population. CHNs may see an unusually high number of people with the same disease, or community members will inform CHNs that they know other people with similar symptoms. Even if a CHN does not suspect an outbreak, reporting contributes to **surveillance**, which is the systematic and ongoing observation and collection of data on disease occurrence to describe phenomena and detect changes in frequency or distribution.

With advanced control of communicable diseases and as individuals live longer, chronic diseases have become the leading causes of death. Currently in Canada, the PHAC monitors communicable diseases. Surveillance incorporates and analyzes data from a variety of sources. Box 16.2 lists 10 commonly used data elements.

List of Notifiable Diseases

The provinces and territories are responsible for maintaining the notifiable (reportable) disease information system. Nationally notifiable diseases (NNDs) are communicable diseases designated by the federal, provincial, and territorial governments as priorities for monitoring and control (PHAC, 2019d). In addition, WHO specifies a number of diseases that must be reported worldwide.

The PHAC determines whether a disease is notifiable based on a variety of characteristics, including:
- Its interest to national or international regulations or prevention programs
- Its national incidence
- Its severity
- Its communicability
- Its potential to cause outbreaks
- The socioeconomic costs of its cases
- Its preventability

BOX 16.2 Ten Basic Data Elements Used in Surveillance

1. Mortality registration
2. Morbidity reporting
3. Epidemic reporting
4. Epidemic field investigation
5. Laboratory reporting
6. Individual case investigation
7. Surveys
8. Use of biological agents and medications
9. Distribution of animal reservoirs and vectors
10. Demographic and environmental data

BOX 16.3 Nationally Notifiable Diseases in Canada

- Acute flaccid paralysis
- Acquired immunodeficiency syndrome (AIDS)
- Anthrax
- Botulism
- Brucellosis
- Campylobacteriosis
- Chicken pox (varicella)
- Chlamydia
- Cholera
- *Clostridium difficile* associated diarrhea (CDI)
- Congenital rubella syndrome (CRS)
- Congenital syphilis
- Creutzfeldt-Jakob disease
- Cryptosporidiosis
- Cyclosporiasis
- Diphtheria
- Giardiasis
- Gonorrhea
- Group B streptococcal disease of the newborn (GBS)
- Hantavirus pulmonary syndrome (HPS)
- Hepatitis A
- Hepatitis B
- Hepatitis C
- Human immunodeficiency virus (HIV) infection
- Influenza, epidemic
- Influenza, laboratory confirmed
- Invasive group A streptococcal disease
- Invasive *Haemophilus influenzae* non-b disease
- Invasive meningococcal disease
- Invasive pneumococcal disease
- Legionellosis
- Leprosy
- Listeriosis
- Lyme disease
- Malaria
- Measles
- Mumps
- Norovirus infection
- Paralytic shellfish poisoning
- Paratyphoid
- Pertussis
- Plague
- Poliomyelitis
- Rabies
- Rubella
- Salmonellosis
- Severe acute respiratory syndrome (SARS)
- Shigellosis
- Smallpox
- Syphilis
- Tetanus
- Tuberculosis
- Tularemia
- Typhoid
- Verotoxigenic *Escherichia coli* infection
- Viral hemorrhagic fevers (Crimean-Congo, Ebola, Lassa, Marburg)
- West Nile virus (WNV)
- Yellow fever

NOTE: This list includes communicable and infectious diseases.
Source: Public Health Agency of Canada (PHAC). (2019d). *List of nationally notifiable diseases.* https://diseases.canada.ca/notifiable/diseases-list

---

- The risk it poses in the public perception
- The need for a public health response
- Evidence that its pattern is changing. (Association of Faculties of Medicine of Canada, n.d.)

All provinces and territories require that diseases identified in the *Public Health Act* be reported to the province or territory (some jurisdictions require the reporting of additional diseases). A reporting mechanism is in place between the provinces/territories and the PHAC to facilitate the surveillance of specific communicable diseases. Some provincial and territorial health authorities also require the reporting of noninfectious diseases that can be caused by environmental hazards, such as poisoning with heavy metals or with carbon monoxide.

Communicable diseases that could pose an immediate, severe threat to the public's health should be reported to the local or provincial department of health by telephone as soon as a case is suspected. Laboratories notify the provincial public health authority of cases of NND when test results are positive. The list of NNDs in Canada is shown in Box 16.3.

Primary, Secondary, and Tertiary Prevention

In the prevention and control of communicable disease, primary prevention seeks to reduce the incidence of disease by preventing it before it happens, and this effort is often assisted by the government. Many interventions at the primary level, such as "no shots, no school" immunization laws in Ontario, Manitoba, and New Brunswick, are population based because of public health mandates (Walkinshaw, 2011). CHNs deliver many of these childhood immunizations in public and community health settings, check immunization records in daycare facilities, and monitor immunization records in schools.

The goal of secondary prevention is to prevent the spread of disease once it occurs. Activities centre on rapid identification of potential contacts to a reported case. Contacts may be (1) identified as new cases and treated or (2) determined to be possibly exposed but not diseased and appropriately treated with prophylaxis. Public health disease control laws also assist in secondary prevention because they require investigation and prevention measures for individuals affected by a communicable disease report or outbreak; for example, the federal *Quarantine Act,* SC 2005, c. 20, Q 1.1, and the *Communicable Disease Act,* RSNL 1990, c. C-26 (Pan-Canadian Public Health Network, 2012). These laws can extend to the entire community if the exposure potential is deemed great enough, as could happen with an outbreak of smallpox or epidemic influenza. Much of the communicable disease surveillance and control work in Canada is performed by CHNs.

Tertiary prevention works to reduce complications and disabilities through treatment and rehabilitation.

The Role of Community Health Nurses in Disease Prevention and Control

Disease prevention is a central focus of community health nursing practice. According to the *Canadian Community Health Nursing Professional Practice Model and Standards of Practice* (Appendix 1), the CHN provides prevention and protection services to address communicable diseases and identifies a range of strategies to prevent disease (Community Health Nurses of Canada [CHNC], 2019). CHNs are involved in administering immunizations for vaccine-preventable diseases, including childhood immunizations and COVID-19, and monitoring the immunization status of patients in clinic, daycare, school, and home settings. CHNs work within immunization programs, which are a shared responsibility between federal, provincial/territorial governments, and local public health authorities. CHNs also work in communicable disease surveillance and control, teach, and monitor bloodborne pathogen control, and advise on the prevention of vectorborne diseases. They teach methods for responsible sexual behaviour, screen for STIs, conduct contact tracing for STIs, and provide HIV counselling, testing, and follow-up. They screen for TB, identify TB contacts, and deliver directly observed therapy (DOT) programs in the community (discussed later in the chapter).

During the COVID-19 global pandemic of 2020 -2021, CHNs played a critical role in contact tracing, administering vaccines, public education, and screening clinics. According to the CNA (2021), some of the major issues that emerged for nurses in Canada during the pandemic included the need for adequate PPE, access to rapid and long-term mental health services for health care workers, and challenges with providing access to harm reduction services.

Vaccine-Preventable Diseases

Vaccines are one of the most effective methods of preventing and controlling communicable diseases. Diseases such as polio, diphtheria, pertussis, and measles, which previously occurred in epidemic proportions, are now controlled by routine childhood immunization. They have not, however, been eradicated, so children need to be immunized against these diseases. In Canada, only three provinces have legislated vaccination policies that apply to children about to enroll in school: Ontario and New Brunswick require immunization for DTP, measles, mumps, and rubella, while Manitoba requires a measles vaccine. However, the legislation includes an exemption

LEVELS OF PREVENTION

Related to Communicable Disease Interventions

Primary Prevention

To prevent the occurrence of disease, the role of the CHN is:
- To provide counselling to individuals on prevention of sexually transmitted infections (STIs)
- To administer immunizations such as influenza vaccine, tetanus boosters, and Pneumovax
- To provide information on safe food-handling
- To provide community education about prevention of communicable diseases
- To notify contacts about their exposure to a notifiable communicable disease
- To advocate for public policy on the prevention of water contamination

Secondary Prevention

To prevent the spread of disease, the role of the CHN is:
- To screen for tuberculosis in health care workers
- To conduct partner notification for STIs
- To offer clinics for testing for HIV
- To advocate for the availability of required screening services

Tertiary Prevention

To reduce complications and disabilities through treatment and rehabilitation, the role of the CHN is:
- To initiate and monitor therapy (e.g., initiate directly observed therapy for tuberculosis treatment)
- To identify community resources for supportive care (e.g., funds for purchasing medications)
- To refer to self-help support groups
- To promote behavioural change to minimize risk factors (e.g., safer sex for adolescents)

clause which allows parents to request exemption from the vaccine on medical, religious, or personal grounds. The policies state that in the event of an outbreak, unvaccinated children will not be permitted to attend public school. Although vaccinations policies do not currently enforce mandatory vaccination, the compliance rates appear to be high in most provinces (Walkinshaw, 2011).

Many infants and toddlers, the group most vulnerable to these potentially severe diseases, do not receive scheduled immunizations on time despite the availability of free vaccines. CHNs who work in regions where groups obtain exemption from immunization on religious or health belief grounds, where immunization is incomplete, or where international visitors are frequent need to be especially alert for communicable disease cases and the need for prompt outbreak control among particularly susceptible populations. Communicable diseases in all age groups can best be prevented through the use of vaccines. Table 16.1 presents a detailed description of vaccine-preventable communicable diseases. The routine immunization recommended for children in Canada is found in Appendix E-4, "Canadian Required Immunization Schedule," on the Evolve website. For some diseases, booster doses are required throughout

TABLE 16.1 Vaccine-Preventable Diseases

Disease	Number of Reported Cases 2012–2019*	Mode of Transmission	Incubation Period	Indicators	Time of Occurrence	Nursing Considerations
Diphtheria	6	Toxigenic strains of *Corynebacterium diphtheriae* cause the disease. The organism (both toxigenic and nontoxigenic strains) may be harboured in the nasopharynx, skin, and other sites of asymptomatic carriers. Transmission is most often spread through person-to-person contact by respiratory means	2–5 days, with a range of 1–10 days	A greyish membrane forms in the respiratory tract with a surrounding inflammation that can lead to respiratory obstruction		Investigate reported cases and initiate control measures for outbreaks, and use every opportunity to immunize
Haemophilus influenzae type B (Hib)	166	Infection enters the body through the nose or mouth; bacteria are spread by respiratory droplets and by direct contact with discharges from the nose or mouth of an infected person	2–4 days	Hib is most commonly associated with bacterial meningitis, but it can also cause pneumonia and inflammation of the skin, joints, bone, throat, and heart; acute-onset fever; vomiting; lethargy; and epiglottitis, bacteremia, and other complications		Educate regarding the importance of immunization, especially in young children
Hepatitis A	1 701	See Appendix 10 ("Viral Hepatitis Profiles")	15–50 days, with an average of 28 days	See Appendix 10	Little seasonal variation	For hepatitis profiles, see Appendix 10
Hepatitis B (HBV)	35 295	See Appendix 10	45–160 days; average 120 days	See Appendix 10	Little seasonal variation.	For hepatitis profiles, see Appendix 10
Influenza (laboratory confirmed)	0 Since 2005, no reported laboratory-confirmed cases of influenza have occurred	It is transmitted by airborne respiratory droplets entering into the nose or mouth or through direct contact with eyes and touching contaminated surfaces	1–4 days, with an average of 2 days	Influenza typically starts with headache, chills, and cough, followed rapidly by fever, anorexia, muscle aches, fatigue, running nose, sneezing, watery eyes, and throat irritation. Nausea, vomiting, and diarrhea may occur, especially in children*	Usually arises from November to April	Counsel regarding measures to prevent spread of influenza. Monitor outbreaks and educate regarding the importance of yearly immunization

Continued

TABLE 16.1   Vaccine-Preventable Diseases—cont'd

Disease	Number of Reported Cases 2012–2019*	Mode of Transmission	Incubation Period	Indicators	Time of Occurrence	Nursing Considerations
Measles (red measles, rubeola)	718 2012 = 9 2014 = 419	Transmission is by droplet spread or direct contact with nasal or throat secretions of an infected person. Less common is airborne spread or transmission by indirect contact with freshly infected articles. In closed areas, infections have been documented for up to 2 hours after the source of infection has been removed; it is one of the most readily transmitted diseases. It is extremely communicable from slightly before the prodromal period to 4 days after appearance of rash; minimal after the second day of rash	7–18 days after contact with person with red measles; fever and cough usually occur 3–4 days prior to the rash; the rash fades in 4–7 days	It is an acute disease with prodromal fever, conjunctivitis, cough, and Koplik's spots on the buccal mucosa. Red blotchy rash appears in 3–7 days, beginning on the face and head and becoming generalized, lasting 3–7 days. Leukopenia occurs; other symptoms include anorexia, diarrhea, lymphadenopathy, and otitis media. It is more severe in infants and adults. It is a systemic infection; the primary site of infection is the respiratory epithelium of the nasopharynx. Bacterial superinfection is a possibility. The case fatality rate may be as high as 25%		Investigate reported cases and initiate control measures for outbreaks; use every opportunity to immunize. Certain groups such as infants and adults become more severely ill when infected with red measles
Meningitis (bacterial)	Since 2000 no new cases have been reported	Transmission occurs by airborne droplets or by direct contact with respiratory secretions	3–4 days, with a range of 2–10 days	Children under 1 and 15- to 19-year-olds are the most affected. It manifests as a sudden onset of fever, headache, and a stiff neck, often accompanied by other symptoms, such as nausea, vomiting, photophobia, and altered mental status	Disease occurs year-round, but there is seasonal variation, with the majority of cases occurring in the winter months	Identify and monitor high-risk groups for outbreaks. Educate regarding the importance of immunization
Mumps	607	It is an acute infectious disease caused by the paramyxovirus. Transmission occurs by inhaling airborne droplets from an infected person or by direct contact with objects contaminated with infected saliva	14–24 days	Chills, headache, anorexia, general malaise, fever, swelling, and tenderness of one or more salivary glands under the jaw and in the cheeks occurs. Deafness may occur in less than one to five cases per 100 000 people; it is usually transient but may be permanent	Disease occurs year-round, but is most frequent in late winter and early spring	Counsel pregnant women that mumps infection during the first trimester of pregnancy may increase the rate of spontaneous abortion. Educate regarding the importance of immunization

Disease	Number of Reported Cases 2012–2019*	Mode of Transmission	Incubation Period	Indicators	Time of Occurrence	Nursing Considerations
Pertussis (whooping cough)	14 905	Respiratory transmission occurs by inhaling airborne droplets from an infected person	5–21 days	The first stage can last 1–2 weeks and includes a runny nose, sneezing, low-grade fever, and a mild cough. The second stage usually lasts 1–6 weeks, but can last up to 10 weeks. A characteristic symptom is a series of rapid coughs, at the end of which the patient has a prolonged inhaling effort characterized by a high-pitched whoop. The patient may turn blue and vomit. The third stage may last for months. The cough usually disappears after 2–3 weeks, but paroxysms may recur with any subsequent respiratory infection		Monitor for outbreaks and educate regarding the importance of immunization
Invasive pneumococcal disease	16 283	Bacteria are spread by close contact with an infected person, coughs and sneezes from an infected person, and articles soiled with respiratory discharges involving secretions from the nose	1–3 days	Pneumococcal pneumonia: an abrupt onset of fever, shaking, chills, chest pain, coughs with sputum production, shortness of breath, rapid breathing and heart rate, and weakness. Pneumococcal meningitis: a sudden onset of high fever, lethargy or coma, nausea and vomiting, and a stiff neck. Fever, vomiting, and convulsions may be the first symptoms in young children. Acute otitis media: Demonstrated by ear pain or red bulging tympanic membrane	Winter and early spring	Identify and educate high-risk groups regarding the importance of immunization
Poliomyelitis (polio)	No new cases have been reported since 1995	Transmission occurs via the fecal–oral route#	6–20 days	Fever, mild headache, sore throat, constipation, fatigue, and stiff neck are usual symptoms; and flaccid paralysis of the legs may occur#		Continue surveillance for possible cases. Educate regarding the importance of immunization

Continued

TABLE 16.1   Vaccine-Preventable Diseases—cont'd

Disease	Number of Reported Cases 2012–2019*	Mode of Transmission	Incubation Period	Indicators	Time of Occurrence	Nursing Considerations
Rabies	1	Transmission occurs through close contact with saliva of infected animals, most often by a bite, scratch, or licks on broken skin or mucous membranes, such as the eyes, nose, or mouth. In very rare cases, person-to-person transmission has occurred when saliva droplets were dispersed in the air.†† Injury to the upper body or face poses the greatest risk of transmission	Can be as short as 5 days or as long as several years, usually taking 20–60 days	First symptoms are usually nonspecific, influenza-like symptoms—fever, tiredness, headache—that may last for a few days. The acute stage, which quickly follows, is indicated by anxiety, confusion, insomnia, agitation, hallucinations, and hyperactivity (furious rabies) or paralysis (dumb rabies). The acute period usually ends after 2–10 days. Complete paralysis develops, followed by a coma. Without intensive care, death occurs during the first 7 days of illness		Provide counselling to patients who are travelling to areas with an increased incidence of rabies. Educate regarding the steps to take to decrease personal risk of rabies. Educate regarding postexposure treatments and monitoring
Rubella (German measles)	6	Respiratory transmission occurs by inhaling airborne droplets from an infected person	12–23 days	Indicators include general malaise, runny nose, cough, painless rose-coloured spots on the roof of the mouth, conjunctivitis, swollen tender lymph nodes on back of neck or under the ears, and a rash that begins on face and neck and then spreads to trunk, arms, and legs, which joins together to form patches. Older girls or women may develop pain and swelling in the joints		Rubella is highly contagious. It is recommended that rubella vaccine not be given to children under 12 months of age or to pregnant women. It is recommended that the vaccine be administered to all female adolescents and to women of child-bearing age (advise to avoid pregnancy for 1 month after vaccination). Counsel pregnant women about congenital rubella syndrome (CRS). CRS can result in miscarriages, stillbirths, and fetal malformations. In all, 85% of CRS cases occur with infection in the first trimester; this is very rare after the twentieth week of pregnancy*

Disease	Number of Reported Cases 2012–2019*	Mode of Transmission	Incubation Period	Indicators	Time of Occurrence	Nursing Considerations
Tetanus (lockjaw)	21	Transmission usually occurs when a skin wound becomes contaminated by a bacterium called *Clostridium tetani*, found in soil and animal feces	3–21 days	Indicators include stiffness of jaw (lockjaw); restlessness; dysphagia; headache; fever; sore throat; chills; muscle spasms; stiffness in neck, arms, and legs; painful muscle contractions; and convulsions		Assess and educate regarding the importance of immunization
Varicella (chicken pox)	2 798	Transmission occurs by direct contact with the virus shed from skin lesions, and oral secretions. Spread can also take place by airborne route. The period of infection is 1 to 2 days before onset of the rash. It lasts until all lesions are crusted over	Symptoms appear in 10–21 days, and usually last 14–16 days	In all, 50% of varicella cases usually occur in children before 5 years old. Indicators include fever, abdominal pain, sore throat, headache, and general malaise 1–2 days before the rash. The rash begins as small, red, flat spots and develops into itchy, thin-walled blisters, usually about 0.5-cm wide, filled with clear fluid and a red base. They appear over 2–4 days. The blister breaks, leaving open sores, which finally crust over to become dry, brown scabs		Investigate cases and initiate control measures for outbreaks and educate regarding the importance of immunization. Severe illness can occur in people with a depressed immune system

Sources: *Public Health Agency of Canada (PHAC). (2019e). Flu (influenza): Flu watch surveillance.* https://www.canada.ca/en/public-health/services/diseases/flu-influenza/influenza-surveillance.html
#Public Health Agency of Canada (PHAC). (2019b). Notifiable diseases on-line. https://diseases.canada.ca/notifiable/
††Public Health Agency of Canada (PHAC). (2015b). Fact sheet: E. coli. http://www.phac-aspc.gc.ca/fs-sa/fs-fi/ecoli-eng.php

the lifespan (PHAC, 2015a). For further information, see the link to the PHAC's "Canadian Immunization Guide" on the Evolve website.

Influenza

Influenza is one of the most common communicable diseases CHNs will encounter. Influenza ("flu") is a viral respiratory infection often indistinguishable from the common cold or other respiratory diseases. The most important factors to note about influenza are its epidemic nature and the mortality that may result from pulmonary complications, especially in older persons.

There are three types of influenza viruses: A, B, and C. Type A is usually responsible for large epidemics, whereas outbreaks from type B are more regionalized; type C epidemics are less common and usually result in only mild illness. Influenza viruses often change in the nature of their surface appearance or their antigenic makeup. Types B and C are fairly stable viruses, but type A changes constantly. Minor antigenic changes are referred to as *antigenic drift,* and they result in yearly epidemics and regional outbreaks. Major changes such as the emergence of new subtypes are called *antigenic shift;* these occur only with type A viruses. Antigenic shift and drift lead to epidemic outbreaks every few years and pandemic outbreaks every 10 to 40 years.

The preparation of influenza vaccine each year is based on the best possible prediction of what type and variant of virus will be most prevalent that year. Because of the changing nature of the virus, yearly immunization is necessary and is given in the early fall before the flu season begins. Flu shots do not always prevent infection, but they do result in milder disease symptoms, especially in healthy population groups. Annually in Canada, it is estimated that influenza cases cause approximately 12 200 hospitalizations and 3 500 deaths (PHAC, 2018a). The Government of Canada has a flu surveillance program called FluWatch, which provides weekly flu reports from across Canada that track and confirm outbreaks (PHAC, 2019e). For further information on seasonal influenza, see Table 16.1.

H1N1 Flu Virus

In the spring of 2009, the H1N1 flu virus (human swine influenza) surfaced in North America. This flu virus differs from the seasonal flu virus in that it is a new strain and most people do not have a natural immunity. Consequently, it has the potential to cause serious illness. The H1N1 vaccine was developed and made available to all Canadians in the fall of 2009. In the initial phase of the H1N1 immunization program, priority vaccinations were targeted for administration to the following groups: children between the ages of 6 months and 5 years; people in close contact with and caregiving for infants under 6 months of age or immunocompromised individuals; people residing in remote communities; health care workers involved with the delivery of essential health services; and people under 65 years of age with a chronic illness. In June 2009, WHO declared the H1N1 flu as a pandemic influenza

(WHO, 2009a). For further information on the H1N1 flu virus, see Table 16.1, the PHAC's Your H1N1 Preparedness Guide web page, and Health Canada's Health Concerns: Influenza (Flu) web page (the links are on the Evolve website). Both online resources provide influenza information for health care providers and consumers.

Smallpox

Smallpox, a severely acute and highly contagious disease caused by the variola virus found worldwide, has been eradicated since 1979. In the 1950s, approximately 50 million cases of smallpox occurred globally each year; however, due to vaccination, this number fell to between 10 and 15 million in the late 1960s. A global campaign to eradicate this deadly and disfiguring disease resulted in its complete eradication. In 1980, WHO declared that smallpox had been globally eradicated, and immunization for smallpox was terminated (WHO, 2009c). Currently, the smallpox vaccine is not available to the general public, but there are stockpiles in Canada and the United States in case of an outbreak. Many health care providers have never seen smallpox; however, they have seen the distinctive scar left on so many shoulders of those who have had the vaccination. CHNs must be especially vigilant because the emergence of only one case of smallpox would need to be recognized immediately as a global epidemic because people are not immunized.

Non–Vaccine-Preventable Diseases

Non–vaccine-preventable diseases are diseases that cannot be prevented by vaccination. TB, a non–vaccine-preventable disease, is of concern globally. An extensive list of non–vaccine-preventable diseases appears in Appendix 9.

Tuberculosis

Tuberculosis (TB) is a mycobacterial disease caused by *Mycobacterium tuberculosis* and is transmitted by airborne droplets. There are different types of TB, such as pulmonary TB, ocular TB, genitourinary TB, military/disseminated TB, and bone and joint TB. TB can be active or latent. Reactivation of latent infections is more common in immunocompromised people, cigarette smokers, underweight and undernourished people, people with diabetes mellitus, and those with silicosis (Health Canada, 2013; PHAC, 2014a).

For most Canadians, the risk of developing TB is very low. However, in 2013 there were approximately 1 640 new active and retreatment cases reported in Canada, so it is important to know the symptoms and how to minimize risk (PHAC, 2014a). The following groups in Canada are at increased risk of developing TB: those who travel to and from countries where TB is endemic; First Nations people living in communities with a high prevalence of TB; homeless people; residents of some long-term care facilities; people in correctional facilities; health care workers; and people with weakened immune systems such as alcoholics, diabetics, those infected with HIV, and older adults.

The PHAC collects and analyzes data on reported cases of TB to improve TB prevention and control. It also engages in surveillance of drug resistance to TB nationally. Screening, diagnosis, and management of TB are well outlined in the PHAC's *Canadian Tuberculosis Standards* (see the link in the Tool Box on the Evolve website). CHNs may administer and interpret TB skin tests, collect specimens, monitor medications, and provide education and support when necessary; therefore, familiarity with current TB guidelines is paramount. A link to the Ontario Lung Association's *Tuberculosis Information for Health Care Providers* is also included in the Tool Box on the Evolve website. The resource covers epidemiology, screening, diagnosis, treatment, and management of TB.

Sexually Transmitted Infections

The diseases that are considered *sexually transmitted infections (STIs)* have also been referred to as *sexually transmitted diseases (STDs)*. Today, the preferred term is *sexually transmitted infection* because the word *infection* implies that symptoms may or may not be present (the word *disease* implies that symptoms are present). The incidence or number of new cases of some STIs, such as syphilis, has been declining, while the incidence of others, such as herpes simplex and chlamydia, is increasing. Moreover, the actual rates of STIs may be twice the reported rate. In Canada, since 1997, there has been a steady increase in the numbers of reported cases of STIs, with chlamydia being the most common, gonorrhea the second most common, and syphilis the least common (Cropp, Latham-Caranico, Stebben, et al., 2007).

CHNs need to be knowledgeable about STIs and their long-term health effects. **Chlamydia** is an STI caused by the organism *Chlamydia trachomatis,* which results in infection of the urethra and cervix. Infections may be asymptomatic and, if untreated, result in severe morbidity. **Gonorrhea** is an STI caused by the bacterium *Neisseria gonorrhoeae,* which results in inflammation of the urethra and cervix and dysuria, or it may result in no symptoms. Common STIs are listed in Table 16.2. The PHAC's "Sexually Transmitted Infections (STI), Sexual Health Facts and Information for the Public" web page provides valuable information on STIs in Canada (see the link on the Evolve website). The PHAC's "Human Papillomavirus (HPV) Prevention and HPV Vaccines: Questions and Answers" web page provides information on HPV, protecting oneself from getting HPV, and vaccination (see the link on the Evolve website).

Generally, community health nursing considerations for all STIs would include the need for diagnosis and confidential treatment for any person, regardless of age; public education about the indicators of STIs, mode of transmission, and the importance of early treatment and follow-up; reporting; and contact tracing follow-up.

HIV and AIDS

Human immunodeficiency virus (HIV) and **acquired immunodeficiency syndrome (AIDS)** continue to have a significant political and social effect on society. AIDS is a syndrome that can affect the immune and central nervous systems and cause infections or cancers. It is caused by HIV. The economic costs of HIV and AIDS result from premature disability and

treatment, and many families become disrupted and lose creative and economic productivity.

It is estimated that approximately 63 110 Canadians were living with HIV (including AIDS) at the end of 2016, with an estimated 2 165 new HIV cases reported in the same year (Haddad, Totten, & McGuire, 2018). Although globally AIDS has been an epidemic, HIV/AIDS infections have decreased due to prevention programs and the HAART treatment regimen. For information on HIV/AIDS globally and in Canada, refer to Boxes 16.4 and 16.5.

Many AIDS-related opportunistic infections are caused by micro-organisms that are commonly present in healthy individuals but do not cause disease in people with an intact immune system. These microorganisms proliferate in those with HIV and AIDS because of a weakened immune system. Bacteria, fungi, viruses, or protozoa may cause opportunistic infections. The most common opportunistic diseases are *Pneumocystis carinii* pneumonia and oral candidiasis.

HIV is not transmitted through casual contact such as touching or hugging someone who has HIV infection. It is not transmitted by insects, coughing, sneezing, office equipment, or sitting next to or eating with someone who has HIV infection. Worldwide, the largest number of HIV infections result from heterosexual transmission. CHNs can provide education on the modes of transmission and be role models for how to behave toward and provide supportive care for those with HIV infection. An understanding of how transmission does and does not occur helps family and community members feel more comfortable in relating to and caring for people with HIV.

The epidemiology, screening, diagnosis, management, treatment, and follow-up of HIV and additional information are well outlined by the PHAC's "Canadian Guidelines on Sexually Transmitted Infections," in the chapter titled "Human Immunodeficiency Virus (HIV) Infections" (the link is in the Tool Box on the Evolve website). CHNs are mostly involved with screening and counselling, follow-up, and providing education and support when necessary; therefore, familiarity with the current HIV guidelines is crucial.

Because AIDS is a chronic disease, affected individuals continue to live and work in the community. They have bouts of illness interspersed with periods of wellness when they are able to return to school or work. The CHN teaches families and significant others about personal care and hygiene, medication administration, routine practices, and additional precautions to ensure infection control, as well as healthy lifestyle behaviours such as adequate rest, balanced nutrition, and exercise. (See the PHAC's "Routine Practices and Additional Precautions for Preventing the Transmission of Infection in HealthCare Settings" web page—the link is on the Evolve website.)

A growing number of services are available for people living with HIV/AIDS. Voluntary and faith-based groups, such as community-based organizations or AIDS support organizations, have developed in some localities to address many needs of people living with HIV/AIDS. Services include

TABLE 16.2 **Common Sexually Transmitted Infections**

Sexually Transmitted Infection	Epidemiology	Mode of Transmission	Incubation Period	Indicators	Nursing Considerations
Chlamydia	Rates have been rising since 1997, with over 121 244 cases reported in 2019*	Oral, vaginal, or anal sex	2–6 weeks	Females: genital discharge, burning feeling while urinating, lower abdominal pain, pain during sex, and abnormal vaginal bleeding Males: burning when voiding, urethral itch, urethral discharge (milky or watery), and pain or swelling in testicles. Often individuals are asymptomatic	Counsel patients on risk factors such as the following: Having sexual contact with a chlamydia-infected partner Having a new sexual partner or more than two sexual partners in the past year Having had a previous STI Having had sexual exposure to vulnerable populations Prevention of chlamydia: Encourage patients to practise safer sex. Screen vulnerable populations (e.g., injection drug users, incarcerated individuals, sex trade workers, street youth, etc.). Assess, treat, and counsel partners of infected individuals. Provide specific screening, treatment, and counselling for pregnant women in the high-risk population. Follow-up: Infected individuals require specific follow-up and education (refer to STI guidelines)
Genital herpes simplex virus (HSV)	Annual incidence in Canada is not known; however, it is increasing globally with country variations. It is more commonly acquired by females*	Most commonly, spread by direct contact with open sores, usually during genital, oral, or anal sex. Although it is rare, pregnant women can pass this infection to their baby during or after childbirth. Herpes infection in infants can be life-threatening	2–21 days; average of 6 days	Tingling or itching in the genital area, painful blisters, fever, and general malaise Females: Sores may occur on the vagina, on the cervix, inside or near the vagina, on the genitals, near the anus, or on the thighs and buttocks; tender lumps in the groin Males: Sores on the penis, around the testicles, near the anus, and on thighs and buttocks; tender lumps in the groin Both males and females can get sores in the mouth or in the genital area after oral sex with an infected person	Counsel regarding the chronic aspects of the disease. Educate about the likelihood of recurring episodes; the potential for infecting partner during asymptomatic periods; care of the infected area and type of clothing to wear; and that antiviral therapy may shorten the duration of lesions and prevent recurrent outbreaks. Counsel regarding safer-sex practices and informing past sexual partners

Sexually Transmitted Infection	Epidemiology	Mode of Transmission	Incubation Period	Indicators	Nursing Considerations
Hepatitis B	See Table 16.1 and Appendix 10 ("Viral Hepatitis Profiles")				
HIV/AIDS	New HIV cases has been steadily increasing from 2 060 in 2013 to 2 344 in 2019*	Exposure to blood or body fluids from an HIV-infected person by sexual contact, IV drug use, HIV-infected blood transfusions, perinatal mother-to-child transmission (throughout pregnancy, during vaginal birth, or through breast feeding, or occupational exposure). HIV is a lifelong infection, but it can be controlled by antiretroviral therapy (HAART)‡	HIV: Can produce antibodies within 3 months	Acute HIV: Fever, arthralgia or myalgia, rash, lymphadenopathy, sore throat, fatigue, headache, oral ulcers or genital ulcers, 5 kg weight loss, nausea, vomiting, and diarrhea Chronic HIV: Oral hairy leukoplakia, unexplained fever (2 weeks), fatigue or lethargy, unexplained weight loss (10% body weight), chronic diarrhea (3 weeks), unexplained lymphadenopathy (usually generalized), cervical dysplasia, dyspnea and dry cough, loss of vision, recurrent or chronic candidiasis (oral, esophageal, vaginal), dysphagia (esophageal candidiasis), red–purple nodular skin or mucosal lesions (Kaposi sarcoma), encephalopathy, herpes zoster (especially if severe, multidermatomal, or disseminated), increased frequency or severity of mucocutaneous herpes simplex infection‡	Screen and counsel high-risk populations; counsel HIV-positive pregnant mothers about the possibility of transmission to their child during pregnancy, at birth, or while breastfeeding; and offer HIV testing. Educate regarding safer sex, not sharing needles, using universal precautions, and informing past sexual partners of HIV status
Human papillomavirus (HPV)	HPV infections are common in both sexes with prevalence usually highest in females less than 25 years, and prevalence in males high at all ages. In Canada, prevalence in females ranged from 14.1 to 46.9% and was highest in those less than 20 years of age living in low-income housing, inner city settings, and Indigenous communities.	Spread through sex, close skin-to-skin contact, or genital area contact with someone who is infected	2–3 months	Warts can appear in clusters like cauliflower. They can be raised or flat and size can vary. Women may present with warts on the vagina, anus, cervix, and vulva. Men can have them on the scrotum or penis. Warts can appear on the lips or mouth after oral sex. Warts may be itchy with discharge or bleeding	Counsel patients regarding transmission through sexual contact and risk factors for disease. Educate about safer-sex practices and the need for regular Papanicolaou tests. Know the provincial/territorial schedule for administration of Gardasil and counsel patients accordingly§

Continued

TABLE 16.2   Common Sexually Transmitted Infections—cont'd

Sexually Transmitted Infection	Epidemiology	Mode of Transmission	Incubation Period	Indicators	Nursing Considerations
Syphilis	The number of new cases of syphilis was on the decline from 1992 to 2000, but recently the number of new cases has been increasing from 3 381 in 2012 to 5 369 in 2019*	Spread during oral, vaginal, or anal sex. Pregnant women with syphilis can transmit syphilis to their unborn child, sometimes causing birth defects and death	1–13 weeks, but typically 3–4 weeks	Primary stage: Painless sore appears on the penis, vulva, or vagina, typically; nontender regional lymphadenopathy Secondary stage: Nonpruritic skin rash 6–12 weeks postinfection, commonly on palms or soles; fever, anorexia, general malaise, enlarged lymph nodes, mouth sores, inflammation of eyes; condylomata lata (raised areas) develop where mucous areas meet skin Latent stage: No symptoms but infection still present Tertiary stage: Cardiovascular syphilis—usually 10 to 25 years after infection—aneurysm, aortic valve leak Neurosyphilis: Benign tertiary syphilis—lumps appear on skin, organs, especially face, scalp, upper trunk and leg, or bones and leave scars	Counsel patients that all partners need to be notified and that there is a VDRL blood test available
Trichomonas	An estimated 170 million cases occur annually worldwide. From 14 to 60% of male infections are associated with an infected female partner†	Spread by sexual contact	3–28 days	Females: Frothy, off-white or yellowish green vaginal discharge Itching and irritation of the genital area Vaginal odour Pain during sex Painful or frequent urination Males: Often asymptomatic Possible symptoms are as follows: Slight discharge from the penis Burning sensation on urination Irritation and redness of the head of the penis	Counsel regarding need for treatment of partner(s).* Educate about safer sex and the chance of increased early delivery or increased low birth weight

Sexually Transmitted Infection	Epidemiology	Mode of Transmission	Incubation Period	Indicators	Nursing Considerations
Ectoparasitic infestations (pubic lice, scabies) sexually transmitted infection	Caused by *Pthirus pubis* (crab louse) and humans are the only reservoir*	Spread by person-to-person contact, including sexual contact Scabies: Contact with mite-infected sheets, towels, or clothing	Pubic lice: Within a few days to 5 weeks Scabies: 2–6 weeks	Pubic lice: Severe pruritus in the pubic area and later in all hairy areas. Light brown insects the size of a pinhead may be seen. Adult lice and small oval white eggs (nits) may be seen attached to hair. Scabies: Severe pruritus in the pubic area A rash with burrows between fingers; on wrists, abdomen, ankles, bend of elbows; or around genitals	Educate patient to do the following: Avoid close body contact with others Avoid scratching because it can lead to secondary infections Obtain treatment to avoid transfer of infection Wash clothes and bed linens in hot water or dry clean and press with a very hot iron Freeze clothes, fabrics, or blankets or store them in an air-tight plastic bag for 2 weeks to destroy the insects and their eggs Inform sex partner(s) and anyone who has shared bed sheets, clothing, or towels, even if they do not have an itch or rash, so that they can seek treatment. Topical medications are recommended. Patients may refer to pubic lice as "crabs."

AIDS, acquired immunodeficiency syndrome; *HIV*, human immunodeficiency virus; *PHAC*, Public Health Agency of Canada; *STI*, sexually transmitted infection; *VDRL*, Venereal Disease Research Laboratories.

Sources: *Public Health Agency of Canada (PHAC). (2019f). *Canadian guidelines on sexually transmitted infections*. https://www.canada.ca/en/public-health/services/infectious-diseases/sexual-health-sexually-transmitted-infections/canadian-guidelines.html
†Public Health Agency of Canada (PHAC). (2019d). *List of nationally notifiable diseases*. https://diseases.canada.ca/notifiable/diseases-list;
‡Public Health Agency of Canada (PHAC). (2012a). *At a glance—HIV and AIDS in Canada*. http://www.phac-aspc.gc.ca/aids-sida/publication/survreport/2012/dec/index-eng.php;
§Public Health Agency of Canada (PHAC). (2014). Canadian guidelines on sexually transmitted infections: human papillomavirus (HPV) infections. Retrieved from https://www.phac-aspc.gc.ca/std-mts/sti-its/cgsti-ldcits/assets/pdf/section-5-5a-eng.pdf
Public Health Agency of Canada (PHAC). (2015a). *Canadian immunization guide*. http://www.phac-aspc.gc.ca/publicat/cig-gci/index-eng.php.

BOX 16.4   Global HIV/AIDS Facts—2017

- 36 900 000 adults and children worldwide are living with HIV
- 1 800 000 new cases of HIV in adults and children
- 940 000 global deaths due to AIDS
- 12 200 000 orphans aged 0 to 17 years old due to parents dying from AIDS
- 75% of people living with AIDS know their status
- 21 700 000 people living with HIV are on ART
- 300 000 estimated TB-related deaths among people living with HIV

Source: Adapted from United Nations AIDS (UNAIDS). (2017). *Global fact sheets: AIDS*. http://aidsinfo.unaids.org

BOX 16.5   HIV in Canada, 2017

- 63 110 Canadians are living with HIV
- The majority of reported HIV cases are among those aged 30–39
- 75.2% of reported HIV cases occurred among adult males
- Females accounted for 24.8% of those newly diagnosed with HIV
- Indigenous people made up 20.1% of new HIV cases
- 60.9% of males were exposed by gay and bisexual individuals and men who have sex with men contacts
- 61.2% of women were exposed by heterosexual contact of which 30.9% of those contacts were from an HIV-endemic country
- 240 infants were exposed to HIV during pregnancy

Source: Haddad, N., Totten, S., & McGuire, M. (2018). HIV in Canada -surveillance report, 2017. Canadian Communicable Disease Reports, 44(12):324-32. https://doi.org/10.14745/ccdr.v44i12a03.

counselling, support groups, legal aid, personal care services, housing programs, and community education programs. CHNs collaborate with workers from community-based organizations in the patient's home and may serve to advise these groups in their supportive work.

INFECTIOUS DISEASES

An **infectious disease** is "a disease caused by a micro-organism and therefore potentially infinitely transferable to new individuals. [It] may or may not be communicable" (Centers for Disease Control and Prevention, 2014). The agent can be a virus, bacterium, parasite, or fungus. If untreated, these diseases are often fatal, so the best approach is to prevent transmission. Examples discussed here are hepatitis, Ebola virus disease, waterborne and foodborne diseases, vectorborne diseases, diseases of travellers, and zoonoses.

Viral Hepatitis

Viral hepatitis refers to a group of infections that primarily affect the liver. These infections have similar clinical presentations but different causes and characteristics. Brief profiles of the types of hepatitis are presented in Appendix 10. The six types of viral hepatitis are hepatitis A, hepatitis B, hepatitis C, hepatitis D, hepatitis E, and hepatitis G. The three that

BOX 16.6   Candidates for Hepatitis A Vaccine

- All household members and sexual contacts of people with hepatitis A virus (HAV)
- All staff of daycare centres if a case of HAV occurs among children or staff
- Household members whose diapered children attend a daycare centre where three or more families are infected
- Staff and residents of prisons or institutions for developmentally disabled people, if they have close contact with people with HAV
- Hospital employees who are exposed to the feces of infected patients
- Food handlers who have a coworker infected with HAV; patrons in unhygienic situations or where food is not heated
- People who travel to countries where the disease is endemic

are most common are hepatitis A virus, hepatitis B virus, and hepatitis C virus. (For specific information on the vaccines available in Canada for hepatitis infections, see the PHAC's "Canadian Immunization Guide" [the link is on the Evolve website].)

Hepatitis A virus (HAV) is a virus most often transmitted through the fecal–oral route. Sources may be water, food, or sexual contact. The virus level in the feces appears to peak 1 to 2 weeks before symptoms appear, making individuals highly contagious before they realize they are ill. The clinical course of HAV ranges from mild to severe and often requires prolonged convalescence. Onset is usually acute with fever, nausea, lack of appetite, malaise, and abdominal discomfort, followed after several days by jaundice.

Although there has been a vaccine for this disease since 1995, HAV infection remains one of the most frequently reported vaccine-preventable diseases. People most at risk for HAV infection are travellers to countries with high rates of HAV, children living in areas with high rates of HAV, injection drug users, men who have sex with men, and people with clotting disorders or chronic liver disease.

HAV is found worldwide. In developing countries where sanitation is inadequate, epidemics are not common because most adults are immune from childhood infection. In countries with improved sanitation, outbreaks are common in daycare centres whose staff must change diapers, among household and sexual contact with infected individuals, and among travellers to countries where HAV is endemic. Box 16.6 lists candidates for hepatitis A vaccine.

Good sanitation, including the prevention of human contact with waste as well as the treatment and proper disposal of sewage and waste water, combined with personal hygiene are the best means of preventing infection. Hepatitis A is associated with the highest mortality and morbidity rates of any vaccine-preventable infection in travellers. Yet, many travellers do not get immunized, resulting in it being the most frequently

EVIDENCE-INFORMED PRACTICE

Liver cancer is a significant health problem in Asia, and it also occurs more frequently in the Chinese population living in North America. Little is known about hepatitis B virus (HBV) and liver cancer control in the Chinese population in Canada. Hislop, Teh, Low, et al. (2007) surveyed a number of Chinese adult immigrants in Vancouver, British Columbia, who have had HBV testing and been vaccinated, to explore their knowledge about HBV. Data collection included a survey using a mailed questionnaire to Chinese households in Vancouver and a random selection of participants for interviews. A total of 504 participants were interviewed (217 men and 287 women). Of these participants, 366 were interviewed in Cantonese, 102 in Mandarin, and 36 in English. Fifty-seven percent of participants had previously had HBV testing; 38% had been vaccinated; and 6% were HBV carriers. Fewer men than women had been tested and vaccinated. The participants' educational levels were associated with HBV testing in women (the higher the education, the more likely the woman was tested). Shorter length of time in North America for both genders was also associated with HBV testing. Over 80% of participants knew that HBV could be spread by people who are asymptomatic and that HBV can cause cirrhosis and liver cancer. However, some confusion existed over the route of HBV transmission—for example, fewer participants knew

that hepatitis B is not transmitted via food (especially males in the sample) and is transmitted during sexual intercourse; approximately 50% did not know that HBV infection is lifelong.

Application for CHNs
The findings of this study strongly suggest that targeted educational campaigns are needed for the Chinese immigrant population about the importance of testing and vaccination for hepatitis B. It is important for CHNs to involve members of the community in all educational campaigns. CHNs need to plan and implement educational campaigns that consider literacy levels, use of interpreters for language translation, and cultural interpretation.

Questions for Reflection and Discussion
1. What type of vaccination campaign would you introduce to encourage the Chinese immigrant population to receive the hepatitis B vaccination?
2. Why are vaccinations important for populations?
3. What recent evidence on vaccination in the Asian population of immigrants in Canada are you able to locate? Use the following keywords: hepatitis B, Asian population, vaccination, health knowledge, practices, immigration.

Source: Hislop, T. G., Teh, C., Low, A., et al. (2007). Hepatitis B knowledge, testing and vaccination levels in Chinese immigrants to British Columbia, Canada. *Canadian Journal of Public Health, 98*(2), 125–129.

occurring vaccine-preventable disease. Hepatitis B is also a disease associated with international travel. In Canada, several preparations are authorized for use, including Twinrix, which is a vaccine that protects against hepatitis A and B.

Hepatitis B virus (HBV) is a virus transmitted through exposure to infected body fluids. Infection results in a clinical picture that ranges from a self-limited acute infection to fulminant hepatitis or hepatic carcinoma, possibly leading to death. The number of new cases of HBV in North America has been decreasing as a result of the use of HBV vaccine. The groups with the highest prevalence are users of injection drugs, people with STIs or multiple sex partners, immigrants and refugees and their descendants who came from areas where there is a high endemic rate of HBV, health care workers, hemodialysis patients, inmates of long-term correctional institutions, and young adults (especially homeless adolescents).

HBV infection can be prevented by immunization, prevention of health care–associated occupational exposure, and prevention of exposure via sex or injection drug use. Vaccination is recommended for people with occupational risk (e.g., health care workers) and for children. Vaccines for HBV authorized for use in Canada include Engerix-B, Infanrix hexa, and Recombivax HB. Hepatitis B immune globulin is given after exposure to provide passive immunity and thus prevent infection. Educating patients about their personal risk for contracting HBV is an essential role for CHNs (see the "Evidence-Informed Practice" box).

Hepatitis C virus (HCV) is a virus transmitted through exposure to infected blood and body fluids. HCV infection was first identified in the late 1980s. This infection has been

called "the silent stalker," since up to 70% of newly infected people experience no symptoms and it may take up to 30 years for symptoms to appear (Harkness, 2003; PHAC, 2015c). Primary prevention of HCV infection includes screening of blood products and donor organs and tissue; risk-reduction counselling and services, including obtaining sexual and injection drug-use history; and infection control practices. Secondary prevention strategies include testing of high-risk individuals, including those who seek HIV testing and counselling, and appropriate medical follow-up of infected patients. HCV testing should be offered to people who received a blood transfusion or an organ transplant before 1992, health care workers after exposure to blood or body fluids, children born to HCV-positive women, and people who have ever injected drugs or been on dialysis. For further information on HCV, see the Canadian AIDS Treatment Information Exchange (CATIE) "Hepatitis C" web page (the link is listed in the Tool Box on the Evolve website).

Ebola Virus Disease

The **Ebola virus disease,** also known as *Ebola hemorrhagic fever,* is a deadly viral illness that is caused by infection with one of the Ebola virus strains from the family of *Filoviridae* genus *Ebolavirus.* Ebola viruses were first discovered in 1976 near the Ebola River in the Congo and, since then, there have been sporadic outbreaks in Africa. It is believed that the virus is animal-borne, especially in bats. The virus is contracted through direct contact with the blood and body fluids of a person who is sick with or has died from Ebola; objects (needles) that have been

CHN IN PRACTICE: A CASE STUDY

Ebola

Susan is an international geography student who has been conducting research on bats in Sierra Leone over the summer semester. She just arrived back in Canada two days ago and is feeling well but is concerned that she has been travelling in a high-risk country for Ebola virus disease. Ten days later, Susan is not feeling well and calls the CHN. Susan describes her symptoms and is immediately told to seek medical advice. Her symptoms include stomach pain, headache, diarrhea and vomiting, weakness, and hypermenorrhea.

Think About It

1. What should the CHN suspect and why?
2. What advice could a CHN give Susan?
3. What is the responsibility of a CHN to promote global health security to stop an infectious disease outbreak?

Source: Centers for Disease Control and Prevention (CDC). (2016b). *2014 West Africa Ebola outbreak communication resources.* http://www.cdc.gov/vhf/Ebola/resources/index.html

BOX 16.7   Identifying Persons Under Investigation for Ebola

A person under investigation has both consistent symptoms and risk factors as follows:

Clinical Criteria
- Fever greater than 38.6°C or 101.5°F
- Severe headache
- Muscle pain
- Nausea, vomiting, and diarrhea
- Unexplained hemorrhage

Epidemiological Criteria
- Contact with blood or other body fluids or human remains of a patient known to have or suspected of having Ebola virus disease
- Travel to an area where Ebola virus disease is active
- Direct handling of bats, rodents, or primates in an endemic area

in contact with the body fluids of a person infected with Ebola; infected fruit bats or primates (apes and monkeys); and contact with semen from a man who is recovering from Ebola. In 2014, a serious outbreak of Ebola occurred in Africa, and the virus spread to many countries around the world. In relation to that outbreak, as of March 30, 2016, Guinea had 3 811 total cases of Ebola, with total deaths at 2 543; Sierra Leone had 14 124 total cases, with total deaths at 3 956; and Liberia had 10 675 total cases, with total deaths at 4 809. As of March 2016, all three countries had been declared free of Ebola virus. Other countries that had confirmed cases but are now Ebola free include the United States (4 cases), the United Kingdom (1 case), and Mali (8 cases) (Centers for Disease Control and Prevention, 2015a, 2016a).

Early recognition of the disease is critical for infection control. Community health nurses can play an important role in identifying patients who may be suspected of having Ebola. Box 16.7 outlines the signs and symptoms that can alert health care providers to the need for further investigation. Persons under investigation (PUI) can be categorized as probable, confirmed, or high risk. See the "CHN in Practice: A Case Study, Ebola" box for a fictitious case of a PUI for Ebola.

Waterborne and Foodborne Diseases

Waterborne pathogens usually enter water supplies through animal or human fecal contamination and frequently cause enteric disease. They include viruses, bacteria, and protozoans. HAV is probably the most publicized waterborne viral agent, although other viruses may also be transmitted by this route (enteroviruses, rotaviruses, and paramyxoviruses). The most important waterborne bacterial diseases are cholera, typhoid fever, and bacillary dysentery. However, other *Salmonella* types, *Shigella*, *Vibrio*, and various coliform bacteria, including *E. coli* O157:H7, may be transmitted in the same manner.

In the past, the most important waterborne protozoans have been *Entamoeba histolytica* (amebic dysentery) and *Giardia lamblia*, but outbreaks of cryptosporidiosis in municipal water in North Battleford, Saskatchewan, in April 2001, and *E. coli* in Walkerton, Ontario, in May 2001, led government and nongovernmental groups to explore how best to safeguard municipal water supplies. Protozoans do not respond to traditional chlorine treatment as do enteric and coliform bacteria, and their small size requires special filtration.

Foodborne illness, or "food poisoning," is often categorized as food infection or food intoxication. Food infection results from bacterial, viral, or parasitic infection of food and includes salmonellosis, hepatitis A, and trichinosis. Food intoxication results from toxins produced by bacterial growth, chemical contaminants (heavy metals), and a variety of disease-producing substances found naturally in certain foods such as mushrooms and some seafood. Examples of food intoxications are botulism, mercury poisoning, and paralytic shellfish poisoning. Table 16.3 outlines some of the most common agents of food intoxication, their incubation period, associated food source, duration, and clinical presentation. Although it is not a hard-and-fast rule, food infections are associated with incubation periods of 12 hours to several days after ingestion of the infected food, whereas food intoxications become obvious within minutes to hours after ingestion. Botulism is a clear exception to this rule, with an incubation period of a week or more in adults. The term *ptomaine poisoning*, often used when discussing foodborne illness, does not refer to a specific causal organism.

Protecting the nation's food supply from contamination by all virulent microbes is a complex issue that would be incredibly costly and time consuming to address. However, much foodborne illness, regardless of causal organism, can be prevented easily through simple changes in food preparation, handling, and storage to destroy or denature contaminants and prevent their further spread. WHO's 10 golden rules for preparing food safely are presented in Box 16.8.

TABLE 16.3 Commonly Encountered Food Intoxications

Causal Agent	Incubation Period	Duration	Clinical Presentation	Associated Food/Source
Staphylococcus aureus	30 minutes–7 hours	1–2 days	Sudden onset of nausea, cramps, vomiting, and prostration, often accompanied by diarrhea; rarely fatal	All foods, especially those likely to come into contact with food-handlers' hands that may be contaminated from infections of the eyes and skin
Clostridium perfringens (strain A)	6–24 hours	1 day or less	Sudden onset of colic and diarrhea, sometimes nausea; vomiting and fever unusual; rarely fatal	Inadequate handling (preparation, storage, and reheating) of high-protein foods such as meats or high-starch foods such as cooked beans and gravies; food contaminated by soil, dust, sewage, and intestinal tracts of animals and humans; multiplication of organisms if exposed to low or no oxygen
Paralytic shellfish poisoning (PSP)	A few minutes–10 hours	2–3 days	Tingling sensation or numbness around lips that spreads to the face and neck; prickly sensation in the fingertips and toes, drowsiness, headache and dizziness and difficulty swallowing*	Seafood such as clams, oysters, and mussels, and the tomalley of lobster and crab
Listeria monocytogenes	24 hours–70 days	24–48 hours	Nausea, vomiting, cramps, diarrhea, severe headache, constipation, persistent fever, and in some cases meningitis, encephalitis; septicemia may develop and can lead to death	Hot dogs; deli meats; soft and semisoft cheeses if made from unpasteurized milk; paté and meat spreads; smoked seafood and fish; raw and undercooked meat, poultry, and fish
Clostridium botulinum	12–36 hours	Usually 2 hours–14 days and maybe longer	Nausea, vomiting, fatigue; dryness in throat and nose to respiratory failure; central nervous system symptoms such as dizziness, double vision, headache, paralysis, and sometimes death	Improperly prepared home-canned low-acid fruits, vegetables, and juices plus salmon; infants under 1 year who have been given honey; consuming improperly prepared raw or parboiled meats from marine animals (e.g., by the Inuit population)
Salmonella	6–72 hours	4–7 days	Fever, chills, nausea, vomiting, diarrhea, abdominal cramps, fever, and sudden onset headache; it may be fatal in high-risk groups	Raw and undercooked meats (especially poultry), unpasteurized daily products, raw fruits and vegetables, fish and shrimp, homemade sauces and salad dressings†
Escherichia coli (*E. coli*)	A few hours–10 days	7–10 days	Severe abdominal cramping, bloody diarrhea; if hemolytic uremic syndrome (HUS) arises, it can cause seizures, strokes, the need for blood transfusions, and kidney failure	Ground beef; raw fruits and vegetables, including sprouts; unpasteurized dairy products or apple juice/cider; untreated water
Shigellosis	Immediately and up to 1 month later	12–50 hours after eating contaminated food	Flu-like symptoms such as nausea, vomiting, fever, diarrhea, stomach cramps	Consuming food or water contaminated by Shigella, such as salads, chopped turkey, raw oysters, deli meats, unpasteurized milk; it can be transferred by flies

Sources: *Canadian Food Inspection Agency. (2012). Marine toxins in bivalve shellfish: Paralytic shellfish poisoning, amnesic shellfish poisoning and diarrhetic shellfish poisoning. http://www.inspection.gc.ca/food/information-for-consumers/fact-sheets/specific-products-and-risks/fish-and-seafood/toxins-in-shellfish/eng/1332275144981/1332275222849;
†Government of Canada (2020). Salmonellosis (Salmonella). Retrieved from. https://www.canada.ca/en/public-health/services/diseases/salmonellosis-salmonella.html.

BOX 16.8   Ten Golden Rules for Safe Food Preparation

1. Choose food processed for safety (avoid unpasteurized foods).
2. Cook food thoroughly (poultry, meat, and eggs are contaminated when raw and need to be cooked thoroughly).
3. Eat cooked food immediately (microbes start growing immediately as cooked foods cool).
4. Store cooked food carefully (to keep food over a period of time, either keep it hot—above 60°C—or cold—below 4°C).
5. Reheat cooked foods thoroughly to ensure a temperature of at least 70°C is evenly distributed in the food.
6. Avoid contact between raw foods and cooked foods (wash and/or use separate food-handling and storage equipment for raw and cooked foods).
7. Wash hands repeatedly (use soap and running water to wash hands prior to food preparation and after every interruption).
8. Keep all kitchen surfaces meticulously clean (use soap and water and clean wiping cloths for food preparation areas).
9. Protect foods from insects, rodents, and other animals (keep foods in storage containers at all times).
10. Use pure water (boil water of questionable quality before adding it to food or making ice for drinks).

Source: Adapted from World Health Organization (WHO). (n.d.). *WHO "golden rules" for safe food preparation.* https://www.paho.org/en/health-emergencies/who-golden-rules-safe-food-preparation

Salmonellosis is a bacterial disease. Although morbidity can be significant, death is uncommon except among pregnant women, infants, older adults, and people who are immunocompromised (Health Canada, 2012). *Salmonella* is the most common pathogen reported to the Canadian National Enteric Surveillance Program in 2012 with 6 979 cases (PHAC, 2012b). Outbreaks occur commonly in restaurants, hospitals, long-term care facilities, and places where children are together. The transmission route is eating food derived from an infected animal or contaminated by the feces of an infected animal or person. Meat, poultry, and eggs are the foods most often associated with salmonellosis outbreaks. Animals are the common reservoir for the various *Salmonella* serotypes, although infected humans may also fill this role. Animals are more likely to be chronic carriers. Reptiles such as iguanas have been implicated as *Salmonella* carriers, along with pet turtles, poultry, cattle, swine, rodents, dogs, and cats. Person-to-person transmission is an important consideration in daycare and institutional settings.

E. coli O157:H7 belongs to the enterohemorrhagic category of *E. coli* serotypes that produce a strong cytotoxin that can cause a potentially fatal hemorrhagic colitis. This pathogen was first described in the 1990s in humans following the investigation of two outbreaks of illness that were associated with the consumption of hamburger from a fast-food restaurant chain. Undercooked hamburger has been implicated in several outbreaks, as have roast beef, alfalfa sprouts, unpasteurized milk and apple cider, municipal water, and person-to-person transmission in daycare centres. Infection with

E. coli O157:H7 causes bloody diarrhea, abdominal cramps, and, infrequently, fever. Pregnant women, children, immunocompromised people, and older adults are at the highest risk for clinical disease and complications (PHAC, 2015b). Hamburger often appears to be involved in outbreaks because the grinding process exposes pathogens on the surface of the whole meat to the interior of the ground meat, effectively mixing the exterior bacteria throughout the hamburger so that searing the surface no longer suffices to kill all bacteria. Tracking the contamination is complicated by the fact that hamburger is often made of meat ground from several sources. The best protection against this pathogen, as with most foodborne agents, is to thoroughly cook food before eating it. The number of *E. coli* O157:H7 cases reported in Canada has declined significantly since 2006, with 484 cases reported in 2012 (PHAC, 2019d).

Vectorborne Diseases

Vectorborne diseases refer to illnesses for which the infectious agent is transmitted by a carrier, or vector, usually an arthropod (mosquito, tick, fly), either biologically or mechanically. With *biological transmission*, the vector is necessary for the developmental stage of the infectious agent. An example is the mosquitoes that carry malaria and the Zika virus. *Mechanical transmission* occurs when an insect simply contacts the infectious agent with its legs or mouth parts and carries it to the host. For example, flies and cockroaches may contaminate food or cooking utensils.

Vectorborne diseases encountered in some parts of Canada are those associated with ticks, such as Lyme disease (*Borrelia burgdorferi*) and Rocky Mountain spotted fever (*Rickettsia rickettsii*) (less common). CHNs who work with large immigrant populations or with international travellers may encounter malaria and dengue fever, which are both carried by mosquitoes. For information on dengue fever, see the PHAC's "Dengue Fever" web page (the link is on the Evolve website). Recently, the Zika virus has become "one of the globalizing emerging infections proliferating beyond previously restricted geographic zones" (Muchaal, 2018, p. 27). Although no longer considered a global health crisis, 16 cases were reported in Canada in 2017, representing an 88% reduction from the previous year when the Zika virus swept through the Western hemisphere. A wealth of resources on vectorborne diseases can be accessed through the PHAC website. CHNs need to be current in their knowledge of the incidence, prevalence, and patterns of known and new vectorborne diseases in Canada.

Prevention of Tickborne Diseases

Measures for preventing exposure to ticks include reducing tick populations, avoiding tick-infested areas, wearing protective clothing when outdoors (long sleeves and long pants tucked into socks), using insect repellent, and immediately inspecting for and removing ticks when returning indoors. Researchers are looking at the effectiveness of using tick-killing acaricides in rodent bait boxes and at deer-feeding stations in areas where Lyme disease is highly concentrated. Ticks require a prolonged period of attachment (6 to 48 hours) before they start blood-feeding on the host; prompt tick discovery and removal can help prevent transmission of the disease. Ticks should be removed with steady, gentle traction on tweezers applied to the head parts of the tick. The tick's body should not be squeezed during the removal process to avoid infection that could be transmitted from resultant tick feces and tissue juices (PHAC, 2018b). When outdoors, permethrin sprayed on clothing and tick repellents containing diethyltoluamide (DEET) can offer effective protection; use of DEET should be avoided on children younger than 2 years because of reports of significant toxicity, including skin irritation, anaphylaxis, and seizures. For further information on Lyme disease, see the PHAC's "Lyme Disease" web page (the link is on the Evolve website).

Diseases of Travellers

Individuals travelling outside Canada need to be aware of and take precautions against diseases to which they may be exposed. The diseases and the precautions depend on the individual's health status, the travel destination, the reason for travel, and the length of travel. People who plan to travel in remote regions for an extended period need to consider rare diseases and take special precautions that would not apply to the average traveller. Travellers should consult the PHAC's "Travel Health" web page (see the link on the Evolve website) and a travel health care provider who can offer specific health information and recommendations for a given situation.

On return from travel abroad, travellers may bring back with them an unplanned souvenir in the form of disease. Therefore, a history of travel should always be closely considered. Even the apparently healthy returned traveller, especially one who was in a tropical country for some time, should undergo routine screening to rule out acquired infections. Likewise, refugees and immigrants may arrive with infectious disease problems ranging from helminthic infections to diseases of major public health significance such as Ebola, Zika, TB, malaria, cholera, and hepatitis. CHNs need to be familiar with these diseases and other infectious diseases. The PHAC's "Infectious Diseases" web page (see the link on the Evolve website) provides a wealth of information on various infectious diseases.

Malaria

Worldwide, malaria is the most prevalent vectorborne disease, occurring in more than 100 countries. In Canada, the incidence of malaria is largely due to newcomers from countries where malaria is endemic and from a small percentage of Canadian travellers to these malaria-endemic areas. Immigrants and visitors from areas where malaria is endemic may become clinically ill after entering this country. CHNs need to be aware of this possibility.

Malaria prevention depends on protection against mosquitoes and appropriate chemoprophylaxis. Medication resistance is an increasing problem in combating malaria. Of the four causes of human malaria, *Plasmodium ovale* and *Plasmodium vivax* result in disease that can progress to relapsing malaria, and *P. vivax* is increasingly drug resistant. *Plasmodium falciparum* causes the most serious malarial infection and is highly medication resistant. Thus, decisions about antimalarial medications must be tailored individually based on the type of malaria in the specific area of the country to be visited, the purpose of the trip, and the length of the visit. The PHAC and WHO publish guides on the status of malaria and recommendations for prophylaxis on a country-by-country basis. At this time, no antimalarial medication is 100% protective and must be combined with personal protective measures (e.g., insect repellent, long sleeves, long pants, insecticide treated mosquito nets). Antimalarials are generally started a week to several weeks before leaving Canada and are continued for 4 to 6 weeks after returning. Despite appropriate prophylaxis, malaria may still be contracted. Travellers should be advised of this fact and urged to seek immediate medical care if they exhibit symptoms of cyclical fever and chills up to 1 year after returning home. CDC provides travellers with detailed information on choosing a medication to prevent malaria (Centers for Disease Control and Prevention, 2015b).

Diarrheal Diseases

Travellers often suffer from diarrhea, so much so that colourful names, such as *Montezuma's revenge, turista,* and *Colorado quickstep,* exist in our vocabulary to describe these bouts of intestinal upset. Some of these diarrheas do not have infectious causes and may result from stress, fatigue, schedule changes, and eating unfamiliar foods. Acute infectious diarrheas are usually of viral or bacterial origin. *E. coli* probably causes more cases of traveller's diarrhea than all other infective agents combined. Protozoan-induced diarrheas such as those resulting from *Entamoeba* and *Giardia* are less likely to be acute, and they are more commonly present once the traveller returns home. Travellers need to pay special attention to what they eat and drink.

As in this country, much foodborne disease abroad can be avoided if the traveller eats thoroughly cooked foods prepared with reasonable hygiene; eating foods from street vendors is not recommended. Trichinosis, tapeworms, and fluke infections, as well as bacterial infections result from eating raw or undercooked meats. Raw vegetables may be a source of bacterial, viral, helminthic, or protozoal infection if they have been grown with or washed in contaminated water. Fruits that can be peeled immediately before eating such as bananas are less likely to be a source of infection. Dairy products should be pasteurized and appropriately refrigerated.

Water in many areas of the world is not potable (safe to drink), and drinking this water can lead to infection with a variety of protozoal, viral, and bacterial agents (including amoebae, *Giardia, Cryptosporidium,* and various coliform bacteria) and can also lead to hepatitis and cholera. Unless travelling in an area where the piped water is known to be safe, only boiled water (boiled for 1 minute), bottled water, or water purified with iodine or chlorine compounds should be consumed. Ice should be avoided because freezing does not inactivate these agents. If the water is questionable, choose coffee or tea made with boiled water, carbonated beverages without ice, beer, wine, or canned fruit juices.

Zoonoses

A *zoonosis* is an infection transmitted from a vertebrate animal to a human under natural conditions. The agents that cause zoonoses do not need humans to maintain their life cycles; infected humans have simply somehow managed to get in their way. Means of transmission include animal bites, inhalation, ingestion, direct contact, and arthropod intermediates. This last transmission route means that some vectorborne diseases may also be zoonoses. Other than vectorborne diseases, some of the more common zoonoses in Canada include toxoplasmosis *(Toxoplasma gondii),* cat-scratch disease *(Bartonella henselae),* brucellosis *(Brucella* species), listeriosis *(Listeria monocytogenes),* salmonellosis *(Salmonella* serotypes), and rabies (family Rhabdoviridae, genus *Lyssavirus).*

Rabies

One of the most feared of human diseases, rabies (formerly *hydrophobia)* has the highest case fatality rate of any known human infection—essentially 100%. Rabies is a significant public health problem worldwide (WHO, 2009b). Rabies in humans in Canada has greatly decreased since the availability of a vaccination for pets. Other carriers of rabies are raccoons, skunks, foxes, coyotes, and bats. Small rodents, rabbits and hares, and opossums rarely carry rabies. Epidemiological information should be consulted for information on the potential carriers for a given geographical region. When the virus spreads from wild to domestic animals, cats are often involved. The best protection against rabies remains vaccinating domestic animals—dogs, cats, cattle, and horses. Human rabies is rare in Canada, and since 1985 there have been only 4 cases reported (Government of Canada, 2018). If an individual is bitten, the bite wound should be thoroughly cleaned with soap and water and a physician consulted immediately. Suspicion of rabies should exist if the bite is from a wild animal or an unprovoked attack from a domestic animal. Even when there is no suspicion of rabies, a physician should be contacted because tetanus and antibiotic prophylaxis may be indicated.

PARASITIC DISEASES

Parasitic diseases are more prevalent in developing countries than in developed countries such as Canada. Contributing factors are a tropical climate and inadequate prevention and control measures. A lack of cheap and effective medications, poor sanitation, and a scarcity of funding lead to high reinfection rates even when control programs are attempted. Parasites are classified into four groups: nematodes (roundworms), cestodes (tapeworms), trematodes (flukes), and protozoa (single-celled animals). Nematodes, cestodes, and trematodes are all referred to as *helminths.*

CHNs and other health care providers need to be aware of the growing numbers of reported parasitic infections in Canada. Knowledge of the true burden of parasitic diseases in Canada is limited, but in 2009 the Food and Environmental Parasitology Network (FEPN) was formed in Canada to bring together researchers, regulators, and public health officials to address this issue (Dixon, Ndao, Tetro, et al., 2014). Some common parasites that cause infections that a CHN might encounter are *Enterobius* (pinworm), *Giardia lamblia, Trichuris trichiura* (whipworm), *Ascaris lumbricoides* (roundworm), and *Taenia solium* (pork tapeworm).

The PHAC's Bloodborne Pathogens Section of the Blood Safety Surveillance and Health Care Acquired Infections Division and the Centre for Infectious Disease Prevention and Control are responsible for evaluating the risks of parasitic diseases in Canada and for conducting surveillance studies. The maintenance of safe blood products is undertaken through evaluating risk and advising on policy direction and changes.

Early detection and intervention by CHNs and other health care providers allows the provision of appropriate treatment and patient education for preventing and controlling parasitic infections. Diagnosis of parasitic diseases is based on a history of travel, characteristic clinical signs and symptoms, and the use of appropriate laboratory tests to confirm the clinical diagnosis. Knowing what specimens to collect, how and when to collect them, and what laboratory techniques to use are all important in establishing a correct diagnosis. Effective drug treatment is available for most parasitic diseases. The high cost of medications, medication resistance, and toxicity are some of the common therapeutic problems. Measures for prevention and control of parasitic diseases include early diagnosis and treatment, improved personal hygiene, safer-sex practices, community health education, vector control, and improvements in the sanitary control of food, water, and wastes.

THE COMMUNITY HEALTH NURSE'S ROLE IN PROVIDING PREVENTIVE CARE

From prevention to treatment, CHNs function as counsellors, educators, advocates, case managers, and primary care providers. Appropriate nursing interventions for primary, secondary, and tertiary preventions are reviewed. The community health nursing process is used to care for patients with communicable and infectious diseases. CHNs are in an ideal position to affect the outcomes of communicable and infectious diseases, and the CHN's influence begins with primary prevention.

Primary Prevention

The goal of primary prevention is to keep people healthy and avoid the onset of disease. This begins with assessing for risk behaviour and providing relevant interventions on how to avoid infection. Health promotion includes education on healthy behaviours.

Assessment

To assess the risk of acquiring an infection, the CHN takes a history that focuses on potential exposure, which varies with the specific organism being studied and its mode of transmission. For example, the specific questions that need to be asked of patients who are at risk for acquiring STIs include obtaining a sexual history and history of injection drug use for patients and their partners. The sexual history provides information that could lead to the need for specific diagnostic tests, treatment modalities, and partner notification. It also facilitates the evaluation of risk factors and is necessary for the CHN to be able to provide relevant education for the patient's lifestyle.

Assessing a patient's risk of acquiring an STI should be done with all sexually active individuals. Such risk assessments should be included as baseline assessment data for those attending all clinics and those who receive school health, occupational health, public health, and home nursing services. To be most effective, the CHN obtaining a patient's sexual history needs to do the following:

- Remain supportive and open to facilitate honesty
- Use terms the patient will understand (be prepared to suggest multiple terms)
- Speak candidly so the patient will feel comfortable talking

A thorough sexual history requires obtaining personal and sensitive information. It includes such information as the types of relationships, the number of sexual partners and encounters, and the types of sexual behaviours that are practised. The confidential nature of the information and how it will be used should be shared with the patient to establish open communication and goal-directed interaction. Most patients feel uneasy disclosing such personal information. The CHN can ease this discomfort by remaining supportive and open during the interview to facilitate honesty about intimate activities. The CHN serves as a model for discussing sensitive information in a candid manner. When discussing precautions, direct and simple language needs to be used to describe specific behaviours. Doing so encourages the patient to openly discuss sexuality during this interaction and with future partners.

CHNs who are uncomfortable discussing topics such as sexual behaviour or sexual orientation are likely to avoid assessing risk behaviours with the patient and may therefore compromise data collection. CHNs can gain confidence in conducting sexual risk assessments by understanding their own values and feelings about sexuality and realizing that the purpose of the interaction is to improve the patient's health. The CHN's comfort in discussing sexual behaviour can be improved by using role-playing to practise assessments of sexual and injection drug-use behaviours and by working with patients to motivate behavioural changes.

Identifying the number of partners for sex and partners for injection drug use and the number of contacts with these partners provides information about the patient's risk. The chance of exposure decreases as the number of partners decreases, so people in mutually monogamous relationships are at low risk for acquiring STIs. This information can be obtained by asking, "How many sex (or drug) partners have you had over the past 6 months?" It is important to avoid basing assumptions about the sexual partner(s) on the patient's sex, age, ethnicity, or any other factor. Stereotypes and assumptions about who people are and what they do are common problems that keep interviewers from asking the questions that lead to obtaining useful information. For example, it should not be taken for granted that if a man is homosexual, he has more than one partner, that an older adult woman is monogamous, or that a business executive does not share drugs. Be aware also that the long incubation of HIV and the subclinical phase of many STIs lead some monogamous individuals to assume erroneously that they are not at risk.

It is important to identify whether the person has sexual contact with men, women, or both. This information can be obtained by asking, "Do you have sex with men, women, or both?" This lets the patient know that the CHN is open to hearing about these behaviours. Asking questions in an open-minded and accepting manner, the CHN is more likely to obtain information that is relevant to sexual practices and risk. Women who are exclusively lesbian are at low risk for acquiring STIs, but bisexual women may transmit STIs between male and female partners. In addition, it is possible for men to have sexual contact with other men and not label themselves as homosexual. Therefore, education to reduce risk that is specifically aimed at homosexual men will not be heeded by men who do not see themselves as homosexual. In such situations, the CHN can inquire with a more general question, such as "When was the last time you had sex with another man?"

Certain sexual activities are more likely to result in exposure to and transmission of STIs. Dangerous sexual activities include unprotected anal or vaginal intercourse, oral–anal contact, and insertion of a finger or fist into the rectum. These activities introduce a high risk of transmission of enteric organisms or result in physical trauma during sexual encounters. The CHN can obtain information about sexual encounters by asking, "Can you tell me the kinds of sexual activities in which you engage? This will help determine what risks you may have and the type of tests we should do." Patients who engage in genital–anal, oral–anal, or oral–genital contact will need throat and rectal cultures for some STIs, as well as cervical and urethral cultures.

Drug use is linked to STI transmission in several ways. Drugs such as alcohol put people at risk because these drugs can lower inhibitions and impair judgment about engaging in risky behaviours. Substance use disorders may cause individuals to perform sexual favours in order to acquire drugs or money to purchase drugs. The result is an increase both in the frequency of sexual contacts and the chances of contracting STIs. Thus, the CHN needs to obtain information on the type and frequency of drug use and the presence of risk behaviours. The administration of vaccines to prevent infection, such as for hepatitis A and C, is an example of primary prevention.

Interventions

Interventions are aimed at preventing specific infections. These interventions can take several forms. For example, an intervention might entail education on how to prevent infection and the availability of vaccines. As another example, based on the information obtained in the sexual history and risk assessment just described, the CHN would identify the specific education and counselling needs of the patient and develop interventions to meet those needs. Community health nursing interventions focus on working with patients to change behaviour and reduce the risk of contracting disease.

Interventions to prevent risky sexual behaviour. Sexual abstinence is the best way to prevent STIs. However, for many people, sexual abstinence is not realistic, and teaching about how to make sexual behaviour safer is critical. Safer sexual behaviour includes masturbation, dry kissing, touching, fantasy, and vaginal and oral sex with a condom. If used correctly and consistently, condoms can prevent both pregnancy and STIs because they prevent the exchange of body fluids during sexual activity. Condoms are not always used correctly. Moreover, alcohol consumption may accompany sexual activity, which also may decrease condom use. Thus, information about proper use of condoms and how to communicate with a partner is also necessary, particularly for those using alcohol or other substances. Condom use may be viewed as inconvenient, messy, or decreasing sensation. The CHN has many opportunities to convey this information during counselling. The CHN can enable patients to become more skilled in discussing safer sex through role-modelling and practising communication skills through role play.

Female condoms can also be a barrier to body fluid contact and therefore protect against pregnancy and STIs. The main advantage of the female condom is that its use is controlled by the woman. Because it is made of polyurethane, it is also useful if a latex sensitivity develops to regular male condoms. Symptoms of latex allergy include penile, vaginal, or rectal itching or swelling after use of a male condom or diaphragm. The female condom consists of a sheath over two rings, with one closed end that fits over the cervix.

Patients should understand that it is important to know the risk behaviours of their sexual partners, including a history of injection drug use and STIs, bisexuality, and any current symptoms. Each sexual partner is potentially exposed to all the STIs of all the people with whom the other partner has been sexually active.

Drug use interventions. Injection drug use is risky because the potential for injecting bloodborne pathogens, such as HIV and HBV, exists when needles and syringes are shared. During intravenous drug use, small quantities of drugs are repeatedly injected. Blood is withdrawn into the syringe and is then injected back into the user's vein. Individuals need to be advised against using injectable drugs and sharing needles, syringes, or other drug paraphernalia. If equipment is shared, it should be in contact with full-strength bleach for 30 seconds and then rinsed with water several times to prevent injecting bleach. People who inject drugs are difficult to reach for health care services. Effective outreach programs include using community peers, increasing accessibility of drug treatment programs combined with HIV testing and counselling, and long-term repeat contacts after completion of the program.

Because of the illegal nature of injectable drugs and the poverty associated with HIV, many people at risk have neither the inclination nor the resources to seek health care.

CHNs need to work to establish programs within communities because the opportunities for counselling on the prevention of HIV and other STIs are increased by bringing services into the neighbourhoods of those at risk. CHNs go into communities to disseminate information on safer sex, drug treatment programs, and discontinuation of drug use or safer drug-use practices (e.g., using new needles and syringes with each injection). Some programs provide sterile needles and syringes, condoms, and literature about anonymous HIV test sites.

Community Education on Communicable Diseases

Using primary prevention, CHNs educate healthy groups about the prevention of communicable diseases. Information about modes of transmission, testing, the availability of vaccines, and early symptoms can be provided to groups in the community and can help prevent the spread of STIs and HIV. Effective and convenient places to hold these educational sessions include schools, businesses, and churches. When talking with groups about HIV infection, the CHN needs to discuss the following:

- The number of people who are diagnosed with AIDS
- The number infected with HIV
- Modes of transmission of the virus
- How to prevent infection
- Common symptoms of illness
- The need for a compassionate response to those afflicted
- Available community resources
- Content about other STIs since the mode of transmission (sexual contact) is the same
- Information on these diseases, including the distribution, incidence, and consequences of the infection for individuals and society

Evaluation

Evaluation is based on whether the risky behaviour has changed to safe behaviour and, ultimately, whether illness is prevented. For example, in relation to interventions to prevent risky sexual behaviour, condom use would be evaluated for consistency if the patient is sexually active. Other behaviours, such as abstinence or monogamy, can be evaluated for their realistic implementation. At the community level, behavioural surveys can be done to measure reported condom use and condom sales, and measures of disease incidence and prevalence can be calculated to evaluate the effectiveness of an intervention.

Secondary Prevention

Secondary prevention includes screening for diseases to ensure their early identification and treatment, and follow-up with contacts to prevent further spread. In general, patient teaching and counselling need to include education about preventing self-reinfection, managing symptoms, and preventing the infection of others.

Testing and Counselling for Patients With HIV

People who have engaged in high-risk behaviours should be tested for HIV. The PHAC's "Canadian Guidelines on Sexually

Transmitted Infections" clearly identify at-risk people who should be offered HIV testing (see the link in the Tool Box on the Evolve website).

HIV pretest and post-test counselling are an important part of care when the **HIV antibody test** is indicated. The ELISA test (enzyme-linked immunosorbent assay) is a laboratory procedure that detects HIV antibodies and is the test commonly used to screen blood for the presence of the HIV antibody. Patients must know that the antibody test is not diagnostic for AIDS but is indicative of HIV infection. Therefore, a positive ELISA test is confirmed using the Western blot test (a confirmatory test). The STI guidelines thoroughly outline the precounselling and postcounselling needed for people with negative and positive antibody test results (PHAC, 2019f).

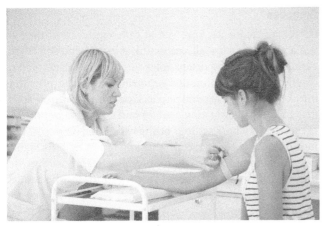

A sexually transmitted infection screening clinic is an example of secondary prevention. (iStockphoto/bluecinema)

Partner Notification

Partner notification, also known as *contact tracing,* is an example of a population-level intervention aimed at controlling infectious and communicable diseases. **Contact tracing** is the process of identifying the relevant contacts of a person with an infectious or communicable disease to inform them of their exposure to that disease. Relevant contacts would include those individuals who were exposed to a disease such as measles, or those who had sex with a person during the infectious period of an STI. Relevant contacts of bloodborne infections would also include those who have shared needles, transfusion recipients, and those who may have been exposed by other means such a needle-stick injury. The term "partner" may not apply in these situations (Provincial Infectious Diseases Advisory Committee [PIDAC], 2009). Partner notification programs usually occur in conjunction with notifiable disease requirements and are carried out by most health units and health authorities. Partner notification is done by confidentially identifying and notifying individuals who have been exposed to people who have reportable diseases. This could result in, for example, family members and close contacts of individuals with TB being given a Mantoux skin test.

Using a case management approach, the CHN can participate in contact tracing by identifying suspected and confirmed cases, and following up with patient education

and counselling. In Canada, all laboratory-confirmed cases of notifiable disease are reported electronically through the Computerized Disease Reporting System (CIDR) and all clinical notifications that are confirmed by a medical practitioner are entered into CIDR by the Provincial Departments of Health (Health Protection Surveillance Centre, 2019). Standard forms for notifiable diseases, including HIV, are available at all local Departments of Health. Once the diagnosis is confirmed, CHNs can work with patients to identify the names and phone numbers of possible contacts so that contacts can be informed of their exposure and obtain the necessary treatment. CHNs can work with patients to notify the contacts but patients may feel more comfortable if the CHN notifies those who are exposed. The CHN would follow up with the patient and contacts to verify that the exposed partners have been examined. If the patient prefers not to participate in notifying partners, the CHN contacts them—often by a telephone and then a home visit—and counsels them to seek evaluation and treatment. It is important during contact tracing that the CHN offers the patient education and counselling services that are culturally sensitive, supportive, and nonjudgemental.

Tertiary Prevention

Tertiary prevention can apply to many of the chronic viral STIs and TB. For viral STIs, much of this effort focuses on managing symptoms and psychosocial support regarding future interpersonal relations. Many patients report feeling contaminated, and support groups may be available to help patients cope with chronic STIs.

Monitoring Care

Patients with tuberculosis. One tertiary intervention is **directly observed therapy (DOT)** programs for TB medication monitoring. The CHN watches individual patients take their TB medications to ensure that they do so and documents the visit. When patients prematurely stop taking TB medications, there is a risk of the TB becoming resistant to the medications. This can affect an entire community of people who are susceptible to this airborne disease. Health care providers share in the responsibility of adhering to treatment, and DOT ensures that TB-infected patients have adequate medication. Thus, DOT programs are aimed at the population level to prevent antibiotic resistance in the community and to ensure effective treatment at the individual level. Many health units and health authorities have DOT home health programs to ensure adequate treatment. The 2014 edition of the PHAC's *Canadian Tuberculosis Standards* discusses the role of the health care worker—often a CHN—in the DOT process (see the link on the Evolve website and refer to Chapter 1 and the section titled "Directly Observed Therapy").

Patients with HIV or AIDS. The management of HIV or AIDS in the home may include monitoring physical and emotional health status and referring the family to additional care services for maintaining the patient in the home. Case management is important in all phases of HIV infection. It is especially important at this stage to ensure that patients have adequate services to meet their needs. This may include ensuring that medication can be obtained by identifying funding resources, maintaining infection control standards, reducing risk behaviours, identifying sources of respite care for caretakers, or referring patients for home or hospice care. Community health nursing interventions include teaching families about managing symptomatic illness by preventing deteriorating conditions such as diarrhea, skin breakdown, and inadequate nutrition.

The importance of teaching caregivers about infection control in home care is vital. Concerns about the transmission of HIV may be expressed by patients, families, friends, and other groups. Whereas fear may be expressed by some, others who care for loved ones with HIV may not take adequate precautions such as wearing gloves because of the concern about appearing as though they do not want to touch a loved one. Others may believe myths that suggest someone they love cannot infect them.

Standard precautions need to be taught to caregivers in the home setting. All blood and articles soiled with body fluids need to be handled as if they were infectious or contaminated by bloodborne pathogens. Gloves should be worn whenever hands will be expected to touch non-intact skin, mucous membranes, blood, or other fluids. A mask, goggles, and gown should also be worn if there is potential for splashing or spraying of infectious material during any care. All protective equipment should be worn only once and then disposed of. If the skin or mucous membranes of the caregiver come in contact with body fluids, the skin should be washed with soap and water and the mucous membranes should be flushed with water as soon as possible after the exposure. Thorough hand washing with soap and water—a major infection control measure—should be conducted whenever hands become contaminated and whenever gloves or other protective equipment (mask, gown) is removed. Soiled clothing or linen should be washed in a washing machine filled with hot water, using bleach as an additive, and should be dried on the hot-air cycle of a dryer.

Supporting Immunization

Because many children receive their immunizations from their family physician, nurse practitioners, or through their public health units or health authorities, CHNs play a major role in the effort to increase immunization coverage of infants and toddlers. Public health nurses track children known to be at risk for under-immunization and call or send reminders to their parents. They help avoid missed immunization opportunities by checking the immunization status of every young child encountered, whether the clinic or home visit is related to immunization or not. In addition, they organize immunization outreach activities in the community that deliver immunization services; provide answers to parents' questions and concerns about immunization; and educate parents about why immunizations are needed, about inappropriate contraindications to immunization, and about the importance of completing the immunization schedule on time.

Engaging in Surveillance of Communicable and Infectious Diseases

CHNs are frequently involved at different levels of the surveillance system for all communicable and infectious diseases. They play important roles in collecting data, making diagnoses, investigating and reporting cases, and providing information to the general public. Examples of possible activities include investigating sources and contacts in outbreaks of measles in school settings or shigellosis in daycare; TB testing and contact tracing; collecting and reporting information pertaining to notifiable communicable diseases; and providing morbidity and mortality statistics to those who request them, including the media, the public, service planners, and grant writers.

> ### STUDENT EXPERIENCE
>
> All provinces and territories in Canada are required to report the occurrences of notifiable diseases. In order to facilitate and monitor specific diseases, a reporting mechanism is in place. The list of NNDs in Canada is shown in Box 16.3, on page 396.
> 1. Find the incidence rate of at least 10 of these notifiable diseases in your community.
> 2. How does the incidence rate of each of the selected diseases compare with the provincial or territorial and national incidence rate?

CHAPTER SUMMARY

16.1 In the 1900s, communicable and infectious diseases were the leading cause of death in Canada. However, improved nutrition, vaccines, and antibiotics have ended the epidemics that once ravaged entire populations. With advanced control of communicable diseases and as individuals live longer, chronic diseases—such as heart disease, cancer, and stroke—have replaced infectious diseases as the leading causes of death. Many communicable and infectious diseases continue to be a concern. CHNs help monitor and track communicable and infectious diseases, and care for patients with these diseases.

16.2 Some of the determinants of health that affect communicable and infectious diseases and sexually transmitted infections (STIs) are health services, poverty, education and literacy, and gender.

16.3 The factors that make up the epidemiological triangle—the (infectious) agent, the host, and the environment—must interact for disease transmission. Effective intervention measures must be aimed at breaking the link or interaction between the agent, host, and environment.

16.4 *Surveillance* is the systematic and ongoing observation and collection of data on disease occurrence to describe phenomena and detect changes in frequency or distribution. An effective surveillance system includes mortality registration, morbidity reporting, epidemic reporting, epidemic field investigation, laboratory reporting, individual case investigation, surveys, use of biological agents and medications, distribution of animal reservoirs and vectors, and demographic and environmental data. Community health nursing actions to prevent and care for people experiencing communicable diseases include assessment of risk, education and counselling, partner/contact notification, testing and documentation of patients complying with drug regime, tracking children at risk for underimmunization, investigating sources and contacts in outbreaks, and sharing that data with other health care providers as needed.

16.5 Common infectious diseases are viral hepatitis, waterborne and foodborne illnesses caused by *Staphylococcus aureus, Clostridium perfringens,* paralytic shellfish poisoning, *Listeria monocytogenes, Clostridium botulinum, Salmonella, Escherichia coli,* shigellosis; vectorborne diseases; diseases of travellers, such as malaria; and zoonoses, such as rabies.

16.6 Parasitic diseases are more prevalent in developing countries than in developed countries such as Canada. Contributing factors are a tropical climate and inadequate prevention and control measures. Diagnosis of parasitic diseases is based on a history of travel, characteristic clinical signs and symptoms, and the use of appropriate laboratory tests to confirm the clinical diagnosis.

16.7 The CHN's role in caring for patients with communicable and infectious diseases involves the three levels of prevention: (1) primary prevention focuses on keeping people healthy and avoiding the onset of disease (e.g., vaccinations); (2) secondary prevention entails the screening of diseases to ensure early identification, treatment, and follow-up of contacts to prevent further spread (e.g., rapid identification of contacts and cases); and (3) tertiary care entails rehabilitation and caring for patients with chronic diseases (e.g., HIV/AIDS and TB).

📋 CHN IN PRACTICE: A CASE STUDY*

Tuberculosis

Li Ming immigrated to Canada from Tibet with her father and brother after her mother's death. During a trip to the emergency department with a fever, hemoptysis, and cough, she was diagnosed with drug-resistant tuberculosis (TB) and placed in directly observed therapy (DOT), which meant a CHN from the local health unit or health authority had to witness her ingesting her medication daily. Ms. Ming found taking the medication a big problem; swallowing the pills caused her to gag. She was embarrassed to have to take them in front of a CHN, and that made the whole situation even harder. Fortunately, the rest of the family had negative Mantoux skin test results and needed to be tested only periodically.

Ms. Ming was thin but not emaciated. She spoke English well enough to communicate with the CHN, Rachel, who told her she could take her time swallowing the medication. They chatted each day about Ms. Ming's life in Tibet and her adjustment to Canada. Ms. Ming worked in a beauty salon washing hair. Although she was 25 years old, her father did not want her to date, and so she never had.

Rachel worked to decrease Ms. Ming's anxiety about taking her pills. She taught Ms. Ming some relaxation exercises that Ms. Ming was able to use. During the first week of visits, it took about an hour for the pills to be ingested. A month later, the pill-taking was down to 15 minutes, and Ms. Ming no longer gagged.

Think About It

1. Explain how you would prepare and administer a Mantoux skin test to Li Ming.
   a. Is the test diagnostic for TB? Explain.
   b. How would you interpret the TB test? Explain.
2. What is the two-step TB testing? When would the two-step TB test be performed?
3. If TB was suspected in one of the family members, what other tests would be performed?
4. Rachel is asked by a nursing colleague if DOT is known to be the best approach for ensuring compliance with the treatment for TB. Find an evidence-informed article that would assist Rachel in responding to her colleague. To assist with your literature, search *The International Journal of Tuberculosis and Lung Disease,* which contains articles on this topic. Other journals also cover this topic.

* This case study was created by Deborah C. Conway and modified by the Canadian authors.

📶 TOOL BOX

The Tool Box contains useful resources that can be applied in community health nursing practice. These related resources are found either in the appendices at the back of this text or on the Evolve website at http://evolve.elsevier.com/Canada/Stanhope/community/.

Appendices

- Appendix 1: Canadian Community Health Nursing Standards of Practice
- Appendix 9: Non–Vaccine-Preventable Diseases
- Appendix 10: Viral Hepatitis Profiles
- Appendix E-4: Canadian Required Immunization Schedule

Tools

Canadian AIDS Information Treatment Information Exchange (CATIE). Hepatitis C. (http://www.catie.ca/en/hepatitis-c)

This web page contains comprehensive information on hepatitis C, including information on prevention, treatment, and healthy living. It also provides a link to information in different languages. The site contains a resource titled *Honouring Our Voices,* which shares personal stories of Indigenous people living with hepatitis C.

Canadian Public Health Association. *Leading Together: Canada Takes Action on HIV/AIDS* (2005–2010). (http://

www.ohtn.on.ca/Documents/Publications/Leading_Together.pdf)

This resource outlines a 5-year action plan that will facilitate implementation of strategies that can be used by many levels of government and other agencies across Canada to address HIV/AIDS in Canada.

Ontario Lung Association. Tuberculosis Information for Health Care Providers, 5th Edition. (https://www.rcdhu.com/wp-content/uploads/2018/12/TB-Information-for-Health-Care-Providers-5th-edition.pdf)

This 2015 Ontario Lung Association publication covers epidemiology, screening, diagnosis, treatment, and management of TB for health care providers.

Public Health Agency of Canada. Canadian Guidelines on Sexually Transmitted Infections. (http://www.phac-aspc.gc.ca/std-mts/sti-its/)

This site is a comprehensive reference for professionals for the prevention and management of STIs and now contains information on at-risk (vulnerable) populations. It is also available as an app for Android and Apple devices.

Public Health Agency of Canada. Flu Prevention Checklist. (http://publications.gc.ca/collections/collection_2011/aspc-phac/HP40-14-2010-eng.pdf)

This one-page checklist from the PHAC provides tips on staying healthy and preventing the spread of seasonal influenza or pandemic influenza. An excellent link is provided for additional information on influenza.

REFERENCES

Association of Faculties of Medicine of Canada. (n.d.). *AFMC primer on population health: Chapter 11 infectious disease control.* https://phprimer.afmc.ca/en/part-iii/chapter-11/.

British Columbia Centre for Disease Control. (2014). *Diseases and conditions: Cryptococcus gattii.* http://www.bccdc.ca/health-info/diseases-conditions/cryptococcus-gattii.

Canadian AIDS Treatment Information Exchange. (2019). *Fact sheets: The epidemiology of hepatitis C in Canada.* https://www.catie.ca/en/fact-sheets/epidemiology/epidemiology-hepatitis-c-canada.

Canadian Food Inspection Agency. (2012). *Marine toxins in bivalve shellfish: Paralytic shellfish poisoning, amnesic shellfish poisoning and diarrhetic shellfish poisoning.* http://www.inspection.gc.ca/food/information-for-consumers/fact-sheets/specific-products-and-risks/fish-and-seafood/toxins-in-shellfish/eng/1332275144981/1332275222849.

Canadian Food Inspection Agency. (2012b). *Salmonella food safety facts: Preventing food borne illness.* https://publications.gc.ca/site/eng/385958/publication.html.

Canadian Food Inspection Agency. (2015). *Canadian food inspection agency confirms Bovine spongiform encephalopathy (BSE) in Alberta.* http://www.inspection.gc.ca/animals/terrestrial-animals/diseases/reportable/bse/cfia-confirms-bse-in-alberta/eng/1423797248015/1423797327027.

Canadian Nurses Association (CNA). (2017). *Code of ethics for registered nurses, 2017 edition.* http://www.cna-aiic.ca/.

Canadian Nurses Association (CNA). (2021). *Nursing issues.* Retrieved from https://www.cna-aiic.ca/en/coronavirus-disease/nursing-workforce.

Centers for Disease Control and Prevention (CDC). (2014). *Emergency preparedness and response: Understand quarantine and isolation.* https://emergency.cdc.gov/preparedness/quarantine/.

Centers for Disease Control and Prevention (CDC). (2015a). *About Ebola virus disease.* https://www.cdc.gov/vhf/ebola/about.html.

Centers for Disease Control and Prevention (CDC). (2015b). *Choosing a drug to prevent malaria.* https://www.cdc.gov/malaria/travelers/drugs.html.

Centers for Disease Control and Prevention (CDC). (2016a). *2014 Ebola outbreak in West Africa—case counts.* https://www.cdc.gov/vhf/ebola/outbreaks/2014-west-africa/case-counts.html.

Centers for Disease Control and Prevention (CDC). (2016b). *2014 West Africa Ebola outbreak communication resources.* https://www.cdc.gov/vhf/Ebola/resources/index.html.

Community Health Nurses of Canada (CHNC). (2019). *Canadian community health nursing: Professional practice model and standards of practice.* https://www.chnc.ca/standards-of-practice.

Cropp, R. Y., Latham-Caranico, C., Stebben, M., et al. (2007). What's new in management of sexually transmitted infections. *Canadian Family Physician, 53*(10), 1739–1741.

Diener, A., & Dugas, J. (2016). Inequality-related economic burden of communicable diseases in Canada. *Canada Communicable Disease Report, 42*(Suppl. 1), S7–S13. https://doi.org/10.14745/ccdr.v42is1a02.

Dos Santos, W. G. (2020). Natural history of COVID-19 and current knowledge on treatment and therapeutic options. *Biomedicine & Pharmacotherapy, 129,* 110493.

Dixon, B., Ndao, M., Tetro, J., et al. (2014). Food and environmental parasitology in Canada: A network for the facilitation and collaborative research. *Food Protection Trends, 34*(6), 376–385.

Drebot, M., Jones, S., Grolla, A., et al. (2015). Hantavirus pulmonary syndrome in Canada. *Communicable Disease Report, 41*(6), 124–131. http://www.phac-aspc.gc.ca/publicat/ccdr-rmtc/15vol41/dr-rm41-06/assets/pdf/15vol41_06-eng.pdf.

Government of Canada. (2015). *Tuberculosis.* https://www.canada.ca/en/public-health/services/diseases/tuberculosis/surveillance.html.

Government of Canada. (2017). *Risks of E. coli (Escherichia coli) infection.* https://www.canada.ca/en/public-health/services/diseases/e-coli/risks-e-coli.html#risks-3.

Government of Canada. (2018). *Fact sheet - rabies.* Retrieved from https://inspection.canada.ca/animal-health/terrestrial-animals/diseases/reportable/rabies/fact-sheet/eng/1356155202013/1356155379445.

Government of Canada. (2019). *Be well aware - information for private well owners.* https://www.canada.ca/en/health-canada/services/publications/healthy-living/water-talk-information-private-well-owners.html.

Government of Canada. (2020). *Salmonellosis (Salmonella).* Retrieved from https://www.canada.ca/en/public-health/services/diseases/salmonellosis-salmonella.html.

Government of Canada. (2021). *Coronavirus disease (COVID-19): Outbreak update.* Retrieved from https://www.canada.ca/en/public-health/services/diseases/2019-novel-coronavirus-infection.html.

Haddad, N., Totten, S., & McGuire, M. (2018). HIV in Canada -surveillance report, 2017. *Canada Communicable Disease Report, 44*(12), 324–332. https://doi.org/10.14745/ccdr.v44i12a03.

Harkness, G. A. (2003). Hepatitis C: The "silent stalker". *American Journal of Nursing, 103*(9), 24–25.

Health Canada. (2012). *Salmonella and salmonellosis.* http://healthycanadians.gc.ca/eating-nutrition/risks-recalls-rappels-risques/poisoning-intoxication/poisoning-intoxication/salmonella-salmonelle-eng.php.

Health Protection Surveillance Centre. (2019). *Notifying infectious diseases.* https://www.hpsc.ie/notifiablediseases/notifyinginfectiousdiseases/.

Hislop, T. G., Teh, C., Low, A., et al. (2007). Hepatitis B knowledge, testing and vaccination levels in Chinese immigrants to British Columbia, Canada. *Canadian Journal of Public Health, 98*(2), 125–129.

Katz, J. R., & Hirsch, A. M. (2003). When global health is local health. *American Journal of Nursing, 103*(12), 75–79.

Lung Association. (2006). *Tuberculosis in Canada today: Resurgence.* http://www.lung.ca.

Marler Clark. (n.d.). *About E. coli: Outbreaks.* http://www.about-ecoli.com/ecoli_outbreaks

Muchaal, P. (2018). Zika virus: Where to from here? *Canadian Communicable Diseases Report, 44*(1), 27–28. https://doi.org/10.14745/ccdr.v44i01a06

National Collaborating Centre for Infectious Diseases. (n.d.). *Notifiable diseases database: factsheet.* https://nccid.ca/publications/notifiable-diseases-database-factsheet/.

Pan-Canadian Public Health Network. (2012). *Guidance for tuberculosis prevention and control in Canada.* http://www.phn-rsp.ca/pubs/gtbpcp-oppctbc/pdf/Guidance-for-Tuberculosis-Prevention-eng.pdf.

Provincial Infectious Diseases Advisory Committee (PICAC). (2009). *Sexually transmitted infectious case management and contact tracing best practice recommendations (ISBN: 978-1-4249-7946-2).* Ontario Ministry of Health and Long-Term Care.

Public Health Agency of Canada (PHAC). (2009). *Polio (Poliomyelitis).* http://travel.gc.ca/travelling/health-safety/diseases/polio.

Public Health Agency of Canada (PHAC). (2012a). *At a glance—HIV and AIDS in Canada.* http://www.phac-aspc.gc.ca/aids-sida/publication/survreport/2012/dec/index-eng.php.

Public Health Agency of Canada (PHAC). (2012b). *Executive summary for the national enteric surveillance program 2012 annual report.* https://publications.gc.ca/collections/collection_2014/aspc-phac/HP37-15-2012-eng.pdf.

Public Health Agency of Canada (PHAC). (2013). *Evaluation of community associated infections prevention and control activities at the Public Health Agency of Canada.* http://www.phac-aspc.gc.ca/about_apropos/evaluation/reports-rapports/2012-2013/ipca-pcia/section-2-eng.php.

Public Health Agency of Canada (PHAC). (2014a). *Canadian tuberculosis standards* (7th ed.). https://www.canada.ca/en/public-health/services/infectious-diseases/canadian-tuberculosis-standards-7th-edition.html.

Public Health Agency of Canada (PHAC). (2014b). *Hantaviruses.* http://www.phac-aspc.gc.ca/id-mi/vhf-fvh/hantavirus-eng.php.

Public Health Agency of Canada (PHAC). (2015a). *Canadian immunization guide.* https://www.canada.ca/en/public-health/services/canadian-immunization-guide.html

Public Health Agency of Canada (PHAC). (2015b). *Fact sheet: E. coli.* http://www.phac-aspc.gc.ca/fs-sa/fs-fi/ecoli-eng.php.

Public Health Agency of Canada (PHAC). (2015c). *Hepatitis C.* http://healthycanadians.gc.ca/diseases-conditions-maladies-affections/disease-maladie/hepatitis-c-hepatite/index-eng.php.

Public Health Agency of Canada (PHAC). (2015d). *Fact sheet on rabies.* https://inspection.canada.ca/animal-health/terrestrial-animals/diseases/reportable/rabies/fact-sheet/eng/1356155202013/1356155379445.

Public Health Agency of Canada (PHAC). (2017). *The FACTS on the safety and effectiveness of HPV vaccine.* Human papillomavirus (HPV) prevention and HPV vaccines: Questions and Answers. https://www.canada.ca/en/public-health/services/infectious-diseases/sexual-health-sexually-transmitted-infections/hpv-prevention-vaccines-questions-answers.html.

Public Health Agency of Canada (PHAC). (2018a). *Flu (influenza): For health professionals.* https://www.canada.ca/en/public-health/services/diseases/flu-influenza/health-professionals.html#a1.

Public Health Agency of Canada (PHAC). (2018b). *For health professionals: Lyme disease.* https://www.canada.ca/en/public-health/services/diseases/lyme-disease/health-professionals-lyme-disease.html.

Public Health Agency of Canada (PHAC). (2019a). *CJD cases by province/territory March 31, 2109.* https://www.canada.ca/en/public-health/services/surveillance/blood-safety-contribution-program/creutzfeldt-jakob-disease/cjd-surveillance-system.html#pycases.

Public Health Agency of Canada (PHAC). (2019b). *Notifiable diseases on-line.* https://diseases.canada.ca/notifiable/.

Public Health Agency of Canada (PHAC). (2019c). *West Nile virus and other mosquito-borne disease report.* https://www.canada.ca/content/dam/phac-aspc/documents/services/publications/diseases-conditions/west-nile-virus-surveillance/2018/november-4-10-week-45/november-4-10-week-45-eng.pdf.

Public Health Agency of Canada (PHAC). (2019d). *List of nationally notifiable diseases.* https://diseases.canada.ca/notifiable/diseases-list.

Public Health Agency of Canada (PHAC). (2019e). *Flu (influenza): Flu watch surveillance.* https://www.canada.ca/en/public-health/services/diseases/flu-influenza/influenza-surveillance.html.

Public Health Agency of Canada (PHAC). (2019f). *Canadian guidelines on sexually transmitted infections.* http://www.phac-aspc.gc.ca/std-mts/sti-its/.

Public Health Agency of Canada (PHAC). (2019g). *Variant Creutzfeldt-Jakob disease (vCJD) in Canada.* http://www.phac-aspc.gc.ca/cjd-mcj/vcjd-faq-eng.php.

Sherman, M., Shafran, S., Burak, K., et al. (2007). Management of chronic hepatitis C: Consensus guidelines. *Canadian Journal of Gastroenterology, 21*(Suppl. C), 25C–34C.

Thunder Bay District Health Unit. (2021). Necrotizing fasciitis "flesh eating disease". Retrieved from https://www.tbdhu.com/health-topics/diseases-infections/diseases-z/necrotizing-fasciitis-flesh-eating-disease.

United Nations AIDS (UNAIDS). (2017). *Global fact sheets: Aids.* http://aidsinfo.unaids.org.

Walkinshaw, E. (2011). Mandatory vaccinations: The Canadian picture. *Canadian Medical Association Journal, 183*(16), e1165–e1166. https://doi.org/10.1503/cmaj.109-3992

World Health Organization (WHO). (1999). *Smallpox eradication: Destruction of variola virus stocks. Fifty-second world health Assembly.* http://apps.who.int/gb/archive/pdf_files/WHA52/ew5.pdf.

World Health Organization (WHO). (2009a). *Influenza A (H1N1): Pandemic alert phase—6 declared, of moderate severity.* http://www.euro.who.int/en/health-topics/communicable-diseases/influenza/pandemic-influenza/past-pandemics/pandemic-h1n1-2009/archive-whoeurope-news-and-updates/influenza-a-h1n1-pandemic-alert-phase-6-declared,-of-moderate-severity.

World Health Organization (WHO). (2009b). *Rabies.* http://www.who.int/topics/rabies/en/.

World Health Organization (WHO). (2009c). *Smallpox: Historical significance.* http://www.who.int/mediacentre/en/.

World Health Organization (WHO). (2011). *NCD country profiles: Canada.* http://www.who.int/nmh/countries/can_en.pdf.

World Health Organization (WHO). (2019). *MERS monthly summary, February 2019.* https://www.who.int/emergencies/mers-cov/en/.

World Health Organization (WHO). (n.d.). *WHO "golden rules" for safe food preparation.* https://www.paho.org/en/health-emergencies/who-golden-rules-safe-food-preparation.

World Health Organization. (2021a). *Considerations for implementing and adjusting public health and social measures in the context of COVID-19.* https://www.who.int/publications/i/item/considerations-in-adjusting-public-health-and-social-measures-in-the-context-of-covid-19-interim-guidance.

World Health Organization. (2021b). *WHO coronavirus (COVID-19) dashboard.* https://covid19.who.int/.

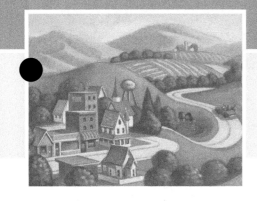

17

Environmental Health

OUTLINE

Environmental Concepts and Principles, 426
 Environmental Risk Factors and Health, 426
 Principles of Environmental Health, 427
The Environment as a Determinant of Health, 428
 Environmental Risk Factors, 428
 Environmental Pollutants, 429
Environmental Health Management in Canada, 430
 Governmental Protection of Environmental
  Health, 430
 Canada's Ecological Footprint, 433
 Canada's Greenhouse Gas Emissions Targets, 433
 Key Areas of Environmental Health Concern: Air, Water,
  and Food, 433
Environmental Epidemiology, 435

Environmental Health Assessment, 436
 Community Health Nursing Assessment and Referral
  Practices, 437
 Risk Assessment, 439
 Risk Communication, 440
Reducing Environmental Health Risks, 441
 Risk Management, 441
The Environment and Children's Health, 442
Community Health Nurses' Roles
 in Environmental Health, 444
 Environmental Ethics and Environmental Justice, 444
 Environmental Advocacy, 445
 The Community Health Nurse and Environmental Health
  Policy, 445

OBJECTIVES

After reading this chapter, you should be able to:

17.1 Define *environment* and describe the four
 environmental principles.
17.2 Explain how the environment, as a determinant of
 health, influences human health and disease.
17.3 Identify Canadian legislative and regulatory policies
 that influence the effects of the environment on health
 and disease patterns.
17.4 Describe environmental epidemiology.

17.5 Describe environmental health assessment, including
 risk assessment and risk communication.
17.6 Describe risk management in relation to environmental
 health.
17.7 Explain why children are more vulnerable than adults
 to environmental hazards.
17.8 Explain the activities of community health nurses
 in environmental health, as well as their roles in
 environmental ethics, justice, and advocacy.

KEY TERMS*

acid rain, 429
built environment, 444
climate change, 426
ecological footprint, 433
economic globalization, 426
environment, 426
environmental epidemiology, 435
environmental ethics, 444
environmental health, 426
environmental justice, 445
environmental scan, 436
environmental standards, 430
global ecological change, 426
greenhouse gas (GHG) emissions, 426
hazardous waste, 429

indoor air quality, 434
monitoring, 428
nonpoint source, 429
outrage, 441
PEEST, 437
point source, 429
poisons, 429
precautionary principle, 440
risk, 426
risk assessment, 439
risk communication, 440
risk management, 441
sink, 429
surveillance, 436
SWOT, 437

*See the Glossary on page 468 for definitions.

In watching diseases, both in private homes and in public hospitals, the thing which strikes the experienced observer most forcibly is this, that the symptoms or the sufferings generally considered to be inevitable and incidental to the disease are very often not symptoms of the disease at all, but of something quite different—of the want of fresh air, or of light, or of warmth, or of quiet, or of cleanliness, or of punctuality and care in the administration of diet, of each or of all of these. (Nightingale, 1859, p. 8)

The quality of the environment in which we live and work can have a major impact on the health of individuals, families, communities and society. Roughly 13.7 million deaths a year are linked to environmental causes, which is 24% of all global deaths (World Health Organization [WHO], 2016, p. 1). Often, we take the environment for granted and fail to see the hazards and risks that can have a negative impact on health. For example, many rural and remote communities in Canada do not have access to safe drinking water, and people living in large urban centres are often exposed to air pollution that can aggravate respiratory disorders such as asthma. In this chapter, we will discuss the environment as a determinant of health and explore the role of community health nurses (CHNs) when people are exposed to environmental risk factors in their homes, workplaces, and communities.

ENVIRONMENTAL CONCEPTS AND PRINCIPLES

Environmental Risk Factors and Health

In order to understand the impact of the environment on health, it is important to understand basic definitions and environmental health concepts. The **environment** can be defined as all that is internal or external to a given host or agent and that is influenced by and influences the host and the agent. It is the sum of all internal and external conditions affecting the life, development, and survival of an organism. CHNs often focus on environmental hazards or risks—in both work and nonwork contexts—that impact individuals, families, and the community. **Environmental health** addresses all the "physical, chemical, and biological factors external to a person, and all the related behaviours" (WHO, 2016, p. 3). It involves assessing and controlling environmental risk factors that can potentially affect health.

In the context of environmental health, **risk** is the chance that a specific health problem will develop in a population because of exposure to certain environmental factors. The goal of environmental health is to reduce environmental risks and create healthy environments that support population health. The WHO has identified nine categories of environmental risk factors that can have an impact on the health of a population (Box 17.1). Unfortunately, the impact of those environmental risk factors most often affects vulnerable populations including the poor, women and children, and Indigenous peoples (Basu & Lanphear, 2019).

An environmental risk factor can be transformed into actual harm to an individual, family, community, or society

---

BOX 17.1   Environmental Risk Factors for Health

- Air pollution (indoors and outdoors)
- Inadequate water, sanitation, and hygiene
- Chemicals and biological agents
- Radiation (ultraviolet and ionizing)
- Community noise
- Occupational risks
- Agricultural practices (pesticide-use, wastewater reuse)
- Built environments (housing and roads)
- Climate change

BOX 17.2   Transforming Environmental Risk into Harm

Factors that transform an environmental risk into a harm include:
- The risk involves toxic chemicals (e.g., contaminants in water) or physical properties (e.g., radiation)
- There is contaminated air, water (surface or groundwater), or soil
- A population lives within the exposure pathway (e.g., living near contaminated soil)
- A route of exposure: inhalation, ingestion, and /or skin absorption
- An adequate amount (dose) of exposure (e.g., chemicals) to result in human harm

---

when certain factors are present and interconnected (Box 17.2).

Climate change has become an urgent environmental concern IPCC (2021). It is defined as "any significant long-term change in current normal climate conditions, such as temperature, precipitation, extreme weather events, snow cover and sea level rise" (Public Health Agency of Canada [PHAC], 2015). According to United Nations Secretary-General, António Guterres, there is no time to lose and the biggest challenge faced by leaders and institutions in relation to climate change is to "show people we care – and to mobilize solutions that respond to people's anxieties with answers" (United Nations, 2019).

Global ecological change is the normal process occurring in the earth's evolution and its response to natural biological shifts. However, global change is a concern because of the unprecedented speed and scale of declines in ecological functioning that are attributable to human activity over the past century, and especially over the last 50 years (Canadian Public Health Association [CPHA], 2015). The effects of global ecological change have been further accentuated by **economic globalization,** which is characterized by rising industrial production, energy extraction (i.e., coal, oil, and gas), international trade, and consumption of material goods and energy (Huwart & Verdier, 2013).

Another environmental problem is **greenhouse gas (GHG) emissions.** Similar to how a greenhouse traps the sun's energy to keep plants warm, gases in the earth's atmosphere trap GHGs that are emitted by natural processes and human activities. In Canada, increases in GHGs are primarily due to human activities such as the use of fossil fuels or agriculture. More industrial activity has meant that huge quantities of GHGs—in particular, carbon dioxide, methane, and nitrous oxide—are accelerating climate change (David Suzuki Foundation, 2014; Previdi, Liepert, Peteet, et al., 2011). Canada's goal is to reduce the 2030 total GHG emissions by 30%, relative to 2005 emission levels. Canada's total GHG emissions in 2018 were 729 megatonnes of carbon dioxide equivalent (Mt CO_2 eq). The most recent data available show that in 2018 emissions were almost equal to 2005 emissions, indicating that Canada still has a long way to go to reach its goal of reducing GHGs emissions (Environment and Climate Change Canada, 2020a).

Environmental health concerns are ever-present, and they have gained attention nationally and internationally, especially in relation to environmental disasters (see Chapter 18). One of the worst environmental disasters related to public drinking water in Canadian history occurred in 2000, when seven people died in Walkerton, Ontario, because of water contaminated with *Escherichia coli* (*E. coli*). In August 2014, a dam at the Mount Polley Mine waste pond in the Cariboo region of British Columbia burst, releasing 10 million cubic metres of waste water and 5 million cubic metres of toxic slurry into nearby creeks and lakes. The magnitude of the water and soil contamination was considered to be one of the largest mining environmental disasters in Canada (Lavoie, 2015).

Principles of Environmental Health

To appreciate how environment risk factors can affect population health, it is helpful to understand four basic principles of environmental health: (1) everything is connected; (2) waste has to go somewhere; (3) impact is proportional to dose; and (4) today's solution may become tomorrow's problem.

Environmental Principle 1: Everything Is Connected

The principle that everything is connected, is the essence of tracking the presence of and exposure to environmental risks. However, in order for an environmental risk to cause harm, there must be a toxic contaminant that causes adverse biological effects, an exposure pathway, and a receptor. For example, a toxic contaminant such as air pollution is present in many urban centres, and the exposure pathway (a route a contaminant may take to come in contact with a receptor) is by air, with the receptors (people) being exposed to the contaminants when they are outdoors. A single contaminant can also follow more than one exposure pathway; for example, contaminants in the soil may be inhaled, absorbed through the skin, ingested directly, or ingested indirectly after accumulating in food grown onsite.

An environmental risk assessment can be conducted to evaluate the contaminant, pathway, and receptor in an effort to determine the resulting risk for specific populations. Air pollution is one environmental risk that, when it is present and people are exposed, has been shown to cause harm and therefore is directly connected to the health of populations. Box 17.3 shows how the environment, specifically the contextual components

---

BOX 17.3 How Your Environment Can Cause Premature Mortality

The neighbourhood in which you live can affect your health. In 2019, researchers Awuor and Melles studied the influence of the environment and health indicators on premature mortality in 140 neighbourhoods in the city of Toronto, Canada. Six environmental variables were examined, including ultrafine particles, carcinogenic and noncarcinogenic pollutants, pollution released into the air, tree cover, and walkability index.

Principle component analysis was applied to an empirical analysis of neighbourhood data to identify patterns and explain variables. Regression analysis was applied to model the relationship between the indices of environmental health and the potential relationship with premature mortality. Premature mortality within neighborhoods was predicted by the presence of the environmental risk factors of air pollution, lack of tree canopy, and a low walkability index. Analysis revealed that there was a significant relationship between a neighbourhood's environmental features and premature mortality, suggesting that these factors can predict urban premature mortality in the city of Toronto.

The implications of these findings include enhancing CHN's understanding of the impact of environmental risk factors with specific populations and implementing strategies to address this risk.

Source: Awuor, L., & Melles, S. (2019). The influence of environmental and health indicators on premature mortality: An empirical analysis of the City of Toronto's 140 neighborhoods. *Health Place*, 58, 102155. https://doi.org/10.1016/j.healthplace.2019.102155

---

of neighbourhoods—such as air pollution and walkability—can predict rates of urban premature mortality.

Environmental Principle 2: Everything Has to Go Somewhere

The principle that everything has to go somewhere means that once products are generated, they must be disposed of by incineration (burning), water discharge, or landfills and soil burial. Burning waste can change the chemical composition through heat, and the products of burning, such as ash and air emissions, must still be controlled and disposed of in a water discharge, placed in a landfill or buried in the soil. To interrupt the exposure pathway, waste products being disposed of in water must be treated to ensure that the dose in the water is not great enough to do harm. When landfills or soil burial are used to dispose of wastes, protections such as liners and leachate pumps and monitors must be put in place, to avoid seepage of harmful doses into groundwater or air. Each of these options for waste disposal is intended to either provide a way to alter the waste product to a less toxic form through chemical intervention (biodegradation) or store the product in a biounavailable form or place (burial). Because each option for disposal can be a problem, reducing waste through such measures as recycling and reuse is more desirable.

One additional point of emphasis is that human effects are intensified in the most sensitive, vulnerable environments, such as estuaries and the nurseries for much of sea and coastal plant and animal life. Some of the most valued food sources are also the most sensitive to pollution. Shellfish are efficient filters of contaminants in the water in which they live. For example, oysters filter and also retain almost all contaminants from the water in which they grow. It is impossible to rid them of contaminants after harvesting. The only protection for humans is to grow oysters in environments free from harmful contamination. Safe seafood depends on clean water. This example leads to the third principle.

Environmental Principle 3: Impact Is Proportional to Dose

The third principle is concerned with the relationship between a dose of (or exposure to) an environmental pollutant and its impact on health. The problem with the application of the principle of dose being proportional to impact is that it is tied to a world view that the environment is a limitless repository for waste. The capacity of large rivers and the ocean to dilute waste may seem boundless, but it is becoming more evident every day that Earth's capacity to assimilate the by-products of human waste is far from limitless. Earth is, in fact, fragile and delicately balanced, and the knowledge and practice about how to live within that balance without doing harm is far from adequate. The fourth principle reflects this insight.

Environmental Principle 4: Today's Solution May Become Tomorrow's Problem

Environmental principle number four states that today's solution may become tomorrow's problem. The brief history of organized environmental protection is filled with examples. Garbage that went from the streets into unlined landfills is now a source of groundwater contamination. Gasoline tanks that were buried underground to avoid an ugly landscape were found to leak over time. Fortunately, new solutions such as lined landfills and double-walled storage tanks with sensors for leaks emerged to address the problems that arose from those previous solutions. Today waste management involves **monitoring**, which is the periodic or continuous surveillance or testing used to determine the level of adherence to statutory requirements or pollutant levels in various media or in humans, plants, and animals. In this way, today's solutions to environmental pollution should not become tomorrow's environmental pollution problems.

THE ENVIRONMENT AS A DETERMINANT OF HEALTH

The physical and psychosocial environments have an impact on the health of the patient. The *physical environment* is the natural and human-built environment and the factors that influence health, such as the quality of air, water, and soil. The *psychosocial environment* refers to psychosocial hazards (factors and situations in one's environment that create or potentiate stress, emotional strain, or interpersonal problems) and other social factors that influence health, such as support networks. The "Determinants of Health" box provides examples of various physical and psychosocial environmental factors in the natural and built environments that influence health.

DETERMINANTS OF HEALTH

Physical and Psychosocial Environments

- Exposure to traffic-related air pollution has been causally linked to negative effects on health, such as asthma.* Prohibiting vehicle engines from running when the vehicle is stopped for longer than 10 seconds (not at intersections) would help minimize the risk of exposure to air pollution.[†] Municipal bylaws designate the exact time vehicles may be idle, and that time varies across the country.
- Respiratory health problems in humans may be due to diesel engines, as they contribute to urban particulate matter, which can carry carcinogens.[‡]
- Agricultural activities have a negative impact on groundwater quality.[§] These activities can result in contaminants such as chemicals, livestock wastes, and fertilizers in surface and groundwater supplies, which can have public health and environmental implications, such as unsafe drinking water supplies and unsafe recreational areas.[ǁ]
- *Salmonella* poisoning can occur through handling or consuming contaminated foods or by contact with pets carrying the bacteria.[**]
- Mercury is a toxic substance that, when released into the environment, causes harmful effects on the neurological, immune, and reproductive systems. In Canada, regulations to minimize mercury exposure have focused primarily on industries such as mining, metal smelting, steel manufacture, cement manufacture, electric power generation and waste disposal. [‡‡]
- Injuries in the workplace are occurring from exposure to hazardous materials and perceived work overload,[§§] CHNs who work in occupational health settings conduct workplace environmental assessments and provide education for employers and workers to prevent workplace injuries.
- Employee perceptions of heavy workload demands, long hours of work, along with increased technological ties to the workplace and multiple personal demands have all caused Canadian workers to report excess worry or stress in the workplace.[##]

Sources: * Brauer, Reynolds, & Hystad, 2013.
[†] Union of Nova Scotia Municipalities, 2011.
[‡] Canadian Centre for Occupational Health and Safety, 2021.
[§] Twarakavi & Kaluarachchi, 2006.
[ǁ] Government of Alberta, 2018.
[**] Finley, Reid-Smith, & Weese, 2006.
[‡‡] Government of Canada, 2020a.
[§§] Breslin, Day, Tompa, et al., 2007.
[##] Blanchflower, 2014.

Environmental Risk Factors

It is important to consider how exposure to environmental risk factors can affect the health of specific populations. Women and children, people who are immunocompromised, and Indigenous peoples are more vulnerable to environmental risk factors than the general population. When assessing a community's environmental health status, it is important for CHNs to review the general health status of the community to identify members who may have higher risk factors and assess their environmental exposure. Nurses must be well-prepared to identify and assess potential environmental health issues related to workplaces, neighbourhoods, houses, and schools (CNA, 2005).

Knowing about the potential environmental health issues related to toxic chemicals in the environment and being able to use that information in practice can seem like a huge task. Fortunately, chemicals can be grouped into families, and it is possible to understand the actions and risks associated within these groups. The following are group examples:

- Metals and metallic compounds such as arsenic, cadmium, chromium, lead, and mercury
- Hydrocarbons such as benzene, toluene, ketones, formaldehyde, and trichloroethylene
- Irritant gases such as ammonia, hydrochloric acid, sulphur dioxide, and chlorine
- Chemical asphyxiants that include carbon monoxide, hydrogen sulphide, and cyanides
- Pesticides such as organophosphates, carbamates, chlorinated hydrocarbons, and bipyridyls

Environmental Pollutants

Many environmental pollutants are known or suspected *neurotoxins*—that is, toxins that destroy nerves or nervous tissue. It is important for CHNs to be aware of environmental hazards in their communities and question the following: Are people in the community eating wildlife, and if so, are they being exposed to toxins such as mercury? (To explore this question further, see the "CHN in Practice: A Case Study, Fishing for Answers" box). What toxic exposures can be identified in homes (e.g., mould)? Do people have access to safe drinking water? What environmental hazards might be present in workplaces? Are workplace and industrial activities producing environmental toxins? Do people use wood-burning stoves in their homes?

CHN IN PRACTICE: A CASE STUDY

Fishing for Answers in Corner Brook

Tami-Lyne, a 28-year-old member of the Qalipu Mi'kmaq First Nation, lives in Cat Arm Reservoir in a small rural community in Newfoundland and Labrador. Her only child, a 10-year-old son named Randy, likes to go fishing for brook trout and for Arctic char with his father. Randy is a healthy young male who enjoys many activities such as biking, fishing, hockey, and spending time with his extended family. Tami-Lyne comes to the community health nursing clinic to talk with the CHN, Lisa, about her recent reading that eating certain fish can cause health problems. She tells Lisa that she and her family eat brook trout and Arctic char at least twice a week and that she has some concerns and questions.

Think About It

1. According to the Government of Canada, what is the maximum amount of Arctic char that Tami-Lyne, her son, and her husband should eat per week? (See https://www.canada.ca/en/environment-climate-change/services/pollutants/mercury-environment/health-concerns/fish-consumption-advisories.html#NF)
2. What symptoms should Lisa ask Tami-Lyne about to determine whether mercury poisoning is present in her immediate family? (See https://www.canada.ca/en/environment-climate-change/services/pollutants/mercury-environment/health-concerns.html)

Toxicology is the scientific study of the poisonous effects of chemicals. **Poisons** are toxic substances that cause injury, illness, or death to humans and other organisms. For example, **acid rain,** precipitation that contains atmospheric pollution (e.g., sulphur dioxide and nitrogen oxides), causes toxic substances such as aluminum to be released into the soil; aluminum is toxic to trees and fish (U.S. Environmental Protection Agency, 2007). The increase in aluminum in lakes and streams can be deadly to aquatic life, and humans who ingest fish with accumulated amounts of aluminum can have adverse health effects. The Environment and Climate Change Canada webpage provides information on what acid rain is, where it is a problem in Canada, and the sources of emissions that contribute to acid rain. For example, eastern Canada is more affected by acid rain (i.e., Ontario, Quebec, New Brunswick, and Nova Scotia) because its geology cannot effectively neutralize acid rain (Environment Canada, 2018).

Pollution sources are also characterized as point or nonpoint sources. A pollutant from a **point source** is released into the environment from a single site, such as a smokestack, a hazardous waste site, hydraulic fracturing or "fracking" site, or an effluent pipe. **Hazardous waste** is any waste material that poses actual or potential harm to the environment and to humans. A **nonpoint source** of pollution is more diffuse; for example, traffic, fertilizer, or pesticide runoff into waterways (whether from large-scale farming operations or from individual lawns and gardens). Another nonpoint source is animal waste from wildlife or confined animal operations for food production (e.g., swine, poultry) that can get into nearby water bodies, resulting in coliform contamination and nutrient overload.

Air pollution and GHG emissions in our environment markedly influence population health. For example, epidemiological studies have concluded that exposure to air pollution increases a population's risk for cardiovascular and respiratory diseases. In Canada, evidence shows that air pollution contributes to more than 14 600 premature deaths, thousands of hospital visits, and millions of days with restricted activity each year (Government of Canada, 2020b). Therefore, it is important for CHNs to understand the health effects of climate change on the health of populations and possible future implications for nursing practice.

As noted earlier, GHGs are naturally occurring gases in the atmosphere that assist in regulating the earth's temperatures for habitation. The GHGs are water vapour, ozone, carbon dioxide, methane, and nitrous oxide. GHGs are also produced by human activities in the agricultural sector, transportation sector, and industrial sectors. A **sink** is a process that serves to remove a greenhouse gas, or a precursor of a greenhouse gas, from the atmosphere (Environment and Climate Change Canada, 2021).

Global warming is an accelerating and urgent environmental and public health issue (Chalupka, 2014; Pinkerton & Rom, 2014). Rapid desertification, chaotic weather patterns, and rising ocean levels are resulting in a massive tide of environmental refugees, people who must leave their homes due to the deep effects of climate change or environmental pollution. The number of environmental refugees is currently greater than the number of refugees from armed conflict. However, environmental issues may also contribute to the conditions of conflict (United Nations High Commissioner for Refugees, 2015). Disaster relief and response are discussed further in Chapter 18.

ENVIRONMENTAL HEALTH MANAGEMENT IN CANADA

Governmental Protection of Environmental Health

Canada is part of the global community, connected through economic interactions, cultural diversity and diffusion, communication exchange through technology, and travel. Environmental impacts currently threaten the health of future generations on all continents. Environmental health indicators have been defined and are tracked by Environment Canada, Statistics Canada, and Health Canada with input from the provinces and territories to measure the relationship between the environment and health (Environment Canada, 2020a). Listed below are environmental indicators that are tracked by the Canadian Environmental Sustainability Indicators program:

- *Air:* Percentage of the population living in areas affected by air pollution.
- *Water:* Drinking water advisories, pulp and paper effluent quality, bisphenol A in water, and sediment.
- *Climate Indicators:* Temperature change, snow cover, and carbon dioxide emissions.
- *Wildlife and Habitat:* The amount and proportion of area conserved, and the amount of timber harvested with the wood supply.

Health Canada has input into the development of environmental regulations and guidelines, and the Minister of the Environment is responsible for the administration of the *Canadian Environmental Protection Act 1999.* That Act regulates pollution prevention and the protection of the environment and human health. It ensures that environmental assessments are completed on all substances not regulated under other Canadian acts. It also ensures that these substances meet Canadian health, safety, and **environmental standards**—governmental guidelines or rules that impose limits on the amount of pollutants or emissions produced. The Act provides the authority needed to effect change in pollution from emissions caused by a variety of toxic substances. Health Canada has total or partial responsibility for several acts—for example, the *Controlled Drugs and Substances Act, Department of Health Act, Food and Drugs Act,* and *Hazardous Materials Information Review Act* (Government of Canada, 2019a).

In Canada, the development of legislation, bills, regulations, and government guidelines and agreements can involve public participation. The CHN needs to be familiar with the many opportunities to become involved in the development of environmental health policies (e.g., through participation in advisory or review committees, CHN position paper writing, general public consultations, petitions). Table 17.1 describes the concepts of legislation, bills, regulations, guidelines, and agreements. It is essential for CHNs to differentiate among them.

Certain federal, provincial and territorial, and local and regional agencies with environmental health responsibilities are presented in Table 17.2. Information on the other responsibilities of these agencies has also been included.

TABLE 17.1   Legislation, Bills, Regulations, Guidelines, and Agreements

Type	Description
Legislation	Legislation, often referred to as *acts* or *statutes*, are written laws. They are passed by the legislative body of government; that is, Parliament. A bill, or draft legislation, when it is brought to Parliament for approval, requires the assent of the House of Commons, the Senate, and the Crown (Governor General) to become law.
Bills	Bills are debated in Parliament by all party members during what are officially known as first reading, second reading, and third reading. Also, bills are presented to a parliamentary committee for appraisal. This committee as a rule asks for the views of interested parties, including the public. Lastly, a bill becomes law (an act) in the course of a formal procedure known as *proclamation,* which is done by the governor in council (Cabinet—i.e., the prime minister and federal ministers).
Regulations	Regulations are made under the authority of an act. Like acts, they are legally binding. Regulations cannot go beyond the act they are associated with. They are the operational part of an act; for example, they describe the meaning of certain terms in the act, as well as actions and procedures that must be followed and standards that must be met to conform to the act.
Guidelines	Guidelines are departmental documents that are used to understand legislation or regulation. Guidelines do not have the force of law, even though they result from legislation.
Agreements	Agreements may also be referred to as *accords, conventions, declarations, final acts, general acts, pacts,* and *protocols.* Some agreements consist of letters of agreement, letters of intent, various types of memoranda, and mutual recognition agreements. Health Canada is involved in a number of mutual and multiparty agreements and planning measures with the intent to achieve defined objectives. Such agreements, depending on their nature, may be legally binding.

Source: Adapted from Health Canada. (2006). *Legislation and guidelines.* http://www.hc-sc.gc.ca/ahc-asc/legislation/index-eng.php

TABLE 17.2 Government Health Agencies With Environmental Health Responsibilities

FEDERAL HEALTH AGENCIES

Agency	Responsibilities	Program, Division, or Branch of Agency	Responsibilities
Health Canada http://www.hc-sc.gc.ca.	• Providing national leadership in the development of health policy, the enforcement of federal health regulations, the prevention of disease, and the promotion of healthy living • Collaborating with other federal departments to reduce health and safety risks • Participating in international knowledge development, surveillance, and regulatory activities	Healthy Environments and Consumer Safety Branch http://www.hc-sc.gc.ca/ahc-asc/branch-dirgen/hecs-dgsesc/index-eng.php.	• Reducing the harm caused by tobacco, alcohol, controlled substances, environmental contaminants, and unsafe consumer and industrial products to assist Canadians to maintain and improve their health by promoting healthy and safe living, working, and recreational environments
		Pest Management Regulatory Agency http://www.hc-sc.gc.ca/ahc-asc/branch-dirgen/pmra-arla/index-eng.php.	• Protecting human health and the environment by pesticide regulation
		Health Products and Food Branch http://www.hc-sc.gc.ca/ahc-asc/branch-dirgen/hpfb-dgpsa/index-eng.php.	• Minimizing health risk factors associated with health products by monitoring for safety, quality, and effectiveness of vaccines, medications, medical devices, natural health products, and therapeutic products • Monitoring the safety and quality of foods • Providing information to Canadians so they can make informed decisions about their health
		Environmental and Workplace Health http://www.hc-sc.gc.ca/ewh-semt/index-eng.php.	• Providing information on many environmental factors that influence health, such as air quality, climate change, noise, occupational health and safety, and water quality
Public Health Agency of Canada http://www.phac-aspc.gc.ca.	• Promoting health • Preventing and controlling chronic diseases and injuries • Preventing and controlling infectious diseases • Preparing for and responding to public health emergencies • Strengthening public health capacity	Health Promotion and Chronic Disease Prevention	• Providing leadership in Canada and globally in health promotion, chronic disease prevention, and control • Coordinating the monitoring of chronic diseases and their risk factors and early disease detection • Developing and evaluating programs addressing common risk factors and concerns for specific aggregates (i.e., older persons, youth) • Educating the public and health care providers • Managing contributions and grants
		Preventative Public Health Systems and Adapting to a Changing Climate Program	• Providing specialized policy advice and coordination • Managing policy partnerships with various stakeholders • Expanding research and further engaging provincial and local public health stakeholders to address climate change impacts • Developing enhanced surveillance methods • Identifying vulnerable groups

Continued

TABLE 17.2 Government Health Agencies With Environmental Health Responsibilities—cont'd

FEDERAL HEALTH AGENCIES

Agency	Responsibilities	Program, Division, or Branch of Agency	Responsibilities
		Infectious Disease Prevention and Control	• Preventing, eliminating, and controlling infectious diseases, including responsibility for pandemic preparedness and response
Environment and Climate Change Canada http://www.ec.gc.ca.	• Protecting and conserving the natural environment • Protecting water resources • Forecasting weather • Monitoring climate change • Promoting sustainable development		• Maintaining the safety and health security of people both nationally and internationally • Providing leadership in health promotion and undertaking programs designed to help Canadians stay healthy, reduce their risks for developing chronic illnesses, and prevent disease progression for those living with chronic diseases • Designing programs to help Canadians stay healthy by reducing their risks of developing chronic illnesses and preventing disease progression for those with chronic illness

Provincial and Territorial Health Agencies

Agency	Responsibilities	Branch of Agency	Responsibilities
Environment ministry	• Ensuring provision of clean, safe drinking water • Protecting air by supporting climate change initiatives • Managing waste to reduce risks to humans and the environment		
Health ministry	Responsibilities of each provincial and territorial ministry, per the *Canada Health Act:* • Administering the health care system • Providing services such as health insurance programs, drug benefits, assistive devices, care for the mentally ill, long-term care, home care, community and public health, and health promotion and disease prevention • Regulating hospitals and nursing homes • Providing medical laboratories • Coordinating emergency health services • Protecting and promoting health, including environmental health	Ministry of labour, which includes occupational health and safety, workplace safety and insurance	Organizing and enforcing workplace health and safety standards for the prevention of workplace deaths, injuries, and disease by setting, communicating, and enforcing standards

Local and Regional Health Agencies

Local and regional boards of health	• Enforcing local bylaws • Conducting complaint investigations and risk assessments • Inspecting premises to ensure adherence to pertinent regulations such as safe food handling, land use, and traffic

Note: Due to variances in titles and contact information, websites have not been included for provincial and territorial health agencies, and local and regional health agencies.

Source: Adapted from Stanhope, J., & Lancaster, J. (2011). Environmental health in Canada. In M. Stanhope, J. Lancaster, H. Jessup-Falcioni, et al. (Eds.), *Community health nursing in Canada* (2nd Cdn. ed., pp. 474–476). Mosby/Elsevier.

Canada's Ecological Footprint

Humans' **ecological footprint** is a measure of the natural resources required to produce the resources we consume and absorb the waste we generate. From 1961 to 2020, Canada's ecological footprint has remained about the same, but its biocapacity has been slowly declining (Global Footprint Network, 2020). *Carbon footprint* is a measure of the amount of carbon dioxide emitted as a result of fossil fuel use (e.g., in travel, during manufacturing). Footprinting allows countries to monitor their annual use of resources to determine whether their consumption of resources exceeds the earth's ability to regenerate. If consumption of resources continues at the current levels, the earth will be unable to meet the resource demands. If interventions are introduced early enough, ecological assets can be used more effectively to sustain the ecosystem. Footprinting also creates a means of measurement for self-awareness and learning regarding individual consumption and habits. For further information on ecological and carbon footprinting, see the Global Footprint Network link on the Evolve website.

Canada's Greenhouse Gas Emissions Targets

At the United Nations Framework Convention on Climate Change held in Kyoto, Japan, in 1997, the Kyoto Protocol was developed with the goal of decreasing GHG emissions globally (Environment Canada, 2012). Canada signed the Kyoto Protocol in 1998 and ratified it in 2002; and in 2005, it became a legally binding agreement (Environment Canada, 2012). Under this agreement, Canada committed to reduce GHG emissions between 2008 and 2012 to a level of 6% below 1990 levels. In 2011, Canada withdrew from the Kyoto Protocol. In 2012, the federal government announced that it would commit to reducing GHG emissions by 17% below 2005 levels by 2020 (Environment Canada, 2012). In the Government of Canada document *Turning the Corner: Regulatory Framework for Industrial Greenhouse Gas Emissions,* additional stringent industrial regulatory targets to reduce GHGs were outlined (Environment and Climate Change Canada, 2021). These targets were set as a result of in-depth governmental (local, provincial, and federal), ministerial, industry, nongovernmental organization, Indigenous peoples, and general public consultations.

Despite its efforts to deal with environmental issues, as of 2016, Canada ranked 14th out of 16 peer countries for its overall environmental performance (Conference Board of Canada, 2020). Only Australia and the United States were ranked lower. Geography and industrial structure were considered to affect the performance of these lower-ranking three countries. Fortunately, Canada's air quality has improved significantly over the past few decades and, according to the WHO, is consistently ranked among the cleanest in the world. According to the Conference Board of Canada (2020), Canada must encourage more sustainable consumption by transitioning residents from the use of wood-burning to heat their homes to the use of hydro or natural gas, where possible. Unfortunately, Canada has a long way to go to address the environmental issues of air pollution, and GHG emissions, but Canada does rank high on low-emitting electricity generation because over half of the country's electricity comes from hydroelectric (water) power.

Key Areas of Environmental Health Concern: Air, Water, and Food

Environmental issues are global issues and are therefore the concern of governments outside of Canada, nongovernmental agencies (e.g., Greenpeace), and Canadian federal, provincial and territorial, and municipal governments. Environmental hazards have the greatest impact on air, water, and food, which, in turn, have an impact on health. The economic impact of environmental hazards is extremely costly because they result in lost productivity, pain and suffering due to illness, health treatment and rehabilitation costs, and cleanup and prevention costs, to name a few.

Provincial and territorial governments have primary jurisdiction over air, water, and land; the regulation of industrial emissions; toxic waste disposal; and the surveillance of environmental health hazards. Local governments are responsible for following provincial or territorial environmental protection acts and federal environmental protection acts; they may also enact bylaws to control environmental health hazards in their own communities. Public health departments are funded by the municipal and provincial or territorial governments; therefore, they follow and enforce the mandated environmental regulations. Environmental hazards may vary from community to community, as do the bylaws that control them, such as pesticide control bylaws. For this reason, it is important for CHNs to stay current on local environmental health issues by using evidence-informed data, which are often available at their local health unit or health authority. The key areas of environmental health issues (air, water, and food) are discussed in more detail here.

Air

Outdoor and indoor air pollution is a major consideration in environmental health. International panels on climate change with representatives from around the world have been established through the United Nations to set goals to manage the adverse effects of climate change and its influence on health.

Outdoor air quality is affected by both natural and human sources. Natural sources are contaminants usually resulting from forest fires and volcano eruptions. People in communities exposed to forest fire smoke may experience health effects; the level and duration of smoke exposure, age, and pre-existing health problems are factors that determine whether a person will be affected (National Collaborating Centre for Environmental Health, 2018). In 2016, wildfires in Fort McMurray, Alberta had a major impact on air quality, causing chemicals such as hydrogen sulphate, ozone, nitrogen dioxide, and carbon monoxide to be released into the air (Landis, Edgerton, White et al., 2017). These well-known environmental risk factors are associated with the development of cardiovascular and respiratory disease.

Human sources of outdoor pollution include transportation, energy generation, industrial energy use, manufacturing, and transboundary air movement (Environment Canada,

2017). Motor vehicles are a major source of air pollution and a key contributor to smog (Government of Canada, 2020d). However, the use of a catalytic converter (an emissions control device) in vehicles, unleaded gasoline, hybrid and electric cars, and public transit have contributed to emissions reductions. Polluted air produced and emitted by certain industries has decreased from projected estimates due to regulations and required changes. However, more changes will be required to meet emissions targets (Environment and Climate Change Canada, 2020b). Air quality and the reduction of emissions remain areas of profound concern that need further research, development, and cooperation. Health effects associated with air pollution include asthma and other respiratory diseases, cardiovascular diseases (including heart disease and hypertension), cancer, immunological effects, reproductive health problems (including birth defects), and neurological problems. **Indoor air quality** is a measure of the chemical, physical, or biological contaminants in indoor air; indoor air quality in the workplace, schools, and homes is a growing concern, especially in relation to children's health (see the "Ethical Considerations" box). Asthma is the most common chronic respiratory disease in children in Canada (The Lung Association, 2020).

ETHICAL CONSIDERATIONS

Indoor Air Quality

A group of CHNs in Corner Brook wanted to know more about the indoor air that children with respiratory diseases were exposed to at a supported housing project. They found that many of the units the children lived in were poorly maintained. They also found that the levels of environmental tobacco smoke were high.

Ethical principles that apply to the environmental health perspective are:

- *Autonomy.* This principle is fundamental to the equality and diversity dimension of health improvement efforts; it covers the protection and promotion of self-respect and self-esteem among individuals, groups, and communities, as part of both promoting a sense of well-being and protecting against unhealthful influences.*
- *Nonmaleficence.* Do no harm; the CHN needs to support environmental preservation and restoration and advocate for initiatives that reduce environmentally harmful practices to promote health and well-being.†

Question to Consider

Given the ethical considerations, what actions should be taken by the CHNs in order to provide "respiratory care" to these children?

Sources: * Tannahill, 2008;
†Canadian Nurses Association, 2017a, p. 19.

The major culprits contributing to poor indoor air are carbon monoxide, dust, moulds, dust mites, cockroaches, pests and pets, cleaning and personal care products (particularly aerosols), lead, and tobacco smoke. It is important for CHNs to assess both the environmental exposures and the human health status in a community. Because most Canadians spend a great deal of time indoors, the quality of indoor air can have a major effect on their health. One of the most harmful indoor air hazards is tobacco smoke. The multiple effects of second-hand smoke have been widely documented (Heffernan & O'Neill, 2013; Keough, 2009; Lajunen, Jaakkola, & Jaakkola, 2013). Recently, major progress has been made in the area of policy development to deal with the effects of second-hand smoke; smoking in public places, parking lots and enclosed spaces is banned across Canada. However, cars and homes remain places where smoking occurs, which is of particular concern, especially when children are present. CHNs are key players in addressing poor indoor air quality issues because they can provide assessments and education to individuals and families.

Drinking Water Quality

People's lives are tied to safe and adequate drinking water. Water is necessary for all life forms. It is also necessary for the production of food. The quality of the soil is affected by its water supply, the chemicals that are intentionally added by humans, and the deposition of pollutants from the air. Soil that is free from harmful contaminants and pathogens is essential for good health. Health Canada (2017) has established *Guidelines for Drinking Water Quality* that specifically address water contaminants that could lead to adverse health effect in humans, such as harmful microorganisms and chemicals. These guidelines identify parameters and provide guidance on how to address some of the contaminants in drinking water, such as *E.coli* and arsenic.

In most parts of Canada, fluoride has been added to municipal drinking water to prevent tooth decay. Some controversy exists about the negative effects of fluoride on health. It is important for CHNs to assess for other sources of fluoride intake. Questions to ask the individual or family would be as follows: Does your drinking water have fluoride (the health unit or health authority would know this answer if the patient does not)? and What other sources of fluoride are you exposed to (toothpaste, mouthwash, fluoride tablets, or drops)?

Discharges into water bodies from industries, industrial animal farms, and wastewater treatment systems can contribute to the degradation of water quality. Water quality is also affected by nonpoint sources of pollution, such as storm water runoff from paved roads and parking lots, erosion from clearcut tracts of land (after timbering and mining), and runoff from chemicals added to soils, such as fertilizers. The chain of potential harm continues with the additives to farm produce and to animal diets, such as antibiotics and growth hormones (which are then consumed by humans).

Food

The safety of food and food production is an ongoing area of concern. In recent years, foodborne illnesses have been associated with *Salmonella* and *E. coli* in chicken, eggs, and hamburger. Good food preparation practices—such as handwashing, washing vegetables and fruits, and cooking at an adequate temperature and for a sufficient amount of time—can prevent foodborne illnesses associated with most pathogens. Other food worries include the presence in food of pesticides and low-level antibiotics (given to beef cattle, pigs, and chickens); the irradiation of food; and the use of genetically modified and genetically engineered crops.

In 2019, a Canada-wide food recall of Rosemount-brand cooked, diced chicken meat was put into place as a result of an outbreak of *Listeria monocytogenes* infections involving three provinces: British Columbia, Manitoba, and Ontario. There were seven confirmed cases of listeria, and six people were hospitalized. The Canadian Food Inspection Agency (CFIA), PHAC, and provincial health partners investigated the outbreak and identified the diced chicken as the source of the outbreak (Government of Canada, 2019b).

Governments need to enhance efforts to deal with environmental threats to food safety. In Canada, the CFIA is the regulatory agency responsible for food, plant, and animal safety. It is "dedicated to safeguarding food, animals and plants, which enhances the health and well-being of Canada's people, environment and economy." The CFIA applies many key strategies to ensure that its goals are met (Canadian Food Inspection Agency, 2020).

ENVIRONMENTAL EPIDEMIOLOGY

As you may recall from Chapter 8, *epidemiology* is the science that helps us understand the strength of an association between exposures and health effects in human populations. For example, the Maternal–Infant Research on Environmental Chemicals (MIREC) national longitudinal study was conducted between 2008 and 2014 with approximately 2 000 pregnant women and their infants through to age 5 from across Canada (Health Canada, 2014). This epidemiological study explored associations between environmental chemical exposure during pregnancy and lactation and a range of child health outcomes.

Environmental epidemiology is the study of the effect on human health of physical, chemical, and biological factors in the external environment. By examining specific populations or communities exposed to different ambient environments, environmental epidemiology seeks to clarify the relationships between physical, chemical, and biological factors and human health. Environmental epidemiology explains risks such as the risk of respiratory illness resulting from exposure to forest fire particulate matter (Moore, Copes, Fisk, et al., 2006); the risk of various cancers in humans related to several pollutants (Boffetta, 2006); and the risk of respiratory disease due to exposure to outdoor air pollutants (Curtis, Rea, Smith-Willis, et al., 2006).

As discussed in Chapters 3 and 8, three major epidemiological factors are agent, host, and environment, which form the classic epidemiological triangle. An *agent* is an animate or inanimate factor (such as a biological or chemical agent) that must be present in an environment in order to produce disease in a susceptible host. A *host* is a living species (human or animal) capable of being infected or affected by an agent. The *environment* is all that is internal or external to a given host or agent and that is influenced by and has influence on the host and the agent (including social and physical factors).

The epidemiological triangle model belies the often-complex relationships among *agent,* which may include chemical mixtures (i.e., more than one agent); *host,* which may refer to a community spanning different ages, genders, ethnicities, cultures, and disease states; and *environment,* which may include dynamic factors such as air, water, soil, and food, as well as temperature, humidity, and wind. This epidemiological triangle, when applied to avian influenza (commonly known as "bird flu"), would depict the initial host as the bird (most common fowl such as ducks, geese, and chickens), the agent as the avian influenza virus H5N1, and the environment as the place of interaction (e.g., a geographical environment such as Fraser Valley, British Columbia). Avian flu may be passed to humans through contact with an infected bird or a contaminated surface. In bird-to-human transmission, the host is the person, the agent is the avian influenza virus H5N1, and the environment is the place of interaction (e.g., China, Indonesia, Thailand, Vietnam, or Egypt). Refer to Table 17.3 for other examples of the application of the epidemiological triangle.

CHNs have an understanding of environmental science; however, it is critical that they also continue to collaborate with environmental experts such as health inspectors, epidemiologists, and microbiologists to address the impact of environmental risk on specific populations.

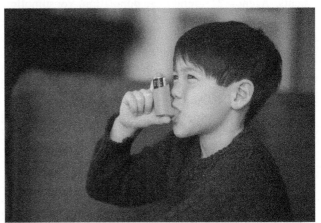
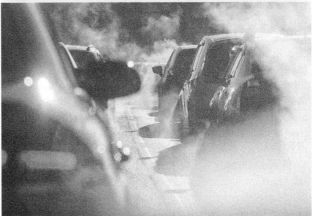

Environmental epidemiology is the study of the effect on human health of physical, chemical, and biological factors in the external environment. Air pollution caused by vehicle emissions and other sources contributes to many health concerns, including the increasing prevalence of respiratory problems such as asthma. (iStockphoto/ FatCamera & iStockphoto/ElCovaLana)

TABLE 17.3	Environmental Health Examples Using the Agent–Host–Environment Triad	
Agent	**Host**	**Environment**
Speeding automobile	Intoxicated drivers	Poor street lighting; unenforced speed limits
Poor-fitting shoes	Older person with impaired vision and decreased muscular agility	Inadequate lighting; stairs
High-powered snowmobiles	Young adult risk-taking males	Early spring unsafe ice conditions on lakes
High-caloric consumption; sedentary lifestyle	Children	Access to high-caloric foods; lack of nutritional information; peer pressure
Tobacco	Youth	Peer pressure; access to tobacco products; unclear health messaging

ENVIRONMENTAL HEALTH ASSESSMENT

In 1992, in Rio de Janeiro, the United Nations Conference on Environment and Development (the Earth Summit) was held, and out of this conference an action plan, called Agenda 21, was proposed and adopted. This plan was to guide future strategies for health and environmental activities and was adopted by over 150 member states of WHO. WHO agreed that "good" health could not be attained or maintained in hazardous or deteriorating environments. Agenda 21 found that population, consumption, and technology are the principal moving forces of environmental change and identified what needs to occur to reduce wasteful consumption patterns in some countries, while encouraging improved but sustainable development in others (United Nations Department of Economic and Social Affairs, 1992).

For sustainability to occur, social, economic, and political issues must all be addressed. An assessment of the impact that these issues have on health is done through an environmental health assessment (also called an *environmental impact assessment*), which is often associated with a health impact assessment. These assessments may be initiated by a local, provincial, or federal agency and implemented by industry, private assessment organizations, or others in order to meet requirements. Environmental health assessments and health impact assessments include factors such as population growth and impact on ecosystems, poverty, unsafe and inadequate amount of drinking water, inadequate shelter, and food insecurity, with risk assessment being a critical part of assessment. These assessments have moved beyond the usual assessment of hazards in air, water, food, and soil and include the impacts that human activity have on other determinants of health.

Health Canada as well as industry and nongovernmental organizations, researchers, CHNs, and interprofessional teams are all involved in environmental health assessments. Health Canada's role is to ensure identification of issues and evaluation of the environment to minimize safety risks to Canadians involved in proposed development projects such as roadways, mines, and energy (Health Canada, 2012). Environmental assessments fall within the mandate of the Canadian Environmental Assessment Agency and

BOX 17.4   Health Canada's Areas of Expertise for Environmental Assessments

Health Canada holds an advisory role with established standards and guidance for provincial and territorial governments in the following areas of the human health and environment connection:

- Human health risk assessment (HHRA)
- Air quality effects
- Contamination of country foods (fish, wild game, garden produce, berries, etc.)
- Drinking and recreational water quality
- Radiological effects
- Electric and magnetic fields effects
- Noise effects

Source: Health Canada. (2015). *Health Canada's participation in environmental assessments under CEAA 2012.* https://www.canada.ca/en/health-canada/corporate/publications/health-canada-participation-environmental-assessments.html

other agencies as directed by the *Canadian Environmental Assessment Act, 2012.* Health Canada makes information available on the areas listed in Box 17.4.

Surveillance is the systematic and ongoing observation and collection of data on disease occurrence to describe phenomena and detect changes in frequency or distribution. CHNs need to be aware of their environment and recognize the value of their observations in contributing to an increased awareness of any abnormal or unusual disease phenomena that may need to be studied further.

An **environmental scan** assesses both the internal and external environments and is often used by researchers to assess population health issues; by organizations to develop, evaluate, and revise programs; and by policymakers to address social, economic, technological, and political issues (Graham, Evitts, & Thomas-MacLean, 2008). It is also undertaken by CHNs to inform their practice. The term *environmental scan* is sometimes used instead of *community assessment.* An environmental scan assesses the internal requirements and assets of a community (micro level) along with assessing the environment external to the community (meso and macro levels). The information provided by an environmental scan is used to identify whether adequate internal resources are available to achieve goals or to identify priorities (see the "CHN in Practice: A Case Study, Understanding Patterns of Air Pollution and Dermatitis" box, which highlights the assessment of patterns of contact dermatitis in a community). The internal environmental scan includes reviewing community resources such as people, education, employment, housing, leisure, geography, and culture. The external environmental scan looks at what affects a community at the following levels: regional, provincial, territorial, national, and global. It should include a **PEEST** analysis: that is, an analysis of *p*olicies, *e*conomic climate, *e*nvironmental factors, *s*ocial (population and lifestyle trends) factors, and *t*echnological factors affecting a situation (PHAC, 2013). A PEEST analysis can be further organized into a **SWOT** format, which identifies *s*trengths, *w*eaknesses, *o*pportunities, and *t*hreats for a community.

CHN IN PRACTICE: A CASE STUDY

Understanding Patterns of Air Pollution and Dermatitis
Thomas is a CHN based at the Corner Brook Community Health Clinic. He conducts outreach to a mineral mining/production town nearby where he has observed a seasonal pattern of dermatitis in the community. It affects the following groups in particular: older persons, retirees, vacationers, and young children. Each summer, when community members are outdoors for longer periods of time, the majority of the population appear to develop the same noninfectious dermatitis that does not appear to affect people working indoors to the same extent. Thomas is concerned about air pollutants or some other potential environmental causes. He is wondering how to advise his patients, who he wants to encourage to participate in outdoor activities.

Think About It
1. a. How would Thomas work with an epidemiologist to conduct an environmental scan?
   b. What other community partners would be involved as team members in conducting an environmental scan?
   c. How could Thomas initiate this collaboration?
2. How and when might Thomas communicate the findings and advise community members?

The nature of environmental health requires an interprofessional approach to assess and decrease environmental health risks. For example, to assess and address a case of contaminated drinking water, the team might include a water treatment operator to assess the associated health risks in the community water treatment facility; clinical specialists to mandate the patients' health needs, and laboratory workers to assess contaminant levels in the patients' blood. This approach could potentially involve the local health department, the provincial department of environmental protection, a rehabilitation setting, and laboratories. The CHN would need to understand the roles of each respective agency and organization, know public health laws (particularly as they pertain to drinking water quality), and work with the community to coordinate services to address the community's needs. The CHN might also set up a community education session to explain the need for a boil water advisory and educate the community on the most current evidence about contamination of drinking water.

Community Health Nursing Assessment and Referral Practices

Assessment activities by CHNs can range from individual health assessments to full participation in community assessment or partnering in a specific environmental site assessment. Referral resources may vary in communities. A starting point may be the environmental epidemiology or toxicology unit of the local or provincial health department or environmental agency—data and interpretation of patterns of disease may already be available to plan interventions.

When environmental exposures are assessed, the environment can be divided into functional locations, such as home, school, workplace, and community. In each of these locations, there may be unique environmental exposures as well as overlapping exposures. For example, ethylene oxide, the toxic gas that is used to sterilize equipment in hospitals, would typically be found only in a workplace. However, pesticides might be found in all four areas. When assessing environments, the CHN determines whether an exposure is in the air, water, soil, or food (or a combination) and whether it is a physical, chemical, biological, ergonomic, or psychological exposure. Refer to Table 17.4 for examples of health hazards found in the home, school, workplace, and community.

HOW TO...

Apply the Community Health Nursing Process to Environmental Health
If, as a CHN, you suspect that a patient's health concern is being influenced by environmental factors, follow the community health nursing process and note the environmental aspects of the health concern in every step of the process as follows:
1. *Assessment.* Include inventories and history questions that cover environmental issues as a part of the general assessment.
2. *Planning.* Look at community policy and laws as methods to facilitate the care needs for the patient; include environmental health personnel in the planning. Establish measurable goals and objectives that can mitigate or eliminate the environmental factors.
3. *Implementation.* Coordinate medical, nursing, and public health actions to meet the patient's needs.
4. *Evaluation.* Document the immediate and long-term responses of the patient to the interventions, as well as the recidivism of the problem for the patient. Document the extent of the accomplishment of goals and objectives.

TABLE 17.4 Environmental Health Hazards

	Physical	Chemical	Biological (Biohazard)	Ergonomic	Psychological
Home	Noise Aerosol sprays Unsafe physical structures Electromagnetic radiation (computers, microwaves)	Bleach Lead paint Paint thinners and solvents Carbon monoxide	Mouse droppings Mould and fungi Dust mites Pet dander	Improper work methods Improper workstations Incorrect techniques Repetition Incorrect posture	Stress Threat of violence Fatigue
School	Noise Laser pointers Poor ventilation Variations in temperature	Asbestos Photocopier ink Perfumes Cleaning solutions	Bacteria Mould and fungi Viruses Dust mites	Repetition Improper play and workstations Incorrect posture	Interpersonal problems Bullying School violence
Workplace	Noise Vibrating equipment Variations in temperature Ionizing radiation (x-rays, etc.) Electromagnetic radiation (computers)	Industrial cleaners Perfumes Carbon monoxide	Viruses Biomedical waste products Latex products	Material handling Improper work methods Improper workstations Incorrect techniques Repetition Incorrect posture	Workplace stress Harassment Job dissatisfaction Shift work Social and physical isolation Inadequate equipment
Community	Noise Variations in temperature Poorly planned structural defects Poorly constructed roads Gas emissions	Pesticides Poorly stored chemicals Chemicals in public pools	Birds and animals Plants Ticks Mosquitoes	Poor community planning and design Poor transit design Lack of traffic control	Violence Unemployment Poverty Lack of housing

LEVELS OF PREVENTION

Related to Unhealthy Environments

Primary Prevention

A CHN works with a community group to prepare a draft proposal for a municipal bylaw change to ban all pesticide use in the community to prevent playgrounds from becoming contaminated with pesticides.

Secondary Prevention

A CHN works with community groups, such as the local hearing society, concerned parents, and school representatives, to organize mass screening programs at local high schools to detect hearing loss in grade 12 students as a result of continual exposure to high-decibel sound related to the use of earphones.

Tertiary Prevention

An occupational health nurse initiates a support group for injured workers.

Exposure to environmental hazards may occur in any settings where people spend time. As a result, CHNs must conduct a complete assessment. Two tools are commonly used to conduct the history-taking of environmental exposure and take the form of a mnemonic. A *mnemonic* is a device such as an acronym, a visual association, or a rhyme to classify or organize information in a systematic manner, and these two were developed to help health care providers remember the questions to ask when taking an environmental history. The first is CH^2OPD^2 (community, home, hobbies, occupation, personal habits, diet, drugs) (Marshall, Weir, Abelsohn, et al., 2002), and the second is I PREPARE (investigate potential exposures, present work, residence, environmental concerns, past work, activities, referrals and resources, educate). Both tools can be used when assessing an individual, family, or community. Box 17.5 explains the I PREPARE mnemonic.

A windshield survey is a helpful first step that CHNs can use to initiate understanding of the potential environmental health risks in a community. If the community is urban, the age and condition of the housing and potential garbage problems (and the associated pest problems) can be easily determined by driving around the neighbourhood. CHNs can also note proximity to factories, dump sites, major transportation routes, and other sources of pollution. In rural communities, attention should be given to the use of aerial spraying and signage regarding types of pesticide and herbicide applications.

See Appendix E-1, "Comprehensive Occupational and Environmental Health History," for a tool that explores environmental risks in the workplace.

BOX 17.5 The "I PREPARE" Mnemonic

An exposure history should identify current and past exposures, have a preliminary goal of reducing or eliminating current exposures, and have a long-term goal of reducing adverse health effects. The "I PREPARE" mnemonic consigns the important questions to categories that can be easily remembered.

I: Investigate Potential Exposures
Investigate potential exposures by asking:
- Have you ever felt sick after coming in contact with a chemical, pesticide, or other substance?
- Do you have any symptoms that improve when you are away from your home or work?

P: Present Work
Ask questions about the patient's present work:
- Are you exposed to solvents, dusts, fumes, radiation, loud noise, pesticides, or other chemicals?
- Do you know where to find material safety data sheets on the chemicals you work with?
- Do you wear personal protective equipment?
- Do you wear work clothes home?
- Do coworkers have similar health problems?

R: Residence
Inquire about the patient's place of residence:
- When was your residence built?
- What type of heating do you have?
- Have you recently remodelled your home?
- What chemicals are stored on your property?
- Where does your drinking water come from?

E: Environmental Concerns
Ask about the patient's living environment:
- Are there environmental concerns in your neighbourhood (i.e., air, water, soil)?
- What types of industries or farms are near your home?
- Do you live near a hazardous waste site or landfill?

P: Past Work
Inquire about the patient's past work:
- What are your past work experiences?
- What is the longest job you held?

- Have you ever been in the military, worked on a farm, or done volunteer or seasonal work?

A: Activities
Ask about your patient's activities:
- What activities and hobbies do you and your family engage in?
- Do you burn, solder, or melt any products?
- Do you garden, fish, or hunt?
- Do you eat what you catch or grow?
- Do you use pesticides?
- Do you engage in any alternative healing or cultural practices?

R: Referrals and Resources
Use these key Canadian referrals and resources:
- Environment and Climate Change Canada (http://www.ec.gc.ca)
- Greenpeace Canada (http://www.greenpeace.org/canada/en/home/)
- National Pollutant Release Inventory (http://www.ec.gc.ca/inrp-npri/)
- Library and Archives Canada (http://www.collectionscanada.ca)
- PHAC (http://www.phac-aspc.gc.ca)
- Disease Surveillance Online (http://www.phac-aspc.gc.ca/dsol-smed/index.php)
- Canadian Centre for Occupational Health and Safety (http://www.ccohs.ca)
- Health Canada (http://www.hc-sc.gc.ca)
- Environmental and Workplace Health (http://www.hc-sc.gc.ca/ewh-semt/index_e.html)
- Local health department, environmental agency, and poison control centres

E: Educate
Use this checklist of educational materials:
- Are materials available to educate the patient?
- Are alternatives available to minimize the risk of exposure?
- Have prevention strategies been discussed?
- What is the plan for follow-up?

Sources: Prepared by Grace Paranzino, RN, MPH, for the Agency for Toxic Substances and Disease Registry (http://www.atsdr.cdc.gov); with additional resources by Heather Jessup-Falcioni and Gloria Viverais-Dresler.

Risk Assessment

One aspect of environmental assessment is risk assessment. **Risk assessment** refers to a qualitative and quantitative evaluation of the risk posed to human health or the environment by the actual or potential presence or use of specific pollutants. In a risk assessment, information on health effects from exposure to various materials in the environment is collected by specific agencies (such as the CFIA) to determine health risks to Canadians. Based on this information, leading authorities, such as Health Canada, the Government of Canada, and Environment and Climate Change Canada, set policies and regulations to protect the public.

Some of Health Canada's activities include developing and providing tools to be used in risk assessments for chemical, radiological, and biological contamination; providing training to governmental departments on risk assessment; developing Canadian soil quality guidelines; and disseminating toxicological reference values used in human health risk assessments (Health Canada, 2019).

The Government of Canada is involved in several aspects of risk assessment and management. Its involvement in risk assessment and management related to chemical substances includes determining how substances get into the environment, registering who is using these chemicals and in what capacity, and implementing relevant tools to address actual and potential risks to humans due to chemicals (Government of Canada, 2016).

Risk assessment in environmental health has focused on characterizing the hazard (i.e., the source), its physical and chemical properties, its toxicity, and the presence of (or potential for) other elements in the exposure pathway—mode of transmission, route of exposure, receptor population, and dose. CHNs should exercise care and caution prior to implementing change that may have ecological harm (there may be insufficient scientific evidence indicating harm). Potential threats should be identified by the CHN and caution exercised before proceeding with the intended action. New products should be proven safe through rigorous research protocols before being introduced onto the market. Some products may not be identified as being unsafe to the environment but may produce symptoms in humans. For example, populations living close to industrial wind turbines have experienced Wind Turbine Syndrome. Some of the symptoms identified are headache, tinnitus, dizziness, nausea, irritability, sleep disturbance, and problems with memory (Pierpont, 2010).

Governmental standards and policy currently incorporate the **precautionary principle,** which suggests that when doubt in the evidence exists, the appropriate action is to err on the side of caution (Chaudry, 2008). For example, in 2009 Health Canada added Bisphenol A (BPA) to the toxic substances list (Mittelstaedt, 2010; Young-Reuters, 2010). BPA is now considered a toxin like asbestos and lead and precautionary policy has been put in place. In Canada, BPA can be found in polycarbonate containers, the lining of some metal-based food and beverage cans, toys, drinking water, and indoor air (Environment Canada, 2020b; Young-Reuters, 2010).

Table 17.5 outlines some of the factors that can affect the perception of risk.

Risk Communication

Risk communication involves consideration of the outrage factors relevant to the risk. These factors and the action to be taken to alleviate them can be incorporated into the message. Action is taken to ensure that safety is increased and unnecessary fear is reduced. **Risk communication** is the exchange of information on the potential harm of health or environmental hazards among risk assessors and managers, the general public, news media, and interest groups. It includes all the principles of good communication in general and the exchange of information about health or environmental risks. It is a combination of:

- *The right information.* Accurate and relevant information in a language that audiences can understand for shaping the message.
- *To the right people.* Communication is directed at those affected and those who may not be affected but are worried. Information about the community is essential: the geographical boundaries, who lives there (demographics), how they get information (flyers or newspapers, radio, television, word of mouth), where they get together (school, church, community centre), and who within the community can help plan the communication.
- *At the right time.* Communication must allow for timely action to allay fear.

As risk communicators, CHNs inform or counsel in areas such as safe drinking water, handwashing techniques, food preparation, risks of pregnancy, communicable diseases (especially sexually transmitted infections), unintentional injury, and personal health-related choices (e.g., smoking, alcohol consumption, diet).

TABLE 17.5	Important Attributes Affecting the Perception of Risk
Involuntary	A risk that is involuntarily imposed (e.g., building an industrial plant without community input) will be judged less acceptable than a risk that is voluntarily assumed (e.g., smoking).
Uncontrollable	The inability to control a risk decreases the judgement of its acceptability.
Industrial versus natural	An industrial risk (e.g., nuclear power) is judged less acceptable than a natural risk (e.g., lightning strike).
Unfamiliar	An exotic or unfamiliar risk (e.g., biotechnology) is judged less acceptable than a familiar risk (e.g., household cleanser).
Memorable	A risk that is embedded in a remarkable event (e.g., airplane crash) is judged to be less acceptable than one that is not.
Dreaded	A risk that is highly feared (e.g., cancer) is judged less acceptable than one that is not (e.g., household accident).
Catastrophic	A catastrophic risk (e.g., airplane crash) is judged less acceptable than diffuse or cumulative risks (e.g., vehicle collision).
Unfair	If a risk is thought to be inequitably or unfairly placed upon a group, it is judged as less acceptable. This is particularly true if that group happens to be children.
Untrustworthy	If the source of the risk is untrustworthy, the risk is judged less acceptable.
Uncertain	A risk that has high uncertainty and that we know little about is judged less acceptable than one that is not.
Immoral	A risk that is deemed to be unethical or immoral is judged less acceptable than one that is not.

Source: Hill, S. (2005). *Appendix A: Some factors affecting the perception of risk. Risk communication literature review: Summary report.* Treasury Board of Canada Secretariat. http://www.tbs-sct.gc.ca. Reproduced with permission.

Environmental hazards often produce fear because they create risk situations and heighten risk perception, which can lead to public feelings of outrage. **Outrage** is the emotional public response to the perception of risk related to an environmental issue; trust in authorities is weak. Outrage is a concept that has been familiar in the United States since the 1970s. Within the past three decades in Canada, interest in public outrage has become more evident. It has escalated particularly because of unforgettable environmental events such as contaminated water in Walkerton, Ontario, and North Battleford, Saskatchewan, and the outbreak of severe acute respiratory syndrome (SARS) in Toronto. Unforgettable environmental events create public awareness and increase the need for information and action on the particular risk associated with the event. The media, in the aforementioned cases, were instrumental in magnifying the risks due to their reactionary reporting of such events, often raising questions of culpability, responsibility, and accountability. As a result, fear was heightened, and outrage resulted from this chain of events. Risk communication harnesses the outrage and fear for health promotion purposes and prevents anxiety and states of crises regarding community health and safety.

REDUCING ENVIRONMENTAL HEALTH RISKS

Preventing problems is less costly than "fixing" them, whether the cost is measured in resources consumed or health effects. Education is a primary preventive strategy. When a CHN is examining the sources of environmental health risks in communities and planning intervention strategies, it is important to apply the basic principles of disease prevention. For a home with lead-based paint, the primary prevention strategy would be to remove that specific source of lead. Good surveillance, a secondary prevention strategy, would not prevent lead exposure, but it might help with early identification of rising levels of lead in blood. For a symptomatic child brought to a health care provider, a system should be in place for specialists familiar with lead poisoning to provide immediate care; swift medical interventions to reduce blood levels of lead can reduce the risk of further harm. This might be a tertiary prevention response.

Risk Management

For workplaces, community health care providers work with a list of precautions for avoiding or minimizing employees' exposure to potentially hazardous chemicals. Once it is established that a human health threat exists, a plan of action needs to be developed to eliminate or manage (reduce) the risk. Risk management should be informed by the risk assessment process. **Risk management** involves the selection and implementation of a strategy to reduce risks. It can take many forms—for example, the "four Rs for reducing environmental pollution," which are as follows, in order of effectiveness:

1. *Reduce.* Reducing consumption lessens waste and unnecessary packaging and nonessentials.
2. *Reuse.* Choosing reusable rather than disposable products creates less waste (e.g., using glass dishes rather than paper

ones or choosing used products such as those found at second-hand stores and yard sales).
3. *Recycle.* The simple activity of recycling paper, glass, and cans to be used to produce new items is one good way to decrease pollution.
4. *Recover.* Recover involves retrieving energy from waste materials such as through the incineration of waste to produce new energy.

In Canada, legislation covers hazardous materials used in the workplace. The Workplace Hazardous Materials Information System (WHMIS) came into effect in 1988 through federal, provincial, and territorial legislations (Canadian Centre for Occupational Health and Safety, 2020). The key elements of the WHMIS are hazard classification, cautionary product labels, the provision of material safety data sheets, and worker education programs on the safe use of hazardous materials used in Canadian workplaces. An example of bringing environmental care to the clinic level can be found in the "CHN in Practice: A Case Study, Bringing Environmental Care to the Clinic" box.

CHN IN PRACTICE: A CASE STUDY

Bringing Environmental Care to the Clinic

Joyce is a primary care nurse practitioner based at the Corner Brook Community Health Clinic in Corner Brook. Occasionally, her clinic also offers a mobile outreach clinic for routine sexually transmitted infections testing, cervical cancer screening, and other routine examinations for high priority patients. Whether in the health clinic or the mobile clinic, Joyce is deeply troubled by the volume of waste produced in her practice. For example, she considers the plastic and disposable speculums and other disposables that will contribute to the environmental problems that impact health. Aware of estimations that residential recycling of plastic, glass, metal, and paper products as well as the composting of organic matter could significantly reduce waste volumes, Joyce wonders about the potential of workplace recycling—as both a practical issue and an issue of role modelling. She raises the topic of recycling at the next clinic council meeting.

Think About It

1. How could a recycling program be implemented at Joyce's clinic?
2. Consider your own residential and workplace recycling:
   a. What are you doing to reduce, reuse, and recycle?
   b. What is your workplace doing to reduce, reuse, and recycle?
   c. What is your community doing to reduce, reuse, and recycle?
3. What more could you be doing?

While reducing waste and material consumption in health care environments is of concern to many groups (Canadian Coalition for Green Health Care, 2020), there are a variety of other forms of risk reduction. One is to reduce the risk from exposure to ultraviolet rays. People should avoid being outside during peak sun hours and need to wear protective clothing or use sunblock. To reduce exposure to dangerous heavy metals, special processes can be employed at water filtration plants that supply the public water. Individuals, communities, and nations can reduce risks; in recent years, there have been global agreements to reduce persistent pollutants and decrease global warming (e.g., agreements by the United Nations Framework Convention on Climate Change).

In 2004, the Government of Newfoundland and Labrador took an ecological approach to the management of drinking water in its province and developed guidelines and strategies to manage risk and ensure the safety of drinking water based on an assessment study of community health needs and resources conducted between 1997 and 2004 (Pike-MacDonald, Best, Twomey, et al., 2007). The study explored the "health beliefs and practices, satisfaction with health and related community services, and community health concerns" for residents residing in various communities in Newfoundland and Labrador (Pike-MacDonald et al., 2007, p. 15). One of the most serious concerns expressed by these study participants was the quality of drinking water. CHNs need to ensure that drinking water is safe (e.g., monitor reports on water quality in their community), partner with communities to inform the public (e.g., work with mass media campaigns to include risks associated with drinking contaminated water), build healthy public policy (e.g., advocate or lobby decision makers), and strengthen community actions (e.g., visually and verbally explain in detail the technique for effectively boiling water). (The authors of the Newfoundland and Labrador study elaborate further on the role of the CHN in environmental health; refer to their article for a greater discussion.)

THE ENVIRONMENT AND CHILDREN'S HEALTH

Children are particularly vulnerable to adverse health effects because of their underdeveloped brains and other organs, undeveloped detoxification systems and more rapid breathing rate, and behaviours such as hand-to-mouth activity. Other factors that put children at risk are their genetic makeup and where they live. The Canadian Partnership for Children's Health & Environment (CPCHE) reports that the overall health of children in Canada is improving; however, some disorders, due in part to environmental exposures, are on the rise. These conditions include asthma, learning and behaviour disorders, some cancers, and obesity (CPCHE, 2008). Children today are also at risk for environmental hazards because of factors such as poverty, lack of access to health care, and the dangerous environmental situations in the communities where they live. Environmental toxins, such as lead, pesticides, mercury, air pollution, solvents, asbestos, and radon, get into homes, schools, childcare centres, and playgrounds (CPCHE, 2008; Fournier & Karachiwalla, 2021).

Children are not just little adults with regard to their responses to environmental exposures. Infants and young children breathe more rapidly than adults and thus have a proportionally greater exposure to air pollutants. While infants' lungs are developing, they are particularly susceptible to environmental toxicants. Because children are short, their breathing zones are lower than those of adults, so they have closer contact with the chemical and biological agents that accumulate on floors and carpeting. Children's bodies also operate differently. Some protective mechanisms that are well developed in adults, such as the blood–brain barrier, are immature in young children, making them more vulnerable to the effects of toxic chemicals. And, finally, the kidneys of young children are less effective at filtering out undesirable, toxic chemicals, which then continue to circulate and accumulate. See the "Evidence-Informed Practice" box for a study on indoor air quality–related health risk factors for children under age 2 in Nunavut.

Toxic chemicals can have different effects, depending on the timing of exposure. During fetal development, there are periods of great sensitivity to the effects of toxic chemicals. During such times, even very small exposures can prevent or change a process that may permanently affect normal development. The brain undergoes rapid structural and functional changes during late pregnancy and in the neonatal period. Therefore, it is extremely important to safeguard women's environments when they are pregnant.

EVIDENCE-INFORMED PRACTICE

Kovesi, Creery, Gilbert, et al. (2006) conducted a pilot study to examine indoor air quality–related risk factors for respiratory infections in Inuit children under the age of 2 years living in Nunavut. The main foci were to assess the indoor air quality in their homes and the children's respiratory health status and to explore risk factors for lower respiratory tract infection (LRTI). This population group is more susceptible to permanent lung injury following a severe LRTI. Young Inuit children are prone to severe LRTIs. Twenty homes in Nunavut were included in this study. A respiratory health questionnaire was used, a structured housing inspection was conducted, and various measures of indoor air quality were taken.

Study findings were: (1) homes were small and single-storey, lacked basements, and were above ground level; (2) several people resided in each home, with young children often sharing a bed for sleeping; (3) many household residents were smokers; (4) air exchange rates were reduced; (5) fungi levels in mattresses were elevated; (6) dust mite levels were minimal; and (7) 25% of the study sample had been hospitalized for chest illnesses. The finding of second-hand smoke in the home and increased LRTIs in young children is well supported in the literature. Also, LRTIs in young children due to exposure to fungi and dampness are also supported in the literature. Many public health suggestions were proposed based on the study findings. It was suggested that additional homes be built with better ventilation systems and the opportunity for less sharing of homes and beds by young Inuit children, that there be more frequent turning of mattresses to reduce the fungi, and that public education be provided to address the issue of second-hand smoke in the home.

📄 EVIDENCE-INFORMED PRACTICE—cont'd

Application for CHNs

The CHN would need to work with this population to develop strategies that are culturally and geographically appropriate to address the findings. CHN interventions that could be offered, in consultation with local community partners, could include providing individual and group educational sessions in the community to reduce the smoking patterns in the home; working with families and community partners to facilitate the acquisition of cribs; working with community partners to address the building standards of the current homes in the community; and working with other community partners, when necessary, to facilitate the acquisition of new housing.

Questions for Reflection and Discussion

1. Which determinants of health are evident in this Nunavut community?
2. What CHN interventions can be implemented to address the identified determinants of health? Elaborate.
3. What type of qualitative research question might you develop to discover what Inuit family members' perceptions are about the air quality in their homes and the respiratory infections of their children?

Source: Kovesi, T., Creery, D., Gilbert, N. L., et al. (2006). Indoor air quality risk factors for severe lower respiratory tract infections in Inuit infants in Baffin Region, Nunavut: A pilot study. *Indoor Air, 16*(4), 266–275.

The PHAC, through its Division of Childhood and Adolescence provides resources for health care providers to help decrease the incidence of death and hospitalizations in Canadian children and youth (PHAC, 2016a). Issues such as the influence of built environments, safe transportation, water and air quality, and toxic substances are addressed by this division.

In 2002, the environment ministers of Canada, Mexico, and the United States agreed to protect children from environmental risks. They set a "cooperative agenda" between the three countries to select and publish a foundational set of indicators for North America of children's health and the environment (Commission for Environmental Cooperation, 2006). The first report, *Children's Health and the Environment in Canada* was released in 2006 as a result of this cooperative agenda; it presents information on available environmental health indicators and measures for Canada. This report contains case studies on subpopulations of children who may be unreasonably affected by environmental contaminants. It also provides extensive information on the environmental health indicators related to GHG emissions, air pollution, the conservation and protection of wildlife and protected natural areas, wastewater management, and legislative and political developments to address environmental health concerns (Commission for Environmental Cooperation, 2019).

A nutritionally balanced diet is important, and fish is a good source of protein; however, the effects of mercury are of extreme concern for Canadians because fish is the main source of mercury. Therefore, Health Canada recommends Canadians consume limited weekly amounts of certain fish, such as shark, tuna, and swordfish. The recommendations for pregnant women, women of child-bearing age, and young children are more stringent (Ontario Ministry of the Environment, Conservation and Parks, 2019). Waterfowl and other wildlife also eat contaminated fish and may be additional sources of mercury to people. Exposure to mercury most often affects the nervous system, the cardiovascular system, the immune system, and the kidneys, with fetal mercury exposure possibly leading to neurodevelopmental problems in children (Health Canada, 2007). Mercury is a metal that occurs naturally, with low levels found in air, water, rocks,

soil, and plant and animal matter, and was used widely in industry with reductions of its use being initiated in the late 1960s (Ontario Ministry of the Environment, Conservation and Parks, 2019). Industrial use of mercury was a source that created residual water contamination; in addition, some quantities of human-made and natural mercury sources currently are entering the aquatic environment from the atmosphere (Ontario Ministry of the Environment, Conservation and Parks, 2019).

Of the many tens of thousands of synthetic chemicals that are in air, water, food, workplaces, and consumer products, only a small percentage undergo toxicity testing. Companies are not required to divulge all the results of their private testing. A full battery of neurotoxicity tests is not even required for chemicals that may be sprayed in nurseries and labour and delivery areas of hospitals, not to mention in our homes. Complicating matters even further, risks from multiple chemical exposures are rarely considered when regulations are drafted. Moreover, evidence indicates that certain groups of chemicals can interact and produce synergistic effects (Silins & Högberg, 2011). Such an omission ignores the reality that children (as well as adults) are exposed to many toxic chemicals, often concurrently.

By contrast, the pesticides used on food supplies are highly regulated in Canada. The Health Canada Pest Management Regulatory Agency is responsible for the regulation of pesticides in Canada. The agency's responsibilities include registering pesticides after they have been stringently tested, re-evaluating pesticides every 15 years to ensure they meet safety standards, and promoting sustainable pest management (Health Canada, 2020a). Several Canadian municipalities have set regulations limiting or banning pesticide use. Health Canada and the CFIA are responsible for guaranteeing the safety of Canada's food supply. CFIA, as previously mentioned, monitors the amount of contaminants in our food supply. The National Chemical Residue Monitoring Program is a surveillance program of the CFIA that monitors the chemicals in our food supply (Health Canada, 2020b). Health Canada is responsible for setting and modifying food standards.

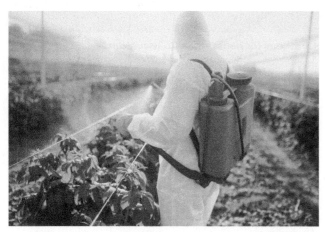

Pest control products are registered; however, the synergistic effects of combined toxic exposure are not well understood. (iStockphoto/ mladenbalinovac)

In 2018 in Canada, unintentional and intentional injuries, including poisonings, resulted in 17 691 deaths and in 2015, unintentional injuries were the leading cause of death among those aged 1 to 34 years (Government of Canada 2020c). Reducing occurrences of injuries would entail redesigning the **built environment**—anything physical in the environment that is built or produced by humans (Lopez, 2012), such as playgrounds—and increasing prevention by teaching about safety in the home and community. Community and neighbourhood infrastructure are considered aspects of built environments, and are important public health interests impacting communicable and noncommunicable diseases, interpersonal and community violence, as well as injury (Cruickshank, 2014; DeGuzman & Kulbok, 2012). Design issues of walkability and access to recreation and greenspace are important health considerations. The built environment also impacts exposure to toxins such as those related to building materials (Muhajarine, 2012).

Built environments can have an impact on all generations and are of particular concern when creating "age-friendly" cities (PHAC, 2016b). Age-friendly cities and communities recognize, anticipate, and respond to age-related needs and preferences (WHO, 2018), such as the need for safe sidewalks, playgrounds, and adequate snow clearing. Age-friendly cities can help to promote built environments that support the needs of all ages and can reduce the impact of environmental risk factors on health.

COMMUNITY HEALTH NURSES' ROLES IN ENVIRONMENTAL HEALTH

CHNs can be and are involved in environmental health in their practice, as an adjunct to existing roles, and as informed citizens. The activities of CHNs in relation to environmental health could include the following:

- *Community involvement and public participation.* Organizing, facilitating, and moderating and making public notices effective, public forums accessible and welcoming of input, information exchange understandable, and problem solving acceptable to culturally diverse communities are valuable

assets CHNs contribute. Skills in community organizing and mobilizing can be essential to a community having a meaningful voice in decisions that affect it.
- *Individual and population risk assessment.* Community health nursing assessment skills are used to detect potential and actual exposure pathways and outcomes for patients cared for in acute, chronic, and healthy communities of practice.
- *Risk communication.* Interpreting and applying principles to practice, CHNs may serve as skilled risk communicators within agencies, working for industries or working as independent practitioners. As risk communicators, CHNs fulfill the roles of educators for patients about environmental risks and possible preventive activities pertaining to the risks. In this role, CHNs must be knowledgeable of community resources and make appropriate referrals.
- *Epidemiological investigations.* CHNs have the skills to respond in scientifically sound and sensitive ways to community concerns about cancer, birth defects, and stillbirths that citizens fear may have environmental causes.
- *Policy development.* CHNs propose, inform, and monitor action from agencies, communities, and organization perspectives.

As CHNs learn more about the environment, opportunities for integration of environmental considerations into their practice, educational programs, research, advocacy, and policy work will become evident. Opportunities abound for those pioneering spirits within the nursing profession dedicated to working upstream and creating healthier environments for their patients and communities. The Canadian Nurses Association released a position statement in 2017 on climate change which stated that nurses have a role in supporting adaptation and mitigation with respect to climate change through nursing practice, research, administration, education, and policy (CNA, 2017b).

Through continued nursing leadership as well as established and new interprofessional partnerships, CHNs can have a positive impact on environmental issues and risks that affect health. Moreover, CHNs screen and educate populations, manage outbreaks, and use surveillance techniques for early detection, harm reduction, and health promotion (Pike-MacDonald et al., 2007).

CHNs need to be environmentally responsible in their practice and encourage and facilitate environmental responsibility in their workplace and community. An international coalition of health care providers, Health Care Without Harm (https://noharm.org/), has a platform of environmentally responsible health care with a focus on environmental issues and their health impact.

Environmental Ethics and Environmental Justice

As discussed in Chapter 6, an understanding of ethics is essential to CHNs, especially when they must justify choices, describe issues and options to patients, and advocate for patients. **Environmental ethics** is a distinct field of ethics that examines the moral relationship of human beings to the environment (Dinkins & Sorrell, 2007). When competing priorities (e.g., jobs versus environmental protection; production versus conservation) are of concern, the skillful CHN can change the discussion from "either/or" to "both" by opening new possibilities for ethical and mutually satisfactory outcomes. Some ethical issues likely to arise in environmental health decisions are:

- Who has access to information and when?
- How complete and accurate is the available information?
- Who is included in decision making and when?
- What and whose values and priorities are given weight in decisions?
- How are short- and long-term consequences considered?
- Is there a conflict of interest?

Recently, consideration of environmental health concerns has included a discussion about environmental justice. **Environmental justice,** from a population health perspective, is the effort to reduce the impact of health inequities and socioeconomic marginalization of persons resulting from environmental conditions that affect adequate nutrition, shelter, sanitation, and safe working conditions (Waldrom, 2020). Environmental justice originated as a social movement in the United States in the 1960s. The concept has gained hold more recently in Canada, in venues such as academia and advocacy movements, especially in relation to the effect of environmental issues on structurally vulnerable people (Waldron, 2020). CHNs can research and share relevant findings that can influence decision making about environmental health; for example, in relation to urban design and issues of the built environment, particularly for racialized and structurally vulnerable groups (Waldron, 2020).

Colonialism, urbanization, and the natural resource economy have most greatly affected and disadvantaged the following populations: resource-dependent communities, which are usually small towns and regions; First Nations communities, which are often affected by close proximity to toxic industries or excluded from the benefits of development; low-income and ethnoracial communities in urban centres, which are often located in deteriorated parts of a city, excluded from easy access to food and green space, and are not part of urban planning and decision making; and biologically vulnerable populations such as older persons and children who are not adequately represented in community health policies and standards (CPHA, 2008).

Bed bugs are one example of an environmental health concern that can affect anyone but disproportionately affects people who are socially and economically disadvantaged. Adverse reactions include skin allergies, secondary infections, and scarring as well as psychological impacts from intense scratching provoked by the insect bites, as well as potential concerns with improper insecticide use that may have lethal effects. This sort of complex environmental health and social justice issue requires a more complex suite of collaborative community health strategies (National Collaborating Centre for Environmental Health, 2015).

Environmental Advocacy

Canadian nurses can be a strong voice for environmental change. As informed citizens, CHNs can take a variety of actions to protect the environmental health of patients. Although every CHN cannot be an expert in environmental health, every CHN does have a basic education in human health and can identify those who may be most vulnerable to environmental problems. Moreover, CHNs' thoughts about the potential effects of new

laws on the health of patients are valuable to legislators. As advocates for environmental issues, CHNs can:

- Write letters to local newspapers responding to environmental health issues affecting the community.
- Serve as credible sources of information at community gatherings, formal governmental hearings, and professional nursing forums.
- Actively participate as committee members on community committees that focus on environmental health issues.
- Volunteer to serve on municipal, provincial, territorial, or federal environmental health commissions.
- Use resources such as those from the CNA's "Nursing and Environmental Health" webpage (see the link on the Evolve website).
- Know and support the zoning and permit laws that regulate the effects of industry and land use on the community, as well as environmental laws that apply to the community.
- Read, listen, and ask questions in order to foster community action to address environmental health threats.

The Community Health Nurse and Environmental Health Policy

The CHN, when working with the community as partner, can facilitate and support environmental health policy development. Policy development usually involves specific goal setting, strategy, and partnering and collaborating with organizations. Conferring with stakeholders (e.g., the community), building capacity for research and communication with the patient, working with designated officials, assessing the environment, gathering and analyzing data, and writing reports are all key tasks in contributing to policy development. Consideration needs to be given to the social, political, and economic costs of a proposed policy. Furthermore, it is important to be aware that some individuals and groups (e.g., certain organizations, agencies, and corporations) may resist the policy and try to prevent it from coming into force or delay it while a "cover up" of the environmental problem occurs. For example, policies to create smoke-free workplaces and public places were resisted by citizens and tobacco companies, who countered health experts' evidence on the negative effects of smoking and second-hand smoke with their own "scientific experts." Legislation for smoke-free public and workplace policy was delayed for many years; however, through the collaborative efforts of concerned citizens in their communities and health care providers, these policies were developed and resulted in laws and bylaws across the country.

As a professional body, the CNA has advocated to promote environmental health and promote healthy public policy. CNA contributions have included passing resolutions on some of the effects of environmental health hazards; creating policy and position statements on the responsibilities of health care providers regarding environmental health activities; and being a member of environmental committees such as the Environmental Health Coalition, the Canadian Coalition for Green Health Care, and the Expert Advisory Board on Children's Health for the Commission for Environmental Cooperation (CNA, 2005). The CNA identifies nurses' involvement at the three levels of prevention in relation to environmental health as outlined in the "Levels of Prevention" box.

LEVELS OF PREVENTION

Related to Environmental Health

Primary Prevention

CHNs:

- Counsel women of child-bearing age about reducing their exposure to environmental hazards
- Support the development of exposure standards for toxins and other contaminants
- Advocate for safe air, water, and soil
- Teach avoidance of ultraviolet exposure and use of sunscreen
- Support programs for waste reduction and recycling, as well as energy conservation in communities and workplaces

Secondary Prevention

CHNs:

- Assess homes, schools, worksites, and communities for environmental hazards
- Review water and soil test results
- Monitor air quality reports

Tertiary Prevention

CHNs:

- Support the cleanup of toxic waste sites and removal of other hazards
- Refer homeowners to approved programs that eliminate contaminants such as lead and asbestos

Source: Adapted from Canadian Nurses Association. (2005). *CNA backgrounder—The ecosystem, the natural environment, and health and nursing: A summary of the issues.* http://cna-aiic.ca/~/media/cna/page-content/pdf-en/bg4_the_ecosystem_e.pdf.

Nurses are taking action on environmental health issues. Through CNA, they have formed a group called Canadian Association of Nurses for the Environment (CANE) (CNA, 2019). CHNs care about the population's health, and ways to convey this are through involvement in environmental health issues, especially policy issues, and by assuming roles in prevention and reduction of environmentally related health concerns.

STUDENT EXPERIENCE

1. What are your beliefs about climate change and the associated environmental issues?
2. What have your contributions been to reduce the ecological and environmental footprint?
3. Refer to the "Reduce Your Carbon Footprint" web page on the David Suzuki Foundation website (http://www.davidsuzuki.org/what-you-can-do/reduce-your-carbon-footprint/). Click on the links for "How We Get Around," "What We Eat," "How We Use Energy in Our Homes," and "The Stuff We Buy." How do you plan to reduce your environmental footprint?
4. Calculate your environmental footprint at the World Wildlife Federation's "Footprint Calculator" (http://footprint.wwf.org.uk/). What were the results? What additional steps were indicated at the website to help reduce your environmental footprint?

CHAPTER SUMMARY

17.1 Environmental health practice comprises health promotion, disease prevention, and health protection. The four environmental principles are (1) everything is connected, (2) everything has to go somewhere, (3) impact is proportional to dose, and (4) today's solution may become tomorrow's problem.

17.2 The environment is a determinant of health because it affects health and disease. In the air we breathe, the water we drink, the food we eat, and the products we use, we are exposed to chemical, biological, and radiological elements that affect our health.

17.3 Federal, provincial, territorial, and municipal laws and regulations exist to protect the health of citizens from environmental hazards. CHNs can work with the community as partner to facilitate and support environmental health policy development.

17.4 Environmental epidemiology is the study of the effect on human health of physical, chemical, and biological factors in the external environment. By examining specific populations or communities exposed to different ambient environments, environmental epidemiology seeks to clarify the relationships between physical, chemical, and biological factors cand human health.

17.5 Assessment of environmental risks is a key part of the nursing process. Risk assessment is a qualitative and quantitative evaluation of the risk posed to human health or the environment by the actual or potential presence or use of specific pollutants. Risk communication is an important skill and must acknowledge the outrage factor experienced by communities with environmental hazards.

17.6 When a CHN is examining the sources of environmental health risks in communities and planning intervention strategies, it is important to apply the basic principles of disease prevention. One form of risk management is the four Rs—that is, reduce, reuse, recycle, recover.

17.7 Children are particularly vulnerable to adverse health effects because of their underdeveloped brains and other organs, undeveloped detoxification systems and more rapid breathing rate, and behaviours such as hand-to-mouth activity. CHN interventions applied specifically to children's environmental health include addressing prenatal toxic exposure, issues related to the built environment that impact injuries and obesity, as well as air pollutants and other causes of asthma.

17.8 Environmental ethics is a distinct field of ethics that examines the moral relationship of human beings to the environment. Environmental justice is the effort to reduce the impact of health inequities and socioeconomic marginalization of persons resulting from environmental conditions that affect adequate nutrition, shelter, sanitation, and safe working conditions. Advocacy skills are important for CHNs in environmental health practice. CHNs must be informed about the environmental health issues affecting their community.

CHN IN PRACTICE: A CASE STUDY

Managing Soil and Water Contamination in the Community

A citizen in Corner Brook calls the local health department to report that his drinking water, which is from a private well, "smells like gasoline." A water sample is collected, and analysis reveals the presence of petroleum products. A nearby rural store with a service station has removed its old underground gasoline storage tanks and replaced them, as required by law. Contaminated soil from the old leaking tank has been removed, and a well to monitor groundwater contamination is scheduled for installation. However, sandy soil has allowed rapid movement of the contamination through the groundwater, and the plume has reached the neighbour's drinking-water well in levels that exceed the standard.

Think About It

1. What are some possible short- and long-term actions to deal with the current situation?

2. If you thought that the drinking water in your community was contaminated from polluted sources, how would you go about verifying your concern? Who would you contact? What would your sources of information be? If you found that you were correct, what steps would you take to remedy this environmental health problem?

3. Think of your community and identify the types of hazardous wastes that are produced. What actions would need to be taken in your community to reduce the amount of identified hazardous wastes?

4. You have been asked to join a municipal environmental health promotion committee newly organized by the mayor's office. You volunteer to determine the health hazards of prominence in your community. What information will you collect from your local public health department? What are the roles of the various public health care providers employed by that agency who work with environmental health issues?

TOOL BOX

The Tool Box contains useful resources that can be applied in community health nursing practice. These related resources are found either in the appendices at the back of this text or on the Evolve website at http://evolve.elsevier.com/Canada/Stanhope/community/.

Appendices

- Appendix 8: CNA Position Statement: "Nurses and Environmental Health"
- Appendix E.1: Comprehensive Occupational and Environmental Health History

REFERENCES

Awuor, L., & Melles, S. (2019). The influence of environmental and health indicators on premature mortality: An empirical analysis of the City of Toronto's 140 neighborhoods. *Health & Place, 58*, 102155. https://doi.org/10.1016/j.healthplace.2019.102155.

Basu, N., & Lanphear, B. P. (2019). The challenge of pollution and health in Canada. *Canadian Journal of Public Health, 110*, 159–164. https://doi.org/10.17269/s41997-019-00175-7.

Blanchflower, D. (2014). The impact of stress in the workplace. *Management Services, 58*(2), 37.

Boffetta, P. (2006). Human cancer from environmental pollutants: The epidemiological evidence. *Mutation Research, 608*(2), 157–162.

Brauer, M., Reynolds, C., & Hystad, P. (2013). Traffic-related air pollution and health in Canada. *Canadian Medical Association Journal, 185*(18), 1557–1558. http://www.cmaj.ca/content/185/18/1557.

Breslin, F. C., Day, D., Tompa, E., et al. (2007). Non-agricultural work injuries among youth: A systematic review. *American Journal of Preventive Medicine, 32*(2), 151–162.

Canadian Centre for Occupational Health and Safety. (2020). *OSH answers fact sheets*. http://www.ccohs.ca/oshanswers/.

Canadian Centre for Occupational Health and Safety. (2021). *Diesel exhaust*. https://www.ccohs.ca/oshanswers/chemicals/diesel_exhaust.html.

Canadian Coalition for Green Health Care. (2020). *The green digest*. https://greenhealthcare.ca/digest/.

Canadian Food Inspection Agency. (2020). *Canadian food inspection agency*. https://www.inspection.gc.ca/eng/1297964599443/1297965645317.

Canadian Nurses Association. (2005). *CNA backgrounder—the ecosystem, the natural environment, and health and nursing: A summary of the issues*. http://cna-aiic.ca/~/media/cna/page-content/pdf-en/bg4_the_ecosystem_e.pdf.

Canadian Nurses Association. (2017a). *Code of ethics for registered nurses*. https://www.cna-aiic.ca/~/media/cna/page-content/pdf-en/code-of-ethics-2017-edition-secure-interactive.

Canadian Nurses Association. (2017b). *Position statement: Nurses and environmental health*. https://www.cna-aiic.ca/~/media/cna/page-content/pdf-en/nurses-and-environmental-health-position-statement.pdf.

Canadian Nurses Association. (2019). *Canadian association of nurses for the environment*. https://cnhe-iise.ca/about.html.

Canadian Partnership for Children's Health & Environment. (2008). *First steps in lifelong health*. https://healthyenvironmentforkids.ca/wp-content/uploads/2021/04/CPCHE_Vision_and_Strategy.pdf.

Canadian Public Health Association. (2015). *Global change and public health: Addressing the ecological determinants of health*. Author.

Chalupka, S. (2014). Climate change and health. *American Journal of Nursing, 114*(8), 67–69. https://doi.org/10.1097/01.NAJ.0000453051.39242.14

Chaudry, R. V. (2008). The precautionary principle, public health, and public health nursing. *Public Health Nursing, 25*(3), 261–268. [Seminal Reference].

Commission for Environmental Cooperation. (2006). *Children's health and the environment in North America: A first report on available indicators and measures.* http://www3.cec.org/islandora/en/item/2272-childrens-health-and-environment-in-north-america-en.pdf.

Commission for Environmental Cooperation. (2019). *2019 annual report at a glance.* http://www.cec.org/files/documents/annual_reports/2019-annual-report.pdf.

Conference Board of Canada. (2020). *Environmental provincial rankings. How Canada performs.* https://www.conferenceboard.ca/hcp/provincial/environment.aspx.

Cruickshank, M. (2014). A web-based survey of residents' views on advocating with patients for a healthy built environment in Canada. *International Journal of Family Medicine,* 458184. https://doi.org/10.1155/2014/458184

Curtis, L., Rea, W., Smith-Willis, P., et al. (2006). Adverse health effects of outdoor air pollutants. *Environment International, 32*(6), 815–830.

David Suzuki Foundation. (2014). *Greenhouse gases.* http://www.davidsuzuki.org/issues/climate-change/science/climate-change-basics/greenhouse-gases/.

DeGuzman, P. B., & Kulbok, P. A. (2012). Changing health outcomes of vulnerable populations through nursing's influence on neighborhood built environment: A framework for nursing research. *Journal of Nursing Scholarship, 44*(4), 341–348. https://doi.org/10.1111/j.1547-5069.2012.01470.x

Dinkins, C. S., & Sorrell, J. M. (2007). The expanding circle of environmental ethics. *Online Journal of Issues in Nursing, 13*(1). http://www.nursingworld.org/MainMenuCategories/ANAMarketplace/ANAPeriodicals/OJIN/TableofContents/vol132008/No1Jan08/EnvironmentalEthics.html.

Environment and Climate Change Canada. (2020a). *Greenhouse gas emissions: Canadian environmental sustainability indicators.* https://www.canada.ca/content/dam/eccc/documents/pdf/cesindicators/ghg-emissions/2020/greenhouse-gas-emissions-en.pdf.

Environment and Climate Change Canada. (2020b). *Canada's greenhouse gas and air pollutant and emission projections.* https://publications.gc.ca/collections/collection_2021/eccc/En1-78-2020-eng.pdf.

Environment Canada. (2012). *A climate change plan for the purposes of the Kyoto Protocol Implementation Act—2012.* https://publications.gc.ca/collections/collection_2012/ec/En11-11-2012-eng.pdf.

Environment and Climate Change Canada. (2020). *Canada's greenhouse gas and air pollutant and emission projections.* https://publications.gc.ca/collections/collection_2021/eccc/En1-78-2020-eng.pdf.

Environment and Climate Change Canada. (2021). *National inventory report 1990-2019: Greenhouse gas sources and sinks in Canada.* https://publications.gc.ca/collections/collection_2021/eccc/En81-4-1-2019-eng.pdf.

Environment Canada. (2017). *Sources of air pollution.* https://www.canada.ca/en/environment-climate-change/services/air-pollution/sources.html.

Environment Canada. (2018). *Acid rain: Causes and effects.* https://www.canada.ca/en/environment-climate-change/services/air-pollution/issues/acid-rain-causes-effects.html.

Environment Canada. (2020a). *Latest environmental indicators.* https://www.canada.ca/en/environment-climate-change/services/environmental-indicators/latest.html.

Environment Canada. (2020b). *Bisphenol A in Batch 2 of the challenge.* https://www.canada.ca/en/health-canada/services/chemical-substances/challenge/batch-2/bisphenol-a.html.

Finley, R., Reid-Smith, R., & Weese, J. S. (2006). Human health implications of Salmonella-contaminated natural pet treats and raw pet food. *Clinical Infectious Diseases, 42*(5), 686–691.

Fournier, B., & Karachiwalla, F. (2021). In *Shah's public health and preventive health care in Canada* (6th ed.). Elsevier Inc.

Global Footprint Network. (2020). *Country trends: Canada.* https://www.footprintnetwork.org/.

Government of Alberta. (2018). *Environmental quality guidelines for Alberta surface waters.* https://open.alberta.ca/dataset/5298aadb-f5cc-4160-8620-ad139bb985d8/resource/38ed9bb1-233f-4e28-b344-808670b20dae/download/environmentalqualitysurfacewaters-mar28-2018.pdf.

Government of Canada. (2016). *Types of chemicals management plan risk assessment documents.* https://www.canada.ca/en/health-canada/services/chemical-substances/fact-sheets/types-chemicals-management-plan-risk-assessment-documents.html.

Government of Canada. (2019a). *Lists of acts and regulations.* https://www.canada.ca/en/health-canada/corporate/about-health-canada/legislation-guidelines/acts-regulations/list-acts-regulations.html.

Government of Canada. (2019b). *Public health notice—outbreak of Listeria infections linked to Rosemount brand cooked diced chicken.* https://www.canada.ca/en/public-health/services/public-health-notices/2019/outbreak-listeria-infections-cooked-diced-chicken.html.

Government of Canada. (2020a). *Mercury and its compounds.* https://www.canada.ca/en/health-canada/services/chemical-substances/chemicals-management-plan/initiatives/mercury-compounds.html.

Government of Canada. (2020b). *Health impacts from air pollution.* https://www.canada.ca/en/environment-climate-change/campaigns/canadian-environment-week/clean-air-day/health-impacts-air-pollution.html.

Government of Canada. (2020c). *Quick facts on injury and poisoning.* https://www.canada.ca/en/public-health/services/injury-prevention/facts-on-injury.html.

Government of Canada. (2020d). *Road traffic and air pollution.* https://www.canada.ca/en/health-canada/services/air-quality/road-traffic-air-pollution.html.

Graham, P., Evitts, T., & Thomas-MacLean, R. (2008). Environmental scans. *Canadian Family Physician, 54,* 1022–1023.

Health Canada. (2006). *Legislation and guidelines.* http://www.hc-sc.gc.ca/ahc-asc/legislation/index-eng.php.

Health Canada. (2007). *Mercury: Your health and the environment.* http://www.hc-sc.gc.ca/ewh-semt/pubs/contaminants/mercur/index-eng.php.

Health Canada. (2012). *Environmental and workplace health.* http://www.hc-sc.gc.ca/ewh-semt/index-eng.php.

Health Canada. (2014). *Maternal–Infant Research on Environmental Chemicals (the MIREC study).* http://www.hc-sc.gc.ca/ewh-semt/contaminants/human-humaine/mirec-eng.php.

Health Canada. (2015). *Health Canada's participation in environmental assessments under CEAA 2012.* https://www.canada.ca/en/health-canada/corporate/publications/health-canada-participation-environmental-assessments.html.

Health Canada. (2017). *Guidelines for Canadian drinking water quality—summary Tables.* https://www.canada.ca/en/health-canada/services/environmental-workplace-health/reports-publications/water-quality/guidelines-canadian-drinking-water-quality-summary-table.html.

Health Canada. (2019). *Human health risk assessment.* https://www.canada.ca/en/health-canada/services/publications/healthy-living/guidance-evaluating-human-health-impacts-risk-assessment.html.

Health Canada. (2020a). *Pest management regulatory agency.* https://www.canada.ca/en/health-canada/corporate/about-health-canada/branches-agencies/pest-management-regulatory-agency.html.

Health Canada. (2020b). *The national chemical residue monitoring program annual report 2014–2015.* https://www.inspection.gc.ca/food-safety-for-industry/chemical-residues-microbiology/food-safety-testing-bulletins/2018-07-11/ncrmp/eng/1530632244911/1530632245212.

Heffernan, T. M., & O'Neill, T. S. (2013). Exposure to second-hand smoke damages everyday prospective memory. *Addiction, 108*(2), 420–426. https://doi.org/10.1111/j.1360-0443.2012.04056.x. https://www.canada.ca/en/health-canada/services/chemical-substances/chemicals-management-plan/initiatives/mercury-compounds.html.

Huwart, J., & Verdier, L. (2013). What is the impact of globalisation on the environment? In *Organisation for economic Co-operation and development, Economic globalisation: Origins and consequences* (pp. 108–125). OECD Publishing. https://www.oecd-ilibrary.org/docserver/9789264111905-8-en.pdf?expires=1626628021&id=id&accname=guest&checksum=0B5D9F0FDE33DB681FDD81A544C283A7.

IPCC (2021). AR6 climate change 2021: The physical science basis. Retrieved from https://www.unep.org/resources/report/climate-change-2021-physical-science-basis-working-group-i-contribution-sixth.

Keough, T. M. (2009). *Adverse effects of second hand smoke exposure in non-smoking women: Maternal and neonatal outcomes (Unpublished master's thesis).* Memorial University.

Kovesi, T., Creery, D., Gilbert, N. L., et al. (2006). Indoor air quality risk factors for severe lower respiratory tract infections in Inuit infants in Baffin region, Nunavut: A pilot study. *Indoor Air, 16*(4), 266–275.

Lajunen, T. K., Jaakkola, J. J. K., & Jaakkola, M. S. (2013). The synergistic effect of heredity and exposure to second-hand smoke on adult-onset asthma. *American Journal of Respiratory and Critical Care Medicine, 188*(7), 776.

Landis, M., Edgerton, E., White, E., et al. (2017). The impact of the 2016 Fort McMurray horse river wildfire on ambient air pollution levels in the Athabasca oil Sands region, Alberta, Canada. *The Science of the Total Environment, 618,* 1665–1676. https://doi.org/10.1016/j.scitotenv.2017.10.008.

Lavoie, J. (2015). *Alaskans to commemorate anniversary of Mount Polley Mine disaster as similar accidents predicted to increase.* July 30. DESMOG.ca. https://thenarwhal.ca/groups-commemorate-anniversary-mount-polley-mine-disaster-similar-accidents-predicted-rise/.

Lopez, R. P. (2012). In *Public health/environmental health: Built environment and public health* (2nd ed.). Jossey-Bass.

Marshall, L., Weir, E., Abelsohn, A., et al. (2002). Identifying and managing adverse and environmental health effects: 1. Taking an exposure history. *Canadian Medical Association Journal, 166*(9), 1049–1055.

Mittelstaedt, M. (2010). *Canada first to declare Bisphenol A toxic.* Globe and Mail. October 13. http://www.theglobeandmail.com/technology/science/canada-first-to-declare-bisphenol-a-toxic/article1214889/.

Moore, D., Copes, R., Fisk, R., et al. (2006). Population health effects of air quality changes due to forest fires in British Columbia in 2003. *Canadian Journal of Public Health, 97*(2), 105–108.

Muhajarine, N. (2012). Built environment health research: The time is now for a Canadian network of excellence. *Canadian Journal of Public Health, 103*(6), S3.

National Collaborating Centre for Environmental Health. (2015). *Bed bugs.* http://www.ncceh.ca/environmental-health-in-canada/health-agency-projects/bed-bugs.

National Collaborating Centre for Environmental Health. (2018). *Public health responses to wildfire smoke events.* https://ncceh.ca/sites/default/files/Responding%20to%20Wildfire%20Smoke%20Events%20EN.pdf.

Nightingale, F. (1859). *Notes on nursing: What it is and what it is not. Harrison.*

Ontario Ministry of the Environment, Conservation and Parks. (2019). *Eating Ontario fish, 2017-18.* https://www.ontario.ca/page/eating-ontario-fish-2017-18.

Pierpont, N. (2010). *Wind concerns Ontario.* http://windconcernsontario.ca.

Pike-MacDonald, S., Best, D. G., Twomey, C., et al. (2007). Promoting safe drinking water. *Canadian Nurse, 103*(1), 15–19.

Pinkerton, K. E., & Rom, W. N. (2014). *Global climate change and public health.* Humana Press.

Previdi, M., Liepert, B. G., Peteet, D. T., et al. (2011). Climate sensitivity in the Anthropocene. *Earth System Dynamics Discussions, 2*(2), 531–550.

Public Health Agency of Canada. (2013). *Key element 1: Focus on the health of populations.* http://cbpp-pcpe.phac-aspc.gc.ca/population-health-approach-organizing-framework/key-element-1-focus-health-populations/.

Public Health Agency of Canada. (2015). *Climate change and public health factsheets.* http://www.phac-aspc.gc.ca/hp-ps/eph-esp/fs-fi-a-eng.php.

Public Health Agency of Canada. (2016a). *Childhood and adolescence.* http://www.phac-aspc.gc.ca/hp-ps/dca-dea/index-eng.php.

Public Health Agency of Canada. (2016b). *Age-friendly communities.* https://www.canada.ca/en/public-health/services/health-promotion/aging-seniors/friendly-communities.html.

Silins, I., & Högberg, J. (2011). Combined toxic exposures and human health: Biomarkers of exposure and effect. *International Journal of Environmental Research and Public Health, 8*(3), 629–647. https://doi.org/10.3390/ijerph8030629

Stanhope, J., & Lancaster, J. (2011). Environmental health in Canada. In M. Stanhope, J. Lancaster, H. Jessup-Falconi, et al. (Eds.), *Community health nursing in Canada* (2nd Cdn. ed) (pp. 474–476). Mosby/Elsevier.

Tannahill, A. (2008). Beyond evidence—to ethics: A decision-making framework for health promotion, public health and health improvement. *Health Promotion International, 23*(4), 380–390.

The Lung Association. (2020). *Asthma and children fact sheet.* https://www.lung.org/lung-health-diseases/lung-disease-lookup/asthma/learn-about-asthma/asthma-children-facts-sheet.

Twarakavi, N. K. C., & Kaluarachchi, J. J. (2006). Sustainability of ground water quality considering land use changes and public health risks. *Journal of Environmental Management, 81*(4), 405–419.

Union of Nova Scotia Municipalities. (2011). *Idle-free toolkit for municipalities.* http://unsm.ca/doc_download/1534-idle-free-toolkit-for-municipalalites.html.

United Nations. (2019). *UN summits to urge "ambition and action" on climate change, sustainable development.* Guterres. UN News. September 18. https://news.un.org/en/story/2019/09/1046712.

United Nations Department of Economic and Social Affairs. (1992). Agenda 21. https://sustainabledevelopment.un.org/outcomedocuments/agenda21.

United Nations High Commissioner for Refugees. (2015). *UNHCR, the environment, & climate change.* https://www.unhcr.org/540854f49.pdf.

U.S. Environmental Protection Agency. (2007). *Acid rain.* https://www.epa.gov/acidrain.

Waldron, I. (2020). *Environmental racism in Canada, the Canadian commission for UNESCO's IdeaLab.* https://en.ccunesco.ca/-/media/Files/Unesco/Resources/2020/07/EnvironmentalRacismCanada.pdf.

World Health Organization. (2016). *Preventing disease through healthy environments: A global assessment of the burden of disease from environmental risks.* https://www.who.int/publications/i/item/9789241565196.

World Health Organization. (2018). *The global network for age-friendly cities and communities: Looking back over the last decade, looking forward to the next.* https://apps.who.int/iris/bitstream/handle/10665/278979/WHO-FWC-ALC-18.4-eng.pdf?sequence=1.

Young-Reuters, J. (2010). *BPA declared toxic by Canada.* CBC News. October 13. http://www.cbc.ca/news/technology/bpa-declared-toxic-by-canada-1.873250.

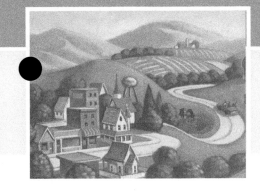

18

Emergency Management and Disaster Preparedness

OUTLINE

Types of Disasters, 452
  Natural Disasters, 452
  Human-Made Disasters, 453
  Biological Disasters, 453
Canada's Emergency Management Framework, 455
Disaster Prevention and Mitigation, 455
Disaster Preparedness, 456
  Personal Preparedness, 456
  Professional Preparedness, 456

Community Preparedness, 457
Influenza Pandemic Preparedness, 459
Public Health Nurses and the H1N1 Outbreak, 460
Disaster Response, 462
  The Role of the Community Health Nurse in Disaster Response, 463
  Emergency Lodging After a Disaster, 463
Disaster Recovery, 464

OBJECTIVES

After reading this chapter, you should be able to:

18.1 Explain the impact of natural and human-made disasters on the health of populations.

18.2 Appraise Canada's emergency management framework.

18.3 Describe considerations for personal, professional, and community preparedness in disasters.

18.4 Compare and contrast the role of the community health nurse in disaster prevention, preparedness, response, and recovery.

KEY TERMS*

Centre for Emergency Preparedness and Response (CEPR), 456
disaster, 452
disaster preparedness, 456
disaster prevention and mitigation, 456
disaster recovery, 464
disaster response, 462

disaster vulnerability, 455
emergency lodging, 463
Emergency Measures Organization (EMO), 458
human-made disasters, 453
influenza pandemic, 459
natural disasters, 452
triage, 463

*See the Glossary on page 468 for definitions.

Individuals, communities, and government must be prepared to prevent and respond to disasters and emergencies, including natural disasters, pandemics, and cyber incidents and terrorism. According to Government of Canada (2019), emergency management and disaster mitigation is a collective responsibility of all federal government institutions and it includes creating plans, procedures, contact lists, and exercises that are undertaken in the event of an emergency or disaster. Some of the most recent major disasters in this century are associated with pandemics, cyber incidents, climate change, global instability, economic downturns, political upheaval with its often-accompanying wars or collapse of governments,

famine, mass population displacements, violence, and civil conflicts (Veenema, 2013). The global pandemic of COVID-19 in 2020, the forest fires that forced a mass evacuation of Fort McMurray in northern Alberta in 2016, the earthquake that destroyed areas of Haiti in 2010, and the earthquake that led to a devastating tsunami in Asia in 2004 illustrate the unpredictable nature of disasters. Although disasters and emergencies are inevitable, there are ways to manage how people respond to them. This chapter considers the types of disasters and emergencies experienced in communities; Canada's emergency management framework (which includes four stages): disaster prevention and mitigation, preparedness, response, and recovery.

TYPES OF DISASTERS

A **disaster** is any human-made or natural event that causes destruction and devastation that cannot be relieved without assistance. The event need not cause injury or death to be considered a disaster. For example, a flood or tornado may cause millions of dollars in damage without causing a single death or injury. Table 18.1 lists examples of natural and human-made disasters.

Although natural disasters cannot be prevented, much can be done to prevent further accidents, death, and destruction after impact. A concise, realistic, and well-rehearsed disaster plan (or *emergency plan*) is essential. So too is open, clear, and ongoing communication among workers and organizations involved in disaster response. Many human-made disasters can be prevented (e.g., major transportation accidents and fires resulting from substance use or illegal drug production).

Disasters can affect a single family or a small group, as in a house fire, or they can kill thousands and result in economic losses in the millions, as with floods, earthquakes, tornadoes, hurricanes, and bioterrorism (which is the use or the threat of use of biological agents to frighten or coerce individuals, groups, or populations as a whole). Disasters such as pandemics, damaging snowstorms, regular droughts and forest fires, the 2013 rail disaster in Lac-Mégantic in Quebec, and the 2013 super flood in southern Alberta have led to the loss of lives, homes, businesses, and even towns and villages. In 2020 the estimated cost of natural disasters worldwide was 75 billion dollars (US), and the estimated insurance loss was 30 billion (Rudden, 2020)

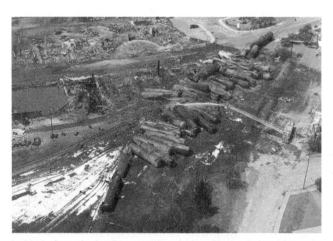

In 2013, the train derailment and explosion disaster in Lac-Mégantic, Quebec, killed 47 people and caused hundreds of millions of dollars of losses. (Transportation Safety Board of Canada)

People in industrialized countries are becoming less self-sufficient because they rely heavily on technology and social and economic systems within their community. Developing countries, however, are most vulnerable to the impacts of disasters because they have fewer resources to adapt—socially, technologically, and financially. A disaster can affect

TABLE 18.1 Types of Disasters	
Natural	**Human-Made**
Meteorological and hydrological	**Conflict**
• Cold wave	• Civil unrest
• Drought	• School violence
• Flood, hail/thunderstorm	• Terrorism/bioterrorism
• Heat wave/cold wave	
• Hurricane/typhoon	**Technological**
• Snow avalanche	• Accident—industrial
• Storm surges	• Accident—other
• Storm—freezing rain	• Accident—transport
• Storm—unspecific or other	• Structural collapse
• Storm—winter	• Computer viruses
• Tornado	
• Wildfire	**Fire**
	• Hazardous chemicals
Biological	
• Epidemic/pandemic	
• Infestation	
Geological	
• Earthquake	
• Landslide/mudslide	
• Tsunami	

the health of all people and their communities in a number of ways, (Veenema, 2013):

- It can cause premature deaths, illnesses, and injuries in the affected community.
- It can destroy the local health care infrastructure and prevent an effective response to the disaster.
- It can create environmental imbalances, thereby increasing the risk of communicable diseases and environmental hazards.
- It can affect the psychological, emotional, and social well-being of the people it affects.
- It can cause shortages of food and water.
- It can displace populations.

Natural Disasters

Urbanization and overcrowding in cities have increased the danger of **natural disasters** (destruction or devastation caused by natural events) because communities have tended to be built in areas that are vulnerable to disasters, such as in known tornado zones or near rivers that are prone to flooding. Natural disasters have led to major increases in insurance payouts in Canada and many other countries in the past several decades. The ice storm of 1998 in the provinces of Ontario and Quebec affected more than 5 million people by creating power outages. The short-term economic cost has been estimated at $1.6 billion (McCready, 2004). The total cost of the super flood in southern Alberta in 2013 is estimated at over $6 billion (Environment Canada, 2014). Many Canadians reside in areas that are prone to natural disasters such as flooding, earthquakes, tornadoes, landslides, and hail (Natural Resources Canada, 2013). Projections suggest that by 2050, populations living in urban areas at risk for natural floods, earthquakes, and severe storms will double, making preventive design and disaster and emergency planning essential for community health and safety (Brecht, Deichmann, & Wang, 2013).

From a global perspective, developing countries experience a disproportionate burden from natural disasters. These countries tend to experience widespread poverty and have limited resources for dealing with the effects of disasters. Natural disasters create the most devastation in developing countries, where the death rate is up to 12 times higher than in developed countries. The poor suffer the most because their houses are less sturdy and they have fewer social security supports. Between 1980 and 2018, the most economic damage worldwide was caused by the 2011 earthquake and tsunami in Japan; and between 1992 and 2017 the most expensive natural disasters were Hurricanes Harvey, Irma, and Maria, which occurred in the Unites States and the Caribbean (Rudden, 2020).

In every region of Canada, there are people who, because of where they live, are more vulnerable in times of natural disasters. For instance, during the 2013 super flood in southern Alberta, those living in Calgary's urban shelters or on the city's streets were more reliant on the rapid implementation of a disaster plan and the creation of new shelters. In May 2016, the forest fires in Fort McMurray destroyed 2 400 buildings, razed nearly 6 000 square kilometres of forest, and forced 80 000 residents to evacuate the area. Residents of Fort McMurray were more vulnerable to the impact of the fires and were either forced to move away or rebuild and were exposed to toxic contaminants in the air. Natural disasters have a significant impact on environmental risk and can create economic and health burdens.

Human-Made Disasters

Urban development and overcrowding have also increased **human-made disasters** (destruction or devastation caused by humans). The stress caused by overcrowding has led to civil unrest and riots. In some parts of the world, modern wars waged over land rights and space have markedly increased the risk of injury and death from disasters.

In Canada and other countries, school violence, a human-made disaster, has increased in intensity and magnitude. In Canada, several violent incidents of school shootings have taken place over the past three decades. The first mass school shooting, referred to as "the Montreal Massacre," occurred in 1989 at the École Polytechnique in Montreal. Fourteen female engineering students were killed by a 25-year-old Montreal man. In 1999, at W. R. Myers High School in Taber, a small town in Alberta, two high school students were shot by a former classmate; the shootings left one student dead and the other seriously wounded. In 2006, a school shooting occurred at Dawson College in Montreal that left one dead and 20 injured. In 2007 in Toronto, a shooting occurred at C. W. Jefferys Collegiate Institute that left a 14-year-old Grade 9 student dead. Most recently, in 2016, a shooting at La Loche Community School in northern Saskatchewan left four dead and four critically wounded. For further information on school violence in Canada, see the RCMP's "School Violence" web page (the link is on the Evolve website).

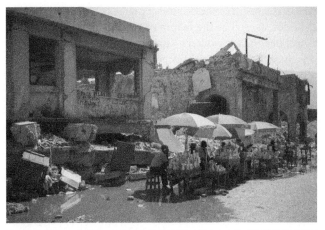

Underdeveloped areas are most at risk after a natural disaster has occurred; their infrastructure and housing quality are often inadequate to begin with, and inhabitants of such areas often have limited resources for coping with a disaster. (iStockphoto/Claudiad)

Biological Disasters

Biological disasters involve the effects caused by the spread of an organism (disease, virus, or an epidemic), or it can be related to the sudden growth of a certain kind of plant or animal (e.g., a locust spread). In 2020, the COVID-19 pandemic swept the globe and caused devastating effects for individuals, families, communities, and society at large. COVID-19 is a mutation of the acute respiratory syndrome (SARS) that also spread globally in 2003 and at that time raised awareness of the enormous human and financial costs that can result from a pandemic. The SARS experience in 2003 led to 8 098 cases worldwide with 774 deaths, and 252 cases in Canada with 44 deaths; including the deaths of two nurses and one physician in Ontario (Frangoul, 2014; Registered Nurses' Association of Ontario [RNAO], 2004).

Unfortunately, the COVID-19 pandemic has had an even greater impact on the health of populations in Canada and around the world. As of July 17, 2021, Canada had 1 422 918 cases of COVID-19 with 26 492 deaths and 1 391 722 cases recovered, while globally there were 191 110 685 cases and 4 103 397 deaths. Canada's response to COVID-19 has included financial support for individuals and businesses, border control measures, travel alerts, education and research, and more (Government of Canada, 2021). The Government of Canada monitors the COVID-19 statistics in an interactive data map that shows cases, deaths, and recovery (see https://health-infobase. canada.ca/covid-19/). Canada has shown a strong response to COVID-19 and has been successful in mitigating the effects of the pandemic.

It is important to understand the history of the response to SARS and how this led to a strong Canadian response to COVID-19. In 2006 the Ontario SARS Commission chaired by the Honourable Archie Campbell released its final report describing the story of SARS as "a system failure." System-wide, there was a lack of preparedness against infectious disease as a result of the decline of public health, and a lack of resources, as well as the failure of systems that are meant to protect health care workers. The report also noted:

- Failures occurred in the occupational safety and infection control systems.
- The health care system failed to provide the necessary resources to manage the outbreak.
- The outbreak resulted in financial costs to the government and health care system; however, the emotional losses related to illness, pain and suffering, separation from support systems, and death need to be recognized.
- One aspect of infection control was related to airborne transmission, and Ontario decided to defer use of protective equipment because scientific evidence on its effectiveness was not available. Campbell refers to this system weakness as ignoring the "precautionary principle" (when doubt in the evidence exists, the appropriate action is to err on the side of caution, which would have meant favouring the use of protective equipment).
- Readiness for "the unseen" is one of the most significant lessons learned from SARS.

SARS was a catalyst for changes to the health care system in preparation for future infectious disease outbreaks (Campbell, 2006). Following the outbreak of SARS, the National Advisory Committee on SARS and Public Health was formed. The committee, led by Dr. David Naylor, produced numerous recommendations on improving public health and the overall capacity of the Canadian public health system to respond to emergencies (Public Health Agency of Canada [PHAC], 2003). The significant changes to the health care system that are a direct outcome of the recommendations in the Naylor Report appear in Box 18.1.

The SARS outbreak in Ontario led to many significant and necessary changes to the management of such disasters in Ontario and other provinces and territories and at the federal level. A number of SARS-related committees at the provincial and federal levels generated noteworthy reports: for example, the Naylor Report, the Campbell Report, and the Walker Report (Mildon, 2004). The recommendations in these reports led to a number of significant changes in the way in which disasters are prepared for and managed in Canada. They also led to the appointment of a minister of Public Safety and Emergency Preparedness and a minister of state for Public Health as well as the creation of the PHAC (Mildon, 2004; PHAC, 2018).

As a result of the lessons learned from SARS, Canada's response to COVID-19 is comprehensive and sweeping and includes consideration of the financial implications of the pandemic, as outlined in Canada's COVID-19 Economic Response Plan, as well as the development of a COVID Alert app, an ethical framework, health care preparedness, border control measures, support for Canadians abroad, public education, and research (Government of Canada, 2021). The response to COVID-19 is in keeping with the federal, provincial, and territorial responsibilities outlined in Canada's emergency management framework.

BOX 18.1   Health Care System Changes That Resulted From SARS

2004	The Public Health Agency of Canada (PHAC) is established. Canada's first chief public health officer, Dr. David Butler-Jones, is appointed.
2004	The Canadian Public Health Network Council is established in collaboration with all levels of government. It provides a forum to discuss key public health issues.
2004	The Global Public Health Intelligence Network—in collaboration with the Canadian Network for Public Health Intelligence, World Health Organization, and United Nations—is launched internationally. It is a secure web-based early-warning system that monitors global media sources for reports of public health significance in seven languages in real time, 24 hours a day. Reports are analyzed by public health officials.
2006	The scope of planning and disaster preparedness is expanded in the revised Canadian Pandemic Influenza Plan, which is coordinated by the PHAC with input from all levels of government.
2006	The Government of Canada stockpiles antiviral medications and secures a domestic vaccine supplier as part of a multifaceted approach to protecting Canadians during an influenza pandemic.
2006	The new *Quarantine Act* is enacted. It enhances the capacity to reduce and prevent the spread of serious infectious diseases by infected individuals entering or leaving Canada through Quarantine Services at key airports across the country.
2007	Multidisciplinary national health emergency response teams are established by the PHAC within the Centre for Emergency Preparedness and Response to be deployed across Canada to provide medical surge capacity caused by a public health crisis.
2011	The Canadian Integrated Outbreak Surveillance Centre is launched. It is a web-based alert system that efficiently provides public health care providers with time-sensitive information on outbreaks.
2012	The capacity of the National Microbiology Laboratory is augmented to be able to respond to outbreaks.
2016	FluWatch, a web-based national surveillance system is launched by the PHAC. FluWatch uses surveillance systems to assess influenza severity, vaccine effectiveness, and antiviral resistance that may be occurring across Canada.

Canada approved the H1N1 vaccine and its distribution to all provinces and territories.

Table 18.2 examines influenza pandemic triggers and actions associated with each of four global phases used to communicate the global view of the evolving picture.

All provinces and territories have an influenza pandemic preparedness plan. These plans are listed on and available through the PHAC's "Pandemic Plans" webpage (see the link on the Evolve website). The Ontario Health Plan for an Influenza Pandemic addresses areas such as roles,

TABLE 18.2 Influenza Pandemic Triggers and Actions

Phase	Triggers	Actions
Interpandemic: The period between influenza pandemics	No new influenza strains are identified in humans	Public education and training Review current publications and human influenza surveillance reports Prepare and/or update educational materials for the general public focused on risks, risk avoidance, universal and respiratory hygiene etiquette, and information on how to reduce transmission Prepare vaccines, treatments, and educational materials for the health care sector, reinforcing recommendations on how to manage patients with respiratory illnesses (e.g., the need for masks for coughing patients) Update infection control procedures and community contact lists Develop fact sheets Educational sessions at workplaces, schools, and community organizations
Alert: Influenza caused by a new subtype has been identified in humans	Novel virus causing human cases is detected somewhere in the world (no transmission or low transmission)	Make preparations to enhance surveillance in Canada Gather data from affected areas Relay information on confirmed cases, and contacts Increase focus on testing, isolating, and treating confirmed cases and their contacts, either in self-isolation at home or in health care setting as a containment strategy Send samples to the National Microbiology Laboratory for confirmation of positive test results
	Novel virus with sustained human transmission detected somewhere in the world	Enhance surveillance Gather data from affected areas Develop specific laboratory diagnostics Continue case reporting and follow-up contact-tracing
Pandemic: The period of global spread of human influenza caused by a new stereotype	Novel/pandemic virus (with sustained human transmission) detected in Canada.	Continue surveillance and data-gathering Activate emergency response protocols Investigate early cases to determine epidemiological and clinical characteristics and inform risk assessment Make arrangements for antiviral access and strategic deployment Provide clinical guidelines and public health advice
	Novel virus detected in provinces, territories, or local jurisdictions	Continue surveillance and data-gathering Implement additional public health measures (e.g., school closures) as appropriate Prepare to distribute, administer, and monitor vaccines
	Demand for service exceeds capacity	Prioritize or triage services Implement broader public health measures (e.g., banning large gatherings)
Transition: Reduction of the assessed risk, resulting in de-escalation of global actions	Waves of influenza and demand for service decline	
	Vaccine available Second influenza wave arrives	Administer and monitor vaccine uptake, safety, and effectiveness Treat cases Continue immunizations Ongoing surveillance to monitor influenza activity, antiviral resistance, and virus strain changes
	Pandemic is over and return to normal activities	Complete pandemic studies and reports Evaluate response and revise plans

Source: Adapted from Government of Canada (2018). Canadian pandemic influenza preparedness: Planning guide for the health sector. https://www.canada.ca/en/public-health/services/flu-influenza/canadian-pandemic-influenza-preparedness-planning-guidance-health-sector/table-of-contents.html#pre

responsibilities, and frameworks for decision making; health care sector communications; surveillance; public health measures; immunization; laboratory and primary care services; and outpatient care and treatment (Ontario Ministry of Health and Long-Term Care, 2013). Similar areas of concern are found in other provincial and territorial influenza pandemic preparedness plans.

Although national, provincial or territorial, and municipal pandemic preparedness plans are in place, when an influenza pandemic occurs, all health care operations are managed at the local or regional level (Tam et al., 2005). The local public health infrastructure needs to be prepared to lead and respond to emergencies, as well as maintain core functions (Johnson et al., 2005). Many workplaces and other institutions such as universities are developing their own influenza pandemic preparedness plans. These plans also need to be documented and shared with local influenza pandemic preparedness planning teams to ensure a coordinated disaster management plan. As well, the Canadian Nurses Association has established a position statement highlighting the role of nursing in disaster management at national, provincial or territorial, and municipal levels (Canadian Nurses Association, 2013).

Locally, mechanisms need to be in place for ill persons and their families to receive needed medical care. Public health units or health authorities in municipalities are taking the lead role in preparing and managing the emergencies related to infectious diseases (Johnson et al., 2005). Public health units or health authorities locally and regionally will "maintain core functions and … lead and support health sector responses to emergencies" (Johnson et al., 2005, p. 412). Some of the core public health functions that are recommended include surveillance activities; preparation for full-scale vaccination programs that would include ensuring that vaccine supplies and staff for mass immunization clinics are available; and specific public health measures, such as reviewing and updating all influenza educational materials and ensuring that resources will be available to handle the many tasks that will be required in a pandemic influenza situation (e.g., case finding, isolation of cases, immunization clinics, and tracking) (Huston, 2004).

CHNs need to continually monitor the latest information on pandemic planning and activities. Available resources may vary in communities. One resource used in Ontario by health care providers is a newsletter published regularly by the Ontario Ministry of Health and Long-Term Care called *The Emergency Preparedness Planner* (see the link on the Evolve website). Resources are also available for workplaces to address pandemic planning. For information on this topic, see the Canadian Centre for Occupational Health and Safety "Pandemic Planning" webpage (the link is on the Evolve website).

DISASTER RESPONSE

Stage 3 of the disaster management cycle is **disaster response,** which refers to activities that are carried out by disaster response teams that consist of police, firefighters, medical personnel, and others during and following a disaster. This is the stage in which disaster plans are implemented. Community residents need to listen to the radio and television to obtain the most current information on the steps to be taken. Depending on the type and severity of a disaster, residents may be advised to remain in their homes and use their emergency kits and supplies or may be directed to certain facilities for safe shelter.

The physical and emotional effects of disasters on people in a community depend on factors such as the type, cause, and location of the disaster; the magnitude and extent of damage; the duration; and the amount of warning provided. For example, no one may die in an earthquake, but the structural damage to buildings and the continuous aftershocks may last for weeks and cause intense psychological stress. In addition, the longer it takes for structural repairs and other cleanup, the longer the psychological effects can last.

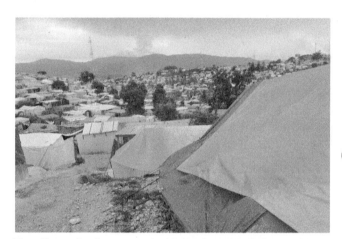

The effects of a disaster can be highly disruptive. In Port-au-Prince, Haiti, over 1 million people were displaced to makeshift tent communities following the 2010 earthquake. (iStockphoto/arindambanerjee)

It is important to be aware that individuals react to the same disaster in different ways, depending on their age, cultural background, health status, social support structure, and general ability to adapt to crises. Box 18.2 describes common reactions of adults and children to disasters. The initial reactions of victims can include fear, distress, anxiety, anger, numbness, difficulty concentrating, and difficulty making decisions (PHAC, 2005). Disturbances in bodily functions, such as gastrointestinal upsets, diarrhea, and nausea and vomiting are also common (PHAC, 2005). Additionally, victims may be fearful of leaving home or loved ones, and fearful of travelling (PHAC, 2005).

During disasters, an existing chronic disease may become exacerbated. For example, the emotional stress of being a disaster victim may make it difficult for people with diabetes to control their blood sugar levels. Grief results in harmful effects to the immune system. It reduces the function of cells that protect against viral infections and tumours. Hormones that are produced by the body's flight-or-fight mechanism

BOX 18.2 Common Reactions to Disasters

Adults
- Extreme sense of urgency
- Panic and fear
- Disbelief
- Disorientation and numbness
- Reluctance to abandon property
- Difficulty in making decisions
- The need to help others
- Anger
- Blaming and scapegoating
- Delayed reactions
- Insomnia
- Headaches
- Apathy and depression
- Sense of powerlessness
- Guilt
- Moodiness and irritability
- Jealousy and resentment
- Domestic violence

Children
- Regressive behaviours (bedwetting, thumb-sucking, crying, clinging to parents)
- Fantasies that disaster never occurred
- Nightmares
- School-related problems, including an inability to concentrate and a refusal to go back to school

BOX 18.3 Populations at Greatest Risk for Disruption After a Disaster

- Persons with disabilities
- Persons living on a low income, including the homeless
- Persons who do not understand the local language
- Persons living alone
- Lone-parent families
- Persons new to the area
- Institutionalized persons or those with chronic mental illness
- Previous disaster victims or victims of traumatic events
- Persons who are not citizens or legally documented immigrants
- Substance abusers

recovery. Assessing emergency health needs can help match available resources to a population's emergency needs. For example, assessments in sudden-impact disasters, such as forest fires and tornadoes, are concerned with ongoing hazards, injuries, shelter requirements, and clean water. A CHN could participate on local committees to help with community emergency preparedness plans that include identifying and preparing shelters for disaster victims. Assessments in gradual-onset disasters, such as famines, are most concerned with mortality rates, nutritional status, immunization status, and environmental health. CHNs could work with communities to assess the need for food banks and evaluate immunization compliance in specific populations.

Ongoing assessments and surveillance reports are just as important as initial assessments of emergency health needs. Surveillance reports indicate the continuing status of the affected population and the effectiveness of ongoing disaster relief efforts. Surveillance continues into the recovery phase of a disaster. Although it is not considered surveillance, the Centers for Disease Control and Prevention (CDC) in the U.S. have developed an epidemiological technique to document and analyze a community's response to an emergency, called the Community Assessment for Public Health Emergency Response (CASPER) Toolkit. This toolkit provides public health leaders, such as CHNs, with information throughout the disaster cycle (preparedness, response, recovery, mitigation). That information generated can be used to initiate public health action; identify information gaps; facilitate disaster planning, response, and recovery activities; allocate resources; and assess new or changing needs in the community (CDC, 2019).

Emergency Lodging After a Disaster

One of the vital areas of assistance that people often require after a disaster is emergency lodging, which is safe, temporary lodging that is provided to people who cannot return home and cannot find alternate accommodations (Canadian Red Cross, 2020). During a disaster, the Canadian Red Cross may open shelters for those affected by the disaster and provides food and lodging to families and disaster workers (Canadian Red Cross, 2020). CHNs may be involved with a variety of

also play a role in mediating the effects of grief. The effects on young children can be especially disruptive. They can resort to regressive behaviours such as bedwetting, thumb-sucking, crying, and clinging to parents (PHAC, 2005). They might also experience nightmares. Box 18.3 lists populations who are at a greater risk for disruption after a disaster. For further information on how to help different groups cope with disasters, see the PHAC's "Responding to Stressful Events" web page (the link is on the Evolve website). See also the National Defence and the Canadian Armed Forces link, which discusses the role of the Canadian military in disaster relief, including the Disaster Assistance Response Team (DART).

The Role of the Community Health Nurse in Disaster Response

Nurses play an important role in all phases of emergency management, including prevention, mitigation, preparedness, response, and recovery (CNA, 2013). CHNs often take a leadership role in helping to plan a comprehensive and coordinated approach to emergency preparedness and response. During the response to disasters, CHNs can be involved in assessing populations' emergency health needs. **Triage** is the process of separating casualties and allocating treatment on the basis of the victims' potential for survival. As a member of the triage team, CHNs must provide accurate information, acquired through assessment, to facilitate rapid rescue and

activities, such as providing first aid, food preparation, record keeping, and maintaining a safe environment.

Although physical health needs are the priority initially, especially among older persons and the chronically ill, many of the predominant problems in shelters revolve around stress. The shock of the disaster itself, loss of personal possessions, fear of the unknown, living in proximity to total strangers, and even boredom can cause stress.

Nurses working in shelters can use the following common-sense approaches to help victims deal with stress (American Red Cross, 2012):

- Listen to victims tell and retell their feelings about the disaster and their current situation.
- Encourage victims to share their feelings with one another, if it seems appropriate to do so.
- Help victims make decisions.
- Delegate tasks (e.g., reading, crafts, playing games with children) to teenagers and others to help combat boredom.
- Provide the basic necessities (food, clothing, rest).
- Try to recover or get needed items (prescription glasses, medications).
- Provide basic compassion and dignity (e.g., privacy when appropriate and if possible).
- Refer a patient to a mental health counsellor if the situation warrants.

⬛ LEVELS OF PREVENTION

Related to Disaster Management

Primary Prevention
A CHN participates with community committee members in developing a disaster plan for the community.

Secondary Prevention
A CHN participates in assessing disaster victims and is involved in triage for care.

Tertiary Prevention
A CHN participates in home visits to uncover dangers that may cause additional injury to victims or cause other problems (e.g., house fires from unsafe use of candles).

Mental well-being is particularly strained for those displaced from their homes following a crisis or disaster (Milligan & McGuinness, 2009). Highly trained mental health counsellors, such as psychologists, psychiatrists, clinical social workers, and nurses are always available in large-scale disasters where shelters are often established to manage victims. Community mental health workers are important members of any disaster team, no matter what the level of disaster, and their services need to be used as often as necessary.

DISASTER RECOVERY

Stage 4 of the disaster management cycle is **disaster recovery,** which refers to activities that focus on rebuilding to predisaster or near-predisaster conditions and on community safety so that the risk of a recurrence of the disaster is reduced. This is the stage in which there is recovery from the physical, psychological, and financial damage. Cleanup, repair, and rebuilding occur in the community. Disaster victims may need community assistance to rebuild their lives and learn to deal with all losses encountered as a result of the disaster. This stage is the best time to start thinking about the lessons learned from the disaster and to consider actions that will decrease vulnerability and mitigate future disasters. Therefore, there is often a willingness to implement mitigation activities to reduce or avoid future similar disasters. Also, disaster plans are reviewed and revisions are made.

Disaster recovery efforts are expensive, and the costs can grow because of the number of people involved and the amount of technology, infrastructure, and physical structures that must be restored. Usually, the government takes the lead in rebuilding efforts, whereas the business community tries to provide economic support to individuals and communities. Many other organizations help with rebuilding efforts, such as religious groups and community service organizations.

The role of CHNs in the disaster recovery stage is to partner with community disaster team members to evaluate the consequences of the disaster. CHNs provide information about what resources are available and accessible to facilitate individual and community recovery. Community cleanup efforts can cause many physical and psychological problems. CHNs should be aware of the potential public health challenges specific to the disaster area. CHNs need to continue to teach proper body mechanics, proper hygiene, make sure immunization records are current, monitor for environmental health hazards (physical, chemical, biological, ergonomic, and psychological), and initiate required actions.

It is important to be alert for environmental health hazards during the recovery phase. During home visits, CHNs may uncover situations such as a faulty housing structure or lack of water or electricity. Objects that have been blown into the yard by a tornado or that floated in from a flood may be dangerous and must be removed. Case-finding and referrals are critical during the recovery phase and may continue for a long time. CHNs and community organizations partner with the victims of a disaster and provide supportive care.

Being prepared for a disaster is of major importance to how disasters are managed. Disaster planning does not guarantee that the management of a disaster will always go as planned, but it does contribute to minimizing the negative physical, psychological, social, and economic impacts related to the disaster. CHNs have many of the necessary skills required to deal with a disaster and need to ensure that they are prepared to respond to a disaster and work with their community to meet the challenges of disaster management.

STUDENT EXPERIENCE

As a nursing student, you have been assigned to a secondary school for your community health nursing clinical experience.

1. Write down your thoughts and beliefs about violence in schools. Questions to consider: In general, how do you feel about school shootings and school violence? Why do you think such violence occurs? What warning signs might violent school-aged children demonstrate? How do you think violence in schools can be prevented?

2. Locate research articles identifying what is known about school violence in Canada.

3. Based on your research findings, write an outline for a teaching package that could be implemented in the school.

CHAPTER SUMMARY

18.1 A disaster can affect the health of all people and their communities in a number of ways, including the following: premature deaths, illnesses, and injuries; destroying the local health care infrastructure, creating environmental imbalances, thereby increasing the risk of communicable diseases and environmental hazards; affecting the psychological, emotional, and social well-being of people; causing shortages of food and water; and displacing populations.

18.2 Canada's emergency framework specifies all-hazards risk assessments and planning activities within all four integrated functions of emergency management, including prevention and mitigation, preparedness, response, and recovery.

18.3 Considerations for personal preparedness include having emergency supplies on hand, such as first-aid supplies; emergency blankets; a flashlight; a radio; medications; ice packs; nonperishable food and water sufficient for at least 72 hours; copies of each person's medical information; local emergency telephone numbers; copies of disaster plans; and copies of important documents such as driver's licenses, birth certificates, and passports. Professional considerations include CHNs being asked to respond to a disaster, which may in turn put them at risk themselves. Community considerations include having a disaster plan that is prepared and ready for implementation if and when a disaster occurs.

18.4 CHNs are becoming increasingly involved in disaster prevention and mitigation, planning, response, and recovery through their local health unit or health authority. Helping patients maintain a safe environment and advocating for environmental safety measures in the community are key roles for the CHN during all stages of disaster management. It is important for CHNs to know about available community resources, especially for vulnerable populations, during the mitigation stage of disaster management to ensure a smooth response and recovery after a disaster.

CHN IN PRACTICE: A CASE STUDY

A Community Health Nurse Is Challenged in a Tornado Zone

Paula, a PHN in a medium-sized public health department in Forest Ridge, was called to serve on her first municipal disaster assignment. Her disaster skills were tested when a tornado hit the next city and its surrounding areas. Paula left Forest Ridge to help manage an elementary-school cafeteria shelter in the tornado-hit zone.

The devastation that Paula saw en route to the school had a negative effect on her. Assigned to help with patient intake, she patiently listened to the disaster victims, referred many of the most distraught patients to the mental health counsellor, and set priorities for other needs as they arose. For example, she found that many of her patients had left their medications behind and needed therapy. Other needs included diapers and formulas for infants, prescription eyeglasses, and clothing. As the days went on, the stress level in Paula's shelter grew. The crowded living conditions and lack of privacy took its toll on the shelter residents. Around the tenth day of her assignment, Paula began to experience pounding headaches and had difficulty concentrating.

She thought she would be fine, but the mental health counsellor said that she was experiencing a stress reaction.

Think About It

1 Which of the following actions would probably be the most useful for Paula to take? Explain your answer.
   a. Share her feelings with the onsite mental health counsellor on a regular basis.
   b. Call home to share her feelings with family members.
   c. Meet the needs of her patients to the best of her ability and accept the fact that stress is a part of the job.

2. Assume that your community has the potential to be hit by a tornado. List the groups that would be most vulnerable. What steps could you take in advance to reduce their vulnerability? What community resources are available? What steps would you take to adequately prepare for the possible disaster? What steps would you take to ensure safety and preparedness for your family and for the patients for whom you care? Whose help would you enlist? To whom would you go for advice?

TOOL BOX

The Tool Box contains useful resources that can be applied in community health nursing practice. These related resources are found on the Evolve website at http://evolve.elsevier.com/Canada/stanhope/community/.

Tools

Canadian Red Cross. Be Ready: Emergency Preparedness and Recovery (https://www.redcross.ca/how-we-help/emergencies-and-disasters-in-canada/be-ready-emergency-preparedness-and-recovery)

This disaster preparedness guide for families and individuals focuses on how to make a plan, get an emergency kit, and what to do during and after a disaster.

REFERENCES

American Red Cross. (2012). *Disaster mental health handbook.* https://www.cuny.edu/wp-content/uploads/sites/4/page-assets/about/administration/offices/ovsa/disaster-relief/hurricanes-harvey-irma/Disaster-Mental-Health-Handbook.pdf.

Booth, C. M., Matukas, L., Tomlinson, G., et al. (2003). Clinical features and short-term outcomes of 144 patients with SARS in the Greater Toronto Area. *Journal of the American Medical Association, 289*, 2801–2809.

Brecht, H., Deichmann, U., & Wang, H. G. (2013). A global urban risk index. *The World Bank Policy Research Working Paper 6506.* https://www.citiesalliance.org/sites/default/files/WPS6506.pdf.

Campbell, A. (2006). *The SARS Commission—Spring of fear: Final report.* http://www.archives.gov.on.ca/en/e_records/sars/report/v2.html.

Canadian Nurses Association. (2013). *Position statement: Emergency preparedness and response.* https://www.cna-aiic.ca/~/media/cna/page-content/pdf-en/ps119_emergency_preparedness_2012_e.pdf?la=en.

Centers for Disease Control and Prevention (CDC). (2019). *Community assessment for public health emergency response (CASPER).* https://www.cdc.gov/nceh/hsb/disaster/casper/docs/CASPER-toolkit-3_508.pdf.

Cross, C. R. (2014). *3-1-1 prepare pamphlet.* http://www.redcross.ca/crc/documents/3-1-1-Prepare-Pamphlet.pdf.

Cross, C. R. (2020). *Red cross services.* https://www.redcross.ca/how-we-help/emergencies-and-disasters-in-canada/get-help-disaster-relief-and-recovery/red-cross-services.

Dwosh, H. A., Hong, H. H., Austgarden, D., et al. (2003). Identification and containment of an outbreak of SARS in a community hospital. *Canadian Medical Association Journal, 168*(11), 1415–1420.

Environment Canada. (2014). *Canada's top ten weather stories for 2013.* https://www.ec.gc.ca/meteo-weather/default.asp?lang=En&n=5BA5EAFC-1&offset=2&toc=hide.

Etkin, D., Haque, E., Bellisario, L., et al. (2004). *An assessment of natural hazards and disasters in Canada: A report for decision makers and practitioners.* Environment Canada. https://www.researchgate.net/publication/259600580_An_Assessment_of_Natural_Hazards_and_Disasters_in_Canada_A_Report_for_Decision-Makers_and_Practitioners.

Frangoul, A. (2014, February 5). *Counting the costs of a global epidemic. CNBC.* http://www.cnbc.com/2014/02/05/counting-the-costs-of-a-global-epidemic.html.

Gebbie, K. M., & Qureshi, K. (2002). Emergency and disaster preparedness: Core competencies for nurses—what every nurse should but may not know. *American Journal of Nursing, 102*(1), 46–51.

Government of Canada. (2015). *Your emergency preparedness guide.* https://www.getprepared.gc.ca/cnt/rsrcs/pblctns/yprprdnssgd/index-en.aspx.

Government of Canada. (2018). *Federal/provincial/territorial public health response plan for biological events.* https://www.canada.ca/en/public-health/services/emergency-preparedness/public-health-response-plan-biological-events.html.

Government of Canada. (2019). *Emergency preparedness.* https://www.canada.ca/en/health-canada/services/health-concerns/emergencies-disasters/emergency-preparedness.html.

Government of Canada. (2021). *Coronavirus disease (COVID-19): Canada's response.* https://www.canada.ca/en/public-health/services/diseases/2019-novel-coronavirus-infection/canadas-reponse.html.

Government of Manitoba. (n.d.). *Manitoba flood facts.* http://www.gov.mb.ca/flooding/history/index.html.

Health Canada. (2012). *Health concerns: Emergencies and disasters.* http://www.hc-sc.gc.ca/hc-ps/ed-ud/index-eng.php.

Health Canada. (2020). *Be prepared for COVID-19 (factsheet).* https://www.canada.ca/en/public-health/services/publications/diseases-conditions/covid-19-be-prepared.html.

Huston, P. (2004). Commentary: Thinking locally about pandemic influenza. *Canadian Journal of Public Health, 95*(3), 184–185.

International Council of Nurses (ICN). (2020). *More than 600 nurses die from COVID-19 worldwide.* https://www.icn.ch/news/more-600-nurses-die-covid-19-worldwide.

Johnson, M., Bone, E., & Predy, G. (2005). Taking care of the sick and scared: A local response in pandemic preparedness. *Canadian Journal of Public Health, 96*(6), 412–414.

Lemyre, L., Gibson, S., Zlepnig, J., et al. (2009). Emergency preparedness for higher risk populations: Psychosocial considerations. *Radiation Protection Dosimetry, 134*(3–4), 207–214.

McCready, J. (2004). *Ice storm 1998: Lessons learned.* British Columbia: 6th Canadian Urban Forest Conference, Kelowna.

Mildon, B. (2004). In The wake of SARS: Structures and strategies. *Community Health Nurses Association of Canada Newsletter, 6*(3), 1–3.

Milligan, G., & McGuinness, T. M. (2009). Mental health needs in a post-disaster environment. *Journal of Psychosocial Nursing and Mental Health Services, 47*, 23–30.

Natural Resources Canada. (2013). *Natural hazards.* http://www.nrcan.gc.ca/hazards/natural-hazards.

Ontario Ministry of Health and Long-Term Care. (2013). *Ontario health plan for an influenza pandemic.* http://www.health.gov.on.ca/en/pro/programs/emb/pan_flu/pan_flu_plan.aspx.

Parry, J. (2003). China is still not open enough about SARS, says WHO. *British Medical Journal, 326*, 1055.

Public Health Agency of Canada. (2003). *Learning from SARS—Renewal of public health in Canada.* Ottawa, ON: Her Majesty the queen in right of Canada. http://www.phac-aspc.gc.ca/publicat/sars-sras/naylor/index-eng.php.

Public Health Agency of Canada. (2005). *Responding to stressful events: Taking care of ourselves, our families and our communities.* http://www.phac-aspc.gc.ca/publicat/oes-bsu-02/comm-eng.php.

Public Health Agency of Canada. (2018). *The Canadian pandemic influenza plan for the health sector.* https://www.canada.ca/en/public-health/services/flu-influenza/canadian-pandemic-influenza-preparedness-planning-guidance-health-sector.html.

Public Health Agency of Canada. (2009). *FluWatch*. https://www. phac-aspc.gc.ca/cpip-pclcpi/assets/longdesc/figure-1-eng.php.

Public Health Agency of Canada. (2018). *Canadian pandemic influenza preparedness: Planning guidance for the health sector*. https://www.canada.ca/en/public-health/services/flu-influenza/ canadian-pandemic-influenza-preparedness-planning-guidance-health-sector/table-of-contents.html#pre.

Public Safety Canada. (2010). *Disaster assistance programs*. https:// www.publicsafety.gc.ca/cnt/mrgnc-mngmnt/rcvr-dsstrs/dsstr-ssstnc-prgrms/index-eng.aspx.

Public Safety Canada. (2014). *Disaster prevention and mitigation*. https://www.publicsafety.gc.ca/cnt/mrgnc-mngmnt/dsstr-prvntn-mtgtn/index-eng.aspx.

Public Safety Canada. (2017). *An emergency management framework for Canada* (3rd ed.). https://www.publicsafety.gc.ca/ cnt/rsrcs/pblctns/2017-mrgnc-mngmnt-frmwrk/2017-mrgnc-mngmnt-frmwrk-en.pdf.

Registered Nurses' Association of Ontario. (2004). *SARS unmasked: Final report on the nursing experience with SARS in Ontario*. http://www.rnao.org.

Rudden, U. (2020). *Natural disaster losses cost worldwide 2000 – 2020*. https://www.statista.com/statistics/612561/natural-disaster-losses-cost-worldwide-by-type-of-loss/.

Tam, T., Sciberras, J., Mullington, B., et al. (2005). Fortune favours the prepared mind: A national perspective on pandemic preparedness. *Canadian Journal of Public Health*, *96*(6), 406–408.

Tam, T. (2018). Fifteen years post-SARS: Key milestones in Canada's public health emergency response. *Canadian Community Disaster Response*, *44*(5), 98–101. https://doi. org/10.14745/ccdr.v44i05a01.

Tam, T. W. S. (2020). Preparing for uncertainty during public health emergencies: What Canadian health leaders can do now to optimize future emergency response. *Healthcare Management Forum*, *33*(4), 174–177. https://doi. org/10.1177/0840470420917172.

Tolomiczenko, G. S., Kahan, M., Ricci, M., et al. (2005). Sars: Coping with the impact at a community hospital. *Journal of Advanced Nursing*, *50*(1), 101–110.

United Nations Office for Disaster Risk Reduction. (2015). *Sendai framework for disaster risk reduction 2015–2030*. https:// www.undrr.org/publication/sendai-framework-disaster-risk-reduction-2015-2030.

Veenema, T. G. (2013). Essentials of disaster planning. In T. G. Veenema (Ed.), *Disaster nursing and emergency preparedness for chemical, biological, and radiological terrorism and other hazards* (3rd ed.). Springer.

World Health Organization (WHO). (2009). *Current WHO phase of pandemic alert for pandemic (H1N1) 2009*. http://www.who.int/ csr/disease/swineflu/phase/en/.

Aboriginal The original inhabitants of a country; in Canada, *Aboriginal* is used to refer to First Nations people, Inuit, and Métis.

absolute homelessness The condition of people who are perpetually homeless; they are sometimes referred to as the *chronic homeless*.

absolute poverty A deprivation of resources that is life-threatening.

accountability Being answerable to oneself and others (patient, profession, and society) for one's own actions; acting in a manner consistent with professional responsibilities and standards of practice.

acid rain Precipitation that contains atmospheric pollution, such as sulphur dioxide and nitrogen oxides.

acquired immunity The resistance acquired by a host as a result of previous natural exposure to an infectious agent; may be induced by passive or active immunization.

acquired immunodeficiency syndrome (AIDS) A syndrome that can affect the immune and central nervous systems and cause infections or cancers. It is caused by human immunodeficiency virus (HIV).

action research A systematic study of practice interventions.

active immunization The immunization of an individual by the administration of an antigen to stimulate active response by the host's immunologic system, resulting in complete protection against a specific disease.

advocacy Interventions such as speaking, writing, or acting in favour of a particular issue or cause, policy, or group of people.

ageism The term used for discrimination toward older persons because of their age.

agent An animate or inanimate factor that must be present or lacking for a disease or condition to develop; part of the epidemiological triangle.

aggregates Groups within a population.

aging The total of all changes that occur in a person with the passing of time.

allophones People whose mother tongue is neither French nor English.

analytical epidemiology A form of epidemiology that examines the etiology (origins or causes) of a disease and associated determinants of health.

Anthrax An acute disease caused by the spore-forming bacterium *Bacillus anthracis*.

anti-oppressive practice Practice that involves not only accepting and valuing people of different cultures, ages, genders, sexual orientation, abilities, and all lifestyles, beliefs, and practices, but also seeking to dismantle the forces and contexts of oppression and colonization.

assessment A systematic appraisal of type, depth, and scope of health concerns as perceived by patients, health care providers, or both.

asset mapping Identifying community-based assets such as individuals, local associations, businesses, public institutions (e.g., schools, libraries, fire stations), nonprofit organizations, the community's physical characteristics.

autonomy This principle is derived from the Greek words *autos* (self) and *nomos* (rule), which means to self-rule. Autonomy means the ability to self-govern and be one's own person. It is based on human dignity and respect for the individual. Autonomy requires that individuals be permitted to choose those actions and goals that fulfill their life plans unless those choices result in harm to themselves or others.

behavioural risk The pattern of personal health habits that defines individual and family health status.

beneficence This principle is complementary to nonmaleficence and requires that health care providers "do good," which is reflected in the provision of high-quality care based in competent, compassionate practice. See also *nonmaleficence.*

best practice guidelines Recommendations pertaining to specific health issues or practice areas based on the most recent research evidence and key expert experiences and judgments.

bias The negative evaluation of one group and its members relative to another.

bioethics A branch of applied ethics concerned about life issues in relation to the principles of autonomy, beneficence, nonmaleficence, and justice.

biological risk A potential health danger for a person who may be prone to certain illnesses because of genetics or lifestyle patterns.

built environment Anything physical in the environment that is built or produced by humans.

Canadian Nurses Association (CNA) The national voice for provincial and territorial Canadian nursing associations and colleges. Its role is to advocate for nursing and health issues.

Canadian Public Health Association (CPHA) A national organization founded in 1910 to deliver and support national and international health and social service programs.

Canadian Red Cross A national organization founded to reduce human suffering through various health, safety, and disaster-relief programs in affiliation with the International Red Cross.

capacity building The process of actively involving individuals, groups, organizations, and communities in all phases of planned change for the purpose of increasing their skills, knowledge, and willingness to take action on their own in the future.

care coordination An essential indirect function that involves linking clients with services.

care planning The community health nurse and patients working together to provide adequate health care service at home.

case fatality rate (CFR) The proportion of persons diagnosed with a particular disease who die within a specified period of time.

case management A collaborative strategy undertaken by health care providers and patients to maximize the patient's ability and autonomy through advocacy, communication, education, identification of and access to requisite resources, and service coordination.

case manager An individual who advocates for the patient, advises the patient, coordinates and facilitates access to suitable health care services in a timely manner, and ensures continuity of care for the patient.

Centre for Emergency Preparedness and Response (CEPR) A federal government agency under the jurisdiction of the Public Health Agency of Canada. This centre is responsible for coordinating services required to handle all health risk and security threats in Canada.

certification A mechanism, usually by means of written examination, that provides an indication of professional competence in a specialized area of practice.

change agent A nursing role that facilitates change in patient or agency behaviour to more readily achieve goals. This role stresses gathering and analyzing facts and implementing programs.

change partner A nursing role that facilitates change in patient or agency behaviour to more readily achieve goals. This role includes the activities of serving as an enabler-catalyst, teaching problem-solving skills, and being an activist advocate.

chlamydia A sexually transmitted infection caused by the organism *Chlamydia trachomatis,* which causes infection of the urethra and cervix. Infections may be asymptomatic and if untreated result in severe morbidity.

circular communication Reciprocal communication between people, whereby each person influences the behaviour of the other.

cisgender Refers to one's gender identity being aligned with their gender assigned at birth (e.g., a cisgender female is a person who was born female, identifies as female, and uses feminine pronouns such as she and her).

climate change Any significant long-term change in current normal climate conditions, such as temperature, precipitation, extreme weather events, snow cover, and sea level rise.

coalition Two or more groups who share a mutual issue or concern and join forces to attain a common goal in reference to addressing the issue.

code of ethics A framework of moral standards that delineate a profession's values, goals, and obligations.

collaboration The commitment of two or more partners (e.g., agency, patient, professional) to work together to address/ achieve a goal.

collaborative patient-centred practice The active involvement of health care providers from various disciplines working together collaboratively to improve patient health outcomes.

colonialism A policy of acquiring or maintaining colonies; it involves a wealthier power controlling and exploiting another society.

commendations Praise from the health care provider to the family for patterns in behaviour that are family strengths within the family unit.

common vehicle Transportation of the infectious agent from an infected host to a susceptible host via water, food, milk, blood, serum, saliva, or plasma.

communicable disease A contagious disease of human or animal origin caused by an infectious agent. Its transmission depends on the successful interaction of the infectious agent, the host, and the environment, the factors that make up the epidemiological triangle.

communicable period The interval during which an infectious agent may be transferred directly or indirectly from an infected person to another person.

communitarianism The theory that maintains that abstract, universal principles are not an adequate basis for moral decision-making; instead, these theorists argue, history, tradition, institutions, cultural heritage, global values and responsibilities, and concrete moral communities should be the basis of moral thinking and action.

community In the context of community health nursing, people and the relationships that emerge among them as they develop and commonly share agencies, institutions, and a physical environment; members may be defined in terms of geography or a common interest or focus.

community capacity building It involves identifying and working with existing community strengths to promote a positive view of the community; therefore, it is focused on helping communities become stronger based on their strengths rather than letting their weaknesses define them.

community competence It is linked to community problem-solving ability and empowerment. A competent community is able to use its problem-solving abilities to identify and deal with community health issues.

community development A process whereby community members identify health concerns or issues affecting their community that require development of capacity-building skills to bring about a needed change; improving the health of the community by engaging the community in working toward community-identified needs.

community forum A meeting, such as a town hall meeting, in which involved parties can gain an understanding of a particular issue of concern to them; it does not involve decision making.

community health The process of involving the community in maintaining, improving, promoting, and protecting its own health and well-being; it involves status, structure, and process.

community health assessment The process of thinking critically about the community and involves getting to know and understand the community client as partner. Assessments help identify community health concerns and identify strengths and resources.

community health concerns Actual, potential, or possible health challenges within a target population with identifiable contributing factors in the environment.

community health nursing Nursing that takes place in and with the community in a variety of practice areas, such as public health, home health, occupational health, and other similar fields.

community health strengths Resources available to meet community health concerns.

community mobilization The use of community capacity to bring about change through an action plan, usually developed and implemented with community partners.

community partnerships A collaborative decision-making process participated in by community members and professionals. It is crucial because community members and professionals who are active participants in such a process have a vested interest in the success of efforts to improve the health of their community.

comprehensive services Health services that focus on more than one health problem or concern.

concurrent disorder When a mental health issue exists in conjunction with addiction or substance use.

confidentiality The duty to not disclose specific patient information.

consequentialism This theory, a type of teleology, holds that the morality of an action is dependent on the outcome of that action. See also *teleology*.

contact tracing The process of identifying the relevant contacts of a person with an infectious or communicable disease to inform them of their exposure to that disease. Relevant contacts would include those individuals who were exposed to a disease such as measles, or those who had sex with a person during the infectious period of an STI. See also *partner notification*.

contracting Making an agreement between two or more parties; it involves a shift in responsibility and control toward a shared effort by patient and health care provider as opposed to an effort by the health care provider alone. It is a vital component of all nurse–patient relationships.

corrections nurse Registered nurse who works in a clinic in a correctional facility providing community health nursing interventions that include direct care, health promotion, disease prevention, inmate advocacy, and crisis intervention.

cultural awareness Self-examination and in-depth exploration of one's own beliefs and values as they influence behaviour.

cultural blindness A denial of diversity and the inability to recognize the uniqueness of individual patients.

cultural competence It is an ongoing process, rather than an outcome. A culturally competent health care provider is aware of their own cultural identity and views on different cultures and is sensitive to and accepting of patients' differing views.

cultural interaction The verbal and nonverbal communication between persons of different cultures.

cultural interpretation Provided by an interpreter, interpretation of spoken words but with additional information about the culture.

cultural knowledge The information necessary to provide nurses with an understanding of the organizational elements of cultures and to provide effective nursing care.

cultural nursing assessment A systematic way to identify the beliefs, values, meanings, and behaviours of people while considering their history, life experiences, and the social and physical environments in which they live.

cultural pluralism The right of groups to maintain their cultural identity.

cultural proficiency The demonstration of new knowledge and cultural skills, including the communication of this information.

cultural safety Gaining an understanding of others' health beliefs and practices so that one's actions demonstrate working toward equity and the avoidance of discrimination. There is a recognition of and respect for cultural identity so that power balance exists between the health care provider and patient recipient.

cultural sensitivity Being able to reflect on the influence of one's own culture on practice, and to appreciate, "respect, and value cultural diversity."

cultural skill The effective integration of cultural knowledge and awareness to meet patient needs.

cultural understanding Continuous reflections on the effects of culture (values, beliefs, and behaviours) for diverse patients.

culture A set of beliefs, values, and assumptions about life that are widely held among a group of people and that differ from those of another group.

culture shock The feeling of helplessness, discomfort, and disorientation experienced by an individual attempting to understand or effectively adapt to another cultural group that differs in practices, values, and beliefs. It results from the anxiety caused by losing familiar sights, sounds, and behaviours.

data collection The process of acquiring existing, readily available information or developing new information about the community and its health.

data gathering The process of obtaining existing, readily available data.

data generation The process of developing data that does not already exist, through interaction with community members. The data are often qualitative rather than numerical.

database The combination of the gathered and generated data.

decolonization The process of undoing the impact of a colonial state.

demonstration project A project funded externally to promote the testing of ideas and hunches.

deontology An ethical theory that bases moral obligation on duty and claims that actions are obligatory irrespective of the good or bad consequences that they produce; the term means "what is due" or "duty." Because humans are rational, they have absolute value. Therefore, persons should always be treated as ends in themselves and never as mere means.

descriptive epidemiology A form of epidemiology that describes health outcomes in terms of what, who, where, and when.

determinants of health Factors that influence the risk for or distribution of health outcomes. They are income and social status, social support networks, education, employment/working conditions, social environments, physical environments, personal health practices and coping skills, healthy child development, biology and genetic endowment, health services, gender, and culture.

directly observed therapy (DOT) A system of providing medications for persons with tuberculosis infection in which the patient is monitored for taking the medication to maximize adherence to the treatment.

disaster Any human-made or natural event that causes destruction and devastation that cannot be relieved without assistance.

disaster preparedness A readiness to respond to and manage a disaster situation and its consequences.

disaster prevention and mitigation Ongoing activities aimed at minimizing or eradicating risks of natural or human-made disasters before the disasters occur.

disaster recovery Activities that focus on rebuilding to predisaster or near-predisaster conditions and on community safety so that the risk of a recurrence of the disaster is reduced.

disaster response Activities that are carried out by emergency response teams that consist of police, firefighters, medical personnel, and others during and following a disaster.

disaster vulnerability The chance that a disaster is likely to occur; considers the ability of a community to avoid or cope with potential disasters.

discharge planning A process that connects patients and services to ensure an appropriate flow or continuity of care after hospital and in the community.

disease The presence of abnormal alterations in the structure or functioning of the human body that fit within the medical model.

disease course The identifiable progression of disease.

disease prevention The activities taken by the health sector to prevent the occurrence of disease, to detect and stop disease development in those at risk, and to reduce the negative effects once a disease is established.

distal determinants of health Determinants that arise from political, economic, and social realities and include colonialism, racism and social exclusion, and repression of self-determination.

distribution The pattern of a health outcome in a population.

distributive justice Requires that there be a fair distribution of the benefits and burdens in society based on the needs and contributions of its members. This principle requires that, consistent with the dignity and worth of its members and within the limits imposed by its resources, a society must determine a minimal level of goods and services to be available to its members. For community and public health care providers, this principle takes on considerable importance.

district nursing A system in early public health nursing in which a nurse was assigned to each district in a town to provide a wide variety of health services to people in need.

diversity In a cultural context, it considers similarities, differences, and power relations across age, gender, race, religion, occupation, sexual orientation, and poverty.

domestic violence Violence, abuse, or intimidation that may be perpetrated by one person over another in a single act or series of acts that form a pattern of abuse which causes fear or physical and/or psychological harm. It includes relationship or dating violence, intimate partner violence, family violence, and gender-based violence.

downstream thinking An approach to intervention that focuses on individual health concerns and treatments without considering the economic, sociopolitical, and environmental factors. It is curative focused. See also *midstream thinking* and *upstream thinking.*

Ebola virus disease Also known as *Ebola hemorrhagic fever,* it is a deadly viral illness that is caused by infection with one of the Ebola virus strains from the family of *Filoviridae* genus *Ebolavirus.*

ecological footprint A measure of how many natural resources are required to produce the resources we consume and absorb the waste we generate.

ecological study A study that bridges descriptive and analytical epidemiology.

ecomap Represents the family's interactions with other groups and organizations, accomplished by using a series of circles and lines.

economic globalization It is characterized by rising industrial production, energy extraction (i.e., coal, oil and gas), international trade, and consumption of material goods and energy, has further accentuated the effects of global ecological change.

economic risk Determined by the relationship between family financial resources and the demands on those resources.

educator A community health nurse who teaches patients or staff for the purpose of facilitating learning.

elimination The removal of a disease from a large geographical area such as a country or region of the world.

emergency lodging Safe, temporary lodging that is provided to people who cannot return home and cannot find alternate accommodations (e.g., after a natural disaster has occurred).

Emergency Measures Organization (EMO) A provincial or territorial organization that assumes the responsibility for developing, coordinating, and managing emergency response plans within the defined area.

emerging infectious diseases Diseases in which the incidence has increased in the past two decades or has the potential to increase in the near future.

empowerment A process that is used to actively engage the patient to gain greater control and involves political efficacy, improved quality of community life, and social justice.

enabling In the context of health promotion, taking action with patients to empower them to gain control over their health and environment with the goal of improving their health.

endemic The constant presence of a disease in a particular population or geographical area.

engagement The beginning of the interview process with a family, where the focus is on the establishment of the nurse–patient relationship.

environment All that is internal or external to a given host or agent and that is influenced by and influences the host and the agent. Environment also includes social and physical factors; part of the epidemiological triangle.

environmental epidemiology The study of the effect on human health of physical, chemical, and biological factors in the external environment.

environmental ethics A distinct field of ethics that examines the moral relationship of human beings to the environment.

environmental health It encompasses all the physical, chemical, and biological factors external to a person, and all the related factors impacting behaviours.

environmental justice From a population health perspective, the effort to reduce the impact of health inequalities and socioeconomic marginalization of persons resulting from environmental conditions affecting adequate nutrition, shelter, sanitation, and safe working conditions.

environmental scan Assesses both the internal and external environments and is frequently used by researchers to assess population health issues; by organizations to develop, evaluate, and revise programs; and by policy makers to address social, economic, technological, and political issues.

environmental standards Governmental guidelines or rules that impose limits on the amount of pollutants or emissions produced.

epidemic The occurrence of a greater number of cases of a disease, an injury, or other condition than expected in a particular area or group.

epidemiological triangle A simple model that depicts the often-complex relationships among agent, host, and environment.

epidemiology The study of the distribution of factors that determine health-related states or events in a population and the use of this information to control health problems.

equality Equal rights under the law, such as security, voting rights, freedom of speech and assembly, and the extent of property rights. It also includes access to education, health care, and other social goods such as economic good and fundamental political rights, and equal opportunities and obligations; involves the whole society.

equity The idea is about fairness. In the context of health care, it means that all persons should have the opportunity through equal access to reach full health potential.

eradication The permanent elimination of a disease worldwide.

ethical courage The courage to stand firm on a point of moral principle in the face of fear or threat to oneself.

ethical decision making The component of ethical thought that focuses on the process of how ethical decisions are made. It involves making decisions in an orderly process that considers ethical principles, patient values and abilities, and professional obligations.

ethical dilemmas Puzzling moral problems in which a person, group, or community can envision morally justified reasons for both taking and not taking a certain course of action.

ethical disengagement A state of ethical detachment that can arise if the disregard of ethical commitments is seen as normal.

ethical issues Moral challenges facing the nursing profession.

ethical (moral) distress Knowing the right thing to do but—for various reasons—being unable to take the right action or prevent potential harm.

ethical problems Conflicts between one or more values and include uncertainty about the right course of action.

ethical uncertainty A feeling of indecision or a lack of clarity about a matter, accompanied by a sense of unease or discomfort.

ethical violation An action or the failure to act that breaches fundamental duties to others, such as patients and coworkers.

ethics A branch of philosophy that includes both a body of knowledge about the moral life and a process of reflection for determining what persons ought to do or be, regarding this life.

ethnicity The state of belonging to a social group that shares common cultural patterns (e.g., beliefs, values, customs, behaviours, traditions).

ethnocentrism A type of cultural prejudice in which one believes that one's own cultural group is the best, is preferred, and is superior to others.

ethnography A qualitative research method used to understand a culture from the emic (insider) perspective.

evaluation The appraisal of the effects of some organized activity or program. Provision of information through formal means, such as criteria, measurements, and statistics, for making rational judgments necessary about outcomes of care.

evidence-informed practice Combining the best evidence from research with clinical practice, knowledge, and expertise, and patient preferences or choices when making clinical decisions.

experimental or intervention studies Include interventions to test preventive or treatment measures, techniques, materials, policies, or medications. Community or clinical trials are examples of such studies conducted in community health.

faith communities Distinct groups of people who acknowledge specific faith traditions and gather in churches, cathedrals, synagogues, or mosques.

family Two or more individuals who depend on one another for emotional, physical, or financial support. Members of a family are self-defined.

family assessment A comprehensive family data-collection process used to identify the health concerns facing the family. It is the cornerstone for family nursing interventions. Family strengths are emphasized as the building blocks for interventions.

family caregiving Support by family members in the home (which may be paid or unpaid) in order to meet the patient's basic needs such as personal hygiene, meal preparation, and medication preparation.

family crisis A situation whereby the demands of the situation exceed the resources and coping capacity of the family.

family demography The study of the structure of families and households and the family-related events, such as marriage and divorce, that alter the structure through their number, timing, and sequencing.

family functions Behaviours or activities performed to maintain the integrity of the family unit and to meet the family's needs, individual members' needs, and society's expectations.

family health The health of a family system that is ever changing and encompasses a holistic focus that includes biological, psychological, sociological, cultural, and spiritual factors.

family nursing Nurses and families working together to ensure the success of the family and its members in adapting to responses to health and illness.

family nursing theory A theory whose function is to characterize, explain, and predict phenomena (events) evident within family nursing.

family resiliency The ability of family members to cope with expected and unexpected stressors.

family strengths Positive behaviours or qualities that help maintain family health.

family structure The characteristics and demographics (gender, age, number) of individual members who make up a family unit.

family systems nursing model A model that takes a holistic approach to assessment of family health. An example is the Calgary Family Assessment Model, which focuses on the family unit as patient and consists of a structural, developmental, and functional assessment of the family.

feminine ethic A belief in the morality of responsibility in relationships that emphasize connection and caring.

First Nations nurses Community health nurses who practice in urban settings as well as semi-rural, rural, and remote settings; this type of nurse works first and foremost with a First Nation Band.

First Peoples A collective term used to refer to the original inhabitants of Canada.

focus group A small group of individuals residing in the community who are brought together to share their beliefs, opinions, and experiences about a selected discussion topic.

forensic nurses Registered nurses who have additional education in forensic science in order to provide specialized care to persons who have experienced trauma or death from violence, criminal activity, or traumatic accidents.

functional families Family units that provide autonomy and are responsive to the particular interests and needs of individual family members.

gender   Refers to a person's identity and social classifications, often based on masculine or feminine qualities and traits.

gender identity   One's personal sense of gender; can be classified as *cisgender* or *transgender.*

genogram   A drawing that shows the family unit of immediate interest. It includes at least three generations of family members with gender and age, their relationships, health status, and mortality, using a series of circles, squares, and connecting lines.

gerontological nursing   The specialty of nursing concerned with assessment of the health and functional statuses of older persons, planning and implementing health care and services to meet the identified needs, and evaluating the effectiveness of such care.

gerontology   The specialized study of the processes of aging.

global ecological change   A normal process in the earth's evolution and its response to biological shifts.

global health   A field of study, research, and practice that places a priority on improving health and achieving equity in health for all people worldwide.

goals   Generally broad statements of desired outcomes. The end or terminal point toward which intervention efforts are directed.

gonorrhea   A sexually transmitted infection caused by a bacterium, *Neisseria gonorrhoeae,* resulting in dysuria and inflammation of the urethra and cervix, or it may result in no symptoms.

greenhouse gas emissions   Emissions into the earth's atmosphere that trap warm air heated by the sun that contribute to the greenhouse effect; various gases, including carbon dioxide, methane, and nitrous oxide, contribute to the greenhouse effect.

grounded theory   A qualitative research method used for theory development.

group   A collection of two or more individuals in face-to-face interactions with a common purpose(s) and who are in an interdependent relationship.

group process   How a group as a unit is working and how group members interact with one another.

Hantavirus pulmonary syndrome (HPS)   An infectious disease caused by the hantavirus that begins with flu-like symptoms that can become life-threatening when the virus affects the lungs and causes respiratory problems.

harm reduction   A strategy used widely in health policy and practice to reduce harm to an individual or society by modifying hazardous behaviours that are difficult, and in some cases impossible, to prevent.

hazardous waste   Any waste material that poses actual or potential harm to the environment and to humans.

health   A positive resource for everyday living that is holistic—that is, it includes physical, social, and personal capabilities.

health advocacy   A combination of individual and social actions designed (either on behalf of or with others) to gain political and community support of the conditions which promote health.

health disparities   Wide variations in health services and health status among certain populations defined by specific characteristics.

health education   Informing people about health promotion, illness prevention, and treatment; it is a common function and practice of community health nurses in any number of roles and settings.

health enhancement   A health promotion strategy that is used to increase health and resiliency to promote optimal health and well-being (the patient can be at any point on the risk continuum).

health inequities   The principal causes of health disparities that are usually not within the typical domain of health, such as the social determinants; these social, economic, cultural, and political inequities result (directly or indirectly) in health disparities; these differences are considered to be unfair and socially unjust.

health literacy   The ability to access, comprehend, evaluate, and communicate information as a way to promote, maintain, and improve health in a variety of settings across the life-course.

health program   Consists of a variety of planned activities to address the assessed health concerns of patients over time and builds on patient strengths to meet specific goals and objectives.

health program evaluation process   The systematic process of appraising all aspects of a program to determine their impact.

health program implementation process   The systematic process of putting the health program's planned activities into action.

health program management process   Addresses health issues of populations and consists of four steps: assessing, planning, implementing, and evaluating a health program, in partnership with the patient.

health program planning process   An organized approach to identifying and choosing interventions to meet specified goals and objectives that address patient health concerns.

health promotion   The process of enabling people to increase control over and improve their health.

health protection   Focuses on health maintenance by dealing with the immediate health risks.

health risk appraisal   The process of assessing and analyzing for the presence of specific factors in each of the categories that have been identified as being associated with an increased likelihood of an illness developing such as cancer, or an unhealthy event, such as an automobile accident.

health risk reduction   The application of selected interventions based on the assumption that decreasing the number of risks or the magnitude of risk will result in a lower probability of an undesired event.

health risks   Factors that determine or influence whether disease or other unhealthy results occur.

healthy community   A community in which people, organizations, and local institutions work together to improve the social, economic, and environmental conditions that make people healthy—the determinants of health.

healthy living   At the population health level, this refers to the practice of health enhancing behaviours that support, improve, maintain, and enhance population health.

healthy public policy   Policy that is developed with the intent of having a positive effect on or promoting health.

hepatitis A virus (HAV)   A virus that is transmitted by the fecal–oral route. The clinical course of hepatitis A ranges from mild to severe and often requires prolonged convalescence. Onset is usually acute, with fever, nausea, lack of appetite, malaise, and abdominal discomfort, followed after several days by jaundice.

hepatitis B virus (HBV)   A virus that is transmitted through exposure to infected body fluids. Infection results in a clinical picture that ranges from a self-limited acute infection to fulminant hepatitis or hepatic carcinoma, possibly leading to death.

hepatitis C virus (HCV)   A virus that is transmitted through exposure to infected blood and body fluids. Hepatitis C virus infection may present with such mild symptoms that it goes unrecognized.

herd immunity   Immunity of a group or community. The resistance of a group of people to the invasion and spread of an infectious agent.

heterosexual   A person who is sexually attracted to people of the opposite sex; see also *sexual orientation.*

hidden homelessness   The condition of people who may be sleeping in their vehicles and/or use the couch or other temporary sleeping cot at a friend's home.

HIV antibody test   A laboratory ELISA (enzyme-linked immunosorbent assay) test that detects HIV antibodies.

holistic care   Care concerned with the body, mind, and spirit in the promotion of holistic wellness.

home visit   The provision of community health nursing care where the patient resides.

homosexual   A person who is sexually attracted to people of the same sex; gay or lesbian; see also *sexual orientation.*

"honour" killing   When a family member or a self-appointed community leader kills another person perceived as having brought dishonour to the family or community by breaking from traditional social conduct (e.g., by dating or having a relationship with someone not approved by the family, being sexually assaulted, identifying too much with Western culture and ideas, defying family guidance or refusing an arranged marriage, pursuing a higher education or career, leaving an abusive spouse).

horizontal transmission   The person-to-person spread of infection through one or more of the following routes: direct or indirect contact, common vehicle, airborne, or vector borne.

hospice   Palliative system of health care for terminally ill persons. It can take place in the home with family involvement under the direction and supervision of health care providers, especially the home care nurse. Hospice care takes place in the hospital when severe complications of terminal illness occur or when the family becomes too exhausted to fulfill commitments.

hospice care   The delivery of palliative care of the very ill and dying, offering both respite and comfort.

host   A living species (human or animal) capable of being infected or affected by an agent; part of the epidemiological triangle.

human-made disasters   Destruction or devastation caused by humans.

illness   An individual's personal experience of, perception of, and reaction to a disease whereby they are unable to function at their desired "usual" level.

immigrant   A person who has chosen to live in Canada and has been accepted by the Government of Canada and may apply for permanent residency.

implementation   Carrying out a plan that is based on careful assessment of health concerns. The third phase of the community health nursing process, which involves the work and activities aimed at achieving the goals and objectives. Implementation efforts may be made by the person or group who established the goals and objectives, or they may be shared with or even delegated to others.

incidence rate   A measure of the number of new cases of a disease or an event in a population at risk over a defined period.

incubation period   The time interval beginning with invasion by an infectious agent and continuing until the organism multiplies to sufficient numbers to produce a host reaction and clinical symptoms of the disease.

Indian   The legal identity of Indigenous people in Canada who are not Inuit or Métis; this term is used in the *Indian Act* and the *Constitution Act*.

Indigenous   A term that means "native to the area"; it is often used by the United Nations to refer to peoples of long settlement and connection to specific lands.

Indigenous peoples   People or groups defined in legislation as having certain rights based on their historical ties to a specific region and their cultural, linguistic, and spiritual distinctiveness.

Indigenous ways of knowing   Approaches to understanding life that underscore the histories, experiences, and teachings of the people who originate from a land.

indoor air quality   A measure of the chemical, physical, or biological contaminants in indoor air.

inequity   Lack of fairness or justice.

infection   The state produced by the invasion of a host by an infectious agent. Such infection may or may not produce clinical signs.

infectious disease   A disease caused by a microorganism and therefore potentially infinitely transferable to new individuals. It may or may not be communicable.

infectiousness   A measure of the potential ability of an infected host to transmit the infection to other hosts.

influenza pandemic   A pandemic that occurs when a new strain of the influenza A virus, to which people have little or no immunity, has a sustained level of transmission that leads to community outbreaks and has the potential to lead to a worldwide outbreak.

informant interviews   Directed conversation with selected members of a community about community members or groups and events; a direct method of assessment.

injury prevention   The use of strategies to help patients prevent and reduce the risk of injury.

interdependent   The involvement among different groups or organizations within the community that are mutually reliant upon one another.

intergenerational trauma   The transmission of a collective emotional and psychological injury over the lifespan and across generations among Indigenous people and continues to affect the health and well-being of young Indigenous men and women.

intermediate determinants of health   The conditions that give rise to the proximal determinants, such as health care systems; educational systems; community infrastructure, resources, and capacities; environmental stewardship; and cultural continuity.

interpretation   The process by which a spoken or signed message in one language is relayed, with the same meaning, in another language.

interprofessional collaboration   A working agreement in which health team members carefully analyze their role and work together to determine the best plan for a patient's care.

interprofessional team   A team that comprises members with expertise in diverse disciplines (e.g., nurses, social workers, dietitians, physiotherapists, and physicians) who work together during the assessment, planning, implementation, and evaluation of patient care; the patient is considered a member of the team.

intervention activities   Means or strategies used to meet objectives, effect change, and break the health concern cycle.

intimate partner violence   The physical or sexual harassment or psychological aggression by a current or former intimate partner (including a spouse, dating partner, or domestic living partner).

intradisciplinary team   A team that comprises members with expertise in the same discipline.

knowledge exchange   A collaborative, problem-solving process in which researchers and decision makers exchange knowledge to solve problems.

leadership   The act of influencing and directing others; it includes assisting the group to meet its goal(s) and maintaining group cohesiveness.

linguistic interpretation   Interpretation of the spoken word only.

menopause   A developmental stage in which the levels of the hormones estrogen and progesterone change in a woman's body.

meta-analysis   A statistical technique that systematically analyzes the results of multiple studies that are comparable to produce a summary of those results.

microaggressions   The subtle, often automatic and unconscious, verbal and nonverbal slights, insults, and disparaging messages directed towards people in relation to their gender, age, disability, and cultural or racial group membership.

midstream thinking   An approach to intervention that addresses the micro-policy level: regional, local, community, or organizational. See also *downstream thinking* and *upstream thinking*.

monitoring   The periodic or continuous surveillance or testing to determine the level of adherence to statutory requirements or pollutant levels in various media or in humans, plants, and animals.

morality   Values of duty, obligations, and conduct.

morals   Shared generational societal norms about what constitutes right or wrong conduct.

morbidity   The number of reported cases or occurrence of disease in a population.

mortality   The number of deaths in a population.

multiculturalism   A notion that recognizes the diverse ancestry of citizens and supports the ideals of equality and mutual respect among the population's ethnic and cultural groups.

multidisciplinary team   A team that comprises members with expertise in diverse disciplines (e.g., nurses, social workers, dietitians, physiotherapists, and physicians) who work independently to make patient-based decisions.

Native   A term that was considered more appropriate in earlier years; it refers to people who originate from a specific place or local territory and is used only in that context.

natural disasters   Destruction or devastation caused by natural events.

natural history of disease   The course or progression of a disease process from onset to resolution.

natural immunity Species-determined innate resistance to an infectious agent.

negative predictive value The proportion of persons with a negative screening test who do not have the disease; it is interpreted as the probability that an individual with a negative screening test actually does not have the disease.

neglect Intentionally or unintentionally not providing care or a lack of services that are necessary for the physical, spiritual, social, and mental health of an older person who is dependent on a caregiver.

newcomer A person who arrives in a new country to settle there for a variety of reasons and with a variety of background experiences.

nonmaleficence A principle, according to Hippocrates, that requires that we "do no harm." It is impossible to avoid harm entirely, but this principle requires that health care providers act according to the standards of due care, always seeking to produce the least amount of harm possible.

nonpoint source A diffuse pollution source (i.e., without a single point of origin or not introduced into a receiving stream from a specific outlet). The pollutants may be carried off the land by storm water. Examples of nonpoint sources are traffic, fertilizer or pesticide runoff, and animal wastes.

nonsuicidal self-injury A term used to describe self-directed, deliberate harm or alteration of bodily tissue without the presence of suicidal intent and includes behaviours such as self-cutting, head banging, burning, self-hitting, and scratching or picking skin or hair to the point of bleeding.

nurse entrepreneur A community health nurse, a registered nurse who is self-employed in the provision of nursing services to patients in the community or in a variety of settings such as workplaces, government agencies, nonprofit agencies, and private businesses; they may be generalists (e.g., a primary health care nurse practitioner working in an independent practice) or specialists (e.g., a nurse offering foot-care clinics).

nurse practitioner A community health nurse and registered nurse with a minimum of graduate-level academic education in advanced practice nursing.

objectives Specific measurable statements of the steps planned to reach the overall health program goal. Each objective includes an expected date of completion.

occupational and environmental health history A series of questions that provide the data necessary to rule out or confirm job-induced conditions and health concerns.

operational health planning A process that is used on a smaller scale and starts with a specific objective in relation to health program planning.

outcome evaluation An assessment of the results of a program. Also, it can be referred to as *summative evaluation*.

outcomes The results or impact of program interventions.

outpost nurse A community health nurse, a registered nurse who works in remote outpost communities.

outpost nursing Nursing care provided in rural and remote communities.

outrage The emotional public response to the perception of risk related to an environmental issue and where trust in authorities is weak.

palliative approach A paradigm of care that seeks to ensure that all patients who need comfort care would receive it early on, while they are still receiving curative therapies, on an as needed but planned basis.

palliative care Alleviating the symptoms of, meeting the special needs of, and providing comfort for dying patients and their families by the community health nurse.

pandemic An epidemic occurring in a geographically widespread area or in a large population.

parish nurse A community health nurse who is a registered nurse with specialized knowledge who is called to ministry and affirmed by a faith community to promote health, healing, and wholeness.

parish nursing Nursing care provided in the faith community to promote whole-person health among parishioners.

participant observation Conscious and systematic sharing in the life activities and occasionally in the interests and activities of a group of persons; observational methods of assessment; a direct method of data collection.

participatory action research An action-oriented research technique used to develop patient-centred interventions and services and to influence policy.

partner notification Also known as *contact tracing*, it is a population-level intervention aimed at controlling communicable diseases that involves identifying and locating contacts of persons who have been diagnosed with a transmissible disease to notify them of exposure and encourage them to seek medical treatment.

partnership A relationship between individuals, groups, or organizations, in which the partners are actively working together in all stages of planning, implementation, and evaluation.

passive immunization Immunization through the transfer of a specific antibody from an immunized individual to a nonimmunized individual, such as the transfer of antibodies from mother to infant or the administration of an antibody-containing preparation (immune globulin or antiserum).

pastoral care staff Faith community leaders, including clergy, nurses, and educational and youth ministry staff.

patient A patient can be an individual, a family, a group or aggregate, a community, a population, or society.

PEEST An analysis of *policies*, *economic* climate, *environmental* factors, *social* (population and lifestyle trends) factors, and *technological* factors affecting a situation.

phenomenology A qualitative research method used to understand the meaning of the lived experience.

point epidemic A concentration in space and time of a disease event, such that a graph of frequency of cases over time shows a sharp point, usually suggestive of a common exposure.

point source A stationary location or fixed facility from which pollutants are discharged; any single identifiable source of pollution (e.g., a pipe, ditch, ship, ore pit, factory smokestack).

poisons Toxic substances that cause injury, illness, or death to humans and other organisms.

population A large group of people who share one or more personal or environmental characteristics.

population health The health outcomes of a population as measured by the determinants of health and health status indicators.

population-focused practice In contrast to individual-focused health care, it emphasizes reducing health inequities of a defined population or aggregate.

positive predictive value The proportion of persons with a positive screening test who actually have the disease; it is interpreted as the probability that an individual with a positive test has the disease.

poverty Having insufficient financial resources to meet basic living expenses.

precautionary principle The principle that suggests that when a credible doubt in the evidence exists, the appropriate action is to err on the side of caution.

prejudice A negative attitude about a person or group without factual data.

prevalence rate The number of persons in a population who have a disease or experienced an event at a specific period (old and new cases included).

primary care The first contact between individuals and the health care system and usually refers to the curative treatment of disease, rehabilitation, and preventive measures.

primary caregiver The health care provider who is primarily responsible for providing for the health care needs of patients.

primary health care Comprehensive care that includes disease prevention, community development, a wide spectrum of services and programs, working in interprofessional teams, and intersectoral collaboration for healthy public policy. Primary health care is comprehensive and addresses social justice and equity issues.

primary prevention A type of intervention or activity that seeks to prevent the occurrence of a disease (based on the natural history of a disease) or an injury. See also *secondary prevention* and *tertiary prevention*.

primordial prevention Activities that focus on preventing the emergence of risk factors that are known to create the conditions for disease.

principlism An approach to problem solving in bioethics that uses the principles of respect for autonomy, beneficence, nonmaleficence, and distributive justice as the basis for organization and analysis.

process evaluation An assessment of a program or activity while it is in development. Also, it can be referred to as *formative evaluation*.

proportion A type of ratio that shows the relationship between the total number and the frequency of occurrence in the case of a particular health event.

proportionate mortality ratio (PMR) The proportion of all deaths that are the result of a specific cause within a specified period.

protective factors Variables that assist in managing the stressors associated with being at risk; examples of these factors include literacy, social support networks, and family support systems.

proximal determinants of health Conditions that directly affect the health of individuals, such as health behaviours, physical environments, employment and income, social status, education, and food insecurity.

public health An organized activity of society to promote, protect, improve, and when necessary, restore the health of its people; it is a scientific discipline that includes the study of epidemiology, statistics, and assessment as well as program planning and policy development.

public health nursing Community health nursing with a distinct focus on and scope of practice; it requires a specific knowledge base. Public health nursing is built on the blending of nursing and the discipline of public health. It is a practice that involves primary, secondary, and tertiary prevention, with a main focus on primary prevention, health surveillance, and at-risk populations. Public health nurses are employed by government agencies to deliver core public health services.

public health surveillance The continuous, systematic collection, analysis, and interpretation of health-related data needed for the planning, implementation, and evaluation of public health practice.

qualitative research A research methodology that explores human experiences. It uses words, text, or themes rather than numbers to describe the experiences.

quantitative research A research methodology that tests hypotheses and uses numbers to describe relationships, differences, and cause–effect interactions among variables.

queer or questioning The umbrella term for individuals who do not identify as heterosexual.

race Primarily a social classification that relies on physical markers such as skin colour to identify group membership. Individuals may be of the same race but of different cultures.

racializing When heterogeneous groups of non-White people are slotted into one category, which ignores class and ethnic differences.

racially visible Racialized peoples. A synonym for the term *visible minority*.

racism A prejudice in which members of one cultural group perceive themselves to be superior to another cultural group.

randomized controlled trials Research method to test the efficacy and safety of interventions. They must have a random sample, manipulation, and a control group.

rate A measure of the frequency of a health event in a defined population during a specified period.

referral process A systematic process of directing a patient to another source of assistance when the patient or community health nurse is unable to address the patient's issue.

refugee A person who was forced to leave their home country because of a well-founded fear of persecution or because of war.

relational ethics An ethical theory that refers to the relational context of practice and asks, What should I be doing for others?

relational practice Practice that is guided by conscious participation with patients using a number of relational skills, including listening, questioning, empathy, mutuality, reciprocity, self-observation, reflection, and a sensitivity to emotional contexts.

relative poverty Individuals and families whose income is considerably less than that of their peers.

reliability The consistency or repeatability of a measure.

residential schools Religious schools established and funded by the federal government to assimilate Indigenous children.

resiliency The capacity of people to cope effectively when faced with considerable adversity or risk.

resistance The ability of the host to withstand infection; it may involve natural or acquired immunity.

risk The probability of some event or outcome occurring within a specified period of time.

risk assessment Qualitative and quantitative evaluation of the risk posed to human health and/or the environment by the actual or potential presence and/or use of specific pollutants.

risk avoidance A disease prevention strategy that is used to avoid health problems and to remain at low-risk level (the patient is at no or low risk on the continuum).

risk communication The exchange of information on the potential harm of health or environmental hazards among risk assessors and managers, the general public, news media, and interest groups.

risk factors Variables that create stress and therefore challenge the patient's health status; those conditions that have a direct effect on the likelihood of an adverse outcome (i.e., they increase the probability of a poor health outcome).

risk management The selection and implementation of a strategy to reduce risks.

risk reduction A disease prevention strategy that is used to reduce or alter health problems so the disease is detected and treated early to prevent moving to high risk level (the patient is at low to moderate risk).

rural Defined either in terms of the geographical location and population density or the distance from or time needed to commute to an urban centre.

screening The application of a test to persons who are at risk for a certain condition but do not manifest any symptoms.

secondary analysis An analysis using previously gathered data.

secondary prevention Activities that seek to detect a disease early in its progression (early pathogenesis), before clinical signs and symptoms become apparent, to make a diagnosis and begin treatment; it relates to the natural history of a disease. See also *primary prevention* and *tertiary prevention*.

secondary victimization When survivors experience further stress or trauma at the hands of health care providers that engage in victim blaming, insensitive communication techniques, delays in care, disbelief, shaming, stigmatization, or minimization of the experience.

self-determination The ability of a group to decide how its needs will be met without the interference of outside governance.

sensitivity The extent to which a test identifies those individuals who have the condition or trait being examined.

severe acute respiratory syndrome (SARS) A disease of undetermined etiology with no definitive treatment. In early 2003, SARS was first reported in China and Hong Kong.

sex workers People who work for street or brothel prostitution, cybersex, pornography, massage parlours, and other areas of the sex industry.

sexual assault Sexual contact with another person without that person's consent. Often, physically abused women are also forced into sex.

sexual assault nurse examiners Community health nurses, registered nurses who have completed specialized education in forensic science. A sexual assault nurse examiner (SANE) assumes a wide range of roles and responsibilities in response to the physical, emotional, and psychological needs of persons who have experienced sexual assault, regardless of age or gender; they provide crisis intervention, assess injuries, provide pregnancy prevention by offering the morning-after pill, test for and treat sexually transmitted infections (STIs), and collaborate with community partners.

sexual orientation   A person's sexual identity in relation to the gender to which they are attracted. An individual's sexual orientation can be said to be *heterosexual*, *homosexual*, or *bisexual*.

sexuality   The way that people experience and express themselves as sexual beings.

sheltered homelessness   The condition of people who need to use emergency shelters either occasionally or regularly for sleeping purposes.

sink   A process that serves to remove a greenhouse gas, or a precursor of a greenhouse gas, from the atmosphere.

Sixties Scoop   A practice of removing or "scooping" large numbers of Indigenous children from their families and either sending them to foster homes or adopting them out, usually into non-Indigenous families in Canada and the United States.

social determinants of health   The social conditions and broader forces (e.g., politics and economics) that interact to influence risks to health and well-being and affect how vulnerable or resilient people are to disease and injury.

social justice   The fair distribution of society's benefits and responsibilities and their consequences. It focuses on the relative position of one social group in relation to others in society as well as on the root causes of disparities and what can be done to eliminate them.

social risks   Risky social situations that can contribute to the stressors experienced by families. If adequate resources and coping processes are not available, breakdowns in health can occur.

society   Systems that incorporate the social, political, economic, and cultural infrastructure to address issues of concern.

specificity   The extent to which a test identifies those individuals who do not have the condition or trait being examined.

stereotyping   The basis for ascribing generalizations about a group to an individual without giving adequate attention to individual values, beliefs, and behaviours.

strategic health planning   Involves matching patient health needs, patient and provider strengths and competencies, and resources.

structural racism   The normalization and legitimization of an interplay of historical, cultural, institutional, and interpersonal dynamics that routinely advantages White people while producing cumulative and chronic adverse outcomes for people of colour.

structural vulnerability   Risks for negative health outcomes because of the interface of socioeconomic, political, and societal hierarchies of dominance and oppression.

subjective poverty   Individuals and families who perceive that they have insufficient income to meet their expenses.

subpopulations   Aggregates within the larger population.

surveillance   A systematic and ongoing observation and collection of data on disease occurrence to describe phenomena and detect changes in frequency or distribution.

survey   Method of assessment in which data from a sample of persons are reported to the data collector.

sustainability   The maintenance and continuation of established community programs.

SWOT   A method of analysis which identifies *s*trengths, *w*eaknesses, *o*pportunities, and *t*hreats involved in a project or venture.

systematic review   A summary of the research evidence that relates to a specific question and to the effects of an intervention.

team   A specialized group working toward a common goal or activity.

telehealth   The use of information technology to deliver health care services at a distance.

telenurses   Community health nurses who are registered nurses with specific nursing knowledge and skill that includes enhanced assessment skills and strong clinical knowledge necessary to provide nursing service to patients using only information technology.

teleology   An ethical theory that explains phenomena by the purpose they serve; the term means the "logic of ends" or consequences.

termination phase   When the purpose of the visit has been accomplished, the community health nurse reviews with the family what has occurred and what has been accomplished. This phase provides a basis for evaluating whether further home visits are needed or referrals to community resources are required.

tertiary prevention   Activities that begin once the disease is obvious; the goals are to interrupt the course of the disease, reduce the amount of disability that might occur, and begin rehabilitation; it relates to the natural history of a disease. See also *primary prevention* and *secondary prevention*.

testicular self-examination (TSE)   Self-examination of the testicles to assess for any unusual lumps or bumps.

three Ds   Dementia (progressive intellectual impairment), *d*epression (mood disorder), *d*elirium (acute confusion).

transgender   Refers to an incongruence in a person's gender identity with the gender assigned at birth (e.g., a transgender male is a person who was born female, identifies as male, and may use male pronouns such as him and he).

transition   The movement from one developmental or health stage or condition to another that may be a time of potential risk for families.

translation   The written conversion of one language into another.

trauma-informed care   Care that attends to a patient's past experiences of violence or trauma and the role it currently plays in their lives.

Treaty   An agreement between Indigenous peoples and government in which Indigenous peoples ceded their rights to land in exchange for reserves, small cash payments, land-use rights, and other considerations.

triage   The process of separating casualties and allocating treatment based on the victims' potential for survival.

United Nations Children's Emergency Fund (UNICEF)   An international organization that focuses on child survival and development, basic education and gender equality, HIV/AIDS and children, child protection, and policy advocacy and partnerships.

upstream thinking   An approach to intervention that looks beyond the individual to take a macroscopic, big-picture population focus. It also includes a primary prevention perspective and is a population health approach. See also *downstream thinking* and *midstream thinking*.

urban   Geographical areas described as nonrural and having a higher population density.

utilitarianism   A form of consequentialism, this theory holds that a morally right action is one that produces the greatest amount of good or the least amount of harm in a given situation.

vaccine   A preparation of killed microorganisms, living attenuated organisms, or living fully virulent organisms that is administered to produce or artificially increase immunity to a particular disease.

vaccine hesitancy   A delay in obtaining vaccines or refusal to get vaccinated, despite the availability of vaccination services.

validity   The accuracy of a test or measurement; how closely it measures what it claims to measure. In a screening test, validity is measured by sensitivity and specificity.

values   Standards or qualities that are esteemed, desired, or considered important, or that have worth or merit.

vector   A nonhuman organism, often an insect, that either mechanically or biologically plays a role in the transmission of an infectious agent from source to host.

veracity   Telling the truth; it is the nurse's duty to tell the truth. Veracity promotes trust in the nurse–patient therapeutic relationship.

vertical transmission   The passing of an infection from parent to offspring via sperm, placenta, milk, or contact in the vaginal canal at birth.

violence   Those nonaccidental acts, interpersonal or intrapersonal, that result in physical or psychological injury to one or more persons. It can be physical, psychological, sexual, financial, or spiritual abuse.

virtual care   Any interaction between patients and members of their circle of care, occurring remotely, using any forms of communication or information technologies with the aim of facilitating or maximizing the quality and effectiveness of care.

virtue ethics This theory asks, What kind of person should I be? Its goal is to enable persons to flourish as human beings.

virtues Acquired, excellent traits of character that dispose humans to act in accord with their natural good.

visible minority A term used by Statistics Canada to describe people of colour; that is, people who are neither Indigenous nor White.

visiting nurse associations Agencies staffed by visiting nurses who provide care where the patient is located, which is most often in the home.

visiting nurses Community health nurses who provide care wherever the patient is located—home, work, or school.

vulnerable populations Specific populations (e.g., groups or communities) that are at higher risk for poor health as a result of the barriers they experience to social, economic, political, and environmental resources, as well as limitations due to illness or disability.

web of causation An explanation of causal relationships; it recognizes the complex interrelationships among many factors, sometimes interacting in subtle ways to increase (or decrease) the risk of disease. Also known as the *web of causality*.

windshield survey An observational method used as a part of a community health assessment that scans the community's physical environment; it can be conducted by walking or driving through a community.

women's health An area of health care that addresses health promotion, health protection, disease prevention, and health maintenance in women.

work–health interactions The influence of work on health based on statistics on employment-related illnesses, injuries, and deaths.

work-site walk-through An assessment of the workplace conducted by the community health nurse, specifically an occupational health nurse.

World Health Organization (WHO) A leading international health organization involved in global health issues.

Canadian Community Health Nursing Standards of Practice

Purpose of Standards of Practice

- Define the scope and depth of community health nursing practice.
- Establish criteria and expectations for acceptable nursing practice and safe, ethical care.
- Provide criteria for measuring actual performance.
- Support ongoing development of community health nursing.
- Promote community health nursing as a specialty and provide the foundation for certification of community health nursing as a specialty by the Canadian Nurses Association.
- Inspire excellence in and commitment to community nursing practice.

Using the Standards of Practice

All community health nurses are expected to know and use these standards when working in any of the areas of practice, education, administration, policy, and research.

- Nurses in clinical practice use the standards to guide and evaluate their own practice.
- Nursing educators include the standards in course curricula to prepare new graduates for practice in community settings.
- Nurse administrators use the standards to direct policy and guide performance expectations.
- Nurse researchers use the standards to guide the development of knowledge specific to community health nursing.
- Nurse policy advisors/advocates use the standards to guide policy recommendations.

A new nurse entering community health practice will likely need at least two years to achieve the practice expectations of these specialty Standards. Strong mentorship, leadership, and peer support, as well as self-directed and guided learning, all contribute to the achievement of the expertise required.

STANDARD 1: HEALTH PROMOTION

Community health nurses integrate health promotion into their practice using the five Ottawa Charter health promotion strategies (build healthy public policy, create supportive environments, strengthen community actions, develop personal skills, and reorient health services). "Health promotion is the process of enabling people to increase control over, and to improve, their health."

The community health nurse …

a. Applies health promotion theories and models in practice, such as change theories, primary health care, population

health model, and social and ecological determinants of health, including Indigenous peoples.

b. Collaborates with patient to do a comprehensive, evidence-informed, and strength-based holistic health assessment, using multiple sources and methods to identify needs, assets, inequities, and resources.

c. Seeks to identify and assess the root and historical causes of illness, disease, and inequities in health, acknowledges diversity and the adverse effects of colonialism on Indigenous people, and when appropriate incorporates Indigenous ways of knowing, including connectedness and reciprocity to the land and all life, in health promotion.

d. Considers the determinants of health, the social and political context, and systemic structures in collaboration with the patient to determine action.

e. Implements appropriate communication approaches such as social marketing and media advocacy to disseminate health information and raise awareness of health issues at the individual and/or societal level.

f. Includes cultural safety and cultural humility approaches in all health promotion interventions.

g. Uses a collaborative relationship with the patient and other partners to facilitate and advocate for structural system change and healthy public policy, using multiple health promotion strategies.

h. Evaluates and modifies population health promotion activities in partnership with the patient.

STANDARD 2: PREVENTION AND HEALTH PROTECTION

Community health nurses use the socioecological model to integrate prevention and health protection activities into practice. These actions are implemented in accordance with government legislation and nursing standards to minimize the occurrence of diseases or injuries and their consequences.

The community health nurse …

a. Participates in surveillance, recognizes trends in epidemiology data, and utilizes these data through population level actions such as health education, screening, immunization, and communicable disease control management.

b. Uses prevention and protection approaches with the patient to identify risk factors and to address issues such as communicable disease, injury, chronic disease, and the physical environment (e.g., air, climate, housing, work, water, land).

c. Applies the appropriate level of prevention (primordial, primary, secondary, tertiary, and quaternary) to improve patient health.

d. Facilitates informed decision making with the patient for protective and preventive health measures.

e. Collaborates with the patient to provide emergency management, including prevention/mitigation, preparedness, response, and recovery.

f. Uses harm reduction principles grounded in social justice and health equity perspectives to identify and reduce risks and increase protective factors.

g. Includes cultural safety and cultural humility approaches in all aspects of prevention and health protection interventions.

h. Engages in collaborative, interdisciplinary, and intersectoral partnerships in the delivery of preventive and protective services, with particular attention to populations who are marginalized.

i. Evaluates and modifies prevention and health protection activities in partnership with the patient.

STANDARD 3: HEALTH MAINTENANCE, RESTORATION, AND PALLIATION

Community health nurses integrate health maintenance, restoration, and palliation into their practice to maintain function, improve health, and support life transitions, including acute, chronic, or terminal illness, and end of life.

The community health nurse …

a. Holistically assesses the health status and functional competence of the patient within the context of their environment, social supports, and life transitions.

b. Supports informed decision making and co-creates mutually agreed upon plans and priorities for care with the patient.

c. Uses a range of intervention strategies related to health maintenance, restoration, and palliation to promote self-management of disease, maximize function, and enhance quality of life.

d. Includes cultural safety and cultural humility approaches in all aspects of health maintenance, restoration, and palliation interventions.

e. Facilitates maintenance of health and the healing process with the patient in response to adverse health events.

f. Evaluates and modifies health maintenance, disease management, restoration, and palliation interventions in partnership with the patient.

STANDARD 4: PROFESSIONAL RELATIONSHIPS

Community health nurses work with others to establish, build, and nurture professional and therapeutic relationships. These relationships promote optimizing participation and self-determination of the patient.

The community health nurse …

a. Recognizes own personal beliefs, attitudes, feelings, and values, including racism and stereotypes and their potential impact on nursing practice.

b. Assesses the patient's beliefs, attitudes, feelings, and values about health and the impact of these on the professional relationship and potential interventions.

c. "Acknowledges that the current state of Aboriginal health in Canada is a direct result of previous Canadian government policies" when working with Indigenous people, as stated in the Truth and Reconciliation Commission of Canada: Calls to Action.

d. Respects and supports the patient in identifying their health priorities and making decisions to address them, while being responsive to power dynamics.

e. Uses culturally safe communication strategies in professional relationships, recognizing communication may be verbal or nonverbal, written or graphic. Communication can occur via a variety of media.

f. Recognizes and promotes the development of the patient's social support networks as an important social determinant of health.

g. Promotes awareness of, and supports linkages to, appropriate community resources that are acceptable to the patient.

h. Maintains professional boundaries in therapeutic patient relationships.

i. Negotiates terminating therapeutic relationships in a professional manner.

j. Builds a network of relationships and partnerships with a wide variety of individuals, families, groups, communities, and systems to address health issues and promote healthy public policy to advance health equity.

k. Incorporates the domains from the National Interprofessional Competencies framework in working with other nurses and health care team members. Domains include 1) interprofessional communication, 2) patient/family/community-centred care, 3) role clarification, 4) team functioning, 5) collaborative leadership, and 6) interprofessional conflict resolution.

l. Evaluates and reflects on the nurse/patient and other community relationships to ensure responsive and effective nursing practice.

STANDARD 5: CAPACITY BUILDING

Community health nurses partner with the patient to promote capacity. The focus is to recognize barriers to health and to mobilize and build on existing strengths.

The community health nurse …

a. Uses an asset approach and facilitates action to support the priorities of the Jakarta Declaration.

b. Enhances the patient's ability to recognize their strengths, their challenges, causal factors, and resources available that impact their health.

c. Assists the patient to make informed decisions in determining their health goals and priorities for action.

d. Uses capacity building strategies such as mutual goal setting, visioning, and facilitation in planning for action.

e. Helps the patient to identify and access available resources to address their health needs.

f. Supports the patient to build their capacity to advocate for themselves.

g. Supports the development of an environment that enables the patient to make healthy lifestyle choices, recognizing relevant cultural factors and Indigenous ways of knowing.

h. Recognizes the unique history of Indigenous people, and incorporates Indigenous ways of knowing and culturally safe engagement strategies in capacity building efforts.

i. Uses a comprehensive mix of strategies, such as coalition building, intersectoral collaboration, community engagement and mobilization, partnerships, and networking, to build community capacity to take action on priority issues.

j. Supports community-based action to influence policy change in support of health.

k. Evaluates the impact of capacity building efforts, including both process and outcomes in partnership with the patient.

STANDARD 6: HEALTH EQUITY

Community health nurses recognize the impacts of the determinants of health, and incorporate actions into their practice such as advocating for healthy public policy. The focus is to advance health equity at an individual and societal level.

The community health nurse ...

a. Engages with the patient using social theory and an intersectional approach from a foundation of equity and social justice.

b. Assesses how the social determinants of health influence the patient's health status, with particular attention to patients who are marginalized.

c. Understands how power structures, unique perspectives, and expectations may contribute to the patient's engagement with health-promoting services.

d. Advocates for and with the patient to act for themselves.

e. Participates with community members and advocates for health in intersectoral policy development and implementation to reduce health equity gaps between populations.

f. Engages with patients who are marginalized in the coordinating and planning of care, services, and programs that address their needs and perspectives on health and illness.

g. Refers, coordinates, and facilitates patient access to universal and equitable health-promoting services that are acceptable and responsive to their needs across the life span.

h. Collaborates with community partners to coordinate and deliver comprehensive patient services, with the goal of reducing service gaps and fragmentation.

i. Understands historical injustices, inequitable power relations, institutionalized and interpersonal racism and their impacts on health and health care, and provides culturally safe care.

j. Supports the patient's right to choose alternate health care options, including "to recognize the value of Aboriginal healing practices and use them in the treatment of Aboriginal patients in collaboration with Aboriginal healers and Elders where requested by Aboriginal patients," as stated in the Truth and Reconciliation Commission of Canada: Calls to Action.

k. Advocates for resources allocation using a social justice lens.

l. Uses strategies such as home visits, outreach, technology, and case finding to facilitate equitable access to services and health-supporting conditions for populations who are marginalized.

m. Advocates for healthy public policy and social justice by participating in legislative and policy-making activities that influence the determinants of health and access to services.

n. Takes action with and for the patient at the organizational, municipal, provincial and territorial, and federal levels to address service gaps, inequities in health, and accessibility issues.

o. Evaluates and modifies efforts to increase accessibility to health and community services, and to advance health equity.

STANDARD 7: EVIDENCE-INFORMED PRACTICE

Community health nurses use best evidence to guide nursing practice and support patients in making informed decisions.

The community health nurse ...

a. Uses professional expertise in considering the best available research evidence, and other factors, such as patient context and preferences and available resources, to determine nursing actions.

b. Seeks out reliable sources of available evidence from nursing and other relevant disciplines.

c. Understands and uses critical appraisal skills to determine quality of research evidence.

d. Understands and uses knowledge translation strategies to integrate high-quality research into clinical practice, education, and research.

e. Uses quality evidence to inform policy advocacy, development, and implementation.

f. Uses a variety of information sources, including acknowledging diverse perspectives and Indigenous ways of knowing.

STANDARD 8: PROFESSIONAL RESPONSIBILITY AND ACCOUNTABILITY

Community health nurses demonstrate professional responsibility and accountability as a fundamental component of their autonomous practice.

The community health nurse ...

a. Assesses and identifies unsafe, unethical, illegal, or socially unacceptable circumstances and takes preventive or corrective action to protect the patient.

b. Recognizes ethical dilemmas and applies ethical principles and the CNA Code of Ethics.

c. Works collaboratively in determining the best course of action when responding to ethical dilemmas.

d. Provides leadership in collaboration with the community to advocate for healthy public policy based on the foundations of health equity and social justice.

e. Identifies and acts on factors that enhance or hinder the delivery of quality care.

f. Participates in the advancement of community health nursing by mentoring students and new practitioners.

g. Participates in professional development activities and opportunities to be involved in research.

h. Identifies and works proactively (individually or by participating in relevant professional organizations) to address health and nursing issues that affect the patient and/or the profession.

i. Provides constructive feedback to peers as needed to enhance community health nursing practice.

j. Documents community health nursing activities in a timely and thorough manner.

k. Advocates for effective and efficient use of community health nursing resources.

l. Uses reflective practice to continually assess and improve personal community health nursing practice, including cultural safety and cultural humility.

m. Acts upon legal obligations (applicable provincial/territorial/federal legislation) to report to relevant authorities any situations involving unsafe or unethical care.

n. Uses available resources to systematically evaluate the achievement of desired outcomes for quality improvement in community health nursing practice.

Source: Adapted from Community Health Nurses of Canada. (2019). *Canadian community health nursing: Professional practice model and standards of practice.* https://www.chnc.ca/standards-of-practice. Reprinted with permission.

CNA Position Statement: Social Determinants of Health

CNA POSITION

- A Health in All Policies approach is best situated to promote health equity. Policies addressing income, employment, education, housing, transportation, and others should be evaluated in their planning stages for their impact on health.
- All facets of nursing[1] practice, in collaboration with others in and outside of the health sector, should strive to reduce, and ultimately eliminate, health inequity.
- Nurses must include the social determinants of health in their assessment and interventions with individuals, families, and communities.
- Nursing education must incorporate the analysis of the social determinants of health, starting with a critical understanding of the political, economic, and social factors that are at the root of health inequities.

CNA BELIEFS

CNA believes nurses have a professional and ethical responsibility to promote health equity through action on the social determinants of health (Canadian Nurses Association [CNA], 2017).

CNA recognizes the important, but limited, influence the health system has on health outcomes and we therefore acknowledge that addressing the social determinants of health needs to be a priority. We believe that a Health in All Policies approach can address inequity because many of the determinants of health are outside the narrow domain of the health-care sector and policies. This approach challenges policy-makers to consider how their decisions will affect the health of the population at all levels and in all areas of governance (WHO, 2014).

CNA believes intersectoral collaboration is a key tool for prioritizing the social determinants of health. We further believe that we must break long-existing organizational silos (de Andrade et al., 2015) by engaging with external stakeholders, such as interest groups, elected officials, municipal and provincial government staff, as well as health care service providers to bring equity to the forefront of the policy agenda (McPherson, Ndumbe-Eyoh, Oickle et al., 2016).

We believe partnership, input, and guidance at the community level are necessary components to policies that address the social determinants of health because community members understand the context and unique challenges where they live (McGill, Egan, Petticrew et al., 2015). This is especially important for Indigenous communities, which are disproportionately affected by the social determinants of health (Kolahdooz, Nader, & Sharma, 2015).

BACKGROUND

The social determinants of health are "the conditions in which people are born, grow, live, work and age. These circumstances are shaped by the distribution of money, power, and resources at global, national, and local levels" (World Health Organization [WHO], 2018, para. 1). They include:
- The conditions of early childhood
- Access to education
- The nature of employment and working conditions
- Access to healthy housing and adequate income
- Social inclusion
- The quality of the built and natural environment in which people reside (American Academy of Family Physicians, 2018; McClintock & Bogner, 2017; WHO, 2008)

Different groups will "have different experiences of material conditions, psychosocial support and behavioural options, which make them more or less vulnerable to poor health" (WHO, 2008, p. 3). Individual choices are constrained or promoted by these conditions (Braveman & Gottlieb, 2014; Mahony & Jones, 2013). Hence, WHO refers to the social determinants of health as the "causes of the causes" (WHO, 2008, p. 42).

Social determinants also affect the ability to access and use health care, which have "consequences for the inequitable promotion of health and well-being, disease prevention, and illness recovery and survival" (WHO, 2008, p. 3).

This relationship between people's health and factors outside traditional health care is being recognized in many forms. For instance, the United Nations' 2030 agenda for sustainable development seeks to improve various conditions such as ending poverty and ensuring quality education (United Nations, 2015; Government of Canada, 2018a and 2018b). The social determinants of health are also being emphasized in the Health in All Policies approach, which considers the health

---

[1]Unless otherwise stated, *nurse* or *nursing* refers to any member of a regulated nursing category (i.e., a registered nurse, nurse practitioner, licensed/registered practical nurse, or registered psychiatric nurse). This definition reflects the current situation in Canada, whereby nurses are deployed in a variety of collaborative arrangements to provide care.

impacts of policies in areas such as finance, education, housing, employment, and transport. In helping policymakers, this approach "takes into account the health implications of decisions, seeks synergies and avoids harmful health impacts in order to improve population health and health equity" (WHO, 2018, p. 2).

The social determinants of health are the primary factor behind health inequities (CNA, 2010). Such inequities represent differences in distribution of health between different populations and are "likely to reinforce or exacerbate disadvantage and vulnerability" (Public Health Agency of Canada [PHAC], 2018, p. 14). Furthermore, health inequities are "inconsistent with Canadian values, threaten the cohesiveness of community and society, challenge the sustainability of the health system, and have an impact on the economy" (PHAC, 2018, p. 13).

The economic impact of health inequities is evident even in a developed country like Canada, where statistics show that approximately one in seven Canadians live in poverty, including almost a quarter of Indigenous people (Citizens for Public Justice, 2020). First Nations, Inuit, and Métis people experience additional barriers to health due to a history of colonization, racism, social exclusion, and the repression of self-determination, both in general society and within health care (Reading & Wien, 2009). While there have been some improvements in absolute values, the relative gap between Indigenous and non-Indigenous people continues to widen across a variety of categories, including education and income (Mitrou, Cooke, Lawrence et al., 2014). As such, challenges remain.

One policy challenge has been the shift from a biomedical to a biopsychosocial model, the latter being a better reflection of the social determinants of health (Tallon, Kendall, Priddis et al., 2017). Furthermore, the determinants have often been poorly defined, in part because they are embedded in a complex web of causation (Baum, Laris, Fisher et al., 2013: Embrett & Randall, 2014). As a result, shorter term policies have taken precedence (Embrett & Randall, 2014).

Approved by the CNA Board of Directors

November 2018

Replaces: *Social Determinants of Health* (2013).

REFERENCES

American Academy of Family Physicians. (2018). *Addressing social determinants of health in primary care: Team-based approach for advancing health equity*. https://www.aafp.org/dam/AAFP/documents/patient_care/everyone_project/team-based-approach.pdf.

Baum, F. E. et al. (2013). "Never mind the logic, give me the numbers": Former Australian health ministers' perspectives on the social determinants of health. *Social Science & Medicine, 87,* 138–146. https://doi.org/10.1016/j.socscimed.2013.03.033.

Braveman, P., & Gottlieb, L. (2014). The social determinants of health: It's time to consider the causes of the causes. *Public Health Reports, 129*(2), 19–31. https://doi.org/10.1177/00333549141291S206.

Canadian Nurses Association (CNA). (2010). *Social justice … A means to an end, an end in itself* (2nd ed.). . https://www.cna-aiic.ca/~/media/cna/page-content/pdf-en/social_justice_2010_e.pdf.

Canadian Nurses Association (CNA). (2017). *Code of ethics for registered nurses.* https://www.cna-aiic.ca/html/en/Code-of-Ethics-2017-Edition/files/assets/basic-html/page-1.html#.

Canadian Nurses Association. (2018). *CNA Position Statement: Social determinants of health.* https://www.cna-aiic.ca/-/media/cna/page-content/pdf-en/social-determinants-of-health-position-statement_dec-2018.pdf?la=en&hash=CCD26634EF89E493DA64F60345A3AAB399089797.

Citizens for Public Justice. (2020). *Poverty trends 2017.* https://cpj.ca/wp-content/uploads/2020/09/Poverty-Trends-2020.pdf

de Andrade, L. O. M. et al. (2015). Social determinants of health, universal health coverage, and sustainable development: Case studies from Latin American countries. *Lancet, 385,* 1343–1351. https://doi.org/10.1016/S0140-6736(14)61494-X.

Embrett, M. G., & Randall, G. E. (2014). Social determinants of health and equity policy research: Exploring the use, misuse, and nonuse of policy analysis theory. *Social Science & Medicine, 108,* 147–155. https://doi.org/10.1016/j.socscimed.2014.03.004.

Government of Canada. (2018a). *The 2030 agenda for sustainable development.* http://international.gc.ca/world-monde/issues_development-enjeux_developpement/priorities-priorites/agenda-programme.aspx?lang=eng.

Government of Canada. (2018b). *Social determinants of health and health inequalities.* https://www.canada.ca/en/public-health/services/health-promotion/population-health/what-determines-health.html.

Kolahdooz, F. et al. (2015). Understanding the social determinants of health among Indigenous Canadians: Priorities for health promotion policies and actions. *Global Health Action, 8*(1), 1–16. https://doi.org/10.3402/gha.v8.27968.

Mahony, D., & Jones, E. J. (2013). Social determinants of health in nursing education, research, and health policy. *Nursing Science Quarterly, 26*(3), 280–284. https://doi.org/10.1177/0894318413489186.

McClintock, H. F., & Bogner, H. R. (2017). Incorporating patients' social determinants of health into hypertension and depression care: A pilot randomized controlled trial. *Community Mental Health Journal, 53*(6), 1–20. https://doi.org/10.1007/s10597-017-0131-x.

McGill, E. et al. (2015). Trading quality for relevance: Non-health decision-makers' use of evidence on the social determinants of health. *BMJ Open, 5,* 1–8. https://doi.org/10.1136/bmjopen-2014-007053.

McPherson, C. et al. (2016). Swimming against the tide: A Canadian qualitative study examining the implementation of a province-wide public health initiative to address health equity. *International Journal for Equity in Health, 15,* 1–18. https://doi.org/10.1186/s12939-016-0419-4.

Mitrou, F. et al. (2014). Gaps in indigenous disadvantage not closing: a census cohort study of social determinants of health in Australia, Canada, and New Zealand from 1981–2006. *BMC Public Health, 14,* 1–9. https://doi.org/10.1186/1471-2458-14-201.

Reading, C., & Wien, F. (2009). *Health inequalities and social determinants of Aboriginal peoples' health.* https://www.ccnsa-nccah.ca/docs/determinants/RPT-HealthInequalities-Reading-Wien-EN.pdf.

Public Health Agency of Canada (PHAC). (2018). *Key health inequalities in Canada: A national portrait.* https://www.canada.ca/content/dam/phac-aspc/documents/services/publications/science-research/key-health-inequalities-canada-national-portrait-executive-summary/hir-full-report-eng.pdf.

Tallon, M. M. et al. (2017). Barriers to addressing social determinants of health in pediatric nursing practice: An integrative review. *Journal of Pediatric Nursing, 37,* 51–56. https://doi.org/10.1016/j.pedn.2017.06.009.

United Nations, Department of Economic and Social Affairs. (2015). *Transforming our world: The 2030 agenda for sustainable development.* https://sustainabledevelopment.un.org/post2015/transformingourworld.

World Health Organization (WHO). (2008). *Closing the gap in a generation: Health equity through action on the social determinants of health.* http://www.who.int/social_determinants/final_report/en/index.html.

World Health Organization (WHO). (2014). *Health in all policies. Helsinki statement. Framework for country action.* http://apps.who.int/iris/bitstream/handle/10665/112636/9789241506908_eng.pdf?sequence=1.

World Health Organization (WHO). (2018). *Social determinants of health.* http://www.who.int/social_determinants/sdh_definition/en/.

SOURCE: Canadian Nurses Association. (2018). *CNA Position Statement: Social determinants of health.* https://www.cna-aiic.ca/-/media/cna/page-content/pdf-en/social-determinants-of-health-position-statement_dec-2018.pdf?la=en&hash=CCD26634EF89E493DA64F60345A3AAB399089797

Declaration of ALMA-ATA

The International Conference on Primary Health Care, meeting in Alma-Ata this twelfth day of September in the year nineteen hundred and seventy-eight, expressing the need for urgent action of all governments, all health and development workers, and the world community to protect and promote the health of all the people of the world, hereby makes the following Declaration:

I

The Conference strongly reaffirms that health, which is a state of complete physical, mental, and social wellbeing, and not merely the absence of disease or infirmity, is a fundamental human right and that the attainment of the highest possible level of health is a most important worldwide social goal, whose realization requires the action of many other social and economic sectors in addition to the health sector.

II

The existing gross inequality in the health status of the people, particularly between developed and developing countries and within countries, is politically, socially, and economically unacceptable and is therefore of common concern to all countries.

III

Economic and social development, based on a new international economic order, is of basic importance to the fullest attainment of health for all and to the reduction of the gap between the health status of developing and developed countries. The promotion and protection of the health of the people are essential to sustained economic and social development and contribute to a better quality of life and to world peace.

IV

The people have the right and duty to participate individually and collectively in the planning and implementation of their health care.

V

Governments have a responsibility for the health of their people, which can be fulfilled only by the provision of adequate health and social measures. In the coming decades a main social target of governments, international organizations, and the whole world community should be the attainment by all peoples of the world by the year 2000 of a level of health that will permit them to lead a socially and economically productive life. Primary health care is the key to attaining this target as part of development in the spirit of social justice.

VI

Primary health care is essential health care based on practical, scientifically sound, and socially acceptable methods and technology made universally accessible to individuals and families in the community through their full participation and at a cost that the community and country can afford to maintain at every stage of their development in the spirit of self-reliance and self-determination. It forms an integral part both of the country's health system, of which primary health care is the central function and main focus, and of the overall social and economic development of the community. It is the first level of contact for individuals, the family, and the community with the national health system bringing health care as close as possible to where people live and work, and it constitutes the first element of a continuing health care process.

VII

Primary health care:
1. Reflects and evolves from the economic conditions and sociocultural and political characteristics of the country and its communities and is based on the application of the relevant results of social, biomedical, and health services research and public health experience.
2. Addresses the main health problems in the community, providing promotive, preventive, curative, and rehabilitative services accordingly.
3. Includes at least education concerning prevailing health problems and the methods of preventing and controlling them; promotion of food supply and proper nutrition; an adequate supply of safe water and basic sanitation; maternal and child health care, including family planning; immunization against the major infectious diseases; prevention and control of locally endemic diseases; appropriate treatment of common diseases and injuries; and provision of essential drugs.

4. Involves, in addition to health sector, all related sectors and aspects of national and community development, in particular agriculture, animal husbandry, food industry, education, housing, public works, communication, and other sectors; and demands the coordinated efforts of all those sections.

5. Requires and promotes maximum community and individual self-reliance and participation in the planning, organization, operation, and control of primary health care, making fullest use of local, national and other available resources; and to this end, develops through appropriate education the ability of communities to participate.

6. Should be sustained by integrated, functional, and mutually supportive referral levels, leading to the progressive improvement of comprehensive health care for all, and giving priority to those most in need.

7. Relies, at local and referral levels, on health workers, including physicians, nurses, midwives, auxiliaries, and community workers, as applicable, as well as on traditional practitioners as needed, suitably trained socially and technically to work as a health team and to respond to the expressed health needs of the community.

VIII

All governments should formulate national policies, strategies, and plans of action to launch and sustain primary health care as part of a comprehensive national health system and in coordination with other sectors. To this end, it will be necessary to exercise political will, to mobilize the country's resources, and to use available external resources rationally.

IX

All countries should cooperate in a spirit of partnership and service to ensure primary health care for all people because the attainment of health by people in any one country directly concerns and benefits every other country. In this context the joint WHO-UNICEF report on primary health care constitutes a solid basis for the further development and operation of Primary Health Care throughout the world.

X

An acceptable level of health for all the people of the world by the year 2000 can be attained through a fuller and better use of the world's resources, a considerable part of which is now spent on armaments and military conflicts. A genuine policy of independence, peace, détente, and disarmament could and should release additional resources that could well be devoted to peaceful aims and in particular to the acceleration of social and economic development of which primary health care, as an essential part, should be allotted its proper share.

SOURCE: Reprinted from Declaration of Alma-Ata, World Health Organization. Copyright 1978. http://www.who.int/publications/almaata_declaration_en.pdf

Ottawa Charter for Health Promotion

The first international Conference on Health Promotion, meeting in Ottawa this 21st day of November 1986, hereby presents this charter for action to achieve Health for All by the year 2000 and beyond.

This conference was primarily a response to growing expectations for a new public health movement around the world. Discussions focused on the needs in industrialized countries, but took into account similar concerns in all other regions. It built on the progress made through the Declaration on Primary Health Care at Alma Ata, the World Health Organization's Targets for Health for All document, and the recent debate at the World Health Assembly on intersectoral action for health.

HEALTH PROMOTION

Health promotion is the process of enabling people to increase control over, and to improve, their health. To reach a state of complete physical, mental, and social well-being, an individual or group must be able to identify and to realize aspirations, to satisfy needs, and to change or cope with the environment. Health is, therefore, seen as a resource for everyday life, not the objective of living. Health is a positive concept emphasizing social and personal resources, as well as physical capacities. Therefore, health promotion is not just the responsibility of the health sector but goes beyond healthy lifestyles to well-being.

Prerequisites for Health

The fundamental conditions and resources for health are peace, shelter, education, food, income, a stable ecosystem, sustainable resources, social justice, and equity. Improvement in health requires a secure foundation in these basic prerequisites.

Advocate

Good health is a major resource for social, economic, and personal development and an important dimension of quality of life. Political, economic, social, cultural, environmental, behavioural, and biological factors can all favour health or be harmful to it. Health promotion action aims at making these conditions favourable through *advocacy* for health.

Enable

Health promotion focuses on achieving equity in health. Health promotion action aims at reducing differences in current health status and ensuring equal opportunities and resources to *enable* all people to achieve their fullest health potential. This includes a secure foundation in a supportive environment, access to information, life skills, and opportunities for making healthy choices. People cannot achieve their fullest health potential unless they are able to take control of those things which determine their health. This must apply equally to women and men.

Mediate

The prerequisites and prospects for health cannot be ensured by the health sector alone. More importantly, health promotion demands coordinated action by all concerned: by governments, by health and other social and economic sectors, by nongovernmental and voluntary organizations, by local authorities, by industry, and by the media. People in all walks of life are involved as individuals, families, and communities. Professional and social groups and health personnel have a major responsibility to *mediate* between differing interests in society for the pursuit of health. Health promotion strategies and programmes should be adapted to the local needs and possibilities of individual countries and regions to take into account differing social, cultural, and economic systems.

HEALTH PROMOTION ACTION MEANS

Build Healthy Public Policy

Health promotion goes beyond health care. It puts health on the agenda of policymakers in all sectors and at all levels, directing them to be aware of the health consequences of their decisions and to accept their responsibilities for health.

Health promotion policy combines diverse but complementary approaches, including legislation, fiscal measures, taxation, and organizational change. It is coordinated action that leads to health, income, and social policies that foster greater equity. Joint action contributes to ensuring safer and healthier goods and services, healthier public services, and cleaner, more enjoyable environments.

Health promotion policy requires the identification of obstacles to the adoption of healthy public policies on non–health sectors, and ways of removing them. The aim must be to make the healthier choice the easier choice for policymakers as well.

Create Supportive Environments

Our societies are complex and interrelated. Health cannot be separated from other goals. The inextricable links between people and their environment constitutes the basis for a socio-ecological approach to health. The overall guiding principle for the world, nations, regions, and communities alike, is the need to encourage reciprocal maintenance—to take care of each other, our communities, and our natural environment. The conservation of natural resources throughout the world should be emphasized as a global responsibility.

Changing patterns of life, work, and leisure have a significant impact on health. Work and leisure should be a source of health for people. The way society organizes work should help create a healthy society. Health promotion generates living and working conditions that are safe, stimulating, satisfying, and enjoyable.

Systematic assessment of the health impact of a rapidly changing environment—particularly in areas of technology, work, energy production, and urbanization—is essential and must be followed by action to ensure positive benefit to the health of the public. The protection of the natural and built environments and the conservation of natural resources must be addressed in any health promotion strategy.

Strengthen Community Action

Health promotion works through concrete and effective community action in setting priorities, making decisions, planning strategies, and implementing them to achieve better health. At the heart of this process is the empowerment of communities, their ownership and control of their own endeavours and destinies.

Community development draws on existing human and material resources in the community to enhance self-help and social support, and to develop flexible systems for strengthening public participation and direction of health matters. This requires full and continuous access to information, learning opportunities for health, as well as funding support.

Develop Personal Skills

Health promotion supports personal and social development through providing information, education for health and enhancing life skills. By so doing, it increases the options available to people to exercise more control over their own health and over their environments, and to make choices conducive to health.

Enabling people to learn throughout life, to prepare themselves for all of its stages, and to cope with chronic illness and injuries, is essential. This has to be facilitated in school, home, work, and community settings. Action is required through educational, professional, commercial, and voluntary bodies, and within the institutions themselves.

Reorient Health Services

The responsibility for health promotion in health services is shared among individuals, community groups, health professionals, health service institutions, and governments. They must work together towards a health care system which contributes to the pursuit of health.

The role of the health sector must move increasingly in a health promotion direction, beyond its responsibility for providing clinical and curative services. Health services need to embrace an expanded mandate which is sensitive and respects cultural needs. This mandate should support the needs of individuals and communities for a healthier life, and open channels between the health sector and broader social, political, economic, and physical environment components.

Reorienting health services also requires stronger attention to health research, as well as changes in professional education and training. This must lead to a change of attitude and organization of health services, which refocuses on the total needs of the individual as a whole person.

MOVING INTO THE FUTURE

Health is created and lived by people within the settings of their everyday life; where they learn, work, play, and love. Health is created by caring for oneself and others, by being able to take decisions and have control over one's life circumstances, and by ensuring that the society one lives in creates conditions that allow the attainment of health by all its members.

Caring, holism, and ecology are essential issues in developing strategies for health promotion. Therefore, those involved should take as a guiding principle that, in each phase of planning, implementation, and evaluation of health promotion activities, women and men should become equal partners.

Commitment to Health Promotion

The participants of this conference pledge:
- to move into the arena of healthy public policy, and to advocate a clear political commitment to health and equity in all sectors
- to counteract the pressures towards harmful products, resource depletion, unhealthy living conditions, and environments, and bad nutrition; and to focus attention on public health issues such as pollution, occupational hazards, housing, and settlements
- to respond to the health gap within and between societies, and to tackle the inequities in health produced by the rules and practices of these societies
- to acknowledge people as the main health resource; to support and enable them to keep themselves, their families, and friends healthy through financial and other means, and to accept the community as the essential voice in matters of its health, living conditions, and well-being
- to reorient health services and their resources towards the promotion of health; and to share power with other sectors, other disciplines and most importantly, with people themselves
- to recognize health and its maintenance as a major social investment and challenge; and
- to address the overall ecological issue of our ways of living.

The conference urges all concerned to join them in their commitment to a strong public health alliance.

Call for International Action

The Conference calls on the World Health Organization and other international organizations to advocate the promotion of health in all appropriate forums and to support countries in setting up strategies and programmes for health promotion.

The Conference is firmly convinced that if people in all walks of life, nongovernmental and voluntary organizations, governments, the World Health Organization, and all other bodies concerned join forces in introducing strategies for health promotion, in line with the moral and social values that form the basis of this charter, Health for All by the Year 2000 will become a reality.

This charter for action was developed and adopted by an international conference, jointly organized by the World Health Organization, Health and Welfare Canada, and the Canadian Public Health Association. Two hundred and twelve participants from 38 countries met from November 17 to 21, 1986, in Ottawa, Canada to exchange experiences and share knowledge of health promotion.

The Conference stimulated an open dialogue among lay, health, and other professional workers, among representatives of governmental, voluntary and community organizations, and among politicians, administrators, academics, and practitioners. Participants coordinated their efforts and came to a clearer definition of the major challenges ahead. They strengthened their individual and collective commitment to the common goal of Health for All by the Year 2000.

This charter for action reflects the spirit of earlier public charters through which the needs of people were recognized and acted upon. The charter presents fundamental strategies and approaches for health promotion which the participants considered vital for major progress. The conference report develops the issues raised, gives concrete examples and practical suggestions regarding how real advances can be achieved, and outlines the action required of countries and relevant groups.

The move towards a new public health is now evident worldwide. It was reaffirmed not only by the experiences but by the pledges of Conference participants who were involved as individuals on the basis of their expertise. The following countries were represented: Antigua, Australia, Austria, Belgium, Bulgaria, Canada, Czechoslovakia, Denmark, Eire, England, Finland, France, German Democratic Republic, Federal Republic of Germany, Ghana, Hungary, Iceland, Israel, Italy, Japan, Malta, Netherlands, New Zealand, Northern Ireland, Norway, Poland, Portugal, Romania, St. Kitts-Nevis, Scotland, Spain, Sudan, Sweden, Switzerland, Union of Soviet Socialist Republics, United States of America, Wales, and Yugoslavia.

SOURCE: Reprinted from *Ottawa Charter for Health Promotion*, Copyright 1986. http://www.phac-aspc.gc.ca/ph-sp/docs/charter-chartre/pdf/charter.pdf

The Giger and Davidhizar Transcultural Assessment Model

CULTURALLY UNIQUE INDIVIDUAL

1. Place of birth
2. Cultural definition
   What is …
3. Race
   What is …
4. Length of time in country (if appropriate)

COMMUNICATION

1. Voice quality
   A. Strong, resonant
   B. Soft
   C. Average
   D. Shrill
2. Pronunciation and enunciation
   A. Clear
   B. Slurred
   C. Dialect (geographical)
3. Use of silence
   A. Infrequent
   B. Often
   C. Length
      (1) Brief
      (2) Moderate
      (3) Long
      (4) Not observed
4. Use of nonverbal
   A. Hand movement
   B. Eye movement
   C. Entire body movement
   D. Kinesics (gestures, expression, or stances)
5. Touch
   A. Startles or withdraws when touched
   B. Accepts touch without difficulty
   C. Touches others without difficulty
6. Ask these and similar questions:
   A. How do you get your point across to others?
   B. Do you like communicating with friends, family, and acquaintances?
   C. When asked a question, do you usually respond (in words or body movement, or both)?
   D. If you have something important to discuss with your family, how would you approach them?

SPACE

1. Degree of comfort
   A. Moves when space invaded
   B. Does not move when space invaded
2. Distance in conversations
   A. 30 to 45 cm (0 to 18 inches)
   B. 45 cm to 90 cm (18 inches to 3 feet)
   C. 90 cm (3 feet) or more
3. Definition of space
   A. Describe degree of comfort with closeness when talking with or standing near others
   B. How do objects (e.g., furniture) in the environment affect your sense of space?
4. Ask these and similar questions:
   A. When you talk with family members, how close do you stand?
   B. When you communicate with coworkers and other acquaintances, how close do you stand?
   C. If a stranger touches you, how do you react or feel?
   D. If a loved one touches you, how do you react or feel?
   E. Are you comfortable with the distance between us now?

SOCIAL ORGANIZATION

1. Normal state of health
   A. Poor
   B. Fair
   C. Good
   D. Excellent
2. Marital status
3. Number of children
4. Parents living or deceased?
5. Ask these and similar questions:
   A. How do you define social activities?
   B. What are some activities that you enjoy?
   C. What are your hobbies, or what do you do when you have free time?
   D. Do you believe in a Supreme Being?
   E. How do you worship that Supreme Being?
   F. What is your function (what do you do) in your family unit/system?
   G. What is your role in your family unit/system (father, mother, child, advisor)?
   H. When you were a child, what or who influenced you most?

I. What is/was your relationship with your siblings and parents?

J. What does work mean to you?

K. Describe your past, present, and future jobs.

L. What are your political views?

M. How have your political views influenced your attitude toward health and illness?

TIME

1. Orientation to time
   A. Past-oriented
   B. Present-oriented
   C. Future-oriented
2. View of time
   A. Social time
   B. Clock-oriented
3. Physiochemical reaction to time
   A. Sleeps at least 8 hours a night
   B. Goes to sleep and wakes on a consistent schedule
   C. Understands the importance of taking medication and other treatments on schedule
4. Ask these and similar questions:
   A. What kind of timepiece do you wear daily?
   B. If you have an appointment at 2 PM, what time is acceptable to arrive?
   C. If a nurse tells you that you will receive a medication in "about a half hour," realistically, how much time will you allow before calling the nurse's station?

ENVIRONMENTAL CONTROL

1. Locus-of-control
   A. Internal locus-of-control (believes that the power to affect change lies within)
   B. External locus-of-control (believes that fate, luck, and chance have a great deal to do with how things turn out)
2. Value orientation
   A. Believes in supernatural forces
   B. Relies on magic, witchcraft, and prayer to affect change
   C. Does not believe in supernatural forces
   D. Does not rely on magic, witchcraft, or prayer to affect change
3. Ask these and similar questions:
   A. How often do you have visitors at your home?
   B. Is it acceptable to you for visitors to drop in unexpectedly?
   C. Name some ways your parents or other persons treated your illnesses when you were a child.
   D. Have you or someone else in your immediate surroundings ever used a home remedy that made you sick?
   E. What home remedies have you used that worked? Will you use them in the future?
   F. What is your definition of "good health"?
   G. What is your definition of illness or "poor health"?

BIOLOGICAL VARIATIONS

1. Conduct a complete physical assessment noting:
   A. Body structure (small, medium, or large frame)
   B. Skin colour
   C. Unusual skin discolorations
   D. Hair colour and distribution
   E. Other visible physical characteristics (e.g., keloids, chloasma)
   F. Weight
   G. Height
   H. Check lab work for variances in hemoglobin, hematocrit, and sickle cell phenomena if Black or Mediterranean
2. Ask these and similar questions:
   A. What diseases or illnesses are common in your family?
   B. Describe your family's typical behaviour when a family member is ill.
   C. How do you respond when you are angry?
   D. Who (or what) usually helps you to cope during a difficult time?
   E. What foods do you and your family like to eat?
   F. Have you ever had any unusual cravings for
      (1) White or red clay dirt?
      (2) Laundry starch?
   G. When you were a child, what types of foods did you eat?
   H. What foods are family favourites or are considered traditional?

NURSING ASSESSMENT

1. Note whether the patient has become culturally assimilated or observes own cultural practices.
2. Incorporate data into plan of nursing care:
   A. Encourage the patient to discuss cultural differences; people from diverse cultures who hold different views can enlighten nurses.
   B. Make efforts to accept and understand methods of communication.
   C. Respect the individual's personal need for space.
   D. Respect the rights of patients to honour and worship the Supreme Being of their choice.
   E. Identify a clerical or spiritual person to contact.
   F. Determine whether spiritual practices have implications for health, life, and well-being (e.g., Jehovah's Witnesses may refuse blood and blood derivatives; an Orthodox Jew may eat only kosher food high in sodium and may not drink milk when meat is served).
   G. Identify hobbies, especially when devising interventions for a short or extended convalescence or for rehabilitation.
   H. Honour time and value orientations and differences in these areas. Allay anxiety and apprehension if adherence to time is necessary.
   I. Provide privacy according to personal need and health status of the patient. (NOTE: The perception of and reaction to pain may be culturally related.)

J. Note cultural health practices.
  (1) Identify and encourage efficacious practices.
  (2) Identify and discourage dysfunctional practices.
  (3) Identify and determine whether neutral practices will have a long-term ill effect.
K. Note food preferences.
  (1) Make as many adjustments in diet as health status and long-term benefits will allow and that dietary department can provide.
  (2) Note dietary practices that may have serious implications for patient.

SOURCE: Davidhizar, R. E., & Giger, J. N. (1998). *Canadian transcultural nursing: Assessment and intervention.* Mosby.

Community-As-Partner Model

The community-as-partner model was developed to illustrate community health nursing as a synthesis of community health and nursing. The model, originally titled *community-as-client,* has evolved to incorporate the philosophy that nurses work with communities as partners. This is congruent with knowing that communities and people change and grow best by full involvement and self-empowerment.

At the heart of the model is the community assessment wheel, which identifies the community's people as partners at the core and incorporates the use of the nursing process to plan nursing care for the community (Vollman, Anderson & MacFarlane, 2016). Without the people there is no community, and it is the people (their demographics, values, beliefs, history) that are of interest to the public health nurse. Surrounding the people: physical environment, education, safety and transportation, politics and government, health and social services, communication, economics, and recreation. These eight subsystems both affect and are affected by each other and the community.

Identifying the strengths in the community is an important step in assessing community health problems and concerns. Community strengths are the lines of defense and resistance that help the community to deal with stressors. Lines of defense are depicted in the community-as-partner model as "flexible" or "normal" to indicate that there are two types of defense: one is the usual or normal "health" of a community and the other is more dynamic or flexible, and changes more rapidly. Two illustrations may assist in clarifying these lines. The flexible lines of defense may be a temporary response to a stressor. For instance, an environmental stressor such as flash flooding or a major fire may call into play resources from within the community and from surrounding areas; these resources are considered the flexible lines of defense. The normal line of defense is the usual level of health a community has reached over time. Examples of normal lines of defense include the immunization rate, adequate housing, or access to Meals-on-Wheels for shut-ins; all of these are normal lines of defense against stressors.

Stressors can affect the community and may be from within or outside the community. Either way, the community's response to the stressors is mitigated by its overall health status, that is, by the strength of its lines of resistance and defense. Learning about these strengths is one of the purposes of a community assessment, which is the first step in formulating a community health nursing diagnosis. In the analysis phase of the nursing process, the CHN will assess the strength of the stressors, as compared to the lines of resistance, and assess the community's degree of reaction to the stressors. This analysis will help the CHN formulate a nursing diagnosis that will give direction to the plan of care, interventions, and evaluation.

One method for formulating a community nursing diagnosis is to state the community health problem or concern and the degree of reaction to the stressor (from which the goal is derived) as related to the stressors. Using this method, an example of a community health nursing diagnosis might be as follows: High risk for communicable diseases (the problem, the degree of reaction) related to poor sanitation, crowded living conditions, poverty, and noncompliance to medical treatment, as manifested by lack of sewage treatment facility, lack of affordable housing, and high incidence and prevalence of TB (the stressors identified in the community assessment) (Figure A6.1). The community's lines of defense could include affordable housing programs and policies, a local community health clinic that provides patient education on communicable diseases, and public schools that have resources to support communicable disease education programs. This example of a community nursing diagnosis has identified some of the stressors arising from two of the community subsystems: the environment and health that are having an effect on the community's flexible lines of defense.

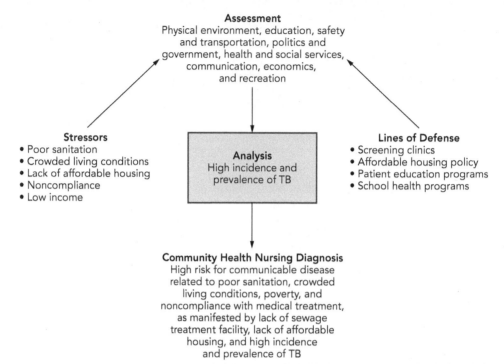

Assessment
Physical environment, education, safety and transportation, politics and government, health and social services, communication, economics, and recreation

Stressors
- Poor sanitation
- Crowded living conditions
- Lack of affordable housing
- Noncompliance
- Low income

Analysis
High incidence and prevalence of TB

Lines of Defense
- Screening clinics
- Affordable housing policy
- Patient education programs
- School health programs

Community Health Nursing Diagnosis
High risk for communicable disease related to poor sanitation, crowded living conditions, poverty, and noncompliance with medical treatment, as manifested by lack of sewage treatment facility, lack of affordable housing, and high incidence and prevalence of TB

FIG. A6.1 Community Assessment and Diagnosis. In summary, the community-as-partner model proposes a systematic approach to assessing and analyzing community health needs and concerns in partnership with the community's people. Using the community-as-partner model could help CHNs formulate appropriate community-focused interventions that would help promote community health. (*Source:* Vollman, A.R. et al. (2016). *Canadian community as partner: theory & multidisciplinary practice* (4th ed., p. 208, Figure 15.3). Lippincott Williams & Wilkins.)

The Calgary Family Assessment Model and the Calgary Family Intervention Model

ASSESSING THE NEEDS OF THE FAMILY: THE CALGARY FAMILY ASSESSMENT MODEL

Family assessment is essential to providing responsive, compassionate, and respectful family care and support. To help families adjust to acute and chronic illness, nurses need to understand the relationships that family members share, what the illness means to the family members, how the illness has influenced family functioning, how the family has been affected by the illness, and the support the family is most in need of (Shajani & Snell, 2019). Box A7.1 lists the particular features of families who should be considered for a family assessment. During an assessment, the nurse, patient, and family relationally and collaboratively engage in conversation to share information with each other and explore family members' experiences of illness, while simultaneously reflecting on issues important to the patient's and family's well-being.

The Calgary Family Assessment Model (CFAM) is a relational, strengths-focused practice model that guides nurses in the completion of a comprehensive family assessment (Shajani & Snell, 2019). The CFAM has received international recognition and has been adopted by schools of nursing around the world. The CFAM focuses on three major categories of family life: structural, developmental, and functional dimensions. Each category has several subcategories; however, not all subcategories will be relevant to every family (see Fig. A7.1). Nurses must decide, on a family-by-family basis, which subcategories are most relevant. Using too many subcategories may result in an overwhelming amount of data and questions for family members; using too few may yield insufficient data, which can distort a family's strengths and/or challenges. The model can be consulted during discussions about family issues.

Structural Assessment

The structural dimension of the family assessment includes:
- *Internal structure*—The people who are included in the family and how they are relationally connected to one another
- *External structure*—The relationships the family shares with people and institutions outside the family unit
- *Context*—The whole situation or background relevant to the family

Internal Structure

The internal structure of the family—the composition and relationships shared by family members—can be further divided into six subcategories: family composition, gender, sexual orientation, rank order, subsystems, and boundaries.

Family composition. *Family composition* refers to the individual members who form the family. The family composition is not limited to the traditional nuclear family; it may include any of the various family forms. It is important to note whether any recent additions or losses to the family composition have occurred.

> *Questions to Ask the Family: Who is in your family? Does anyone else live with you, for example, grandparents, boarders? Has anyone recently moved out, married, or died? Can you think of anyone else who is like a family member but is not biologically related?*

Gender. *Gender* is the set of beliefs about or expectations of masculine or feminine behaviours and experiences. These beliefs are fundamental to intimate relationships and are influenced by culture, religion, and family. It is useful to understand how male and female members of a particular family may view and experience the world differently.

> *Questions to Ask the Family: How have your parents' ideas about masculinity and femininity affected your own? Have your ideas about gender been challenged in any way since you become parents? Do you have expectations of your children on the basis of their gender? Is the division of labour at home based on gender roles?*

Sexual orientation. *Sexual orientation* refers to the heterosexual, gay, lesbian, bisexual, or transgendered orientation. Heterosexism, a belief that male–female bonding is the only legitimate type of bonding, is a form of bias that can affect families and health care providers. Discrimination based on sexual orientation remains a problem. Unless relevant to the patient's or family's presenting concern, the nurse does not usually ask questions about sexual orientation but avoids stereotyping or making assumptions when asking general questions.

Rank order. The order of children by age and gender is called *rank order*. The birth order, gender, and distance in age between siblings are important considerations because they may influence roles and behaviours. The child's characteristics and the family's idealized "program" for the child (going

---

BOX A7.1 Features of Families Who Should Be Considered for a Family Assessment

Families who may benefit most from a family assessment include those who:

- Are experiencing emotional, physical, or spiritual suffering or disruption caused by a family crisis (e.g., acute, chronic, or life-threatening illness, injury, death, addiction, and/or suspected family violence)
- Are experiencing emotional, physical, or spiritual suffering or disruption caused by a developmental milestone (e.g., birth, marriage, child leaving home)
- Define a problem or illness as a family issue (e.g., the impact of chronic illness on the family)
- Have a child or adolescent whom they identify as having difficulties (e.g., cyberbullying at school, fear of cancer treatment)
- Are experiencing issues that are serious enough to jeopardize family relationships (e.g., terminal illness, abuse, addictions)
- Have a family member who is about to be admitted to the hospital for psychiatric or mental health care
- Have a child admitted to the hospital

Source: Adapted from Shajani, Z., & Snell, D. (2019). *Wright and Leahey's Nurses and Families: A Guide to Family Assessment and Intervention* (7th ed., p. 5). Philadelphia: F.A. Davis Company. Reprinted with permission.

---

to school, college, university, work, getting married, and so forth) are also important.

> *Questions to Ask the Family: How many children are in your family? What are the children's ages? Do you have distinct expectations for the oldest and younger children?*

Subsystems. Subsystems are smaller groups of relationships (i.e., based on generation, interests, skills, or gender) within a family. For example, a family could have a sibling subsystem, a husband–wife subsystem, and a parent–child subsystem. Each family member usually belongs to several subsystems, and in each subsystem, they play a different role, use different skills, and have a different level of power (i.e., a teenager behaves differently with her younger sister than she does with her father). Adapting to the demands of different subsystems is a necessary skill for each family member.

> *Questions to Ask the Family: What groups have you noticed in your family? Are there times when disagreements occur among and between the subgroups in your family? If your family had more or fewer subgroups, what effect do you think that might have? What might you most like to change about the subgroups in your family?*

Boundaries. Boundaries define family subsystems and distinguish one subsystem from another. They influence how members participate in each subsystem. For example, a child in a parent–child subsystem may be given certain responsibilities and power but is not expected to be involved with family decision making. Boundaries can be weak, rigid, or

flexible, and they change over time as family members age or are gained or lost.

> *Questions to Ask the Family: Who do you talk with when you feel happy? Who do you talk with when you feel sad? Does the family have any "unwritten" rules about topics never to be discussed outside of the family?*

External Structure

External structure refers to the connections that family members have to persons outside the family. Two subcategories to external structure exist: extended family and larger systems.

Extended family. *Extended family* includes the family of origin, and current generation, and step-relatives. How each member sees themselves as an individual, yet also as part of the family, should be critically assessed. The nurse should note whether family members make many references to the extended family during the interview and inquire about the nature of the relationships shared with extended family members.

> *Questions to Ask the Family: Where do your parents live? How often do you have contact with them and your siblings? Which family members do you see or speak with regularly? Who in your extended family are you closest to? Have members of your extended family been helpful to you during this time of illness? In what way?*

Larger systems. *Larger systems* are groups with whom the family has meaningful contact. Groups include health care organizations, work, religious affiliations, school, friends, and social agencies such as public welfare, child welfare, foster care, and courts. Usually, contact with such larger systems is helpful. However, some families have difficult relationships with individuals from these groups, which can create stress for the family.

> *Questions to Ask the Family: How many health agencies regularly interact with you? What agency professionals are involved with your family? How have they been helpful or not helpful to your family? How are you hoping the nurse might support you differently than other professionals involved in your family's care?*

Context

Context refers to the situation or background relevant to the family. A family can be viewed in the context of ethnicity, race, social class, spirituality and religion, and environment.

Ethnicity. *Ethnicity*, which is the concept of a family's cultural, historical, geographic, linguistic, and ethnic heritage, can greatly influence family interaction. Ethnicity often influences a family's functioning, structure, perspectives, values, health beliefs, and philosophies. Cultural and ethnic heritage can affect, for example, religious practices, child-rearing practices, recreational activities, and nutrition. Individually focused assessment is important, as different members of an

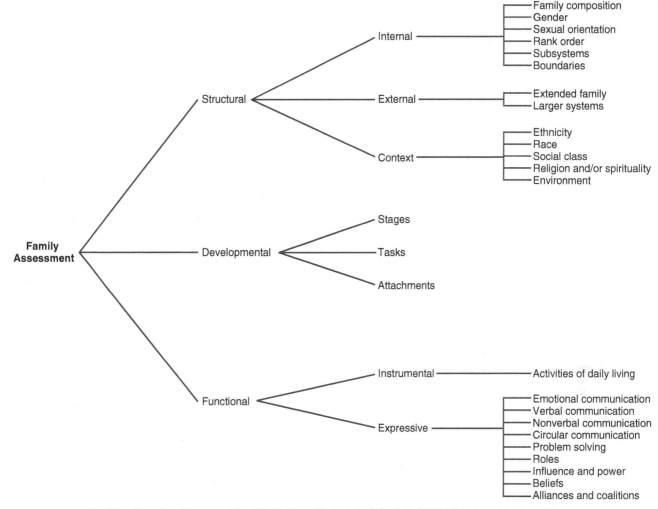

Fig. A7.1 Branching Diagram of the CFAM. (From Shajani, Z., & Snell, D. [2019]. Wright and Leahey's Nurses and Families: A Guide to Family Assessment and Intervention [7th ed.]. F.A. Davis.)

ethnic group may subscribe to differing beliefs, traditions, and restrictions, even within the same generation.

Questions to Ask the Family: Do you think of your family as having a strong ethnic identity? Has your ethnic background influenced your health care? Could you tell me about ethnic traditions you practise? How are these traditions helpful to your family?

Race. *Race* (biological characteristics such as skin and hair colour) influences individual and group identification and is closely connected to ethnicity. Family members' interactions among themselves and with health care providers are influenced by racial attitudes, stereotypes, and discrimination. If ignored, these influences may constrain the nurse and family's relationship.

Questions to Ask the Family: If you and I were of the same race, would our conversation be different? How?

Social class. *Social class* is shaped by education, income, and occupation. Each class has its own values, lifestyles, and

behaviours that influence family interaction and health care practices.

Questions to Ask the Family: What is your job? How many hours a week do you work? How does this affect your family life? Does anyone in the family work shifts? How does that influence your family functioning? What level of education have you completed? Does your family have economic challenges at this time?

Religion and spirituality. Family members' spiritual or religious beliefs, rituals, and practices can influence their ability to cope with or manage an illness or health concern (McLeod & Wright, 2008; Walsh 2010a, 2010b; Wright 2005, 2008; Wright & Bell, 2009). Spirituality is often an underused resource in family nursing. Increasingly, families choose to explore the spiritual beliefs and practices that best fit their multifaith lives, beliefs about spirituality, and relationships. Spiritual assessment and support will therefore be highly individualized within an inquiry-oriented approach (Hartrick Doane & Varcoe, 2006; Walsh, 2010a).

Questions to Ask the Family: What spiritual practices does your family have? What priority do these practices hold in your family? Have your family's spiritual beliefs changed or been challenged in any way during this illness? Are you involved in a particular church, temple, mosque, synagogue, group, religious, or spiritual community? Would you discuss a family problem with anyone from your place of worship? Do you consider your spiritual beliefs a resource? A source of stress?

Environment. The family *environment* refers to the larger community, neighbourhood, and home contexts. Environmental factors that may affect family functioning include availability or lack of adequate space and of access to schools, day care, recreation, and public transportation.

Questions to Ask the Family: What are the advantages and disadvantages of living in your neighbourhood? What community services does your family use? What community services would you like to learn about?

Structural Assessment Tools

The CFAM encourages nurses who work with family members to create genograms and ecomaps to facilitate documentation and understanding of the family structure and its contact with outside individuals and organizations. A *genogram* is a sketch of the family structure and relevant information about family members (see Fig. 12.4 in Chapter 12). Some agencies have genogram forms, but genograms can also be sketched on other forms, such as admission forms and records. The genogram becomes part of the documentation about the client and family. An *ecomap* is a sketch of the family's relationship with persons and groups outside of the family (see Fig. 12.5 in Chapter 12). The family members who share the household are depicted in the centre of the ecomap, and various important extended family members or larger systems are sketched in to show their relationship to the family.

Nurses are encouraged to draw genograms and ecomaps for families with whom they will be involved for more than one day. Information for brief genograms and ecomaps can be gleaned from family members during the initial assessment of the family structure. The most essential information for genograms includes data about ages, occupation or schooling, religion, ethnicity, and current health status of family members. For a brief genogram, the nurse focuses only on information that is relevant to the family and the health problem. The shared creation of a genogram by a nurse and family can be an important time for the nurse to engage with the family, forming a relational connection between family members and the nurse. Engagement can be facilitated through the use of humour, curiosity, and invitations for family members to describe the strengths they see in one another. For example, the nurse might ask a child (8 years old), "What do you most like about your dad?"

Developmental Assessment

Families, like individuals, change and grow over time. Although each family is unique, all families tend to go through certain stages that require family members to adjust, adapt, and change roles. Each developmental stage presents challenges and includes tasks that need to be completed before the family can successfully move on to the next stage. Family development is more than the concurrent development of children and adults. It is the interaction between an individual's development and the phase of the family developmental life cycle that can be significant for family functioning. Therefore, in addition to understanding family structure, nurses need to understand the developmental life cycle of each family.

In their articulation of the expanded family life cycle, McGoldrick, Garcia Preto and Carter (2016) described the emotional process of life cycle transition, as well as the family development tasks for different stages. The family life cycle stages they describe include "Emerging Young Adults, Couple Formation: The Joining of Families, Families with Young Children, Families with Adolescents, Launching Children and Moving on at Midlife, Families in Late Middle Age, and Families Nearing the End of Life" (pp. 24–25). Additionally, the unique challenges faced by lone-parent, lesbian, gay, bisexual, and transgender families, as well as those facing transitions related to divorce, are discussed. Understanding family development theory can help nurses to promote health during expected family life cycle transitions and experiences of illness. For further information, please see *The Expanding Family Life Cycle: Individual, Family, and Social Perspectives* (5th ed.). (McGoldrick et al, 2016).

Functional Assessment

A *functional assessment* focuses on how family members interact and behave toward each other. Nurses assess family functioning by closely observing the interactions of family members in two subcategories: instrumental and expressive functioning.

Instrumental Functioning

Instrumental functioning refers to the normal activities of daily living, such as preparing meals, eating, sleeping, and attending to health needs. For families with health problems, these activities often become a challenge. Roles may change as family members cope with a relative's illness and disability. Within the context of illness, nurses and other health care providers play an important role in accessing practical and financial resources to support family members' instrumental needs (e.g., financial resources for medical supplies that parents need to care for an ill child at home).

Questions to Ask the Family: Who is usually responsible for housekeeping and childcare? Do other family members help with these tasks? Does anyone in the family require help with activities of daily living? Who usually provides this help?

Expressive Functioning

Expressive functioning refers to the ways in which people communicate. The significance of communication within the family cannot be emphasized enough, for it has a profound impact on a family's adjustment to illness and on their resiliency in the face of developmental and illness-related challenges. Illness and disability often alter expressive functioning within the family. A diagnosis may cause intense feelings of anxiety or grief, both within the person being diagnosed and within other family members. Nurses should encourage families to explore their understanding of illness and how it impacts their lives. Nurses may need to assist family members with these difficult conversations, given the emotional intensity of this communication. There are 10 subcategories of expressive functioning: emotional, verbal, nonverbal, and circular communication; problem solving; roles; influence and power; beliefs; and alliances and coalitions.

Emotional communication. *Emotional communication* encompasses the range and types of feelings that are expressed by the family. Most families express a wide range of feelings. However, families with problems may have rigid patterns with narrower ranges of emotional expression (e.g., a family coping with a father's cancer diagnosis may be anxious and unable to express optimism or hope for the future). Family roles and gender may affect emotional expression. For example, brothers and sisters who have a sibling with a life-threatening illness may not express their own experiences of suffering because they want to protect their family from further distress and worry.

Questions to Ask the Family: How can you tell when each member of your family is happy, sad, or under stress? How do you express happiness, sadness, or stress? When you are sad or worried, who in the family do you most like to spend time with or talk to about that?

Verbal communication. Nurses should observe a family's verbal communication, focusing on the meaning of the words in terms of the relationship. Is communication among family members clear and direct, or is it vague and indirect? The nurse should also ask family members about how well the family communicates.

Questions to Ask the Family: Which family member communicates most clearly? How might your family members communicate with each other more effectively? Families sometimes find it helpful to talk with one of the nurses about their life at home after learning about an illness. Do you think your family would find that helpful?

Nonverbal communication. *Nonverbal communication* consists of messages conveyed without words, including body language, eye contact, gesturing, crying, and tone of voice. An example of nonverbal communication is children's body language regarding each other or in response to their father's abuse of alcohol.

Questions to Ask the Family: How do you think your daughter feels when your son rolls his eyes while she is talking? Who shows the most distress when talking about dad's drinking? What are some of the nonverbal signals that indicate your daughter is distressed when talking about her dad's drinking?

Circular communication. *Circular communication* refers to reciprocal communication between family members; that is, each person influences the behaviour of the other. Circular communication can be adaptive or maladaptive. For example, an adaptive communication pattern is when a parent comforts a child when the child cries. Because the parent responds to the child, the child feels safe and secure. An example of a maladaptive communication pattern is when a parent criticizes a teenager for not phoning home. The teenager is angry for being criticized and avoids the parent, and then the parent becomes angrier and criticizes more.

Questions to Ask the Family: You mentioned that your teenage daughter does not phone home. What do you do then? What do you think your daughter is thinking when you criticize her?

Problem solving. *Problem solving* refers to how a family thinks about actions to take to resolve difficult situations.

Questions to Ask the Family: Who first notices problems? How does your family tend to deal with problems? Is one member more proactive than others about solving problems?

Roles. *Roles* are established patterns of behaviour for family members, often developed through interactions with others. Formal roles include those of mother, husband, friend, and so forth. Informal roles can include, for example, those of "the softy," "the angel," or "the scapegoat." In the context of illness, family members must often take on new roles, such as medical caregiver.

Questions to Ask the Family: Who is the "good listener" … who is "the angel" in your family?

Influence. *Influence* refers to methods of affecting or controlling another person's behaviour. Influence may be instrumental (e.g., rewards for behaviour such as the promise of candy, computer time), psychological (communication to influence behaviour such as praise, admonishment), or corporal (the use of body contact, such as hugging, hitting).

Questions to Ask the Family: What method does your mom use to get you to go to bed on time? How does your grandma get your brother to attend school when he refuses?

Beliefs. *Beliefs* are individual- and family-held fundamental ideas, values, opinions, and assumptions (Wright, Watson, & Bell, 1996). Understanding the core beliefs (Wright & Bell, 2009) of family members is central to understanding their suffering and to facilitating healing in the context of illness (Wright et al., 1996; Wright & Bell, 2009). Beliefs influence behaviour and how the family adapts to illness. For example, if a family believes that vaccinations may cause disabilities, the parents may decline vaccinating an infant. Beliefs may also influence how a family responds to another member's depression or chronic pain.

> *Questions to Ask the Family: What do you believe is the cause of your husband's depression? What do you believe would be the effect on your chronic pain if you choose to participate in that treatment?*

Alliances and coalitions. *Alliances and coalitions* involve the directionality, balance, and intensity of relationships among family members or between families and nurses.

> *Questions to Ask the Family: If the children are playing well together, who would be most likely to get them to start fighting? Is there anything that you were hoping we would talk about today that we haven't spoken about?*

FAMILY INTERVENTION: THE CALGARY FAMILY INTERVENTION MODEL

After assessment, nurses intervene to help families meet their needs, face challenges, and appreciate their strengths. A range of family nursing interventions can be offered to families in the context of a therapeutic relationship. Some, such as parent education and caregiver support, are general; others are specific and require therapeutic communication and family interviewing skills. The ultimate goal is to help family members discover solutions that may lessen or alleviate emotional, physical, and spiritual suffering. Whether caring for a patient with the family as context or directing care to the family as patient, the aim of nursing interventions is to enhance family members' abilities in certain areas, to remove barriers to health care, and perform actions that the family cannot perform for itself. The nurse guides the family in problem solving, provides practical services, and conveys a sense of acceptance and caring by listening carefully to family members' experiences, concerns, suggestions, and questions.

Interventions for each family must be individualized and focus on particular areas of family functioning (cognitive, affective, behavioural) (Shajani & Snell, 2019). Nurses can only *offer* interventions and must not instruct, or insist, on a particular kind of change or way of family functioning. Nurses need to sensitively attend to ideas or interventions that the family perceives as being most helpful (Shajani & Snell, 2019).

The Calgary Family Intervention Model (CFIM) is a companion model to the CFAM and can be used as a guide for nursing intervention with the family (Shajani & Snell, 2019). The CFIM focuses on promoting and improving family functioning in three domains: cognitive, affective, and behavioural. Interventions may affect functioning in any or all of the three domains. For example, when a clinic nurse informs a wife that her husband who has amyotrophic lateral sclerosis, is still capable of large gross motor movement, the nurse can suggest he could help with chores in the house, such as bringing the laundry upstairs. This intervention may challenge the wife's thinking that her husband is incapable of work, influence her to feel less depressed over her husband's declining physical capacity, and lead her to change her behaviour by including her husband when performing other household chores.

The CFIM recommends many relational nursing practices that promote family health and functioning, including asking interventive questions, offering commendations, providing information, validating emotional responses, encouraging illness narratives, supporting family caregivers, and encouraging respite. Central to this interventional practice is the nurse's engagement with family members in a thoughtful, purposeful relation (Table A7.1). Within CFAM and CFIM, as well as the Illness Beliefs Model (Wright & Bell, 2009; Wright et al, 1996), nurses are guided to continually attend to the cultivation of a relationship that is collaborative, responsive, and nonhierarchical. Within this relationship, there is a privileging of family expertise and a commitment to listening deeply to the concerns, suffering, and questions of family members.

The guidance provided by Hartrick Doane and Varcoe (2005, 2015) in their discussion of relational inquiry is another helpful resource for your relational engagement with the families you encounter in your practice.

Asking Interventive Questions

One of the most effective ways that nurses can help families is by engaging in therapeutic conversations with families and asking them questions. Questions lead the family to reflect on their situation, clarify opinions and ideas, and understand how they are affected by their family member's illness or condition.

TABLE A7.1 The ABCs of Engaging Families		
A	**B**	**C**
Assume an active, confident approach.	Begin by providing structure to the meeting (time frame, orientation to the context).	Create a context of mutual trust.
Ask purposeful questions that draw forth family assessment data.	Behave in a curious manner, and take an equal interest in all family members, whether present or not.	Clarify expectations about your role with the family.
Address all who are present, including small children.	Build on family strengths by offering commendations to the family.	Collaborate in decision making, health promotion, and health management.
Adjust the conversation to children's developmental stages.	Bring relevant resources to the meeting (list of agencies, phone numbers, pamphlets).	Cultivate a context of racial and ethnic sensitivity. Commend family members.

Source: Adapted from Levac, A.M.C., Wright, L.M., & Leahey, M. (2002). Children and families: Models for assessment and intervention. In J.A. Fox (Ed.), *Primary health care of infants, children, and adolescents* (2nd ed., p. 111). Mosby.

By hearing their own responses to questions, as well as the responses of others, family members can better understand themselves and each other and perhaps discover new possibilities for health and healing. Interventive questions also elicit information important to the nurse.

There are two types of interventive questions: linear and circular questions (Tomm, 1987, 1988). *Linear questions* elicit information about a patient or family. They explore a family member's descriptions of an illness or life challenge. For example, linear questions may be used when exploring a couple's perceptions of their daughter's anorexia nervosa: "When did you notice that your daughter had changed her eating habits?" "Has she been hospitalized in the past for this problem?" These questions inform the nurse of the daughter's eating patterns and illuminate family perceptions or beliefs about eating patterns.

Circular questions help determine changes that could be made for a patient's or family's life. They help the nurse understand relationships between individuals, beliefs, and events and elicit valuable information to help create change. In this way, circular questions often help patients make new cognitive connections, paving the way for changes in family behaviours. For example, with the same family, the nurse could ask, "Who is most worried about Cheyenne's anorexia?" or "How does Ellen show that she's worrying the most?" Although linear questions may imply that the nurse knows what is best for the family, circular questions facilitate change by inviting the family to discover their own answers. Linear questions tend to target specific yes-or-no answers, thereby limiting the options for the family; for example, "Have you tried time-out to discipline your 3-year-old?" An alternative circular question might be, "Which type of discipline seems to work best for your 3-year-old?"

Several types of circular questions exist, and each can affect the cognitive, affective, and behavioural domains. These types include difference questions, behavioural effect questions, hypothetical or future-oriented questions, and triadic questions (Tomm, 1987, 1988; Shajani & Snell, 2019) (see Table 12.6 in Chapter 12).

Offering Commendations

Families do not always view themselves as having inherent strength and resilience. The nurse can help the family become aware of its own unique strengths, thus increasing their potential and capabilities. A *commendation* is a conversational statement that emphasizes family strengths and abilities. While spending time with the family, the nurse may observe many instances in which the family displays strengths. It is important to acknowledge these with the family so that they can recognize and appreciate their capabilities. By commending a family's strengths and capacities, nurses can offer family members a new view of themselves, and this may invite a change in how they view their health challenges. The nurse should look for patterns of behaviour to commend, rather than a single occurrence. For example, the nurse may say, "Your family has shown courage living with your wife's cancer for 5 years" or "I'm impressed with how the family worked together during

the crisis." Families coping with chronic, life-threatening, or psychosocial problems frequently feel hopeless in their efforts to overcome or live with the illness. Therefore, nurses should offer as many truthful, genuine commendations as possible. In a qualitative research study exploring the practice of commendations, family members shared their belief that commendations were part of the "special, meaningful, and caring relationships that they developed with the therapists [nurses]. Commendations were not techniques ... but *a way of being with people in the world*" (Hougher Limacher, 2008, p. 99).

Family strengths include clear communication, adaptability, healthy boundaries, support and nurturing among family members, and the use of crisis for growth. The nurse can help the family focus on these strengths rather than on weaknesses.

Providing Information

Families need information from health care professionals about developmental issues, health promotion, and illness management, especially if the illness is complex (Hartrick Doane & Varcoe, 2015). Accurate, timely information is essential for the family to make decisions and cope with difficult situations. Health education is a process by which information is exchanged between the nurse, patient, and family. Family and patient need for information may be elicited through direct questioning but are often far more subtle. In this role of education, the nurse may recognize, for example, that a new father is fearful of cleaning the newborn's umbilical cord stump or that an older woman is not using her cane safely. Respectful communication is required. Nurses often share information subtly: "I notice you are trying to not touch the umbilical cord stump; I see that a lot with other new parents" or "You use the cane the way I did before I was shown a way to keep from falling or tripping over it; do you mind if I show you?" When the nurse assumes a humble, caring position instead of coming across as an authority on the subject, this attitude often decreases the patient's defences and invites the family to listen without feeling embarrassed.

Validating or Normalizing Emotional Responses

Validating intense emotions can alleviate a family's feelings of isolation and loneliness and help family members make the connection between a family member's illness and their own emotional response. For example, after a diagnosis of a life-shortening illness, families frequently feel powerless or frightened. It is important for nurses to validate these strong emotions as normal and reassure families that they will adjust and learn new ways to cope. Nurses may do this by sharing experiences they have had with other families who have faced a similar situation.

Encouraging Illness Narratives

Too often, patients and family members are encouraged to talk only about the medical aspects of their illness rather than the emotional aspects. An *illness narrative* is the person's story of how the illness affects their whole being, including the emotional, intellectual, social, and spiritual dimensions (Kleinman, 1988; Wright & Bell, 2009). Hearing the person's illness narrative helps the nurse understand the person's/family's strengths and challenges, and the beliefs they hold about their illness experience. This information enables the nurse to offer commendations to the family. Many people also find that the telling of their story helps them better understand themselves, their experience, and their family's experience. Families also benefit from listening to one another's illness narratives. Prior to meeting with their nurse, families may not have had the opportunity to hear and understand how other family members have suffered in living with illness.

Communicating what it is like to live with individual, separate experiences, particularly the experience of illness, is a powerful human need (Wright, 2005). Frequently, nurses believe that listening entails an obligation to "fix" whatever concerns or problems are raised. However, showing compassion through deep listening and offering commendations are usually more therapeutic or helpful than offering solutions to problems (Hougher Limacher, 2008; Wright & Bell, 2009).

Encouraging Family Support

Family functioning is enhanced by encouraging and assisting family members to listen to each other's concerns and feelings. This assistance can be particularly useful if a family member is embracing some constraining beliefs when a loved one is dying or has died (RNAO, 2015; Wright & Nagy, 1993). For example, a family may believe that talking with the ill person about death and dying would hasten the person's death.

Supporting Family Caregivers

Family members are often afraid of becoming involved in the care of an ill member without a nurse's support. One way the nurse can best provide care is through supporting family caregivers. Without preparation and support, caregiving can be stressful, causing a decline in the health of the caregiver and the care receiver or the development of abusive relationships.

Despite its demands, caregiving, whether one spouse caring for the other or a child caring for a parent, can be a positive and rewarding experience (Duxbury, Higgins & Schroeder, 2009). The interpersonal dynamics between family members influence the ultimate quality of caregiving. Nurses can play a key role in helping family members develop better communication and problem-solving skills needed for caregiving.

Researchers have identified variables, such as caregiver and care recipient expectations, that influence caregiving quality. Carruth (1996) studied the concept of *reciprocity*, in which care recipients acknowledged the importance of the caregiver's help, and contributions to a caregiver's self-worth. When the caregiver knows that the care recipient appreciates his or her efforts and values the assistance provided, the caregiving relationship is healthier and more satisfying.

Encouraging Respite

Nurses should encourage respite for caregivers, who may feel guilty about or not even recognize their need to withdraw, even temporarily, from caregiving tasks. Sometimes an ill person may be encouraged to accept another person's temporary assistance so that family members can take a break. Whatever

the situation, the nurse should remember that each family's need for respite varies.

Providing care and support for family caregivers often involves using available family and community resources for respite. Caregiving burden can be lessened by the use of a caregiving schedule when multiple family members are participating, the sharing of any financial burdens posed by caregiving, and communication of support from extended family members who live at a distance. However, it is important to understand the relationship between potential caregivers and care recipients. If the relationship is not a supportive one, community services may be a resource for both the patient and family.

Services that may be beneficial to families include caregiver respite, caregiver support groups, housing and transportation services, food and nutrition services, housecleaning, legal and financial services, home care, hospice, and mental health resources. Before referring a family to a community resource, it is crucial that nurses be aware of the community services themselves, understand the family's dynamics, and know whether such support is desired or welcomed. A family caregiver may resist help, feeling obligated to be the sole source of support to the care recipient. Nurses must be sensitive to family relationships and help normalize the demands of caregiving and the need for respite.

Source: Excerpted from West, C. H., & Jakubec, S. L. (2019). Family nursing. In B. J. Astle & W. Duggleby (Eds.). *Canadian fundamentals of nursing* (6th ed., pp. 312–320). Elsevier Canada.

REFERENCES

Carruth, A. K. (1996). Development and testing of the caregiver reciprocity scale. *Nursing Research, 45*(2), 92–97.

Duxbury, L., Higgins, C., & Schroeder, B. (2009). *Balancing paid work and family caregiving responsibilities: A closer look at family caregivers in Canada. Human Resources and Skills Development Canada.* [Seminal Reference].

Hartrick Doane, G., & Varcoe, C. (2005). *Family nursing as relational inquiry. Developing health promoting practice.* Lippincott, Williams & Wilkins. [Seminal Reference].

Hartrick Doane, G., & Varcoe, C. (2006). The "hard spots" of family nursing: Connecting across difference and diversity. *Journal of Family Nursing, 12*(1), 7–21. https://doi.org/10.1177/1074840705284210. [Seminal Reference].

Hartrick Doane, G., & Varcoe, C. (2015). *How to nurse: Relational inquiry with individuals and families in changing health care contexts.* Wolters Kluwer/ Lippincott, Williams & Wilkins.

Hougher Limacher, L. (2008). Locating relationships at the heart of commending practices. *Journal of Systemic Therapies, 27*(4), 90–105. https://doi.org/10.1521/jsyt.2008.27.4.90. [Seminal Reference].

Kleinman, A. (1988). *The illness narratives: Suffering, healing, and the human condition.* Basic Books. [Seminal Reference].

Levac, A. M. C., Wright, L. M., & Leahey, M. (2002). Children and families: models for assessment and intervention. In J. A. Fox (Ed.), *Primary health care of infants, children, and adolescents* (2nd ed.) (p. 111). Mosby.

McGoldrick, M., Garcia Preto, N., & Carter, B. (Eds.). (2016). *The expanding family life cycle: Individual, family, and social perspectives* (5th ed.) Pearson.

McLeod, D. L., & Wright, L. M. (2008). Living the as-yet unanswered: Spiritual care practices in family systems nursing. *Journal of Family Nursing*, *14*(1), 118–141. [Seminal Reference].

Registered Nurses' Association of Ontario (RNAO). (2015). *Person- and family-centred care*. Author.

Shajani, Z., & Snell, D. (2019). *Wright and Leahey's nurses and families: A guide to family assessment and intervention* (7th ed.). F.A. Davis Company.

Tomm, K. (1987). Interventive interviewing: Part II. Reflexive questioning as a means to enable self-healing. *Family Process*, *26*(2), 167–183.

Tomm, K. (1988). Interventive interviewing: Part III. Intending to ask lineal, circular, strategic or reflexive questions. *Family Process*, *27*(1), 1–15.

Walsh, F. (2010a). Spiritual diversity: Multifaith perspectives in family therapy. *Family Process*, *49*(3), 330–348. https://doi.org/10.1111/j.1545-5300.2010.01326.x. [Seminal Reference].

Walsh, F. (2010b). *Spiritual resources in family therapy* (2nd ed.). Guilford Press. [Seminal Reference].

West, C. H., & Jakubec, S. L. (2019). Family nursing. In B. J. Astle, & W. Duggleby (Eds.), *Canadian fundamentals of nursing* (6th ed.) (pp. 312–320). Elsevier Canada.

Wright, L. M. (2005). *Spirituality, suffering, and illness: ideas for healing*. F. A. Davis. [Seminal Reference].

Wright, L. M. (2008). Softening suffering through spiritual care practices: one possibility for healing families. *Journal of Family Nursing*, *14*(4), 394–411. [Seminal Reference].

Wright, L. M., & Bell, J. M. (2009). *Beliefs and illness: A model for healing*. 4th Floor Press. [Seminal Reference].

Wright, L. M., & Nagy, J. (1993). Death: The most troublesome family secret of all. In E. I. Black (Ed.), *Secrets in families and family therapy* (pp. 121–137). W. W. Norton. [Seminal Reference].

Wright, L. M., Watson, W. L., & Bell, J. M. (1996). *Beliefs: The heart of healing in families and illness*. Basic Books. [Seminal Reference].

CNA Position Statement: "Nurses and Environmental Health"

CNA POSITION

The environment is an important determinant of health and has a profound impact on why some people are healthy and others are not.[1] There is a role for every nurse to promote and support actions to optimize the health of the environment because of the link to human health.

The Canadian Nurses Association (CNA) *Code of Ethics for Registered Nurses* supports registered nurses' engagement in environmental health issues as part of their work for social justice. The code suggests that, as part of ethical practice, registered nurses may undertake the ethical endeavours of "supporting environmental preservation and restoration, and advocating for initiatives that reduce environmentally harmful practices in order to promote health and well-being [and] maintaining awareness of broader global health concerns such as… environmental pollution." (CNA, 2017, pp. 20–21)

Canadians trust nurses[2] and value their expertise (EKOS, 2007). CNA believes that the public expects nurses to be aware of and know how to promote Canadians' health in the context of environmental health issues. This is accomplished through nurses' roles in clinical practice, education, research, administration, and policy. Nurses are also in a strong position to advocate for those who are particularly vulnerable to health effects from the environment, as a result of "physical differences, behaviours, location and/or control over their environment" (Health Canada, 2011, para 1).

The role of nurses in environmental health includes:

- Assessing and communicating risks of environmental hazards to individuals, families, and communities
- Educating patients, families, and communities about environmental health and how to address key environmental health issues
- Collaborating with interdisciplinary colleagues to identify and mitigate environmental health risks in practice environments

- Advocating for policies that protect health by preventing exposure to those hazards and promoting sustainability
- Producing nursing science, including interdisciplinary research, related to environmental health issues
- Promoting the development of natural and built environments that support health

Understanding and applying environmental health principles should be a part of every nurse's practice. CNA values the work that nurse leaders, educators, and students are doing to integrate and bolster nursing knowledge and skills related to environmental health. We advocate for further inclusion of concepts that support ecoliteracy in basic and continuing nursing education, strengthened (where necessary) and taught in both academic and workplace settings. Rather than taught as a specialized area of practice, environmental health can be integrated into all areas of nursing practice.

Nurses are uniquely qualified to advise the public on how to protect themselves from and mitigate environmental exposures. They have the assessment skills to identify potential hazards, the scientific background to inform interventions that promote environmental health, and the communication skills to clearly explain environmental exposure and risk reduction.

Nurses are valuable contributors as principal investigators and co-investigators in interdisciplinary environmental health research. Their participation in nursing science related to environmental health supports all areas of nursing practice and ensures that nursing roles and perspectives are incorporated.

The health of the environment affects human health, and CNA values actions that prevent or reduce harm to the environment. CNA expects that, as nurses become more ecoliterate, they will increasingly focus on reducing the environmental impact of the health setting in which they work (and of their personal activities), and thus promote environmental health and sustainability.

CNA endorses the use of the *precautionary principle* as a fundamental tenet of practices that affect the environment. The effects of any future environmental health changes due to human impact are unpredictable, and precautionary principle establishes that "in the case of serious or irreversible threats to the health of humans or the ecosystem, acknowledged scientific uncertainty should not be used as a reason to postpone preventive measures" (Martuzzi & Tickner, 2004, p.1).

Protecting human health and preventing disease and death must be the first priorities for environmental legislation and regulations. All levels of government in Canada have a

---

[1] This position statement does not address health care work environments. For positions on this topic, please see joint CNA/CFNU Position Statement: *Practice Environments: Maximizing Clients, Nurses and Organizations*, 2015.

[2] Unless otherwise stated, *nurse* or *nursing* refers to any member of a regulated nursing category, i.e., a registered nurse, licensed/registered practical nurse, registered psychiatric nurse, or nurse practitioner. This definition reflects the current situation in Canada whereby nurses are deployed in a variety of collaborative arrangements to provide care.

responsibility to manage environmental hazards through various governance instruments. Nurses and nursing organizations must work with governments to improve environmental policy and to advocate for healthy public policies and health-supporting environments.

CNA believes that intersectoral and interdisciplinary collaboration, within and outside of the health system, are crucial to nurses' work in environmental health. It is also important for health care professionals to consider environmental health impacts outside the clinical care context and lead the focus on environmental health, since "we cannot have healthy people on a sick planet" (Health Care Without Harm, 2014, p. 2).

BACKGROUND

The World Health Organization (WHO, 2017) defines environmental health as all the physical, chemical, and biological factors external to a person, and all the related factors impacting behaviours. It encompasses the assessment and control of those environmental factors that can potentially affect health. It is targeted towards preventing disease and creating health-supportive environments. This definition excludes behaviour not related to environment, as well as behaviour related to the social and cultural environment, and genetics (para. 1)

To supplement this definition, we should also see environmental health as influenced by the social determinants of health (including social and psychosocial factors in the environment, and cultural and genetic factors). The environment supports human health and survival, and humans and environmental health "co-benefit" from the interactions between people and the environment, such as engaging in physical activity outdoors (Coutts & Hahn, 2015, p. 9788). This expanded definition is useful to guide nurses to include environmental health in practice, since it includes determinants of health that nurses already routinely address (biological and psychosocial factors, including income inequity) and adds others they may not (physical and chemical factors). Addressing environmental health and promoting ecoliteracy within the nursing profession enhances work in which nurses are already engaged, rather than introducing a new specialty area, and guides areas of nursing intervention (assessing, correcting, controlling, and preventing) that are part of theories and conceptual frameworks used by nurses.

Environmental Factors and Health Effects

The connections between health and the environment, including air, water, and food quality, are well known. However, the health effects from the environment are constantly changing. The recent understanding of the ways that multiple environmental factors influence health is essential for nurses to consider in their practice. For example, the average amount [of time] that individuals spend indoors is increasing, and indoor air quality may be considerably lower than it is outdoors,

depending on the emissions from cooking and building and from material products like plastics (El-Batrawy, 2013). Toxic substances in the environment (e.g., air, water, and soil) are causes and hastening agents of diseases and conditions such as cancer, affected by poor outdoor air quality (resulting in increases in mortality and morbidity from both cardiovascular and respiratory diseases), chemicals (implicated as a cause of cancer, neurotoxicity, developmental setbacks, as well as reproductive, respiratory, cardiopulmonary, psychological, hepatic, urinary, among other systematic diseases. Nurses are in a unique position to advocate for the adoption of health practices (e.g., physical activity) and interventions (e.g., reducing unnecessary medical and nonpharmacological products) that benefit the environment. Recent research on the impact of releasing medication and antibiotics into the waste stream revealed increases in antibiotic-resistant organisms in aquatic wildlife and humans (Wigle, 2003).

Practice and Policy Implications

The effects of climate change on the environment and human health are significant to understand because of their implications in practice and policy. Climate change has affected the health of Canadians through soil and coastline erosion, ozone depletion, increases in seasonal temperatures, longer seasons for vector-borne diseases (e.g., West Nile virus and Lyme disease), increases in precipitation linked to the increased risk of water-borne diseases, and more intense weather events such as thunderstorms, floods, and heat waves. Some of the health effects associated with these changes can include heat stress, water- or vector-borne disease, mental health afflictions, cardiopulmonary-respiratory disorders, and death[3] (Public Health Agency of Canada, 2015).

The Built Environment

The natural world is only one aspect of the environment that influences human health. Recent understandings of the built environment and urbanization and its impacts on health should be considered and incorporated into planning and policies. Noise, traffic, and light pollution are consequences of human-built environments that can be mitigated through advocacy and interdisciplinary collaboration. Incorporating public transportation, natural green spaces, areas for physical activity, quality housing and building materials, as well as effective water and waste treatment systems support the health of individuals as communities grow (Thompson, Kent, & Lyons, 2014). Since outdoor environmental changes are linked with those that occur indoors, and populations in the developed world may spend up to 90% of their time indoors, indoor workplaces can also be a source of exposure to environmental hazards, including chemical, gaseous, microbial,

---

[3]For more information on the diverse impacts of climate change, including health impacts, see the Climate Atlas online (https://ncceh.ca/content/blog/climate-atlas-canada-resource-environmental-public-health).

thermal, physical, moisture, pollution, and indoor ozone (Fisk, 2015).

Advocacy and Ecoliteracy

Nurses have a history of advocating for patients and for other issues of public policy such as sanitation, birth control, safe work environments, women's suffrage, and women's rights, as well as for environmental health issues such as regulations to restrict pollution and tobacco use (CNA, 2013). Environmental health issues related to climate change that nurses are engaged in include advocating for clean air regulations, environmental social justice, and addressing disparities in wealth among nations and vulnerable populations. Nurses also take action at work and in their personal lives by reducing greenhouse gas emissions and waste, using (and encouraging others to use) less toxic products, increasing the use of reusable and recyclable products, and moving away from consumerism toward understanding the impact of our resource use and waste production on global well-being.

Ecoliteracy in nursing education (basic and continuing) enables nurses to consider environmental factors that may be contributing to poor health and to know the health impact of environmental hazards. Ecoliteracy also promotes an understanding of how individuals and communities provide environmental stewardship and guides nurses in making recommendations to reduce or prevent exposures to environmental hazards and conducting research on environmental health issues.

Nursing Research

Nursing research in environmental health focuses on identifying environmental exposures that pose a risk to human health as well as human activities that affect environmental health. This research also evaluates the effectiveness of nursing interventions to reduce the impact on human health and involves assessing which populations are most vulnerable to what exposures, and which strategies are most effective in reducing those risks.

Vulnerable Populations

WHO reports that, while diseases linked to the environment are a global burden, the heaviest impact is on vulnerable populations living in low- and middle-income countries. In all countries, these vulnerable populations—which include families living in poverty, women, children, elderly people, and migrant workers—are more likely to be exposed to environmental hazards and to experience greater negative health effects from the same (Prüss-Üstün, Wolf, Corvalán et al., 2016). In particular, fetuses, infants, and children are at greater risk for health effects from environmental influences because of their increased needs for oxygen and nutrients to support their development. Also, due to changes in industrialization waste, urbanization, and pollution, and considering they do not have control over their environmental exposure (pre- or postnatal and in their younger years),

children are more likely to be exposed to greater levels of chemical, heavy metals, and environmental threats (Miller, Marty & Landrigan, 2016). Environmental changes, like climate change, are accelerating the effects of harmful environmental exposures for all populations. Canada's First Nations and Inuit peoples have a particularly high risk for (1) environmental effects related to poor housing and indoor air quality, (2) lack of adequate drinking water and sanitation systems, and (3) climate changes affecting permafrost and ocean ice, which affects food sources (Health Canada, 2014).

Environmental Health Principles and Position Statements

The *Canadian Environmental Protection Act* employs the precautionary principle and other environmental protection principles.[4] Even though there is no scientific certainty of harmful health effects of exposure, nurses can apply this principle to their work in supporting health for the environment and for individuals, families, and communities. Although the precautionary principle was developed to protect the environment, it can also be used to guide health protection activities. Nurses can use the precautionary principle to support measures that reduce the risk of environmental hazards through advocacy, health promotion, education, public safety controls, and collaboration with sectors within and outside of health care that focus on health in industry, occupational safety, and urban planning.

Nursing associations in Canada and the United States have outlined environmental health principles and position statements for nurses. The American Public Health Association (2015) released a position statement about health and climate change for public health nurses; the Canadian Occupational Health Nurses Association (2013) and Community Health Nurses of Canada (2019) have standards for occupational and community health nurses that address environmental health; CNA (2015) has an online nurse framework that incorporates the environment as a key assessment and metaparadigm in nursing practice; and the American Nurses Association (2007) has environmental health principles for nurses. The November 2015 UN Paris climate conference highlighted numerous collaborative actions that are urgently needed by multiple countries and sectors, which focus efforts to reduce harm to the environment for subsequent reductions in health effects for all.[5]

Approved by the CNA Board of Directors
June 2017
Replaces: Nurses and Environmental Health (2009)

---

[4]For more information on the health implications of the Canadian *Environmental Protection Act*, see the Health Canada website (https://www.canada.ca/en/environment-climate-change/services/canadian-environmental-protection-act-registry/related-documents.html).
[5]For more information on the Paris Agreement, see the United Nations *Framework Convention on Climate Change* (https://unfccc.int/resource/docs/2015/cop21/eng/l09.pdf).

REFERENCES

American Nurses Association. (2007). *ANA's principles of environmental health for nursing practice with implementation strategies.* https://www.nursingworld.org/~4afaf8/globalassets/practiceandpolicy/work-environment/health--safety/principles-of-environmental-health-online_final.pdf

American Public Health Association. (2015). *Public health opportunities to address the health effects of climate change.* https://www.apha.org/policies-and-advocacy/public-health-policy-statements/policy-database/2015/12/03/15/34/public-health-opportunities-to-address-the-health-effects-of-climate-change.

Canadian Nurses Association. (2013). *One hundred years of service.* https://www.cna-aiic.ca/~/media/cna/page-content/pdf-en/cna_history_book_e.pdf?la=en.

Canadian Nurses Association. (2015). *Framework for the practice of registered nurses in Canada.* https://www.cna-aiic.ca/~/media/cna/page-content/pdf-en/framework-for-the-pracice-of-registered-nurses-in-canada.pdf?la=en.

Canadian Nurses Association. (2017). *Code of ethics for registered nurses.* Author.

Canadian Occupational Health Nurses Association. (2003). *Standards of practices for occupational health nursing.* http://cohna-aciist.ca/wp-content/uploads/2017/03/Occupational-Health-Nursing-Practice-Standards-2003.pdf

Community Health Nurses of Canada. (2019). *Canadian community health nursing: Professional practice model and standards of practice.* https://www.chnc.ca/standards-of-practice.

Coutts, C., & Hahn, M. (2015). Green infrastructure, ecosystem services, and human health. *International Journal of Environmental Research and Public Health, 12*(8), 9768–9798. https://doi.org/10.3390/ijerph120809768.

EKOS. (2007). *Public views of environmental health issues and nursing: a qualitative study.* Unpublished paper prepared for CNA.

El-Batrawy, O. (2013). Indoor air quality and adverse health effects. *World Applied Sciences Journal, 25*(1), 163–169. https://doi.org/10.5829/idosi.wasj.2013.25.01.7614.

Fisk, W. J. (2015). Review of some effects of climate change on indoor environmental quality and health and associated no-regrets mitigation measures. *Building and Environment, 86,* 70–80. https://doi.org/10.1016/j.buildenv.2014.12.024.

Health Canada. (2011). *Environmental and workplace health: Vulnerable populations.* http://www.hc-sc.gc.ca/ewh-semt/contaminants/vulnerable/index-eng.php#ap.

Health Canada. (2014). *A statistical profile on the health of First Nations in Canada: Determinants of health, 2006 to 2010.* https://www.sac-isc.gc.ca/eng/1585414580249/1585414609942

Health Care Without Harm. (2014). *Global reach enduring change: 2014 impact report.* noharm-uscanada.org/sites/default/files/documents-files/3428/HCWH%202014%20Impact%20Report%20%28Web%29.pdf.

Martuzzi, M., & Tickner, J. A. (Eds.). (2004). *The precautionary principle: Protecting public health, the environment and the future of our children.* WHO Regional Office for Europe. http://www.euro.who.int/__data/assets/pdf_file/0003/91173/E83079.pdf?ua=1.

Miller, M. D., Marty, M. A., & Landrigan, P. J. (2016). Children's environmental health: Beyond national boundaries. *Pediatric clinics of North American, 63*(1), 149–165. https://doi.org/10.1016/j.pcl.2015.08.008.

Prüss-Üstün, A., Wolf, J., Corvalán, C. et al. (2016). *Preventing disease through healthy environments: A global assessment of the environmental burden of disease from environmental risks.* World Health Organization. http://apps.who.int/iris/bitstream/10665/204585/1/9789241565196_eng.pdf?ua=1.

Public Health Agency of Canada. (2015). *Climate change and public health factsheets.* https://www.canada.ca/en/public-health/services/health-promotion/environmental-public-health-climate-change/climate-change-public-health-factsheets.html.

Thompson, S., Kent, J., & Lyons, C. (2014). Building partnerships for healthy environments: Research, leadership and education. *Health Promotion Journal of Australia, 25,* 202–208. https://doi.org/10.1071/HE14039.

Wigle, D. (2003). *Child health and the environment.* Oxford University Press.

World Health Organization. (2017). *Environmental health.* http://www.searo.who.int/topics/environmental_health/en/.

SOURCE: Canadian Nurses Association. (2017). *Position statement: Nurses and environmental health.* https://www.cna-aiic.ca/~/media/cna/page-content/pdf-en/nurses-and-environmental-health-position-statement.pdf

Non–Vaccine-Preventable Infectious Diseases

Epidemiology	Mode of Transmission	Incubation Period	Indicators	Time of Occurrence	Nursing Consideration
Avian Influenza (AI)					
There have been no confirmed cases of human infection in Canada. World Health Organization (WHO) reports that there has been a total of 24 laboratory confirmed cases of A (H5N6) from China since 2014.*	Human infection with the A (H5N6) or A (H7N9). Humans acquire the infection primarily through direct contact with live or dead poultry or a contaminated environment. This is especially possible during slaughter, butchering, or preparing the bird for consumption.†	Incubation period can range from 2–5 days and possibly as long as 10 days.	Symptoms are usually mild or subclinical and they can resemble those of human influenza: high fever (greater than or equal to 38°C), cough, followed by symptoms of lower respiratory tract involvement, including sore throat, dyspnea or coryza. Other symptoms include nausea, vomiting, bleeding from the nose or gums, encephalitis, and chest pain. Complications include respiratory failure, mutli-organ dysfunction, septic shock and bacterial and fungal infections.		Counsel individuals who will be travelling to areas where there are outbreaks of the disease. Provide education to high-risk groups and general population regarding preventive measures. Identify possible cases and report to the appropriate authority.
Creutzfeldt-Jakob Disease (CJD)					
CJD has been found in all developed nations. The incidence of definite and probable CJD cases in Canada in 2019 was 32.§	Not known to spread by contact from person to person or by the airborne or respiratory route; however, transmission can occur during invasive medical interventions.	Incubation period can extend up to 30 years	Progressive dementia including confusion and memory loss; progressive unsteadiness and clumsiness; visual disturbances such as dizziness, double vision, and blurriness; and muscle twitching, fatigue, and a variety of other neurological symptoms. The affected person is usually mute and immobile in the last stages; in most cases, death occurs within a few months of onset of symptoms. This disease always results in death as there is no treatment.		Educate public regarding indicators of the disease.
Ebola					
No reported cases in Canada. The 2014–2016 outbreak in West Africa was the largest outbreak since 1976. In 2018–2019 another outbreak occurred in the eastern Democratic Republic of the Congo.‖	The virus is transmitted to people from wild animals and spreads to the human population through human-to-human transmission through direct contact (broken skin or mucous membranes) with contaminated blood and body fluids of a person who is sick with or has died from Ebola; objects that have been contaminated with body fluids (blood, feces, vomit) from a person sick with Ebola, and infected animals (fruit bats, primates, forest antelope, or porcupines). Burial ceremonies with the body of the patient can also contribute to transmission.	Incubation period is 2 to 21 days.	Fever greater than 38.6°C or 101.5°F, severe headache, muscle pain, nausea, vomiting and diarrhea, unexplained hemorrhage, contact with blood or other body fluids or human remains of a patient know to have or suspected of having Ebola, travel to an area where Ebola is active, direct handling of bats, rodents, or primates from a disease-endemic area		Early recognition of the disease is critical for implementation of strict infection control procedures.

Disease	Transmission	Incubation	Signs and symptoms	Season	Role
Hantavirus Pulmonary Syndrome (HPS) Since 1989 there have been 109 confirmed cases and 27 deaths in Canada.****	Direct contact with rodents or their droppings or inhalation in areas with large number of rodent droppings. No person-to-person transfer has been found. Hantavirus is found in urine, feces, and saliva of rodents. Workers in agricultural or rural settings (e.g., farmers, grain handlers) are at the highest risk.	3–60 days; average is 14–30 days	Fever, chills, headache; may develop gastrointestinal symptoms. Five days after onset of symptoms, cough and shortness of breath develop—this may be severe within hours due to pulmonary edema and deterioration of cardiopulmonary function.	Often occurs in spring	Provide information and education to the public regarding potential infection with virus when in contact with rodents or their droppings. Educate target groups about preventive measures.
HIV and AIDS See Table 16.2					
Lyme Disease The number of cases reported in Canada has more than doubled since 2016, with 992 cases increasing to 2025 cases in 2017.**	The bacterium that causes Lyme disease is normally carried in mice, squirrels, birds, and other small animals. The bacterium is transmitted to ticks when they feed on these infected animals and then to humans through the bites of the infected ticks.	3–32 days after tick exposure	Three stages: **First stage:** Red spot or rash at site of tick bite (*erythema migrans*), fatigue, chills, fever, headaches, joint pain, and swollen lymph nodes **Second stage:** Occurs if disease is left untreated and can last for months. Development of *erythema migrans* on other areas of the body; central and peripheral nervous system disorders, e.g., Bell's palsy, heart arrhythmias, arthritis and arthritic symptoms, and feelings of extreme fatigue **Third stage:** Chronic arthritis, neurological symptoms, i.e., problems with memory, speech, and sleep	Summer and early fall	Educate public regarding preventive measures that can be taken when entering into a possible tick-infested area. Educate public about what action to take in the event of being bitten by a tick. Assist in the surveillance of the disease.
Malaria Canada is not considered a country at risk for the transmission of malaria; however, Canada sees an average of 488 malaria cases per year and worldwide in 2015 there were 214 million cases and 438 000 deaths.††	Transmitted to humans through a bite of an infected female mosquito. Very rarely, it can also be transmitted by transfusion with infected blood, or by shared needle use, or from a mother to her unborn child.	Varies, from 7–30 days	Fever and influenza-like symptoms such as headache, nausea, vomiting, muscle pain, malaise, shaking and chills, and spleen enlargement. *Plasmodium falciparum* can cause cerebral malaria leading to delirium, confusion, seizure, coma, kidney or respiratory failure, and even death.		Provide information for travellers who are visiting malaria-affected regions. Educate regarding measures that can be undertaken for prevention. Educate regarding symptoms of disease so that individuals can recognize if they may have become infected.

Continued

Epidemiology	Mode of Transmission	Incubation Period	Indicators	Time of Occurrence	Nursing Consideration
Noroviruses About 300–400 outbreaks are reported each year in Canada.‡‡	Found in the stool or vomit of infected individuals while they are ill and up to at least 3 days after recovery. May be contagious for as long as 2 weeks after recovery. Infection can occur by direct contact with a person who is ill or has recently been ill or through indirect contact by touching surfaces contaminated with the virus, such as door handles, or by eating contaminated food or drinking contaminated water.	24–48 hours (median in outbreaks 33–36 hours), but cases can occur within 12 hours of exposure	Nausea, vomiting, diarrhea, and stomach cramps. Sometimes, people may have a low-grade fever, chills, headache, muscle aches, and fatigue. The illness often begins suddenly, about 24–48 hours after exposure.		Educate public regarding the importance of preventive measures such as handwashing. Monitor the number of cases occurring in the area.
Severe Acute Respiratory Syndrome (SARS) In 2003 in Ontario, 351 cases were identified and 44 deaths occurred. By the end of July 2003, it had spread to 8 098 people in 30 countries, killing 774 people. The WHO declared the end of the epidemic in July 2003.§§	Person-to-person contact (direct mucous membrane contact) with infectious respiratory droplets and/or direct contact with infected body fluids. Also can be transmitted through blood transfusions or sharps injuries.	2–14 days	Fever >38°C, myalgia, malaise, chills, nonproductive cough and rigor. After 2–7 days followed by respiratory symptoms—cough, shortness of breath, difficulty breathing, or pneumonia		Educate public regarding indicators of SARS. Provide information and education about prevention and spread of the virus. Use vigilance in the assessment of possible cases and report any suspicions immediately. Clinical management relies mainly on providing supportive care.
Tuberculosis (TB) In 2017 the rate of active TB in Canada was 4.9 per 100 000. There were 1 796 cases of active TB reported in Canada, with foreign-born individuals and Indigenous peoples accounting for the majority of cases.‖‖	Airborne transmission from infected person	Varies from weeks to years	Cough lasting 2 weeks or longer, especially with hemoptysis, fever, weight loss, night sweats, and anorexia		Identify high-risk groups and provide information and education. Provide information for travellers who may visit high-risk areas.

	Transmission	Incubation	Symptoms	Season	Prevention
West Nile Virus In 2018, there were 427 human cases of West Nile virus reported in Canada.##	Transmission by bite of a mosquito that has ingested the blood of infected birds	2–15 days	Infected individuals may be asymptomatic or have only mild symptoms. Symptoms vary but include fever, headaches, body aches, mild rash, and swollen lymph nodes. Individuals with weakened immunity can develop more serious conditions such as meningitis, encephalitis, or acute flaccid paralysis.	Mid-April to October	Educate public regarding measures to avoid being bitten by mosquitoes. Identify high-risk areas and reinforce need for preventive measures.
Anthrax No reported cases for humans. Usually, livestock are infected through eating food contaminated with the anthrax spores.***	Transmission by inhalation (pulmonary), ingestion (gastrointestinal), or skin contact (cutaneous)	1–7 days; usually 2–5 days	Skin infection: small painless bump that blisters and then develops an ulcer with a black centre. This is the most common type of infection. Stomach infection: fever, loss of appetite, vomiting, and diarrhea Lung infection: fever, sore throat, and general malaise, followed by dyspnea after several days. This is the most serious type of infection.		
Clostridium difficile In 2011 there were 3 472 reported cases in Ontario, Canada.#	Direct contact with feces or objects contaminated with feces	1–10 days	Watery diarrhea, fever, anorexia, nausea, and abdominal pain		Educate and reinforce proper handwashing techniques as prevention in general public and in occupational settings, especially health care.

AIDS, Acquired immunodeficiency syndrome; _HIV_, human immunodeficiency virus.

Sources: *World Health Organization (WHO), 2019a.
†WHO, 2018.
§Public Health Agency of Canada (PHAC), 2019a.
‖WHO, 2019b.
#Provincial Infectious Disease Advisory Committee, 2013.
**Government of Canada, 2018.
††Government of Canada, 2016.
‡‡PHAC, 2015.
§§PHAC, 2011.
‖‖PHAC, 2019b.
##PHAC, 2019c.
***Canadian Food Inspection Agency, 2009.
****Government of Canada, 2019.

REFERENCES

Canadian Food Inspection Agency. (2009). *Anthrax*. http://www.inspection.gc.ca/animals/terrestrial-animals/diseases/reportable/anthrax/eng/1330045348336/1330045807153.

Government of Canada. (2016). *Surveillance of malaria*. https://www.canada.ca/en/public-health/services/diseases/malaria/surveillance-malaria.html#a4.

Government of Canada. (2018). *Surveillance of Lyme disease*. https://www.canada.ca/en/public-health/services/diseases/lyme-disease/surveillance-lyme-disease.html.

Government of Canada. (2019). *Surveillance of hantavirus related diseases*. https://www.canada.ca/en/public-health/services/diseases/hantaviruses/surveillance-hantavirus-related-diseases.html.

Provincial Infectious Disease Advisory Committee. (2013). *Testing, surveillance and management of clostridium difficile*. https://www.publichealthontario.ca/-/media/documents/cdiff-testing-surveillance-management.pdf?la=en.

Public Health Agency Canada (PHAC). (2011). *Pathogen Safety Data Sheets: Infectious Substances—Severe acute respiratory syndrome (SARS) associated coronavirus*. https://www.canada.ca/en/public-health/services/laboratory-biosafety-biosecurity/pathogen-safety-data-sheets-risk-assessment/severe-acute-respiratory-syndrome-sars-associated-coronavirus.html.

Public Health Agency of Canada (PHAC). (2015). *Norovirus*. http://www.phac-aspc.gc.ca/fs-sa/fs-fi/norovirus-eng.php.

Public Health Agency of Canada (PHAC). (2019a). *Creutzfeldt-Jakob disease surveillance system report*. https://www.canada.ca/en/public-health/services/surveillance/blood-safety-contribution-program/creutzfeldt-jakob-disease/cjd-surveillance-system.html.

Public Health Agency Canada (PHAC). (2019b). *Tuberculosis monitoring*. https://www.canada.ca/en/public-health/services/diseases/tuberculosis/surveillance.html.

Public Health Agency Canada (PHAC). (2019c). *Surveillance of West Nile Virus*. https://www.canada.ca/en/public-health/services/diseases/west-nile-virus/surveillance-west-nile-virus.html.

World Health Organization (WHO). (2018). *Influenza (Avian and other zoonotic)*. https://www.who.int/news-room/fact-sheets/detail/influenza-(avian-and-other-zoonotic.

World Health Organization (WHO). (2019a). *Influenza at the human-animal interface*. https://www.who.int/influenza/human_animal_interface/Influenza_Summary_IRA_HA_interface_27_09_2019.pdf?ua=1.

World Health Organization (WHO). (2019b). *Ebola virus disease: Key facts*. https://www.who.int/news-room/fact-sheets/detail/ebola-virus-disease.

Viral Hepatitis Profiles

	Hepatitis A (HAV)	Hepatitis B (HBV)	Hepatitis C (HCV)	Hepatitis D (HDV)	Hepatitis E (HEV)	Hepatitis G
Incubation period in days	Range: 15–50 Average: 28	Range: 40–160 Average: 120	Range: 17–175 Average: 45	Range: 14–43 Average: 28	Range: 15–60 Average: 40	Unknown
Mode of transmission	• Fecal–oral route • Contaminated environment or objects • Contaminated food or water	• Percutaneous or mucosal contact with infected biological fluids • Mother-to-newborn child at birth (rare in Canada)	• Infected blood and blood products • Mother-to-newborn child at birth (vertical) • Sharing personal items	• Most often by exposure to contaminated needles • Sharing personal items contaminated with the virus • Unprotected sex with multiple sex partners	• Fecal–oral route	• Infected blood and blood products • Sharing personal items contaminated with the virus • Mother-to-newborn child at birth • Various sexual activities
Incidence in Canada	0.68 per 100 000 in 2016*	4 905 cases 192 cases of acute (0.5 per 100 000) 4 086 cases of chronic (11.4 per 100 000 in 2017)†	11 592 cases 31.7 per 100 000 in 2017‡	Extremely low in Canada§	Rarely seen in Canada	Found in 1–4% of the Canadian blood donor population‖
Persons at risk	• Travellers to HAV endemic countries • Residents of certain institutions such as correctional facilities • Men who have sex with men (MSM) • Households or close contacts of persons who have HAV • Hemophiliacs • Injection drug users sharing needles	• Infants exposed during child birth to mothers who are carriers • Injection drug users sharing needles • Households with HBV carriers • People at risk for sexually transmitted infections (STIs) • Immigrants from countries where virus is prevalent • Hemodialysis clients	• Injection drug users sharing needles • Hemodialysis clients • Those who receive tattoos or body piercing done with unsterile equipment • Those who have sex with an HCV carrier • Babies born to mothers who have HCV • Health care workers	• Injection drug users sharing needles • Those who have unprotected sex with multiple partners • MSM and bisexual men • Immigrants from countries where virus is prevalent • Residents of certain institutions such as correctional facilities • Hemophiliacs • Hemodialysis clients • Health care and emergency care workers	• People living in subtropical areas • People with low SES, living in areas where virus is prevalent • People on maintenance dialysis • Injection drug users • People who have other viral bloodborne infections • Travellers to areas where the virus is prevalent	• Recipients of blood and blood products • Hemodialysis clients • Injection drug users • People who receive tattoos, acupuncture, or body piercing with unsterile equipment • Clients with impaired immune response • People who engage in prostitution • MSM
Chronic carrier state	No	Yes Less than 5% of residents have markers and less than 1% are carriers	Yes	Yes	No	Yes Carrier rate of between 2 and 5% of general population

	Hepatitis A (HAV)	Hepatitis B (HBV)	Hepatitis C (HCV)	Hepatitis D (HDV)	Hepatitis E (HEV)	Hepatitis G
Indicators	• Acute onset • Fever • Nausea • Lack of appetite • Malaise • Abdominal discomfort • Jaundice	• Mild influenza-like symptoms • Fever • Nausea • Extreme lethargy • Joint pain • Jaundice	• Fatigue • Anorexia • Malaise • Weight loss • Right-sided pain • Occasional jaundice	• Mild influenza-like symptoms • Fever • Nausea • Extreme lethargy • Joint pain • Jaundice	• Jaundice • Uneasiness • Loss of appetite • Abdominal pain • Inflammation of the liver	• Almost no cases have symptoms like the other hepatitis viruses
Method of diagnosis	Serological test (anti-HAV), viral isolation	Serological test (HBsAg), viral isolation	Serological test (anti-HCV)	Serological test (anti-HDV), liver biopsy	Serological tests (anti-HEV)	None currently
Sequelae	No chronic infection	Chronic liver disease; liver cancer	Chronic liver disease; liver cancer	Chronic liver disease; liver cancer	No chronic infection	Rare or may not occur
Vaccine availability	Yes; vaccination recommended for health care workers, preschool children, travellers to endemic regions, MSM	Yes; vaccination recommended for health care workers, infants, individuals with exposure risks, MSM	No	No	No	No
Control and prevention	Personal hygiene, proper sanitation	Pre-exposure vaccination, reduction of risk behaviours for exposure	Screening of blood and organ donors; reduction of risk behaviours for exposure	Pre-exposure or post-exposure prophylaxis for HBV	Protection of water systems from fecal contamination	Unknown

Nursing considerations	• Educate client about mode of transmission and preventive measures
	• Recommend prophylactic immune globulin when there is exposure through close contact with an infected individual or contaminated food or water
		• Recognize chronic HBV symptoms:
		  • Anorexia
		  • Fatigue
		  • Abdominal pain
		  • Hepatomegaly
		  • Jaundice
		• Educate client about mode of transmission and preventive measures
			• Assess high-risk clients for presence of HCV
			• Offer blood testing as indicated
			• Educate client about mode of transmission and preventive measures
				• Educate client about mode of transmission and preventive measures	• Educate client about mode of transmission and preventive measures	• Educate client about mode of transmission and preventive measures

HbsAg, Hepatitis B surface antigen; *SES*, socioeconomic status.

Note: Data are Canadian unless otherwise specified.

Sources: *Public Health Agency of Canada (PHAC), 2018

†PHAC, 2017

‡PHAC, 2017

§PHAC 2015

‖PHAC, 2004.

REFERENCES

Public Health Agency of Canada (PHAC). (2004). *Hepatitis G fact sheet*. http://www.phac-aspc.gc.ca/hcai-iamss/bbp-pts/hepatitis/hep_g-eng.php. [Seminal Reference].

Public Health Agency of Canada (PHAC). (2015). *Surveillance of hepatitis D*. https://www.canada.ca/en/public-health/services/diseases/hepatitis-d/surveillance-hepatitis-d.html.

Public Health Agency of Canada (PHAC). (2017). *Report on hepatitis B and C in Canada*. https://www.canada.ca/content/dam/themes/health/publications/diseases-conditions/report-hepatitis-b-c-canada-2017/report-hepatitis-b-c-canada-2017.pdf.

Public Health Agency of Canada (PHAC). (2018). *Reportable cases in Canada—Notifiable diseases on line*. https://diseases.canada.ca/notifiable/charts?c=pl.

INDEX

Page numbers followed by *f* indicate figures; *t*, tables; *b*, boxes.

A

Aberdeen, Lady, 33t
Aboriginal. *See* Indigenous
Aboriginal Diabetes Initiative (ADI), 261
Aboriginal Head Start in Urban and
    Northern Communities (AHSUNC),
    107
Aboriginal health advocacy actions. *See*
    Indigenous health advocacy actions
Aboriginal Nurses Association of Canada
    (ANAC), 333
Aboriginal people, 148. *See also* Indigenous
    people
  in Canada, definitions of, 325
  cultural considerations for, 326b
  determinants of health in, 334–336
    distal, 335–336
    intermediate, 335
    proximal, 334–335
  females, missing and murdered, 332f
  health, 324–350
    case study for, 336–345, 345b
  health advocacy actions of, 332
  health issues of, historical and legislative
    context in, 327–330
    colonization in, 327–328
    First Nations Peoples Treaties,
      328–330, 330f–331f
    Indian Act, 330
    key events and legislation in, 328,
      328t–329t
    precolonization, 327–328
  health status of, 326–327
  human rights and community health of,
    8–9
  nursing, in Canada, 332–333
  population snapshot of, 325–326
  projected life expectancy of, 326
Absolute homelessness, 358
Absolute poverty, 356
Abuse
  elder, 269–270
  violence as form of, 361–364
Acceptability, 71
Access and equity
  in CCHN Standards, 157
  standards of practice, 203b
Accessibility, 71
  of primary health care, 9
Accidents, injuries and, in child and
    adolescent health, 256–257, 256b
Accommodating, for conflict resolution,
    317t
Accountability, 138
  professional, 480–481
  standards of practice, 203b
Achieving Health for All, 4

Acid rain, 429
Acquired immunity, 394
Action research, 124
Active immunization, 394
Adequacy, 239t–240t
ADI. *See* Aboriginal Diabetes Initiative
    (ADI)
Adjourning, in group development, 312
Adolescents
  common health concerns in, 250t
  developmental stages of, 251t
  sexual behaviour of, and pregnancy,
    375–377
    early identification of, 376
    factors contributing to, 377b
    special issues in caring for, 376–377
Adult health, 259–266
  men, 264–266
  women, 259–264
Adults, older, fall-prevention program for,
    236f
Advanced practice nurse (APN), 29
Advocacy, 109, 139–140, 140f
  conceptual framework for, 140
  ecoliteracy and, 506
  in environmental health, 445
  health, 54, 55b
  practical framework for, 140
Affordability, 71
Age
  cancer cases and, 265t
  as risk factor, 356
Age-adjusted death rates, 196
Ageism, 266
Agent, 66
  in epidemiological triangle, 185, 186b,
    435
  host, and environment, 394–395
  of infection, 394, 394b
Agent-host-environment triad, 436t
Age-related changes, in body systems, 267t
Aggregates, 14, 310
Aging, 266
Aging population, 147–148, 148f
Agreements, 430t
AHSUNC. *See* Aboriginal Head Start in
    Urban and Northern Communities
    (AHSUNC)
AIDS, 405–410
  Canadian information on, 410b
  epidemiology and transmission of,
    399t–403t
  global information on, 410b
  patients with, 419–420
  testing and counselling for clients with,
    418–419
Air, climate and, 430, 433–434

Air pollution, 429, 437b
Alliances, in family, 500
Allophones, 152
Alma-Ata Declaration, 90–92, 485–486
ANA House of Delegates, 129
Analytical epidemiology, 177
Analytical studies, 193
  comparison of, 194t
Anderson, Helen, 36f
An Inclusion Lens, 104t
Anthrax, 391
  letters, 179–180
Anticolonial knowledge, 336
Antismoking programs, 257–258
Apathy, 360
APN. *See* Advanced practice nurse (APN)
Applied ethics, 131
Appropriate technology, of primary health
    care, 10
Assault, 364–366
  sexual, 364–366
Assessment
  behavioural risk, 299
  biological risk, 295–297
  community health, 213–218
  congenital and genetic predisposition,
    377–378
  contraceptive, 259
  defined, 233
  environmental health, 436–441
  environmental risk, 297–299
  family, 287–290, 293–294
    models and approaches in, 287–290
  issues, 218
Asset mapping, 103, 212
Atherosclerosis, 252–253
At-risk populations
  and homelessness, 359–360
  for mental illness, 367–368
Attitude scales, 238–239
Attributable risk (AR), 185t
Authoritarian leadership style, 314–315
Autocratic leadership style, 314–315
Autonomy, 133, 133b
Availability, 71
Avian influenza (AI), 183
Avoidance, for conflict resolution, 317t

B

Baby Friendly Initiative (BFI), 106
Bacillus anthracis, 391
Bed bugs, 445
Behavioural approach, 101, 102t
Behavioural risk, assessment in, 299
Beliefs, of family, 499–500
Beneficence, 133, 133b
Best practice guidelines, 118
Betty Neuman's system model, 206

BFI. *See* Baby Friendly Initiative (BFI)
Bias, 160
Bills, 430t
Bioethics, 131
Biological and infectious hazards, 66, 66b
Biological disasters, 453–454
Biological risk, assessment of, 295–297
Biological transmission, 414
Biological variations
  in Giger and Davidhizar Transcultural
    Assessment Model, 165
  in Transcultural Assessment Model, 491
Biology, as determinant of health, 5
Biomedical approach, 101, 102t
Bisphenol A (BPA), 440
Blended family, 278t
Botulism, 412
Boundaries, in family structure, 496
Bovine spongiform encephalopathy (BSE),
  392
Breast cancer, 259, 263
Breast self-examination, in women's health,
  259
BSE. *See* Bovine spongiform
  encephalopathy (BSE)
Building healthy public policy, 105–106,
  487
Built environment, 444, 505–506
Bullying, 361

C
Calgary Family Assessment Model
  (CFAM), 276, 287, 495–502, 497f
  branching diagram of, 279f
  structural assessment in, 495–498
    context, 496–498
    external structure, 496
    internal structure, 495–496
    tools for, 498
Calgary Family Intervention Model
  (CFIM), 276, 300–301
Canada Health Act, 3
Canada's Dietary Guidelines, 253
Canada's ecological footprint, 433
Canada's emergency management
  framework, 455
Canada's greenhouse gas emissions targets,
  433
Canadian Childhood National
  Immunization Survey, 258
Canadian Collaborative Mental Health
  Initiative (CCMHI), 15
Canadian community health agencies, 3
Canadian Community Health Nursing:
  Professional Practice Model and
  Standards of Practice, 3, 14, 85
Canadian Community Health Nursing
  Standards of Practice (CCHN
  Standards), 3, 20–25, 20t, 21f, 22t–24t,
  57, 157–159, 478–481
  capacity building and, 479–480
  evidence-informed practice, 480

Canadian Community Health Nursing
  Standards of Practice (CCHN
  Standards) *(Continued)*
  health equity, 480
  health maintenance, restoration and
    palliation and, 479
  health promotion and, 88b, 478
  health protection in, 87b
  prevention and health protection and,
    478–479
  professional relationships and, 479
  professional responsibility and
    accountability and, 480–481
Canadian Community Health Survey
  (CCHS), 193, 207
Canadian Environmental Protection Act,
  430, 506
Canadian family, 277–280, 277f
Canadian Healthy Communities project,
  103
Canadian Heart Health Initiative, 103
Canadian Hospice Palliative Care
  Association (CHPCA), 61
Canadian Human Rights Act, 155
Canadian Indigenous Nurses Association
  (CINA), 68–69
Canadian Institute for Advanced Research
  (CIFAR), 94
Canadian Institute for Health Information
  (CIHI), 207
Canadian Institutes of Health Research
  (CIHR), 3
Canadian Mental Health Association
  (CMHA), 368
Canadian Nurses Association (CNA), 29,
  57, 100, 118, 129, 209, 256
  Code of Ethics for Registered Nurses, 504
  in global health efforts, 8b
  in injury prevention, 256b
  position statement, 504–505
Canadian Pandemic Influenza Plan, 459
Canadian Public Health Association
  (CPHA), 34, 104
Canadian Red Cross, 36
  role in disaster, 456
Cancer
  diagnosis, 263
  in women, 263–264
Capacities, as intermediate determinant of
  health, 335
Capacity building, 21–25, 104, 211t,
  479–480
  in CCHN Standards, 157
  standards of practice, 203b
Car accidents, 455
Carbon footprint, 433
Cardiovascular disease
  smoking, 257
  women, 261
Care at home, 59
Care coordination, 60
Caregiver stress, 120b

Caregiving roles, 270
Care planning, 60
  with families, 303
    mutual goal setting and, 303–304
    phases of, 303t
Case control, study design, 194t
Case fatality rate (CFR), 183, 183t
Case management, 54–57, 56b
  central activities, 56t
  historical perspective, 55
  models and strategies, 55–57
Case manager, 55
Cause-specific mortality rate, 183t
CCBT. *See* Community Capacity Building
  Tool (CCBT)
CCDIC. *See* Centre for Communicable
  Diseases and Infection Control
  (CCDIC)
CCMHI. *See* Canadian Collaborative
  Mental Health Initiative
  (CCMHI)
Centenarians, 266
Centre for Communicable Diseases and
  Infection Control (CCDIC), 391
Centre for Emergency Preparedness and
  Response (CEPR), 456
Certification, 57
Cervical cancer, 264
CFAM. *See* Calgary Family Assessment
  Model (CFAM)
CFIM. *See* Calgary Family Intervention
  Model (CFIM)
CFR. *See* Case fatality rate (CFR)
CH^2OPD^2, 438
Change agent, 221–222
Change partner, 221–222
Charette, 237
Chemical asphyxiants, 429
Chemical hazards, 66, 66b
Chicken pox, 399t–403t
Child and adolescent health, 248–258
  assessment of, 250b
  common health concerns of, 250t
  Comprehensive School Health Approach
    in, 254–256
  developmental stages in, 251t
  injuries and accidents in, 256–257
  nutrition in, 252–254
  overweight and obesity in, 251–252
  physical activity in, 252
Child development, 247–248
Childhood experiences, as determinant of
  health, 4
Child poverty, 248
Childhood obesity
  determinants of, 124
  managing, 252b
Children
  and mental illness, 367
  vulnerability, 375–377
Children's health, environment and,
  442–444, 444f

Chlamydia, 405, 406t–409t
CHN. *See* Community Health Nursing (CHN)
CHNAC. *See* Community Health Nurses Association of Canada (CHNAC)
CHNC. *See* Community Health Nurses of Canada (CHNC)
Cholera death rates, 178t
CHPCA. *See* Canadian Hospice Palliative Care Association (CHPCA)
Chronic homeless, 358
CIHR. *See* Canadian Institutes of Health Research (CIHR)
Circular communication, 301, 301t
  of family, 499
Cisgender, 154
Citizenship Act, in 2015, 149
Civil Marriage Act, 153
CJD. *See* Creutzfeldt-Jakob disease (CJD)
Climate
  change, 426
  indicators, 430
Clinical judgement, 304–305
Clinical practice guidelines, 121–122
Clinical question
  examples of, 120b
  formulating, 119–120
Closing the Gap in a Generation: Health Equity Through Action on the Social Determinants of Health, 6
Clostridium botulinum, 413t
Clostridium perfringens, 413t
CNA. *See* Canadian Nurses Association (CNA)
CNA Code of Ethics: An Ethical Basis for Nursing in Canada, 129
Coalitions, 210
  community, 210
  in family, 500
Code of ethics, 129, 137
  community health nursing and, 130b, 138–139
Code of Ethics for Registered Nurses, 137, 504
Cohabiting partners, 278t
Collaboration, 15, 53–57
  for conflict resolution, 317t
  definition of, 320
Collaborative patient-centred practice, 320
Collected data, routinely, 195
Colley, Kate Brighty, 34–35
Colonialism, as distal determinant of health, 335–336
Colonization, 327–328
  consequences of, 330–334
  waves of
    administrative, 327
    ideological, 327
    legal, 327
    negative impact of, 327t
Colorectal cancer, 263–264
Commendations, 301, 501

Commission on Social Determinants of Health, 7
Common vehicle, 395
Communicable disease, 394–396
  agent, host, and environment in, 394–395
  definition of, 394
  development of, 395
  ethical considerations of, 396b
  historical perspectives of, 391–392
  non-vaccine-preventable, 404–405
  notifiable diseases and, 396–397, 397b
  prevention of, 397–398, 416–420
  spectrum of, 395–396
  surveillance of, 396–410, 396b
  transmission of, 395
  vaccine-preventable, 398–404, 399t–403t
Communicable period, 395
Communication
  in Giger and Davidhizar Transcultural Assessment Model, 165
  strong, 317
  in Transcultural Assessment Model, 490
Communitarianism, 134
Community, 14
  action, 103–105
  building, 103
  concepts of, 203–204, 204t
  cultural considerations, 206b
  defined, 203–204
  and determinants of health, 206–207, 207b
  family nursing, 276–277
  implementation in, 221–222
  as partner, 204–207
  preparedness, 457–459
  resources and facilities of, and violence, 361, 361b
  working with, 202–226
    ethical considerations, 205b
Community-as-partner model, 204–207
Community assessment, 436–437
Community Assessment for Public Health Emergency Response (CASPER) Toolkit, 463
Community-based strategies, 103–104
Community capacity
  building of, 211–212
  features of, 212t
  mapping, 212
Community Capacity Building Tool (CCBT), 25, 340
Community coalitions, 210
Community competence, 212–213
Community development, 53, 103, 211–213
  components of, 211t
  outcomes of, 212–213
  strategies, 103–104
Community education, in communicable diseases, 418
Community exclusion, 104t
Community-focused perspectives, 98–100
Community forum, 217, 235t

Community health, 207–209
  assessing, 213–218
  concept of, 208t
  evaluating intervention for, 222–223
  human rights and, 8–9
  planning for, 218–221
  process, 208–209
  status, 207–208
  strategies to improve, 209
  structure, 208
  substance use and, 372–375
Community health assessment, 336–337
  data sources, summary of, 235t
Community health concern, 214, 222
  identifying, 218
  priority, 220t
  in Stanfield Township, 220t
Community health index, 239
Community health nurses (CHNs)
  agency resources for, 379
  capacity building and, 479–480
  collaborative role of, in community mental health care, 369–372
    in crisis intervention and prevention, 369–370
    with law enforcement, 369
  corrections nurse as, 73
  in disease prevention and control, 398, 416–420
    assessment of, 416–417
    evaluation of, 418
    interventions in, 417–418
  environmental health roles of, 444–446
  evidence-informed practice, 480
  First Nations nurse as, 76
  forensic nurse as, 73–75
  health equity, 480
  health maintenance, restoration and palliation and, 479
  in health program, 228
  health promotion and, 85
  and mental illness, prevention of, 367–368
  nurse practitioner as, 72–73
  occupational health nurse as, 65–68
  older persons, caring for, 268–270
  outpost nurses as, 68–72, 75
  parish nurse as, 76
  prevention and health protection and, 478–479
  prevention and mitigation, 455
  professional relationships and, 479
  public health nurse as, 62–65
  relationship with patient and, 379
  resources for, 270–271
  role of, 221–222, 380–383
    community health concern and, 221–222
    in disaster response, 462–464
    social change process and, 222
  rural nurse as, 68–72
  settings, functions, and roles of, 57–77, 57f

Community health nurses (CHNs)
  (Continued)
    sexual assault victims and, 364–366
    street nurse as, 75
    and structural vulnerabilities, roles and
        levels of prevention for, 377–384, 382b
    and suicide, prevention of, 370–372
    telenurse as, 75–76
Community Health Nurses Association of
    Canada (CHNAC), 38–39
Community Health Nurses of Canada
    (CHNC), 20, 39, 315
Community Health Nursing (CHN), 1–28,
    47–82
  Aboriginal peoples and, 148
  aging population in, 147–148, 148f
  assessment issues, 218
  in Canada
    evolution of, 29–46, 30b
    milestones of, 33–44, 33t
  collaborative practice of, 25b
  cultural competence and, 159–163
    inhibitors to, 160–163
    responsive care in, 160
  cultural humility and, 164
  cultural nursing assessment and,
      165–167
  cultural safety and, 163–164
  cultural skill and, 167–170
  culture in, 146–147
  demographic groups for, 147–149
  diversity in, 146–147
    abilities, 154–155
    approaches to, 157–159
    as determinants of health, 156–157,
        157b
    disability, 154–155
    ethnic, 149–152
    linguistic, 152–153
    religious, 153
    sexual, 153–154
    types of, 149–155
  epidemiological studies, use of, 192–195
  ethnicity, 146–147
  evidence-informed practice in, 117–127
    appropriateness and applicability of, 125b
    best practice guidelines in, 118
    case study in, 126b
    clinical practice guidelines in, 121–122
    cultural considerations in, 123b
    determining which evidence is best to
        inform practice, 125–126
    ethical considerations in, 121b
    systematic review in, 122
  examples of, 11
  functions and practices, 48–57
    care and counselling in, 48–49
    case management in, 54–57
    community development, 53
    consultation, decision-making,
        leadership, and followership in,
        53–54

Community Health Nursing (CHN)
  (Continued)
    continuity of care in, 49
    discharge planning in, 50–52
    health advocacy in, 54
    health education in, 52–53
    historical perspective in, 55
    literacy and health literacy assessment
        in, 52–53
    outreach in, 49, 49f
    referral in, 49–52, 50t–51t
    research and evaluation in, 54
    risk assessment and response in, 49
    screening and surveillance in, 54
    team building, community
        development, and collaboration
        in, 53–57
  for health program planning, 228–229
  immigrant population and, 148–149,
      149f
  Indigenous peoples and, 148
  inequities, 156–157
  interpreter in, 168–170
  newcomer populations and, 167
  nursing code of ethics and, 137
  practice areas of, 16–19, 16f, 17t–18t
  practice, characteristics of, 207–210
  practice model for, 21f
  practice of, 15–19
  process, 204
  relational practice in, 165–167
  roles and functions of, 16, 19t
  standards of practice, 87b
  steps in investigating disease outbreak,
      177b
  student experience in, 199b
Community health patient, 14, 14f
Community health strengths, 214
Community Helpers program, 109
Community inclusion, 104t
  cultural consideration in, 105b
Community infrastructure, as intermediate
    determinant of health, 335
Community mental health, 366–372
  community health nurse's collaborative
      role in, 369–372
  in crisis intervention and prevention,
      369–370
  with law enforcement, 369
Community mental health nurses
    (CMHNs), 368
Community milieu, 125
Community mobilization, 103, 212
  framework, 98–100
Community organizing, 103
Community partnerships, 210
Community preparedness, 457–459,
    458b–459b, 459f
Community resources, 305
Commuter family, 278t
Comparison groups, 196
Competing, for conflict resolution, 317t

Composite database analysis, 214
Composition, in family structure, 495
Comprehensive School Health (CSH),
    approach in, 254–256
Comprehensive School Health Framework
    (CSHF), 254
Compromising, for conflict resolution, 317t
Concurrent disorder, 372
Confidentiality, 138, 138f, 218
Conflict
  group, 316
  intergroup, 316
  interpersonal, 316
  intrapersonal, 316
  transformation, 315–317
Connectedness, 427
Consequentialism, 131
Consultation, 53–54
Consumption, tuberculosis and, 34
Contact tracing, 419
Continuity of care, 49
Contraceptive assessment, 259
Contraceptive counselling, 259
Contracting, 60
"Cooperative agenda", 443
Coping skills, as determinant of health, 5
Coronavirus disease. See COVID-19
Corrections nurse, 17t–18t, 73
  definitions of, 73
  functions and roles of, 73
  levels of prevention in, 73b
  practice settings for, 73
COVID-19, 32b, 39, 155, 451
  aging population, 39–40
  biological disasters as, 453–454
  emergency management and disaster
      plans, 458
  evidence-informed practice, 354b
  health inequities, 352–353
  personal preparedness, 456
  professional preparedness, 456
  risk communication, 49
  secondary prevention, 65b
  virtual care, 75
CPHA. See Canadian Public Health
    Association (CPHA)
Creutzfeldt-Jakob disease (CJD), 392, 393f
Crimean War, 31–32, 178
Criminal Code, 364
Critical thinking, 304–305
Cross-sectional, study design, 194t
Crowe, Cathy, 359–360
Crowe, Heather, 109f
Crude mortality rate, 183t
Cultural blindness, 160
Cultural competence, 159–163
  attributes of, 161t–162t
  dimension of, attributes and, 161t–162t
  responsive care in, 160
  steps to developing, 159b
Cultural considerations, 123b, 168b

Cultural continuity, as intermediate determinant of health, 335
Cultural humility, 164
Cultural interpretation, 168
Culturally responsive care, 160
    inhibitors to, 160–163
Culturally unique individual, in Giger and Davidhizar Transcultural Assessment Model, 165
Cultural nursing assessment, 165–167
Cultural pluralism, 146
Cultural safety, 163–164
Cultural skill, 167b
    in community health practice, 167–170, 167f
Culture, 146–147
    definition of, 147
    as determinant of health, 5, 167
    features, 147
    levels of prevention in, 167b
    literacy and, 167b
Culture shock, 160
Cumulative effects, life course approach, 188
"Custodial" care, 59–60
Cyberbullying, 361

D
d'Aiguillon, Duchesse, 33t
Database, 214
    analysis, composite, 214
Data collection, 213–214
    direct data of, 214–217
    methods, 214–218
Data gathering, 214
Data generation, 214
Death rates, age-adjusted, 196
Decision-making, 53–54, 56b
Decolonization, 333–334, 333b
DEET, 414–415
Delirium, 269
Dementia, 269
Democratic leadership style, 315
Demographic groups, for community health nursing
    Aboriginal peoples in, 148
    aging population in, 147–148, 148f
    First Nations people in, 148
    immigrant population in, 148–149, 149f
    Indigenous peoples in, 148
    Inuit people in, 148
    Métis people in, 148
Demography, family, 277–278, 278t
Demonstration project, of Canadian Red Cross, 36
Dental health, 355–356
Deontology, 131
Department of Health, 34
Depression
    in older adult, 267f
    in women, 263
Dermatitis, air pollution and, 437b
Descriptive epidemiology, 177

Descriptive studies, 193
Determinants of health, 3–6, 156–157, 157b, 355, 355b
    communicable diseases and, 392–394, 393b–394b
    community and, 206–207, 207b
    consideration for, by community health nurse, 383
    early child development as, 247–248
    environment as, 428–430, 428b
    family-level, 278–280, 279b
    Indigenous, 334–336
        distal, 335–336
        intermediate, 335
        proximal, 334–335
Developmental theory, 283t–284t
Diabetes mellitus, in women, 261–262
Diarrheal diseases, 415
Diffusion
    of innovation theory, 98
    misconception against, 99t
Diphtheria, 399t–403t
Direct data, collection of, 214–217
Directly observed therapy (DOT), 419
Disability, 154–155, 156f
Disaster, 452, 452f
    biological, 453–454
    children in, 455–456
    chronic disease during, 462–463
    common reactions to, 463b
    disruption after, 463b
    emergency lodging after, 463–464
    human-made, 453
    levels of prevention for, 464b
    natural, 452–453
    preparedness, 451–467
    reactions to, 463b
    Red Cross's role in, 456
    types of, 452–454, 452t
    vulnerable populations and, 458
    warning of, 458
Disaster Assistance Response Team (DART), 462–463
Disaster plan, 452
Disaster preparedness, 456–462
Disaster prevention and mitigation, 455–456
Disaster recovery, 464–465
Disaster response, 462–464
    role of community health nurse in, 463
Disaster vulnerability, 455
Discharge planning, 50–52
Disease, 86, 395
    course, 86
    elimination of, 394
    foodborne, 412–414
    injury prevention, 11
    natural history of, 189
    prevention, 86, 88f
    resistance to, 394
    screening criteria for early detection of, 191b

Disease (Continued)
    specific protection against, 189
    spectrum, 395–396
    waterborne, 412–414
Dish With One Spoon Wampum, 328
Distal determinants of health, 335–336
    colonialism as, 335–336
    racism and social exclusion, 336
    self-determination as, 336
Distribution, 177
Distributive care, 13
Distributive justice, 133, 133f, 133b
District nursing, 32, 35f
Diverse abilities, 154–155
Diversity, 146–147
    abilities, 154–155
    approaches to, in community health nursing practice, 157–159
    as determinants of health, 156–157, 157b
    disability, 154–155
    ethnic, 149–152
    linguistic, 152–153
    multiculturalism and, 152
    population projections and, 150
    power of, 316
    religious, 153
    sexual, 153–154
    types of, 149–155
    visible minority population and, 146
Domestic violence, 362–363
Downstream thinking, 13b
Drinking water quality, 434
Drug use, interventions in, 418
Dyke, Eunice, 34, 35b
d'Youville, Marguerite, 33t
Dysfunctional families, 280–281

E
Early child development, 247–248
Early Learning and Child Care (ELCC), 254
Ebola hemorrhagic fever, 411–412
Ebola virus, 391, 411–412
Ebola virus disease, 179–180, 411–412, 412b
Eco-epidemiology, 198
EcoHealth, 8
Ecoliteracy, 506
Ecological footprint, 433
Ecological models, in health promotion, 100–101
Ecological studies, 193
Ecomap, 298, 298f
Economic development, 485
Economic globalization, 426
Economic risk, 297
Ectoparasitic infestations, 406t–409t
Education
    as determinant of health, 4
    health, for vulnerable populations, 383–384
    interprofessional, 320–321
    as proximal determinant of health, 334

Educational systems, as intermediate determinant of health, 335
Educator, 64
Effective Public Health Practice Project (EPHPP), 122
Egalitarianism, 134–135
ELCC. *See* Early Learning and Child Care (ELCC)
Elder abuse, 269–270
Electronic cigarettes (E-cigarettes), 257–258
Elimination, of disease, 394
Emergency lodging, 463–464
Emergency management, 451–467
  in Canada, 455
  community health nurse, role, 463
  framework, 455
Emergency Measures Organization (EMO), 458
Emergency plan, 452
Emergency preparedness and response, 11
Emerging infectious diseases, 391
EMO. *See* Emergency Measures Organization (EMO)
Emotional abuse, 362
Emotional communication, of family, 499
Employment
  as determinant of health, 4
  as proximal determinant of health, 334
Employment Equity Act, 146
Empowerment, 21–25
  family, 302
Enabling, 85
Endemic, 182, 395
Engaged interaction, 136
Engagement, in family home visits, 291–293
Entamoeba histolytica, 412
Enviro-mechanical hazards, 66, 66b
Environment, 4, 394–395, 435
  agent, host and, 394–395
  children's health and, 442–444, 444f
  community health nurses' roles in, 444–446
  definition of, 426
  as determinant of health, 428–430, 428b
  in epidemiological triangle, 185, 186b
  factors and health effects, 505
  family and, 498
  physical, 428
  psychosocial, 428
  risk factors and health, 426–429, 426b
Environmental advocacy, 445
Environmental concepts, 426–428
Environmental control, in Transcultural Assessment Model, 491
Environmental epidemiology, 435, 435f
Environmental ethics, 444–445
Environmental hazards, 438t, 441
Environmental health, 425–450
  assessment of, 436–441
  in Canada, 430–435
  definition of, 426
  governmental protection of, 430, 431t–432t

Environmental health (*Continued*)
  hazards, during disaster recovery, 464–465
  issues, 433
  key areas of, 433–435
  principles and position statements, 506
  principles of, 427–428
Environmental health risks
  assessment of, 439–440
  reduction of, 441–442, 441b
Environmental impact assessment, 436, 436b
Environmental justice, 444–445
Environmental pollutants, 429–430
Environmental principles, 427–428
  principle 1, 427
  principle 2, 427–428
  principle 3, 428
  principle 4, 428
Environmental protection, 189
Environmental risk assessment, 297–299, 427, 427b
Environmental scan, 436–437
Environmental standards, 430
Environmental stewardship, as intermediate determinant of health, 335
"Environmental tobacco smoke", 257
Enzyme-linked immunosorbent assay (ELISA), 192
EPHPP. *See* Effective Public Health Practice Project (EPHPP)
Epidemic, 182, 395. *See also* Pandemic
Epidemiological applications, 176–201
  evidence-informed practice, 182b, 198b
Epidemiological measures, in community health nursing, 180–185
Epidemiological models, and approaches, 185–189
Epidemiological research, basics of, 192–196
Epidemiological studies
  specific, original data collected for, 195–196
  types of, 192–195
Epidemiological triangle, 66, 66f, 185–186, 186f, 435
  client situations using, 187f
Epidemiologists, 179–180
Epidemiology
  analytical measures of association in, 185t
  basic measures, 192–196
  community health nurses use, 196–199
  definition of, 177
  environmental, 435
  history of, 178–180
  measures of, 180–185
  overview of, 177–178
  risk factor approach to, 198
Episodic care, 13
Epp Report, 4, 38, 93
Equality, 7, 135

Equity, 7, 135
  social justice and, 8
Equity seeking, 352
Eradication, of disease, 394
Escherichia coli (E. coli) O157:H7, 392
Ethical courage, 130b
Ethical decision-making, 129–130
Ethical dilemmas, 129–130
Ethical disengagement, 130b
Ethical (moral) distress, 130b
Ethical issues, 129–130
Ethical principles, 132–135
  for effective advocacy, 140b
Ethical problems, 130b
Ethical reflection, 131t
Ethical uncertainty, 130b
Ethical violations, 130b
Ethics, 6–7, 7b
  advocacy and, 139–140
  of care, 136–137
    decision process, 137b
  case study in, 141b–142b
  codes, 139
  in community health nursing practice, 128–144
    evidence-informed practice in, 139b
  definitions of, 130–131
  environmental, 444–445
  ethical decision-making in, 129–130
  nursing and, history of, 129
  nursing code of, 137
    and community health nursing, 138–139
  principles of, 130–131
  public health interventions and, justification of, 140–141
  standards of, 139
  student experience in, 141b
  theories of, 130–131
Ethnic diversity, 149–152, 150f–151f
Ethnicity, 147
  family and, 496–497
Ethnocentrism, 160
Ethnocultural population, 149–150
Ethnography, 124
Evaluation, 54, 222–223, 342, 418
  in family home visits, 294
  group, 318f–319f
  process, for health program, 237–241
Evidence-based practice, 64
Evidence for Policy and Practice Information Coordinating Centre (EPPI-Centre), 123
Evidence-informed practice, 117–127, 480
  action research in, 124
  appropriateness and applicability of, 125b
  assessing evidence in, 121–125
  best practice guidelines in, 118
  case study in, 126b
  choices in, patient, 125
  clinical practice guidelines in, 121–122
  clinical question in

Evidence-informed practice (*Continued*)
  examples of, 120b
    formulating, 119–120
  in community health nursing, 117–127
  community health nursing in Canada
      and, 30b
  community milieu in, 125
  cultural considerations in, 123b
  determining which evidence is best to
      inform practice, 125–126
  epidemiological applications, 182b, 198b
  ethical considerations in, 121b
  experiences in, patient, 125
  gathering evidence in, 121–125
  global historical roots in, 32b
  knowledge exchange in, 125–126
  meta-analysis in, 122
  meta-synthesis in, 124
  participatory action research in, 124
  PICO approach in, 119
  preferences in, patient, 125
  process, 118–126
  professional knowledge and experience
      in, 121
  public health nurses, 64b
  puzzle, 119f
  qualitative approaches in, 124
  qualitative research in, 120
  quantitative research in, 120
  randomized controlled trials in, 123–124
  scientific knowledge in, 122–125
  student experience in, 126b
  systematic review in, 122
  values in, patient, 125
  vulnerable populations, 354b
Evolution of health, 91f
Exercise and wellness program,
    development of, for Indigenous
    women in Northern Creek, 336
  background for, 336
  community health assessment in,
      336–337, 338t
  community health nursing intervention
      for, planning for, 337–345
  evaluation of, 342
  evaluation report in, 342–345, 343t–344t
  health promotion and risk reduction in, 338
  implementation of, 342, 342t–344t
    preparing for, 339–342, 340t
  planning for, CHN considerations in,
      338–339
  primary prevention in, 338
Existential theoretical perspectives, 101
Experimental/intervention studies, 193–195
Exploitation, 269–270
Expressive functioning, of family, 499
Extended family, 278t
  in family structure, 496

F
Facebook, 49, 456
Faith communities, 76

Fall-prevention program, for older adults,
    231f, 236f
Families, 20t, 59
  care planning with, 303
  as component of society, 281
  as context or structure, 281
  definition of, 277
  four views of, 281f
  as patient, 281
  supporting, through difficult news, 306b
  as system, 281
  working with, 275–308
Family assessment, 293–294
  families considered for, 496b
  models and approaches in, 287–290
    Calgary Family Assessment Model, 287
    Friedman Family Assessment Model
        (Short Form), 287
    McGill Model of Nursing, 287
    McMaster Model of Family
        Functioning, 288
    relational practice, 288–290, 289b
Family caregiving, 59, 502
Family communication, in resilient
    families, 303
Family crisis, 302
Family demography, 277–278, 278t
  in determinants of health, 278–280
  structure in, 278
Family empowerment, 302
Family forms, examples of, 278t
Family functions, 297
Family health, 280–281
  functionality and, 280–281
  risk and capacity, appraisal of, 295–299
    behavioural risk assessment in, 299
    biological risk assessment in, 295–297
    environmental risk assessment in,
        297–299
  risk reduction, 301–302
Family home visits, 290–295, 290f
  cultural considerations in, 293b
  engagement in, 291–293
  evaluation in, 294
  family assessment in, 293–294
  interventions in, 294
  planning for, 290–291, 291b–292b
  postvisit documentation in, 295
  safety concerns and precautions for, 294b
  stages and activities of, 292t
  termination in, 294
Family interventions, 299–305
  Calgary Family Intervention Model,
      300–301, 500–502
  planning, factors to consider in, 300b
  tips, 300b
Family member accord, in family resiliency,
    302
Family nursing, 276–277
  four approaches to, 281, 282f
  theoretical frameworks for, 281–287
  theory, 281

Family resiliency, 302–303
Family strengths, 300
Family structure, 278, 279f
Family support, 502
Family time, in resilient families, 303
Fear, 360
Female genital mutilation, 363–364
Feminist ethic of care, 137
Financial abuse, 362
Financial management, in resilient families,
    303
First Nations and Inuit Health (FNIH), 330
First Nations and Inuit Health Branch
    (FNIHB), 3
First Nations Health Authority (FNHA),
    39, 326
First Nations nurse, 76
First Nations people, 3, 148. *See also*
    Indigenous people
  suicide rate in, 370
First Nations Peoples Treaties, 328–330,
    330f–331f
First Peoples, 325
Flesh-eating disease, 392
Flexibility, in family resiliency, 302
FNHA. *See* First Nations Health Authority
    (FNHA)
FNIH. *See* First Nations and Inuit Health
    (FNIH)
FNIHB. *See* First Nations and Inuit Health
    Branch (FNIHB)
Focus groups, 110, 215, 235t
Followership, 53–54
Food
  adequate, access to, as proximal
      determinant of health, 335
  insecurity, 353
  intoxications, 413t
  poisoning, 412
  safe preparation of, 414b
  safety, 434–435
Foodborne diseases, 412–414
Forensic nurse, 17t–18t, 73–75
  definition of, 73
  functions and roles of, 75
  practice settings for, 73–74
Forming, in group development, 312
Four *Ps* of social marketing, 108
Four *Rs*, 441
"4 *Hs*", in assessing substance use patterns,
    374
Frankel, Lee, 34
Friedman Family Assessment Model (Short
    Form), 287
Functional families, 280–281, 280t
Funding applications, 110

G
Gantt chart, 236f
Gay, Lesbian, Bisexual and Transgendered
    (GLBT) Community Organization,
    212

GDM. *See* Gestational diabetes mellitus (GDM)
Gender, 154
    as determinant of health, 5
    in family structure, 495
    identity, 154
Genetic endowment, as determinant of health, 5
Genogram, 295, 296f
German measles, 399t–403t
Gerontological nursing, 266
Gerontology, 266
Gestational diabetes mellitus (GDM), 262
Giardia lamblia, 412
Giger and Davidhizar Transcultural Assessment Model, 165
Gilligan, Carol, 136–137
Global ecological change, 426
Global health, 8
    equity and social justice, 8
    organizations involved, 8b
Global Health Council, 8b
Global warming, 429–430
Goals, 220–221, 221t, 234–235
Gold standard, 192
Gonorrhea, 405
Governmental protection, of environmental health, 430
Gradual Civilization Act, 330
Gradual Enfranchisement Act, 330
Grandparent-led family, 278t
Greco–Roman civilization, 31
Greenhouse gas (GHG) emissions, 426–427
Greenhouse gas emissions targets, 433
Grey Nuns, 33t
Grounded theory, 124
Group-building roles, 313t
Group cohesion, 312
Group conflict, 316
    ethical considerations in, 316b
    resolution strategies for, 317f, 317t
Group development, 312–313, 312b
    adjourning in, 312
    forming in, 312
    norming in, 312
    performing in, 312
    storming in, 312
Group evaluation, 317
    form for, 318f–319f
Group interaction, 311
Group involvement, 311
Group process, 311–312, 311f
Group productivity, 312
Group roles, 313t
Group rules and standards, 313–314
Groups, working with, 309–323, 310t, 310b–311b
    case study, 321b–322b
    definition of, 310
    physical and emotional climate of, 311
Guidelines, 430t

H
Habitat, 430
H1N1 flu virus, 404
H1N1 outbreak, public health nurses and, 460–462, 461t
Haemophilus influenzae, 399t–403t
Hantavirus pulmonary syndrome (HPS), 391–392
Harm reduction, 75, 88, 89f, 372–373
    prevention strategies, 373–375
Hazardous waste, 429
HBV. *See* Hepatitis B virus (HBV)
HCV. *See* Hepatitis C virus (HCV)
Health
    advocacy, 54, 55b
    community, 207–209
        assessing, 213–218
        evaluating intervention for, 222–223
        goals and objectives, 220–221
        planning for, 218–221
        process, 208–209
        status, 207–208
        strategies to improve, 209
        structure, 208
    definition of, 86
    determinants of, community and, 206–207
    governments' responsibility for, 485
    poverty and, 356–358
Health care
    in Canada, 3
    Indigenous women, 33
Health care system, as intermediate determinant of health, 335
Health care team, working with, 317–321
Health communication, 108–109
Health concern
    analyzing, 218–219
    assessing and defining, 233–234, 234b
    priorities, identifying, 219–221
    weighing, solution options, 237
Health disparities, 352
Health education, 52–53, 383–384
    levels of prevention in, 52b
Health enhancement, 87
Health equity, 480
Health index, community, 239
Health inequities, 6, 352–353, 355–356
    identifying, 6b
Health literacy, 53, 107–108, 107b
    assessment, 52–53
Health maintenance, 479
    restoration and palliation, in CCHN Standards, 157
Health nurse's role, community, 221–222
    health concern and, 222
    social change process and, 222
Health nursing, community, process, 203–204
Health palliation, 479
Health policy, environmental, community health nurse and, 445–446

Health Products and Food Branch (HFPB), 3
Health program, 228
    evaluation
        considerations, 237b, 239t–240t
        criteria, 239–241
        sources, 238
        types of, 238t
    goals and objectives, 234–236
    implementation process, 228
    management process, 227–228
    planning, 228–229
        models, 229–232
        process, 228, 232–237
Health promotion, 21–25, 83–116, 89f, 478
    activities to facilitate, 108–109
    approaches, 101–102, 102t
        behavioural approach in, 101
        biomedical approach in, 101
        socioenvironmental approach in, 101–102
    Canadian framework for, 93
    capacity, 111t
    in CCHN Standards, 157
    developments in, 85–86, 93–94
    evidence-informed practice in, 110b
    evolution of, 90–96, 90b, 91f
        Alma-Ata Declaration in, 90–92
        Epp Report in, 93
        international health promotion conferences in, 95–96
        Lalonde Report in, 90
        Population Health Promotion Model in, 94–95, 94f
        summary of, 96
    foundational concepts in, 86–90
    landmark initiatives in, 90b
    models, theories and frameworks, 96–101
        community-focused perspectives in, 98–100
        ecological models, 100–101
        individual-focused perspectives in, 97–98
        public policy-focused perspectives in, 100
    Ottawa Charter for, 92–93, 487–489
    of primary health care, 9
    programs, 11
    skills, 109–110
        focus groups as, 110
        funding applications as, 110
        health promotion capacity as, 110, 111t
    standards of practice, 87b–88b, 203b
    strategies, 102–109
        activities to facilitate, 108–109
        advocacy, 109
        building healthy public policy as, 105–106
        community action as, 103–105
        creating supportive environments as, 106

Health promotion (Continued)
  developing personal skills as, 106–107
  health literacy, 107–108
  mutual aid, 109
  reorienting health services as, 108
  World Health Organization principles
    of, 92
Health protection, 86
  prevention and, 478–479
  programs, 11
  standards of practice, 87b, 203b
Health Protection and Promotion Act, 63
Health restoration, 479
Health risk appraisal, 295–299, 301–302
Health services, as determinant of health, 5
Health status, 485
Health surveillance, programs, 11
Healthy behaviours, as determinant of
    health, 5
Healthy Cities/Healthy Communities, 209
Healthy communities, 209
Healthy Environments and Consumer
    Safety Branch (HECSB), 3
Healthy lifestyle, promotion of, 373
Healthy living approach, 246–247
Healthy public policies, 87
  building, 105–106
Heart disease, in women's health, 260–261
Hébert, Marie Rollet, 33t
HECSB. See Healthy Environments and
    Consumer Safety Branch (HECSB)
Helminths, 416
Hepatitis A vaccine, 410b
Hepatitis A virus (HAV), 410
  epidemiology and transmission of,
    399t–403t
Hepatitis B virus (HBV), 406t–409t, 411
  epidemiology and transmission of,
    399t–403t
Hepatitis C virus (HCV), 411
Herd immunity, 394
Herpes simplex virus (HSV), genital,
    406t–409t
Hertzman, Clyde, 188–189
Heterosexual, 153
HFPB. See Health Products and Food
    Branch (HFPB)
HHN. See Home health nurse (HHN)
Hidden homelessness, 358
Hippocrates, 178
Historical roots, global, of public health,
    32b
Historical trauma, consequences of,
    330–334
HIV/AIDS, 391, 395, 405–410
  Canadian information on, 410b
  epidemiology and transmission of,
    399t–403t
  global information on, 410b
  patients with, 419–420
  testing and counselling for clients with,
    418–419

HIV antibody test, 419
Holistic care, 76
Home health nurse (HHN), 16, 17t–18t,
    58–62, 58f, 58b
  care and counselling, 60
  definitions of, 59
  functions and roles of, 59–61
  hospice palliative care, 61–62, 61b
  practice settings for, 59
Homelessness, 188f, 358–360
  at-risk populations and, 359–360
  concept of
    evaluation of, 359b
    understanding of, 358–359
  contributing factors to, 358b
Homeless Partnering Strategy (HPS), 210
Home visit, 291, 291b
Homicide, 360
Homosexual, 153
"Honour"-based violence, 364
Honour killings, 364
Horizontal transmission, 395
Hormone replacement therapy (HRT), 260
Hospice, 61
Hospice care, 61
Hospice palliative care, 61–62, 61b
Host, 394
  agent, and environment, 394–395
  in epidemiological triangle, 185, 186b,
    435
Housing instability, 358–360
  health and, 359
HPS. See Hantavirus pulmonary syndrome
    (HPS); Homeless Partnering Strategy
    (HPS)
HRT. See Hormone replacement therapy
    (HRT)
Humanistic theoretical perspectives, 101
Human-made disasters, 453
Human papillomavirus (HPV), 406t–409t
Human rights, community health and, 8–9
Hydrocarbons, 429
Hypertension, 359

I
I PREPARE, 439b
ICN. See International Council of Nurses
    (ICN)
Illness, 86
Illness narratives, 501–502
Illness trajectory, 86
Immigrant, 167–168
  population, 150
Immunity, 394
Immunization, 258, 258f
  passive, 394
  supporting, 420
Implementation, 342
  in community, 221–222
  planning for, 236–237
Incidence, measures of, 182
Incidence rate, 181t

Income
  as determinant of health, 4
  as proximal determinant of health,
    334
Incubation period, 395
Indian, 325
Indian Act, 330
  Bill C-31, 330
Indian Health Service, 30
Indigenous, 325
Indigenous groups, median age of, 151t
Indigenous health advocacy actions, 332
Indigenous people, 148
  in Canada, definitions of, 325
  cultural considerations for, 326b
  determinants of health in, 334–336
    distal, 335–336
    intermediate, 335
    proximal, 334–335
  females, missing and murdered, 332f
  health, 324–350
    case study for, 336–345, 345b
  health advocacy actions of, 332
  health issues of, historical and legislative
    context in, 327–330
    colonization in, 327–328
    First Nations Peoples Treaties,
      328–330, 330f–331f
    Indian Act, 330
    key events and legislation in, 328,
      328t–329t
    precolonization, 327–328
  health status of, 326–327
  human rights and community health of,
    8–9
  nursing, in Canada, 332–333
  population snapshot of, 325–326
  projected life expectancy of, 326
  social determinant of health, 152
Indigenous women
  gestational diabetes mellitus in, 262
  health care, 33
Individual-focused perspectives, 97–98
Individual-oriented roles, 313t
Indoor air pollution, 433–434
Indoor air quality, 433–434
Industrial Revolution, 31
Inequalities, 352–353
Inequities, as determinants of health,
    156–157
Infant
  common health concerns in, 250t
  developmental stages of, 251t
  immunization, 259f
Infant malnutrition, 219
  in Stanfield township, 220t
Infant mortality rate, 180–181, 183t–184t
Infection, 395
Infectious disease, 410–416. See also
    Communicable disease
Infectiousness, 394
Influence, of family, 499

Influenza, 404
  epidemiology and transmission of,
    399t–403t
Influenza pandemic preparedness, 459–460,
  461t
Informant interviews, 214–215, 215b
Injury
  accidents and, in child and adolescent
    health, 256–257, 256b
  prevention, 86
Innovation, 98
Institutional racism, 162–163
Instrumental functioning, of family, 498
Instrumental problems, 288
Integrated Pan-Canadian Healthy Living
  Strategy (HLS), 246–247
  framework of, 248f
Intellectual capacity, 267
Interactional theory, 283t–284t
Interdependent environment, 136, 204
Interdisciplinary, community health
  practice, 10
Intergenerational trauma, 335–336
Intergroup conflict, 316
Intermediate determinants of health, 335
  community infrastructure, resources,
    and capacities as, 335
  cultural continuity as, 335
  educational systems as, 335
  environmental stewardship as, 335
  health care systems as, 335
International Conference on Primary
  Health Care, 485
International Council of Nurses
  (ICN), 129
  Code of Ethics for Nurses, 129, 130b
  founding of, 34
  in global health efforts, 8b
International health, 8
"International Health Partnerships", 210
International health promotion
  conferences, 95–96
Interpersonal conflict, 316
Interpretation, 213–214
  session, 169b
Interpreter, 168–170
  working with, 170b
Interprofessional
  collaboration, 62
  community health practice, 10
  education, 320–321
  partnerships, 319–320
  team, collaborating in, 14–15
Intersectoral
  collaboration, 210
    of primary health care, 10
  community health practice, 10
  networking, 211t
Intervention activities
  to assess infant developmental levels in,
    222t
  identifying and prioritizing, 221

Interventions
  experimental/intervention studies,
    192–193
  in family home visits, 294
  principles for justification of, 140–141
  smoking, 257
Intimate partner violence, 363
  risk and resiliency factors for mental
    health problems after, 362b
Intrapersonal conflict, 316
Inuit peoples, 148
Invasive pneumococcal disease, 399t–403t
Irritant gases, 429

J
Jakarta Declaration, 95
Job security, 6
Justice, 134–135

K
Key informants, 235t
Key stakeholders, 233
Knowledge exchange, 125–126
Koch, Robert, 178

L
Laissez-faire leadership style, 315
Lalonde Report, 9, 38, 90
Language, 152–153
Larger systems, in family structure, 496
LAT. See Living apart together (LAT)
Latent effects, life course approach, 188
Law enforcement, collaboration with, 369
Leadership, 53–54
  behaviours, 314–315, 314b
  participative, 317
  styles of, 314
    autocratic, 314–315
    democratic or participative, 315
    Laissez-faire, 315
    shared, 315
  transformational and transactional,
    comparison of, 315t
Legislation, 328, 328t–329t, 430t
Lesbian, gay, bisexual, transgender, queer
  or questioning, and two spirited
  (LGBTQ2), 153
Levels of prevention, 13b, 189
  cardiovascular disease, 197b
  communicable disease, 398b
  community health nurse and, 107b,
    383–384
    primary, 383
    secondary, 383
    tertiary, 383
  in corrections nurse, 73b
  culture and, 167b
  environmental health-related, 438b, 446b
  in ethical decision-making, 138b
  family interventions, 300b
  in health education, 52b
  health program planning and evaluation-
    related, 241b

Levels of prevention (Continued)
  in home health nursing, 60b
  in nurse practitioner, 73b
  in occupational health nursing, 68b
  in outpost nursing, 72b
  in public health nursing, 65b
  in rural nursing, 72b
  for unhealthy environments, 438b
Liberal democratic theory, 134
Libertarian theory, 134
Liberty rights, 134
LICOs. See Low-income cut-offs (LICOs)
Life course approach, 188–189
Life course epidemiological approach, 188
Life expectancies, 265t
Lifespan, health and wellness across,
  245–274
  in adult, 259–266
  child and adolescent, 248–258
  Comprehensive School Health approach,
    254–256
  in early child development, 247–248
  healthy living approach, 246–247
  immunization in, 258
  in men, 264–266
  nutrition in, 252–254
  in older person, 266–271
    community health nurse in, 268–270
    ethical considerations in, 268b
  overweight in, obesity and, 251–252
  physical activity in, 252
  resources for, 270–271
  student experience, 270b
  tobacco use in, 257–258
  unintentional injuries and accidents in,
    256–257
  in women, 259–264
    breast self-examination, 259
    cancer, 263–264
    diabetes mellitus, 261–262
    heart disease, 260–261
    menopause, 260
    mental illness, 262–263
    obesity, 264
    reproductive issues, 259–260
Linguistic diversity, 152–153
Linguistic interpretation, 168
Listeria monocytogenes, 413t, 435
Lister, Joseph, 178
Literacy
  assessment, 52–53
  as determinant of health, 4
Living apart together (LAT), 278t
Local area development, 211t
Lockjaw, 399t–403t
Low-income cut-offs (LICOs), 356
Lung cancer, 263
Lyme disease, 414

M
Mad cow disease, 392
Maintenance role, 313, 313t

Malaria, 415
Male attendants, as first nurses, 33t
Malnutrition, infant, 219
    in Stanfield township, 220t
Mance, Jeanne, 33t
MAPP. *See* Mobilizing for Action through
    Planning and Partnerships (MAPP)
McGill Model of Nursing, 287
McMaster Model of Family Functioning
    (MMFF), 288
Measles, red (rubeola), 399t–403t
Measures of association, 184–185, 185t
Media, in Milio's framework, 100
Medicine healers, 160
Meningitis, 399t–403t
Menopause, 260
Men's health, 264–266
Mental health
    community, 366–372
        community health nurse's collaborative
            role in, 369–372
    definition of, 366
    determinants of, 369
    problems, risk and resiliency factors for,
        after intimate partner violence, 362b
Mental Health Commission of Canada
    (MHCC), 367
Mental illness, 366
    at-risk populations for, 367–368
        children as, 367
        older persons as, 367–368
        youth as, 367
    people with serious and persistent, 368
    potential consequences of, 367b
    in women, 262–263
Mental well-being, 464
MERS-CoV, 392
Meta-analysis, 122
Meta-ethics, 131
Metallic compounds, 429
Metals, 429
Métis people, 148
Metropolitan Life Insurance Company, 34
MHCC. *See* Mental Health Commission of
    Canada (MHCC)
Microaggressions, 152–153
Middle East respiratory syndrome (MERS),
    391
Midstream thinking, 13b
Milestones, of community health nursing in
    Canada, 33–44, 33t, 40t–43t
    1970 to 1999, 38–39
    2000 to present, 39–44
    late 1800s to early 1900s, 34–35
    post-World War I, 35–37
    post-World War II, 37
    remarkable legacies in, 35
Milio's framework, 100
Military nurse, 17t–18t
Mitigation, disaster, 455–456
Mobilizing for Action through Planning
    and Partnerships (MAPP), 229, 230t

Monitoring, 428
"Montreal Massacre", 453
Morality, 130–131
Morals, 130–131
Morbidity, 180–185
Mortality, 180–185
    premature, 427b
    rates, 178t, 183–184, 183t
        age-specific, 183t
        age-standardized, 179t
        cause-specific, 183t, 184
        common, 183t
        crude, 183t
        infant, 183t
        standardized, 183
Motor vehicles, air pollution and, 433–434
Multiculturalism, 152
Mumps, 399t–403t
Mutual aid, 109
Mutual goal setting
    advantages and challenges of, 303–304
    for care plan, 303
    phases of, 303t
Mutual respect, 136
Mycobacterium tuberculosis, 404
Myocardial infarction, web of causation for,
    187f

N
National Chemical Residue Monitoring
    Program, 443
National Longitudinal Survey of Children
    and Youth (NLSCY), 193
Nationally notifiable diseases (NNDs), 396
National Microbiology Laboratory (NML),
    460
National policies, governments and, 486
Native, 325
Natural disasters, 452–453, 453f
Natural history of disease, 189, 190f
Natural immunity, 394
Necrotizing fasciitis, 392
Negative predictive value, 192
Neglect, 269–270, 362
Neisseria gonorrhoeae, 405
Neonatal mortality rate, 183t
Neurotoxins, 429
Newborn
    common health concerns in, 250t
    developmental stages of, 251t
Newcomer populations, 167
New Perspective on the Health of Canadians,
    4
Nightingale, Florence, 31, 129, 203
    development of epidemiology and, 178f
NLSCY. *See* National Longitudinal Survey
    of Children and Youth (NLSCY)
Noddings, Nel, 136–137
Noncompliant families, 280–281
Nonfunctional roles, 313t
Nonmaleficence, 133, 133b
Nonpoint source, 429

Nonsuicidal self-injury (NSSI), 370
Non-vaccine-preventable diseases, 404–405
Nonverbal communication, of family, 499
Normative ethics, 131
Norming, in group development, 312
Northern Creek, 336–337
Northern Creek Fit and Active Program,
    343t–344t
Notifiable diseases, 396–397, 396b
NSSI. *See* Nonsuicidal self-injury (NSSI)
Nuclear family, 278t
Nurse entrepreneur, 17t–18t, 76–77
Nurse practitioner, 72–73
    functions and roles of, 72–73, 72b
    levels of prevention in, 73b
Nurses
    emergency management, 463
    role of, 456f
Nursing assessment, in Transcultural
    Assessment Model, 491–492
Nursing research, 506
Nutrition, in child and adolescent health,
    252–254

O
Obesity, 251–252
    adolescent, 86–87
    consequences of, 252
    factors, 251
    managing, 252b
    in women, 264
Objectives, 220–221, 221t, 234–235
    SMART, 236t
Occupational health nurse (OHN), 17t–18t,
    65–68
    functions and roles of, 67–68
    practice setting for, 65–67
    services provided by, 68b
Occupational health nursing
    competency categories, 67b
    definitions of, 65
    levels of prevention in, 68b
    occupational and environmental health
        history in, 67
    work–health interactions, 65
    work-related diseases in, 67t
    work-related hazards in, 66b
ODARA. *See* Ontario Domestic Assault
    Risk Assessment (ODARA)
Odds ratio (OR), 185t
OHN. *See* Occupational health nurse
    (OHN)
Older persons
    fall-prevention program for, 231f, 236f
    mental illness, 367–368
Older persons' health, 266–271
    changes in, physiological, 267t
    community health nurse, role of,
        268–270
    depression in, 267f
    ethical considerations in, 268b
One Health, 8

INDEX 529

Ontario Domestic Assault Risk Assessment (ODARA), 363
Operational health planning, 228–229
Oral rehydration therapy (ORT), 189
ORT. See Oral rehydration therapy (ORT)
Osteoporosis, 260
Ottawa Charter for Health Promotion, 3–4, 85, 92–93, 487–489
Outcomes, 234
Outdoor air pollution, 433
Outdoor air quality, 433
Outpost nurses, 17t–18t, 68–72
    definitions of, 68–69
    functions and role of, 70–72, 71b
    practice setting for, 69–70
Outpost nursing, 36
    key findings about, 69b
    levels of prevention in, 72b
Outrage, 441
Outreach, 49, 49f
Outreach nurse, 75
Overt racism, 162–163
Overweight, 251–252
    psychosocial disadvantages of, 252

P
Palliation
    health, 479
    standards of practice, 203b
Palliative approach, 61
Palliative care, 61
Pandemic, 182, 395
    influenza pandemic, preparedness, 459–460, 461t
    preparing for, 459–460, 461t
Papanicolaou (Pap) test, 189
PAR. See Participatory action research (PAR)
Parallel testing, 192
Paralytic shellfish poisoning (PSP), 413t
Parasites, 416
Parasitic diseases, 416
Parish nurse, 17t–18t, 76
Parish nursing, 76
Parish nursing associations, 38
Participant observation, 215
Participative leadership, 317
    style, 315
Participatory action research (PAR), 124
Partner notification, 419
Partnerships, 210, 319
    definition of, 319
    effective and sustainable, 320b
    interprofessional, 319–320
    in social marketing, 108
    spirit of, 486
Partners, working with, 309–323
    case study, 321b–322b
Passive immunization, 394
"Passive smoking", 257
Pasteur, Louis, 178
Pastoral care staff, 76

PATCH. See Planned Approach to Community Health Model (PATCH)
Paternalistic leadership style, 314–315
Pathway effects, life course approach, 188
Patient
    choosing best solution for, 237
    defined, 310
    health concern
        assessing and defining, 233–234
        stages used, 234b
PEEST analysis, 436–437
Performing, in group development, 312
Personal preparedness, 456
Personal skills, developing, 106–107, 488
Persons under investigation (PUI), 412
Pertussis (whooping cough), 399t–403t
Pesticides, 429
PHAC. See Public Health Agency of Canada (PHAC)
Phenomenology, 124
PHNs. See Public health nurses (PHNs)
Physical abuse, 362
Physical activity, in child and adolescent health, 252
Physical environment, 428
    as determinant of health, 4
    as proximal determinant of health, 334
Physical hazards, 66, 66b
PICO approach, 119
Pine Ridge, 229
Planned Approach to Community Health Model (PATCH), 229, 230t
Planning models, health program, 228
Planning process, health program and, 228
Plans of action, governments and, 486
Plasmodium falciparum, 415
Plasmodium ovale, 415
Plasmodium vivax, 415
Pneumococcal disease, 399t–403t
Point epidemic, 182
Point source, 429
Poisons, 429
Policy
    holder, in Milio's framework, 100
    influencers, in Milio's framework, 100
    in social marketing, 108
Policy, Regulatory and Organizational Constructs in Educational and Environmental Development (PROCEED), 230–232
Polio, 399t–403t
Poliomyelitis (polio), 399t–403t
Pollutants, environmental, 429–430
Pollution, 429
Population, 14
    boundaries, 234
    characteristics of, and violence, 360
    at risk, 180
Population-focused practice, 3–4
Population health, 3–6, 14, 21–25
    approach, 95f
    assessment, 11

Population health promotion model, 4f, 94–95, 94f
Population projections, 150
Positive outlook, in family resiliency, 302
Positive predictive value, 192
Postneonatal mortality rate, 183t
Postvisit documentation, in family home visits, 295
Potential years of life lost (PYLL), 185t
Poverty, 356–358
    child, 357–358
    definition of, 356
    health and, 356–358
    homelessness and, 358
    women and, 357
Precautionary principle, 440, 504
PRECEDE. See Predisposing, Reinforcing, and Enabling Constructs in Ecosystem Diagnosis and Evaluation (PRECEDE)
PRECEDE-PROCEED model, 100–101, 230–232, 231f, 232t–233t
Precolonization, 327
Predictive values, 192t
Predisposing, Reinforcing, and Enabling Constructs in Ecosystem Diagnosis and Evaluation (PRECEDE), 230–232
Pregnancy, and adolescent sexual behaviour, 375–377
    early identification of, 376
    factors contributing to, 377b
    special issues in caring for, 376–377
Pregnancy counselling, 376
Prejudice, 162
Preparedness
    community, 457–459
    influenza pandemic, 459–460, 461t
    personal, 456
    professional, 456–457
    team, 458
Preschooler, 253t
    common health concerns in, 250t
    developmental stages of, 251t
Prevalence rate, 181t, 182–183
Prevention
    of communicable diseases, 397–398, 416–420
    crisis intervention and, 369–370
    fall-prevention program for older adults, 231f, 236f
    health protection and, 478–479
    and health protection, in CCHN Standards, 157
    levels. See Levels of prevention
    and mitigation, disaster, 455–456
    standards of practice, 203b
Primary care, 9
Primary caregiver, 64–65
Primary health care, 485
    interprofessional collaboration in, 11b
    principles of, 9–10, 10t

Primary health care nurse practitioner (PHCNP), 17t–18t
  practice settings for, 72
Primary prevention, 13, 189, 416–418
  of communicable diseases, 397–398
  services, 383
Primordial prevention, 13, 255
Principlism, 132, 133b
Priority criteria, community health concern, 219–220
Probability, 353
Problem solving, in family, 499
PROCEED. *See* Policy, Regulatory and Organizational Constructs in Educational and Environmental Development (PROCEED)
Process dimension, 209
Professional accountability, 480–481
Professional preparedness, 456–457
Professional relationships, 479
  in CCHN Standards, 157
Professional responsibility, 480–481
  and accountability, in CCHN Standards, 157
Program feasibility, 234
Program Logic Model, 229, 231f
Program records, 239
Proportion, 180, 181t
Proportionate mortality ratio (PMR), 183t
Prospective cohort, study design, 194t
Protective factors, 89
Provisional Society of the Canadian National Association of Trained Nurses (CNATN), 34
Proximal determinants of health, 334–335
  adequate food, access to, 335
  education as, 334
  employment, income, and social status as, 334
  health behaviours as, 334
  physical environments as, 334
PSP. *See* Paralytic shellfish poisoning (PSP)
Psychological abuse, 362
Psychosocial environment, 428
Psychosocial hazards, 66, 66b
Ptomaine poisoning, 412
Public
  in Milio's framework, 100
  in social marketing, 108
Public health
  advocacy, 139
  definition of, 11
  efforts in Canada, 32–33
  global historical roots of, 31–32, 31t, 32b
  interventions, justification of, 140–141
Public Health Agency of Canada (PHAC), 3, 62, 179–180, 246–247
  communicable diseases, 391
  elements of, 95, 95f
Public health nurse, 9f, 12, 12b, 17t–18t, 29, 62–65, 62b
  ethical considerations of, 87b

Public health nurse *(Continued)*
  functions and roles of, 63–65
  Health Protection and Promotion Act for, 63
  practice setting for, 63
Public health nursing
  in Canada, milestones of, 33–44, 33t, 35b, 40t–43t
  definitions in, 62
Public Health Nursing Discipline Specific Competencies Version 1.0, 12, 39
Public health practice, 11–15
  principles of, 12–14
Public health surveillance, 195
Public participation, of primary health care, 10
Public policy-focused perspectives, 100
Purse strings, in social marketing, 108

Q
Qualitative research, 120, 124
Quantitative research, 120
"Quick Stats" sheet, 197
Quit4Life smoking cessation program, 257–258

R
Rabies, 399t–403t, 416
Race, 147
  as determinant of health, 5
  family and, 497
Racializing, 146
Racially visible, 146
  Canadian population, 151t
  median age of, 151t
Racism, 147, 162–163, 352
  as determinant of health, 5
  as distal determinant of health, 336
Random allocation, 123–124
Randomized controlled trials (RCTs), 123–124
Rank order, in family structure, 495–496
Rape, 364
Rate, 180, 181t
Ratio, 180–182, 181t, 185t
RCTs. *See* Randomized controlled trials (RCTs)
Recovery, disaster, 464–465
Referral, 49–52, 50t–51t
  practices, community health nursing assessment and, 437–438
  resources, 437
Refugee, 167–168
Registered Nurses of Canadian Indian Ancestry, 38
Regulations, 430t
Relational capacities, 166
Relational ethics, 136, 136t
Relational practice, 165–167, 288–290, 289b
  application of, 166b
  good communication skills in, 165–166
Relative poverty, 356
Relative risk (RR), 185t

Relevance, 239t–240t
Reliability, 191
Religion, family and, 497–498
Religious diversity, 153
Reorienting health services, 108, 488
Reported data, collection of, 217–218
Reproductive issues, in women's health, 259–260
Residential school, legacy of, 330–332
Resiliency, 89
  factors
    for mental health problems in, after intimate partner violence, 362b
    promotion of, 373
  family, 302–303
  in vulnerable populations, 353
Resistance, to disease, 394
Resistant families, 280–281
Resources, as intermediate determinant of health, 335
Responsibility
  professional, 480–481
  standards of practice, 203b
Retrospective cohort, study design, 194t
Risk, 185t, 426
  assessment, 439–440
  avoidance, 87
  management, 441–442
  reduction, 87, 301–302
  and resiliency factors, 362b
Risk communication, 49, 440–441
Risk continuum, 88f
Risk factors, 89
  in vulnerable populations, 353
Risk perception, 440t
  attributes affecting, 440t
Rituals, in resilient families, 303
Robert's Rules of Order, 314
Rocky Mountain spotted fever, 414
Roles, 313t
  in family, 499
Routinely collected data, 195
Routines, in resilient families, 303
Rubella (German measles), 399t–403t
Rule ethics, 131–132
Rural, 70
Rural health, 70b
Rural nurses, 68–72
  definitions of, 68–69
  functions and role of, 70–72, 71b
  practice setting for, 69–70
Rural nursing, levels of prevention in, 72b

S
Salmonella, 413t, 414
Salmonellosis, 414
Same sex partners, 278t
SANEs. *See* Sexual assault nurse examiners (SANEs)
SARS. *See* Severe acute respiratory syndrome (SARS)
Schizophrenia Society of Canada, 368

Schoolchild
  common health concerns in, 250t
  developmental stages of, 251t
Scientific knowledge, 122–125
Screening, 54, 189–192, 191b
Secondary analysis, 217
Secondary prevention, 13b, 189, 418–419
  activities, 383
  of communicable diseases, 397–398
Secondary victimization, 362
Second-hand smoke, 257
Self-care, 59–60
Self-determination, as distal determinant of
  health, 336
Self-help, 109
Self-management, 48–49
Sendai Framework for Disaster Risk
  Reduction 2015–2030, 455
Sensitivity, 191, 192t
Series testing, 192
Severe acute respiratory syndrome (SARS),
  3, 29, 40t–43t, 179–180, 182, 392, 395,
  441, 453–454
  biological disasters as, 453
  evidence-informed practice, 457b
  health care system, 454b
  system failure as, 453–454
Sexual abuse, 362
Sexual assault, 364–366
Sexual assault evidence kit (SAEK), 366
Sexual assault nurse examiners (SANEs),
  54, 73, 74f
  case study, 74b
Sexual diversity, 153–154
Sexual history, 155b
Sexuality, 153
Sexually transmitted diseases (STDs), 405
Sexually transmitted infections (STIs),
  405–410, 406t–409t
Sexual orientation, 153
  in family structure, 495
Sex workers, 360
Shamans, 160
Shared leadership, 315, 317
Shared recreation, in resilient families, 303
Shared responsibility, power of, 316
Sheltered homelessness, 358
Shigellosis, 413t
Sink, 429
Sixties Scoop, 332
"Skills Online", 195
Skipped generation family, 277, 278t
Smallpox, 32, 404
SMART acronym, use of, 236t
Smoking
  cessation, 97t
  in child and adolescent health, 257
Snow, John, 178
  cholera death rates by, 178t
Social change process, 222
Social class, family and, 497
Social determinants of health, 5–6, 5t

Social Determinants of Health: The
  Canadian Facts, 93
Social Determinants of Health: The Solid
  Facts, 6
Social development, 485
Social environments, as determinant of
  health, 4
Social exclusion, as distal determinant of
  health, 336
Social justice, 7–9, 7b, 135
  equity and, 8
Social marketing activities, 108–109
Social media, 49
Social organization
  in Giger and Davidhizar Transcultural
    Assessment Model, 165
  in Transcultural Assessment Model,
    490–491
Social risks, 301
Social status
  as determinant of health, 4
  as proximal determinant of health, 334
Social support, networks, as determinant of
  health, 5
Socioecological frameworks, in
  determinants of health, 4
Socioeconomic resources, 377
Socioenvironmental approach, 101–102,
  102t
Solidarity, power of, 316
Sources of data, 195–196
Space
  in Giger and Davidhizar Transcultural
    Assessment Model, 165
  in Transcultural Assessment Model, 490
Specificity, 191, 192t
Spirit of partnership, 486
Spirituality, 267–268
  family and, 497–498
  in family resiliency, 302
Spousal violence, 362
Stages of change model, 97–98
Standard population, 196
Standards of practice, 203b
  Canadian Community Health Nursing,
    20–25, 87b
  health promotion and, 88b, 203b
  health protection and, 87b
Staphylococcus aureus, 413t
Statistical indicators approach, 235t
4-Step Planning Process, 229, 230t
Stereotyping, 162
STIs. See Sexually transmitted infections
  (STIs)
Storming, in group development, 312
Strategic health planning, 228–229
Street nurse, 75
Street or outreach nurse, 17t–18t
Stress, 270
Structural and social determinants of health
  (SDOH), 352–353
Structural dimension, 209

Structural racism, 162–163
Structural violence, 353
Structural vulnerabilities, 352. See also
  Vulnerable populations
Structure-function theory, 281–287,
  283t–284t
Subjective poverty, 356
Subpopulation, 14
Substance use, 372–375
  education for, 373
  families and, 375
  problems, 374
    assessing socioeconomic concerns
      resulting from, 374b
Subsystem, in family structure, 496
Suicide, 370–372
  in Aboriginal communities, 370
  in Indigenous communities, 370
  protective factors for, 371b
  rates of, 372b
  risk factors for, 372b
  warning signs of, 371
Supportive environments, creating, 106,
  487–488
Support networks, in resilient families, 303
Surveillance, 54, 195, 436
  of communicable diseases, 396–410,
    396b, 420
Survey, 217–218
  of existing community agencies, 235t
  of residents of the community to be
    served, 235t
Sustainability, 212–213
SWOT format, 436–437
Syphilis, 406t–409t
Systematic review, 122
"System failure", 453–454
Systemic racism, 162–163
Systems theory, 283t–284t

T
Targeting Outcomes of Planning (TOP),
  230t
Task roles, 313, 313t
TB. See Tuberculosis (TB)
Team
  building, 53–57, 317–319
  working with, 309–323
    case study, 321b–322b
Telehealth, 75
Telenurse, 17t–18t, 75–76
Telenursing, 75
Teleology, 131
Termination
  in family home visits, 294
  in mutual goal setting, care planning
    and, 304
Tertiary prevention, 13, 189, 419–420
  activities, 383
  of communicable diseases, 397–398
Testicular self-examination (TSE), 266f,
  266b

Tetanus (lockjaw), 399t–403t
The Chief Public Health Officer's Report on the State of Public Health in Canada 2009: Growing Up Well-Priorities for a Healthy Future, 248
"The Children and Adolescent Trial of Health (CATCH)", 255
The Human Face of Mental Health and Mental Illness in Canada, 367
The Nightingale Pledge, 129b
Theory of planned behaviour, 97
The Pan-Canadian Gold Standard for Palliative Home Care, 61
Three Ds, of intellectual impairment, 269
Tickborne diseases, 414–415
Time
    in Giger and Davidhizar Transcultural Assessment Model, 165
    in Transcultural Assessment Model, 491
Tobacco, in child and adolescent health, 257–258
Toddler, 253t
    common health concerns in, 250t
    developmental stages of, 251t
TOP. *See* Targeting Outcomes of Planning (TOP)
Toxic chemicals, and children's health, 442
Toxicology, 429
Traditional knowledge holders, 160
"Train the trainer" sessions, 106–107
Transcultural Assessment Model, 490–492
Transgender, 154
Transitions, 287
Translation, 168
Transmission, of disease, 395
Transtheoretical model, 97–98, 97t
Trauma-informed care, 334, 334b, 353
Travellers, diseases of, 415
Treaty, definition of, 328–330
Triage, 463
Triangle, epidemiological, 185–186
Trichomonas, 406t–409t
Truth and Reconciliation Commission of Canada (2015), 333
TSE. *See* Testicular self-examination (TSE)
Tuberculosis (TB), 30, 187f, 391, 404–405, 419
Turning points in life, 250
Twitter, 49, 456

U

UBC. *See* University of British Columbia (UBC)
Unhealthy environments, levels of prevention for, 438b
Unintentional injuries, accidents and, in child and adolescent health, 256–257, 256b
United Nations Children's Emergency Fund (UNICEF), in global health efforts, 8b
Unit of care, 203b

University of British Columbia (UBC), 35–36
Unmotivated families, 280–281
Upstream thinking, 3, 13b
Urban health, 69b
Urban populations, 69–70
Utilitarianism, 131

V

Vaccination programs, 33
Vaccine, 394
Vaccine hesitancy, 258
Vaccine-preventable diseases, 398–404, 399t–403t
Validating or normalizing emotional responses, 501
Validity, 191–192
Values, 130–131
Varicella (chicken pox), 399t–403t
Vector, 395
Vectorborne diseases, 414–415
Veracity, 132
Verbal communication, of family, 499
Vertical transmission, 395
Victimization, secondary, 362
Victorian Order of Nurses (VON), 16, 29, 38f
Violence, 360–366
    assault and, 364–366
    bullying and, 361
    by dating partner, 363
    definition of, 360
    domestic, 362–363
    and female genital mutilation, 363–364
    as form of abuse, 361–364
    homicides, 360
    "honour"-based, 364
    indicators of, 361b
    intimate partner, 362b
    sexual assault and, 364–366
    social and community factors that influence, 360–361
        community resources and facilities as, 361
        population characteristics as, 360
    spousal, 362
Viral hepatitis, 410–411
Virtual care, 75
Virtue ethics, 135–136, 135b
Virtues, 135
Visible minority, 146
    population, 150f
Visiting nurse associations, 36
Visiting nurses, 36, 57
Vital records, 195
VOICE. *See* Voluntary Organizations Involved in Collaborative Engagement (VOICE)
Voluntary Organizations Involved in Collaborative Engagement (VOICE), 104
VON. *See* Victorian Order of Nurses (VON)

Vulnerability, 352–356
    of children and youth, 375–377
    disaster, 455
    factors predisposing people to, 355–356
Vulnerable populations, 506
    congenital and genetic predisposition of, assessment for, 377–378
    intervention for, 379b–380b
    working with, 351–388
        case study for, 354b, 357b, 359b, 375b, 377b, 385b
        community health nurses in, roles and levels of prevention, 377–384, 382b

W

Wakefield District immunization, 235
Wald, Lillian, 34
Water, 430
Waterborne diseases, 412–414
Waterfowl, 443
Web of causality/causation, 186–188
    for homelessness, 188f
    for myocardial infarction, 187f
Weighing health concern, solution options, 237
Weiss's framework, 100, 101b
Welfare rights, 134
Western blot, 192
West Nile virus (WNV), 392
WHMIS. *See* Workplace Hazardous Materials Information System (WHMIS)
WHO. *See* World Health Organization (WHO)
Whooping cough, 399t–403t
Wiisokotaatiwin Palliative Care Program, 124
Wildlife, 430
Windshield/walking survey, 206, 215f–217f, 438
WNV. *See* West Nile virus (WNV)
Women, and poverty, 357
Women's health, 259–264
    breast self-examination, 259
    cancer, 263–264
    diabetes mellitus, 261–262
    heart disease, 260–261
    menopause, 260
    mental illness, 262–263
    obesity, 264
    reproductive issues, 259–260
Work–health interactions, 65
"Working for", 100
"Working on", 100
"Working with", 100
Workplace Hazardous Materials Information System (WHMIS), 441
Work-related diseases, 67t
Work-site walk-through, 68

World Health Organization (WHO), 85
  disability rates, 155
  environmental health, 505
  Fourth Global Conference on Health
    Promotion, 95
  in global health efforts, 8b
  health promotion, 92, 92t
  healthy cities movement, 209
  Second Global Conference on Health
    Promotion, 93–94

World Health Organization (WHO)
    (Continued)
  Seventh Global Conference on Health
    Promotion, 96
  Sixth Global Conference on Health
    Promotion, 95–96
  on social determinants of health, 6
  Third Global Conference on Health
    Promotion, 94

Y
Youth
  mental illness, 367
  risk factors and protective factors, for
    substance use, 372b
  vulnerability, 375–377

Z
Zoonoses, 416

AA	Alcoholics Anonymous
ACNP	acute care nurse practitioner
AIDS	acquired immunodeficiency syndrome
ANA	American Nurses Association
ANAC	Aboriginal Nurses Association of Canada
AND	allowing natural death
AR	attributable risk
ATOS	alcohol, tobacco, and other substances
BFHI	Baby-Friendly Hospital Initiative
BFI	Baby Friendly Initiative
BMI	body mass index
BPA	Bisphenol A
BSE	breast self-examination OR bovine spongiform encephalopathy
CAHN	Canadian Association for the History of Nursing
CAPC	Community Action Program for Children
CAPNM	Canadian Association for Parish Nursing Ministry
CASA	Canadian Agricultural Safety Association
CATIE	Canadian AIDS Treatment Information Exchange
CCAC	Community Care Access Centre
CCBT	Community Capacity Building Tool
CCHS	Canadian Community Health Survey
CCMHI	Canadian Collaborative Mental Health Initiative
CCOHS	Canadian Centre for Occupational Health and Safety
CDC	Centers for Disease Control and Prevention
CEPR	Centre for Emergency Preparedness and Response
CESI	Canadian Environmental Sustainability Indicators
CFAM	Calgary Family Assessment Model
CFIA	Canadian Food Inspection Agency
CFIM	Calgary Family Intervention Model
CFR	case fatality rate
CH^{2}OPD^2	community; home, hobbies; occupation; personal habits; diet, drugs
CHARGE	coloboma, heart defects, atresia choanae, retarded growth and development, genital hypoplasia, and ear abnormalities
CHMS	Canadian Health Measures Survey
CHN	community health nurse
CHNC	Community Health Nurses of Canada
CHPCA	Canadian Hospice Palliative Care Association
CHR	community health representative
CHS	Canada Health Survey
CIAR	Canadian Institute for Advanced Research
CIHI	Canadian Institute for Health Information
CIHR	Canadian Institutes of Health Research
CIS	Canadian Incidence Study of Reported Child Abuse and Neglect
CJD	Creutzfeldt-Jakob disease
CMA	Canadian Medical Association OR Census Metropolitan Area
CMHA	Canadian Mental Health Association
CMHN	community mental health nurse
CNA	Canadian Nurses Association
CNPS	Canadian Nurses Protective Society
COHNA	Canadian Occupational Health Nurses Association
COPD	chronic obstructive pulmonary disease

CPCHE	Canadian Partnership for Children's Health & Environment
CPHA	Canadian Public Health Association
CPHI	Canadian Population Health Initiative
CPNP	Canada Prenatal Nutrition Program
CPR	cardio-pulmonary resuscitation
CPRN	Canadian Policy Research Networks
CPSP	Canadian Pediatric Surveillance Program
CRaNHR	Centre for Rural and Northern Health Research
CSH	Comprehensive School Health
CSHF	Comprehensive School Health Framework
CULTURE	C = commonly, U = understood, L = learned, T = traditions, U = unconscious, R = rules of, E = engagement
CVA	cerebrovascular accident
CVD	cardiovascular disease
D.A.R.E.	Drug Abuse Resistance Education
DART	Disaster Assistance Response Team
DEET	diethyltoluamide
DNA	deoxyribonucleic acid
DNAR	do not attempt resuscitation
DNR	do not resuscitate
DOH	determinants of health
DOT	directly observed therapy
E. coli	Escherichia coli
EAD	Environmental Assessment Division
EICP	Enhancing Interdisciplinary Collaboration in Primary Health Care
ELCC	Early Learning and Child Care
ELISA	enzyme-linked immunosorbent assay
EMO	Emergency Measures Organization
EPD	early postpartum discharge
EPHPP	Effective Public Health Practice Project
EPPI-Centre	Evidence for Policy and Practice Information and Coordinating Centre
FAAR	family adjustment and adaptation response
FASD	fetal alcohol syndrome disorder
FGM	female genital mutilation
FNIH	First Nations and Inuit Health
FNP	family nurse practitioner
FSN	family systems nursing
GAS	group A streptococci
GDM	gestational diabetes mellitus
GHG	greenhouse gas
GLBT	gay, lesbian, bisexual, and transgendered
HAV	hepatitis A virus
HBV	hepatitis B virus
HCV	hepatitis C virus
HERT	Health Emergency Response Teams
HHN	home health nurse
HIA	health impact assessment
HIV	human immunodeficiency virus
HPS	hantavirus pulmonary syndrome OR Homelessness Partnering Strategy
HPV	human papillomavirus
HR	human resources
HRT	hormone replacement therapy
HUS	hemolytic uremic syndrome
IAFN	International Association of Forensic Nursing
IALSS	International Adult Literacy and Skills Survey